A STUDY ON
MATERIA MEDICA

BY

N. M. CHOUDHURI, M.D.

Principal and Senior Professor of Materia Medica,
Bengal Allen Homœopathic Medical College
and Hospital, Calcutta, and Editor,
"Home & Homœopathy."

B. Jain Publishers Pvt. Ltd.
New Delhi (India)

Reprinted 1988

© B. Jain Publishers (P) Ltd.

Price : Rs. 60.00

Publishers :   B. Jain Publishers (P) Ltd.
1921, Chuna Mandi, 10th Street,
Paharganj, New Delhi - 110055.
Post Box 5775

ISBN 81—7021—039—9

Printed in   : J. J. Offset Printers
India by   Pharganj, New Delhi-110055

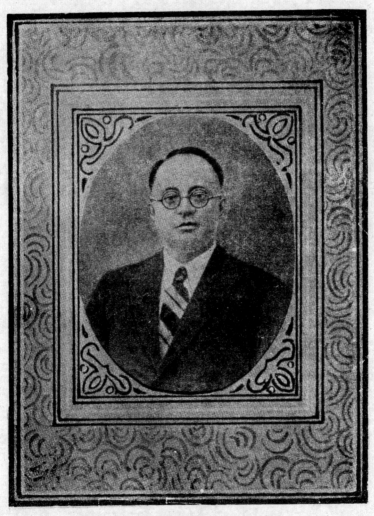

Dr. N. M. Choudhury, M.D.

Dr. N. R. Crombridge, M.D.

PREFACE TO THE SECOND EDITION

—·••◆•·—

THE First Edition of "*A Study on Materia Medica*" is exhausted and a Second Edition of the book has taken the place of the First. We are enjoined to do the best we can according to the light that is thrown on us. Judging from this standard, I feel that the First Edition has been a success.

In accordance with the newer light and the fresher revelations to the soul, the New Edition of the book has been so reformed and altered that it might as well have been a different book with a new nomenclature. It is a great improvement on the First, inasmuch as it covers a vastly bigger field and embodies the experience of the last twenty years of my practice. The remedies have been arranged in alphabetical order, and great endeavour has been made to rectify many of the defects of the previous Edition. Almost all the known remedies have been embodied in this volume with the exceptions of a few, a very few minor ones of empirical and unauthenticated nature.

In my capacity as the Principal of the Bengal Allen Homœopathic Medical College I have to deal very largely with *Materia Medica*, and this treatise, properly speaking, is the outcome of the lectures delivered to the students.

It has therefore done its day's work in the propagation of the principle of "*Similia*." I too have been amply repaid for the night after night of toil by the satisfaction it has already afforded me, that though the way has been long and dreary, it has been traversed in the wake of the immortals—of my loving preceptors here as well as abroad, whose standard it has been my good fortune to carry in the field of their glory.

A short and a concise *Repertory* has been affixed to help in the study of the *Materia Medica*. The method followed has been the usual one of the organs in order of their natural arrangement. Kent, Kneer, Lippe, Bœnning-hausen, Bœricke, Conant and other popular authors have been consulted. A great deal of unnecessary and un-authenticated matter has been left out, to make the Repertory portion useful and easy of reference.

The reason why a Repertory has been added to this volume is because practical Homœopathy is identical with Repertory practice. Negligence and inaptitude in handling Repertory are frequently the causes of unsuccess of many amongst us. The proper understanding and management of the Homœopathic Materia Medica is a stupendous task. As has been mentioned repeatedly, it is a philosophy and a science combined in one. It needs the best brain, the coolest judgment, and an untiring and endless endeavour to master it even partially, and Repertory forms a valuable aid in achieving this object. It has been my utmost endeavour, in this volume, to so elucidate this complex subject as to bring it within the compass of the commonest intelligence, to ingrain and imprint the knowledge of the remedies in the heart of every homœopath, to impress on the serious nature of this study, and finally to point out the proper method of study that helps essentially in the real under-standing and absorption of the Homœopathic Materia Medica.

Finally, it gives me great pleasure to have this oppor-tunity to express my heart-felt thanks to some of my colleagues for the valuable service rendered by them, chief among whom must be mentioned the names of Doctors K. M. Banerji, J. N. Hazra, and M. N. Banerjee. To Dr. K. M. Banerji is due great credit for many of the practical suggestions I received from him. Drs. J. N. Hazra and M. N. Banerjee have great claim on me for the untir-ing devotion, zeal and earnestness with which they have served me during these tedious months of hard mental labour.

CALCUTTA:
The 1st June, 1929.   N. M. CHOUDHURI.

PREFACE TO THE FIRST EDITION

--- ◆◆◆ ---

THIS work on *Materia Medica*, the result of years of patient labour, has its origin in my by-gone student-days, when, as an alumni of the Hering Medical College, that fountain, since dried up, of true and pure Homœopathy, I used to sit at the feet of apostles like Doctors Allen, Taylor, Tom Hagen and Farrington. The principle of differentiation and assimilation then inculcated in me by these expounders has been given the greatest importance in this work. I will consider myself satisfied and my duty fulfilled, if I in my turn can impress on students and practitioners on this side of the hemisphere the essential importance of this most pivotal principle of this true science of the Healing Art.

To the teachings of those Masters of the West I have added many important practical hints from my preceptor Dr. P. C. Majumdar, with whom I had the good fortune to spend a few years of my early career.

I have further enriched this volume with the experiences of our Eastern Masters such as Doctors B. L. Bhaduri, Salzer and M. L. Sarkar. I have not only clothed many of the abstract principles of the *Organon* in flesh and blood but given them rich and attractive apparel in the form of illustrations and anecdotes to make them interesting and impressive.

I must acknowledge my obligation to the following authors, whom I consulted often and from whom I picked up many valuable information:—Doctors H. C. Allen, T. F. Allen, J. H. Clarke, H. N. Guernsey, J. B. Bell, C. M. Conant, N. B. Bose, E. M. Hales, J. T. Kent, E. B. Nash, Samuel Lillienthal, P. C. Majumdar, Salzer, Constantine Hering and E. A. Farrington. I have also taken many hints from the American Homœopathic Pharmacopœia.

In this connection I like to add that my heart-felt obligation is due to Kali Pada Pathak, but for whom this book would never have seen light and to whose whole-hearted devotion, sincere love and patient helpfulness I owe not only this treatise on Materia Medica but a great part of my personal comfort and a big share of my energy.

Finally, let me mention that I cherish no anxiety about the future of this volume, for a fate worse than what has been predicted by a great friend and sincere well-wisher of mine, " It will at least be popular amongst vermin if not amongst human being," can never befall this volume.

CALCUTTA :

The 1st December, 1916.   N. M. CHOUDHURI.

A STUDY ON

MATERIA MEDICA

———•—•◄•———

ABIES CANADENSIS.

Our **Abies can.**, a remarkable remedy in the treatment of chronic gastric affections and uterine disorders, is prepared from the fresh bark and young buds of the Canada Pitch. It is called Hemlock Spruce and it belongs to the natural order of Coniferæ. It produces a kind of catarrhal condition of the stomach. Although imperfectly proved, we have records of numerous instances of cures effected with this remedy. These patients suffer from great debility and there is a strong desire to lie down and rest most of the time. A sort of languor is to be found in **Gelsemium** also. It is easy, however, to differentiate between the two remedies. In **Abies can.** it is debility pure and simple due to mal-assimilation of food whereas in **Gelsemium** it is only a muscular debility and a want of tone in the muscular system.

The most prominent symptoms to guide us in our selection of **Abies can.** are to be found in the gastric region. Canine hunger is present most of the time. It is a cruel hunger that gnaws in the stomach causing a sort of fainting feeling at the epigastrium. In his hunger he does not know how much he eats and very often there is excessive loading of the stomach which causes distention of stomach and abdomen with severe palpitation of the heart.

It is also applicable in uterine displacements. The patient complains of a sore feeling at fundus of uterus and relief is obtained by pressure. Chilliness, prostration and the peculiar cravings when associated with the abovementioned gastric symptoms will make its application almost a certainly.

H. M. M.—1

ABIES NIGRA.

Abies nigra, called the Black or Double Spruce, is prepared from the gum of the plant, a native of the northern part of North America. It is undoubtedly a grand remedy in dyspepsia especially of the aged, habituated to excesses of tobacco and tea. They are generally low-spirited and dull and have wakeful nights. This remedy has a symptom which has been verified repeatedly and which can be described as the most characteristic indication of Abies Nigra. This keynote symptom consists of a sensation of a lump in the cardiac end of the stomach. The patient describes this as a feeling as though he had swallowed some indigestible substance which had stuck in his stomach. It is like a continual distressing constriction just above the pit of stomach, as if every-thing was knotted up and this would neither go down nor come up. Sometimes it is described as a sensation of hard-boiled egg lodging in the stomach. Severe pain in stomach is felt after eating. Symp-toms like these are to be encountered daily and a few doses of. **Abies nigra** will nip the trouble in the bud.

In this connection we may compare Abies Nigra with **Bryonia, Calcarea carb, China, Lactic Acid, Nux vom., Natrum mur.** and **Zincum.**

ABROTANUM.

Artemisia Abrotanum is prepared from the fresh leaves and stems of Lady's Love. I have used this remedy with great success in cases of marasmus of infants. They look puny, wrinkled, cross and depressed. The emaciation is more marked in the lower limbs. Malnutrition is evident from progressive atrophy inspite of ravenous hunger. The prostration is so great that they cannot even hold up their heads. They are very subject to alternate diarrhœa and constipation. Protruding hemorrhoidal tumors with a burning pain when touched, oozing of blood and moisture from the navel, dis-tention of abdomen, constant pain in stomach making the child irritable and ugly, a sort of hectic fever with painful inflammatory rheumatic swellings in different parts of the body, flabbiness of skin hanging in folds are symptoms to be always encountered in an Abrotanum baby.

Abrotanum, however, is not our only remedy for marasmus of children. **Æthusa, Antim. crud., Baryta carb., Calcarea carb,**

Cina, Iodium, Naturm mur., Petroleum, Sarsaparilla, Silicea and Sulphur are important remedies to be remembered in this connection.

In Æthusa with the emaciation we have immoderate vomiting of milk immediately after nursing. The same emaciation, the same want of power to hold the head up are present but the great intolerance of milk should always be our guide in its selection.

In Antimonium crudum we have the vomiting of food and drink, we have the watery diarrhœa, but the ugliness and peevishness of the child, the want of animal heat and the heavy milky or the milk-white coating of the tongue should help us in our selection.

Baryta carb is indicated when in addition to the general emaciation we have the immature and dwarfed mental condition of the child to think of. A general tendency towards swelling of cervical and other glands is also to be noticed in this remedy.

In Calcarea carb the emaciation is more marked in tissues other than adipose. The muscles and the bones suffer before the fatty tissues are affected. There is a general deceptive appearance of plumpness about this child. Profuse sweat especially in the head, crusta lactea, engorgement of glands, especially the mesenteric, sour pungent clayey diarrhœa and great craving for eggs are prominent symptoms.

Cina is inferior to none in marasmus but the itching of the anus, the wetting of the bed, and presence of worms in the stools, the beastly temper, the constant picking of the nose and a strong desire on the part of the child to be constantly rocked are guiding indications.

Iodium is indicated when the hunger is excessive and the child wants to eat constantly. In addition to this we have swelling and induration of the mesenteric glands.

Natrum mur, a great remedy at all times, is particularly indicated in marasmus when atrophy is more marked in the throat and neck of children. The mapped tongue, herpes labialis, marked repugnance to bread, sadness, profuse sweating, palpitation and constipation are sure indications for Natrum mur.

Petroleum is indicated in marasmus when the patient is subject to a peculiar type of diarrhœa, harassing all day long but mostly absent at night time. The other prominent symptoms are a marked odour of garlic in the breath and fæces of the patient, aversion to fresh air, a marked tendency for eczema, excoriating cracks and bleeding rhagades.

We use **Phosphorus** in children growing over-tall but slender The pot-belliedness, the pale waxy countenance, the delicate eye-lashes and soft hair, a frequent tendency for diarrhœa where stools pour away like water from a hydrant, the great tendency for affection of bones, the strong craving for cold iced drinks are symptoms too definite to be misleading.

Sarsaparilla is generally called for in very pronounced cases of marasmus where the disease is fully developed. The emacia-tion is extreme, the face looks shrivelled, the skin lies into folds, eruptions are prone to appear on tongue and roof of mouth. Offensive sweat about genitals, restlessness before passing of urine, passing of great quantity of sand in the urine are also cha-racteristic of this remedy.

Silicea is indicated in nervous, irritable, timid children wh though wasting everywhere present an exceedingly large head. Malnutrition is marked everywhere in **Silicea.** A great aversion to mother's milk is also noticed.

Sulphur though coming last in this list is not second in im-portance to any. In fact it is used oftener than many of the other remedies mentioned in this list. No body can mistake a Sulphur baby. There is nothing inviting about him. The skin is dry, harsh and wrinkled giving the child an old man look. Eczema, itch, eruptions, enlargement of the glands, obstinate constipation and persistent diarrhœa, a never-to-be-forgotten nauseous smell, dirt and filth speak of an ugliness that is only to be encountered in **Sulphur.**

ABSINTHIUM.

This drug is prepared from the Common Wormwood, a plant very well known because of the famous liquor extracted from it. The tincture is made from the chopped leaves and blossoms of this plant, macerated in two parts by its weight of alcohol.

Many symptoms of this remedy have been obtained from persons indulging too freely in this deleterious drink. This liquor is consumed very extensively in Switzerland and France. In the latter country the consupmtion of **Absinth** has assumed such pro-portions that it has been truly esteemed a grave national evil. The symptoms of over-indulgence are muscular quiverings, emaciation, melancholy look, giddiness, tingling in the ears, hallucinations of sight and hearing, loss of brain power and eventual idiocy.

In homœopathic therapeutics this remedy is used extensively in epileptiform seizures. A large number of fits occur in the same day in rapid succession. Trembling, tremor and terrific hallucination precede the attack and it is mostly followed by motor and sensory paralysis. An obtuse state of the mind prevails after the attack is over.

In delirium calling for **Absinth** we notice great restlessness as manifested by a desire to walk about; they cannot stop in one place because of the terrible visions that come to them. In the typhoid state it is prescribed for sleeplessness when sleeplessness is suspected to be due to congestion of the base of the brain.

We must not forget the vertigo of **Absinthium.** It is characterized by a tendency to fall backwards. It is also accompanied by general constipation and spasmodic twitching of the facial muscles.

ACALYPHA INDICA.

Acalypha Indica is a common weed growing in the East Indies. It belongs to the natural order of Euphorbiaceæ. This drug has a marked action on the respiratory organs. This is one more of our new remedies which I cannot, for sake of decency, overlook. I have used this remedy with great satisfaction in hemoptysis of phthisis. There is dullness of chest on percussion. Patients complaining of severe pain in chest, progressive emaciation, night sweat, evening rise of temperature, all indicating a serious stage, have been helped by the administration of **Acalypha.** The cough of **Acalypha** is dry and hard and each time it is followed by hemoptysis. The blood ejected is bright red in the morning, dark and clotted in the afternoon. We also have a spluttering diarrhœa with forcible expulsion of noisy flatus in this remedy. Rectal hæmorrhage, too, is not uncommon.

It belongs to the same category as **Hamamelis, Ipecac, Millefolium, Phosphorus** and **Aconite.**

This remedy was first proved by Dr. P. C. Mozumdar of Calcutta.

ACETIC ACID.

It is common vinegar. It produces a sort of anemia with
debility, loss of flesh, cough, dropsical swelling and hæmorrhage
and is, therefore, a very remarkable therapeutic agent in many
cachectic conditions arising from cancer, phthisis, fever, diphtheria,
croup and diabetes. The patient presents a pitiable condition. He
is pale, waxen, and emaciated. Wasting is excessive and progressive. Thirst is very intense. Nausea, retching and sour rising
are frequent symptoms. It has been known to palliate intense
gnawing, ulcerative pains of cancer in the stomach with great
burning and profuse diarrhœa. Dropsical swellings common in the
later stages of the above complaints also find in **Acetic acid** a great
help. We have hæmorrhage from every outlet of the body. These
are all very serious symptoms but they come well under the influence of **Acetic acid**.

Case.—A few years since, a young lady, in easy circumstances, enjoying
good health, was very plump, had a good appetite, and a complexion blooming with roses and lilies. She began to look upon her plumpness with suspicion, her mother being very fat, and she was afraid of becoming like her.
Accordingly she consulted a woman who advised her to drink a small glass
of vinegar daily; the counsel was followed, and the plumpness soon diminished
She was delighted with the success of the remedy and continued it for
more than a month. She began to have a cough, but it was at first dry,
and regarded as a cold that would subside. But from being dry, it was
presently moist. A slow fever came on, with difficulty of breathing; her
body became lean and wasted away; night sweats, with swelling of the
parts succeeded; and a diarrhœa terminated her life. On examination all the
lobes of the lungs were found filled with tubercles, and somewhat resembled
a bunch of grapes.—"The London Medical Gazette," 1838-39.

ACONITE NAPELLUS.

This is a very strong poison. It is commonly known as the
Monkshood or Wolfsbane. It grows over bare rocks in various
parts of Europe and Asia. The tincture is prepared from the
whole plant when beginning to flower. It was introduced into
our Materia Medica by Hahnemann.

No single word expresses the general character of **Aconite**
better than "tension." Every fiber of the **Aconite** patient is an
illustration of this condition. The great anxiety, fear and restlessness illustrate his emotional tension. His intellectual tension
is evidenced by the great acuteness of all his senses. His senses

of smell, sight, touch and hearing become exceedingly active, which it will not take long for the most casual observer to find out. His pulse is another proof of his acute, over-sensitive and highly-strung condition. It is full, hard and bounding.

Another important point that should not escape our attention is the intensity, the acuteness and rapidity of all the symptoms of **Aconite**; for example, the fever, for which **Aconite** is the remedy, is rapid in its onset, intense in its character and overwhelming in its nature. It runs up to an extreme temperature of 104° or 105° in a very short while and his internal turmoil manifests itself by the intense agonising restlessness, the great but inexplicable anxiety, apprehension and fear.

The appearance of the **Aconite** patient during fever is very characteristic. We notice redness and heat of one and coldness with paleness of the other cheek. Sometimes the face looks red while lying down but becomes deathly pale on rising up, and he becomes faint or giddy and falls over. This is accompanied with vanishing of sight and unconsciousness. The heat is dry and burning in character and is accompanied by intense and excessive thirst. Water tastes very sweet and he drinks large quantities at a time. During sweat he wants to be covered up. The sweat is warm and profuse and is over the entire body. The ætiology of the **Aconite** fever is very important and should be borne in mind. The ailment is the result of an exposure to dry cold wind while in perspiration or getting wet.

Aconite is very rich in mental symptoms. He is impatient and his impatience makes him restless. He throws himself about and constantly changes his position. The true reason of this restlessness is to be found in a state of internal turmoil and anxiety and agony; that is why he cannot continue long at one thing or at one space. He moans and laments he screams and shouts not knowing what to do and how to find consolation. Fear is a prominent factor in his life and this fear is mostly about the safety of his own life. He fears to go out where there is an excitement or any congregation of people. At times this fear assumes the aspect of clairvoyance and he predicts the time of his death. He also seems to be conscious of things that are happening far away.

He is extremely sensitive mentally and physically. He gets vexed at trifles and takes things seriously even when meant in joke. Physically this sensitiveness is manifested by his extreme susceptibility to pain. He makes a bad patient. He makes mountain of a molehill. Even when the pains are slight and bearable, due to his extreme susceptibility he exaggerates them to such an extent that his own imagination of the enormity of his complaint overpowers him.

The **Aconite** patient is also inclined to be hysterical. We notice great variation of mood and temperament. He is cheerful this minute, he weeps the next. He is sad and taciturn now, he is gay and loquacious the next moment. The expression of his face is anxious and one of extreme fear. It is also livid, at times getting almost blackish. A great victim to giddiness on rising from a recumbent posture, his red face gets deathly pale and he becomes dizzy and falls.

Congestion being an integral part of **Aconite,** our patient is a martyr to severe throbbing headaches with great fulness and heavy feeling in the brain; he feels as if everything is about to be pushed out of the forehead. The carotids throb and the head feels hot while the rest of the body becomes cold. Neuralgia of the Trigeminus with fiery red face, restlessness and anguish is a frequent occurrence.

Aconite has strong action over mucous membranes where it causes severe inflammation. In the eyes we use it in conjunctivitis, sclerotitis and ophthalmia, when symptoms are over-acute, pain extra-severe, and redness and photophobia are extreme. Chemosis, hyperæmia, heat, dryness, profuse lachrymation and copious inflammatory discharges from the nose are common. We also notice fluent coryza, roaring in the ears and frequent sneezing, the effect of exposure to a draft of dry cold wind. If not checked in time it travels downwards and the inflammatory process may give rise to serious type of laryngitis. Hoarseness, rattling, suffocative spasms, husky voice, crowing croupy cough, dryness in the wind pipe, wheezing sawing breath, indicate serious complications. It may also extend to the respiratory tract and we may have a serious case of bronchitis or pneumonia to deal with. Tightness of the chest, a sense of oppression and a feeling of great weight ought to put us on our guard. Severe stitching pain lancinating through the chest, difficult breathing, violent chill, blood-streaked sputa should draw our attention at once to **Aconite.**

Together with **Spongia** and **Causticun, Aconite** forms an important trio for such affections of the respiratory troubles as cough and croup. The cough is more of a croupy nature. It is dry, hoarse and suffocating. Sometimes we hear a ringing, whistling sound on expiration. The child grasps its throat with every attempt at coughing. In this connection we may compare it with **Hepar sulph** and **Sambucus.** The former remedy should be given when the cough is aggravated towards morning and on uncovering. There is regular rattling of mucus in throat as in **Antim tart.** In the latter remedy nervous symptoms such as spasms of the glottis are noticed. The breathing is more of a wheezing crowing character; the trouble is almost worse after midnight and on lying with head low. The patient can inspire better; expiration is hard and difficult.

In pleurisy we may think of **Aconite** in the very first stage before exudation has set in. Sharp stitches are felt on chest with chill and fever. It is specially indicated when the trouble has arisen from exposure or a checked perspiration. Right here we will also speak of **Aconite** in pneumonia. It is used in the first stage when symptoms of engorgement of lungs are very prominent. The cough is hard, dry and painful. The expectoration is blood-streaked. The mental phenomena, so charactristic of **Aconite** are ever present.

Aconite is an important remedy in many affections of the heart, such as neuralgia, hypertrophy, pericarditis, angina pectoris and many other varieties of inflammatory processes. Violent hyperæmia with severe anxiety about the præcordia, stitches at the heart, numbness in the left arm and tingling in the fingers, quick pulse and fainting are important indications calling for **Aconite.**

We use **Aconite** very extensively in diarrhœa, specially of infants, during summer. The stools are green like chopped herbs. It is attended with colic that forces them double. **Aconite** is still our remedy when this green stool turns bloody and there are intense urging and other inflammatory symptoms, such as high fever, intense pain, distended abdomen, etc.

It is one more of our hemorrhagic remedies but the hemorrhage that we find under **Aconite** is active hemorrhage—the blood passed being pure and profuse. We use it in menorrhagia, metrorrhagia, hemoptysis, epistaxis, hematemesis and hematuria when accompanied with the moral symptoms stated above.

Pregnancy and parturition call for **Aconite** in impending cases of abortion when induced by fright and vexation.

The labor pains of **Aconite** are very violent and distressing; progress is slow, the contraction being insufficient. The patient, red, thirsty and sweating, keeps shrieking on account of the overwhelming but ineffectual pain. It is called for even in convulsions due to excessive cerebral congestion. Milk fever and other varieties of child bed fevers can be helped with **Aconite**, provided we have frequent tense hard pulse, fearful, wild, staring, glittering eyes, dry tongue and great thirst.

We will now discuss the indications of **Aconite** in febrile affections. It is a remedy par excellence in the treatment of fevers, especially in fevers of inflammatory types. The heat is very great with agonised, tossing about. It is generally a dry radiating heat. The thirst is great. Chilliness is experienced on slightest movement. The patient shudders on lying down. With the chill we also have internal heat, anxiety and red cheeks. Sometimes the redness in only to be seen in one cheek only.

Aconite is very useful in cholera, both in the congestive stage and in the stage of collapse. The violence of the attack and the mental symptoms should be powerful factors in our decision. It is recommended even as a preventive measure during severe epidemics of cholera, when the atmosphere gets surcharged with fear and anxiety, every body dreading to be the next victim.

Sulphur is the chronic of **Aconite**; where **Aconite** partially helps, **Sulphur** finishes the cure.

Case 1.—Pleurisy from sitting at an open window. Stitches at the right side of the chest, through the lungs in different directions, causing her to cry out; the least motion causes great pain; breathing short and rapid; restlessness, and although the movement of her body increases the pain. One dose of **Aconite** 50,000, dry, on the tongue, relieved the pain for a few hours, when it returned in all its force. Six pellets of the same preparation, dissolved in water, acted better; after the first teaspoonful she fell asleep, awoke in a profuse, warm perspiration, and by next morning felt entirely relieved. —Dr. Lippe.

Case 2.—Mrs. H., aged forty-nine, after a fatiguing walk, sought a cool retreat to rest. She soon began to feel rigors passing down her back, which were followed by shuddering and indescribable aching, from the head to the lower extremities. She could scarcely endure contact with the bed clothing, and this sensitive and sore feeling was all over the body. She had great thirst, a thick, white coating upon the tongue; a tumefied countenance, expressive of much pain. Her pulse was not much accelerated. Chilliness and heat in rapid alternation, with this intolerable aching, thirst, and dry skin, continued all night. Prescribed **Arsenicum** 3 trituration; called in the afternoon, and found that her pains had been frightful, tending more to her head. Prescribed **Aconite** 3. The first dose had a quieting effect; her pains became diminished; her skin moist; sensitiveness to contact was removed; her thirst diminished; and, finally, she fell into a quiet slumber, and rested well until morning. She soon recovered.—Dr. A. E. Small.

ACTÆA RACEMOSA.

This is also called the Black Cohosh or Cimicifuga Racemosa. Its main sphere of action lies in the female sexual system especially upon the uterus and ovaries. It works on the muscular system as well, as we will find out in a short while. It is most useful in difficult labor due to rigidity of os as in **Caulophyllum** but the extreme severity of pain—pain that brings on fainting is the differentiating feature. The patient in the first stage of labor suffers from fits of shivering, a sort of nervous chill, shaking her through and through. Given during the last month, it shortens labor. Also it is a protection against false labor pains and prevents sickness of pregnancy and after pains. The symptom to indicate it in the last condition has been very aptly described by Dr. Lippe as a sensation as if the recently delivered uterus becomes actually jammed in the pelvis with great pain. It is also a great remedy for uterine neuralgia, the pain shifting from side to side. There is also a bearing down sensation as if everything is being pressed out and this sensation is somewhat relieved by the patient lying down. The mense may be either profuse or scanty although it is generally scanty and during each menstrual period the patient suffers from strong labor-like pains. During menses the patient becomes hysterical or suffers from epileptic spasms. The mental symptoms, of which there are a great variety and which we will discuss presently, undergo strange aberrations and aggravations during this period. In this connection we may as well mention that it is a great remedy for reflex pain; we use it in sharp lancinating electric like pains in various parts of the body when in sympathy with ovarian irritation or due to reflex from uterus.

As may be easily imagined this patient is sad and morose. There is a great abundance of sighing as in **Ignatia**. Mental depressions sometimes take the form of suicidal mania. She is constantly afraid of becoming crazy and we notice that she has to exert great control to prevent her from committing suicide.

This depression is so great that everything in **Actæa** looks covered with a death-like pall. She feels as if a heavy black cloud has settled over her and enveloped her head, so that all were darkness and confusion. This intensified gloom often leads to real mania, of which she is so constantly afraid, and we find her imagine all sorts of strange things. She imagines strange objects about her bed and sees rats and sheep roaming everywhere. At times there is the illusion of a mouse running from under her chair. She avoids company and wanders on from place to place evading questions asked. Then again we find her suffering from a great fear, as if everybody around her would conspire and kill her. She gets so suspicious of everybody and everything that she would not take medicine if she knew she was taking it.

It is a great remedy for headache but the headache is of uterine origin; due to great rush of blood to head, the brain feels too large for the cranium. This congestion to head is the effect of suppression of uterine discharges or suddenly ceasing of neuralgic pains. It is felt even in the eye-balls and is increased by the slightest movement of head or eye-balls. This headache is better in open air. We have also neuralgic pains affecting malar bones and ciliary neuralgia under **Actæa.** The pain extends from the temple to the eye-ball and is so severe as to drive her almost crazy.

Now we will discuss its application in rheumatism. There is general aching all over the limbs and the muscular soreness is excessive. We think of it in stiffness in joints, experienced early in the morning as if he had walked hard the day before. **Actæa Racemosa** is particularly applicable in rheumatism affecting the bellies of the muscles. We also have sensitiveness of spine with a feeling of great weight in the lumbar and sacral regions.

It has been recommended in insipient tuberculosis when the peculiar "**Actæa cough**" is present. It is mostly a noctural cough and although dry there is at times an expectoration of a viscid stringy mucus. The cough becomes particularly harassing when he attempts to speak. There is also a persistent diarrhœa which unless checked at the proper moment, will lead the patient on to a maze of suffering, ending ultimately in tuberculosis of lungs.

Case 1.—Mrs. C., dark complexion, dark brown eyes, has had for years uterine troubles; cancer of the left mamma, and was taking medicines for these general ailments. In the course of treatment she caught cold, and exhibited the following condition: Headache in occiput and right temple; intermittent. Eyeball aches and feels as if there were "a shot in it." Darting in right eye at intervals during the day, but in both eyes, and much more severe at night. She says "I shall go crazy." Involuntary twitching of eyelid. Worse from light especially from glass-light. Worse from least noise, as others walking, etc. Gave **Spig.** 30. No relief. I then studied **Cimicifuga,** of which I gave two doses of the 30th. The neuralgia was well the next day and with it the following improvement: A heavy pain in the right ovary disappeared. She could lie on right side, which she hadn't done before for two months, and a troublesome leucorrhœa of several month's standing, ceased entirely.—Dr. E. A. Farrington.

Case 2.—(Spinal congestion from a Railroad injury.) H. V. aged twenty, single, was admitted to the hospital December 7, 1876. One year ago was crushed between two cars, the bumpers catching him in the left hypochondriac and inferior mammary regions. He did not think the injury would end seriously, and allowed to go without treatment. He now complains of very severe pain and hyperæsthesia of the whole left side; aggravated by lifting, but relieved by walking about. A light slap on the leg induces severe cramps and simply touching him on the breast over the cardiac region, will almost immediately bring on a fit of crying; has pain commencing in the cardiac region and extending downward, and sometimes sharp, twitching pain in the lower extremeties, which extends upward. On passing the finger along the spinous process of the vertebræ, we find excessive sensitiveness from the fourth dorsal vertebra to the sacrum. Has some headache; bowels regular; but the stool causes some pain. Sleeps only two or three hours each night, and the little rest he does get is taken in a chair. Has not been in bed for nine or ten months. As soon as he attempts to lie down he is taken with severe cramps, which are unrelieved until he rises and moves about. Pulse 76; temperature 98½; Arn. 30. December 8. No better; changed prescription to **Cimicif. rac.** 200; 10th, improving; 13th, is gaining rapidly; 15th, went to bed last night after considerable urging and slept soundly for twelve hours, which was the first sleep he had enjoyed in bed for over ten months. January 18, continued gaining under **Cimicif. rac.** 200, above, and was this day discharged cured.—Dr. B. G. Carleton.

ACTÆA SPICATA.

This is a rheumatic remedy and it has special affinity for smaller joints, particularly the wrist. The patient goes out feeling well but after a slight exercise the joints start aching and swell compelling him to hurry home in disgust. Affected joints are swollen and motion is rendered absolutely impossible. In the affected limb great weakness is felt as if paralysed. Extreme tenderness to touch, nocturnal aggravation, weakness and tingling are some of the cardinal symptoms.

It bears great resemblance to **Viola odorata, Caulophyllum, Sabina, Colc.** and **Sticta** in rheumatism.

It is particularly suited to old people. The aggravation is noticed from motion and change of weather.

ADONIS VERNALIS.

It is a popular home remedy for heart troubles and it is of the same type as **Convallaria** and **Digitalis.** It is reputed to be serviceable in cases of endocarditis, valvulitis and other heart affections secondary to Bright's disease. The symptoms are, rapid and feeble action of the heart, dropsy, irregular and intermittent pulse, œdema of the legs, ascites and dyspnœa. Hale reports of a beautiful cure in a labourer suffering from chronic valvular disease of the heart with dilatation under the action of **Adonis.** The heart became diminished in size, the congestion of the lungs disappeared, the œdema of the legs vanished, the palpitation of the heart and the dyspnœa stopped. This drug has not been proved in its potency.

ÆSCULUS HIPPOCASTANUM.

Æsculus is the common horse chestnut, a native of Asia but cultivated extensively in Europe and America. It was proved by Dr. Cooly of the New York State.

It is one our of great hemorrhoidal remedies. Its efficacy in the treatment of this trouble is indisputable.

The action of **Æsculus** is mostly centred on the rectum and the rectal mucous membranes. It causes great plethora in that neighbourhood. This plethora leads to a sensation of fullness which is one of our keynote symptoms of this remedy. Another very noted symptom of **Æsculus** is dryness—a dryness that renders defæcation extremely painful and it is this dryness that is mainly responsible for the splinter-like pain so characteristic of the remedy. Extreme heat, a sense of constriction, a feeling of thickening of the rectal mucous lining obstructing defæcation, intense unallayed pain are sure indications of **Æsculus.** Sometimes we have a real blockage of the rectum due to the presence of innumerable hemorrhoidal knobs. When to such a condition is added the difficult task of a passage of a large hard, dry, knotted stool, the agony becomes simply indescribable. A portion of the anus protrudes and with it a bundle of piles looking like a bunch of grapes. Another great characteristic symptom of this remedy is lumbo-sacral backache. The patient feels as if his back is almost breaking and no position relieves. It feels almost like a knife sawing up and down along the passage. **Æsculus** has been known to bring immediate and instantaneous relief, in such cases. Pain and lameness in each sacro-iliac symphisis, paralytic feeling in arm, feet and spine, fullness in various parts of the body, as if containing an undue amount of blood, heaviness and lameness are indications that will rarely betray any confidence reposed on Æsculus.

It may be compared with **Carbo veg., Lachesis** and **Muriatic acid** in respect of the bluish colour of the piles.

ÆTHUSA CYNAPIUM.

Æthusa is prepared from a very common weed of Europe known as the Fools Parsley. It is a great friend of the children as it helps us to cure many of their ailments. I would like to give it a very important place amongst the remedies we use to check vomiting of milk in infants. This intolerance of milk is due to a peculiar gastric irritation frequently met with in children during dentition. As soon as the child drinks its milk, up it comes with great gush and in big quantity. If the milk is kept down for a little while it is vomited out in the form of big, thick, greenish curds. It thus resembles **Ant. crud., Nat. mur., Silicea, Sulphur** and **Valeriana;** but the utter prostration, great sleepiness, the peculiar woe-begone, anxious, pain-stricken, drawn look of **Æthusa** speak in language too plain for even a beginner to make a mistake. These children are too weak to stand and even when held up, their heads droop down as in **Abrotanum.** After the exertion of vomiting, the child falls into a sort of helpless slumber from which it wakes up, crying with violent hunger, to eat and to vomit again. Very often this is complicated with diarrhœa of a light yellow bilious colour. If this is not checked by the timely administration of **Æthusa,** it may run on to cholera infantum and hydrocephalus.

Æthusa is equally great in convulsions in which the thumbs are clenched and the eyes are turned downward. The appearance of the patient is very striking. His eyes look sunken with a peculiar pearly whiteness of all that portion of the face bounded by the upper lip and two distinct lines drawn from two orifices of the nose to the angles of the mouth. This is called **Linea nasalis.** This is more characteristic of **Æthusa** than any other remedy that I know of.

Dr. Clarke recommends it highly in patients suffering from want of the power of concentration. He mentions of a young undergraduate in whom with **Æthusa** he helped to bring back his long-lost power of concentration.

Æthusa is wanting in thirst like **Pulsatila** and **Apis.**

AGARICUS MUSCARIUS.

Agaricus Muscarius belongs to the natural order of Fungi. I am afraid I shall not be far wrong in according **Agaricus** an important place in our Meteria Medica. Owing to present-day allurements and excesses, hundreds of our young men fall easy victims to drink and debauchery, and stand in need of remedies like **Agaricus.** After a whole night of debauch, our victim wakes up the next morning with a big and swollen head. Confused ideas, great giddiness, irritability of temper, depression of spirit, disinclination for exertion of any kind are accompanying symptoms. A few drops of **Agaricus** will soothe his over-excited brain and nerves, and herald a normal functioning of all the organs, rendered topsy-turvy, by his night's intemperance.

It is also very useful in headaches of those who are subject to chorea, or who readily become delirious in fever or with pain. It is very helpful in vertigo arising out of the above mentioned causes. The patient feels a great weight in his head and constantly feels like falling backward

We notice a great tenderness, soreness and aching in the lumbar and sacral regions. Symptoms of chorea varying from simple involuntary motions to a regular dancing of the whole body, are also very common, but what characterises these involuntary movements in **Agaricus,** is that they are only present while the patient is awake, ceasing during sleep. Great sexual excitement both in the male and in the female is also noticeable. Great desire for an embrace, voluptuousness and a marked debility after coitus are important indication of **Agaricus.**

Locomotor ataxia finds in **Agaricus** a ready remedy. There is the uncertainty of the gait, the patient stumbling over everything in his way. The symptom that makes **Agaricus** very efficacious in such complaints is a terrible pain in the heels, as if they have been bitten. Another characteristic indication of this remedy is that the parts pain, as if touched or pierced by needles of ice.

On the skin we find many miliary eruptions, the parts looking red and swollen with intense burning as in frost-bite.

It is very rich in mental symptoms. The patient sings and talks but does not answer questions. There is a lascivious desire to kiss. Great loquacity, convulsive movements of the facial and cervical muscles of the right side, bringing the head down to the shoulder are symptoms that indicate **Agaricus** in delirium, insanity, idiocy, softening of the brain and various kindred ailments.

Case 1.—Albert L., aged ten years, slender, well grown, with a lively, sanguine temperament and merry disposition, had an attack of St. Vitus' dance when he was four years old, which was then cured by iron-powders. Four months before I was called to see him, he had another attack of the same disease. It commenced this time with an impediment of speech; he ceased to talk intelligibly. After this he began to drag his right foot; he could not walk in a straght line, nor did the muscles of his right arm obey his will. He could not use it for eating, because his hand would go everywhere but to his mouth. The same symptoms soon extended to the left side, particularly of his face; and when I first saw him his limbs were in incessant motion, with the distinct character of involuntary jerking, pushing or pulling in various directions. These motions lasted all day, and during the first period his mother had to use some violence to keep him in bed; but as soon as he has once fallen asleep, all motion ceases entirely, and he sleeps quietly. His appetite is very strong, and his bowels are in good order. He passed a couple of long worms some time ago. His speech is entirely unintelligible to every stranger; his tongue is not subject to his will, and the same phenomenon extends to the muscles of deglutition; the food he eats and the water he drinks fall out of his mouth again, before he is able to swallow them. He walks in a jumping, jerking way, as if were pushed by some invisible power, in one or the other direction, different from that of his will. His mind is not impaired at all, and his disposition exceedingly merry and playful, inclined to fun and mischief. The latter circumstances which struck me as a prominent symptom of the case, decided my choice among the indicated remedies in favour of **Hyoscyamus**. But to my astonishment, this remedy did not show the least effect in the course of one week; whereupon I prescribed **Agaricus muscarius 3**. This exhibited a slow but decided action upon all the symptoms at the end of the first week after commencing it. It was therefore continued, and four weeks later, I made the following memorandum. Improvement steadily progressing; he walked out alone for the first time to-day; has dressed himself without assistance; he can drink alone; he jerks his mouth, which, when talking he opens in the form of a fish-snout; his speech is much better, but he still makes involuntary motions with his hands and feet, particularly in a backward direction. **Agaricus muscarius 40** was persevered in for some time longer, and gradually restored the boy, who at the same time was growing and rapidly gaining perfect health.—Blœde in the "U. S. Jour. of Hom." Feb. 1861.

Case 2.—Hon. Mr.———,aged about forty; robust, ruddy and plethoric; large head and massive chest; sedentary; a free liver, and habitual but not immoderate user of tobacco and stimulants. Since two years, frequent attacks of vertigo, with the usual heaving and whirling of objects about him; tendency

H. M. M.—2

to fall forward; partial amaurotic blindness, with floating muscæ and vibrating spectra, and partial numbness of the left side of the tongue; temporary constipation; exciting debate or protracted mental application invariably brought on the attacks, which were accompanied by slight nausea but no unusual change of color, coolness of extremities nor heat of scalp. **Nux, Bell., Ig., Glo.,** and **Cocc., in medium and high potencies,** in connection with cathartics when constipated, were given, without relief. Finally, I prescribed ten or fifteen drop doses of the tincture of **Agar.,** three times daily, whenever the symptoms appeared, and also directed its use for three or four days after the attacks passed away. Each successive attack was greatly diminished in severity and duration, they became less frequent, and in less than three months wholly disappeared. Nearly two years have elapsed since the last attack.—Dr. G. W. Pope.

AGAVE AMERICANA

It is also called the American Aloe. The tincture is prepared from fresh chopped leaves. This remedy has not been given a thorough scientific proving but as it is reputed to have a great curative value in hydrophobia, it will not do to leave it out of our Materia Medica. We have a nice instance of a cure of hydrophobia with **Agave** reported in "The Homœopathic Recorder." A boy developed symptoms of hydrophobia four months after the bite. Quarrelsomeness, inability to swallow, desire to bite anybody near about, were symptoms that were thoroughly relieved by the boy partaking in crude juice of the plant that was simply thrown at him. Since then it has been used in similar instances on similar symptoms and numerous cures have been recorded as effected by **Agave.**

AGNUS CASTUS.

The tincture is prepared from the berries of the Chaste tree, a plant growing extensively on the shores of the Mediterranean Sea. Its chief action is felt over the sexual sphere and the nervous system. It belongs to the same category as **Selenium, Staphysagria** and **Acid phos,** although properly speaking it typifies a condition more desperate than that presented by any one of those remedies.

We think of **Agnus** when the sexual life is entirely annihilated, due to abuses and excesses of former years. The sexual desire is very much lessened, at times it is almost lost. The penis is so relaxed that voluptuous fancies excite no erection. The testes get cold and the spermatic fluid is absolutely thin. We should think of this remedy in impotence particularly brought about by frequent attacks of gonorrhœa. A short comparison of **Agnus castus** with **Caladium, Conium, Lycopodium, Phosphorus, Sulphur** and **Thuja** will not be out of place here.

We think of **Caladium** in impotence where voluptuous excitement is present but not attended with proper erections.

Conium and **Phosphorus** are remedies in impotence, the result of undue continence.

Lycopodium and **Sulphur** are similar to **Agnus** in respect of coldness of the sexual parts and smallness of the sexual organ.

We should think of **Thuja** in impotence after gonorrhœa same as **Agnus.**

Agnus is equally applicable in hysterical women suffering from maniacal lasciviousness, although generally it is oftener indicated in cold women suffering from sterility and entire loss of sexual desire. The sexual parts are extremely relaxed and we have a transparent leucorrhœal discharge passing imperceptibly from the relaxed parts.

This decay of one's sexual life is further portrayed in his premature old age, melancholy apathetic indifferent look, loss of power of sight and a constant fear of death. This fear of death is not as in Aconite, due to some catastrophe immediately impending but to a vague and remote apprehension of approaching end.

Agnus patients suffer from illusion of smell. They complain of an imaginary odour as of herring or musk always sticking to their nose.

Case 1.—A woman of loose virtue, who had borne out the child, now ten years old, applied to me for something to renew her almost extinguished venereal appetite. She suffered with an incorrigible womb-disease which had been treated by a dozen doctors without result I had her under my care for six months, and effected positively nothing. The whole uterus was engorged and thickened, extensive ulceration occupied the os and even reached into the interior of the womb. The menses, exceedingly profuse (probably free hæmorrhages), generally occurred twice a month. One specialist injected a solution of chromic acid into the cavity. Several of them scarified the os every week or two for months at a time. The menses were exceedingly painful and she was terribly tormented with ovarian neuralgia. She had abandoned all treatment in despair. Although very thin and haggard, she was still beautiful, and ostensibly kept a mistress, she had more lovers than one. She came to me, as I said, for something to renew her sexual vitality. Coitus had been somewhat painful for years, but now it was absolutely abhorrent. She seemed utterly fagged and worn out in that respect. She had lost interest in everything, could hardly ever be persuaded to dress herself and go out for a little air. She was indifferent to persons and things, and described herself as feeling stupefied, benumbed and dead to all excitements. Taking the physical and moral symptoms into consideration, I prescribed **Agnus castus, 1st dec. dil.,** ten drops three times a day In a month she reported herself better, and her decidedly improved appearance confirmed the statement. Another month passed, with only one dose daily, and the menses had appeared only once and without pain, and not preceded or followed, as usual, by ovarian neuralgia. The medicine was discontinued. The next monthly period was retarded ten days, and the flow was perfectly natural. She had become so much larger about the hips, breast and abdomen that she fancied she was pregnant. I saw her lately and was astonished at the change. She is about fifteen pounds heavier than she was when she began the treatment. She rarely has any pain, and feels as well, she affirms, as she did before her marriage, which occurred eleven years ago.—Dr. Holcomb, "The Am. Homœopathist," January, 1878.

Case 2.—Gonorrhœa in a gentleman who had frequent attacks. The inflammatory symptoms had been subdued by **Gels.,** and there now remained a purulent discharge, staining the linen yellow. **Agn. 3** cured in three or four days.—Hoyne.

AILANTHUS GLANDULOSA.

The common name of this plant is the Tree of Heaven. It is a native of China. It is cultivated very extensively in the United States as a shade tree.

It is better that we should know something about this remedy. It is very helpful in some of those obstinate cases of malignant sorethroat accompanying scarlatina, measles and other eruptive diseases. It was in such a case that I first tried **Ailanthus.** The result exceeded my most sanguine expectations. The fever was very high and the patient was in a state of stuporous delirium. His whole body was covered with a sort of a dark miliary rash. The inside of his throat was swollen and livid. The tonsils looked immensely large and were studded with ever so many angry-looking ulcers discharging a sort of a fetid ichorous humour. The tongue looked equally bad—it was cracked, dry and parched. The teeth were covered with a brown sordes. The cellular tissues around the neck were infiltrated. Through the nostrils there flew a thin ichorous bloody discharge. All symptoms pointed towards a fatal end. His prostration very marked from the beginning progressed with leaps and bounds. This sudden and great fall in vital force, so characteristic of **Ailanthus,** first drew my attention to it and as it covered most of the symptoms of the patient, it was administered.   The cure was speedy and marvellous.

It may be very aptly compared with **Apis, Carbolic acid, Crotalus, Lachesis, Lycopodium, Merc. cyan., Nitric acid** and **Phytolacca**—remedies equally adapted to those serious types of malignant sorethroat and diphtheria.

Apis is generally applicable in those forms of throat complaints where the disease starting, as it does so insidiously, without much pain and inconvenience is not thought of seriously in the beginning.   It is a right-sided remedy and the right tonsils are studded with deep, gray looking ulcerations exuding a scanty and putrid discharge.   Œdema of throat and uvula is a marked feature of this remedy.   Fetidity of breath, thirstlessness, painful and scanty micturition, intense sense of suffocation and a very high fever are characteristic indications of **Apis.**

Carbolic acid, like **Apis,** is marked by an absence of pain but unlike **Apis** we have a low adynamic fever.   The stench from the mouth is almost unbearable, and we have an extensive area of glandular involvement.

Crotalus is mostly adapted to cases marked with a persistent hæmorrhage from the orifices of the mouth and nose.   Gangrenous destruction of tissues of the fauces and tonsils, great thirst, excessive prostration, are prominent indications of **Crotalus.**

Lachesis has marked asthenia from the start.   It is a left-sided remedy as most of its complaints start from that side.   It is the very reverse of **Apis** inasmuch as we have intense pain accompanying an apparently small amount of inflammation.   Deep redness of fauces, constant desire to put the tongue out of the mouth which trembles like that of a snake, infiltration of the cellular tissue about the neck, cardiac debility, aggravation from hot and relief from cold drinks are the cardinal symptoms of **Lachesis.**

Lycopodium is eminently a right-sided remedy with a desire for warm drinks which are grateful to the throat.   Tendency to cellular paralysis, dropping of lower jaw, rapid rattling breathing, brownish redness of fauces and aggravation from sleep are the cardinal symptoms of this remedy.

Merc. cyanatus is particularly adapted to throat troubles of putrid and adynamic character.   The fetor oris is most marked. The tenderness of the salivary glands is great.   The nasal cavities, mouth, fauces, pharynx and larynx are covered by dark, grey or thick greenish leathery exudations. Profuse epistaxis, incessant salivation and abundant perspiration are highly characteristic of **Merc. cyan.**

Nitric acid is mostly indicated in nasal diphtheria. There is chilliness with aversion to heat. Nose-bleed, distress and uneasiness in stomach with total rejection of all food, stinging splinter-like pains, excessive salivation are most marked in **Nitric acid**.

Phytolacca is indicated when we have a feeling in throat as if it were a large empty cavern. Aggravation from hot fluids, pains in head, neck and limbs, difficulty of swallowing, each attempt being followed by sharp shooting into ears, are important landmarks of this remedy.

Case 1.—Whilie, aged ten years, has been subject to epileptic fits for nine months past. The attacks recur about once a week, in the morning, between the hours of 4 and 6 o'clock. They are announced by no premonitory symptoms. During the paroxysms, he struggles violently, his breathing is embarrassed, his face turgid, and livid, his hands are clenched and he foams at the mouth. The convulsive movements continue about fifteen minutes, when he falls into a deep sleep, from which he awakes in one or two hours, remembering nothing of what occurred during the fit. November 13, 1875. Prescribed **Ailan. gland.,** two drops of the mother tincture in two teaspoonfuls of water, morning, noon and night. December 20. Has had but one slight convulsion during the five weeks past; looks and feels much better. **Ailan.** continued morning and night. April 28, 1876. Patient had had slight twitchings of the facial muscles three times, in the morning, during the last four months, but no convulsions. He has been so well that his mother discontinued the use of the remedy two months ago.—Dr. George W. Richards.

Case 2.—Maggie N., aet. twelve, complained, December 17, of chilliness, headache, sore throat, etc., **Bell. 30.** December 18. Delirium all night; wants to go home; screams that the house is on fire; falls back exhausted. Rash fully out, but of a dusky color; tongue dry, fissured, with brown sordes; teeth covered with brown slime; edges of lips fissured; eyes sensitive to light; the whole body, especially the head, burning hot; involuntary urination; lies in bed in a semi-stupor, and when spoken to, recognizes the speaker and tries to answer correctly, but becomes again semi-comatose; great thirst for cold water. **Bell 30,** in water, every three hours. December 19. Worse; great restlessness, alternating with fear; bad all night; complains of her piercing headache; otherwise, same. **Bell. 30.** Late in the evening raging; eyes brilliant (usually a mild child); struggles to get up; bloated around eyelids. **Apis. 200,** in water, through the night. December 20. Same; **Ailan. 3,** in water, every two hours. Improvement began with the first dose and continued steadily till recovery was complete.—Dr. S. Lilienthal.

ALETRIS FARINOSA.

The tincture is prepared from the Star Grass. It is said to be a very bitter substance.

It is generally indicated in anæmic patients, especially in females suffering from protracted ailments or defective nutrition. Great debility is characteristic of this remedy. The patient is tired all the time and suffers from prolapsus, leucorrhœa, sterility and rectal discomfort. Great weariness of mind and body, anorexia, nausea and a sensation of weight in uterine region are important indications of **Aletris.**

It is reputed to be as good a remedy for constipation as **Alumina**—an inveterate constipation due to complete atony of rectum. Defecation is accompanied by terrible pain.

ALLIUM CEPA.

The tincture is prepared from the common red onion. It is one of our great catarrhal remedies. We have catarrh of the eyes, nose, throat and even of the bronchial tubes. This catarrhal inflammation of the mucous membrane leads to increased secretion. Thus we have profuse watery and acrid discharge from the eyes, nose and throat with violent sneezing. Due to a similar inflammation in the larynx the voice gets set and the cough becomes incessant. The cough is associated with intense pain in the throat. The patient grasps his throat every time he coughs as if to save it from being torn to pieces.

Thread-like pains are very characteristic of **Cepa.** Such a pain in any part of the body ought to remind us of this remedy. We use it in paronychia when red streaks run up the arms and is accompanied with a thread-like pain. **Cepa** patients are always better in a cold room and open air. Other similar catarrhal remedies are **Euphrasia, Arum trif., Arsenic,** etc.

Case 1.—December 19, 1877. Mr.——caught cold during the first week of December, with frontal pain; lachrymation; pain in left eye; weakness, and loss of appetite. For these symptoms he took **Sep.** On the 14th, he went out of doors, there being a cold wind. His cold improved, but the eye became worse. On the 15th, had pain and lachrymation of the left eye, with running from left nostril. Took **Euph.**, with relief. On 16th, at noon, the pain returned, with watering from left eye and left nostril. This lasted till 7 p.m., then went off. On 17th, the symptoms returned, at 12 or 12-30 p.m., Again took **Euph,** and in the evening, then went off suddenly. Yesterday the attack came on at 1 p.m. lasting till 5 p.m., then decreasing. Today, eye felt nearly well in morning, except photophobia. There had been a little lachrymation during the night. At 1 p.m., aching pain in left eye and left brow. After thirty minutes, bland lachrymation, heat and redness of the left eye, with running from left nostril. This lasted till 5 p.m., then decreased. Accordingly I gave one dose of **Cepa.** 200 (Leipzig) at 6-30 p.m. 20th. No redness or return of paroxysms; not the slightest pain to-day till 2-30 p.m., and then it was very slight; a little lachrymation, at times. 21st. No paroxysms, but only a little pain in eye about 1 p.m., and then it was less than yesterday; a feeling of lachrymation, and still a little photophobia. 24th. Much better; afterward, eye remained a little sensitive to cold air for a few weeks, but subsequently recovered.—Dr. E. W. Bridge.

Case 2. (Traumatic Sciatica after Amputation).—Amputation of lower third of thigh, made necessary by the results of an abscess in the popliteal space. Union by first intention followed, and everything proceeded most favourably up to the point of complete restoration to health, except a neuralgic condition of the sciatic nerve, which had been involved in the abscess. A burning, stinging pain began to be felt running up the thigh and down to the sole of the foot as soon as the abscess began to form; it increased in severity, and was not relieved by amputation. There was no sleep or rest. The patient became desperate, and no proper relief was given by any of the remedies administered, except from half-drachm doses of **Amm. muriat.** Nearly three months after the operation, the patient picked up a scrap or printed paper, and his eye met a little paragraph, on raw onion in neuralgia. He resolved to try it, and ate a whole one at bed time. All pain immediately ceased, and he slept quietly that night. **Allium 200** was given without effect, but ten-drop doses of the tincture were taken for two days, since which there has been no pain.—Dr. C. S. Shelton.

ALLIUM SATIVA.

It is the garlic of our everyday use and is adapted to high livers and fleshy people who consume an enormous quantity of food and suffer from indigestion as a result of their gluttony. Their bowels are apt to be disturbed by the slightest deviation in diet. The least change in their usual manner of living increases the dyspepsia. Heartburn, belching, copious flow of saliva after eating, wind colic, great distention and pressure in epigastrium and transverse colon are important symptoms.

These people, as is very often the case with high livers, are martyrs to rheumatism. The pain, however, is mostly in hip, as well as in iliac muscles.

Its cough is very similar to that of **Capsicum** in as much as it is associated with very fetid breath. It is aggravated after smoking.

ALOES SOCOTRINA.

To write a Meteria Medica without **Aloes** is to write a novel without a hero. Its importance and usefulness become evident as soon as we launch in our business of curing the sick. Its chief and the most important action is seen in the large intestines. Taken in a big dose it increases the intestinal secretion and its peristaltic action. It also produces sensation of heat, fullness, heaviness and throbbing in the rectum. In the homœopathic therapeutics, **Aloes** justly assumes an important place in the treatment of diarrhœa. I would like to give it the very first place in those peculiar cases where the **Aloes** characteristics are present. As homœopaths we have got no surer guide and no simpler process than to be guided by those characteristics. They are :—

Firstly, a great feeling of weakness and loss of power of sphincter ani. This leads to a sensation of insecurity in the rectum. They are afraid to pass flatus for fear stool will escape. In this **Aloes** resembles **Oleander, Phosphorous, China, Hyosc, Opium** and **Acid phos.** The urging for stool is great; he runs for the bath room, but unfortunately even before he gets to it, his clothes are all soiled.

Secondly, a great feeling of fullnes and weight in the pelvis as though the rectum were full of fæcal matter which would fall out if not for the extreme caution.

Thirdly, loud rumbling and gurgling in the abdomen as though water were running out of bottle. This symptom when present in dysentery becomes a great characteristic.

Fourthly, the aggravation of the condition after each meal as in **Arsenic, China, Lycopodium, Podophyllum, Thromb, Croton tig.** and **Ferrum.**

Aloes causes great portal congestions and as is usually the case in all such remedies we notice a great depression, lassitude and languor clouding their mental atmosphere. They are fleshy and phlegmatic, highly dissatisfied and angry about themselves. They consider life as almost a burden and carry on their existence in a sad dispirited sort of way. They are inclined to suffer from congestion of the head and hence a dull frontal headache with heaviness of the eyes is common. Sometimes the headache alternates with lumbago. They suffer from pain deep in the orbits and have yellow vision. The congestion of the portal system referred to above gives them a sensation of constant fullness and heaviness in the abdomen. Rumbling in the abdomen, constant discharge of flatus, a feeling of weakness in the abdomen as if diarrhœa would set in, great cutting, griping pain in the right and lower portion of abdomen, a sensation of plug between symphisis pubis and os coccyx, urging to stool, constant bearing down in rectum are symptoms that ought to be very carefully remembered. The character of the **Aloes** stool also is equally striking. It is mostly transparent, jelly-like in dysentery and yellow semi-liquid fæcal in diarrhœa. This diarrhœa is always worse while walking or standing and is often followed by great prostration and fainting spells.

The hemorrhoids of **Aloes,** the result of the same portal congestions, protrude like a bunch of grapes. Constant backache, the same bearing down sensation in the rectum, the sensation of fullness described above should be our important landmarks in the selection of the remedy. The hemorrhoids are mostly moist due to constant mucous secretion from the anus. They are very tender, sore, hot, itchy and are generally relieved by washing it with cold water.

In this connection we may think of **Bromium** and **Mur. acid,** two remedies equally great in hemorrhoids. It differs from the former in the fact that **Bromium** piles are relieved by application of saliva and from **Mur. acid** by its relief from application of **warm** water.

The constipation of **Aloes** is equally prominent because of the same want of confidence in the sphincter ani. I remember quite vividly a case of a little boy about five years old that was brought to our college clinic years ago, when I was a student in the Hering Medical College of Chicago. He used to soil his clothes at all odd times with hard lumpy stools, which his mother ascribed to sheer wickedness on his part. When cane failed and the trouble grew worse, he was brought to the clinic. A few doses of **Aloes** put an end to all his unintentional villainy.

Aloes is a deeply anti-psoric remedy and it is of special use in chronic cases when the above symptoms are well marked.

Case 1.—A German woman, aged seventy-two, had been a hard worker; married nearly fifty years, and had reared a large family of children. Complained of severe pain in abdomen. Her husband called, and not being able to talk English, the doctor derived but little information. Gave **Nux vom.** and **Diosc.,** to be given alternately. Two weeks later, patient's daughter called, reporting her mother no better. Doctor called to see her, found pulse over 100, full; skin hot and dry; tongue, covered with heavy white fur and quite dry; lips dry and sore; much thirst, desire for cold and sour. Had been a habitual cider drinker. Anything cold aggravated the complaint, causing more frequent passages and pain. Stools were very frequent, especially from 4 to 10 a.m., consisting of stringy mucus of yellow color, and occasionally mixed with foul material. Desire for stool came on suddenly; could hardly get off her bed quick enough before some of the stool would escape. Any attempt to pass urine, would be accompanied with flow of stool. Stools accompanied with much flatulence, and were preceded with much pain in hypogastrium and sacrum, which was relieved by passage of stool. Symptoms all worse in forenoon. Patient was irritable, and angry because she was sick. **Aloes**, 20th trit., every two hours. Two days later, found patient worse, very much prostrated, and fever still present. First dose of **Aloes** was followed with intense head-ache, tearing and pressing in character, confined to left side of head and worse in fore part of the day; relieved somewhat by tying a handkerchief tightly about the head. Regarding this as aggravation of the remedy, two doses were ordered to be given daily of the same remedy. Three days later, the patient was found to be much better in every respect.—Dr. G. J. Jones.

Case 2.—Mr. C. H. B., aet. fifty-five, gentleman. July 13. Has been troubled excessively for six years with what he termed "moist piles," for which he had in vain tried allopathic and homœopathic treatment, here and in Europe. He complained of his linen being constantly stained by a mucous discharge from the anus; bowels generally moved once a day; stool covered with slime; after stool, feels "played out"; is always worse after bathing; at times, the discharge is so disagreeable and annoying that he feels like shooting himself. Prescribed **Ant. crud. 1m.,** which was repeated in August, and again on October 17, when he wrote me: "The whole thing has experienced a great change for the better since taking your few powders; for while, formerly, the spongy substance was most always passing off, there is only now and then some of this mucous whitish stuff, which is easily wiped off." Very little if any, improvement followed until January 3, 1875, when I prescribed **Aloes 30,** to be taken in water a teaspoonful, night and morning. for one week, the indications being "gob-like evacuations of clear jelly, with faintness for hours afterward, and anxiousness on account of health; a kind of chill running through the system, with pressure on the bladder, chill disappearing at once after making water." **Aloes** relieved markedly until February 4, when the prescription was repeated. May 27. My patient came again, after having been troubled for six weeks, and at this time he gave me another indication for **Aloes,** viz., "always much worse during hot, damp weather." **Aloes 5c.,** one dose every day, was followed by rapid improvement, and now (August 3) my patient considers himself radically cured.—Dr. C. Mohr, Jr.

ALUMEN.

This is our common Potash Alum. The trituration is prepared from pure crystals. It is a great astringent and is in great use amongst our people for common sore-throat on account of its astringent properties. This remedy is not in very great demand, but when the demand comes it is almost invaluable.

I shall give one or two leading characteristics of this remedy; one is found in its stools. The evacuations are exceedingly hard and knotty like stones, and they happen at very long intervals —say once or twice a week. These hard lumps, as they pass, leave the rectum intensely sore and tender, and it pains for a long time afterwards. Such inveterate constipation is also to be met with in **Ammon carb, Antimonium crud, Bryonia, Lach., Plumbum, Sepia** and **Sulphur.**

The second characteristic of this remedy is found in its peculiar hæmorrhage of a large mass of coagulated blood, putrid, disintegrated and of a dark colour, so often seen in the latter stages of typhus.

The **Alum.** patient is very sensitive to cold. We find aggravation during sleep, and on turning on the right side.

These patients are predisposed to tonsillitis and various forms of affections and inflammations of the buccal cavity. It is particularly indicated in chronic sore throat and pharyngitis. The veins about the fauces are distended. The relaxed and the ulcerated condition of the throat and spasmodic constriction in œsophagus make swallowing very difficult. The voice is entirely lost.

Case 1.—Young lady, twenty-one years old. This patient had seen me several times in my office, during which time she complained of a sore throat. The left tonsil was much inflamed and enlarged, and she experienced great difficulty in swallowing. I thought at the time that it was only a case of tonsillitis and prescribed **Belladonna.** Finally I was called again to visit her at her home, and, on examining her throat, found the left tonsil and the back part of the throat covered with a grayish white membrane. The most prominent symptoms were: violent head-ache; vomiting; excessive prostration; difficult deglutition; pains through the chest; expectoration of a large quantity of mucus, which was thick stringy; sleeplessness; fever every night, and all the symptoms aggravated toward evening; loss of appetite; great fetor, which was intolerable; great thirst, the patient constantly asking for cold drinks. I commenced treatment with **Aconite** and **Mercurius iodatus.** The second day found my patient about the same, or perhaps worse, the membrane spreading to the right side of the throat; continued **Mercurius iodatus,** as she remarked that her throat was not quite so painful. On the third day there was no marked improvement. I then stopped **Merc. iod.,** and gave **Nitric acid.** On the fourth day there was some little improvement; the head-ache had left and she could take some nourishment, such as beef-tea and chicken-broth. I imagined that the false membrane was shrinking, and at all events a portion of it had peeled from the right tonsil. On the sixth day the patient was no better. She complained of excessive prostration; had no sleep, was restless and desponding; on examining the throat I found that the membrane had changed from a grayish-white to a dark gray, almost black in some parts. The prostration was so great on this day, that my patient's voice became almost extinct. Her pulse could hardly be felt, and I warned the family of the danger she was in. I have in my library twenty volumes of an old French Journal, published by the Royal Academy of Medicine, Paris. In Vol. III., I found a long report, directed to the Academy, by Brettonneau, on diphtheria, in which he mentions his success, as well as that of Dr. Arctree, during an epidemic at Lyons in 1819. During this epidemic it seems that all the cases subjected to the antiphlogistic treatment died, and Dr. Arctree decided to try **Alum** which was the remedy employed by the ancient physicians as far back as the 16th and 17th centuries. They prepared a paste of alum and water, and applied this paste with the handle of a spoon immediately to the affected parts of the throat and at the same time gave calomel. Dr. Arctree gives a long list of cases in his report, and says that from the time he commenced this treatment he saved every patient. This decided me to try **Alum** as a last resort. I accordingly dissolved some **Alum** in water and gave a tea-spoonful of the solution every hour. I did this because my patient would not allow me to apply it topically, for fear that I would make her gag and vomit. On the following day I saw my patient about noon, and upon examining her throat found that every particle of the membrane had disappeared. She said she felt better than at any time since she had been taken sick. She is now convalescent. Three other cases in which **Alum** was used with promptly beneficial effect are to be added to the above report.—Dr. J. G. Houard, "Hahn. Monthly," March, 1875.

Case 2.—Cough acquired in the cold season, would last till warm weather came, unless relieved by medicine. Worse in the evening and at night. The night previous she had coughed all night long; aggravated on getting up in the morning, likewise from laughing, lasted a long time before any sputa was raised, and the longer she coughed the greater was the inclination; it was ameliorated by lying flat on the face. The top of the head was painful during an attack, and paroxysms made her feel very weak. Voice weak and hoarse, the latter increased in the morning. Nose was red; mouth moist and lips dry. Breathing somewhat wheezy. She was very nervous and easily laughed or cried. **Alumen 30,** daily, cured in a week.—Dr. C. P. Norton in "Am. Homœopathist," 1877.

ALUMINA.

Alumina is prepared from Oxide of Aluminium, a kind of clay, white in color, soft to touch, inodorous, tasteless and insoluble in water. It was introduced into our Materia Medica by Hahnemann.

This great anti-psoric is best suited to old and emaciated constitutions and to young girls at puberty suffering from chlorosis, also to weak undeveloped infants raised on artificial food and lacking in strength and vitality.

The characteristics of **Alumina** that appeal to me as being of predominant importance are paralysis of the involuntary muscles and depletion of life-force in many of the organs of the human system. This is seen in the atony of the intestinal tract that gives rise to a peculiar constipation for which **Alumina** is famous; it is a constipation in which the patient loses all desires for stool and every ability to pass it out. It is indeed a job with these patients to get a stool. They grasp the seat of the closet tightly and strain hard and strain continually till they succeed in getting rid of a few hard knotty laurel-berry balls covered with mucus as in **Graphites.** Even when the stools are soft like clay the same exertions and the same straining are necessary. There are remedies like **Anacardium, Platinum, Silicea** and **Veratrum** where we find a similar state of affairs, but they differ in other characteristic points. Sometimes the **Alumina** patient has to stand up to be able to defecate. In this **Alumina** resembles **Causticum.** The **Alumina** constipation is very often to be met with in women during pregnancy, in old people and also in bottle-fed babies.

A further illustration of the paralytic action of **Alumina** is seen in the loss of power of the internal rectus muscle causing squint.

Alumina is just as good a remedy for ptosis as **Gelsemium** and **Causticum.** This property of **Alumina** to cause paralysis and also to cure it makes it an admirable remedy in the treatment of that dreaded disease, locomotor ataxia. Bœnninghausen cured four such cases with **Alumina** on the following symptoms:—Formication, inability to walk in the dark or with eyes closed, sensation as if there is a cobweb on the face or as though the face were covered up with the white of an egg, pain in the spine as if hot iron were thrust into it and numbness of the heel when stepping.

Leucorrhœa, to which our **Alumina** patient is a constant subject, is another illustration of the depletion of the vital force. It is acrid and so profuse that it runs down the thigh clear to the heels. They are very afraid to go out into society and amongst friends for fear of this exhausting continual and debilitating leucorrhœa. The leucorrhœal discharge is transparent, ropy and tenacious.

Mentally they are low-spirited, melancholy and lachrymose. They are constantly troubled with an apprehension as if they will go crazy. A suicidal trait is sometimes noticed specially when they see blood or knife or something of that sort. Lassitude, languor, indifference are constantly present. They are very slow in accomplishing anything; time moves on very slowly with them— half a day seems like half a month.

They suffer from an abnormal craving for all kinds of absurd things such as chalks, charcoal, mud, etc.

They suffer from disorder of digestion as a result of which they are constantly belching.

Alumina is considered a very valuable remedy in typhoid fever. We use it when the patient passes clots of solid blood that look like little pieces of liver. Potatoes disagree.

Another symptom the result of great exhaustion and of profound prostration is involuntary spasdomic twitching of the lower jaw. The upper lip is covered with numerous little blisters and is dry and cracked. The teeth are covered with sordes. The urine is passed with great deal of difficulty.

All symptoms of Alumina are worse at new moon and full moon.

AMBRA GRISEA.

Ambergris is a fat-like substance found in the intestines and among the excreta of the spermwhale.

A remedy so useful as this should hardly be over-looked. The red strand of this remedy is found in its bashfulness, embarrassment and nervousness. It is thus like **Cepa** another remedy great in bashfulness. All his troubles are aggravated when he gets upset and nothing upsets him more than company. He cannot pass stools when somebody is present. The cough also starts troubling him when he goes among strangers or gets excited in any other way. The **Ambra grisea** cough is very peculiar and should

be specially remembered. It is a cough that is followed by eructations of wind. Only a few remedies such as **Sulph. acid, Arnica,
Sanguinaria** and **Veratrum** can come up to it when this symptom
is concerned. It is spasmodic in nature and is worse from talking,
and writing.

Ambra grisea has a marked action over the female genital
organs. During menses the leg becomes quite blue from distended
varices and also painful. As in **Bovista** we find a slight show
of blood between periods. Every little accident or a little over
exertion such as straining at stool or indulging in walk little longer
than usual brings it on. In this it is very similar to **Calc. carb.**
Another point of semblance between these two remedies consists
in a sensation of coldness felt mostly in the abdomen.

The leucorrhœa of Ambra grisea is thick and bluish white in
color. It occurs only at night as in **Causticum, Mercurius** and
Nitric acid.

Ambra grisea is a good remedy for sleeplessness due to nervousness and business embarrassment. He feels sleepy but as soon
as his head touches the pillow he wakes up.

AMMONIUM BENZOICUM.

This is the Benzoide of Ammonia, a salt exetremely useful in
albuminuria complicated with gout. The appearance is particularly characteristic; the eyelids are swollen and the face is bloated. The urine which is smoky and scanty is full of albumen. Its
other indications are pain across sacrum with urgency to stool,
sensation of internal soreness on pressure in the region of right
kidney and gout with fluid in large toe joints.

AMMONIUM CARBONICUM.

It is called the sal volatile or smelling salt. It is particularly
adapted to stout, plethoric women addicted to sedentary habits and
constantly tired though doing nothing.

Ammon. carb. acts very strongly on the blood. It generally
leads to a dissolution of red blood corpuscles due to poor oxygenation. Hence, gangrenous ulcerations, flabbiness of the muscles,
spongy consistency of the gums and other similar changes of tissues
are very common in this remedy. Due to degeneration of blood
tissue, the hæmorrhage to which these patients are frequent
subjects, is characterised by dark, strumous clotted blood. They

are, due to the very same reason, constantly chilly and are averse to fresh and open air. Washing, wet applications, cold wet weather aggravate all their complaints.

Mentally these patients are very restless and lethargic and they get more so during a wet stormy weather. A symptom to which they are constantly subject, is a sensation of oppressive fullness near the bridge of the nose as if everything inside would burst. All the head troubles are particularly located in this region. The headache may be pulsating, beating, pressing but it is always located in the forehead.

Ammon. carb. acts on the mucous membrane as well. Hence it is such an important remedy in nasal catarrh. We particularly think of it in coryza in hysterial females. The symptom that is considered most characteristic is the stoppage of the nose mostly at night times. The patient must open his mouth and breathe through it, as breathing through the nose is apparently impossible; hence it is such an important remedy in snuffles of children.

On the throat its action is no less marked. It is applicable in ordinary sore throat as well as in putrid sore throat of scarlatina and diphtheria. The tonsils are enlarged and highly inflamed and look almost bluish. Gangrenous ulceration of the tonsils is not uncommon. The stoppage of the nostrils leads to frequent waking up and is a source of great uneasiness and discomfort to the patient. We have also involvement of the neighbouring glands and there is great swelling of the neck. The cervical lymphatics as well as the parotid glands are engorged. Great burning is felt in the throat and in oesophagus as from alcohol. This picture is very similar to that of **Lachesis** but the difference consists in that **Ammonium carb.** is a right sided remedy whereas in Lachesis the left side is affected. The sensitiveness of **Lachesis** is also wanting.

The cough of **Ammonium carb.** is dry and tickling, almost always associated with hoarseness and great deal of oppression due to accumulation of mucus in the chest. The cough is always aggravated at 3 o'clock in the morning. Great tickling is felt in the larynx and throat as from a feather, and the patient is disturbed with a constant titillating cough which at times becomes almost asthmatic, due to great rattling as in emphysema. In fact, it is a great remedy in emphysema. The peculiar ashy paleness of the lips, the shortness of breath and palpitation after every excitement, somnolence—all pointing to carbolic acid poisoning of the blood—

are very characteristic of **Ammonium carb.** and will lead to great relief of suffering if applied in proper potency and in right time.

Now we shall discuss its actions in the female sexual organs. It is indeed a capital remedy in many of the affections of the females pertaining to those organs. First of all we should think of it in hysteria, when it is due to unnatural excitement of the sexual organs especially of the clitoris. The course is generally anticipated by six days. The blood, as is everywhere the case in **Ammonium carb.** is blackish and clotted. It is also extremely acid so as to make the thighs sore. The leucorrhoeal discharge also is excoriating and leads to ulceration in vulva. It is extremely profuse and sets up irritation, itching, burning and consequent swelling of the pudenda. The patient suffers from all sorts of aches and pains, particularly toothache and colic during catamenia.

They are particularly exhausted during the menstrual period. They complain of great fatigue, especially of the thighs, and they yawn and stretch with chilliness. A very important symptom of **Ammonium carb.** and one that is particularly characteristic of this remedy is the cholera-like diarrhoea at the commencement of catamenia.

It is extensively used in whitlow and panaritium. The finger is extremely inflamed and deep seated periosteal pain is felt and red streaks run up to the axilla from the inflamed area. We also have inflammation and pain in the ball of the great toe which looks red and swollen.

Lastly, we shall examine its action on the skin. It is a great remedy for malignant scarlatina, but the rash is unlike the rash of **Belladonna,** a miliary rash. It is accompanied with putrid sore throat, somnolence, palpitation, parotitis, involuntary defecation and stertorous breathing.

It is inimical to **Lachesis** and is antidotal to **Rhus** poisoning and stings of insects.

Case 1.—Mrs. B., aged forty-six. August 4, 1871. Pain at epigastrium, like a weight, constantly present; worse after food, especially meat; sinking immediately after food; weight over eyes; tongue looks clean, but feels foul; bad, acid taste; no relish, but can take food; thirst; catamenia every fortnight, black, coagulated, profuse; very much milky leucorrhoea, with itching of vulva and backache, especially before and after the catamenia; water reddish; flow often interrupted; flushes, **Amm. carb, 200,** three times to-day. August 8. All the symptoms better; the weight seems to be raised higher up than the epigastrium; water better quality, and does not intermit. Sac. Lac. August 15. Much better; has had a burning heat all over the body, but this has ceased; very little leucorrhœa. Sac. Lac. Cured without repetition of the medicine.—Dr. R. M. Theobald.

Case 2. (Inflammation of left big toe).—By a fall from the horse, a gentleman sprained his left big toe. Since then, he has had several attacks of inflammation of the joint of this toe, which kept him usually in bed for six weeks, under the continual alternate use of **Sulphur** and **Nux vom.** The inflammation sets in suddenly, without apparent cause; the toe-joint becomes red, hot, painful, and so sensitive to touch that he cannot bear the pressure of the bed-cover. He has the continual sensation as if the toe were sprained. **Amm. carb.,** 200 in water, every three hours, one table spoonful, cured in twenty-four hours; no relapse afterward.—Dr. Landesmann.

AMMONIUM CAUSTICUM.

It is the hydrate of Ammonia, or in other words Ammonia. This powerful drug is a strong cardiac stimulant. It is caustic in nature and produces burning in throat, gullet and rectum. It strongly affects the mucous membrane causing œdema and ulceration.

It is one of our best remedies in aphonia. Its strongest indication is the burning rawness in the throat. Spasm of the glottis, suffocation, pain in œsophagus are its characteristic indications. Great exhaustion and muscular debility prevail.

AMMONIUM MURIATICUM.

It is otherwise called Sal ammoniac. The very first thing that strikes us about the **Ammon mur.** patient is the ugly want of proportion between the upper and lower limbs. Above the waist line he is corpulent, fleshy and very coarse, while the legs are disproportionately thin.

This remedy has a very strong action over the mucous membrane of the human system. Its action on the nasal mucous membrane is manifested by a watery acrid coryza. The discharge is very profuse and it corrodes the inside of the nose as well as the upper lip. The nose gets quite blocked at night time. In this respect it is in no way inferior to **Aconite, Allium cepa, Arsen., Arum triph, Euph,** and **Sabadilla.** In the mouth and throat we find an extra accumulation of viscid saliva which is difficult to throw out. The cough of this remedy is peculiar in as much as the cough excites the salivary glands and while coughing the mouth fills up with saliva. I do not know of any other remedy with a similar cough.

Ammon mur. has a very important action over the tendons and fibrous tissues about the joints. The patient complains of a peculiar tense contracting pain. On this indication we use this remedy in old chronic sprains and also in rheumatic and other troubles when there is noticed a peculiar tension and a sense of contraction in tendons and fibrous tissues of any of our joints. It has helped in many cases of lameness due to contraction of the hamstrings muscles.

I have not yet touched upon the symptom that I consider most important in **Ammon mur.** It is seen in its action over the female genital organs. The menses come on too early with a severe tense contracting pain in the groin so much so that the patient walks bent. The menstrual time is at all times an ugly time with our patient. It is accompanied with diarrhœa and vomiting. Sometimes the stools are bloody. The menses flow more profusely at night time. In this respect it is very similar to **Bovista** and **Magnesia carb,** in both of which remedies we find a profuse flow at night when lying down—very little during the course of the day when the patient is on her feet walking about.

Cyclamen has a similar symptom viz., menses flow less when moving about. **Lilium tig.,** on the other hand, has exactly the opposite symptom—the menses flowing only when she is moving about, ceasing when lying down.

As regards diarrhœa, we can compare **Ammon mur.** with **Ammon carb.** In the latter remedy it has not only diarrhœa, but symptoms very similar to cholera appear during the menstrual period—and it is further associated with a great aching of the thighs, fatigue, sadness, yawning, toothache and a great chilliness. For menses during day time only we should compare it with **Causticum** and **Pulsat. Phel.** has menses in the evening only. **Sepia** and **Carbo animalis** are to be thought of in menses appearing in the day, specially in the hours of morning.

It is also indicated in leucorrhœa when it is of an albuminous nature following every urination.

The constipation in **Ammonium mur.** is an important feature of the remedy. The stools are hard requiring great exertion in expelling and they crumble as soon as they come near the verge of the anus. As a consequence these patients suffer a great deal from piles and we notice great burning in the rectum, during and after such painful acts of defecation.

I must mention, before closing, one more important symptom noted under this remedy. It is a sensation of icy coldness on the back between the shoulder blades, not relieved by warm clothing; I further like to emphasize that the symptom that stikes me as being the most characteristic is the contractive tensive pain—a symptom that makes it applicable in any disease when present.

Case 1.—Chronic eruption of the face and upon the lower part of the back. The skin presented an intensely red appearance, and was covered with a fine brownish exfoliation. There was intense burning, relieved only by the constant application of cold water. Even in order to procure sleep the cold wet cloth had to be renewed from time to time. The patch on the back never changed during two years. **Arsenic** alone gave some other relief, other remedies failed entirely. **Amm. mur., 12th dilution,** four doses cured the face in the course of a month; the spot on the body also disappeared slowly. There was no return of the trouble for a year; the cure, therefore, is likely to be permanent.—Dr. C. W. Boyce.

Case 2. (Chronic Ulcer of the Leg).—A case of the above, with sharp stinging pains at night, was cured in three weeks by **Amm. mur.**—Dr. M. Preston.

AMYGDALA AMARA.

Amygdala amara is prepared from bitter almonds. It is very akin to Hydrocyanic Acid, consequently many of its symptoms are similar to those of Hydrocyanic Acid. The glossy brilliance of the eyes, the dark red colour of the faces, difficult in swallowing and jerky speech are common to both the remedies.

This remedy has been used with great success in diphtheria and tonsillitis. Dr. Farrington reports of a case of diphtheria where **Amygdala** was of incalculable value and he prescribed it on the indication of a deep dark glossy redness of the whole fauces with sharp shooting pains on each attempt at swallowing. Prostration is also very marked.

AMYLENUM NITROSUM.

It is a yellowish etherial liquid having the odor of over ripe pears and an aromatic taste. One part by weight of this substance is dissolved in nine parts by weight of alcohol.

The Allopaths use it in all conditions where blood vessels are spasmodically contracted as in angina pectoris, epilepsy and asthma, in the form of an inhalation of 2 to 5 minims on a handkerchief. Within a very short time of such inhalation, the patient experiences a " sensation of heat, fulness, throbbing of the face and head, immediately followed by an indescribable and most distressing commotion within the chest, the heart beating fast and furiously and the breathing being panting and hurried." The relief following due to relaxation of the spasm and contraction is immediate and complete.

Our principle of Similia is more than verified in the case of this remedy. When the above symptoms are present due to some diseased condition we prescribe **Amyl nitrate** irrespective of any disease by name. Our application, however, in those troubles are based on the following indications:—Præcordial anxiety, cardiac oppression, stitching pains and a feeling of constriction in the cardiac region, great dilatation of carotids, fluttering of the heart at the slightest excitement, tremulousness of hands and stiffness and numbness of fingers and profound and repeated yawning.

This remedy is very similar in its action to **Glonoin** and **Belladonna** as it causes an intense surging of blood to head and face. To make way for this great rush of blood, the arteries dilate.

The red strand of this remedy is found in the blushings and flushings to which these patients are frequently subject. At the least excitement the face looks flushed and pulsation is felt over the entire body. The heart's action becomes intensified and almost tumultuous. Intense throbbing of the carotids is also noticed. Præcordial anxiety, oppression, sensation of swelling of the front of chest, great craving for fresh air, a bursting out feeling in ears, sensation of constriction in throat and heart, tremor, are a few of its trustworthy symptoms. Two other peculiar symptoms are a constant smacking of lips as if in the act of tasting and a constant movement of the lower jaw as in chewing.

ANACARDIUM ORIENTALIS.

This medicine is prepared from the crushed seeds of the marking nut. It was introduced into our Materia Medica by the master himself.

Its importance and usefulness will be apparent after we make a study of it and learn to use it in the proper manner. It has a few very characteristic symptoms which we will do well to remember :—

1. Sudden loss of memory for which it is a remedy par excellence. Everything is forgotten; confusion reigns supreme; they do not seem to be fit for business any more.

2. They suffer from a very peculiar and contradictory state of mind such as laughing at serious matters and serious over trifling things. We also notice an irresistible desire to curse and swear in persons never addicted to such habits. They also suffer from fixed ideas such as the following :—As if their mind and body are separate; as if they are double; as if a demon sits on their neck; as if they have two wills, one commanding them to do certain things, the other hindering them from doing it; as if some one is pursuing them. They suspect everybody and everything around them. They are also subject to illusions of hearing and smell.

3. A peculiar sensation of a hook or a pin on the surface of the body as also a sensation of a plug causing a pressing penetrating pain are very characteristic of **Anacardium.** These sensations whenever present and in whatever ailment will make it a first rate remedy.

It is a remedy for bad effects of strenuous mental exercise and over wrought mental state due to prolonged application. The mind is in a state of fatigue and the slightest mental exercise brings on a dull headache as of a pressure with a plug on upper border of right orbit extending into brain. The strangest part of this headache is relief after eating. Great disinclination for walk and aggravation from motion characterise this headache. We also think of it in headache of gastric origin i.e., in headaches of dyspeptics who suffer from constant fulness and distention of abdomen with hypochondriacal humour.

Anacardium although a great remedy for dyspepsia is much neglected. **Nux vom.** is used in great many cases where **Anacardium** should be thought of. Such a mistake is due to great similarity between the two remedies. In both of them we notice ineffectual desire for stool. In **Nux** it is due to an irregularity of peristalsis whereas under **Anacardium** it is the effect of a paralytic condition of the rectum. Further in **Anacardium** this desire for stool is produced by a sense of a lump or a plug in anus, which he tries to get rid of. These two remedies differ in the fact that the **Anacardium** patient is almost always better after eating, whereas **Nux** is always worse after eating. **Anacardium** patient feels an uneasiness when the stomach is empty. It is a sort of an all-gone feeling experienced as soon as the stomach gets empty and is always better by eating.

The action of **Anacardium** on the skin is quite prominent and should be carefully noted. It produces eruptions that are umbilicated. They may occur in the face as well as other parts of the body. They are extremely irritable. The itchiness is so great that the patient very frequently brings on bleeding by excessive scratching; even then no relief is found.

It is also used in spinal affections when the following symptoms are present: A great tired feeling of all the limbs, incomplete palsy of the voluntary muscles, trembling, cramps in calves when walking, stiffness and lassitude in knees as if paralysed and a sensation of bandage in the legs.

Case 1.—Lady, aged seventy, was affected with ulcers on the feet, and vertigo, causing her to fall from the chair frequently. One year after an apoplectic fit, the following symptoms set in: Her memory had been strikingly decreasing for several days in succession; on a morning the coffee-cup fell out of her hands, her head worked forward upon the chest; her features were distorted, her looks staring; did not recognize those around her; muttered unintelligible sounds; breathing easy; skin cold; pulse full. When urged to rise, she did so, but fell back upon the chair immediately; forgot to swallow what she had in her mouth, and did not swallow it until requested. **Anac 1,** and recovery in a few hours. The remedy also prevented a new attack, the precursory symptoms of which came on after the lapse of ten months.—Hygea.

Case 2.—Frequent tenesmus for many days, without being able to pass anything; great and urgent desire for stool, but on sitting down to stool, the desire immediately passed away, without any evacuation; the rectum seemed to be powerless, with a sensation as if plugged up; she had to strain, though the stools were soft. This is the case of an old lady who had been afflicted for years with hæmorrhage when at stool. At the present time, eighteen days had passed without an evacuation, though the above symptoms were almost constantly present. Enemas had been used but returned without bringing any fæcal matter. A powder of **Anac. 20,** dissolved in three teaspoonfuls of water, and given in teaspoonful doses every four hours, produced an evacuation in twelve hours.—Dr. W. E. Payne.

ANGUSTURA VERA.

The tincture is prepared from the bark of a plant known as Galipea Cusparia, a native of Venezuela. It belongs to the natural order of Rutaceæ. Its action is centred principally on spinal motor nerves and mucous membranes, hence it makes an admirable remedy in rheumatic affections and paralytic complaints. Fatigue of arms on movement bordering almost on paralysis and cracking in joints are some of the symptoms to indicate it in the above complaints and therefore it should be studied in close comparison with **Bryonia** and **Rhus tox.**

One grand characteristic of **Angustura** is the strong craving for coffee. It is at times almost irresistible; also aversion to meat especially pork, is very marked. We further notice a great desire for warm drinks.

The second characteristic point is the over-sensitiveness. It is present everywhere and we will have ample illustrations of this later on. This sensitiveness makes itself manifest even in the mental condition of the patient; the slightest offence, a mere trifle, irritates him.

Here we have a remedy that resembles **Nux** and **Ruta** to a great extent. Its similarity to the former remedy consists mainly in the mental condition of the patient, for in **Angustura** we have to deal with a patient just as irritable and oversensitive as **Nux vomica.** He is always in ill-humour and discontented, but what enables us to discriminate is the pusillanimity of the **Angustura** patient. He is more of the nature of a coward. He wants the tenacity, obstinacy and the overbearing self-confidence of **Nux vomica.**

It resembles **Ruta** in its action over the muscles and the bones. We notice a sort of a bruised sore feeling as after a blow. The muscles and the joints too, feel sore and tense. It has special affinity for the long bones such as the humerus, femur, tibia, etc. We think about **Angustura** specially in carious affections of these bones and in exostosis and necrosis of lower jaw. The carious ulcers pierce the bones down to the marrow and we find little chips of dead bones thrown out occasionally.

Another complaint, for which **Angustura** is specially needed, is tetanus, either traumatic or otherwise. It is indicated when there are twitching or jerking of muscles, excitability to touch and noise, wasting of the soft parts and catalepsy.

Angustura like **Ambra grisea** is a remedy in which cough is followed by hiccough and belching. This remedy was proved by Hahnemann.

Case No. 1.—Stiffness in the elbow joints and the paralytic heaviness in arms, making him unfit for any kind of work, in consequence of holding the arm for a long time upward, during sitting as model for a picture. A great many things had been applied without benefit. **Ang. Cort. 3.,** smelling gave great relief at once, and cured in two weeks by taking five globules, night and morning, for that length of time.—Dr. Landesmann.

Case No. 2.—A lady ran a pin into her foot; two weeks after she was taken with tetanic pains, striking from the point injured to the back of the heel, then up the limb and up the back; she had darting spasmodic pains from the nape of the neck to the neck of the jaws, both sides; jaws stiff, not closed; the pains began to be terrific. **Ang. 3rd dec.,** was given every half hour. In an hour the pains abated, and she gradually recovered in the space of four days.—Dr. Hubbard.

ANTHRACINUM.

Anthracinum, a nosode is the alcoholic extract of the anthrax poison extracted from the spleen of cattle infected with the disease Dr. G. A. Waber used this remedy very extensively in the cattle plague and he cured every case with it. Also, men poisoned by the contagion were benefited by it. **Anthracinum** is the homœopath's knife that helps him to tide over many a difficult case, called surgical. Cases of carbuncles, malignant pustules, septic wounds, gangrenous degenerations, where the most up-to-date surgeon feels his limitation, have been cured without number by the administration of this remedy. But there, as elsewhere, the same law of **Similia Similibus Curantur** holds good.

The characteristic symptoms are:—A horrible burning pain; presence of sepsis as indicated by rapid loss of strength, sinking pulse, delirium, fainting, and sloughing; red lines from the area of infection marking out the course of the lymphatics; induration of the cellular tissue; rapid spread of infiltration and œdema of the cellular tissue; abundant ichorous offensive pus; gangrenous ichor of horrible smell; dark brown redness in face; loss of appetite; excessive thirst with inability to swallow; increased salivation and offensive odor from the mouth.

I remember with pride how on these symptoms after **Arsenic** and **Lachesis** had failed, I saved a man's arm from amputation. His troubles started with an ordinary felon. Alarming symptoms very soon made their appearance and his whole hand from the elbow joint to the finger tip became one huge mass of swelling. Amputation was the only thing they thought that might possibly sa e the man's life. Under the action of **Anthracinum** within an incredibly short time the swelling got dispersed, the pains vanished, the sloughing stopped and he became his old self minus the loss of half of his big finger which had sloughed off before he came to the homœopath.

ANTIMONIUM ARSENICUM.

It is the Arsenite of Antimony and has been advocated greatly in emphysema characterized by excessive dyspnœa and cough. After pneumonia and pleurisy when all the acute symptoms have subsided and only dyspnœa remains a few doses of **Antimonium ars.,** will be very helpful. This drug has not been verified often. With time and experience I feel sure, it will be more and more popular.

ANTIMONIUM CRUDUM.

Antimonium crudum, the sulphide of antimony, a great antipsoric is prepared from black antimony, a mineral found in various places of Europe. It is an acquisition to the homœopathic Materia Medica and every homœopath is proud of it. In all ages and climes, in every stage of life beginning from the puny little baby to the decrepit old man, **Antimonium crudum** finds lot to do. Its field of action is immense and great and when prescribed on proper indications its effects are nothing short of the marvellous. Mentally, these patients are very morose, downhearted and gloomy. We notice almost a loathing of life in these patients. Often in their sadness and desperation they are driven to commit suicide especially by drowning themselves. Very often this sadness, intermingled with a strange amativeness, sentimentality and emotion, plays an active part in their make up. Ecstatic fancies, exalted ideas of love and friendship make them act very foolishly at times. An irresistible desire to talk in rhymes and verses, especially in the moon light when their ecstatic fancies are fumed to flame is a guiding characteristic of **Antimonium crudum.** Fretfulness plays no mean part in their behaviour, We find them extremely ugly and impatient and in cases of children it becomes extremely difficult to distinguish it from **Chamomilla.** The baby whines and cries and nothing pleases him. He does not wish to speak or being spoken to. He would rather be left alone. Every attempt to pacify him, each offer of friendship, are spurned away.

The gastric symptoms of **Antimonium crudum** are perhaps most marked of all its symptoms. Great uneasiness prevails in the whole of the digestive tract beginning from the tongue down to the rectum. In the first place the tongue is absolutely covered with white fur so much so that it looks almost white washed. Sometimes, though we find this coating of white interrupted with little tinges of yellow we must not be misled. The other symptoms of nausea, vomiting, impaired appetite, colic, loseness of the bowels and ptyalism should rivet our attention on **Antimonium crudum.** This indigestion in **Antimonium crudum** is the result of indulgence in bad sour wine, pastries, fat food and other varieties of indigestible articles. The vomiting is frequent and constant and the patient brings up large quantities of food eaten in a sort of half digested acid state. The patient belches incessantly and it is accompanied with the taste of what has been eaten. Violent cutting colic in abdomen with a feeling of oppression coming from stomach, indisposition to work, diarrhœa the effect of his gluttony, protrusion of rectum with the loose bowels are symptoms too prominent to lead us astray.

Hæmorrhoidal complaints due to constant over-indulgence is not an infrequent occurrence in the life of the **Antimonium crudum** patient. The pile is a mucous pile. There is a constant oozing of mucus from the rectum, staining the linen yellow and emitting a sort of disgusting odor.

There is another constitutional peculiarity which we should closely observe. Horny structures of the human system are defective in their growth in this remedy. The nails are brittle and they crack and crumble easily. There is also noticed a tendency towards callositis, corns and other horny excrescences on the body, especially on the soles of the feet and palms of hands. Skin also is unhealthy as in **Silicea, Hep. sulph.,** and **Graphites.** Cracks and fissures especially in the commissures of the body are very common.

Eruptions of **Antimonium crudum** are thick and scabby. Honey colored fluid sometimes looking almost greenish oozes through cracked crust of many of these eruptions. Tetters, fistulas, ulcers, deep spongy sores, warts and pustules looking like varicella are numerous. Yellow crusted eruption on cheek, cracking of the nostrils, are common in **Antimonium crudum.**

The action of **Antimonium crudum** on the female genital organs should not be overlooked. It is useful in prolapsus uteri with tenderness over ovarian region when such has been brought about by indiscriminate bathing in cold water during catamenia. The leucorrhœal discharge containing little pieces of lumpy substance is extremely acrid and causes a smarting sensation along the thighs. It acts admirably in over-excitement of the sexual organs giving rise to conditions of nymphomania due to suppression of catamenia from cold bathing.

Antimonium crudum is thought of in the vomiting of curdled milk in children. In this respect it is like **Æthusa** from which it differs in its want of sleepiness and prostration.

Case 1.—In the case of a certain child there had been noticed from his birth an occasional whistling sound during respiration, which usually occurred after waking from sleep, but also during the waking hours, and was always accompanied with loss of breath. At the sixth month, the symptoms were: General convulsions; spasmodic contraction of the arms, hands and feet, of the muscles of the face and eyes; then coma and trembling of the hands followed by restlessness of the arms and head with staring of the eyes. These attacks came on suddenly every hour and lasted several minutes. He had a large head and open fontanelles. **Ignatia 39** relieved these attacks at last. When the child was fifteen months old, the whistling sound during breathing, already mentioned, came on more frequently and breathing was interrupted for a longer time. This showed itself after each waking from sleep and after every mental excitement. The child is backward in every sense of the word. Fontanelles still open. The attacks are nearly constant and take the following form: Spasmodic contraction in closing the mouth firmly; stertorous breathing with danger of suffocation. After going to sleep it jerks all over, moans constantly and has a croupy respiration. **Hepar, Calcarea, Sulphur, Ipecacuanha, Belladonna, Tartar emetic** were given without relief. Basing the prescription upon the whole history of the case, **Antimonium crudum 2**, was given twice a day with immediate improvement and a final cure.—Dr. Parsenow in the "Allg. Hom. Zeitg.," iii, 124.

Case 2. (Polyuria).—F., aged four years, passes large quantities of urine, which is as clear and odorless as distilled water; much of it passes involuntarily; drinks often and much at a time; eyes are both inflamed—conjunctiva quite red, cornea dim—they are both very dry and he keeps them closed; nostrils are very sore; mouth is very dry; tongue clear, cracked transversely; skin very dry; emaciated to a skeleton; keeps the bed, and sleeps much during the day; craves sour food; exceedingly irritable; strikes and scolds; no sugar in urine. **Phos. ac., Natr. mur., Lyc.** and **Sulph.** of no use. The mother says the boy cannot bear to be looked at. **Ant. crud. 6** cured.—Dr. C. Bernreuter.

ANTIMONIUM TARTARICUM.

It is a salt well known by the name of Tartar Emetic. It i commonly prepared by boiling together in water Antimonium Oxide and acid potassium tartrate (cream of tartar) and obtaining the resulting double tartar by crystallization. It is a colorless transparent substance of a sweetish metallic taste. It becomes opaque white on being exposed to air. One part by weight of this substance is dissolved in 99 parts by weight of distilled water.

It is a cardiac depressant and it stimulates secretion. It causes intense nausea and vomiting. It is also a powerful irritant when applied to the skin where it produces an eruption which though papular at first turns soon into a pustular kind.

In **Antimonium tartaricum** we have an excellent remedy as every homœopath will testify. Its range of action as has been hinted before is extensive and very often the relief obtained by it is instantaneous and astonishing. At times when a cure is not possible and relief is all that is expected, **Antimonium tartaricum** will bring the desired relief.

Very recently I was called in to do my last service to an old lady writhing in the agony of death. Aged and decrepit, she was in the last stage of phthisis. Her pale blue face was covered with cold perspiration. The excessive accumulation of phlegm in the throat, which she was too weak to expel, was making a coarse rattling sound choking her almost every minute, drowsiness was great, amounting almost to coma. The hands of death were too tight on her for human skill to relieve. The indicated remedy did what it was possible to do, that is, made her expectorate the phlegm and relieved the choking and the rattling sound. The last few moments were passed in peace and quiet. The remedy was **Antim tart.**

Antimonium tartaricum, like **Apis**, **Belladonna** and **Sulphur** is extremely useful in cases of suppressed eruptions when the bad effect of such suppression show itself in cerebral symptoms. In measles. scarlatina and pox when the rash does not appear after a primary show and the patient gets drowsy and delirious, and looks bluish and purple, twitches and starts, and when respiratory symptoms become visible. **Antimonium tartaricum** will frequently restore the eruptions and cure the case.

Antim. tart. is a splendid remedy for bronchitis and pneumonia when we notice loud rattling of mucus in chest. We use it also in threatened paralysis of lungs. A few other remedies that should be thought of in this connection are **Ipecac, Kali hydriodicum** and **Carbo veg.**

Ipecac frequently precedes **Antim tart.** Loud rales are heard. Very little phlegm is raised on coughing, though each attempt is attended with gagging.

In **Kali hydriod.** there is great rattling of mucus in chest accompanied with œdema of lungs. The little sputa that is raised, is greenish and frothy.

In **Carbo veg.** the rattling is accompanied with symptoms of collapse, such as cold breath. coldness of the hands and cold sweat.

It is equally invaluable in cough and pertusis. Attacks recur more when the patient is asleep and the cough is provoked every time the child gets angry. This symptom can be considered a charactertistic symptom. There is quite a lot of orthopnœa as is evident by constant dilatation of nostrils and rapid movement of thorax. The patient wants to be supported in bed in a sitting posture. Such oppression of breathing is generally relieved by expectoration of phlegm. It also relieves asphyxia from mechanical causes as in drowning.

The cough is also provoked by crying, eating and drinking. Sometimes the fit is so severe and the cough so uninterrupted that we have vomiting of bloody, frothy masses. The patient springs up in bed and clings to those around him. Another important symptom is gaping and coughing consecutively. In addition to all these the most important thing for every homœopath to remember is that there is great accumulation of phlegm in the chest and in the bronchial tubes but that the expulsive power is feeble and wanting. Every time the patient coughs there appears to be a large collection of mucus in the bronchial tubes and that, volumes would be expectorated but nothing or little comes up.

It is helpful in certain varieties of gastric derangement especially in dyspepsia. We notice a great disgust for food and constant nausea and relief is only obtained after vomiting. Desire for acids, fruits and cold drinks are equally characteristic. Now this vomiting in **Antimonium tartaricum** is as severe as in **Ipecac.** He vomits until he faints and each attempt is attended with drowsiness and prostration. It is a long continued and tormenting nausea frequently reminding one of **Ipecac,** but it wants the gagging of the latter remedy. With this vomiting we notice a great præcordial anxiety, pressure and distention in hypochondriac region. The patient breaks out into cold sweat while vomiting. All these indications lead one to believe that it will make an excellent remedy in cholera morbus which indeed it is. Sharp cutting colic before stool, burning at anus after each stool, tenesmus during and after loose stools, drowsiness and coma, profuse perspiration leading on to collapse, hardly perceptible thread like pulse and ever increasing prostration, make it a capital remedy in that complaint. In this connection we will look into the tongue of **Antimonium tartaricum.** It is a tongue that has a coating of white fur but the papillæ are red and prominent and edges are characterised by a band of red all around it. At times it has a red band running longitudinally along the centre of the tongue. The tongue is dry, sometimes ulcerated and has the imprint of teeth on its borders.

Antimonium tartaricum as has been hinted before produces pustules very similar to those of small pox and hence according to our principle of Similia, it makes an admirable remedy in that complaint. It is particularly adaptable to that stage and condition where after one batch drying up, a fresh lot makes its appearance and as some get dry, others mature. Intense backache, the teasing rattling cough, the persistent headache make its indication a certainty.

Antimonium tartaricum is a sycotic remedy; we have warts behind the glans penis, a symptom that has been verified frequently by many eminent physicians. It is also used in secondary orchitis the effect of checked gonorrhœa and as such should be compared with **Pulsatilla.**

The mental symptoms of **Antimonium tartaricum** are characterized by bad humour, apathy and indifference. If it is a child, it whines and cries and nothing can be done to please him. It is, therefore, very much like **Cina, Ant. crud.** and **Chamomilla.**

Case 1.--A little son of C. P. K., Esq., aged two years, became hoarse and croupy from almost any exciting cause. His father was an asthmatic subject, and his mother was feeble and cachectic, and their little son was, on the whole, far from being strong and vigorous. His nurse had observed for some days that he was indifferent about his playthings, and wanted to be held in her arms, and yet he ate and slept as usual. Without any previous exposure, a severe attack of croup came on in the middle of the night; all at once he became hoarse and coughed frequently. Being called immediately, I observed that his breathing was very labored, and that a profuse perspiration was standing upon the face, and that the trachea and larynx were rapidly contracting. Gave **Tart. emet., 3rd. trit.** about five grains in half a tumbler of water, and a teaspoonful every ten or fifteen minutes. The effect was almost magical, as the disease seemed to be arrested at once. The medicine was continued for more than an hour, when the little fellow went to sleep. He breathed better and better, until he awoke quite relieved. He had attacks subsequently, which the same remedy speedily removed.— Dr. A. E. Small.

"The indications for this remedy in croup are based on the predominating symptoms of partial paralysis of the pneumogastric nerve. The short, hoarse, nearly suffocative breathing is accompanied by a whistling noise, heard even at a distance, whilst the thorax expands only with the greatest muscular effort, and the greatest anxiety and uneasiness, together with great prostration, are manifested. The head is thrown backward; face livid and cold."

Case 2.—Pustular eruption leaves ugly, bluish-red marks on the face, also similar eruption on genitals and thighs; so painful, can neither sit nor walk. Sleepless from pain and irritation. **Tart. Emet. 2** cured.— Dr. Dudgeon.

Pustules with red areola, which leave large scars behind; crusts brown; eruption very painful; decided drowsiness, with nausea; longing for acids, with aversion to milk; the eructation tastes like sulphur; severe colic pains; short breathing, and rattling respiration; do not like to be touched.

APIS MELLIFICA.

This medicine is prepared from the poison of the honey bee. It was first introduced into our Materia Medica by Dr. Humphreys of New York. The preparation is very simple. Live bees are put into a bottle and shaken violently. Upon them is poured five times their weight of dilute alcohol. After saturation and shaking the tincture is poured off and strained.

Apis acts on cellular tissue and causes œdema of skin and mucous membranes. Erysipelatous inflammations, dropsical effusions, acute inflammation of parenchymatous tissues are some of the pathological conditions of this remedy. This inflammation of **Apis** is asthenic in character. It lacks the virulent tension of remedies like **Belladonna** and **Aconite**. The inflamed area is pale and œdematous and more inclined to gangrenous degenerations.

I have to confess that years ago, while a little boy, I unwittingly became a subject of verification of **Apis** toxicology. At the advice of a mischievous friend, for the sake of fun, which I had in abundance, I innocently threw a stone at a bee-hive. The fun commenced immediately after in the shape of hundred stings in different parts of my body. The whole body became swollen and œdematous with a rosy pinkish hue of the skin. The stinging, burning, lancinating pain became unbearable and fever soon supervened. The swelling of some parts of the body underwent resolution in a short while, but others progressed on to phlegmonous erysipelas.

Now I will enumerate the most important characteristic symptoms of **Apis** in order of their importance. The first and the foremost is the pale waxy œdematous swelling due to accumulation of serum in cellular tissue. The swelling has a red rosy hue. Such serous accumulation may also happen in the various cavities of our body, such as the synovial cavity, the ventricles of the brain, and the hollow space of the abdomen. It thus becomes a splendid remedy in synovitis, hydrocephalus, ascites, dropsy and hydrothorax; of course, in all these troubles the characterisctic symptoms of the remedy must be present to make the prescription an infallible one.

The next great characteristic of the remedy is the extreme sensitiveness to touch. This is almost an universal symptom in **Apis.** We notice it in every ailment where **Apis** is indicated. Thus in cholera, diarrhœa and dysentery, because of the extreme sensitiveness, the patient would not tolerate any pressure on the abdomen. In rheumatic and gouty complaints a similar dread of touch is noticed; even the hair is too sore to be touched. A similar tenderness noticed in uterine and ovarian regions is a further illustration of our point.

A burning, stinging, sore pain, suddenly migrating from one part of the body to another, occupies the third place. The shrill piercing sudden cry in meningitis, the occasional shrieks that break through the monotony of the stuporous delirium, point to the existence of such a fleeting stinging pain.

Extreme but rapid prostration as shown by trembling, a deathly faint feeling, loss of consciousness, premonition of approaching death, slow beat of heart and imperceptibility of pulse, are a few more features of **Apis.** With regard to the burning it resembles **Arsenicum,** but the burning of **Apis,** unlike that of **Arsenic,** is always relieved by application of cold. The restlessness of **Apis** is merely a fidgetiness, due perhaps to a general nervous feeling.

Apis is a right-sided remedy; either most of their complaints are on that side or they start from the right side and travel to the left. **Apis** is further thirstless.

Mentally **Apis** is somewhat like our **Pulsatilla** patient. She is tearful and lachrymose. Dread of death, apathy, jealousy, awkwardness and impaired memory are a few other traits of her mental sphere.

The dread of death takes the form of apprehensiveness. Apathy is almost as prominent in **Apis** as in **Lili. tigrinum** and **Sepia.** The patient lies in bed absolutely indifferent as to what is happening around. Sometimes this indifference is merely the fore-runner of unconsciousness and a soporous condition. He lies in bed absolutely languid and listless, complains of nothing and mutters away all the time by himself.

Jealousy in **Apis** is as marked as in **Lachesis.** All her ideas and actions are centred around this. This frequently leads her on to suspect everybody and she keeps on entertaining ideas of being poisoned. The natural pose of her mind, thus lost, brings on a terrible awkwardness. She drops everything out of her hand and breaks them. Impatience gradually makes itself manifest and she gets extremely restless, constantly changing about from one kind of work to another.

In **Apis** we have quite a lot of congestion to head and face in consequence of which a general aching through the brain is complained of. This violent congestion may lead to meningitis and meningeal irritations. The gradual increase in torpor, the sudden shrill cries, squinting, grinding of teeth, boring of the head in pillow, ought to keep us on our guard and warn us of the terrible breakers ahead. A few doses of **Apis** in this condition may clear up the whole case. Other symptoms indicating **Apis** are twitching of one side of the body, the other side remaining in a state of semi-paralysis; scantiness of urine; turning up of the big toe; offensive odor from the mouth; thirstlessness or extreme thirst and soreness of the tongue.

These symptoms remind one of **Belladonna, Bryonia** and **Helleborus,** but a little care on our part enables us to differentiate between them easily. In **Belladonna** the skin is hot and the face is red, whereas in **Apis** paleness and œdematous conditions prevail. The congestion of **Belladonna** is violent as evidenced by the throbbing of the carotids and the injected condition of the eyes. True, the jerkings and twitchings are present in both remedies and cerebral cries are common but the adynamia of **Apis** is absolutely wanting in the great violence and tension of the other. In **Apis** the twitchings and tremblings are more of a nature of nervous fidgetiness.

Bryonia resembles **Apis** in the suppression of eruptions bringing on this cerebral effusion. The patient is certainly drowsy but it lacks the total involvement of the sensorium as in **Apis** and **Helleborus.** The face is dark red showing a tolerable amount of congestion. The thirst in **Bryonia** is indeed very great and each movement speaks of great bodily aches and pains.

Helleborous, a great remedy in meningitis, is indicated when the mental torpor is complete. The nervous fidgetiness of **Apis** and the irritation of **Bryonia** give way to entire and complete torpor. The wrinkled forehead, dilated pupils, the dropping of the lower jaw and automatic motion of one arm and one leg, the suppression of urine, the chewing motion of the mouth, the dark shooty nostrils, the constant picking of nose, lips and bed clothes make confusion impossible even to the merest novice.

Apis is very useful in intermittent fever when the characteristic at 3 p. m. chill is present. Here let me caution my readers against a very common mistake. Inspite of general thirstlessness in **Apis,** the patient at this stage complains of great thirst and a general feeling of oppression in chest. In the following two stages of heat and sweat, thirst is characteristically absent although the feeling of oppression continues. After the stage of chill is over, the patient breaks out in profuse urticaria, and falls into a sort of dull slumber.

Apis is also very serviceable in fevers of cerebral and exanthematic forms, that is, in fevers complicated with suppression of eruptions. These are cases that generally prove very trying. The brain, as a result of such suppression, soon becomes cloudy. Delirium, not of an active type, soon appears. Violence is not a feature with these patients; they are in a state of stupor and they mutter constantly. Their tongue, ulcerated, cracked and blistered, trembles as soon as it is protruded. The prostration is so great that they frequently slide down in bed. Tenderness and bloated condition of abdomen, foul smelling diarrhœa, incontinence of urine, moist cough, a pale waxy colour of the skin, great sleepiness with occasional piercing shrill cries, are a few more important symptoms.

Another symptom, that I consider very important, is unequal distribution of heat on the surface of the body. Some parts of the body are burning hot, while others are unnaturally cool. The blistered tongue is very often covered with a tough tenacious mucus that requires to be wiped away from the tongue as they are unable to spit it out. Cases, so critical and prostrated, remind us also of **Acid mur, Arnica, Baptisia, Helleborus, Opium** and **Lachesis.**

The disease, where **Apis** has done the most good and earned the greatest renown, is diphtheria. **Apis** diphtheria is characterised by an insidious progress and absence of pain inspite of intense and extensive inflammation. In those cases where pain is present it is only trifling and negligible. The right side is more often affected than the left side. The whole throat, when examined carefully, looks painted with a strong glossy red varnish. Great œdema of throat and uvula which looks like a bag of water makes swallowing excessively painful. In some cases the breath is very offensive. Along with this we notice all the other characteristic features mentioned above.

Apis has a very strong action on the female genital organs. It aggravates sexual desire in widows, driving them to masturbation. **Apis** also checks the tendency to abortion at or before the third month. It is very serviceable in ovaritis, especially when the right one is affected. The pain is of a stinging burning character with great tenderness and soreness. Sometimes the pain travels down the thigh of the same side. It is accompanied with a feeling of tightness across the chest on coughing.

Lastly we shall discuss its indications in abdominal complaints. It is helpful in a wide range of affections beginning from common irritation to peritonitis. The sorness that has been spoken of as marked characteristic of **Apis** is prominently present. Intestines feel bruised and the abdomen is very tender to touch, even to the pressure of the bed clothes, and sensation of bloatedness in the abdomen accompanied with a feeling of tightness, causing difficulty of breathing, is also to be seen. We also have copious watery, almost black motions; sometimes the stools are olive green and full of bright red lumps like chopped beets. The stools are generally involuntary escaping continuously from the wide open anus which does not close even after the stool is over. The patient complains of the anus feeling raw and sore. Hæmorrhage from the bowels may also be present. The above symptoms may be complicated with hæmorrhoids when the stinging, burning and the soreness already complained of assume a fiercer form. Varices protrude causing intolerable smarting, burning and stinging; we may even have bloody exudation.

As a general rule, we may say that the **Apis** patients are always relieved by cold applications and they are worse in a warm room. **Apis** is inimical to **Rhus tox.**

Case 1.—B. H., aged nine years, very scrofulous by inheritance from both parents. Patient had a fair skin and was always pale; blue eyes; red hair. Had lost, in his sixth year, the use of his legs, but, after a tedious course of treatment, had regained their use, so he could walk with considerable ease. We found the child with a high fever, sore throat and scarlet rash. **Aconite** was indicated and was given. He was very ill, but did passably well until the fourth day, when the eruption commenced to disappear and, at the same time, alarming changes took place. The fever became continuous; the countenance bore an expression of stupor, increased by the drooping of the lower jaw; the nose looked pinched; the teeth were covered with dirty, sticky slime; discharge of foul matter from the secretion. It seemed as if the vital forces had completely surrendered themselves to the poison, which evidently penetrated the whole system. At first, **Cuprum met. 30** was given, with the view of bringing out the disappearing eruption. The patient growing worse, **Apis 2** was prescribed without producing any change. The symptoms remained the same; the tongue became sore, cracked, bleeding; the discharge from the nose became very irritating; the bowels became hard and were tender to touch; diarrhœa set in. Remedies were changed as seemed best, the patient apparently sinking. œdema of the feet and limbs then set in, with painful and scanty emissions of urine. At that time **Arsenic 30** was given, but without producing any effect, when we concluded to give **Apis 30** until the patient got better or died. This was strictly followed out during the six weeks of sickness following. He was on the verge of death for weeks. General dropsy developed itself; suffocation threatened one day to end his life, from effusion in the thorax; hydrocephalus had all but declared itself on the next; the glands of his neck swelled; his ears discharged; his face was bloated, so he could not see; at last the abdominal dropsy became so threatening that I proposed tapping as a last resort to save his life, the parents objecting. At that time we changed to the second attenuations of **Apis**; the change was followed by excellent effects upon the kidneys. Within forty-eight hours enormous quantities of urine were passed, relieving the patient very much. Under the action of **Apis** for it alone was given, alternating weekly the lower triturations with the higher dilutions of the drug, one symptom after the other disappeared. Occasional aggravations showed themselves, but on the whole the little fellow gained ground inch by inch. All during the succeeding summer, he was more or less of an invalid, but by the first of October, his father brought him to the office, having walked the entire distance from his home, and looking fresher and healthier and feeling better than he had for many years. The cure was permanent; and he seemed ever after in perfect health.—Dr. C. J. Hampel, and H. R. Arndt.

Case 2.—A boy, four years old, a son of German parents, was given up by the attending allopathic physician as a case of hopeless hydrocephalus. When first seen, the child was lying on its back, with eyes wide open, extreme squinting, dilated pupils, rolling eyeballs without winking. He gave no evidence of seeing when the finger was thrust toward the eye; when pricked with a pin, no sign of feeling; when water was put into his mouth no effect at swallowing was made. The left side had been entirely motionless for two days, but he moved the right arm and leg occasionally. He had passed no water for forty-eight hours and the region of the bladder showed very slight distension. Drugs had produced no stool for several days. At the commencement of his illness, he complained of pain in the occiput with occasional sharp shrieks. He had been blistered with cantharides from the nape of the neck to the lumbar region two days previously, since which time he had passed no water, and given no evidence of seeing, hearing or feeling. **Apis 30.** After five days he had so far recovered that he sat up in bed; he moved both sides of the body equally well, and all his senses were restored.—Dr. W. P. Wesselhœft.

Case 3—Was called in consultation to see Miss M., who was thought to be near dying. I found the patient in great distress, **panting respiration,** unable to speak only in a whisper, and each word uttered separately from the next by several respirations. She had great **pain shooting** all through her chest, from front to back. She had informed me she could not long survive, as **each breath seemed as if it would be her last one.** She had **no thirst, scanty urine,** and had **not slept** for two days. Percussion over her chest gave a clear and healthy sound. Auscultation revealed permeatibility of air through her lungs, but a very loud bronchial rale. No other remedy has this combination of symptoms excepting **Apis.** My choice fell on the 40m potency for the reason that she was too ill to bear a lower potency of a large dose of the material. Directions were given to repeat **Apis 40m** in water every hour till she seemed a little better, then to cease giving entirely till we saw her in the morning. After the third dose she became quiet, fell asleep for two hours and remained quiet all night, sleeping at intervals till morning. Contrary to instructions, the medicine was repeated every time she awoke, till 9 in the morning, when she received the last dose remaining, soon after which she became as bad as on the previous evening. We saw her at 10-30 a.m., and found her about the same as on my first visit. Now what was to be done. The same remedy was still indicated, and it was very evident that she had been overdosed, therefore **Sac. lac.** was given during the day, and when we saw her at 6-30 p.m., she was again more comfortable. **Sac. lac.** was given till 10-30 the next morning, when we found her still more comfortable. Next day still better, and still **Sac. lac.** So day after day showed that, on the whole, she was improving and she made a perfect recovery without a further dose of medicine.—Dr. H. N. Guernsey.

APOCYNUM CANNABINUM.

This medicine is prepared from the Indian Hemp, a tree with tuff fibre utilized in the making of strong cordage.

Apocynum has very strong action over the kidney. It causes increased functional activity of that organ and thus helps elimination. It is reputed to be a very good remedy for dropsy, hydrocephalus and ascites, and as such it occupies a place as important as that of **Apis**. It is indicated mostly in uncomplicated cases of dropsy. The symptoms are, low-spiritedness, confusion of mind and bewilderment, great thirst with intolerance of water, distention of abdomen, oppression about the epigastrium and chest with irresistible disposition to sigh, loose rattling in chest, diarrhœa of a loose bilious character and profuse uterine hæmorrhage. Urine is generally scanty.

In hydrocephalus the head looks large and bulging, fontanelles are wide open. Squinting and in txtreme cases blindness, constant and involuntary motion of one arm and leg and sometimes paralysis of one side of the body, are all important symptoms.

It is easy to differentiate this remedy from **Apis** for it lacks the cephalic cry of that remedy. It is generally indicated in more serious cases where **Apis** fails.

The sinking feeling at the stomach is very characteristic. It is a feeling difficult to describe. It is more like a sensation of oppression about the stomach and the chest. The patient cannot tell what it is and does not know how to get relief. He finds it difficult to get a deep breath or even to speak. With this oppression we have great irritability of the stomach, so that even a small quantity of water cannot be retained. He vomits and becomes drowsy and then vomits again. Great thirst is felt, but he cannot drink as water causes pain and is thrown out immediately. The face which is usually bloated and has a bluish leaden hue is expressive of great anguish. All these point to **Apocynum** as a great cardiac and a renal remedy.

ARALIA RACEMOSA.

Our authority of this remedy is Dr. S. A. Jones, who experimented with it on himself. It brought on him symptoms of asthma, loud wheezing respiration, spasmodic cough on lying down, tickling in the throat, constriction of chest and a feeling of foreign body in the throat. Its principal action, therefore, is to be seen over the respiratory organs. The characteristic cough occurs at about 11 p.m., generally after a short sleep. The respiration is dry, wheezing and worse from lying down on back.

There is a sensation of constriction in chest; it feels, as if a foreign body were in the throat.

These patients are extremely susceptible to the least current of air which causes frequently sneezing with copious excoriating nasal discharge. The patient perspires profusely while asleep.

ARANEA DIADEMA.

Aranea diadema is one more of our fever remedies. I cannot with justice pass it over as I know of instances where it has rendered yeoman's service and where but for **Aranea** it would have meant the confirmation of the popular belief, of the futility of the Homœopathic system of therapeutics in the treatment of ague and marsh fevers. As far as this remedy is concerned, two symptoms must be mentioned in letters of gold, for in no other remedies are they so well marked and characteristic as here. One is the aggravation of all complaints and symptoms by exposure to damp and cold. The patient feels exceedingly well on a bright and sunny day. He is always at his best in a dry climate. Nothing goes amiss with him so long as he keeps away from moisture, cold and dampness; but as soon as the weather turns cold, rains commence, or as soon as business takes him away to a damp swampy place, his troubles come in swarms. Thi is exactly what Grauvogl means by hydrogenoid constitution. In this abnormàl sensitiveness to damp and cold places, **Aranea** is at the top of our list of similar remedies. The second symptom is the unvaried, unchanging, periodicity of this remedy. Complaints ppear with great regularity at precisely the same hour every day, every other day, every week. or every month as the case may be. This precision is almost tragic and clock-like, and like the hand of fate it steps in at the fixed hour. Both these symptoms make it a great remedy, as I have said before, in the treatment of malarial fevers. The fever may be quotidian or tertian. The chill is very long-lasting. It is a severe shaking chill, felt in the bones. He feels almost frozen. Nothing relieves this chilliness.

The spleen is often enlarged, but what makes this remedy very characteristic, is the frequent absence of heat and sweat, or if they are at all present, they are very slight and imperceptible. Such periodicity is also marked in **Cedron, Chin. sulph., Cina,** and **Gels.** In this connection I cannot do better than to cite the case of a sea-master who developed ague with great stiffness, tiredness, and sick-feeling, after a night spent on wet straw, in the bar-room of a hotel in Germany, on a winter night as reported by Grauvogl. I would cite the great Homœopath's own language: "Chill began at 7 p.m., and lasted till precisely 8 in the morning, every day at the same hour, without heat or sweat, with cough, loss of appetite, sleeplessness and great exhaustion, which distressed him most next day, and interfered with his occupation; being unskilled in Homœopathy and not having the least confidence in fever and ague, I gave him two-grain doses of quinine every two hours at first, then every hour during the day until he had taken 40 powders without the least improvement; on the contrary his general weakness had increased. I now consulted the original proving and found that according to the law of similarity **Aranea** must be the remedy. He received 5 drops of the second dec. attenuation every hour. Next day the patient exclaimed, 'Now you have hit the right medicine. After the second hour I felt warmth again in my whole body and for the first time for three weeks I slept some hours at night again without any chill.' Cure was completed in six days and for 17 years he had no relapse." My object in citing this case is not so much to emphasise the indication of **Aranea** as to draw your attention to the fact that quinine is not a panacea in all cases of malaria.

Quinine only cures where it is indicated, and it is only indicated where the three states are well marked; particularly the stage of heat and sweat. It is also my intention to prove that Homœopathy is as certain a cure in malaria, as it is in other troubles, and it is up to us to prove that we as Homœopaths suffer from no limitations.

I have just one or two more symptoms to add. It is very efficacious in head-ache and confusion of head brought about and aggravated by smoking. The **Aranea** head-ache is greatly relieved by the open air.

The tooth-ache of this remedy is very peculiar. It starts as soon as the patient goes to bed at night time. That other characteristic of periodicity stamps its mark on tooth-ache as well as elsewhere. It appears invariably at the same hour and at a certain fixed time. I will close my lecture on this remedy with one additional symptom, namely, the patient often wakes up from sleep with a peculiar sensation of some part of the limbs feeling enlarged and augmented.

Case 1.—Mrs. J. G. M., aged forty-eight. Sanguineous temperament, regular in her monthly courses, and mother of nine children; has always enjoyed good health, and having been her physician for twenty-five years, have never observed any other alternations in her health except those consequent to child-birth, and occasionally a slight eruption of her face, which made its appearance in cold weather. About three months ago in consequence of a cold, she complained of a violent pain in her abdomen with a great deal of rumbling in the bowels, and loose stools. **Cham. 200,** repeated several times, and **Ars. 200** relieved the pains somewhat; but after studying her case more carefully, I finally observed that every day, at 4 o'clock in the morning, the pain would return with great violence, with the rumbling noise and diarrhœa; also a sensation of numbness of the superior and inferior limbs; then the pain would subside, and she would sleep until 7 or 8 o'clock. After getting up, she would feel restless and unwell during the day; no appetite, when she partook of food the pains increased at night. I then gave a few doses of **Diadema** with the happiest results, and she remained perfectly cured. Several medicines have some of the symptoms mentioned above but none of them except **Diadema** have the characteristic symptoms of colic, with rumbling bowels, liquid stools, and numbness of the arms and legs at the hour indicated.

Case 2.—Mrs. J. P. G., aged twenty-two; lymphatic temperament and weak constitution; suffered, at the age of puberty, from an attack of amenorrhœa, with all the symptoms usually experienced in this disease, which was treated by the rational means employed in Homœopathy in these cases. In four months she was restored to health, which she continued to enjoy until she married, two years ago, since when she commenced to be irregular in her courses; they appeared at times too soon, and at others too late; she experienced, in the course of eight months, two attacks of menorrhagia, which lasted, more or less abundantly, about two weeks, and was thought to be an abortion. She was treated allopathically after her marriage, and had tonics, antispasmodics and lastly, Anzola water and sea bathing, without any good results; on the contrary, after returning from the sea shore, she suffered from terrible pains in the stomach, which came on every day, regularly, at dinner time, on going to bed, and on rising in the morning. After making a thorough examination of her case, we collected the following symptoms: Dejected countenance and pale face; dark circles under the eyes; lips blanched; dull expression of the eyes, deep melancholy, inexplicable malaise, with a constant desire to lie down, and a crawling sensation over the whole body; after partaking of a few spoonfuls of soup, and especially after eating a very little food, she would experience violent convulsive pains in the stomach, with nausea, oppression of the chest and repeated gaping; the convulsive movements of the stomach, in a short time, would become general, with trembling of the whole body; great pain in the stomach, obliging her to move constantly while sitting and her mind would become confused; the pain would, at times, return, although with less intensity, on going to bed and on rising in he morning. **Diadema 200** cured.—Dr. J. G. Howard

ARGENTUM METALLICUM.

Argentum met. is prepared from Precipitated Silver. It is mainly a left-sided remedy like **Lach.** It is generally indicated in tall, thin and irritable persons; patients with hollow eyes, pale skins and with a tendency to caries, cancers and deep ulcerations. They are as a rule extremely forgetful. Restlessness, anxiety, ill humour and disinclination to talk are marked features of the patient.

It affects the cartilages, joints and bones. Hence, it is a great remedy in rheumatic affections. We think of it especially in arthritic rheumatism, when swollen parts feel bruised on pressure. The pains are tearing in nature. There are sometimes electric-like shocks, in joints and limbs.

The muscular system is likewise affected in **Argen. met.** Cramps are special features here. The parts feel stiff and numb. Calf muscles feel too short when going downstairs.

Argent. met. acts upon the mucous membranes as well. It produces copious exudation of mucus in the larynx. The mucous exuded is white and starchy. There is burning and rawness in the larynx.

We think of this remedy principally in epileptic attacks where such attacks are followed by delirious rage. The patient, as soon as the attack is over, jumps about, striking those near by. It is especially indicated in nervous, hysterical women and men who have lost a good deal of seminal fluid.

It is a good remedy in frontal headaches of businessmen. The headache increases gradually and when at its height, ceases suddenly. There is vertigo on entering a warm room after a walk, very similar to what we find in **Pulsatilla.**

It has a strong action over the urinary organs. There is frequent desire to urinate with profuse discharge of urine. Extreme dryness of the mouth, great hunger after a full meal and thirst make **Argent. met.** an admirable remedy in diabetes, where it is particularly indicated, if in addition to the symptoms mentioned above, there is swelling of the ankles.

There is one symptom that I have not touched or, if I have, I must have done so very lightly and that is, the indication of **Argent. met.** in impotence. This impotence is the effect of onanism. The organ is shrivelled up and atrophied. In testicles there is a bruised feeling.

There is also hoarseness in this remedy, especially of singers and speakers; talking and laughing aggravate. There is also aggravation after sleep, lying on back and on entering a warm room.

ARGENTUM NITRICUM.

This irritant poison is commonly known as Lunar Caustic and Nitrate of Silver. It was first proved by Hahnemann. The first potency is made by adding one part of this substance to nine parts by weight of distilled water.

In **Arg. nit.** we have a patient prominent by reason of his ugliness. The dried withered and haggard look, the general emaciation specially of the lower limbs as in **Ammon mur,** the peculiar nervous mental state are features too striking to escape notice.

Our **Argentum** patient is in constant hurry, fearful lest delay will spoil everything. When she is to go somewhere, she starts early and even then worries as if she would not arrive in time. In spite of all this hurry, she accomplishes little. She is nervous. This is illustrated by the fact that when about to go to church or opera or ready to appear before an audience, her over-excitability of mind brings on a kind of nervous diarrhœa. In this she is very much like **Gelsemium.**

She is further very apprehensive, constantly borrowing troubles. She is afraid to consult a doctor for fear of being told that she is subject to some incurable disease. She constantly feels as if her doctor is concealing facts and that his assurances are not to be relied on. To crown all she suffers from a peculiar type of suicidal mania. When about to cross a bridge, she gets an irresistable desire to jump over. Memory too is faulty.

Our patient is also a subject to frequent errors of perception. While walking through the street she dreads the corners as they seem to her to be projecting out and she feels afraid she will be bumping against them. The structures on the sides of the street seem to her as if about to stumble down and crush her. All this is due to imperfect co-ordination of the ocular muscles.

The **Argentum nitricum** patient is extremely sad, gloomy, and taciturn. She feels as if she is neglected and despised by everybody, and hence finds no pleasure in life. She is not only melancholy but apprehensive as well, and is constantly worried about some serious disease overtaking her.

Another key-note feature of this remedy is flatulence. The wind rumbles in the abdomen which the patient finds hard to expel. When at last she succeeds in doing so, it comes out in an enormous volume and with great noise. Stomach feels as if it would burst. In this respect **Argent. nit** is similar to **Carbo. veg., Lycop., Nux mosch.** and **Iodium.**

It thus occupies an important place in the therapeutics of dyspepsia. The **Argent. nit.** dyspepsia is characterised by gastrodynia. The pain is referred to the pit of the stomach, and from this spot it radiates into all directions. It is a pain that increases and decreases gradually. This pain is generally the result of over-indulging in ice-cream and other cooling dainties. When the pain becomes excessive, the patient vomits glairy stringy mucus.

We notice belching after every meal, and belching which usually is a difficult piece of business with her, is always violent. Eructation usually relieves a big portion of her uneasiness; nausea is violent and deathly.

Prescribed on such symptoms, it also cures gastric catarrh and ulceration of stomach. In this connection we should remember that it is very useful in the ill-effects of a long 'spree.'

It is one of the best remedies we have for hemicrania. Most pressive screwing throbbing pain is felt in the frontal protuberance. It is so excessive that the patient lies in a dazed condition with her eyes closed. Trembling of the body accompanies this condition, and at the very height of the pain, the patient brings up a kind of watery bilious substance. As in **Belladonna** and **Glon.**, we notice a great congestion of the brain. The arteries, especially the carotid arteries, throb obliging her to loosen her clothings about neck. To this intense congestion is also to be ascribed the sensation of expansion of the head. The head feels much bulged and she has a feeling of top-heaviness. It is in consequence of this rush of blood to brain that we find her particularly anxious to have a tight bandage about her head.

Bandaging keeps out the great on-rush of blood and thus indirectly brings relief. It is also a good remedy for gastric headaches of literary men where the least mental exercise aggravates the headache. Photophobia is excessive, so he wants door and windows shut.

We should specially think of **Argent. nit** in purulent conjunctivitis and ophthalmia. The discharge is thick and profuse. Cornea is sometimes involved. The conjunctiva looks excessively red like a piece of raw beef. Œdema and agglutination of the lids and extreme photophobia, are characteristic.

We use **Argent. nit** in metrorrhagia from uterine fibroid. Leucorrhœa is copious yellow and corroding; it is due to ulceration of os or cervix uteri.

We think of **Argent. nit.** in women, when coition becomes painful and is followed by bleeding from the vagina.

Argent. nit. is very useful in epilepsy. The indications are: Dilatation of pupil for days or hours before the attack, great restlessness following the attack and trembling of the hands.

Before closing let me mention one more important indication of **Argent. nit.** It consists in a sensation of splinter. Such a sensation may be felt in the throat, uterus and other parts of the body. In this it resembles **Dolichos, Nitric acid, Hepar sulph** and **Silicea.**

Lastly we will discuss the action of **Argentum nitricum** on the bowels. The stools are generally green like chopped spinach; while not green, they turn so after they are allowed to remain on diaper for some time. The diarrhœa is oftentimes brought about by over-indulgence in candy and sugar. Sometimes they pass masses of epithelium connected by muco-lymph as in **Aloes.** The bowels are apt to move as soon as any food or drink is taken. It is also indicated in diarrhœa from fright, excitement and apprehension, as has been mentioned before.

Case 1.—Feb. 18, 1880. J. B. C., of La Porte, Ind., has for five years, had a constant sensation in right side of throat, of a hair hanging down into larynx, causing a constant titillation, and a hoarse gasping cough, followed by a slight whitish or yellowish expectoration. The cough is always much worse at night, preventing sleep; must get up and walk the room to obtain relief. Invariably relieved by smoking a cigar. Has been in the habit of smoking at least five or six cigars a day for a number of years; several years ago, had a serious affection of the heart, and is now suffering at times with a sharp pain in præcordial region accompanied with an irregular, intermittent pulse. The chief diagnostic symptom ·in the case is **the amelioration from smoking** a cigar, when the cough and irritation at night are so severe as to prevent sleeping. The law of narcotism is that "every narcotic palliates the symptoms it produces "; and here we have the direct irritation of the drug expending its force on the laryngeal mucous membrane. The ,sensation, as "though a hair or string" were hanging down the throat from the base of the tongue, which the patient affirms is the cause of his cough, is a symptom not unfrequently met with in cases of laryngeal irritation. In this case a careful exploration of the throax by the stethoscope and by percussion reveals no organic disease of the heart or lungs, and we must decide this to be case of functional disturbance alone, caused by excessive use (for him) of tobacco; prohibited the use of tobacco at once, prescribed **Arg. nit. 200**, a powder once a day. March 3, 1880. Reported by letter: Coughs much less and consequently sleeps much better; "but has burning sensation in the stomach after taking each powder." Sac. Lac. once a day. April 7. Has used no more tobacco since it was prohibited. No cough, throat or heart trouble now, and considers himself cured.—Dr. H. C. Allen.

Case 2.—A young man of twenty commenced six or eight years since to have frequent attacks of pain in his stomach, probably in consequence of mistakes in diet, or from getting wet or chilled in hunting. When he confined himself principally to a light vegetable diet, he was much better, but as this did not satisfy his immense hunger, he had hearty food and meat. This and immoderate drinking increased his disease. His physician supposed he had a tape-worm, and administered a regular tape-worm treatment, but no worm passed off. Status præsens: continuous **pressing** pain in the fundus ventriculi, as if from a stone, at times better, at times worse; better after, worse before eating; the more he eats at a meal, the longer the amelioration continues, and the more hungry he is, the worse the pain. It is better when lying, worse when sitting, still worse when moving. When perspiration is produced by exercise, or when he gets warm in bed, the pain is better, and sometimes entirely absent. Now bread with butter, or meat, causes more pain and sometimes entirely absent. Appetite good; slight constipation. Diagnosis probably erosion of the mucous membrane. **Arg. nitr. 3,** four times a day, and simple nourishing diet, not much meat. At night a wet compress over the bowels. Cured in a few months.—Dr. Mossa.

ARNICA MONTANA.

The common name of this plant is Leopard's bane. It grows plentifully in the mountainous districts of Europe. Two parts of the root, one part of the herb and one part of the flower are pounded together and mixed with two parts by their weight of alcohol and then the tincture is extracted.

Dr. Hering and other authorities enjoin on us strictly the use of the roots alone as the tincture prepared from the flowers is very often adulterated with foreign bodies, specially insects generally found concealed in the petals of the flowers.

Arnica is the king of our traumatic remedies. We use it in injuries of the muscles, fractures of the bones, contusion of the periosteum and in sub-cutaneous and external hemorrhage due to mechanical injuries. Other remedies such as **Conium Calendula, Anacardium, Hypericum, Ledum, Rhus tox, Ruta, Staphysagria, Sulph. acid** and **Symphytum,** are also useful in cases of injury. Out of these the indications of **Calendula, Rhus tox, Ruta** and **Staphysagria** have been discussed elsewhere, and here we will go through the relationship of the rest of the drugs.

Conium is thought of in indurations of glands, such as the mammæ, testicles, etc, the result of contusions or bruises. We think of this remedy in these cases specially when the hardness becomes very intense.

Hypericum is indicated when the nerves are injured along with the soft parts as in treading on nails, needles, pins, splinters, in bites of insects and animals. The damage to the nerves is indicated by the presence of intolerable pain.

Anacardium is especially thought of, when tendons are affected.

Symphytum is a great remedy for mechanical injuries due to a blow with a blunt instrument. We think of it specially in injuries of flat bones. It may be administered in cases of irritable stump after amputation.

Ledum is useful in injuries inflicted with pointed instruments; the punctured wound feels cold to touch and to the patient. This intense coldness is the red strand of this remedy.

We shall now enquire into some of the most characteristic features of **Arnica.** Intense sensitiveness due to excessive pain is in my opinion the greatest feature of this remedy. We notice it in gout, rheumatism, traumatic injuries and other affections of

Arnica. They are in constant dread of people approaching them. They fear, through inadvertence they may touch or strike them and thus bring about intense agony.

Arnica patient is sore, lame and bruised all over, as if beaten. His whole body aches and pains. It is because of this that he dislikes lying down; everything on which he lies seems hard and uncomfortable. He constantly keeps on changing from side to side and from bed to bed in search of a soft place. This is an oft verified symptom.

Many a time and oft have I used **Arnica** in typhoid fever on such pointers as these. It is indeed an admirable remedy in typhoid, typhus and other ailments of equally debilitating type. In **Arnica** apathy and stupefaction are apparent from the beginning. Breath becomes foul-smelling, and ecchymotic spots, sometimes yellow green spots on skin soon become visible. Unconsciousness, involuntary stool and urination, distention of abdomen, rumbling and gurgling during stool, bruised feeling, intense heat of head with coolness of the rest of the body, confusion of ideas, slow delirium, great restlessness, are some of the guiding symptoms of **Arnica** in such cases.

It is at times really difficult to differentiate **Arnica** from **Baptisia** and **Acid phos.** In all these three remedies the patient so easily falls asleep while answering questions that one is apt to be confused as to the correct prescription. The restlessness, the tossing about, the universal complaint of the bed feeling too hard, are symptoms calculated to increase the doctor's confusion. The apathy, the indifference, are equally marked in all three of them; but **Arnica** combines a great sensitiveness with this apathy. There is also in **Arnica** the great difference in the temperature of the body and the head—a symptom of such towering importance that it will very easily enable the experienced prescriber in finding out his bearings.

It is equally great in the treatment of malarial and intermittent fevers. In the prodromal stage, the patient complains of drawing pains in the periosteum and thirst for large quantities of cold water. The chill soon starts from the pit of stomach with sore bruised pain in muscles of back and extremities. We should take note of the unequal distribution of heat in the **Arnica** patient. The head and face are generally hot and rest of his body feels cool to touch. One cheek is red and feels hot to touch, while the other is pale and cold. Thirst is present in the stage of chill. When this chill gives way to heat, the soreness of flesh becomes more intense and in consequence he becomes more restless. The heat of his body is sometimes internal and it is intolerable. In great agony he throws his covers off, but feels chilly as in **Nux vom** and **Apis,** and has to cover again. The sweat that follows is sour, fetid and offensive. The taste is putrid as of rotten eggs.

The effect of **Arnica** on skin is very well-marked. It produces crops of small boils all over the body. They are very painful to touch. One crop after maturing is followed by another crop. I have verified this symptom repeatedly. It is used on corns externally and is supposed to give permanent relief.

It is extremely useful in erysipelatous inflammations. The part affected looks dark and blue. Numerous semi-transparent vesicles with red basis merge together and the whole area becomes phlegmonous. Extreme tenderness, presence of numerous bullæ, heat, swelling and shining hardness give it almost the appearance of septicemia.

Arnica is considered as great a remedy for dyspepsia as **Nux vom** and **Carbo veg.** The tympanitis is excessive, and the abdomen feels full to bursting. Belching is loud and continuous. He is a great subject to obstinate constipation. Rectum is loaded with fæces, but they are not expelled easily; when they do come out after excessive straining they look flat and ribbon like. This is due either to enlargement of prostate or to retroverted uterus. The stools as well as the flatus are extremely offensive. The discharge too is frequently involuntary. The stools contain particles of undigested food and is associated with violent belly-ache. It is fluid, foamy and highly acrid.

In dysentery its most prominent indication is the long interval between the stools. The frequency of stools of the various preparations of **Mercurius** is absent. The patient gets a copious discharge of dark, venous blood at intervals of several hours relieving him of his uneasiness for an appreciable period. Ischuria or tenesmus of neck of bladder, a bruised sensation in the anus, a painful prolapsus of the rectum, are some more of its indications.

Its action on the urinary organs is quite important, and hence should not be overlooked. We not only use it in bladder and kidney affections after mechanical injuries, but in primary lesions of those organs as well. It is an admirable remedy in nephritis. The symptoms are violent chill followed by extreme nephritic pain

with nausea and vomiting—the pain extending from right hypochondrium down to the groin. It almost feels like knife plung-
ing into the kidneys. It is accompanied by frequent desire for
urination, but he has to wait a long time for urine to pass. Very
often urine is full of blood with a heavy admixture of pus.

My task will not be complete, if I omit to emphasise the importance of **Arnica** in pregnancy. It is one of our great stand-by
for threatened abortion due to falls and shocks. We also think of
this remedy in ineffectual labor pains. The pains though violent do
but little good. The patient complains of great sore, bruised feeling in the neighbourhood of the pelvis, and also of the whole body.
I use **Arnica** almost invariably after parturition, and I am confident,
it removes all the evil effects of labor and promotes proper contraction of uterus and expulsion of any foreign substance such as portions of placenta or membranes that might have been left behind.
It has been used with as great success in checking hemorrhage
after parturition as **China, Belladonna** and **Secale.**

Before I finish let me add one very odd symptom of **Arnica** and
that is great coldness of the nose. Clarke reports to have cured
a case of facial neuralgia with **Arnica** being guided to it by this
symptom alone.

Arnica locally used produces an extraordinary growth of hair.
Arnica oil is, therefore, considered useful in baldness.

Arnica is quite an important remedy in whooping cough and
its most characteristic symptom is that the child cries before
coughing, as if aware of the soreness it will cause. The paroxysm
is so violent that it brings on ecchymotic spots in the eyes and it
is often followed by nose-bleed. The expectorated fluid also is full
of foamy blood. The cough is excited by a sensation of creeping
and soreness in trachea, bronchi or larynx.

Case 1.—German, aged thirty, a brewer, visited beer vaults on a hot day
while perspiring freely, and drank freely; a sudden suppression took place,
resulting in a severe cold, followed with severe laryngeal and pulmonary
cough, ranging through a period of several weeks. Constant cough day
and night, great and almost insupportable titillation in the larynx and trachea;
rawness and scraping in the bronchi. Expectoration offensive, green and
purulent, streaked with blood. After each coughing spell would belch up
volumes of gas so offensive as to drive everyone out of the room and so
violent in its force as to raise the patient up almost bodily. Was emaciated
and prostrated; had profuse cold night sweats, offensive papescent stools,
at times involuntary, emitting much the same odor as that accompanying the
emissions of gas. Urine scanty, dark brown, with brick-dust sediment.
Repugnance to food generally, although craving sour things. Tips of the

fingers and end of the nose usually cold. After a number of remedies without benefit. **Arnica 3** was given every three hours with cure in six weeks.—Dr C. H. Von Tagen.

Case 2.—H. felt badly for several days, had an attack of fever on June 9th, and again on June 11th. Symptoms: Yawning, shivering, aching of bones, great thirst. In about an hour the shivering culminated in a hard shake with cold hands and heat **in the head and face.** The craving for water was less violent. After about an hour. there was great heat of the entire surface of the body, but the slightest motion in bed, turning or uncovering, caused a return of the shake. Gradually the hot stage terminated in a copious, sour-smelling perspiration. He had also pains in the extremities, as if they were bruised; loss of appetite; desire for stool with scanty evacuation, pain in the left hypochondrium upon deep pressure; restless and unrefreshing sleep, peevishness and an anxious, troubled state of mind. Prescribed four doses of **Arnica 6** during the apyrexia. On June 13th he had a slight paroxysm, without any aching in the limbs, no attack on June 15th. He remained well.--Hencke in "All. Hom. Zeitg." Vol. LIV, 126.

ARSENICUM ALBUM.

Arsenicum album is another of our Master's immortal monuments. It is a remedy we cannot very well afford to do without and most of our Homœopathic practitioners will, I am sure, say the same thing about it, for as a remedial agent it is of great and extensive application.

Arsenic is a highly brittle metal of a steel-grey color. It is used in the manufacture of small shots as an alloy to lead. Also it is added to iron and steel in the manufacture of chains and ornaments for the resulting combination takes on a brighter polish. Arsenic is also utilized in the manufacture of glass.

But the **Arsenicum album** of our Materia Medica is the Arsenious Acid of the chemists. It is called an acid because of its power of combining with alkalies. It is one of our great metallic poisons. It has scarcely any taste; hence it can very advantageously be used for criminal purposes. Arsenic poisoning, therefore, is very common and many of the symptoms of the remedy are derived therefrom.

The quantity of this poison required to destroy life may be assigned at from two to three grains and the period at which death takes place from large doses of Arsenic varies from eighteen hours to three days.

We will now study a case of Arsenic poisoning in its entirety. Poisoning by Arsenic may be either acute or chronic. In the former variety the attack comes on with great violence and is ushered in by nausea, a sense of fainting and a great depression of spirit. This is soon followed by vomiting and great burning pain in the epigastrium with sensitiveness to pressure. The pain in the abdomen becomes more and more severe till at last we find the patient purging most violently. This purging is very often associated with pronounced straining. The vomiting is violent and incessant and is excited by the least thing taken into the stomach. The pulse becomes small and imperceptible and the body covered with cold and clammy perspiration, thus presenting a perfect posture of collapse. Tetanic convulsions, and even coma and paralysis may close the last hours of agony of the unfortunate patient. Great restlessness and thirst are two of the most prominent symptoms that characterize the Arsenic poisoning.

Chronic poisoning is marked by a gradual falling off of the appetite, an undefined feeling of uneasiness, paleness due to the destruction of the red blood corpuscles, a suffused condition of the conjunctivæ, impaired muscular power sometimes amounting to real paralysis, and a sort of a vesicular eruption on the skin, commonly designated the eczema arsenicale. Strangury, jaundice and salivation are also noticed in Arsenic poisoning. It has been said that persons handling Arsenic get ulcerations of the scrotum and penis.

Now let us peep into the chamber of pathology and see the havoc caused by this poison on the vital organs of our system. The organs bearing the brunt of the poison are the stomach and the intestines. The mucous membrane of the stomach becomes inflamed and presents a dark scarlet color. Here and there the lining membrane thickens into fungoid forms with pasty arsenic imbedded in the holes. In rare cases we find ulceration and still rarely gangrene and perforation. The mucous membrane of the small intestines may be inflamed throughout, but mostly do we find it so in the region of the deodenum. In the large intestines the inflammation is mostly confined to the rectum.

Now a few words about the history of this poison. It has been utilized for medicinal purpose from very ancient times. We find this drug mentioned in the writings of Dioscorides and in the ancient Hindu literature. Three compounds of arsenic were used by the Hindus of old, such as arsenious anhydride or white arsenic, red sulphide of arsenic or realgar and the yellow sulphide or orpiment. Of these three, orpiment and realgar were of larger use while the white arsenic has been in use only since the time of the Bhabaprakasa and the Tantras.

White arsenic, in the Hindu system of medicine, is known by various names such as Sankha Visha, Darumuch and Sambalakshara. It was employed in a great variety of combinations for varied ailments, such as intermittent fever, remittent fever, malarial cachexia, diarrhœa, cholera, anæmia, asthma, pulmonary tuberculosis and so forth. In Europe the use of arsenic was not popular till very lately when the English physicians took it up. Amongst them Fowler was very prominent, to commemorate whose memory a preparation of arsenic still goes by the name of Fowler's solution. Arsenic again got into disuse and was much neglected till, be it said to the credit of homeopathy, Dr. Charge of Marseilles proved its wonderful efficacy and brought it back to use. Dr. Boudice, chief of the military hospital of that city, through his suggestion, used it with great deal of success in the treatment of intermittents among soldiers returning from the African moors. Since then Arsenic is enjoying uniform popularity.

Now a few words about the preparation of this remedy will not be out of place. One part by weight of vitreous arsenous acid is boiled to complete solution in sixty parts of water. This is filtered and more distilled water added till it is raised to ninety parts. To this is added ten parts of ninety-five p. c. alcohol.

Arsenic is very rich in mental symptoms and they are so clear cut and well defined that there is hardly any possibility of confusion of mind. The remedy is really forced upon us. Who can mistake the great restlessness of this irritant poison? And it is not simply a physical restlessness, for underlying it we find great mental turmoil almost bordering on anguish. He wants to move from one bed to another thinking he will feel a bit easy after the change. But alas! this search after ease and quiet is simply a mirage. There is no relief anywhere and in any position. He does not know what to do or where to go. Even when the patient is too weak to move, this internal restlessness manifests itself by a constant movement of the limbs and when that is not possible, by a sort of woe-begone desperate look that tells of the tumult within him.

Another important characteristic is fear. The patient thinks it is useless to take medicine as his disease is incurable. We find a similar state of mind in **Acon.** but the difference is that in the latter remedy it is more of a nervous kind whereas in **Arsen.** the anxiety is caused by the real critical state of his sickness. With this fear is mixed a certain amount of indifference.

We find under **Arsen.** a great desire for suicide. In fact it is almost as marked as in gold. This desire of doing away with one's own self is mostly seen in cases of mania. Insanity, to which **Arsenic** is homœopathic, comes from long physical suffering and consequent exhaustion. The patient suffers from all kinds of hallucinations. He is afraid of ghosts, thieves; he sees all kinds of vermin on his bed, throws handful of them away and tries to escape from them. Very frequently the insanity takes the form of religious melancholia, hopelessness and despair. He despairs of his salvation; life holds out no charm for him. This disgust for life is manifested by great anguish and restlessness and he tries to kill himself, especially by hanging.

Other remedies we can think of with a similar suicidal tendency are **Alum, Agn, Aur. met, Ant. crud** and **Nat. sulph.** Though similar they are characteristically different and it will pay us to study this minutely.

Alum is a low-spirited sort of patient; he is conscious of his personal identity being confused. He doubts if he is himself. He is conscious of his weak-mindedness. Evil ideas come to him inspite of his will and he wants to make short of his intolerable existence by cutting his throat.

Agnus castus is indicated mostly in puerperal insanity with suicidal tendencies. The most prominent feature of this patient is her aversion to her husband, babe and to all sexual intercourse.

Aurum met. is a sovereign remedy for insanity with suicidal ideas. Time and again have I verified this in my personal experience. He indulges in the gloomiest of ideas and the most depressing of emotions, having a syphilitic or syphilo-mercurial constitution as the back of it all. He has a special hankering for shooting himself or throwing himself from a height.

Antim. crud works miracles in sentimental insanity. We call these people moon-struck. They constantly indulge in an ideal love for some ideal female. From non-gratified craving they get gloomy and peevish and want to end their miseries by shooting and drowning themselves.

Nat. sulph is another great remedy for suicidal mania. He is in constant need of restraint lest he will do himself bodily harm. Such patients have got to be constantly watched. They dread music, for music makes them melancholy. This insanity is to be traced to a jar or a knock on the head or a fall or to some sort of injury about the brain.

A great deal has been said about the fear and anguish of this patient; but this fear is to a great extent modified by a sort of calm indifference. He is afraid that his case is going to be fatal and yet he accepts it as inevitable. The dread of death is more noticeable when alone or on going to bed.

Another important feature of this remedy, that will help us in many difficulties, is the great prostration to which our patient readily becomes a subject. This is quite guiding. Some cases take on bad turn from the beginning. Although the suffering is not much and the duration of sickness is only small, the vital power of the patient sinks rapidly. This sinking is explained by the des tructive process that is going on inside and unless this process is stopped by the timely administration of **Arsenic,** our case will proceed deathward. And yet we must remember, as Dr. Farring ton has cautioned us, that this remedy must not be used early unless needed.

This process of destruction of tissues and consequent weaken ing of vital power, has always been a great guide for me. Some time ago I had a case of inflammation of the left big toe in a working man. The whole leg was a mass of swelling, hot and bluish in color, and the old school's advice was amputation below knee joint. The prospect of a wooden leg was not naturally liked by him and he tried homœopathic treatment. The burning pains coupled with the rapid progress towards gangrene decided me in the selection of this remedy and the result more than exceeded my expectations. This principle is exemplified also in typhoid and typhus, in paralysis, in pernicious anæmia, in diarrhœa, in enteritis, in cholera and in a host of other complaints.

Irritability is another important characteristic of our drug. This is marked almost everywhere. The stomach is irritable and it rejects food and water inspite of hunger and thirst. The skin is rritable—it itches, but scratching is impossible due to great irrita bility. The mental condition is just as irritable and we notice that our patient is low-spirited, exceedingly sensitive, despondent, weeping, the least trifle filling her with care and solicitude.

But the symptom that I consider the most guiling, is the midnight aggravation of all the symptoms of this remedy. On this one symptom alone, have I repeatedly cured the most desperate cases and its importance will be equally testified to by many other practitioners of this most reliable system of medicine.

It will be inexcusable if I omit to mention another characteristic symptom—I mean that one pertaining to its pain and its amelioration. The pain of **Arsenic,** in whatever part or organ it may be, is always burning in nature. It feels that it has been set on fire. The general rule is that the parts that have become abnormally heated, cool down on cold application and that sensations of heat are ameliorated by cold appliances; but **Arsenicum** is an exception to this rule. The universal burning of **Arsenicum** is always relieved by hot applications wherever the sensation of burning may be; the patient is constantly calling for hot water bottles, hot fomentations and so on, for heat is the only thing that temporarily relieves. But a few words of caution will not be out of place here. It will be a mistake to use **Arsenicum** for a mere sensation of heat, for such sensations may arise from nervous causes only. The burning pain in **Arsenicum** is really due to destruction of tissues either progressing or impending. Hence its need in gangrene, in sloughing diseases and in carbuncles, where its action is undeniable and invaluable.

Before I run on to another subject, I think it is wise to differentiate between **Arsenicum** and **Secale,** for in the latter remedy the burning is just as prominent as in the former. **Secale** too is just as restless with his intense burning, but he is constantly calling for cold application and this constitutes the difference between the two great " burners."

Thirst is another important feature of **Arsenicum** but water molests the patient; every time he drinks he vomits it up. That is why, inspite of his unquenchable craving for water, he drinks little at a time. In respect of unquenchable thirst **Arsenicum** stands on the same level with **Acon, Bry, Calc ost, Caps, Cham, China, Dig, Eup. perf, Iod, Merc, Nat. mur.** and **Phos.**

Now that we have gone through the general outline of this remedy, we will go in detail into its symptomatology. It is called for in a very obstinate type of frontal headache, when that is accompanied by vertigo. The head feels pressed as from a heavy load on the brain; this sensation is temporarily relieved by cold washing and permanently by a walk in the open air. The scalp is so very sensitive that it can scarcely bear the hair to be touched.

Arsenicum is called for in a serious type of vertigo that emanates from malaria. He complains of great heaviness in the head and humming in the ears. It goes off in the open air but returns again as soon as he enters the room.

The efficacy of **Arsenicum** in the treatment of the diseases of the eye is invaluable and extensive. The symptoms, too, are so very clear-cut and precise that there is hardly any chance of mistake. **Arsenicum** has been reported to cure cases of pterygium, scrofulous ophthalmia, chronic trachoma, parenchymatous keratitis. keratitis punctata, kerato-iritis, iritis rheumatica, retinitis albuminurica and so on. The eyelids are so swollen and œdematous that they look as if distended with air; they are spasmodically closed. The internal surface of the lids are very sore and the conjunctiva looks like a piece of raw beef; when opening the eyes, the patient complains of intense burning sticking pains.

The photophobia is intense; lachrymation is excessive and scalding. This corrosiveness is characteristic of all the discharges of this remedy. In diarrhœa the stools excoriate the anus; in otorrhœa the whole auditory passage gets raw and inflamed owing to the corrosiveness of the discharge; in cold, the nose gets red and scalded; the leucorrhœa also is burning. The photophobia is so intense that he lies in bed with his face buried in the pillow. The hot and scalding lachrymation causes an eczematous eruption on that part of his cheek over which the tears flow.

Arsenicum is a good remedy for horizontal half-sights. He can only see objects in the lower part of his field of vision and that is why he lifts his head high and throws it somewhat backward when looking at a distant object. Sometimes his whole vision is dim and objects look as if he has been looking through white gauze.

Arsenicum has another important symptom which may be invaluble to us on certain special occasions. Everything he looks at seems green to him. In this place we will consider about a few other remedies like **Caps, Actæa spic, Camph, Ruta** and **Cina.**

In **Caps** all objects look black.

In **Actæa spic** on the other hand everything he looks at seems blue.

In **Camph** the patient tells us that everything about him is bright and glittering.

In **Hyos** he finds red spots before his eyes whereas in **Ruta** candle-light seems surrounded by red halo.

Last of all we come to **Cina.** It is a great remedy for xanthopsia or yellow seeing. There is a yellow tint imparted to landscapes and objects looked at, an effect perhaps most comparable to that of looking through yellow glass.

I will cite here a very instructive case of keratitis punctata that Schlosser cured with **Arsenicum.** "The outer segment of the conjunctiva was enormously swollen; the iris was discolored, reacting sluggishly. Posterior synechiæ was well marked with some exudation into the pupil. The pain in the upper part of the orbit was excruciating and burning in character. There were nocturnal aggravation and copious secretion of scalding tears." All the symptoms pointing to **Arsenicum** he administered a few doses of this remedy with marvellous effect.

Before I take up another symptom it would be advisable to differentiate between **Arsen, Apis** and **Rhus tox,** as these remedies are somewhat similar. We find œdematous swelling in all three of them but in **Apis** it is merely a puffiness in **Rhus** it is dependent upon the infiltration of the connective tissues and sometimes there is suppurative inflammation of the deep structures of the eye, whereas in **Arsenicum** the swelling is the outcome of the deep **Arsenic** cachexia.

The pain of **Apis** though apparently similar is essentially different, for in **Apis** it is relieved by cold applications.

The burning hot lachrymation of **Apis** is similar to that of **Arsenicum** but it is not acrid and excoriating as in the latter remedy. Besides we must not forget that the affections of **Arsenicum** are periodic in their nature commencing every fall and often alternating from one part to the other.

Arsenicum is indicated in otitis externa diffusa when we find great burning and itching and oozing of a corrosive watery discharge. The tissues of the meatus themselves become the seat of innumerable burning pustules which later on turn into painful ulcers.

Arsenicum is useful in mumps especially with metastasis to the testicles.

In **Arsenicum** we find a splendid remedy for fluent coryza The nose feels stopped up although it flows freely and the discharge is corrosive and excoriating. As a result of this the nose and its surrounding parts become raw and inflamed.

Toothache is a trifling ailment but there are occasions when the poor patient will do anything to get relief and **Arsenicum** helps in those cases which are peculiarly its own. The toothache is very severe indeed and it is mostly in the first lower bicuspid. It is excited by cold weather and is aggravated by the sound of other's talking. In this last respect it is somewhat similar to **Therid,** where we find the toothache to be caused by shrill noise. The **Arsenicum** toothache is relieved by heat of stove, sitting up in bed, and by striking head.

There is another important condition where it helps and that is when toothache is associated with dysmenorrhœa and also when toothache precedes menses. **Calc. ost, Cham, Lach, Phos, Sepia** and **Staph,** also have toothache during menstruation.

Homœopathy would have been far less enchanting and its field of action greatly curtailed, had it not been for **Arsenicum album;** treatments of fevers specially of different types, would have been far less satisfactory affording chance to our antagonist friends to feel jubilant over failure of Homœopathy; but fortunately for us this great legacy of the great Master has supplied the greatest ingredient towards the perfection of his science. In the hands of the homœopath **Arsenicum** proves a more powerful drug than crude quinine—that great object of vaunting to our regular friends—for when quinine fails **Arsenicum** cures.

Arsenicum is useful in quotidian, tertian, quartan and double tertian fevers-also in typhoid, typhus and all other varieties of septic fevers, but only when it is indicated. With this remedy I have cured the most obstinate type of malarial fevers. For intermittents contracted in the salt marshes, near the sea shores and the Assam valleys, it is a capital remedy. The most appropriate time for the paroxysm is between 1 to 2 p.m. and 12 to 2 a.m. Periodicity as I have said before, is a prominent feature of these paroxysms. They come every fourteen days and sometimes we get yearly return of the complaint. **Arsenic** paroxysms are anticipating in nature and the period is one hour every other day. For a few days before the paroxysm the patient complains of weariness, lassitude and languor and then with an immense lot of gaping, stretching and yawning, as in **Rhus tox,** the chill starts. The state of chill is irregularly developed and vaguely defined. The patient while feeling chilly complains of heat. There is little, if any, thirst during chill and even when thirsty he prefers hot drinks which he takes little at a time but often.

We must not also forget to mention that drinking in **Arsenicum** patient increases his chill and causes vomiting. This absence of thirst during chill and preference for hot drinks when thirst is at all present, are considered very important indications of **Arsenicum** and their absence a counter indication by Dr. Guernsey. Sometimes the chill gradually increases to a shaking rigor and he shivers and shudders specially when walking in the open air.

In some cases of malaria of the perinicious variety during the cold stage we notice colic, loose stool, nausea, and unconsciousness. I will cite here a very interesting case that I treated sometime ago and which brought me quite a big share of renown— a thing that comes easily to a cautious, studious, and patient homœopath. It was in a young man of thirty-two, hailing from one of the malaria-infected areas of Bengal. I found him in a semi-unconscious state, covered up to the head with a blanket and purging most violently. He was highly restless and the profuse stools were a mass of blood. He received **Acon** 6 which beyond checking the bloody stools did no other good. He also received **Euphorbium** on the ground of cholera like symptoms during fever and that did not do him much good either. The patient responded very sympathetically to a dose of **Arsen. cm.** which cured him radically.

The hot stage of Arsen is long lasting (two to four hours) and is very prominent. The burning is intense. He feels as if boiling water were flowing through his veins. The thirst at this stage is insatiable. He wants tumblersful of water. Sometimes we find him drinking little at a time but often vomiting each time after drinking. The restlessness is very great and this is partly due to burning and partly to the anguish to which he is subject.

The next stage is the stage of sweat. The sweat is cold, clammy and prostrating. The thirst continues but the peculiarity of thirst at this stage, unlike the thirst of chill and heat, is that he drinks quantities at a time. A sort of an icterus is very often noticed after the fever. The skin is pale, cold and parchment-like. During apyrexia the patient manifests a craving for refreshing drinks such as wine, coffee, lemonade, etc.

Before I close my remarks on fever I cannot do better than reiterate the statements of Dr. Wurmb concerning the indications of **Arsenicum** in intermittent fever, for no other man in the history of medical literature has so graphically and vividly described the intermittent cachexia and its relation to **Arsenicum.**

" **Arsenic** is indicated in cases which are distinguished not only by weakness in the vital power and deterioration of the organic substance, but also at the same time by symptoms of excitation of the circulation or of the nervous system alone or of both together. Again it seems to be more especially indicated, the more malignant the influence from which the disease has sprung. Marsh miasm is the chief of these influences; in this originate the most serious and most dangerous cases of fever and in these **Arsenic** is often the only remedy that will rescue the patient. Again, the longer the disease has lasted, the more is **Arsenic** generally indicated, because the more deeply have the organs and tissues been affected, the more nearly has the patient's condition approached that what is known as the intermittent cachexia and which so nearly resembles the arsenical cachexia. Especially is this the case where the liver and the spleen have swollen.

"The intermittents which find their homœopathic remedy in **Arsenic** present in their paroxysms the following peculiarities.

"The paroxysms are general, violent and of long duration, the stages are either distinctly doveloped and equally proportioned to each other, or else as is most frequently the case, one of the stages is absent or is very feebly present; if the latter be the case, it is generally the cold stage which fails and the hot is all the more violent. The more intense the heat, the longer it continues, the higher the degree of development of the accompanying excitement in the vascular system, the more burning and insatiable the thirst, the better is **Arsenic** indicated. The sweating stage may be altogether wanting, or the perspiration may be very copious; it breaks out generally several hours after the hot stage and lasts a long time."

I will cite a case here from my practice just simply to confirm the above statement. A gentleman, aged about 45, who had contracted the marsh malaria for the past 3 years, came under my treatment sometime ago. His spleen was enormously swollen and hard, abdomen big and distended with the hypertrophied spleen— the rest of his body presenting a sad contrast to the mid segment. The anemia was appalling, the prostration very great. Diarrhœa peeped occasionally. The vital organs all proved to be at their lowest ebb. In fact a worse picture of deviated health could not be imagined. Three years of Allopathic treatment had left him a wreck—economical and physical. Symptoms of **Arsenic** were many and precise and **Arsenic** rescued him. Since then he has

turned a great admirer of Homœopathy. A stauncher believer an-
a nobler monument of Homœpathy than him cannot be found in
the whole of India. Glory be to Hahnemann and his immortal
science of therapeutics!

Arsenicum makes a capital remedy for typhoid fever when it
assumes a slow protracted form. Delirium is mild with suspension of consciousness. Restlessness inspite of exhaustion is very
great. The face is hippocratic and distorted; eyes are glistening,
staring, sunken or closed with sticky matter in them; cheeks are
burning hot with circumscribed redness. The lips are dry and
cracked and covered with a fetid black sordes. He is very thirsty,
and the water drunk descends audibly into his stomach. The stools
are watery, foul and involuntary. The aphthæ in mouth bleed
easily. The pulse gradually gets weaker more rapid and intermittent showing that the life-force is waning fast. The breathing
is short, anxious and labored. The skin is dry and parchment-
like—that gloss and smoothness, the usual accompaniment of
health is gone. Very often this dry surface becomes covered with
cold and clammy sweat which gives a sort of pungent sensation
to the touch. Our patient slides down in bed and his lower jaw
keeps hanging down. These symptoms indicate great gravity of
the case, but **Arsenic** will even then rescue such cases when indicated.

Arsenic has a wide range of action over the heart and it is
gratifying to notice the marvellous effect it produces when indicated. It is used in hydropericardium, endocarditis, valvular diseases,
hypertrophy and fatty degeneration of the heart. Palpitation is
a very frequent complaint and it is so violent that even the chest
wall heaves up and down and his whole frame shakes and the sound
becomes audible to those near about. This is accompanied by
anguish and dyspnœa. The dyspnœa and anguish are always
aggravated at night and by lying on back. In extreme cases
general œdema manifests itself beginning with puffiness in eyes
and swelling of feet.

Arsenic is of great use in rheumatism of the heart. Dr. Nash
has reported a case of a girl of sixteen summers who
was suddenly taken ill with severe pain in the region of
the heart. The pains were very excruciating causing her to
cry out with every breath. I will cite the doctor's own words—
"Inspite of the best prescribing I could do, the case progressed
from bad to worse until the following condition was present— viz:

Great dyspnœa, could not lie down at all. Violent beating of the
heart, shaking visibly the walls of the chest. With first beat of
heart very loud bellows sound. Waxy paleness of skin. Feet
œdematously swollen up to knees. Great restlessness, wanted to
be moved from place to place. Great thirst for small quantities
at a time. Pulse 110 to 120. **Arsenicum** 30, four doses of a watery
solution, one hour apart and then waited. Immediately improvement started; the dyspnœa, swelling of feet, restlessness, and in
short all the above symptoms except the blowing sound of the heart
were removed."

Angina pectoris is another affection which **Arsenicum** may
cure and in those desperate cases where no cure is possible it will
help. I remember the case of a gentleman of about 50, who was
relieved and benefited by **Arsenicum** to such a great extent that the
agonizing pain in the pericardial region, the sense of tightness
around the heart, anxiety, difficult breathing, dyspnœa, and fainting
spells, disappeared. The peculiar symptom he had was relief from
sitting, either bent forward or head thrown back.

Hartmann regards **Arsenicum** almost as a specific in this
disease when it is unattended by any structural disorganization of
the heart or of the larger vessels. He says " In my opinion and
according to the experience I have had **Arsenicum** is the chief
remedy more especially if the angina is a pure neurosis; its curative power is of course problematical, if the angina is complicated
with disorganizations which we cannot cure and where we only
expect a palliative influence. In this respect no remedy can be
more certainly relied upon than **Arsenic.**"

Besides **Arsenicum** we find Hartmann advocating **Plumbum,
Sambucus, Angustura, Lactuca virosa, Veratrum alb, Asafœtida** and
Sepia, but we must not forget that the totality of the symptoms
is our sole and the only guide in the selection of the remedy.

Arsenicum has got a wide range of applications in ailments
of the respiratory system. It affects the larynx, the bronchi and
the lungs. We use it in laryngitis when the voice becomes hoarse,
weak, trembling and uneven, sometimes amounting to real aphonia.
This is accompanied by a burning pain in tne larynx. There is
also a constant titillating cough induced by a sensation of sulphur
vapor in the larynx. The spasm of the glottis too may also be
present. In very advanced cases where there is extensive ulceration, we notice a sort of an acrid sero-purulent discharge from the
throat.

Arsenic is a capital remedy for asthma. I have often relieved asthmatic paroxysms with **Arsenic.** We use this remedy both in acute and chronic asthma specially when it is periodic in nature. Often we notice co-existence of emphysema and cardiac affections with asthma; the dyspnœa is particularly aggravated by lying down. One symptom that strikes us as being very peculiar is that the paroxysms almost always come on at about mid-night when with anguish and suffocation he hurries out of bed and keeps panting and wheezing, bathed in profuse perspiration—his limbs cold and stiff as if he is going to breathe his last. The paroxysms abate as soon as he begins to cough and throw off mucus of a tenacious viscid character.

Arsenicum is an invaluable remedy when the asthma results from suppression of eruptions and in children of enfeebled and impaired constitutions. The **Arsenic** asthma is always worse from exertion, talking, laughing and atmospheric changes.

Ferrum met. comes very close to **Arsenicum.** In this remedy also we find a similar mid-night aggravation when the poor patient is compelled to sit up or walk slowly about. He talks slowly and keeps his chest uncovered for these manœuvres bring him decided relief. These patients flush very freely and they are frequent subjects of epistaxis.

Another similar remedy is **Graphites.** The paroxysms come on at mid-night when our patient has to hurry out of bed with anguish and suffocation and hold on to something for support. He feels very hungry at such times and a few morsels bring him untold relief.

Now let us consider a sister ailment—Phthisis and the relationship of **Arsenicum** thereto. There is scarely a remedy in our entire Materia Medica that has proved more serviceable in phthisis either in its stage of incipiency or in the most advanced stage than **Arsenicum album.** Many cases of Phthisis in its incipient stage and quite a few cases in the advanced stage have been cured by the timely and judicious application of this great anti-psoric. Its indications are very clear-cut and well defined. The first symptom to attract our attention is the gradual and progressive emaciation. The patient eats well but he does not thrive much. This is also characteristic of **Nat mur.** and **Iod.** He also complains of frequent,.acute, sharp, stitching, darting pain in apex and through upper third of right lung. This is accompanied by a sense of constriction which is more noticeable on going up hill. The expectoration is mainly frothy and this is considered an important characteristic of the remedy, although sometimes we may notice a tenacious, viscid, yellowish green and blood-stained sputa. Hemoptysis may also be present.

There are some cases of diarrhœa where **Arsenicum is** peculiarly applicable and where none but **Arsenic** will help. The stools are watery, brownish, copious, painless and cadaverous smelling. Generally it is very scanty but prostrating. This offensive nature of the discharge is a guiding feature. The smell is very aptly described as a carrion-like smell. You have just got to smell it once to remember it all your life long. Of course this is not the only remedy where the stools stink so badly. We may also add **Bapt, Carb veg, Asaf, Graph, Lach, Psor, Scill** and **Sulph** to the list but every one of them has its own peculiar characteristic difference to save the prescriber from confusion and mistake.

Another symptom that I have verified again and again in my practice and which I consider very important is the dark color of the stool. Sometimes it is real black. This peculiar color either points to putrefied blood in the stool or to defective function of the liver and **Arsenicum** is admirably suited to both these conditions. There are a few other remedies with black stools and I like to mention them in this connection.

One of them is **Bromium.** The stools of **Bromium** are intensely black but the diarrhœa in **Brom.** is mostly brought about by oysters. These patients are prone to painful blind varices and we find them very averse to the application of warm or cold water, for water in either form produces terrible aggravation. When the pain becomes unbearable we find them wetting their varices with saliva for that is the only process that relieves.

A second remedy is **Leptandra.** The stools are jet black, almost like tar and the patient complains of a severe aching burning sensation in the region of the liver. There is quite a good bit of cutting pain and distress near the umbilicus and in the epigastrium. I have used this remedy with great deal of satisfaction in infantile liver and cholera.

Another remedy that I can think of is **Psorinum.** The stools are black and there is no mistaking about the odor. It is also a valuable intercurrent remedy when well-chosen remedies fail to act.

It will be very unjust indeed not to give **Scilla** a place in this list. The stools are very offensive and black, but it lacks the great debility of **Arsenic.** The consistency of the stools in this remedy is a bit different from that of **Arsenicum** in as much as it is full of froth. The stools are mostly involuntary.

In **Stramonium** the stools are black and fluid and it is very often called for in typhoid conditions.

I will not feel satisfied unless I mention the bearing of this remedy on Asiatic Cholera. We need it very often in the stage of collapse. I cannot do better than quote from the writings of my Mentor in Homœpathy, that true and universally revered follower of Hahnemann, the late Dr. P. C. Majumdar.

"**Arsenicum** is a very important remedy in the collapse stage of cholera. Its pathogenetic symptoms are so closely similar to Asiatic cholera that an arsenical poisoning case may be easily mistaken for a cholera case. It has a vast range of action and we have repeatedly verified its curative power in most serious cases of the disease. It is for this reason that I select it as a prototype of collapse remedies. Its symptoms are very marked and unmistakable.

"Great irritability associated with profound exhaustion is the most prominent characteristic of **Arsenic.** The patient's pulse is vanishing, he is so weak as to be unable to utter a single word and is yet restless, anxious and irritable.

"Great anxiety and restlessness, fear of death, great prostration of strength, sunken eyes, distorted face, pointed nose, cold and clammy perspiration, burning of the whole body, retching and vomiting, unquenchable thirst, drinking frequently but small quantities at a time and vomiting immediately after drinking, violent burning of stomach and abdomen, urine completely suppressed, are some of the indications of this remedy.

"When a patient gets an attack of cholera after eating fruits and drinking ice-water, living in a damp place, exposed to the influence of putrefactive and offensive smells, **Arsenic** is the remedy."

Arsenic is used in acute and chronic inflammation of the kidneys. The urine is scanty, turbid and thick like beer. In severe cases it looks almost dark like dung-water. The smell is terribly fetid. Great œdema and dropsy, irritable stomach and bowels, great thirst, intense burning during micturition, are some of the symptoms. We use it in cystitis both acute and chronic. The bladder becomes greatly distended and sometimes paralysed, and the patient finding it very difficult to urinate. In very chronic cases we fiind pus mixed with blood.

Arsenicum is a valuable remedy in retention of urine due to atony of bladder after parturition. The atony is complete. The patient feels no desire whatsoever to pass water. We can fully rely upon this remedy and rarely have to employ any other. But if **Arsenic** fails, **Caust** and **Hyos** will do the work.

Arsenicum is frequently needed in the treatment of syphilis and syphilitic bubo. The ulcer on the genitalia is serpiginous in character and sometimes even gangrenous. The granulations are florid and unhealthy and they bleed on the slightest touch. From this ulcer oozes out a watery, corrosive, and offensive secretion. Constitutional syphilis with indescribable feeling of weakness and dropsy finds a ready remedy in **Arsenicum.** Coffee-colored eruptions on the skin are very often present.

In the female sexual sphere **Arsenic** is indispensable for ailments like ovaritis, ovarian dropsy, metritis, uterine cancer and menorrhagia, when they all take on a serious type and present symptoms of **Ars.**

In uterine cancer of **Arsenicum** we have great swelling of the womb, and hardening of the os. The pain is agonizing; it is burning and lancinating in character and oh, the smell of the thin ichorous secretion from the diseased uterus! It makes her life unbearable. She is a frequent subject of fainting fits because of the excessive debility and emaciation. The leucorrhœa, too, of which she is a frequent subject, is corroding and profuse.

We use **Arsenic** in gastritis, gastralgia, ulceration and cancer of stomach. The pain in epigastrium and stomach is unbearable and can better be felt than described. But here also the characteristic of the pain remains the same. His stomach, as he describes it, "burns like fire," and this symptom of burning, whatever the complaint may be so long as **Arsenicum** is the remedy, stands out prominently and should always attract our attention. He also complains of great heaviness and pressure in stomach. It feels as if there is a load or a stone. These are accompanied by serious gastric symptoms—such as irritability of the stomach as manifested by nausea and vomiting, water brash, eructations and loss of appetite. The thirst is intense, burning and unquenchable. He drinks much but little at a time and drinking does not refresh him. The stomach is so very irritable that the least food or drink taken into the stomach is thrown out instantly. In gastric ulceration and in cancer of stomach we find even vomiting of blood. He gulps out big mouthfuls of tar-like substance with clots of blood in it. Oftener we notice a sort of coffee-ground substance. These are very serious symptoms and should at once draw our attention to **Arsenicum**.

Before closing my remarks on **Arsenicum** I should like to say a few words about its action on the skin. Like the deep structures the skin also is affected profoundly and the kind of skin that we consider pre-eminently an **Arsenic** skin, is the scaly, pale, dry, waxy parchment-like skin, so often met with in serious ailments. The eruptions too that we find here are bran-like, dry and scaly with intense itching and burning. Ecchymosed spots like those found under **Acid sulph** and **Arnica** are frequent. It is rarely used in vesicular and pustular eruptions, but for ulcers of cancerous character with elevated edges having great burning as their characteristic **Arsenic** is almost a specific. These ulcers keep on secreting a thin watery, bloody fetid pus. Sometimes they become gangrenous attended with great sloughing of the neighbouring parts.

The **Arsenic** gangrene has a special affinity for certain parts of our system such as buccal cavity, the scrotum, the sexual parts and the lower limbs.

It would pay us to remember also that **Arsenicum** is of very great use in ailments from chewing of tobacoo, alcoholism, seabathing, sausage poisoning, dissection wounds, anthrax poison, and in diseases caused through dainties like ice-cream.

Case 1.—G., aged thirty-seven, has been ill for two weeks. Cause, exposure and intemperance. Has a dry cough, aggravated at night, especially from 10 to 11 pm., expectorates a frothy sputa; sharp, shooting pains in the left side; respiration labored and hurried; Dyspnœa was so marked that he could not assume the recumbent position; hurried respiration; slight dullness over both lungs, especially over the lower lobes. Small mucus rales, most marked over the inferior regions of the chest; sordes on lips and teeth, tongue small and dry, along its median portion a blackish coat, and in protruding, its blackish, stringy mucus was seen extending from roof of mouth to the tongue; mouth dry and parched, constant desire for small quantity of water; has eaten little the past six days; stomach sore and sinsitive; constipation; has dull pain in the lumbar region; urine scanty, high-coloured, and frequent calls to urinate, which on examination, revealed pus corpuscles, and about one-half per cent. of albumen. Pulse 120; small, weak, and almost imperceptible; œdema of extremities, hands cyanotic. **Ars.** 30 cured in two weeks. Dr. B. G. Carleton.

Case 2.—H. F., aged twenty-eight years, tall, slender, narrow-chested, had bleeding from the lungs. The blood was arterial, fresh, and the quantity lost during each attack was enormous. He was wasted to a skeleton, his pulse was thread-like and showed, far more than seven months, an average of 98 beats per minute. He had also: a constant dry, hacking cough, continuing night and day, without tickling the throat, hectic fever, lasting all day, followed at night by profuse sweat; deathly pallor of the face; bright, red spots on one and on both cheeks; great dryness of the mouth and throat; tormenting thirst; ravenous hunger; tedious voiding of dark red urine, which was scanty and scalding; occasionally long-continued suppression of urine; agonizing restlessness day and night; sharp, shooting, burning pains in the chest; extreme dyspnœa, still further aggravated at night. Great fetor of breath. Expectoration of fetid, dark, greenish, solid lumps of matter. The attacks of bleeding recurred every three or four weeks. He had been treated and given up to die by several prominent physicians of different schools. The patient was treated with **Arsenicum** 3, 6, 12, and discharged, seemingly well, after about ten months of constant treatment. He received a very occasional dose of China and Phosphorus. He enjoyed good health for several years, when he again exposed himself in a very imprudent manner, and, I am told, died of pneumonia.

ARSENICUM HYDROGENISATUM.

It is a preparation of **Arsenicum** obtained by dissolving it in distilled water or in other words it may be called Arseniuretted Hydrogen. A certain amount of experiments were conducted with this by Dr. Drysdale in 1849 in the treatment of asiatic cholera. In this preparation of **Arsenicum** we have a more accentuated action of the remedy. Great disorganisation of blood, hemorrhages from the different mucous membranes of the body, suppression of urine, coldness, prostration, weakness, nausea, and violent vertigo are some of the symptoms that may be added to the whole host of symptoms of **Arsenicum album** to which it has almost an equal claim.

ARSENICUM IODATUM.

It is the Iodide of Arsenicum and as a remedy it is very useful in all kinds of chronic inflammatory conditions of the lungs, bronchial tubes and the mucous membranes of the human system. The great keynote of this remedy is to be found in the character of its discharge. It is profuse, greenish-yellow, and pus-like and is persistently excoriating. It irritates every portion over which it flows, and hence we use it in ordinary coryza as well as in chronic nasal catarrh. It may be used in otorrhœa, diarrhœa, hay fever or in any other complaint with the characteristic scalding discharge.

It is extremely useful in tubercular and phthisical affections of the lungs. It is indicated by a hoarse racking cough with profuse expectoration of purulent nature, great emaciation and weakness, constant fever, sweat, persistent diarrhœa and a tendency for general glandular involvement.

It has been used successfully in the treatment of tumors, and even epithilioma has been known to be cured with **Arsenicum Iodatum.** Dr. L. B. Wells cured with it a case of hard tumor in the left axilla of a lady aged 49. The gland which was of the size of a hen's egg and from which exuded a sort of fluid that formed into a crust on drying responded to **Ars. Iod.** Not only the tumor disappeared but the left breast which was enlarged and indurated as a sort of secondary affection also became normal.

Lastly we will discuss the action of **Arsenicum iod.**, on the skin. It is a remedy par excellence in psoriasis and in ichthyosis. The most significant symptom is marked exfoliation of skin in large scales which leaves raw, bleeding surface underneath. The strumous or psoric diathesis in conjunction with **Arsenic** symptoms should always an invaluable guide in the selection of the remedy.

ARTEMISIA VULGARIS.

The tincture is prepared from the root of worm-wood belonging to the natural order of Compositæ. This remedy has been handed down to us from a very ancient time by the Romans and the Greeks, who used to employ it in epilepsy and spasms. We are also much indebted for our knowledge of this remedy to the dominant school. Many of their observations and remarks have helped us in determining the proper valuation of this remedy in various ailments.

The principal action of **Artemisia** seems to be confined to the nervous system and the uterus and we are going to discuss in this chapter mostly symptoms pertaining to those organs.

It is a principal remedy for epilepsy, catalepsy, spasmodic twitching as is seen in cholera, hysterical fits, eclampsia and convulsion of various types such as occur in hydrocephalus, teething etc. **Artemisia** is specially indicated in epilepsy after a fright or grief or a blow on the head. The attacks are frequently repeated to be followed by a long interval of rest. It is also indicated in epilepsy due to menstrual disturbances. It has been used also with success in epilepsy coming on after a long fit of dancing. In **Artemisia** we have several attacks of epilepsy in the same day. After the attack the patient remains well for several days, but when it does occur again, it is repeated several times in the course of the same day.

In this connection I would like to remark that epilepsy runs a chronic course and it will be sheer folly to claim to cure it by the administration of a few doses of any medicine attained proportionately more fortunate results than that obtained by other system of treatment in vogue in present days.

The causative factor of the disease should be removed first if possible; menstrual derangements, helminthiasis, excessive nocturnal emission, selfabuse and other causative factors, if found out, should be removed first, if at all the disease has to be combated with success. It is said, the disease can be warded off, where the aura is distinctly marked, by tying a ligature to the extremity where the aura appears. Great care must be taken to protect the patient from all possible injuries, for these patients indeed run grave and serious risks. Meat should be scrupulously avoided. My object in mentioning these points is to impress on all practitioners the need of care and caution, if success is at all to be courted. Indicated remedies are indispensable no doubt, but I consider the other valuable adjuncts more important with regard to the achievement of success. Success in medical line depends more on plodding perseverance, care, attention and observation than on lightning-like acumen and supernatural genius, same as elsewhere. As far as the medical treatment of epilepsy is concerned we have a whole list of remedies to choose from; the most important ones amongst them are the following:—

Cuprum—It is particularly useful in epileptic paroxysms breaking out at night time.

Plumbum is useful in epilepsy with a well defined aura where paralytic symptom, and entire or partial loss of consciousness remain for some time even after the attack. It is generally useful in chronic cases of epilepsy where structural changes have taken place in the brain.

Cal. carb is useful in cases of children particularly in epilepsy occurring in scrofulous diathesis.

In **Bell** the epileptic convulsions are mostly due to an intense surging of blood into the brain during and between paroxysms.

Cicuta Virosa is indicated by strange movements of head and trunk, lockjaw, bluish countenance, portrusion of the eyes, vomiting, a weak and scarcely perceptible pulse, great venous congestion of the abdominal viscera and convulsion occurring during the act of parturition.

Opium—This is a great remedy in epilepsy occurring during sleep at night, and for epileptic convulsions in insane persons. Other remedies used with partial success in epilepsy are—**Agaricus, Cocculus, Hyos, Stram., Lyc., Acid nitric, Ranunculus, Cina., Digit., Ignatia, Indigo, Ipecac, Lachesis, Nux vom., Pulsatilla, Stannum, Sulph, Verat. album, Zincum** and **Bufo.**

One characteristic symptom of **Artemisia,** that I have forgotten to mention, is the peculiar fetid, cadaverous odour resembling the odour of garlic found in all its discharges.

ARUM TRIPHYLLUM.

.This is the Indian turnip. It is one of our sovereign remedies for an acute cold. The nose feels stopped up inspite of a constant watery discharge. Sneezing is incessant. The discharge is quite acrid and makes the nostrils sore. The lips become swollen and cracked and look as if they are chaffed. The skin of the lips peels off. Submaxillary and parotid glands are also swollen. The tongue too looks cracked.

From the above symptoms it is apparent that **Arum triph.** is a splendid remedy for bad cases of scarlatina complicated with sore throat and diphtheria. The whole of buccal cavity looks raw and sore. Salivation is excessive. The cavity of the mouth is covered with numerous diphtheric deposits and ulcerations. He refuses food and drink on account of soreness of throat and intense burning caused by contact of food. Even voice becomes hoarse and uncertain. But the most important characteristic of this drug—a characteristic that frequently leads to its application in graver affections, such as typhoid fever, meningitis and the like, consists of constant tendency to pick at the nose. He keeps on boring with his finger into his nose till it draws blood. Suppression of urine, prostrating diarrhœa, unconsciousness, restlessness, tossing about in bed, desire to escape and apathy, are symptoms worth noticing.

Case 1.—February 3, 1878, I added to an already severe "cold" by being obliged to wade around in deep snow; the horse which I was driving being "stalled" in a snow drift. I suffered from neuralgic pains through the head, coryza, smarting and rawness at posterior nares, hoarseness, etc., for which I took **Nitric acid** with but little benefit. February 5. At 5-30 p.m. I started to go home by cars, but on arriving at Syracuse at about 8 o'clock, I was in such pain that I stopped over there, not wishing to risk adding to my unpleasant and painful symptoms by a night on the sleeping-car. Here I drove directly to the office of my good friend Dr. H. V. Miller, and requested him to prescribe for the following condition. A decayed and broken malar in my lower jaw, left side, was ching, a hard continual pain, which had been much relieved (as had my general condition) by getting my face (and myself) very warm, while in the car. From this point some fugitive pains extended to the eye, temple and throat. A hard pain, not sharp, was felt at location of the left tonsil. Continual soreness and pain in the larynx, worse when talking and when swallowing. Voice uncertain. Could not speak with a decided effort. Nose obstructed, notwithstanding a considerable watery discharge. On examination, no inflammation in the pharynx or about the tonsil. Touching the tooth caused pain along the whole left side of the lower jaw, not very severe. **Arum triphyl. 200** was given. In half an hour after the first dose, without having been able to avail myself of the palliative influence of the warmth, the pain in the tooth ceased and has not returned since. Three doses of medicine were taken that night. February 6. After a good night's sleep, I found myself better in every respect. Voice still hoarse, but decidedly improved. February 8. Continued improvement. Hoarseness quite disappeared in the course of the day. Improvement continued to a pleasant recovery without a change of medicine (the dose had not been repeated since the first night) Dr. C. W. Butler.

Case 2. Scarlatina.—High fever with delirium; excessive restlessness; nose obstructed and dry; much mucus in the posterior nares; lips peeling off in large patches. Corners of the mouth cracked; violent cough apparently caused by some mucus which accumulated above the larynx; the violent paroxysms of cough compelled him to sit up and to hold his abdomen with his hands; mouth and throat felt very sore, so that he refused to drink; tongue very red; papillæ, especially on the edges, very elevated; diphtheritic deposits in the throat; pulse 160; eruption livid; profuse pale urine. **Arum triph. 20m,** dry on tongue. Being no better next day, he received **Arum 40m,** ten pellets in four ounes or water, a teaspoonful every two hours. A perfect cure. His brother showed on the fifth day the following symptoms: Fever worse every afternoon at 4 p.m.; nose obstructed; corners of mouth cracked and bleeding; the tongue slightly coated at the root, the tip and edges red; diphtheritic deposition on the much-swollen tonsils; breathing rapid and rattling, as if all the bronchial tubes were filled with mucus; pulse hard, small, 140; urinary secretion diminished. Cured by **Lycopod. 10m,** and **Arum triph. 40m.** Dr. Ad Lippe.

Case 3. Biting the finger Nails.—C. W., a child æt, three years, with light hair and eyes; though not decidedly scrofulous, has suffered about a year and a half from the habit—which has been constantly increasing—of biting the finger nails; he would bite them until the fingers would bleed, and it had become very annoying and troublesome. The parents had tried various mechanical means without any benefit, and although firm believers in homoeophthy, thought it useless, or worse than useless, to think of correcting what they were pleased to term, " a mere habit," by internal medication. Like many of our professional brethren they clung with a tenacity worthy a better cause to their faith in the material nature of disease. Guided by the similiarity of symptom, "picks the lips till they bleed," he was given **Arum Triph. 3.** and an immediate improvement followed. In two weeks he was well and has had no return of the "habit." Dr. H. C. Allen.

ASAFŒTIDA.

Here is a remedy which in common language is called the Devil's Dung, a name very appropriate because of the very offensive smell. A tincture is made of the gum-resin obtained from Narthex asafœtida, a plant growing very largely in Persia where it is used as a condiment for flavouring sauces and food.

It was introduced in our Materia Medica by Franz in 1822 and Hahnemann himself contributed to the proving. Its influence is most marked on the nervous system, producing hysteria, chorea and neuralgia. Of the many remedies that come to our mind in that most puzzling of women's complaints hysteria, **Asafœtida** stands very high. It is marked by a great sensitiveness to external impressions, especially to excitement and noise, together with a great distention of the abdomen with flatulence, which only passes upward, rarely downward. It is particularly useful in hysteria from suppression of habitual discharges, such as the sudden checking of a long standing expectoration, or of a chronic diarrhœa or menses. Like **Ignat** it has the globus hystericus very well marked. She feels as if a ball or a large body ascends from stomach to œsophagus, making her constantly swallow and which relieves the sensation. With this we have distention of the abdomen, and a sensation as if the peristaltic motions were reversed attended with disgusting eructations smelling like garlic. Here is a very faithful picture of **Asafœtida,** which will cure many a case of obstinate hysteria and earn for the homœopath the laurel of success and fame.

Asafœtida is oftentimes very useful in supraorbital neuralgia where the patient feels a severe boring, throbbing pain across the brows This pain is worse at night and better from rest and pressure.

It is also indicated in extensive ulceration of the cornea with burning, stitching and pressing pains from within outwards; here also is to be noticed the same characteristic feature of relief from rest and pressure and aggravation at night.

Asafœtida has cured quite a few cases of iritis when due to abuse of mercury and syphilis. It has saved many people from the terrible ravages of syphilis but its use needs especial discrimination.' Ths superior homœopathic prescribing always depends on fine and delicate differentiation and discrimination. It acts on the bones, especially the shin bones, where it produces periosteal inflammation which generally leads to ulcerations. These ulcers are very sensitive and that is why these patients cannot put on any dressing. They discharge a thin fetid ichorous fluid.

Now we will close with a few words on its stomach symptoms. The patient feels a strange pulsation in the pit of the stomach with an empty, all-gone feeling at about 11 A.M. In this it resembles **Sulphur.**

ASARUM.

Asarum Europœum is notable for its over-sensitiveness of nerves. This is so great that the mere scratching of linen or crackling of paper puts him on the jump. The very thought of such noise seems to send through him a thrill of the most disagreeable kind that arrests all his actions and thoughts. It can thus be compared with **Borax, Ferrum, Nux moschata, Coffea, Belladonna** and **Opium.**

The next important point in **Asarum** is seen in its sensitiveness to cold. It is a chilly patient that we have to deal with in this remedy. This chill is mostly nervous; it is not relieved by warmth or covering. He suffers from coldness of hands, feet, knees and abdomen even during the hottest part of the weather. These patients are excessively timid and nervous.

Another characteristic symptom is seen in the relief of most of its symptoms by the application of cold water. Pain in the eye and headache due to overuse of the organ of vision are relieved by bathing the eyes with cold water.

The nervousness already mentioned tinges the mental aspect of the **Asarum** patient. He is over excitable. The least emotional disturbance sends up cold shivers through him.

Another peculiar symptom is a morbid exaggeration of the power of imagination. He imagines himself too light and seems to hover in the air like a spirit as in **Lac caninum** and **Valerian.**

An unconquerable longing for alcohol is extremely characteristic of **Asarum.**

Case 1.—Woman, two months after confinement, applied for medicine for dysentery, saying that she had stools of mucus, with pain in the belly. **Merc.** and **Puls.** did not do any good. I found that the stool was a long, yellow, twisted string of inodorous mucus. **Asar. 2,** three doses, cured.—**Am. Jour. Hom. Mat. Med.**

ASCLEPIAS TUBEROSA.

Another name for this is Pleurisy-root on account of its action over the muscles of the chest where it causes sharp, stitching and pricking pain like that happening in pleurisy. This pain is almost always aggravated by movements, such as drawing a deep breath, motion of hands, walking, and muscular exertions of any kind. It is therefore, very similar to **Bryonia.** Rheumatic pains affecting the body are not infrequent. These pains run diagonally. They are aggravated in cold and damp weather. The cough is usually dry and hacking with expectroration of very little mucus. A similar catarrhal irritation of the larynx is manifested by hoarseness and tightness of breathing.

It is also useful in pneumonia of a sub-acute type. Pain in chest, specially located at the base of the left lung, shoots downward from the left nipple. The pain in the lungs is relieved when he bends forward.

A group of symptoms similar to those described above also indicate it in sub-acute pericarditis. Slight dyspnœa, acute pain in the chest on inspiration and movement of arms, indescribable uneasiness in shoulder and arms, tenderness and pressure over the region of heart, are sure guides to the indications of this remedy in the above complaint.

ASTERIAS RUBENS.

This medicine is prepared from Star-fish belonging to the natural order of Radiata. It has been utilised for medicinal pur-pose from the time of Hippocrates downwards. It is a powerful remedy with great possibilities. It affects the head as well as the mind causing profound sanguinous congestion to the brain. This leads to a sensation of intense heat in the brain and a feeling as if the whole head is surrounded by an atmosphere of hot air. There is the intense throbbing of the carotid arteries and a general feeling of fulness in the brain. The patient awakens with great distress at night time as from electric shocks in the brain. The face looks flushed and swollen. Everything speaks of the great on-rush of blood and portends apoplexy. A few doses of **Asterias rub.** will bring on a moderation in the circulation and avoid the great catastrophe. It thus resembles some of our great congestion re-medies like **Belladonna, Aconite, Verat. vir** and **Glonoine.**

It has important bearings on the female sexual organs where it causes great excitement and a consequent increase of the venereal appetite about the early hours of the morning making the patient ill-humoured and hysterical throughout the day.

Its greatest action, however, is to be seen in the hard cancer-ous tumors of the breast. Numerous cases are on record where **Asterias** brought not only palliation but a radical cure of cancer of mammæ even in the ulcerative stage. It is generally indicated in the cancer of the left breast. The tissues around the nipple get indurated and hypertrophied and the nipple sinks into a cavity, the skin all around being strongly adherent to the hard cancer-ous tissues underneath. The lancinating pain, the swelling of the axillary glands, the pulling sensation in the breast, the neuralgia of the breast and arm have been known to disappear under the action of this remedy.

Asterias removes the disposition to pimples at adolescence.

AURUM METALLICUM.

Gold, the source of so many trials and tribulations of mankind, has been potentised into a very useful drug. Its most important characteristic is found in its profound melancholy—a melancholy that almost overpowers. She looks at the dark side of everything and keeps pining away. Hopelessness, despondency and a sense of utter wretchedness are her constant companion. Weary of life and devoid of all ambition she looks for a ready redemption in death. This idea of suicide haunts her constantly, and it is suicide, she longs for. We have got to be on constant watch, for fear, she will do herself harm. Loquacity, tendency to pray constantly, changeability of mood, dread and anxiety, anguish of mind, loss of self-confidence, quarrelsomeness and sensitiveness, complicate the complex texture of her mind. Other mental phenomena of **Aurum met.** are found it its intolerance of contradiction and a tendency to brood over suppressed grief, disappointment, anger, fright and unfulfilled longings.

It develops conditions bearing strong resemblence to syphilitic and mercurial affections. We are in the dark as to how it simulates syphilis and venereal conditions, but the fact remains that it does do so, as is manifested by wide spread affections of the bony system of the human body, and arthritic inflammations of the various joints. The nocturnal boring pains, the carious destruction of the hard tissues, the exostosis of the skull and other bones, indicate the substrata of syphilis and mercury, and applied on such, sure indications, **Aurum met.** puts on a certain check to the deleterious process of the devastating influence of the syphilitic poison. It is, therefore, an anti-syphilitic remedy of high repute. The bones principally affected by **Aurum met.** are the nasal, palatine and mastoid bones. The discharges in this remedy are very putrid.

Its actions on the eye are equally prominent. We use it in ophthalmia, syphilitic iritis, coreo-retinitis, opacity of cornea, pannus and a large variety of other ocular troubles. Photophobia is extreme and there is profuse lachrymation on opening eyes. The tears scald as they come out. We have horizontal half vision in **Aurum met.,** the upper half being invisible. The patient is unable to see the upper half of a room or of any large object though the lower half is clearly visible. We also have greenish vision in this remedy. The pain of **Aurum met.** is of a burning character and is better by the application of cold water. In iritis the pain around the eye is intense and seems to be deep in the bones.

Obstinate fetid otorrhœa, with strong indication of caries of mastoid process, scrofulous and syphilitic affections of bones of nose, face and palate, ulcerated and agglutinated condition of the nostrils, redness and swelling of the nose, thick yellow offensive discharge, constant presence of toothache at night, foul breath of mouth, indicate the constitutional havoc wrought by that vilest of the vile poison we call syphilis, and **Aurum met.,** used with judgment and discretion may rectify matters even if they look too fargone and seem to be beyond redemption.

Now we must look to the male and female sexual organs and take note of ravages done in these parts. It is used in epididymitis, orchitis, balanitis and induration of testes, the effect of syphilis and its secondary consequences. Frequent discharge of prostatic fluid the effect of onanism, while associated with settled melancholia and suicidal mania point to **Aurum met.** as their sure remedy.

It causes a kind of passive congestion of the female womb. The whole viscera feels hard and swollen and it presses down giving rise to a sensation of prolapsus—a feeling almost chronic with these patients. A kind of bruised pain generally worse after lifting a heavy load associated with constant, profuse, corroding leucorrhœa and back-ache indicate it in these affections of the uterus.

Aurum met. should not be over-looked in its action over the heart where it causes great cardiac hypertrophy and a sort of fatty degeneration of that organ. Loud endocardial bruits, visible beating of carotids and of temporal arteries, repeated attacks of anguish about the heart, tremulous fearfulness, constant inclination towards self-destruction and hurried desire for mental and bodily activities, are clear cut indications of **Aurum met.**

Case 1.—Mr. M., æt, fifty-two, of a healthy family, had always enjoyed good health. Had been actively engaged for twenty years as a manufacturer of edge tools, and was in financial matters independent. He first became despondent, then melancholy, thought his business affairs were in bad shape, and that he was coming to poverty. From this stage he thought he had committed some great wrong, and could not obtain forgiveness. Next he was in mortal fear of being deserted by his wife (who never left him for a day during his illness), and frequently wept on account of it. A terrible insomnia troubled him from the beginning, and anodyne prescribed for his sleeplessness only made him worse. He had the best allopathic advice, but the medicine appeared to make him worse instead of better, and he soon declined very positively to take any more. Then change of air was advised, and he was taken to the seaside, and from one watering-place to another, but after a time he no sooner reached a place than he wanted to leave again, at some even declining to remain overnight. He was first attacked in March, 18 0, and it was now September—six months—and he was steadily growing worse, so that an insane asylum was now advised as a **dernier resort**. Fifteen powders of **Aurum met.** 12th trit., was sent, and one every morning was given in his food. His wife wrote that "From the first time the powder was given she noticed a change. He slept better from the first day the remedy was exhibited, so that when nine powders were taken he was almost as well as ever, and the medicine was discontinued. "He remained well for three years, when a slight return was again promptly relieved by **Aur.,** and he has continued in good health ever since. Dr. H. C. Allen.

Case 2.—Mrs. A., aged thirty-two, Norwegian by birth, first came to the hospital for treatment early in July, 1877. Three years before (1874) she had a large ulcer on the leg, which was treated allopathically for many months and finally healed, leaving a large cicatrix. Soon after, or a little over a year ago (1876), another ulcer made its appearance upon the other leg in the neighbourhood or the ankle, which was continued to grow in circumference. Three months before she came to the dispensary (April, 1877), the nose became affected and ulceration soon took place. I elicited the fact that some years ago she had few little sores about the external genital organs, which disappeared after a time, she meanwhile using some sort of ointment. The ulceration about the nose involved, to a certain extent, the nasal bones. The skin of the face, especially under the eye and in the immediate neighbourhood of the large ulcer, has a coppery-red color, resembling somewhat an erysipelatous inflammation. This color is not confined to the left side of the face, but passes over the nose and is most marked just below the right eye. There is no pain or tenderness anywhere except when slight pressure is made over the nasal bones. Although the ulceration is confined to the left side of the face and nose, slight pressure over the bone upon the right side occasions some pain, showing that that side is involved to a certain extent. In the mouth another large ulcer on the hard palate which also involves the bone and, at one time, communicated with the nasal passage. The patient at first complained of a discharge into the mouth through this opening—the discharge consisting of nasal mucus and pus. This is no longer the case now as the opening or sinus seems to have become obliterated. We have two other ulcers, a large and small one upon the ankle. When we first saw this sore, it presented an indolent appearance, was covered with a thick, lardaceous matter, with pale, flabby granulations; had a foul smell and showed no disposition whatever to heal. In fact it was constantly extending in circumference. **Nitric Acid 30.** Slight improvement followed this prescription. I now selected as being specific to syphilitic affections of the nasal bones, **Aurum m.,** which was given in the 6th three times a day. Under the influence of this remedy the patient improved from week to week, so far as the face and nose were concerned. On July 22, a piece of bone about as thick as the thumb nail, and three-eighths of an inch square, was exfoliated and discharged through the nasal opening. Ever since then this ulcer has radually been growing smaller until now when it is about two-thirds the ze of the original sore. This patient was still improving under this prescrip- on the last time we saw her. Hoyne.

AURUM MURIATICUM.

It is the chloride of gold, a great sycotic remedy, which causing uppressed discharges to reappear. These patients like all other ycotic patients are subject to great depression of mind. They uffer from an insermountable mental and bodily restlessness. Like **Ignatia** and **Staphy.,** we use the remedy in ailments from vio- ent chagrin.

It has pronounced action on the heart causing over-activity of hat organ. It is a favourable remedy for angina pectoris and ndocarditis and rheumatism. Beating of the heart is violent ausing great anxiety and sleeplessness. Irregularities of heart eat, severe sense of constriction of the chest, sometimes throb- ing of the carotids and temporal arteries are important symptoms.

It affects the bones and periosteum of the human body causing aries and exostoses. Swellings and indurations of glands and nuscular tissues are also very common. The swellings are cha- acterised by heat, hardness and tension. Lips, nose, tongue, terus, liver, spleen—all show signs of indurations. Of course, we nust never forget the under current stain of syphilis, present in hese cases. The vaginal discharge with its unbearable odor, the ncient appearance in spite of the young age, condylomata at the nus, excrescences on scrotum, necrosis of long bones are all ndications of the vile poison contaminating his blood. **Aur. mur.** is articularly valuable in hæmorrhages from the womb at the cli- nacteric age and after, in sycotic constitutions.

AURUM MURIATICUM NATRONATUM.

This medicine is prepared from the double chloride of gold nd sodium. It is very useful in chronic and sub-acute indurations f the womb and ovary and in chronic suppurations of the glands nd bones.

Old cases of rheumatism and gout have been helped on the ndication of aggravation of all symptoms from rest. This remedy works better in mercuro-syphilitic constitutions.

The most important symptom of this remedy, however, is oring pain felt all over the body but mostly in the skull, tibia and

other bony structures of the human system. These pains are
invariably worse in the cold wet weather. Owing to the above-
mentioned stain and stigma in their blood they are prone to
scrofulous manifestations. They suffer from malignant cancerous indurations, ulcers and various kinds of warty growths in
various parts of the body. The organ, however, that suffers mostly
is the uterus and its appendages.   Enormous distention of the
ovary with corroding leucorrhœa has been helped with this remedy
It is particularly useful in sub-acute metritis, ovaritis, endo-cervicitis and ulceration of uterus.

In men we also have chancers on internal surface of
pepruce and below in the folds of groin due however to the undercurrent stain mentioned above.

It should be carefully compared with **Merc. iod., Conium, Kal**
bichro and **Thuja** to all of which remedies it bears resemblance.

AZADIRACHTA INDICA.

This medicine is prepared from the bark of a tree that grows
extensively in India and is known as the **Neem** tree.   It is a great
favourite of the Indian people who love to grow it in their own
yard as its effect is supposed to purify atmosphere of all impurity
The Indians also use it locality in the form of a decoction for
various kinds of skin troubles.

We are indebted for this medicine to Dr. P. C. Mozumder of
Calcutta who is our chief authority on this.

It causes a sort of an afternoon fever starting from
about 3 to 4-30 P.M. with a slight chill and subsiding at about
7-30 P.M. The patient experiences a sort of a glowing heat
in face, eyes, palms of hand and soles of feet in open air. It is
particularly useful in cases maltreated with quinine and as such
should be compared with **Cedron, China, Arsenic, Nat. mur.,** and
Nux vomica.

BADIAGA.

This remedy is prepared by triturating the fresh water sponge.
The most characteristic symptom of **Badiaga** is soreness—
a soreness that is general and extensive. Integuments, bones and
muscles feel as if they have been beaten to pulp.

Another keynote indication of **Badiaga** is seen in the induration of the cellular and the glandular structure of the system. We
use it in syphilitic bubo, and in other scrofulous indurations.
Its tendency is to absorb the swelling and this it invariably does
in the first stage of the trouble. Even after fluctuation is noticed,
it has been known to have brought about absorption.

Badiaga has been successfully used in headaches associated
with inflammation of the eyes. This headache is better at night but
after sleep it returns violently. It is worse from motion.

Dr. Biegler reports of a case of persistent headache, lasting
off and on for months in a lady, which baffled him till the following
symptoms led him to prescribe **Badiaga** with great success. It
was a severe pain in the right eyeball extending thence to forehead
and temples and it made her whole scalp excessively sore.

I have found it extremely satisfactory in the treatment of
chronic chancres specially after they have been tampered with,
which left them more disfigured and obdurate.

The respiratory symptoms of **Badiaga** are worth noticing.
An oft verified symptom is the sudden flying out of mucus from
mouth and nose on coughing. It shows the spasmodic nature of
the cough. Also the cough of **Badiaga** is followed by sneezing;
there is also a profusion of catarrhal symptoms accompanying this
cough.

On the skin we notice quite a lot of freckles and rhagades.

BAPTISIA TINCTORIA.

This is commonly known as Wild Indigo, a plant that grows
abundantly throughout the United States. The tincture is prepared from the fresh root and the bark of this plant.

The pathogenesis of this remedy is so similar to that of typhoid
fever that it has been regarded as a great remedy in that complaint. But it would be a mistake to use it indiscriminately in all
cases of typhoid and typhus. Used on proper indications and in
proper manner it cuts the disease short. Dr. Nash reports of but

one case of typhoid fever during the whole term of his practice that ran its full course inspite of the application of Baptisia. Dr. Farrington also expresses a similar opinion.

It is such a deep acting remedy and so elaborate in its pathogenesis that it may be used in all the stages of that disease. In the premonitory stage we are led to **Baptisia** by the predominence of gastric symptoms such as pain in the ileocecal region, putrid loose stools, great and sudden prostration, indifference, apathy and a general bedimmed condition of the sensorium. Later, in the course of the disease, when it takes on a more fearful turn, as exhibited by extreme putridity of the alvine discharges and unconscious evacuation, when the already bedimmed sensorium becomes totally blunt, and indifference and apathy merge into stupor and coma, when the face becomes flushed, heavy and besotted, when that calm and placcid stupor becomes disturbed with the ripples of peculiar illusions, we still think of **Baptisia.**

The tongue looks dry, heavy, brown and heavily coated, edges still remaining red. The teeth are covered with sordes. The breath is fetid. Urine becomes scanty and offensive and sweat smells disgusting.

In cases, like above where the vital fluid is undergoing evident decomposition and rapid disintegration, a few doses of **Baptisia** will work miracles. I have forgotten to mention one very important indication of this remedy that should be specially looked for in every case of **Baptisia.** It is a great tenderness and a general sore feeling that pervade the whole system.

Baptisia bears a great semblance to **Gelsemium** especially in the primary stage. The drowsiness, tender and sore feeling, and the chilliness may naturally suggest **Gelsemium;** but very soon the intensity, the severity and the disintegrating nature of the disease will prove our mistake and suggest the administration of deeper acting **Baptisia.**

The intense restlessness, the brown tongue and the muscular soreness, may point towards **Rhus tox,** which is often a remedy in the first stage of the disease but very soon the kelidoscopic changes of symptoms will render the administration of Baptisia necessity.

Arnica closely resembles **Baptisia,** but in the former the involvement of the brain is more pronounced, the stupor and apathy more profound and there are presence of ecchymotic spots due to breaking up of capillary **vessels.**

The remedy that bears a still closer semblance to **Baptisia** is **Lachesis.** It has the same putridity of the discharges and the exhalations of the body, the same depraved condition of the vitality, the same benumbed sensorium, but it differs from **Baptisia** in its aggravation after sleep, in its tendency towards hemorrhage and in its sensitiveness to touch, specially of the neck and the waist.

Last of all we will discuss the relationship of **Baptisia to Mur. acid.** The two remedies so closely resemble each other that differentiation becomes very difficult at times. It will be of great value however to remember that the prostration of **Mur. acid** exceeds that of any other remedy that we know of. The patient constantly slides down in bed; the jaw hangs down; evacuations are constant and unconscious. In fact the patient is on the very brink of the grave. To the credit of Homœopathy be it said that **Mur acid** often brings on the most satisfactory solution of such grave situations in life.

Case 1,—September 10, 1878.—I saw a well-nourished and ruddy-looking old man of seventy years, who had suffered for the last five months with convulsive contraction of the œsophagus and cardiac orifice, so that at times the fluid food would remain in the stomach and easily regurgitate. Some days the fluid-food entered the stomach without hinderance, and digested well. At other days patient was compelled to be fed by means of an œsophagus bougie. I could not find any diseased state; only that patient admitted that he always liked to eat very hot food. On examination I found the mucous membrane of the œsophagus very much reddened and granulated. **Bapt. 12,** a few powders, one to be dissolved in a half a glass of water, three to four doses per day. In the course of a week I received information that three days after taking the remedy, food entered the stomach without difficulty, and patient considered himself well.—"Schweitzer Volksarzt."

Case 2. Shivering; restless sleep; yellow cheeks, with central deep flush; tongue yellow-white, deeply furred; pulse 110, variable and thready; sleeplessness and wandering of mind; occasional diarrhœa; frequent sweats; critical sweat on forehead and face; hopeless of recovery and certain of death. Semi-comatose; unable to swallow; unconscious evacuations; urine alkaline and offensive; aphthæ in mouth, tongue ulcerated; sordes on teeth and lips; spitting out of liquids put in the mouth; mucus rattle in throat; sinking down in bed; lying with head thrown back; jaw dropped; chokes even with a half-spoonful of water, cannot swallow, pain in the articulation of lower portion of zygoma; rigidity of the muscles of the jaw; the effort to swallow produced violent pain; uvula inflamed and somewhat elongated; tonsils enlarged; mouth full of thick, viscid saliva, neither able to swallow nor expectorate. **Bell., Merc. viv. et biniod.** failed. **Baptisia** cured.—Dr G. F. Butman.

Case 3.—G. G. , aged six, had recently recovered from pertussis, when on November 11, 1865, he played about all day in the hot sun and was seized in the evening with violent headache and vomiting, considerable fever, quick pulse, and somewhat dilated pupils. I gave him **Gelsemium** 6, every two hours. Nov. 12. High fever and delirium during the night; this morning he is conscious, but the tongue has become foul and yellow; the fever continues, with occasional vomiting, and all the symptoms indicate the commencement of a regular attack of gastro-enteric fever. Baptisia lx was ordered every two hours, and by the 16th, i.e., in four days, the boy was quite convalescent. I have known so many cases of this sort which, under allopathic treatment, have dragged out a weary length of many weeks, that I feel well satisfied with the curative action of **Baptisia.** At the end of the summer of 1864-65, viz.,from March to May, gastric fever was very prevalent at Brighton, a suburb of Melbourne, and I treated several cases with **Baptisia**...All those whom I saw from the commencement recovered rapidly.

BARYTA CARB.

This medicine is prepared by triturating pure Carbonate of Barium, a substance found in nature in the form of yellow grayish crystals of rhomboid prisms.

In **Baryta** we have one of our great anti-scorfulous remedies. It affects all the glands of the human system. We find enlarge ment of tonsils, testes, parotid, axillary, próstate and mesenteric glands. Like all anti-scrofulous remedies it is characterised by great sensitiveness to cold and exposure. Every exposure to cold or damp brings on headache, sore throat, diarrhœa, cough and a series of other complaints.

It suits the two extremities of human life—the childhood and the old age. Many of the complaints at these stages find in **Baryta** a ready help. Sometime ago a young boy was brought to me suffering from chronic tonsillitis. He was dwarfish mentally and physically. With a high swollen pot-bellied abdomen, a bloated face and an idiotic vacant look, he made a very sorry figure. The most cursory examination revealed deficiency of memory. Forgetful and inattentive, he could not be taught anything. Every feature and trait suggested **Baryta.** He is making rapid progress and **Baryta** promises to put him right. These patients are, as a rule, very shy and afraid of strangers. They know their limitations. They consider themselves the observed of all observers and the subject of criticism of every body. Sometimes we notice certain ebullitions of anger, but this anger is almost always associated with cowardice.

Baryta carb is also used in mania during pregnancy. There is a sort of loquacity, but there is hardly any coherence in her talk. Another feature, rather an important feature, is a great tendency to go out of the house. We also notice a great amount of irresoluteness in these patients; they can hardly make up their minds to do anything. Another peculiar symptom mentioned by Dr. Talcott is that the patient thinks his legs are cut off and that he is walking on his knees. This symptom needs further verification.

There is a certain amount of unhealthiness of the skin though not to the same extent as in **Silicea.** Moist eruptions on head and behind the ears are common. These lead to falling off of hair. Tumors on scalp are common. The face is disfigured with rough dry eruptions. Another symptom worth remembering is a sense of tension of the whole face as if white of egg had dried on it.

We will next discuss the most important feature of **Baryta carb.** namely its action on the palate and the throat. No where do we find such extensive connective tissue proliferation as in this locality. The tonsils are always in a state of chronic induration. On the slightest exposure to cold and damp, the tonsils tend to suppurate. The submaxillary and parotid glands get tender and swollen which naturally leads us to think of **Belladonna.** The absence of bright redness of the latter remedy and acute inflammatory symptoms should be of great help in the selection of **Baryta carb.**

It is an invaluable remedy in that dread disease of old age, the hypertrophy of the prostate gland. Only those know what it is to suffer from this, that really go through the tortures of the enlarged and indurated prostate. **Baryta carb.** is almost a god-send to those people. There are various other conditions of old age where **Baryta carb.** is equally indicated. It is quite an important help in old age, where due to atrophy of the cranial matters the patient goes into his second childhood. Sexual weakness becomes quite marked amounting almost to impotence. Penis becomes inordinately relaxed and coition becomes impossible due to premature emission.

Baryta carb. is one of the best remedies we have for the prevention of the recurrence of tonsillitis. It checks, as has been mentioned before, the tissue proliferation and rectifies to a great extent the strumous diathesis. As such it bears a close resemblance to **Calc. carb., Calc. phos.,** and **Calc. Iod.**

It should not be lost sight of in suffocative catarrh of old people. The great accumulation of phlegm threatens paralysis of the lungs. In this respect it is similar to **Antim. tart.** a remedy to which it acts as a valuable adjunct. The sensation is, as if the lungs are full of smoke, and that further respiration is impossible.

It is indicated in a peculiar type of cough that becomes chronic in scrofulous constitutions. The swollen and enlarged glands all over, the hypertrophied tonsils, the excess of phlegm, the presence of fatty tumors in various parts of the body, the fetid foot sweat the occurrence of night sweats and the dwarfish stunted growth make **Baryta carb.** a valuable remedy.

BARYTA MURIATICUM.

It is the Chloride of Barium. Its symptoms are very similar to those of **Baryta carb.** The same disposition to enlargement of glands, the same predisposition for tonsillitis are marked. It has however, a few symptoms particularly characteristic of the muriate element in it which is our object to study just now. It has particular action on the cardiac orifice of the stomach where it causes induration as well as narrowing. The result is great epigastric tenderness as well as over-sensitiveness of the stomach. Considerable hardness is felt over the region of the stomach.

It also causes induration of the pancreas with profuse flow of saliva from the mouth as in mercurial poisoning. Like its sister remedy it is a great help in abdominal aneurism. The patient writhes in agony and rolls on the floor with attacks of anxious dyspnœa.

Another symptom particularly characteristic of **Baryta mur.** is the irritation it causes and hence cures in the female sexual system. It increases the sexual desire to an inordinate extent and has been recommended very highly in all forms and kinds of mania with increase of sexual passion.

It is also useful in multiple sclerosis of the brain and the cord. There is entire loss of voluntary muscular power, the sensibility remaining in tact. It has been used with success in attacks of epileptic convulsions characterized by the retention of full consciousness.

BELLADONNA.

Belladonna is a herbaceous perennial plant that grows to the height of four or five feet in the sandy parts of Europe and Asia. The flowers are pendulous, bell-shaped and purple in colour and are followed by purple-black berries. The juice is extracted from the entire plant before it flowers and then mixed with an equal part by weight of alcohol.

It is also called the Deadly Night shade. It belongs to the natural order of Solanaceæ. It was known to the medical profession as early as 1500 A.D., but the first Homœopathic proving was made by Samuel Hahnemann. It comes from two Latin words **bella donna,** which mean the beautiful lady, from the circumstance that the Venetian ladies of old used it as a cosmetic to brighten the eyes and flush the cheeks. Its properties are due to the alkaloids **atropin** and **belladonnin.** Physiological experimentation shows that **Belladonna** affects the sensory nerves, especially their extremeties, thus causing cutaneous anæsthesia. The Allopaths, therefore, make use of it locally in ointments, liniments and plasters as anodyne for external pains. It also affects the motor nerves causing peripheral paralysis; hence it is also utilized by our brethren of the other school as an antispasmodic. They use it in rigidity of the os uteri during labor. **Belladonna** further excites the sympathetic nervous system as is manifested by the dilatation of the pupil when locally applied. We must not forget a fourth action of this drug. I mean the arrest of secretions especially of the salivary glands and the skin. This phenomenon, too, is made use of by the allopaths, in hidrosis of the hands and feet, in salivation, in checking the secretion of milk where that is necessary; but they apply it locally.

Mentally these patients are very excitable. Mirth and hapiness easily give way to anger and misery. Fretfulness and irritability of temperament make them very unsociable. They are ordinarily extremely averse to noise and company, hence we find them preferring solitude and dark places to mirth and gaiety.

Constitutionally these patients are rather fleshy, phlegmatic, and plethoric; hence they are similar to the **Calcarea carb.** patients; the difference consisting mainly in the congestion of the former and the pallor of the latter remedy.

Belladonna is the prince of our congestion remedies. This congestion may take place anywhere—head, chest, uterus, joints,

skin, in fact any part of our organism, but the most peculiar
feature about this congestion is its vehemence and its suddenness.
Ther are other remedies such as **Acon., Bry., China, Ferr, Merc.,
Nux v., Puls., Phos.,** and **Sulph.,** where we find great rush of blood
to single parts, but in none of them do we notice the lightning-
like rapidity that characterizes **Belladonna.** The suddenness and
this violence characterize all the symptoms of **Belladonna.** The
baby goes to bed hale and hearty, but in the dead of night it
wakes up with sudden convulsions. Just so in pains, in inflammations and in troubles of all kinds. The violence, the suddenness, the over-whelming intensity point to **Bell.** as the indicated
remedy.

Sometimes this rush of blood to brain is so intense that our
patient turns delirious. His eyes become injected, his carotids
throb violently. Although he is sleepy, he is unable to sleep; he
keeps his head rolling from side to side; at other times he is wide
awake with pupils widely dilated. More frequently these two
states alternate, that is at times the patient is drowsy and falls
into a heavy slumber from which he wakes up with a cry or a
jerk or start and keeps looking at things around him in a strange
fashion. Even these slumbers are not undisturbed slumbers. He
dreams of falling and that is why he starts as if in a fright clutching at the air. Sometimes he dreams of murders, of robbers, of
fires, and tries to get away from them. In some cases the delirium assumes a fierce form and the patient breaks into fits of
laughter, then gnashes his teeth, strikes and bites every body
around him. Sometimes he sees ghosts, hideous faces, monsters,
black dogs and various insects. At other times he keeps picking
at bed clothes as if looking for some thing lost with confused
muttering.

It is not always very easy to distinguish **Belladonna** from
Hyoscyamus and **Stramonium.**

In **Stramonium** the congestion of the brain is not so well
marked: the violence and the intensity too are not at par with
those of **Belladonna.** Furthermore, in **Stramonium,** the incoherent
loquacity, the praying and the beseeching attitude, the desire
for light and company always help to mark out the lines of
demarcation.

Belladonna scores very high in mania. He calls for his food
and when he gets it, instead of making good use of it he bites
his spoons into two then gnaws at his dish and snarles and barks

like dog. He tries to throttle himself and begs those around him
to kill him.

Symptoms like these are often seen in hydrophobia and on
such indications **Belladonna** has been known to have made
wonderful cures.

Cantharides is another well-known remedy in hydrophobia.
There is furious delirium with crying, barking, bleating, confusion
of head and anxious restlessness. Paroxysms of rage alternate
with convulsions and convulsions are excited by the slightest touch
on the larynx, by pressure upon the abdomen and by the sight of
water. There is also excessive desire for sexual intercourse with
constant painful erections.

Cuprum met is sometimes usefully employed where during
delirium the patient howls and mutters, is afraid of every one
who approaches him and shrinks away from the intruder. The
other similar remedies are **Lyssin, Hyoscyamus, Lachesis, Scutellaria, Tanacetum vulg** and **Vipera.**

Moaning is a great characteristic of our remedy. Well or
ill we find him constantly indulging in this. Garrulity is also
present. His speech and actions are rapid and hasty. We find
him often uttering inarticulate confused sounds which carry
absolutely no meaning. Another characteristic of **Belladonna** that
should be remembered is a desire to escape and hide. Either in
his insanity or in his delirium he shows a great anxiety to escape
attention and tries to hide himself either in his bed or behind
some furniture in the room. This might have been induced by
fear which is almost a red strand of **Bell.** He fears imaginary
things and wants to run away from them. When closing his eyes
even before he has fallen asleep, he sees fierce wicked-looking,
large animals with horns and bushy heads. These conditions
call for **Belladonna** wherever found and in whatever ailment they
may be present.

Due to congestion of the brain our patient is a victim to
constant headache. The pain which is of a throbbing nature, is
worse on the right side and is associated with intolerance of
light and noise. Any position that throws him out of the per
pendicular, makes him worse, consequently we generally find him
sitting propped up with pillows. We recognise the **Belladonna**
patient instantly we enter the sick-room; we find the doors and
windows closed, and the room is perfectly dark and quiet. Then
again we have to be very cautious as we walk, for the least jar.

noise and shaking make him distinctly worse. He complains of a sensation as if the brain were pressed to the forehead and the sensation disappers quickly on bending the head backward. In walking he feels as if the brain rose and fell in forehead. The nature of the pain is of a kind that we have already mentioned. It is very violent, it comes suddenly, lasts indefinitely and goes just as suddenly.

Other remedies with similar congestive headaches are **Amyl nitrate, Aurum met., Crotalus, Ferrum met., Glonoine, Magnesia mur.,** and **Nux vom.** In Amyl Nitrate the surging of blood to head and face is very intense; he craves fresh air; so intense is his craving that he opens his clothings, throws his bed coverings away and opens the doors and windows. There are the flushings and the blushings which are temporary and circumscribed unlike the turgid face of our **Belladonna** patient.

Aurum met. is good for congestive headaches in syphilitic patient with exostoses on and gummata inside the skull. He feels as if a current of air were rushing through his head; he sees sparks before his eyes. All his symptoms are aggravated by the least mental exertion. The profound melancholy, the great key-note of Aur. met, is always a guiding indication.

In **Crotalus** the headache which is congestive in nature is worse on the right side; like **Bell.** it is worse lying down but the **Crotalus** headache is mostly to be found in patients suffering from zymotic or septic diseases.

In **Ferrum met.** the headache is just as intense as in **Belladonna.** The pain is hammering, beating, and pulsating; it gets worse after midnight. The face, generally pale, becomes red and flushed during the headache. The intensity is there, but it is not the over-whelming intensity of **Bell.,** while the suddenness is entirely wanting. It is a continuous hammering pain in anæmic patients, that we have to contend against in **Ferrum met.**

Glonoinum has more a sun-headache than a congestive headache. There is a crushing weight across the forehead with throbbing which is synchronous with every beat of the heart.

Magnesia mur is good for congestive and hysterical headaches. The patient gets the sensation of boiling water in the head. The headache is better from firm pressure, from moving about and worse from quiet.

The congestive and abdominal headache of **Nux vomica** comes after debauch, after drinking coffea, every morning on walking.

after eating and in the open air. Although the headache is very severe and gives the patient the sensation as if his skull would split, there is very little danger of a confusion between the two remedies.

Belladonna is a handy remedy in apoplexy. As every case of apoplexy is preceded by violent cerebral hyperæmia, we have the use of this remedy confined to the preliminary stage of the trouble. It is not likely that this remedy will have any direct influence over the extravasated blood, hence its use is limited and so it is prescribed with in the first ten or twelve hours of the attack. There is yet another affection where we use **Belladonna** with great advantage and that is inflammatory affection of the membranes of brain. Here also, as in apoplexy, the remedy is useful in the early stage before inflammation has progressed far to the stage of exudation.

All the senses in **Belladonna** become more acute. This irritability and impressionableness of the senses are evident from the exalted sensibility of all the organs. He tastes and smells everything more acutely than others. The sense of sight and hearing is keener; even the mind is more easily moved and the thoughts are more active. He catches cold easily. The least draught or breeze blowing anywhere is felt by him, even when nobody else notices it.

Belladonna is no doubt our main remedy in convulsions; it is particularly indicated in robust corpulent children with unmistakable symptoms of cerebral congestion. In cases of poisoning with Belladonna we get the exact symptoms of convulsions which demonstrate with remarkable accuracy the truth of the principle of simila as a therapeutic maxim. It is equally useful in puerperal eclampsia, where many of its symptoms are present.

Now we will discuss its application in epilepsy. It requires great power of observation to treat such causes successfully. We must find out the exciting cause if any. We have to take notice of the aura—where it begins, how it travels, where it ends, its nature and many other important details which help us to individualise the case. **Belladonna** is used in recent cases with decided brain symptoms. The aura is peculiar; it feels like mouse running over an extremity or as if fear is rising from the stomach. The convulsions commence in upper extremities and extend to the mouth. There is also a peculiar clutching sensation at the throat during the fit, which makes it difficult for him to swallow. The spasms are excited by the least touch. **The sensation** of mouse running over is also to be seen in **Sil., Sulph., Ign., Calc. ost.,** and **Nitric acid.,** but the totality of symptoms will help us to decide.

In **Nux vom** too we find convulsions brought about by least touch, but it is a convulsion with consciousness.

We have next to speak of the action of **Belladonna** on the skin. There is at first an erythema, a condition midway between hyperæmia and inflammation, of the skin which becomes bright red, glossy, and exceedingly sensitive to touch. The part becomes hot and imparts a burning sensation to the examining hand. This condition becomes general and we have an uniform scarlet redness of the entire surface of the body.

The heat, the redness and the restlessness are also to be found in **Aconite** but the uniform, smooth and glossy appearance of the skin always points to **Belladonna.**

This erythema may pass on to real inflammation. The parts around the neighbourhood become œdematous; suppuration soon intervenes and burrows deep into the cellular tissue. **Belladonna** is still our remedy and the symptoms on which the prescription should be based are the violence and suddenness of the symptoms, the sharp lancinating, stinging pains associated with great deal of throbbing, high fever, and cerebral complications. Here is a true picture of phlegmonous erysipelas. When the inflammation passes on to mortification, we have other remedies to think about such as **Lach., Crotalus hor., Ars., Sec.,** and **Carb. veg.** But before this stage is reached, it may be necessary to think of remedies like **Apis** and **Rhus tox** which should come in after the stage of Belladonna is over but before gangrene has set in. They are, therefore, adapted to an intenser stage of the disease than **Belladonna.**

In **Rhus** we have a copious vesication over the inflamed area; the fever, though very intense, assumes an adynamic type. The tongue becomes dry, and the great nervous excitement becomes superseded by a sort of soporous stupefaction. Apis is useful in the œdematous variety of erysipelas especially of the face, travelling from the right to the left side.

Belladonna is a capital remedy in boils, abscesses and carbuncles. In this it is similar to **Arn., Hep sulph.,** and **Merc.**

In **Arnica** we have crops of small boils and they are extremely painful to touch.

Hep. Sulph. promotes suppuration in boils which are about as sensitive.

Merc. has a dual function. It helps suppuration as well as promotes absorption. We use it after pus has formed or is about to be formed.

Belladonna in its application in throat troubles deserves careful attention. The throat feels raw and sore and looks red and shining. There is intense lancinating and throbbing pain; the cervical glands become inflamed suddenly. There is great dryness of the mouth with constant desire to swallow, but swallowing hurts, as the throat feels too narrow for anything to pass through it. That is why we get impeded deglutition or entire inability to swallow, even liquids which are ejected by the nose. These symptoms remind us of **Acon, Amygdala amara, Canth., Sulphur,** and **Ignatia.** All of these are noted for phlegmoncus angina but every one of them is good in its own individual sphere.

In **Aconite** the burning, the contraction of the throat during deglutition, the high fever and the great sensitiveness of the throat to touch, are as marked as in **Belladonna,** but the dry heat, the burning unquenchable thirst, the great restlessness, the fear are alone sufficient to establish the undisputed indentity of the remedy.

Amygdala amara is very similar to Belladonna, and it has cured many cases where **Belladonna** was inffectively used. It causes a dark red injection of the fauces, uvula and tonsils, marked prostration and sudden sharp pains during swallowing.

It is easy to differentiate **Belladonna** from **Cantharis.** The latter is useful in more advanced cases where the gangrenous process has commenced. Here too, as in **Belladonna,** the symptoms come on with great rapidity. Swallowing is just as difficult, for here also the liquid drunk is returned by the nose. The constriction is just as marked, but the great heat and the intense burning of **Cantharis** are wanting in Belladonna. The highly inflamed throat of **Canth.** feels as if on fire and it is covered over by a layer of plastic lymph.

Hepar sulphur represents a condition far too similar to **Belladonna.** The smarting, the roughness, the rawness of the fauces, the heat and scraping sensation in throat, the great sensitiveness to pain, to atmospheric changes, to cold and draught, the swelling of the tonsils and cervical glands are all to be found here but the great distinctive symptom, the sensation of pins or splinters in throat, is wanting in **Bell.**

In **Ignatia** our "remedy of contrasts", we meet with many points of similarity and dissimilarity. The pains extending to ears are worse between the acts of deglutition and are better by swallowing solids.

Belladonna is useful in affections of the larynx as well. We use it in acute laryngitis, croup and diphtheria. The symptoms calling for it are: Hoarseness and roughness of voice amounting to complete aphonia. The vocal chords look bright red. He can hardly swallow on account of soreness and a sensation of fullness in the dry larynx. This irritable and inflammatory condition of the larynx and trachea gives rise to a paroxysmal dry cough. It is excited by a sort of tickling sensation. The child cries before coughing as each paroxysm means great deal of pain. The cough frequently ends with sneezing.

We next come to that portion of **Belladonna** that deals with the female sexual system. It is useful in uterine displacements. This displacement becomes manifest by means of its symptoms of pressure in pelvis as though everything is coming down through the external genitals, particularly in the morning. Great heat and dryness of the vagina are felt. We naturally expect this bearing down sensation to get worse in a perpendicular position, but the strange feature about it is, that it feels better standing and gets worse lying down. We have prolapsus of the uterus also in the **Actea race., Lilium tig., Nat. mur.,** and **Sepia** and some differentiation is necessary.

In **Actea race** the bearing down sensation is to be found in patients of neuralgic or of rheumatoid diathesis.

In **Lilium tig** the bearing down sensation is very intense, so much so that she has to put her hand on the vulva to prevent everything from coming out through the vagina. She dates all her troubles and pains from a miscarriage.

The **Nat. mur** patient has to sit down every morning to prevent prolapsus. She is also troubled with a violent headache every morning as she awakes. She imagines there are robbers in the house at night and nothing short of a thorough search of the house will quieten her. This speaks of a nervous temperament.

Last of all we come to **Sepia.** The bearing down sensation is, indeed, very marked here. She feels she must cross her legs to prevent the organs from coming out of the vagina. The aggravations and the ameliorations are just the reverse of those in **Belladonna..**

Belladonna is most indispensable in cases of metritis associated with marked tympanitis. The abdomen swells up like a drum and extreme sensitiveness is manifested. The least jar hurts. The bearing down sensation just mentioned is also present. The marked cerebral irritation, the sudden appearance and disappearance of pain, the high fever, the involuntary urination, point most decidedly to **Belladonna.** Hartman says "If the inflammation sets in after confinement, the lochial discharge is arrested, the placenta adheres or is discharged in the shape of an ichorous fetid liquid with violent burning and a sensation of fullness in the vagina, the employment of Belladonna is called for so much more pressingly."

Very often during nursing, the mother's breast cakes up on account of excessive accumulation of milk; and unless the milk is dispersed inflammation is sure to set in. The breast feels heavy and hard, and we find red streaks running like radii from a central point. The throbbing pains are very torturing. A few doses of **Belladonna** will clear the whole thing up like magic.

Belladonna is one of our hemorrhagic remedies. The blood is bright red and hot; at times it is offensive with clots of dark decomposed blood. We have to use it often in bad cases of dysmenorrhœa, when these symptoms are present. Under Belladonna the menses are early, copious and bright red. It is also attended with severe bearing down pain in the back. It feels as if the back would break. The patient is exceedingly sensitive and can bear neither touch, pressure or jerk.

It is an exceptionally good remedy in parturition when the labor pain is deficient, ineffectual and spasmodic. It is particularly efficacious when the muscles of parturition become rigid, and instead of promoting, hinder the expulsion of the fœtus. For this same reason it is invaluable in the labor pains of grown-up people where naturally we have great rigidity of the muscles. It also checks hæmorrhage after confinement or after miscarriage. It is also extremely efficacious in puerperal peritonitis, especially at its onset, when the temperature becomes very high and gives a sort of steaming sensation to the hand.   Convulsions, cramps, eclampsia, and mania after child-birth, come under its influence when many of the above-mentioned symptoms are present.

We have yet to deal with the fever of **Belladonna.** It begins with a chill of a congestive nature. Violent, bursting frontal headache, dilated pupils, dread of light and noise, accompany the chill. The feet become icy cold and the face looks flushed and bloated. There is scarcely any thirst during this stage.

The stage of heat is extremely violent. The thirst is great and the water seems to taste cold. There is great burning of the whole body, internal and external. The pungent heat of the **Belladonna** patient gives us the sensation of steaming vapour. The congestion already noticed becomes more severe. We have violent throbbing of the carotids, with red face, delirium and rest-lessness. Inspite of this heat the patient is sensitive to the least draught of air. He is always covered up, and we notice sweat on covered parts only. The pulse is full, bounding and globular. It is like the stroke of a small hammer against the examining finger. The tongue, too, is quite charateristic of **Belladonna.** It is dry and covered with a white clammy fur and much tenacious yellow-ish white mucus. Sometimes the tongue becomes inflamed and looks quite swollen with prominent red papillæ.   Often we meet the straw-berry tongue so characteristic of Bell.

Belladonna is highly useful in gastritis, gastralgia, and other kindred troubles. The symptoms calling for it are pressure in the stomach, especially after a meal, nausea and vomiting. The pain is violent, recurring and transient. It is also pressing and cramping, and the patient finds relief by bending backwards.

It is equally useful in inflammatory affection of the abdomen, such as peritonitis. Great distention of the abdomen, high fever, extreme sensitiveness of the abdomen to touch, are its indications. This sensitiveness is so acute that the patient can hardly bear the bed-cover and the pressure of the clothing.   During pain the transverse colon protrudes like a pad all the way across the abdo-men.

We must not overlook **Belladonna** in dysentery. The stools are thin, greenish, bloody or papescent white. They are small in quantity, frequent and involuntary. Sometimes during dentition of children, and in summer complaints of babies. Bell. comes in very handy where **Cham.** and **Podo.** fail. I remember a case of infantile green diarrhœa that I was called on to treat in the beginning of my practice. It was one of those persistent cases that one meets with in the course of one's practice. The stools were green and the period was that of dentition.

The child's abdomen was highly tympanitic. His diarrhœa was worse precisely after each meal and the irritability of temperament was great. He seemed to suffer from an abnormal appetite. **Arg. n., Arsenic, Cham., Colocynth, Mag. c., Merc. v., Crot. tig.,** and **Sulphur** were all tried, but in vain. The diarrhœa, inspite of all attempts continued for about two, months, when one fine morning to my surprise, I found the child pretty nearly cured. The stools were gone and I was told that for the first time during this long period of sickness the child had a nice night's rest. Of course, I attributed this to the last remedy prescribed by me and felt jubilant over my success. I have not yet mentioned that the child's father was a good homœopathist himself and had previous to that morning taken the liberty of prescribing a dose of **Belladonna** 200. I need hardly mention that though my happiness was great, my exultation over my supposed success was somewhat lessened. I mention this story to show the folly of a routine practice. The totality of symptoms must always be our only and the sole guide in the selection of the remedy.

We must not forget the action of **Belladonna** over the kidneys and the bladder. We use it in nephritis when the quantity of urine becomes greatly diminished and it looks turbid like yeast. It is also used in cystitis when the urine becomes extremely hot and fiery-red. A peculiar sensation like that of a ball rolling inside is felt in the bladder. Tenesmus of the bladder, strangury, frequent desire to urinate with scanty discharge of urine are a few more of its symptoms. We also have involuntary micturition as well as retention of urine in **Belladonna.** The former due to paralysis of the sphincter muscles and the latter to paralysis of the walls of the bladder. The vesicular region is extremely sensitive to pressure and jar. For involuntary micturition we should compare **Belladonna** with **Arnica., Caust., Nat. m., Pulsatilla,** and **Rhus tox** and for retention of urine it ought to be differentiated from **Nux v., Opium** and **Stramonium.**

Case 1.—M. A., girl of fourteen years, dark hair and complexion, was first affected with epilepsy at the age of twelve years. She was usually attacked during the afternoon, preceded by sleepiness and sullenness of disposition. There was no aura epileptica; but she gave the usual shriek, and fell to the floor convulsed, with great tossing about, rolling of the eyes, and snapping of the teeth, so that the tongue was frequently lacerated. One symptom was constantly present. **The right hand persistently clutched at the throat.** I commenced giving the patient Belladonna 3, twice a day, and continued for about a month. I then changed to Belladonna 30, once every three days; and after three months' treatment with these potencies, gave her Belladonna 200, after every severe attack. The improvement under this remedy was marked from the beginning. The attacks first began to diminish in severity, then in frequency, and in one year they had ceased altogether. The menses came on in due time, and although at first very painful, the remedy seemed to influence them in the direction of health to such an extent, that in time they caused no inconvenience.—Dr. J. Martin Kershband. The Medical Investigator, March, 1874.

Case.—S., a stout woman: after cathartic pills had convulsions during labor. Skin moist and warm; rush of blood to face; vessels resembling cords; eyes rolled up and back; head and spine curved backward; pupils were much dilated; abdomen thrust forward and upward; trembing, shuddering, groaning, the contortions and jerkings of dreadful clonic spasm; thumb and wrist inverted; spasm lasted five minutes, followed by deep coma; no spasm during expulsive efforts, but several minutes after, two labor pains during free intervals. Bell. 200. No spasm for one hour; pain increases; child born in two hours; only one more severe spasm.—Dr. O. P. Baer.

BELLIS PERENNIS.

Bellis Perennis is our common everyday daisy. It belongs to the natural order of Compositæ. It has been used as household remedy from a very long time for bruises and injuries. Its common name " Bruise-wort " clearly testifies to its usefulness in such conditions. We are greatly indebted to Dr. Burnett for our knowledge of **Bellis.** He had been its chief exponent and had conducted extensive provings to give **Bellis** a solid position in our Materia Medica of the vulnerary remedies.

Its action is chiefly centred in the muscular fibres of the blood vessels. We find as much muscular soreness and lameness in Bellis as in **Arnica.** It is not only superficial muscles but the deeper tissues that are involved due to mechanical causes and as such it belongs to the same category of remedies as **Vanad., Arnic., Calend., Hyper., Con., Ham.,** and **Sulph. acid.**

" Stasis and fag " mark the keynote of Bellis. Exudations and swellings of all kinds, varicose veins, cerebral stasis as manifested by giddiness in elderly people, engorgement of breast and uterus in women, come under its influence.

I had occasion to use Bellis once in the case of a lady in an advanced stage of pregnancy. She was troubled badly with varicose veins and a great soreness located in the region of the pelvis, so much so, that she could hardly walk. **Bellis** did not disappoint me. The soreness disappeared and movement became much easier. At times this soreness is located in the pelvis, extends up to the abdominal wall, and stitches and pains are felt even there.

It is pre-eminently a left-sided remedy. It is also eminently indicated in ill effects of cold or iced drinks when overheated.

Traumatism of the pelvic organs, due either to mishandling or false steps or accidents also call for **Bellis.** The patient complains of a sore, bruised feeling in the pelvis.

Boils are numerous and they are sensitive to touch.

BENZOIC ACID.

The most important characteristic of this remedy is found in its urinary symptoms. The urine is highly offensive. It smells strongly of ammonia. The color of the urine too is very dark. We have also in this remedy enuresis nocturna of delicate children. It is also good for dribbling of urine in old men with enlarged prostate. In every case, of course, we are guided by the strong characteristic odor of urine. This offensive odor reminds us of **Nitric acid, Calcarea carb, Asafoetida** and **Moschus.**

We find a very characteristic diarrhœa in **Benzoic acid.** The stools are profuse, exhausting and entirely watery, running right through the diaper as in **Podophyllum.** The smell resembles that of burnt gun-powder. This brownish watery stool contains little pieces of fæcal matter that look like tiny portions of sponge.

I have forgotten to mention that this remedy is mostly indicated in people of rheumatic tendency with syphilitic and gonorrhœal history. There are deposits of gouty concretions in different joints of the body, in consequence of which they make cracking noise on motion. The pains in the joints are tearing and stitching in character. Inflammation frequently accompanies the pains. This remedy should be studied along with **Colchicum.**

Before I close, let me add that Benzoic acid is one of our remedies for ganglion of the wrist.

Case.—The patient was a gentleman, forty-five years old, who had suffered from frequent returns of asthma for more than twenty years; venesection on his first attack had doomed him to long continued suffering, and he had tried all possible rational and irrational remedies. Saltpeter no longer relieved him. I found him ill; his lower extremities much swollen (œdema), and his strength much diminished. The urinary secretion was almost suppressed, and the very small quantity of urine passed by him but twice in twenty-four hours, was of a dark color and of a very disagreeable, pungent smell. Guided by this well-known symptom of acidum benzoicum I gave him one dose of the remedy. Very shortly afterwards he had the worst paroxysm of asthma he ever experienced; the attacks then became less frequent and less severe. After three days the urine became quite profuse, with considerable sediment but without the former pungent smell, and much paler. After ten days more, the urine again becoming dark and slight attacks of asthma returning during the early morning hours, I administered another dose of benzoicum acidum 11000 (Fincke). He improved, progressed well, and was, some weeks later restored to full health.

Case.—In the case of a gentleman seventy-two years of age, (who had suffered long from gout and asthma, which latter generally appeared on the 4th of July, and always left him with a violent attack of gout), the same urinary symptoms led me to give him benzoicum acidum. The asthma had always been worse after lying down, and especially after midnight, when he was compelled to sit until morning in a chair inclined forward; there was no anxiety or restlessness present, the absence of which symptoms counterindicated arsenicum, which might otherwise have been selected as the homœopathic curative agent. Two doses of benzoicum acidum 11000 cured the case, and no gouty symptoms followed, as in the previous attacks.—**Hahnemannian Monthly, Sept., 1887.**

BERBERIS VULGARIS.

Berberis belongs to the natural order of Berberidaceæ to which order also belongs Caulophyllum and Podophyllum. It contains an alkaloid called Berberina.

It occupies a very important place in our Materia Medica. The main influence of this remedy is found on the kidneys. It has been used with miraculous success in renal calculi. We notice stitching cutting pain in the left renal region that follows the course of the ureter into bladder and thence into the urethral canal. This pain sometimes shoots all through the pelvis into the hip and down into the testicle of the affected side, which seems drawn up. The urine is greenish, bloody, turbid and full of slimy mucus. Every movement brings on or increases the pain. A bruised pain with stiffness, lameness and numbness in the small of back which renders movement difficult often accompanies these urinary symptoms. On such symptoms it has repeatedly relieved the agonising distress of gravel in many instances.

We also use it in biliary calculi when jaundice follows the colic. Violent stitching pains are felt in the right hypochondriac region that cause him to hold his breath. The stools become clay colored. This is sometimes complicated with fistula in ano and a troublesome short cough.

The appearance of Berberis is striking as well as characteristic. Every feature of the patient speaks of constant pain and suffering. The checks are sunken and the eyes are deeply imbeded in their sockets with a deep blue margin around them. The complexion is pale, gray and earthy. Mentally they are extremely anxious, fretful and full of worry. They are also afraid of twi-light, because at that hour, when light merges into darkness signalling the death of day, they are troubled with terrifying apparitions. All sorts of images crop up at that hour, and put fear and dread into their mind.

Two symptoms are particularly characteristic of this remedy. One is wandering, radiating pain. It rarely stops where it begins, starting in the kidney it radiates into the bladder and then along the hip into the thighs. When the location of the trouble is the liver, and the remedy is Berberis, we find the characteristic sticking pain radiating from the liver under the border of the false ribs on to the right side and into the abdomen. The other important characteristic already referred to is a peculiar bubbling feeling as if water were coming through the skin. Similar bubbling sensations are felt in the joints and other parts of the body. A third symptoms worth noticing is a sensation of tight cap pressing upon the whole scalp.

It also is used in complaints of females, particularly when menstrual symptoms are associated with urinary difficulties. The sticking, radiating pain, so characteristic of this remedy, is constantly present. This remedy also has a great sensitiveness and soreness of the vagina.

It is a great remedy in lumbago. The pain extends, as elsewhere, from the back round the body and down the thigh. It is greatly aggravated by movements and fatigue. Dr. Simmons reports of a cure of a case of lumbago in a gentleman with a single dose of Berberis. The symptoms were: "After he had walked a short distance he was compelled to stop from a feeling of intense weariness, heaviness, lameness and stiffness of the legs, which felt sore as if bruised." Dr. Guernsey's admirable summing up of Berberis is worth reading and is as follows: "Affects particularly the lumbar region; kidneys; uterus. The patient is sometimes unable to tell the exact locality but the pain is somewhere in the back and shoots up the back; or into spermatic cord, or testes, bladder, buttocks, or legs. The pain may shoot up or down or both ways. Pains may be felt all over the body, emanating from the back; the pains are of a sticking, pricking, lancinating or jerking character, flying about, now here and now there. There is often a bubbling sensation in the region of the kidneys, this sensation may occur elsewhere, but it is usually found here."

Case 1.—Bright's Disease of the Kidneys.—Mr. W., æt forty-nine, dark complexion, of slender stature, carpenter and hard worker, January, 1872. Had dizziness or a sensation of whirling in the heel; bruised pain in the region of the kidneys when stooping or moving about; general weak feeling and want of energy. In March commenced passing bloody urine; accompanied with dull, aching pain in the renal region, and a drawing cramp-like sensation in the direction of the left ureter, extending to the bladder; urine thoroughly mixed with blood and voided without difficulty. During the summer was under homœopathic, allopathic and electric treatment without good result. Nov 1. The urine consists of a dark red or blackish fluid, thoroughly mixed with blood, which, after standing, deposits a sediment resembling burnt umber mixed with oil. In decanting, it adheres to the vessel like paint; at times it is bright red, and deposits a sediment of pure blood; at other it is the color of strong chocolate, with a sediment like brick-dust. He passes three pints of this urine per diem without difficulty; tenderness to pressure over renal region, with burning, smarting sensation, as if a hot poultice was applied to the parts; dull pain in back; contractive pain in region of left ureter, preventing him from straightening the body; vertigo, when lying quiet in bed; head feels as large as a half-bushel; palpitation of the heart, relieved by change of position; sharp pains in region of kidneys; sensation of constriction across the epigastrium; jerking of the lower extremites at night, so violent as to almost throw him out of bed; frequent shocks through the whole body; very wakeful, does not sleep five minutes some nights; much reduced in strength and flesh; good appetite, no thirst, bowels slightly constipated, stools scanty and very dark colored; skin pale and anæmic. **R. Tereb. 6,** three doses daily; passed clear while taking this. **R. Natrum mur. 30.** Nov. 23. Sleeplessness; pain and stiffness in back, with restlessness; Urine the same. **R. Rhus tox 30.** Dec. 4. Little change; bad sleep; passes large clots of dark coagula with urine. R. Lycop 20, night and morning for a week. Dec. 21. Sleeps better, burning, smarting in kidneys; dizziness; palpitation and fluttering of the heart. **R. Hepar a. c. 30.** January 6. No better. Epithelial casts in urine. Nitric acid test shows albumen; very weak; cannot rest nights; renal pain worse; hands and fingers swollen, still; œdema of upper eyelids. R. Arsen. 30 continued about the same hours. various remedies till April 10, when **R. Berb. vulg 20,** every six hours. On the third day after taking this remedy, the patient was seized with a severe drawing pain in the region of the right kidney (had never experienced any pain, on this side before) which extended down the course of the ureter to the bladder and testicles, with frequent desire to urinate, passing small quantities of clear urine. While suffering thus, several dark cylindrical pieces about an inch and a half in length, and of the diameter of a rye straw, were discharged with the urine, after which the pain subsided, and with it all traces of albumen which had been so abundant; applied the Nitric acid test, but could discover none whatever; urine still remains bloody. R. Sac. lac. April 19. Improving. May 9. Urine clear of blood or albumen. June 28. Cured.—Dr. J. D. Johnson.

Case 2.—Urethral Stricture.—Urinary tenesmus when not urinating, felt just above fossa navicularis; worse when standing and when walking; smarting in fossa navicularis after micturition; urinates freely except just before the close, when the stream suddenly stops; afterward a few drops escape involuntarily; urine dark; profuse sweat of the parts when walking; varicocele of left side; soreness in left inguinal region and thigh, extending to the left testicle; feels drowsy all the time; has not been exposed to gonorrhœa. During three weeks, various remedies were administered unsuccessfully. August 9, 1869. Additional symptoms recently developed; constant burning sensation in left testes, epididymis, spermatic cord and urethra; emission of semen premature during coitus. Cured with Berberis.—Dr. H. V. Miller.

BISMUTH.

The main characteristic of this drug is found in its extreme anguish of mind. He sits, he walks, he lies down, but nothing brings him any ease and comfort. In this **Bismuth** resembles **Arsenicum** . Another point of similarity is found in the great irritability of stomach. He vomits water as soon as he drinks it. He can retain solid food to a certain extent. Sometimes however a different condition is noticed. The patient retains both solids and liquids, but after an interval of many days when food has filled the stomach, he brings out an enormous quantity of substance taken, both digested and undigested.

The facial appearance of the patient betokens of great exhaustion and profound loss of vitality. He is pale, cold and earthy. Blue rings round the eyes are also visible. The feature becomes entirely hippocratic. In fact, everything points to a serious derangement

Bismuth exerts a very strong influence on the stomach. We frequently notice a distressing pressure and burning pain in the region of the stomach. It feels like a load in one spot. Other symptoms are an intense convulsive gagging, great nausea, purging, vomiting and prostration. These symptoms lead to its indication in cholera, gastritis, gastralgia, headache and cancer of stomach.

It is useful in toothache, when cold water in mouth begets relief, but the relief only lasts till the water gets warm in the mouth.

One mental symptom of **Bismuth,** worth remembering, is a great desire for company. This is particularly noticeable in children. They hold on to their mother or the nurses for company. Solitude is unbearable.

Case 1.—A lady twenty-five years of age, had facial neuralgia of some weeks' standing. Worse in the morning. The pain was excruciating, burning, greatly aggravated by warmth. She could only obtain relief by holding cold water in the mouth and moving about. **Bismuth 200** gave immediate and permanent relief.—Dr. G. M. Ockford, ("**Am. Hom.,**" Nov., **1879**).

Case 2.—Dyspepsia.—A gentleman, aged thirty-four, was unable to partake of any solid food for many weeks, on account of the distress which followed in his stomach and bowels. He suffered at the time from pains in his head, abdomen, upper and lower extremities, that made him very restless. Bowels sometimes loose, passing considerable bloody water; greatly prostrated; craves cold water. **Arsenicum** and **Nux vomica** without relief. **Bismuth,** three doses, cured him entirely in four weeks.—Dr. A. E. Small.

BLATTA ORIENTALIS.

Blatta Orientalis is prepared from **Talapoka,** the Indian cockroach, an insect found abundantly in dwelling houses. Its properties were accidentally found out by a gentleman, a chronic martyr to asthma, who after taking tea, in which through inadvertence of the servant lots of these insects were boiled down, was wonderfully relieved from all his distressing symptoms. Later on Dr. D. N. Ray of Calcutta made a thorough proving of the drug and recorded his experience in the **Homœopathic Recorder** of 1890, to whom we are indebted for our knowledge of this drug to a great extent. It acts better in acute cases and in corpulent constitutions. It has saved many cases from threatened suffocation due to excess of mucus in bronchi. Oppression of breathing, restlessness, profuse perspiration and aggravation from lying down are some of the symptoms.

This drug should not be confused with **Blatta Americana,** another drug prepared from the American cockroach, and greatly used in cases of dropsy and jaundice.

BORAX.

In **Borax** we have to deal with a very dirty and unclean sort of a patient, a patient whose hair is constantly tangled and knotted, whose eyelids are loaded with a gummy exudation, whose nostrils are always crusty and inflamed, from constant flowing of an excoriating coryza, whose mouth is full of aphthous sores that prevent eating and whose tongue is cracked and dry.

Further these patients are very nervous. They get frightened from the least noise as of coughing, sneezing and lighting a match.

The skin too partakes of the same unhealthy tone as is common everywhere in this remedy. Least injury brings on suppuration as in **Hepar sulph, Mercurious, Silicea, Calendula, Fluoric acid, Sulphur** and **Petroleum.** Inspite of such semblance between these remedies, the individuality of **Borax** is easily marked out by a great dread of the downward movement, a symptom that is considered the grand keynote of the remedy. It is found in almost all complaints where **Borax** becomes indicated. We notice this in the child, when the nurse puts it down on the couch, the child cries and clings to the nurse. We notice this in the grown-up man, when he goes down the lift. All downward motion brings on a kind of shudder.

Borax helps in the red nose of young women.

Two really important symptoms—symptoms highly characteristic of **Borax**, have been omitted. One is great irritability and fretfulness of mind before the almost natural afternoon stool. She feels lively, contented and cheerful after the stool is over. The second point is a restlessness through the afternoon. She finds it difficult to settle down to any definite work. She changes from one work to another and roams about indefinitely. This restlessness cannot be accounted for in any way.

It abounds with a whole array of symptoms pertaining to the female sexual system. In the first place we will talk about its menstruation. The menses generally are, too profuse and during this period the nervousness is on the increase. It is not only profuse but early as well, and is accompanied with stitching and pressing pain in the groins. There is profuse, white, albuminous, acrid leucorrhœal discharge appearing between catamenia which irritates the labia and inflames the Duverney's glands. The leucorrhœal discharge, as it runs down the thigh, feels like warm water,

There is one more symptom that needs attention, and that is a disagreeable sensation of emptiness in mammæ after sucking the child. A contractive pain is also felt in the left breast as the child nurses the right.

Case 1.—I had a very pretty proving of Borax several weeks since. A few days after having discharged myself from an obstetric case, I was again summoned to prescribe for the baby, which the mother said was "so nervous," and also said that she noticed this nervousness chiefly in one symptom, that the child (a girl) "was exceedingly afraid of falling;" she said this symptom was so noticeable that her husband and others had observed it. I, of course, at once thought of **Borax**. and was about looking into the little one's mouth in search of further indications. At this juncture the mother of the child informed me that "the baby had not a sore mouth, as the nurse had given it a washing out twice a day with **Borax** to prevent it, and had also washed the baby all over with the preparation every day to make its skin healthy." Suspecting a **Borax** proving, I determined to confirm my suspicions and give no medicine. I accordingly stopped the nurse's work and gave **Sac. Lac.** enough to last three days. Calling at the end of that time, I found that the child was too well to need any antidote. I should also state that I found a slight inflammation of the mouth on the first inspection, which would doubtless have developed into something more troublesome. I cannot say whether this was also a "proving" or a mere chance symptom, but believe the former as it also disappeared with the other. Dr. William Jefferson Guernsey.

Case 2.—I was called to see a child about six months old. Aug. 7, 1867. Symptoms: Screaming; fever and hot head; all worse at night; starts in sleep, as if frightened. At the time I called in the evening, the child was very pale. It had light-colored and green, slimy discharges from bowels. The light-colored part appeared to be undigested milk. Discharges more frequent during afternoon and evening. While talking with the mother, the child being asleep upon her arm, she bent forward to pick something from the floor. The child immediately threw up its hands. Upon questioning her, she said the child appeared to be afraid of falling, and she "didn't see how a child so young should know anything about falling." This led me to inquire whether the child had had a sore mouth. I was informed that, about a mouth previous, the mouth had been sore, and had been cured, as she supposed. Here seemed to be but one remedy indicated, although, until the symptom came out, "fear of falling from downward motion"—**Belladonna** was the remedy; now the whole is changed, and **Borax** is the remedy. I gave one dose 1m Fincke's. The next morning the child was well.—Dr. H. N. Martin.

BOTHROPS LANCEOLATUS

Bothrops Lanceolatus is an Ophidian of the family of Crota-lidæ. It is an inhabitant of the island of Martinique. It is also called the yellow Viper. We are grateful to Dr. Ch. Ozanam for our knowledge of this remedy. Its symptoms are not many but the few, we have, are important and it will be worth our while to remember them.

The best way to study this remedy is to have a visual image of case of bite by this dangerous reptile. It resembles a case of septicæmia of the worst type.

The bitten limb swells speedily to an enormous size. It becomes soft and flabby as if full of gas. The whole limb becomes infiltrated with a bloody serum—the infiltrated limb looking discoloured with blotches of blue. Very soon extensive suppuration sets in, the skin and flesh coming off in bits. The result is an alarming process of moist gangrene, exposing the bones, tendons and the harder tissues. The whole limb is dissected alive. Colliquation succeeds and if the patient does not already die from effects of purulent absorption, fatal syncope sets in.

One remarkable feature about **Bothrops** poisoning is that the blood becomes extremely fluid and dark, and sometimes spouts out in jets. This feature should constantly be borne in mind, as it constitutes an important land-mark in **Bothrops**. In this respect **Bothrops** is very similar to our other snake remedies **Crotalus horid., Elaps, Naja** and **Lachesis**.

BOVISTA

It is prepared from the Warted puff-ball, a fungus, eaten in Italy, and is a handy remedy in the treatment of old maids, who are naturally nervous and awkward. One must not be led to feel that we have stereotyped remedies for certain classes of people; all we mean is that **Bovista** corresponds to a certain type whom circumstances of life have made intensely awkward and ill at ease. This awkwardness is manifested by a constant tendency to drop things. They drop cups, saucers and various other objects and break them constantly inspite of great carefulness and firm determination not to do so. This is partly due to weariness and weakness of joints and partly to intense nervousness.

Another peculiarity with these patients, is that they are somewhat bloated. They are more or less puffy, and the integument about them is somewhat velvety. The result is that they can not handle anything tight without having distinct marks left about them.

A third and an important characteristic is a sensation of enlargement——a feeling of hugeness. The ovaries feel too large; the uterus seems enormous. A sensation of this description is a sure call for **Bovista,** and numerous cures have been effected on this symptom alone.

A fourth point to remember is that the discharge, be it from nose, throat, vagina, or any other orifice, is tough and tenacious. The skin is without doubt very unhealthy. It is leathery. The eruptions may be either dry or moist. Warts and corns are to be found everywhere. Urticaria covers nearly the whole body. There is one particular locality, a special cite in Bovista where we find intense itching and that part is the tip of the coccygeus. She scratches till it bleeds and even then there is no relief.

Bovista is a hemorrhagic remedy as well. We think of it in hemorrhage from the gums after extraction of teeth. We also have hemorrhage from nose, specially in the morning after awaking or during night when asleep. It stops hemorrhage from other wounds as well.

It is a good remedy in menorrhagia where the flow takes place at night only, as in **Magnesia carb,** and **Natrum mur.** In **Sepia** the flow takes place only in the morning hours. In **Phel.** it happens in the evening.

Bovista patient suffers from diarrhœa before and during menses as in **Ammon carb, Ammon mur,** and **Veratrum album.** This remedy also has occasional show of menstrual blood every few days between periods. This is an soft verified symptom. I cured an old maid, who used to get her mense every fifteen days, with painful bearing down sensation and diarrhœa with **Bovista.**

It has a pronounced leucorrhœa. The discharge may be like the white of an egg or yellowish green. It is profuse, acrid, corrosive and tough.

In diabetes mellitus it is an excellent remedy provided of course the indications are present. The desire to urinate is frequent. The urine is yellow-green or turbid like lime water.

We also think of it in colic, either flatulent or renal. The patient doubles up with pain as in **Colocynth,** but unlike **Colocynth**

there is relief after eating. During colic the patient passes red
urine. There is great intolerance of tight clothing about the waist.
     It has some important application in certain abnor-
malities of vision. We use it with great success in amaurosis and
the peculiarity is that it is worse after sun-rise.

Case 1.--Metrorrhagia.—"A married lady had always menstruated profusely. After bearing children her catamenia became a fearful menorrhagia,
completely exhausting her.   There was nothing particularly characteristic,
further than a wonderful flow of blood, and an amelioration during the day
time when on her feet, and an aggravation at night when lying down. This
condition continued for months, under allopathic treatment. **Bovis.** cured her.
During the prevalence of this trouble, her attendant advised her to become
pregnant, which seemed impossible, although during thirteen months, to use
her own words, "we never tried to prevent." Three months after taking
Bovis. she became pregnant when they did try to "prevent." She was
delivered at full term of a fine, healthy boy, and has continued well, it now
being nearly two years since I first saw her." Dr. Isaac Cooper.
     Case 2.—Girl, æt. twenty-one, pale and cachectic, had been affected with
spasms for a long time; they occurred previous to the menses or after mental
emotions, and were preceded by tearing and stitching from the left shoulder
to the elbow, which was especially violent at night and when at rest. Spasms
sometimes twice a day. First was seized with constant yawning, followed
by stitching in the throat, sensation as if the tongue were cut through with
a knife, accompained with painful tensions in the mouth, and convulsions of
all the facial muscles, after which spasmodic weeping and laughter, with
suffocation, constriction or distention of the throat, and lastly with spasms
of chest and dark red face.—**Bov. 18** cured. Archiv.

BRACHYGLOTTIS REPENS

This plant hails from New Zealand. It is called by the native
Maories Puke Puke, and it belongs to the natural order of
Eupatoriaceæ. We are indebted for this remedy to Dr. C. L.
Fischex. Although none of its symptoms has been clinically verified,
it is spoken of very highly in certain affections of the kidneys,
specially albuminuria. The urgency in voiding urine is very great.
He must pass the urine at once or else, he feels he would not be
able to retain same. He passes a big quantity of pale urine of low
specific gravity containing mucous corpuscles, epithelium, albumen
and casts. Great pain is experienced in neck of the bladder, urethra,
and penis if the desire is not attended to immediately. A very
important indication is a fluttering or a swashing sensation in the
bladder. In its action it resembles **Acid phos., apis,** and **Helonias,**
and hence a comparative study will be of benefit to the students of
Materia Medica.

BROMIUM

Bromium is a dark red or more correctly reddish-brown liquid found in the water of many salt springs. Its principal action is found in its tendency to cause induration and enlargement of the glands of the body. Hence it is one of our favourable remedies in scrofula. We think of it in inflammation of the parotid gland, when the swelling is of stony hardness with a tendency towards suppuration. It is equally useful in induration of the glands of the axilla. It has been used in swelling of the testicles after suppression of gonorrhœa and in goitre.

The most important action of this remedy, however, is seen in diphtheria, membranous croup, laryngismus stridulus and other serious affections of the throat. I will speak of laryngismus stridulus first. The hale and hearty child, all on a sudden, turns blue in the face, and his body is thrown into violent convulsions due to the spasm of the glottis. **Bromium** works like a charm in such cases. It relieves the spasm and prevents the repetition of such occurrence.

In diphtheria, the membranes starting in the larynx spreads upward and covers the whole fauces; inspiration becomes extremely difficult; breathing becomes hoarse and rattling, and sounds as though it has been obstructed by a sponge or certain other loose substance, vibrating in the passage. He cannot inspire deep enough. He further complains of a sensation of coldness in the larynx. **Bromium** is extremely serviceable in these cases.

The mental symptoms of **Bromium** need close attention as we have a few characteristic points to note. A peculiar form of anxiety is felt by these patients. It is a sort of a dread of something, or someone turning up unexpectedly before them. It is a feeling that some one is looking from the back whom they dread to meet and hence would not look back for fear of encountering this strange imaginary person.

It has a peculiar vertigo. It is a sensation felt deep in the brain, as if vertigo or apoplexy would come on. This giddiness is always worse on looking at running water hence our Bromium patient is very unwilling to go over a bridge. The vertigo is relieved by nose-bleed showing the congestive nature of this giddiness.

We have discussed the applicability of **Bromium** in diphtheria. We will now consider its usefulness in croup and pneumonia. The cough is wheezing and rattling as in **Antim tart.**

The voice gets hoarse amounting sometimes to complete aphonia. In pneumonia the lower lobe of the right lung is particularly affected. Great oppression of breathing is experienced and although the rattling shows great accumulation of mucus, very little is expectorated.

Coming to the female sexual system we have loud emission of flatus from the vagina. Other symptoms, which are not very important may be omitted.

Before closing, it is only proper that I should mention something about the hæmorrhoids of Bromium as they are a bit out of the common. They are blind and intensely painful during and after stool. Washing with cold or warm water renders them insupportable. Relief is only possible by the application of saliva. Another symptom is that the stools in **Bromium** are generally black fecal stools.

Case 1.—About two years ago, being challenged to show some evidence of the effects of homœopathic remedies in a curative directions, I was given a case of bronchocele to treat, that had been in a progressive state for at least fifteen years, in the person of a married woman, æt. forty six, and the mother of six living children. She enjoyed excellent health, with the exception of this deformity. The enlargement was in the right lobe, and was bounded superiorly by the inferior margin of the body of the lower maxillary, extending from the symphisis to the angle, and inferiorly by the clavicle— filling completely the intervening space, and presenting externally as much convexity as might be equivalent to the concavity naturally existing within the boundaries above described. Not wishing to show any want of confidence in my remedies, I told the parties interested, if they would give me six month's trial, I would furnish the proof desired. Being reasonable people, and all patrons of the system, they told me I might have a year, and longer if I considered it necessary. I can assure you, I felt an unusual responsibility, knowing how much might depend upon the result should it prove a failure. The tumor gave no inconvenience, except to a very slight degree in the movement of the head, so I had no keynotes to guide me. I decided to give **Bromine**, and accordingly directed that ten to fifteen pellets, saturated with the second decimal dilution, be taken every night. About this time I was a frequent visitor to the house professionally, but gave no special attention to the case, except to replenish the remedy when required. About the expiration of the third week, my attention was particularly called to the fact that the tumor was diminishing. The medicine was then given on alternate nights, and during the latter part of the second month the tumor had decreased to such an extent that the remedy was given twice a week, until the expiration of the third month. At this period, so little deformity remained that the medicine was discontinued. I saw the patient a few days since, and could not detect the slightest remains of what was, until the administration of **Bromine**, a deformity indeed. Dr. A. H. Allen.

Case 2.—I was called to a child about two years of age, who had been treated for five or six days for diphtheria, which, not withstanding repeated cauterizations and vomitings, had attacked the larynx. The last consultation, held by three allopathic physicians, was to discuss the propriety of tracheotomy as a last resource. The child was breathing with fearful difficulty, voice wholly extinguished, circulation flagging, skin cold and blue. They determined not to operate, as they considered death imminent and certainly inevitable. Under these circumstances I was called to take charge of the case. I wasted about twelve hours in trying **Kali bichromicum** 2d dec., and then **Kaolin 6th.** My experience with diphtheritic croup had not been pleasant or favourable, and I hardly knew where to turn for a remedy which I believed would be strictly homœopathic to the case. At last I ordered **Bromine,** one drop to four ounces of glycerine and water (equal parts), one teaspoonful every half-hour. In a few hours improvement was decided, and the interval lengthened to two hours, and afterward to three times a day. Convalescence went on rapidly, and the child made a beautiful recovery, although he did not recover his voice for two weeks. This case ought to have convinced our three allopathic friends of the truth of **similia similibus;** but there are minds that would not, indeed, could not, believe, "though one rose from the death."—Dr. Holcombe.

Case 3.—A girl, twenty-nine years old, whose mother had died in her thirty-eighth year from cancer in the breast, noticed, some four years ago, scirrhous indurations in the left breast, which increased in spite of treatment and were finally removed with the knife. A year later, the right breast became similarly affected. The greater portion of the right breast is as hard as marble, the surface uneven, knotted, and a rope-like induration extends into the axilla. The induration adheres firmly. Periodic, lancinating pains, especially at night; she cannot bear external pressure. Grayish, dingy color of the countenance, great mental depression and hopelessness. Menstruation ceased several years ago. She used to have constant itching and irritation of the skin. **Sulphur 200** was followed by slight general improvement; **Phosphorus 200** relieved the pain somewhat. **Bromine 30,** two doses each day. Remarkable improvement after four doses, followed by a complete cure after taking eighteen doses. (**Gauwerky, Allg. Hom. Zeitg. xliii. 241.**)

BRYONIA.

The tincture of **Bryonia** is prepared from the thick fleshy succulent roots of wild hops, a climbing perennial plant growing along hedges and fences in Germany and in France. The juice is expressed from the fresh root before the plant is in bloom and then mingled with an equal part by its weight of alcohol.

Bryonia occupies a place second to none in our Materia Medica. We need it in our everyday practice. It produces sharp pains and causes inflammation in various parts of the body, particularly serous membranes and the lungs. Hence it is considered essential in various affections of the respiratory system and in rheumatic ailments. But here, as elsewhere, our treatment is based on symptomatology. We will therefore, investigate into the main points of this important remedial agent.

The first and the foremost is the aggravation of its symptoms from motion. Whatever may be the affection, this symptom is prominently present. Thus in headache, the patient wants to keep absolutely quiet, for shock and jar aggravate his troubles. In pneumonia we find him resting on the painful side; in pleurisy we notice him pressing his chest tightly while coughing,—all to avoid jar and the motion. Even in diarrhœa he wants to be absolutely quiet for motion brings on increased urging for stool. So in rheumatism, synovial troubles, lumbago, muscular pain, asthma, cough, this desire for quiet and dread of motion are characteristically present. Another valuable modality of **Bryonia** is amelioration from pressure; but this is simply because pressure retards motion.

Great dryness, of all the mucous surfaces of the body, constitutes the second important characteristic of **Bryonia.** This is due to lack of secretion of the numerous glands, embedded in the mucous tissues. Commencing from the lips, this excessive dryness is to be found, throughout the entire alimentary tract down to the rectum. The lips are parched and cracked. The tongue too is equally devoid of moisture, and is covered with a white dark-brown coating. A similar condition prevails in the stomach, as is evident from the excessive thirst for large quantities of cold water to which we find our **Bryonia** patient a constant subject. The hard, burnt, knotted stools, indicate a similar dryness of the intestinal tract. Urine, except in rare cases, is scanty.

Stitching pain, in various parts of the body, is the third important point. It feels like needle poking into the affected part. Such pains are frequently met with, in pleurisy and pleuro-pneumonia. **Bryonia** thus becomes useful in the treatment of those complaints.

The typical Bryonia patient is choleric and bilious in his temperament. It is not the keen business man that we find in **Bryonia** ——one that is forever thinking, planning and concocting, ever on the watch for opportunity, intellectual and masterful, but a thin, irritable subject, very prone to muscular pains and aches and ever ready to catch cold. It is a shallow disposition that we have to contend with in **Bryonia.** The mood is uncertain. He does not know what he wants, and not knowing his own mind, he finds it extremely hard to please himself. He wants various things, which when offered, are refused. Though he resembles **Nux vom** to a great extent, the similarity is only superficial. As has been mentioned before, inspite of his ugliness of temperament, he is no match for the **Nux vom.** patient. The latter combines with his bilious mood, a real mental strength and an intellectual stamina. He is peevish and hasty in his disposition. There is also an undercurrent of despondence that colors his entire being. This at times, takes on the form of anxiety about the future. A sort of a doubt, as to whether there will be enough to live on, persists in his mind. This feature of Brvonia, is particularly noticeable, in women during lying-in period. Another equally characteristic symptom, particularly noticeable in cases of delirium, is a conviction, that they are away from home. Great unhappiness is felt, and a constant hankering expressed to be conveyed home, where they would be better looked after and cared for.

Anger and ill-humour, always, have a deleterious influence on the human system, and no where is this better proved than in the case of **Bryonia.** After a fit of bad humour, he gets a severe attack of neuralgia, diarrhœa, indigestion or giddiness. Although in this respect, **Bryonia** resembles **Colo., Ignatia,** and **Staphi.,** it is to be differentiated from them, by the fact, that Bryonia feels inordinately chilly, after such an occurrence.

In **Bryonia** the sensorium is not too bright. He feels a sort of stupefaction of the head. This feeling turns into real giddiness, when he sits up from a recumbent posture. It is a kind of whirling sensation that he feels, accompanied with nausea and giddiness. Even when he is in bed, he feels as if he is sinking deep down. This giddiness, is often, associated with a sensation of fulness and heaviness in the forehead. It feels, as if the brain is being pushed out. A certain amount of congestion is at the root of this feeling, as is evidenced by occasional epistaxis. Call it a heaviness or headache, as you like, but the modality must never be lost sight of. Stooping, coughing talking or any exertion meaning the slightest jar, aggravates this headache. Even the slightest movement is avoided. He lies with his eyes closed, for even the attempt of opening the eyes, leads to this oppressive headache. Sometimes the **Bryonia** headache closely resembles the headaches of **Gels.** and **Nat. mur.** It starts in the morning as he rises from bed, and keeps getting worse as the day advances, ending at last with the vomiting of bilious fluid. Mental exertion too is avoided, as that even leads to an aggravation. Constipation is always a guiding feature of **Bryonia** and it is invariably present with this headache.

Bryonia is useful in all kinds of fevers, although we find it indicated oftener, in certain varieties than others. It is applicable in the ordinary intermittent fevers, when due to exposure, there is irritation and inflammation of the mucous and serous membranes. Symptoms, spoken of before, of which there is hardly any need of recapitulation, lead to its application. In the more severe types of fevers, such as typhoid and typhus, we find it indicated, in the early as well as in the later stage. There is certainly a great depression, though not usually a total eclipse of the senses. The patient is somewhat sleepy, and during sleep, he shows symptoms of mild delirium. He picks at his dry and parched lips and makes them bleed. Gradually as the depression increases, his confusion of mind becomes more pronounced, and he rambles in his talk. His sleep is more or less interrupted, with dreams, and he gradually loses his bearing, and his talks partake more of the nature of hallucination. Generally he dreams about his household affairs and business he has transacted during the day. He is extremely thirsty and calls for frequent drinks, which he takes with great avidity. When his delirium is at its deepest and he is getting drowsy and comatose, we find him frequently getting up in bed and trying to get out. He says he wants to go home. I have repeatedly seen **Bryonia** giving a thorough turn to the case and the delirium subsiding as if by magic. Gastric symptoms are not infrequent. Great tenderness is complained of in the region of the liver. Transient stitches are felt in the right hypochondrium, with each cough and movement. The tongue which is usually dry, is coated white and yellow, and the taste in the mouth is bitterish. Sometimes the tongue gets so intensely dry that it becomes almost cracked. It trembles also, like the tongue of **Acid mur.**, though the trembling is ever so much lighter, due to the vitality being less profoundly affected. Nausea, as has been hinted at before, is quite a guiding symptom. The least movement brings it on so we find him lying extremely quiet. He does not get evacuation, for days together, and when after prolonged absence it really comes, it has to be expelled with great difficulty, necessitating continuous straining and a consequent rush of blood to head with confusion. From this we must not rush into conclusion, that soft stools are an improbability in **Bryonia**. In very severe cases we have soft, pasty, and mushy stools. The stools cause soreness and boring pain in the rectum. The smell is putrid like that of old cheese. It may also be involuntary. Distention in abdomen, rumbling, tenderness are also present.

Bryonia as a remedy, is greatly abused, in catarrhal inflammations such as coughs, colds and bronchitis. Quite an indiscriminate use is made of **Bryonia**, irrespective of its symptomatology. It is also indicated in fluent coryza, beginning with violent and frequent sneezing, and associated with stitching headaches and hoarseness. It generally follows and not precedes **Aconite**.

In bronchitis great pressure is felt over the sternum. Quite a lot of dyspnœa is experienced. The cough, which is dry, teasing and constant causes, great deal of stitching pain in head and chest. During cough the patient presses his chest with his hands, as a sort of protection against pain. It is considered the remedy in pleurisy, but is to be used after exudation has started. **Aconite** has preferrence in the inflammatory stage. The fever which in **Aconite** was at its intensity, has calmed down, to a great extent and the starting of the friction sound, showing that the stage of effusion has set in calls for the application of **Bryonia**. It misses the restlessness of Aconite, although the facial expression still retains the look of agony.

Its application in pneumonia is generally confined to the croupous variety and to pleuro-pneumonia. The constriction in the chest, the stitching pain, the scanty expectoration, high fever, profuse perspiration, intense thirst and the bloody sputa are all too clear indications for **Bryonia**.

Bryonia is particularly useful in synovitis. The affected joint is red, but not that vermilion red of **Belladonna**, nor the rosy red of **Apis mel.** It absorbs all effusion off the synovial sac. I

remember the case of a rich merchant of this city, who had to give
up riding and all other exercises, due to a chronic inflammation
of his knee-joint. Everything was tried but in vain, and the poor
man had to be satisfied with a tight knee-cap and a prognosis,
that was just as lame as his damaged knee-joint. To his utter
surprise every bit of that fluid dried up under the action of Bryonia
and in an incredibly short time he became his old-self again.

It affects the muscular system profoundly. It causes and
hence cures the muscular soreness. Acute articular rheumatism
also comes under its curative agency. The symptoms are very
clear-cut and need no further enumeration.

We will now discuss the action of **Bryonia** on the female
sexual organs. It is useful in menstrual difficulty, when the flow
is too early and too profuse and is accompanied with intense backache and a splitting headache, but more particularly is it useful,
when the normal flow has been suppressed, giving way to a
certain other vicarious form of discharge. Thus, for example,
when it is time for the menses to appear, the patient gets epistaxis
or a flow of milk from the breast or a running from the ear.
Bryonia also removes severe pain in the region of right ovary
as from a sore spot. The pain is stitching in character and is,
like all other Bryonia pain, aggravated on taking a deep inspiration. It is also helpful in puerperal fever, particularly when the
breasts are distended with milk. I have had the most satisfactory result in incipient mammary abscess, where the absence
of all violent symptoms, precluded Belladonna and yet where
the induration was quite hard and of a pale red colour.

Lastly, we will discuss its relation to the skin and various
forms of eruptive diseases. It has been recommended in nettlerash, erysipelatous inflammations and various other forms of
cautaneous eruptions; but mostly do we think of **Bryonia** in the
slow development of rash in eruptive fevers or in sudden receding
of rash. Whenever we find the child getting drowsy, and the
fever more persistent and the disappearing of rash, we should think
of Bryonia. A few doses of **Bryonia** will cause the rash to
reappear and with this will ensue a gradual subsidence of all
complications. Tardy appearance or a suppression of rash is not
a thing to be neglected; many a baby is carried to an early
grave because of this. **Bryonia** is only one amongst a long list
of remedies, serviceable in such contingency, and should be
studied in comparison with the following remedies——**Apis mel.**

Belladonna, Cup. met., Helleborus, Zinc. met., Sulphur and **Gelsemium.**

Apis mel. is a remedy when receding eruption comes in, long after **Bell.** and **Bryonia** have done their bit. The stage of congestive excitement is over, having been superceded by cerebral symptoms, the result of much effusion. The eruptions, what little is left, are of a pale œdematous type.

Antim. tart. finds application in suppressed eruptions, particularly of the type of variola. It is characterised by great drowsiness and a distinct involvement of the lung tissue which practically gets choked up with phlegm resulting in bluish appearance of the face and a rattling breathing.

Belladonna comes in the first stage of the disease, when inspite of great febrile excitement, the rash does not appear. It throws up the fever still higher and coaxes up the smooth scarlet rash.

Cuprum met. is indicated, when as a result of suppressed eruptions, cerebral symptoms show themselves. Convulsions with screaming, clutching of the thumb into the palm of the hand, boring of the head into the pillow, and spasms of the flexor muscles are the chief indications.

Gelsemium is indicated, when due to defective reaction the rash does not appear and the child becomes dull and listless. It is more an apathy than a torpor induced by cerebral conditions.

Helleborus is a great remedy and means a pronounced cerebral involvement. It closely resembles **Apis,** only the sensations are more completely benumbed, the apathy having given place to a real stupor. The dark sooty nostrils, the suppression of urine, the constant chewing motion of the mouth, the everpresent cephalic cry, the wrinkled forehead, the dilated pupil and the dropping of the lower jaw really speak of a desperate condition.

Sulphur is our great stand-by in repercussion of chronic eruptions. It modifies the entire constitution of the patient, and is not merely a temporary measure.

Zincum met. is an invaluable remedy where due to defective vitality, the constitution does not throw up any rash properly, and we come face to face with all the evil consequences of such suppression.

Case 1.—Lady, aged twenty-four, on the seventh day of her second childbed, complained in the evening, after having been out of bed for too long a time, and probably having eaten too much, of a chill, followed by much heat, soreness of the abdomen, which was worse when pressing on it; pulsation (beating) and stitches in the abdomen when moving or inhaling a deep breath; considerable thirst; mouth dry; tongue yellowish; quiet, as motion much increases the pain; lochia not suppressed; face red; skin hot; pulse 120, full, hard; sleepless. **Bry. 200,** one dose cured in three days.—Dr. A Lippe.

Case 2.—Tumor. Mrs. S., aged sixty, observed for two weeks a smooth, hard swelling at the left angle of the lower jaw; the integument is soft, slightly red and moveable; it appears as if the tumor beneath the skin were firmly adherent to the jaw; slightly painful; much weakness and general feeling of discomfort and illness. Prescribed **Bry. 6.** The swelling diminished for the next two weeks, when it was less than half its original size. A poultice was applied, and opening appeared and a slight amount of pus discharged. It soon healed.—Dr. C. Wesselhœft.

BUFO

This remedy is prepared by triturating with sugar of milk, the poison thrown out by the dorsal glands of the toad, through the skin. It was proved by Dr. Carl Hencke of Germany.

It produces an important train of symptoms such as imbecility, impotence and a great tendency towards masturbation. They frequently seek privacy, to indulge in this suicidal habit. This habit thus practised gradually ushers in symptoms, that simulate those of epilepsy. **Bufo** thus becomes an important remedy in the treatment of epilepsy. Its chief laurels have been won, in those cases where the aura starts from the sexual organs, or from solar plexus (**Artem, Calc. carb, Nux vom, Silicea.**)

It is our particular remedy for epilepsy, in which the fits occur during coition or are worse at times of menses and during sleep. These symptoms are almost always preceded by great irritability of the mind. The convulsions are usually followed by profound sleep.

I have had very gratifying results from **Bufo** in epilepsy, in a negro girl aged about 17 or 18 years. The least pressure on the right hypogastric region used to throw her into violent fits. From her shy, downward look, listlessness, indifference I had cause to suspect that she was a great victim to this vicious habit. Since she has been put on **Bufo,** she has kept free from any further attack.

Bufo causes a strong craving for alcohol. Our desires and aversions are the resultant tangents of various forces working within us. Any abnormality, means, therefore, a corresponding abnormality in the working forces and a proper adjustment is only possible by the most accurate regulation of the vital force, which alone, by reason of its omnipotence, can direct the proper flow of the tide of life. Any system of treatment that does not take proper cognizance of these details, is liable to get ship-wrecked on the shoals of hidden rocks. Like the ripples on the surface of water the symptoms tell us of the depth and condition of the submerged soil. Like the navigator, the physician has to take note of these ripples of symptoms. The only system of treatment that takes notes of these details, considered unimportant by our friends of the other school, inspite of all claim to scientific accuracy, is the system of treatment propounded by Samuel Hahnemann.

Bufo has a strong action on female sexual organs, especially the ovaries. It cures swelling and tenderness of these organs. Even hydatids of the ovaries, have known to have been cured with **Bufo.**

We should never lose sight of **Bufo** where, after an injury the whole of the lymphatic course is found to be affected. In panaritium, where the pain runs in streaks all the way up the area, it points always to **Bufo.**

CACTUS GRANDIFLORUS

It is specially applicable to sanguinous persons of plethoric habits.

The symptom that stands out most prominent in **Cact.** which you will do well to remember always, is a sensation of constriction in heart, as if an iron band prevented its normal movement. This sensation of constriction is not only present in the heart but is marked everywhere. It is felt in the throat, chest, bladder, rectum and vagina. We must not think that there is no other remedy except **Cact.** that has got this symptom of constriction. What is meant is that whenever we have this symptom of constriction, particularly in a case of heart-complaint, our attention should be primarily directed to **Cactus. Acon, Amyl nit, Aurum met, Calc. carb, Chelid, Cuprum, Iod, Ignatia, Lilium tig, Lycop, Lach, Moschus, Phos,** and **Naja,** can boast of a similar sensation of constriction to a certain extent. The essence of homoeopathic prescribing consists in making differentiations and we have a big list before us to consider.

Cact. is somewhat similar to **Acon.** in respect of congestive violence. Both of them throws blood with terrific rapidity to the affected part. In both, the pains are unendurable. Both **Amyl nit**

and **Lil. tig** have constrictive aching pain around heart; in **Ignat.** the constrictive pain, which appears more during menstrual period, with palpitation, is accompanied with anxiety, sadness and sighing; in **Arsen.** and **Calc. carb** the constriction is felt more while ascending steps; in **Calc. carb** this sensation of constriction is greatly relieved by the patient drawing his shoulders back; **Cuprum met** is characterised by constriction from anger and after drinking; in **Mosch.** the differentiating feature is a sensation of trembling in the heart found associated with this constriction. We have constriction in **Phos.** particularly while the patient is coughing.

Now that we have done our homage to the most important indication of **Cactus,** let us have a peep into the mental atmosphere of this remedy. Fear of death, despondence about cure, a great apprehension about some impending calamity, sadness, taciturnity and an irresistible desire to cry, are symptoms to be noted. Profound hypochondriasis, a great unwillingness to speak and an unusual melancholy are symptoms to be always noticed in these patients. In fact, all heart remedies present, more or less similar symptoms. Truly courage in human being has always been associated with a sound heart, and the reverse, to weak, diseased, disorganised cardiac organs.

Cact. presents some very important head symptoms. We notice a heavy pain like a weight on the vertex. This pain is relieved by pressure, and is aggravated by sounds of talking and least noise. It is more like a pressing pain in the head. There is quite a great deal of cerebral congestion, in consequence of which, strong pulsations are noticed in the temples. He feels, as if his skull would burst. This continued, and tormenting pulsations in the temples and in the ears, cause him great annoyance, and bring on hypochondriasis. Very often this annoying pulsation and pain cause him to cry out. In this respect **Cact.** can be compared well with **Acon, Apis, Aloes, Alum, Bell, China, Ferr, Glon,** and **Natrum mur.** In all these remedies great amelioration is noticed from pressure.

He suffers from flushes of heat in the face. Sometimes, especially in cases of cardiac rheumatism, he may present a pale deathlike countenance.

Before proceeding any further, let us study its action over the heart. As has been mentioned before, nowhere does it appear to a better advantage than in its relation to affections of the heart. It is an important cardiac stimulant. It does not affect the heart by acting on the centres as in **Dig.** It increases blood pressure by quickening and strengthening the heart-beat through direct action upon its nerves. The Allopaths recommend it highly in aortic regurgitation and relative cardiac incompetency and functional weakness of the heart. We, on the other hand, prescribe **Cact.** like all other remedies not on pathological basis but on strange, characteristic indications presented by the disease. It has been used with great success in cardiac rheumatism, carditis, acute and chronic angina pectoris, fatty degeneration of the heart, hypertrophy, cardiac dropsy, mitral regurgitation, aneurism of heart and large arteries, stenocardia, valvular diseases of the heart and in various other affections, provided the symptomatology calls for it. The patient complains of constant pain in the region of heart with a sensation, as if the heart were compressed or squeezed by an iron hand.

The pain is sometimes so excruciating, that the patient has to forego the slightest movement of the body. It impedes his breathing; it causes oppression, and it prevents him from lying down. It is so acute and so intense that he frequently bursts out into weeping. Sometimes, the pain starting from the apex of the heart, shoots down along the left arm to the end of fingers. Œdema, cyanosis, feeble intermittent pulse and palpitation of the heart are frequent symptoms. The latter symptom, palpitation, is almost constant, causing great restlessness and uneasiness. The slightest physical or mental exertion brings it on. It is frequently associated with vertigo, loss of consciousness, and dyspnœa. It is generally worse while walking, at night and on lying on left side. Sometimes it is so violent that it brings on suffocating spells.

Dig. on the other hand, is used for a condition exactly the reverse to that of **Cac.** It stimulates the muscular fibres in the cardiac and arterial walls, and, at the same time, slows down the heart's action by stimulating the ends of the vagus. We use it in subacute inflammation of the heart and in cases where we have direct manifestations of the gradual failing power of that most important organ known as the heart. Directly we suspect the loss of compensation from symptoms, such as feeble and quick beat of the heart, irregularity of the pulse, dyspnœa, œdema of the feet and the ankles. **Dig.** should be commenced to regulate the constriction of the heart and to increase the intravascular pressure. We will come to a full discussion of this later on, when we take up **Dig.**

Heart is such an important organ, and its affections are generally so serious, that it would not be out of place to discuss, in this connection, the relationship of **Cact.** in palpitation, to remedies such as **Aur. met, Ambra, Antim. tart, China, Conium, Cuprum, Crotal, Dig, Kali carb, Lach, Nat. mur, Opium, Phos, Spig, Sepia, Staph,** and **Sulph.** All of these have palpitation to a greater or to a lesser extent. But they all have their peculiar distinguishing features.

Ambra and **Staph.** are both noted for the peculiar symptom of palpitation brought on by listening to music. Music therefore is not always such a desirable subject with them.

Ant. tart and **Sulp.** have palpitation while the patient is having stools, whereas in **Conium,** palpitation comes after defecation is finished.

China is not inferior to **Cac.,** or to any other remedy in palpitation. But in this remedy palpitation comes on before an attack of chill.

Crotal. hor. and **Lach.** have palpitation especially marked during menopause.

In **Dig.** and **Sepia** the bad effects are more marked after coition; we think of **Dig.** and **Opium** in palpitation from grief and after fright.

Kali carb is an important heart-remedy; most of the troubles here are due to distorted cardiac valve due to deposits. Heart's action is weak and he has a feeling as if the heart were hanging by tightly drawn hands.

In **Nat. mur.** on the other hand, we notice palpitation during chill. He feels a great weakness of the heart as if life were ebbing away.

Phos., a great cardiac remedy, is especially applicable in the fatty degeneration of the heart, and where due to destruction of the **muscular** fibre of that organ, the heart becomes devitalized, impotent and insufficient. This is an important remedy to be thought of in those cases of palpitation where the patient is unable to have sexual intercourse, as each attempt at coition brings on most dire results. We use it also in palpitation of old maids, who are generally so nervous, that even the entrance of an unexpected visitor into the room, brings on palpitation.

Nat. Mur. is in no way inferior to any remedy we have discussed so far. We think of this in cases of overworked heart, and where there has been a great abuse of quinine, with consequent enlargement of the spleen and hypertrophy of the heart. The heart's pulsation here is an important feature. It shakes the whole body. These patients complain of a feeling of coldness about the heart. Palpitation is brought on, and aggravated by mental exertion and lying on the left-hand side.

Spong. like **Cac, Cuprum, Nat. mur,** and **Sepia,** has aggravation of palpitation before menses. She is unable to lie on her back with her head low which brings on a spell of suffocation. She is often roused from sleep as if something is stirring and sits up with anxiety, dread and fear of death. Pressing pain in præcordial region, pneumonic complications such as cough, violent gasping breath etc. are frequently present.

Sulph. patient frequently complains of palpitation when going upstairs or when climbing a hill. There is violent orgasm of blood in chest and a sort of a sensation of boiling in that region, and a great tremor in his right arm. A great craving for fresh air, with a desire to have all doors or windows open, is a marked characteristic of this remedy.

Spigelia has palpitation from exertioin, during deep inspiration and from leaning forward of the chest. Dyspnœa in this remedy is marked at every change of position. The pains are very sharp, shooting through heart to back or radiating from the heart down the arm or over the chest.

Cactus is an important hæmorrhagic remedy. But we think of it, only, when the hæmorrhage is associated with some cardiac disorder. The hæmorrhage is of an active type with fast action of the heart as in **Acon.**, but unlike Acon., it is wanting in anxiety and excitement. Menses in **Cact.** is black and pitch-like. Dr. Herring used this remedy in pneumonia where in an interval of every 4, 6, 7 or 8 hours, the patient expectorated a large quantity of blood. **Cact.** not only relieved but stopped the bleeding permanently.

It is used with success in pleurisy and diaphragmitis. We use it, when the patient complains of a feeling of a cord, tightly tied round the lower part of the chest. This feeling causes difficulty of breathing, continued oppression and uneasiness.

Case 1. Cardiac Dropsy.—Mrs. B.———, a lady aged sixty years, was attacked on the first day of July, 1878, with violent palpitation of the heart, accompanied with very distressing dyspnœa. Upon examination I found evidence of structural change of the mitral valves, with regurgitation, and congestion of the lungs. These symptoms continued two weeks, when general dropsy supervened. At this juncture I gave an unfavourable prognosis, and commenced a course of treatment, looking more for palliation than a cure. The breathing became more and more labored, and it was impossible for the patient to assume the recumbent position. Two weeks later, the extremities became œdematous. I succeeded in relieving the effusion temporarily with large doses of Indian Hemp and Digitalis. But very soon the dropsical symptoms increased, with an aggravation of all the distressing symptoms. I then gave the most powerful drastic cathartics and diuretics, until the bowels and kidneys utterly failed to respond to any of them, whereupon I advised my patient to "set her house in order," expecting at every subsequent visit to see what physicians are so often compelled to meet, viz., crape on the door. At this time, while visiting another patient, I was asked to see a cactus in block. The flower was given me, and from it I prepared a tincture and gave my patient four drops every three hours, which decidedly aggravated her symptoms. I then gave the third decimal dilution, with slight amelioration only. Following that I gave the 29th dilution, and it was like "throwing water on fire." It is now the 1st of October, and my patient is well. During three months' treatment the **Cactus** was the first drug that restored the bowels and kidneys to a healthy action. Every vestige of the dropsy has disappeared; the regurgitation has ceased, and there are no abnormal symptoms remaining, except slight valvular murmur. Dr. E. J. Morgan.

Case 2.—Mrs. C., aged twenty-eight, tall, dark hair and eyes. Rheumatism of all joints of the extremities, great deal of pain, stiffness and swelling; worse in the evening, and again in the morning on first rising; aggravation while at rest, on beginning to move, and from a change of weather, especially if the change be a cold, damp one; amelioration from continued but gentle motion; since some weeks constant pain in the region of the heart, with sensations as if the heart were "bound down," or "had no room enough to beat," or "as if bolts were holding it"; paroxysms of violent, stitching pain in the heart, with icy coldness of the limbs; cold sweat, particularly on the forehead; sense of constriction of the chest; with suffocation; fainting; pale, death-like countenance; violent, turbulent action of the heart—it beats violently for a short time, then ceased entirely; pulse feeble, intermittent, or entirely gone; screaming with the pains, or complete loss of consciousness. These attacks occur several times daily, and are brought on by any emotion, excitement, or upon attempting to exercise; also lying on left side at night excites them; oedema of lower extremities; loss of appetite; restless sleep; emaciation, pale face; despondent; thinks she will not recover; weeps much. Physical examination realed valvular disease, the second sound of heart being replaced by a harsh murmur. **Cactus** 800 F, one dose, followed by rapid improvement, since which time has had no return of symptoms.—Dr. Goodno

CADMIUM SULPH.

Cadmium sulph is an important remedy and should have an important place in every book on Materia Medica. It is a metal found very often in nature in conjunction with **Zincum.** The first real proving was made in 1854 by Petroz; later on in 1878 a more thorough proving was made by Doctor Hardenstein of Vicksburg, who used it with great success in the then prevalent epidemic of yellow-fever. It is an antipsoric of high rank.

Although of great curative value, **Cadmium sulph** unfortunately is not often used by medical men, the reason being want of knowledge. I have seen this remedy omitted in many a treatise on Materia Medica, which accounts for the negligence, it so often receives, at the hands of numerous homœopathic practitioners. The profound action of **Cadmium sulph** is found mostly on the stomach, where it causes intense burning and sharp cutting pains. The intense retching gagging and bringing up of tough mucus, bring **Cadmium sulph** into close proximity with **Ipecac, Tabac., Tart emet.** and **Arsen.** This nausea is so intense that the least thing touching the lip excites vomiting. The qualmishness is deathly. The patient must lie absolutely quite to ward off the vomiting. It has been found effective when the other remedies mentioned above have failed. The next important feature of **Cadmium sulph** is the profound exhaustion it produces. In this respect again, it is similar to **Arsen.** Dr. Clarke in his Dictionary has very aptly described it as a cross between **Bryo.** and **Arsen.**

The third grand characteristic consists in its chilliness. We notice aggravtion of all symptoms from cold and draught of cold air. There is icy coldness even when near a fire. We have horripilation after drinking, in **Cadium sulph.** This feature points to its usefulness in malarial fevers and in other ailments of similar nature. Dr. Hering in his guiding symptoms, cites a cure of a half-sided rheumatic paralysis of face, appearing suddenly, in a man in France, who rode in a sharp North-West wind. This patient was treated for four weeks by many eminent physicians of the old school without success. This patient got weil in 8 days after two doses of the 12th potency. This further shows that **Acon** is not our sheet-anchor in such instances.

The symptom that in my opinion ought to occupy the fourth place of importance is the black vomiting. This was the indication that led Doctor Hardenstein to prescribe this remedy, with success, in that fatal epidemic of yellow-fever. The taste in the mouth is almost pitchy. He feels as if he has a piece of metal in his mouth, all the time. This pitchy or metallic taste is probably due to accumulation of decomposed blood in the stomach, which imparts blackish colour to the substance vomited.

It acts well with drunkards and in women during pregnancy.

Now coming back to stools, I must say that the alvine evacuations are almost gelatinous, of a yellowish green semifluid character. This indication, together with that of incessant vomiting has made it a first rate remedy in cholera infantum.

Lastly, before finishing, I must not omit to mention that it is of value in palpitation of heart, when such palpitation is associated with constriction of chest. There is only one more remedy I know of and that is **Kali chlor.** where palpitation of heart is associated with constriction in chest.

CAINCA.

Caina, a Brazillian plant, used as a specific for dropsy, has been proved by Lippe. Its urinary symptoms are very well-marked and it is clinically similar to **Apocynum.** It is useful in dropsy when associated with dryness of skin. An important symptom, is a severe pain in the region of kidneys in the morning. The pain is so intense that the patient is unable to change his position. It is usually described as a sort of stiffness of the back. Urine is passed copiously and often day and night. This polyuria is particularly marked while travelling. It also removes fatigue from too long riding on horseback.

CAJUPUTUM.

Cajuputum is derived from leaves of Melaleuca leucadendron. It belongs to the natural order of Myrtaceæ. Our friends of the Old School use it as a local application in rheumatism and dysmenorrhœa but its homœopathic proving reveals a lot of reliable symptoms which lead to its application in headache, hiccough and stricture of œsophagus.

The keynote indication is a feeling of enlargement. Head feels as large as a bushel. We have also hiccough that starts at the slightest provocation in **Cajuputum.** It is also noted for a persistent sensation of choking as in hysteria. It is a first rate remedy for stricture of the œsophagus and hence should be studied in comparison with **Arsenic, Baptisia, Baryta carb.** and **Nat. mur.** There is a constant inclination to spit, and he hawks up large quantities of tough mucus drawn from the nares. Urine smells like cat's urine.

CALADIUM.

Caladium is a splendid remedy for that troublesome affection known as pruritus vulvæ. It is so bad as to induce onanism. This complaint usually becomes frequent during pregnancy.

We also think of it in sexual debility and impotence. It is the result of masturbation. Nocturnal emissions are frequent and they occur without dreams. The penis remains relaxed during an embrace.

Caladium proves of great service in a special type of fever where the patient falls asleep every evening during the paroxysm, and wakes up after it is over. The sweat smells sweet and at-tracts flies.

CALCAREA CARBONICA.

This remedy is prepared by triturating the inner snow-white portion of the oyster shells. This is regarded as one of our great constitutional remedies. It is specially adapted to the leuco-phlegmatic constitutions. They are corpulent and unwieldy. It is not a healthy regular growth that we find in **Calcarea** but an accumulation of undue and disproportionate amount of fat that serves only to make the patient weak, fragile and incapable of sustained exertions. Like all fat people they sweat profusely all over the body, though it is more pronounced on the head and nape of the neck. While sleeping, their pillows get wet far around. It is so profuse that it rolls down the face in large bead-like drops. It is copious and exhausting. The smell of the **Calcarea** sweat is sour. This acid smell is found everywhere in **Calcarea**. The taste of the mouth is sour; the diarrhœa is sour; in fact the patient is sour all over.

The remedy is characterised by defective assimilation and imperfect ossification. The bone tissues take long time to develop and even after maturing, they remain fragile. This is why curvature of the bones is such a common feature in **Calcarea**, and that the **Calcarea** child takes so long in learning to walk The bones of the leg give way under the heavy weight of the body; so knock-knees and bow legs are often to be met with in **Calcarea** babies.

Fontanelles and sutures take long to close. The head is too large for the body and the enlargement is. in many cases. hydrocephalic in nature. The abdomen is hard and protuberant, due to enlargement of the mesenteric glands. Flatulence plays an important part in this distention. The navel is sore and full of moist excrescences. The walls of the abdomen are very thin.

Great enfeeblement of mind is to be found in **Calc. carb.** The mind is so confused, that it does not apprehend or understand, even the simplest problems of life It is true that they listen most carefully or read, but their intellect does not seem to absorb even a portion of what they hear or read. At times the mind becomes complete blank, and fear is entertained by the patient's friends and relatives, of a complete state of imbecility, coming on the patient. This defective intellect, is quite in keeping with the general state of malnutrition, to be observed all throughout their sys tem. We must not, however, expect this state of mind in every **Calcarea** patient. Often the reverse state prevails. Inspite of bodily defect, the mind is seen to be in a state of over-activity as in **Opium** and **Nux. vom.** Thoughts rush in such quick succession, that they prevent sleep. They are in an utter state of apprehension about the present and the future. The mind is never at rest, due to a sort of fear of some impending calamity. This fear and anxiety, make them low-spirited and melancholy, and in consequence. we find them larchrymose. Sometimes this fear takes a peculiar form in the shape of a dread of insanity. They are afraid of losing their reason and are in a constant state of caution. lest people would find out the confusion of their mind. This anxiety and this dread are particularly worse in the evening. Sometimes they take the form of despair and hopelessness of ever getting well.

This is one of the first remedies we think of in scrofula. A great tendency towards glandular enlargement is noticed everywhere and nutrition becomes more and more defective. Inspite of the unwieldy mass of fat in undue places he is emaciated and shows signs of marasmus everywhere. His appearance is one of bloatedness rather than health.

The skin is unhealthy . The least scratch suppurates. Eruptions, ringworms, eczema, papules, pustules, acne, blisters, ulcers, encysted tumors. cystic swellings, lipoma and warts are everywhere to be seen

One thing to remember always in **Calc. carb.,** is the presence of glandular swellings. As in **Silicea.** a sister remedy. we find thick crusts forming. the result of dried secretions.

The eruptions are generally scaly with thick yellow pus underneath. It is a great remedy for fibroid tumors and numerous cures, have been reported through its agency.

The **Calcarea** patients are very susceptible to cold. The least bit of cold air goes right through them and brings on all kinds of ailments. A symptom, worth remembering and one that topples over many others, is a sensation of coldness felt in single part of the body, such as head, stomach, legs, feet etc. They find it very hard to keep them warm. Their appetite is uncertain and peculiar. We notice a great longing for boiled eggs, raw potatoes and flour. There is great aversion to meat and smoking.

It is a great remedy in defective dentition in children. They look fat and chubby, but are very slow in teething. These children, as is always the case in **Calcarea carb.,** are scrofulous and they are a constant subject to sour diarrhœa. Tardy development of bony tissues, lymphatic enlargements, open fontanelles, curvature of bones, profuse perspiration over the head, tendency to obesity with pot belliedness are guiding symptoms. **Belladonna,** though always useful in these conditions, does not go deep down to set the constitutions right. Undoubtedly, it helps the temporary derangement but the real spadework of setting the constitution right, is to be left to **Calc. carb.,** a great constitutional remedy at all times.

Calcarea carb., being the chronic of **Belladonna,** the presumption is, that we are likely to meet with a certain amount of congestion in the head, same as in **Bell.** The face is red and puffed and the patient complains of a concussive, stitching, pulsating, and throbbing pain in head, beginning in occiput and spreading to the top of the head. Great burning is felt in vertex as in **Sulphur** and **Phosphorus.** Confusion of senses and dullness of the whole head are marked indications. A still more characteristic indication, however, is a feeling of icy coldness in some parts of the head, as if a piece of ice is lying against it and this inspite of all the congestion mentioned beforehand. The strangest symptom of all is, that inspite of this coldness, we have copious, exhausting sweats over the head. So profuse is this sweat that it rolls down the face in large bead-like drops.

Being a scrofulous remedy, there is no dearth of scrofulous ailments of the eyes, ears, and nose in **Calcarea carb.** It is used in keratitis with great photophobia and morning agglutination of lids. There is stinging pain in eyes, worse from candle lights. The pupils are usually dilated. It is also used in scrofulous and arthritic ophthalmia. The lids are red, swollen, painful and itching. The conjunctiva is inflamed as well. There are numerous vesicles with pus on cornea. Of course we must not forget the light hair, blue eyes, the distended abdomen and the enlargement of gland on neck and elsewhere. It is a well-known remedy in cataract as well with chronic dilatation of pupils. Lachrymal fistula, induration after styes also come under its influence.

On the ear, it produces thickness of the tympanum, with all symptoms of defective hearing. Ringing, buzzing, singing, hissing and thundering noise in ears lead to many perversion of hearing We also have muco-purulent otorrhœal discharge, due to ulcera tion with accompanying inflammation of the parotid glands.

On the nose its influence is no less marked. It is a great remedy for chronic nasal catarrh, which is, at all times, a barometer indicating scrofulous diathesis. The wings of the nose are thickened and there is an offensive discharge which is both purulent and bloody. It works admirably in polypus of nose as well as of the ears.

A great trait which we must not lose sight of in **Calcarea carb,** is a constant tendency to diarrhœa. It is of frequent occur- rence. Inspite of all precautions, at all odd times, it comes on to the great annoyance of the patient. The stools are of varying character although we mostly find them to be whitish, sour, fetid and undigested. Sometimes to start with, they are hard and then become pasty and finally absolutely liquid. It is extremely use- ul in diarrhœa of psoric children, specially during dentition. The pit of stomach becomes swollen, and looks like an inverted saucer. The stools are involuntary and foamy. A great characteristic s intolerance of milk; as soon as it is taken, it is either vomited out in sour curds or ejected through rectum in white curdled lumps. Appetite gets ravenous. On these indications, it may be used in summer complaints of children, or in genuine cholera in- antum. Prolapsus ani are of frequent occurrence. The abdomen s sensative to pressure, due to heavy accumulation of flatus. colicy pains about umbilicus, certain amount of nausea, great gurgling in right side of abdomen, swelling and hardness of the mesenteric glands, clay-colored evacautions, ascites, general emaciation (except in abdomen), enlargement of liver and finally pressure and pain in the hepatic region, aggravated by every movement are symptoms, too guiding to lead us astray.

In constipation the stools need mechanical assistance as in œ, **Sanicula, Selenium, Sepia,** and **Silicea.** The constipation, is generally complicated with hæmorrhoidal affections and it is mostly mucous hæmorrhoids that we find in **Calcarea carb.**

Calcarea carb., with such extensive influence on the human economy, affects the sexual aspect and revolutionises the sexual life of the man and the woman. On the male it increases the sexual desire and provokes emission. It also makes up for the evil consequence of onanism and too frequent indulgence. It removes lassitude and weakness and stops frequent involuntary nocturnal emissions. The condition for which it is particularly useful is where the sexual life, though on the wane, is not utterly dead. Lascivious fancies excite desires, but the organ has become too frail for an erection, and emission takes place too soon with consequent weakness of limbs and excitement of nerves. It also rectifies induration of testicles, inflammation of prepuce, warty growths on sexual organs, smelling like old cheese and herring brine.

On the female sexual system a similar condition is observed and there is undue excitement leading on to nymphomania. It is particularly useful in flabby, plethoric girls who grow too rapidly and in whom menstruation starts too early, flows very profusely, and lasts too long. The flow is provoked by over-exertions and emotions. Therefore these patients are practically never without a show of their period. A little physical exercise or the least excitement, as that caused by any emotion, ushers in a return of profuse catamenia. They feel none too well before menstruation. Headache, aching of backs and hips, pain and swelling of breasts, leucorrhœa, mental excitability and amorous dreams are particularly troublesome at this period and even when menstruation stops, they linger on. Sometimes the flow is so excessive as to amount to a regular hæmorrhage. These hæmorrhages are very often due to abnormal growths in the uterus or a such fibroid tumor or a polypus. Calcarea patients are particularly troubled with leucorrhœa, especially between menses. The discharge may be thick yellowish, but it is specially indicated in leucorrhœa occurring before puberty and in infants. In this connection we might as well mention that it is a great remedy in chlorosis in young girls. They look apparently healthy but it is really plethora more than health. They look robust, as if beaming with health, but on examination it is found that they are sadly lacking in red blood corpuscles. Suppression of menses, in women of such leucophlegmatic temperament, generally leads to lung complications, which may be easily avoided by the timely administration of the deep acting **Calcarea carb.**

Calcarea carb. profoundly influences the urinary organs. It is applicable in diabetes, albuminuria, polypi and varices of the bladder and hence we come across all kinds of urine in **Calc. carb.** It may be clear, milk-white, or full or blood, but the one outsanding feature is the strong odor. Once smelt, it is always remembered. The desire for urination is quite frequent. The patient has to run and pass a few drops of urine several times within the course of an hour. Trickling of urine after micturition, involuntary passage of urine on every motion, nocturnal enuresis may also be present.

Calcarea carb. exercises a very useful function in putting right many of the deviations occurring during pregnancy. In the first place it helps conception. In many instances, when all the organs of conceptions, are found to be tolerably in good condition, and still where conception does not take place, due to some constitutional dyscrasia, **Calcarea carb.** causes conception to take place readily. Then again, when menses continue, still after pregnancy, it cheeks the flow and prevents miscarriage. Like **Nux.,** it also checks vomiting and toothache during pregnancy. Cramps in toes and soles of feet, a frequent occurrence during pregnancy, give in readily under the influence of **Calc. carb.** We use it also in false labor pains, when they run upward. Unless stopped, these pains prove particularly deleterious, and serve only to reduce the strength of the mother. Under the influence of **Calcarea** we see these obnoxious symptoms disappear and child-birth becomes a matter of ease and safety. Then again **Calcarea** comes in as a great help in phlegmasia alba dolens. It removes the inflammation, reduces the pain and dispels the swelling. It also becomes useful in various disorders, relating to secretion of milk after child-birth. It is almost like a panacea in all such disorders, arising out of excessive or deficient secretion of milk. It checks galactorrhœa as well as helps to remove scantiness of the flow of milk. It goes even further, and improves the quality of the mother's milk. Often we find, due to a disagreeable nauseating taste, the child would not take to the breast. It cries itself hoarse and still would not suck. A few doses of **Calcarea** given to the mother sweetens the milk and the child devours greedily what he disliked so utterly only a while ago.

We will now study its action on the respiratory organs. It is useful in all varieties of complaints beginning from ordinary bronchial catarrh to pneumonia and phthisis. It is particularly useful in chronic bronchitis when complicated with emphysema. The sputa is yellow, lumpy and sweetish and when thrown into water, it resembles a falling star, as the heavier portion while setting at the bottom, draws behind it a long trial of mucus. It is a very useful remedy in phthisis in all its stages. We use it in the prodromal stage when the patient, generally of leuco-phlegmatic constitution, emaciates rapidly and complains of such symptoms as sour eructations, diarrhœa with prolapsus recti, palpitation, nocturnal emissions, irregular or profuse menstruation, spasmodic cough, clammy extremities, chilliness and sweating of palms of hands and soles of feet. It may be used in the advanced stage as well when large cavities have formed specially in the middle third of the right lungs and all the symptoms described above have become more pronounced.

Before closing I would like to emphasise on a piece of caution, dropped by Hahnemann, which is, that this remedy should not be used before **Nitric acid** or **Sulphur,** as it is likely to bring on unnecessary complications.

We will last of all discuss the application of **Calcarea carb.** in fevers of various types. It is indicated in the Intermittent fevers of potters, brickmakers, gardeners, fruitgrowers, and those other people, whose occupation in life, makes exposure a matter of everyday necessity. It is not the type of exposure found in **Aconite, Rhus tox.** and **Bryonia..** It rather resembles **Dulcamara** where the patient has to work, standing in cold water. As a result of such occupation, the patient starts with a sensation of drawing pain in all the joints and great heaviness of the head and the limbs. These prodromal feelings are followed by a distinct sensation of chill, beginning in stomach, accompanied with an agonising sensation of weight, increasing with the chill and disappearing with it. The limbs feel icy cold and the patient finds it very difficult to get them warm, though covered warmly. The stage of heat is free from thirst. Great orgasm of blood, gives a sensation, as if the patient had been drenched with hot water. During this period he is tortured with anxiety, and a heavy despair, regarding his life which he finds difficult to shake off, inspite of all his determinations to do so. The next stage which is the stage of sweat is characterized by want of thirst. The constitutional symptoms, the psoric cachexia, should never be lost sight of, in the selection of **Calcarea carb.**

It is equally indicated in typhoid fever at its very onset. The symptom that leads to its indication is a state of utter sleeplessness due to over-activity of mind. At first it may look like **Opium, Nux** and **Bryonia** from which remedies it ought to be closely differentiated. The over-activity of mind in **Calcarea** takes a peculiar form. He finds no rest because of some disagreeable idea, always lingering in his mind, and rousing him, as often as he falls into a light slumber. He sees horrid visions before his eyes. In his delirium he plays with cats and other animals and talks about fire, mice and murder. Palpitation, a tremulous pulse, anxiety, exhaustion and weakness are determining symptoms.

It is recommended in epilepsy, where immediately before the attack, the aura starts, with a sensation of something, running in arms, or from pit of stomach down through abdomen into feet. Vexation, fright, onanism and suppression of chronic eruptions are principal important idiopathic factors.

Case 1.—D, aged forty-five, quarrelled with his aliopathic doctor, who advised preparing for death. Breathing heavy and difficult; face waxy pale; face and head bathed in perspiration, running off in little streams; violent palpitation of the heart; lower extremities cold, so much so that all summer he had slept with a feather bed over him, while his body was bathed in perspiration, especially the head. Vertigo on going up stairs, or up a hill; bloating in the region of the stomach, compelling him to open his clothing; appetite poor, with an aversion to meat and a craving for boiled eggs. **Calc. c.** 6m, three times daily, cured in five weeks.—Dr. W. D. Hall.

Case 2.—W., paper-hunger, had a fit three months ago, followed in six weeks by three more in succession, remaining insensible for twelve hours after them. Day before I saw him, had three more which left his mind confused. Pale and haggard; mouth half open; eyes starting; starting at the least noise; hands cold, clammy and trembling; he continually interrupted his wife saying, "let me tell," and then would seem to forget and say, "yes, yes, yes"; words seemed to stick in his mouth as if his tongue was too large. The fits of yesterday had convulsions only on left side; began with a cold feeling in the hand which crept up the arm to the cheek, when a gush of ice-cold water came from his mouth, which water "gave the mouth a nasty state." The peculiar sensation was repeated three or four times before the fit. During—left side of face red; right side—hands and feet cold and white. After—complained of ringing in the ears as of a hundred bells. **Calc. c. 2000** cured.—Dr. T. F. Allen.

Case 3.—Dr. R. aged thirty-five, taken sick yesterday, with great prostration, great heat all over, strong desire to sleep with sleeplessness; pain in all the limbs; want of appetite and aversion to light. He took **Bell. 200,** one dose. Next day,—had not slept, mind was too active, but they were always the same ideas which disturbed him; continued hacking cough, from tickling in bronchia, aggravated and excited by motion or talking; expectoration, tough green mucous; cough caused violent stitches in head; head pained all over, felt numb; tongue white, showing imprints of teeth; pulse small—empty, frequent, 94-106; no appetite and slight thirst; great prostration; lowspirited and taciturn; no stool for forty-eight hours; urine scanty and seldom. **Calc. c. 200**, one dose (prescribed by Dr. Hering and self in consultation) cured in five days.—Dr. Ad. Lippe.

CALCAREA FLUORATA.

Calcarea Fluorata is our Calcium Fluoride. It was proved by Dr. J. B. Mell on himself and others in 1874. It is found in the surface of bones and in the enamel of teeth. Homœopathic literature is replete with instances of bony growths and various other diseases of the bones having been cured with this remedy. It is also efficacious in indurated glands.

I have used this remedy with great satisfaction in opacity of the cornea. The patient's vision is blurred, and he has flickering and sparks before his eyes.

In osseous growths and in suppuration of bones, it acts favourably after **Silicea** and **Calc. phos** have failed. Dr. Farington cured a case of necrosis of the lower jaw in a lady with **Calc. fl.** after everything had failed.

The relation of homœopathy to surgery is a very delicate one. That surgery is useful and beneficial is undeniable. To gainsay this would be utter folly; but still I have come across people, who vaunt of curing every surgical case with homœopathic medication. This great faith owes its origin to some marvellous cures effected by homœopathy. We must not forget that surgery has got its own domain. There will be cases when surgical interference will be absolutely necessary. The case, referred to by me just now, is such as to excite great confidence in the mind of the homœopath and make him justly forget the delicate line that divides homœopathy from surgery. I can do no better than cite the case in Dr. Farrington's own language. " This summer a lady came to my office, with what the dentist had pronounced to be necrosis of the lower jaw on the left side. The teeth had been removed by him, but the patient, instead of getting better, grew worse, and there was a continual discharge from the cavity. The molar, just back of the one taken out, had been filled with gold, which I found on examination to be rough at its root, and when she would press her jaws together tightly, there would ooze, apparently from its fangs, a fluid which was offensive, dark and bloody, and mixed with fine pieces of decayed bone. The gum around the bone was purple and offensive in itself. The dentist had said that a surgical operation was necessary. The first remedy given was **Silicea,** which seemed to have some effect. This was followed by **Fluoric acid.** These two remedies are complementary, and you will frequently find in bone diseases that you will have to give one after the other. **Fluoric acid** is especially indicated when **Silicea** has been used. It is also indicated when **Silicea** apparently does some good but fails to complete the cure. Now in the case I have just related, Fluoric acid also helped for a while, but improvement again came to a stand-still, and now I noticed a swelling of the bone on the outer surface. This led me to think that **Calcarea fluorica** would act better, and I gave it in the sixth trituration. This she has been taking since the first of August. A week ago, the discharge had entirely ceased. The tooth which had been filled with gold was no longer painful. Pink granulations were springing up all over the gums. The probe can no longer detect bone which is diseased."

Dr. W. P. Wesslehœft has reported two cures of syphilitic periosteal swelling—one on right radius and one on left ulna with **Calc. fl.** cm. potency. Dr. Hate, too, has cited several cures of osseous tumours with **Calc. fl.** in lower potency. The great Dr. Constantine Hering has cited a case of a rough hard bony swelling, covering the whole width of shin-bone in a young lady, who was formerly treated for periostitis of the humerus. **Calc. fl.** cured the case in three weeks. Other bone affections, such as swelling of the lower jaw-bone, swelling of the elbow joint, osseous tumors on the spine, of scapula, affection of the phalanx, tarsal and carpal indurations, have all been cured with this wonderful remedy.

The discharges in **Calc. fl.** are offensive, thick and greenish-yellow. Hence it finds its application in catarrhal affections as well.

CALCAREA HYPOPHOSPHOROSA.

This is Hypophosphite of lime. This salt was originally proved by A. R. Barret, who took one grain of the 2x trituration. The main symptoms experienced, were heavy pressure on top of the head, feeling of oppression around the heart, dyspnœa, profuse sweat and pallor of the skin.

Personally I cannot speak very much in favour of or against this remedy. My reason for taking it up, is that I have been vastly impressed with the cure that Dr. Nash made with this remedy in a person, who had several abscesses in and around the knee-joint—ugly abscesses that had gone as far as the tibia and had eaten away half of the bone exposing the ragged necrosed osseous tissue underneath.   Here is another instance of a cure that leads the homœopath on to a firmer faith in his science.   Cases similar to this are not infrequent, and they are the ones to beguile the homœopath into pronouncing hard, unscientific dictum on surgery; not that they do not believe in the usefulness of surgery, not that they can dispense with it altogether, but that circumstances in their own life and in the life of other brother practitioners of their own school, had shown them, time and again, that where surgery was deemed absolutely essential, and that where even surgery wavered, Homœopathy snatched away the laurel with the greatest of ease and nonchalance. Dr. Nash's language in this connection is very impressing— " The little fellow was greatly emaciated and had no appetite, and was as pale as a corpse. I told the mother that I thought this was a case for the surgeon, but I would try to get him in better condition for the operation. I remembered reading once before, of the cures of abscesses by this remedy, made by Dr. Searles of Albany, and empirically concluded to try it in this case.

I put him upon the first trituration, a grain a day. Called in a week and found a great change for the better. The mother exclaimed as I came in: " Ah, Doctor, the boy is eating us out of house and home." Under the continued use of the remedy he made a complete and rapid recovery, except that the tibia was a little bent. I have since used the remedy in some very large swellings, where pus had formed, with the effect of complete absorption of the pus and no opening of the abscess on the surface. One was a case of hip-joint disease which had been pronounced incurable by a specialist on ulcerations. (How is that for a specialist, regular at that). The different combinations of the Calcareas ought to be so thoroughly proven as to enable us to put them each in their exact place. So, also, with the Kalis, Magnesias, Natrums and Mercuries, etc."

CALCAREA PHOSPHORICA.

This is phosphate of calcium. The component ingredients are lime and phosphorus. It is a great remedy in defective nutrition. Hence, it is often used in children, who are predisposed to glandular and bony diseases, slow development of teeth and spinal curvature. Children who suffer from rickets, who are slow to grow. and who, though well-fed, never assmiliate and in consequence look puny, pot-bellied and unhealthy, whose fontanelles and sutures take long in closing, whose skulls are soft, thin and fragile, are the ones to come under the influence of this remedy. The neck is so thin and weak that it cannot support the head. It is, therefore, a grand rejuvinator. It puts new life into such diseased atoms and renovates, rebuilds and redirects the flow of vitality into the proper channel; it transforms such scrap materials into splendid structures, into—what we call happy, healthy and forceful individuals. Mentally these children are as deformed as their physical bodies. There is lack of memory. They are dull and obtuse. Hence **Calc. phos.** becomes particularly useful in bad effects of mental strain, such as headaches in school children of a weak intelligence.

The digestive system is just as wrong. The child vomits milk persistently, whether it is breast-fed or brought up on artificial food. Colic is a constant companion. There is stomachache on every attempt to eat. Incipient tabes of mesenteric glands are frequent complications with these children. They are as equally prone to diarrhœa as our **Calc. carb.** patient. The stools are green. slimy, undigested, hot, watery, spluttering, and extremely offensive During stool there is emission of much offensive flatus. The child has an anxious expression on its face. Sleep is restless; but still the child is drowsy all day. The emaciation is so great that child looks old and wrinkled. It is better indicted in those moribund cases of chronic diarrhœa in children where constant, continuous and persistant purging has led on to a hydrocephaloid condition. Grauvogl recommends it very highly in chronic hydrocephalus. He even advocates it as a preventive in hydrocephalus. It has been recommended as a prenatal remedy during pregnancy to women who have given birth to hydrocephalic children.

Calc. phos has many important symptoms of the sexual system both in the male and in the female. Sexual desire is increased; erection is painful, it occurs even while riding in a carriage. In the female we notice nymphomania with incessant desire, particularly before catamenia. The sexual parts feel alive with blood. She feels pulsations in the parts with an increase of sexual desire. Even urination brings erection of the clitoris. There is leucorrhœa which is of a creamlike consistency. The menses are profuse and the patient is weak and consumptive. The catamenial flow is dark. We notice labour-like pain before and during catamenia. Throbbing, stinging, tickling and pressing pains in the genitals, going up towards symphysis and downwards to the thighs are mostly present.

We must not forget the characteristic craving in this remedy. There is desire for salt, smoked neats and for bacon. The tongue is white, furred, with disgusting bitter taste in the morning, when waking up. Hunger is more felt at the special hour of 4 P.M.

It has been recommended in Diabetes Mellitus where the lungs are implicated. It is of great service not only to the lungs but also in diminishing the quantity of urine and lowering its specific gravity.

Case 1.—Miss S. G.—, thirty-one years old, of a delicate texture and blonde complexion, with large blue eyes, and highly nervo-lymphatic temperament. She is of a small delicate frame and a strumous constitution, where lymph predominates. About fifteen years ago, she took a severe cold, which resulted in pneumonia of the left lung; since then, she has suffered more or less every winter with pulmonary trouble, which has increased until it resulted in a true case of scrofulous pneumonia. Muco-purulent phthisis set in permanently some years ago. Such was the history of the case. The crepitant rales were heard all over her left lung, with dullness on percussion. The cheesy expectoration, indicative of yellow tubercle, the slow but steady progress of the disease, the pain in the lungs and great loss of strength, appetite and flesh, with fever at intervals, though yet able to be out, more or less, and generally quite comfortable in summer; the enormous expectorations of a viscid, yellow-white character—these peculiarities belong to scrofulous phthisis. When I examined her the first time, I found her left lung entirely hepatized, with the exception of a few spots; her voice was hoarse, and the breathing bronchial. This lung was much contracted, with little expansion in breathing. The right lung I found in a better condition, but crepitating under the axilla, and painful at times. The pulse was natural in the morning; high in the afternoon, till about 9 P.M. At night she was restless; the cough being paroxysmal and very distressing. After **Acon., Hyos., Puls.,** and other remedies, I finally prescribed **Calc. phosph.** 3d dec., one powder of two grains, every two hours. After a few days I found her expectoration much diminished in quantity and more liquid; the crepitant rale became less audible, the sonorous rhonchus disappeared and the sibilant rale here and there was often heard. The voice became stronger and less tremulous; fever disappeared; the nightsweat also became less troublesome; her appetite also improved; her diet consisted of oysters and beef-tea, with raw pounded beef in old whisky, to be taken three times a day. At intervals I used hypophosphite of lime by inhalation, which seemed to answer very well. As she became anæmic, I prescribed hypophosphite of iron and Arsenicum. The **Calc. phos.**, even in this desperate case, proved a very efficient remedy.

Case 2.—A child was cured, after the failure of other remedies by **Calc. phos.** 2c on the symptoms of "longing for bacon, ham-fat," etc. Dr. E. A. Farrington.

CALCAREA PICRICA.

It is the Picrate of Calcium. This remedy too has not been well proved, but we have a few important clinical indications worth remembering.

It is a remedy, par excellence, in peri-follicular inflammation. Like **Arnica** and **Picric acid** it is helpful in painful boils, in the meatus of the auditory canal.

CALCAREA SULPHURICA.

It is the Sulphate of Calcium, from which we get our supply of Plaster of Paris. This remedy has not been proved sufficiently; but what proofs we have had lead us to the conclusion that it is a kindred remedy to **Hepar sulph** and **Silicea.** Dr. Clarke advises its application in cases where pus has already found a vent. It differs from **Hepar sulph** in its sensitiveness to atmospheric changes. **Hepar sulph** cannot stand the draught, the same as **Bell** and **Psorinum** where **Calc. sulph** is distinctly better in open air.

My experience of this remedy has been very limited. I have used it once or twice in abscesses after **Hepar sulph** had failed. There was no special indication to guide me to it except that **Hepar sulph** did not do its work. Dr. Nash, who used this remedy with signal success, in a case, where there was a great discharge of pus in the urine, and which was diagnosed by a Chicago specialist as a case of Bright's disease, had also no particular indication, to give us as a guide.

CALENDULA.

It is our favourite Marigold. The tincture is prepared both from the flower and the leaves. It belongs to the same category of remedies as **Arnica, Rhus tox, Hyper, Staphi, Ledum** and **Symph.** It is thus an important member of our homœopathic vulneraries. I have used this remedy most extensively in my practice and I find it intensely soothing and antiseptic. It restores the vitality of the injured parts, and acts as an impregnable barrier to infections and germs. It prevents suppurations where suppuration should be prevented, and it brings on healing with wonderful promtitude. It is suitable to all cases of injury where the skin is broken and where the soft parts have been lacerated. I have used it, times without number, in carbuncles and ulcerations and all varieties of septic wounds. It has been used by me as a compress (an ounce in a pint), both hot and cold. After surgical operations, it promotes healthy granulation and arrests gangrene. It can be used both internally and externally, and it is an excellent hæmostatic

Case 1.—On Sunday, Mr. S. found occasion to throw stones at a troublesome cat that interfered either with his siesta or his devotional frame of mind. Be that as it may, on the following Tuesday he experienced intense pain in the right shoulder and arm. Pain comes on in paroxyms, worse on moving the affected arm; relieved by lying perfectly at rest and on walking about the room. Part sensitive to the touch. Tongue slightly furred, bowels constipated, pulse and temperature normal. Neither **Rhus.**, **Bry.** nor **Arn.** gave any relief, though used in different potencies. Hot applications relieved for a short period, but soon lost their good effect. On the evening of the third day of treatment, the pain was so excruciating that I was tempted to inject morphine, but gave **Calendula** 3x, and was rewarded by a good night's rest on the part of the patient, who only suffered one severe paroxysm after taking the remedy. The recovery was rapid and satisfactory.—Dr. H. M. Dayfoot.

Case 2.—A boy, aged ten, fell on the stairs, his chin coming in contact with a chair standing upon the landing at the bottom of the flight. The lower lip was divided, and a deep incised wound made in an oblique direction for three inches, to the angle of the jaw. There was not much hæmorrhage, considering the extent of the injury. Five sutures were required to draw the two sides of the wound into apposition. A pledget of lint, soaked in the tincture of **Calendula,** was applied, and although the whole of the lower part of the face was much ecchymosed from the force of the fall, the wound healed by the first intention, and has left but a slight linear cicatrix, which is scarcely discernible at a short distance from the lad. We have no doubt that plastic surgical operations would be more successful if this preparation were more generally used.

CAMPHORA.

Camphor is obtained from Laurus Camphora, a very handsome plant growing plentifully in China, Japan, Isle of Formosa and a few other adjacent places. This drug too, like many others, was first introduced into our Materia Medica by Samuel Hahnemann.

Living, as we do, in the cholera zone of the world, it will be unwise to leave **Camphor** out of our Materia Medica. It typifies the collapse stage of Asiatic cholera. It is indicated when the patient sinks low, and still keeps on sinking, till at last his face hangs and his whole body becomes icy cold and blue. His face grows hippocratic and pinched; cold sweat stands in drops on his face; his voice turns husky and his sight becomes bedimmed. Even the tongue of **Camphor** is cold. The voice is almost lost. If he can at all speak, the voice is either high-pitched or husky. We have also cramps in **Camphor** but it is less pronounced than in **Cup. met.** There is marked nausea in **Camphor** and the expression is one of utter despair and intense agony. Difficult breathing, due to spasm of pulmonary arteries, is markedly present. The nose becomes cold and looks almost pointed. The cold tongue looks flabby and almost trembles. We have insatiable burning thirst. The collapse of **Camphor** is sudden and overwhelming and is not as in **Veratrum alb.,** due to excess of purging and vomiting. In fact it often comes on after the cessation of vomiting and diarrhœa and can be only accounted for, by a profound disturbance of the nervous organisation.

A great characteristic of **Camphor,** that often helps us to differentiate it from other remedies, is a great dislike to be covered, notwithstanding the icy coldness of the entire body.

It is an important remedy in mania with melancholy. Violent rage is characteristic of **Camphor.** The patient scratches, bites, and tears her clothes and foams at the mouth. Great precaution is necessary or else she would throw herself out of the window. We also have incessant fits of crying in **Camphor,** which the patient is hardly able to explain. The whole condition is one of indescribable wretchedness.

Camphor, as has been mentioned before, is an excellent remedy in summer diarrhœa, cholera infantum and Asiatic cholera. The attacks are very sudden and are characterized by sudden sinking of strength. The stools may be rice-water stools or blackish like coffee-grounds. The urine is either scanty or suppressed.

Intense burning is felt during urination. The pulse is weak, almost imperceptible.

It is a great remedy in shocks. We think of it particularly in asphyxia of new-born children. It is good to remember that like **Cuprum, Zinc,** and **Gelsemium** it is an important remedy in re-percussed eruptions.

Camphor is serviceable in pernicious fevers. The stage of chill is long lasting and without thirst. Icy coldness of the body, death-like paleness of the face, excessive sensitiveness to cold air, dislike of covering, slight heat without thirst and profuse cold exhausting sweat are the indications.

One great characteristic of **Camphor,** that I have omitted to mention, is that most of its pains are felt when the patient is oblivious of it. A distinct improvement is noticed as soon as the patient starts thinking about his complaint.

CANNABIS INDICA.

Cannabis indica is our Indian hemp. It grows most plenti-fully in the sub-division of Nowgong in the district of Rajshahi. It is much used by the natives of India, Arabia and neighbouring countries as an intoxicant. It is collected in three forms; the flowering tops of the female plant are known as Ganja, the leaves supply what is called Bhang, and the resin exuding from the plant supplies the world with Charas. This resin, in combination with opium and other narcotics, makes up what in Arabia goes by well-known name of Hashish. A decoction made from the leaves, is a beverage with many of the inhabitants of this country. The effect produced is, an inebriation of an agreeable character. It excites the individual to sing and laugh, and causes pleasant and gor-geous visions, hallucinations, and a sense of ecstasy. It produces a sort of temporary delirium During intoxication, the sensual propensities of the individual are stimulated.

The effect produced by **Cannab. ind**. varies considerably ac-cording to the mode of administration. When the fumes are in-haled, the effects are more lasting. Taken into the stomach in the form of a beverage, its action is slow and temporary. It is an anodyne and antispasmodic and as such it ranks with **Opium.** It is not a dangerous drug, but one which gets stronger and stronger hold of the individual and gradually drags him down to the lowest strata of degradation The man gets thin and emaciated; muscles and fat gradually deteriorate. In the habitual smoker of Ganja, the voice becomes harsh, discordant and grating. It is a sedative. It has proved of value in the aged, when the mental faculties are weakened and when restlessness and sleeplessness have become prominent symptoms.

In the homœopathic therapeutics it is a remedy of considerable value. The most important characteristic of **Cannab. ind.** is the state of exultation. This makes **Cannab. ind.** very rich in mental symptoms. We notice great gaiety and disposition to laughter at the merest trifle. There is sudden transition from one fantasia to another. He uses enthusiastic language and is full of loquacity. Ideas flow in quick succession in his brain and he is ever busy making theories.

Hallucinations and imaginations are most active. He feels as if his body is swelling and he is becoming larger and larger. He hears numerous sweet sounding bells ringing all around him. He seems to float in an atmosphere of music. As soon as he shuts his eyes, he gets lost in the most delicious thoughts and dreams.

Exaggeration of time and space is a prominent feature. A few seconds seem an age; a few yards seem an immense distance; time to him is interminable, and space illimitable. This excess of imagination makes him incoherent in his behaviour. He is full of fun and mischief. He laughs till his face becomes purple and his aching in loins.

These symptoms are not all. Forgetfulness crowns the list of his folly. He begins a sentence but cannot finish because he forgets what he intends saying. This last symptom of forgetfulness has been verified by Dr. Nash who prescribed it with great success in a lady, who after being relieved of the superfluous dropsical fluid, found herself unable to talk. This inability to talk was due to utter forgetfulness. With **Canna. ind.** she rapidly recovered her power of expressing herself.

CANNABIS SATIVA.

This is the European and American hemp. It belongs to the same natural order as **Cannab. ind.** It is practically the same plant as the other one, but due to difference of soil, the properties are different. In this remedy the genito-urinary symptoms are most prominent. It causes acute inflammation of the mucous membranes of the urethral passage. The most chracteristic indication is the extreme sensitiveness of the urethra. The patient cannot walk in a healthy, normal way. Due to the inflammation having spread through the urethra into the bladder, there is pain with frequent desire to pass urine which is usually bloody. It is thus a splendid remedy in the treatment of gonorrhœa, especially in the inflammatory stage when the above mentioned symptoms are usually in existence. Phimosis is an oft present indication. The penis is swollen. There is thick purulent discharge. Urine is difficult to pass. It is passed very slowly and in small quantities. It causes intense burning and obstruction and interferes with free urination due to spasm of the passage. Priapism, nocturnal emissions of bloody substance, redness, swelling and sensitiveness of the prepuce and pressing, dragging sensation in testicles when standing, are symptoms to be constantly bourne in mind. A peculiar dropping sensation of the heart is also to be met with in **Cannab. sat.**

Case 1.—June 28. Mrs.—was confined May 15, and had much hemorrhage; since then very weak; giddiness when walking, with feeling of falling (once she actually fell forward), and at the same time feeling as if she would lose her senses; every day pain in right temple and vertex, as if opening and shutting; it begins when she wakes and lasts all day, off and on; it is worse from noise; head feels as if it would fall in all directions; for last week, voices, including her own, seem to come from a distance; her own voice seems strange, as if it were somebody else speaking from a distance; memory bad; forgets when speaking what she is going to say; forgets what she has to do if she does not make a note of it; appetite poor; does not like meat, of which she used to be fond; time seems prolonged, especially for last week or two; every day faint feeling, sometimes faints right off; cannot follow long what persons say to her; seems to be in a dream, as if things were not real; feels at times as if she were somebody else; sometimes feels as if she did not know where she was; objects seem strange; nasty taste in mouth on washing; it goes off after cleaning teeth, but returns after meals; when writing repeats or omits words; after looking long mistiness before eyes, so that she cannot see well. **Cann. sat.** 1000 (Jenichen) cured.—Dr. E. W. Berridge.

Case 2.—Threatened abortion from Gonorrhœa.—A robust lady, æt. fifteen, in her first pregnancy, in the eighth month, discharged blood from vagina, until apprehension of premature confinement was excited, after **Sabin.**, passed clots of blood; neither **Secal.** nor **Pulsat.** improving. She finally confessed to suffer a burning in making water, while with it a purulent matter passed off. **Can. sat.** 6 restored her within a week. It was discovered that her husband had gonorrhœa before she was ill.— Dr. M. L. Sircar.

Case 3.—An old gentleman, a clergyman, of nervo-lymphatic temperament, having been for years afflicted with stricture of the urethra, was finally much relieved by bougies. There remained however, an obstinate urging to urinate which was irresistible. He was often obliged to run out of the house to answer this irrepressible spasm of the bladder. He was cured in about a week by **Cannabis 30**, four pellets every night.—Dr. J. C. Morgan.

CANTHARIDES.

This medicine is prepared from the Spanish fly, an insect about an inch long and yellow-green in color; it thrives on the leaves of poplar, ash, elder, etc. It is killed, dried in the sun and then reduced to a coarse powder. Five parts by its weight of alcohol is added to it and after a certain period of saturation the tincture is poured off and filtered.

The symptoms of **Cantharides** that should be written in flaming characters on our memory, are constant intolerable urging towards urination and a furious burning cutting pain in the urethra before, during, and after micturition. This needs a little explanation. The feeling, that he must urinate, is constantly on him. Oftentimes this is so exaggerated and intensified that it becomes simply impossible for him to withstand the desire; but the idea of the suffering, that micturition brings on, makes him shudder. We have simply to see such a case to appreciate the immensity of the suffering. Urine does not come out with its natural flow. There is a constant dribble and every drop feels like molten lead. I remember treating a case of this kind in an engine driver years ago; the suffering of the man, was so utterly unbearable and agonising, that it even now, seems to be an occurrence of yesterday. The urine itself is frequently bloody and the straining to expel the few drops of this bloody accumulation is intense. We find him passing urine every two or three minutes. Fibrinous casts, epithelial cells and little pieces of mucous membrane, from the lining of the bladder and the tubules of the kidneys, are plentiful in the urinary secretion. These symptoms when present would indicate **Cantharides**, in diabetes, cystitis. stricture, gonorrhœa prostatitis, renal colic and other ailments.

On the sexual system the influence of **Cantharides** is equally prominent. It increases the sexual desire to such an extent that sleep is disturbed at night and frightful satyriasis, painful priapism with voluptuous and frequent nocturnal emissions become common. These painful and persistent erections often bring on cutting pain along the spermatic cord to the testicles, which feel as if drawn up.

On the skin the action of **Cantharides** is prominently marked. When applied locally, it produces inflammation rapidly developing into vesication. These vesicles fill up with yellowish white serum. These bullæ, as they are called, are so large that the parts look as if burnt or scalded. On these indications it may be applied in burns. It thus becomes a very important remedy in burns as well. Hering recommended that the injured parts should be bathed constantly with a solution of **Cantharides.** He has challenged septics to burn their fingers and then immerse them in a solution of **Cantharides.** This, we feel certain, will lead to a cure of all their septicisms and a confirmation in the immutable law of similars. We use it in psoriasis, pemphigus, eczema and variola, when vesicles are numerous and the affected parts look burnt as if from fire, as often happens from a local application of the drug. It is particularly useful in erysipelas, especially of the vesicular type when it begins on nose and thence spreads over the cheeks and other parts.

The stools of **Cantharides** in dysentery are of white or pale red tough mucus. They look like the scrapings of the intestines, as we have seen in **Carbolic acid.** .The patient experiences, violent colic and urging before stool; during stool there are burning and cutting in anus extorting cries from the patient; after the stool the colic is alleviated, but the tenesmus continues. The most important point in this dysentery is the association of the tenesmus with dysuria. This last named symptom, helped me to score a decisive victory in a case of dysentery in a child of three. Physicians of both denominations, allopathic as well as homœopathic, treated the child for months without success. They forgot to notice that the child had to strain considerably, every time it wanted to evacuate its bladder. A few doses of **Cantharides** brought a very speedy cure.

The mental symptoms of **Cantharides** are worth noticing. It is useful in mania and delirium when we have violent paroxysms of rage, tearing of clothes, biting and kicking. They bark like dogs. Amativeness is also very characteristic. Aggravation is caused by bright dazzling objects and touch.

CAPSICUM.

This remedy is prepared from the Cayenne or the red pepper. The most striking symptom of **Capsicum,** is its intense burning and smarting as if Cayenne pepper were sprinkled on the parts. It is generally indicated in people of phlegmatic diathesis, who are fat and indolent, averse to exercise of any kind and who are exhausted very easily. They are constantly chilly and consequently dread open air. It thus resembles **Belladonna, Hepar sulph., Nux vomica, Psor., Calcarea** and **Baryta carb.**

It affects, principally the mucous membrane of the body, where it produces a sensation of constriction. It also affects bones, particularly the bone of the face.

A very great characteristic of the remedy is a burning pain, same as what is produced by the application of red pepper on the skin. This burning is aggravated by the application of cold water and by the slightest draught of cold air.

Mentally, **Capsicum** is very taciturn, peevish and obstinate. Great clumsiness and awkwardness, somewhat similar to what is found in **Bovista,** is present in **Capsicum** and this is more perceptible when the patient is suffering from a bad headache. It is our principal remedy for home sickness. Sleeplessness, a desire to commit suicide, and a gradually deepening melancholia follow in the wake of this home sickness. Red cheeks and the characteristic sensation of hot feeling in fauces, also characterize this home sickness. Dr. Clarke cured with a few doses of **Capsicum,** an Australian girl who had come to study in London and was quite incapacitated by it.

Capsicum is an excellent remedy, in diseases of the middle ear, specially in caries of mastoid process. At my hand it has given instantaneous relief, to the intense pain and burning, so frequently, associated with such cases. It is equally efficacious in many of the affections of the throat such as angina faucium, diphtheria and gangrene. The odor from the mouth is unbearable and almost carrion-like. Mouth becomes exceedingly dry and the tongue has a coating of tough, yellow mucus. A similar accumulation of congealed mucus obstructs the posterior larynx. Elongated uvula, burning smarting pain in fauces associated with a sensation of constriction of throat, intense dark redness of fauces and pharynx, are constantly present. Pain is not altogether absent and is mostly felt not while swallowing but between the acts of deglutition. A symptom particularly characteristic of **Capsicum** is a sensation of shuddering felt by the patient while drinking.

Bell calls **Capsicum** one of the royal remedies for dysentery. The stools are full of mucus and blood. In some cases, the slime becomes adhesive, with occasional presence of numerous streaks of black, coagulated blood. Every stool is followed by thirst and every drink by shuddering. Tenesmus and burning in anus continue far after the stool is over. It resembles **Cantharis** in the simultaneous presence of tenesmus of the bladder and rectum, but it lacks in the other keynote symptoms of **Cantharis**. One more important symptom that accompanies this dysentery is backache. Commonly this is expressed as a drawing pain in the back.

Regarding its action on the urinary organ, we notice burning in the bladder, burning in the whole channel, and the orifice of the urethra. The patient suffers from frequent unsuccessful desire to urinate. When passed the urine scalds and smarts. It is also useful in the second stage of gonorrhœa, when the discharge assumes a creamy appearance, and when the chrodee is so violent that the patient is compelled to seek relief by immersing the parts in cold water.

The cough of **Capsicum** is very peculiar and should have our special attention. It is nervous and spasmodic. Everytime he coughs, there escapes a volume of pungent fetid air from his mouth. Another point is that the patient feels pain in distant parts when coughing such as bladder, knee, legs, ears, etc.

Capsicum is a valuable remedy in intermittent fever. The thirst commences long before the chill comes on as in **Eupatorium** and **Natrum mur,** but it is wanting in the bone pains of the two remedies. The chill commences on the spine between the scapulæ, with great thirst, but drinking water causes shivering and increases chilliness. This chill is relieved by hot iron or jug of hot water to the back and by walking out of doors. During this stage of chill he becomes sensitive to noise. Irritability particularly too becomes more prominent at this time.

Both the stages of heat and sweat are without thirst.

Case 1.—An hysterical woman received quinine for chills, owing to the difficulty in getting symptoms. They stopped, but returned in two weeks. After three weeks of unsuccessful treatment, she said: " Isn't it strange, every time the chill is going to come on, I begin to d ink"? **Capsicum 2 c.** one dose, cured; she had only one chill after. —Dr. R. W. Martin.

Case 2.—Mrs. B., æt. sixty-one, of nervous temperament and full habit, by exposure too soon after an attack of chills and general congestion, had a relapse, with symptoms of pleuro-pneumonia in the extreme lower anterior portion of the right lung. Respiration labored, and about 60 per minute; breath a little fetid; pulse 115, dry, hacking cough, and great nervous excitement. The administration of ordinary remedies indicated, for three or four days, relieved some symptoms, and modified others. The breath at times became quite fetid, and there came a distinctive cough in sudden paroxysms at intervals of one to two hours; nervous, spasmodic, very explosive cough, convulsing the whole body. At each such explosive effort, and at no other time, there issued from the lungs a volume of air, of a most pungent, fetid odor, with an offensive taste in the mouth. Whenever such a coughing spell occurred, the air of the room became so badly tainted, that the daughter, who attended the patient, was obliged to leave the room. At other times, the breath and eructations from the stomach gave out no fetor. Expectoration of a dirty brown, but not rusty color. With each cough there was a "catching pain" in the region of the liver and lower portion of the right lung. Natural movement of bowels every day. In no place could I find anything like such a cough described, except in Jahr's old unabridged Symptomen Codex, under **Caps. an.** "When coughing, the air from the lungs causes strange, offensive taste in the mouth. When coughing, a badly smelling breath rushes out of the lungs." I gave the first dose of **Caps.** at an evening visit (one dose only for the night), and the next morning was informed that there had been no paroxysm of the cough during the night, to the great joy and relief of the patient. The cough returned, however, at various intervals, for a period of two weeks, when there was an entire recovery from it under the administration of **Caps.** Several times I omitted the Caps., and gave other remedies that seemed indicated by other symptoms, and invariably noted that the fetor and cough returned very soon after the effect of the **Caps.** had passed off. I also noticed that after each administration of the **Caps.**, the effect lasted about twelve hours, and not more than fifteen. The only attenuation used was the 200th.—Dr. A. R. Wright.

CARBO ANIMALIS.

This valuable remedy is prepared from Charred ox-hide. It is specially adapted to the scrofulous diathesis, venous constitutions, and in old people, who after some debilitating disease, have become greatly enfeebled. A marked disintegration of tissue is seen everywhere. Poorness of circulation and bad oxygenation of blood are manifested by the blue color of the limbs in general. Hands and feet look blue with distended veins showing through everywhere.

A great feature of this remedy consists of utter debility felt particularly after menses. It is so over-powering that she can hardly talk or walk. Another important symptom is a sensation of coldness felt in different parts of the body. The weakness, so characteristic of this remedy, is felt even in the ankles. They sprain easily from the slightest exertion. It is a great remedy with us for weak ankles in children whose feet turn under them while walking.

The most prominent action of the remedy, however, is seen in its action over the glands which get inordinately indurated and hypertrophied. This involvement of the gland is universal. We have serious indurations in the mammæ, induration of the axillary and inguinal glands, as well as other glands and organs, of the human body. In mammary cancer, the gland becomes stony, hard, and there is a dirty, bluish, loose appearance of the skin covering it. The axillary glands in the affected side become indurated and the patient complains of a burning drawing pain through the mammæ. We use it in old maltreated syphilitic buboes that inspite of surgical operation and cauterization refuse to heal, and keep on secreting offensive discharge

In relation to the female sexual organ, it is important inasmuch as it is a valuable remedy in chronic metrorrhagia of cold cachectic women, who suffer from periodical hæmorrhage with great lameness of thighs and legs and yawn constantly with chilly waves running through them. This hæmorrhage, on digital examination is found to be the result of induration of the uterus and malignant ulceration of the os uteri. Leucorrhœal discharge is constant and it stains the linen yellow.

Carbo animalis is usually indicated in the last stage of pneumonia and phthisis pulmonalis, when huge cavities have taken place due to extensive destruction of lung tissue. Suffocative hoarse cough that shakes the entire brain, with expectoration of green, purulent, offensive mucus, and pus should draw our attention to this remedy I have been able to verify this symptom in the case of a young lady of twenty-five or twenty-six, who was suffocating to death, as a sequel of stagnation of the air cells in the lung tissue with extremely ichorous, offensive sputa which was being raised occasionally, but not in sufficient quantity, to bring actual relief. Dyspnœa was marked. The patient was covered with fœtid sweat, which was also staining her covering yellow. After great deliberation, even then with a certain amount of doubt as to the ultimate issue, **Carbo animalis** was prescribed. The result exceeded the fondest expectation. She recovered and is alive now, a healthy buxom woman of 35 summers.

Carbo animalis is used in far-sightedness.   While walking along the street, objects seem to be far off.   Another important symptom which I have omitted to mention is a sensation of looseness felt in various parts of the body.   Eyes feel as if they were lying loose in their sockets.   Even the brain feels loose when he coughs

Case 1. Struma Aneurismatica.—A woman, forty-six years old, complains since her first confinement, which took place at the age of twenty, of a swelling of the thyroid gland. At first it was scarcely observable, but has grown since to the size of a common apple. It is tense, uneven and pulsates clearly. If she wears a dress which is in the least narrow around the neck, it causes dizziness, and difficulty of breathing. External and internal application of **Iodine** had not had the least effect, and to be operated upon she could not assent, as the desired result could not positively be promised. Finally, she consented to try homœopathy.   Since two months she has missed her courses but instead, is troubled with a profuse leucorrhœa of a yellow-greenish color. For this I gave her **Sepia 10,** night and morning. Ten weeks after, the leucorrhœa was cured, but the swelling of the neck remained the same. As a mere experiment **Carb. an.** 6 was prescribed, one powder every fourth evening. The woman came not back. More than a year later, however, she came to express her thanks, and on examining her neck, there was not a trace left of the former swelling.—Dr. Payr.

Case 2.—Von H., aged thirty-three, in poor circumstances, of weakly constitution, pale and cachectic, very feeble, of constipated habit, with a poor appetite and a slimy, coated tongue, consulted me in April, 1831, for a severe pain in the back, which extended into the hip, burning pain in the bowels below the umbilicus, deranged menstruation, and very profuse discharge of slimy, ill-colored blood, accompanied by labor-like pains, which had, of late, made their appearance. Examination showed a considerable enlargement and induration of the uterus. After relieving the hæmorrhage and the most urgent symptoms by ordering laxative remedies and perfect quiet in the horizontal position, **Carbo animalis** was given in doses of three grains, three times each day. This treatment was continued throughout the following summer. Later, baths were ordered and the patient sent upon a pleasure trip. The enlargement and the induration gradually lessened, menstruation became regular, the countenance assumed a healthy look and the other symptoms disappeared altogether. A year later (1832) she again became pregnant, gave birth to a healthy child and has since then enjoyed a very high degree of health.—Dr. Schmalz in **Frank's Magazine, Vol. iv.**

CARBO VEGETABILIS.

"Lowitz, a German, discovered the properties of vegetable charcoal to deoderize and arrest putrefaction. It was first employed in medicine with success, externally, to fetid ulcers and eruptions, afterwards internally for flatulence—its employment all the while being based upon its chemical influence. It was left to Hahnemann to find out its real curative value on the principle of similia, by proving the triturated vegetable charcoal on healthy persons and then applying it in practice. His experiments were made on twenty or thirty different persons, who were strictly aloof from all medicinal influences. The cruder preparation failed to produce any symptoms of importance, but after potentization was carried further on, a steadily increasing number of symptoms was produced in sensitive persons and in animals. He used the **Carbo ligni betulæ,** but assures us that well prepared charcoal acts in the same manner, irrespective of the kind of wood used. The provings by Adams, Gersdrof and Caspari in the Materia Medica Pura, contained 1189 symptoms. We have had no provings since, excepting one by C. Neidhard, with the second centesimal trituration. The charcoal contains carbonate of potash."

This is a desperate remedy for a desperate condition, a condition where the vitality has been drained to the very bottom. Every feature of this patient speaks of the great drain, his system has undergone. The face is hippocratic, pale and ashy gray. It is covered with cold sweat; the eyes are dull and lustreless; he sees black spots floating before the field of vision, a sign of intense debility and profound prostration. The facial appearance speaks of great anxiety; memory is weak; flow of idea is slow; indifference and lassitude mark his behaviour everywhere; nothing affects him pleasantly or **unpleasantly.**

His great weakness, renders him an easy subject to vertigo. When he wants to move, he has to hold on to something for support or else he falls. A sensation of whirling is constantly experienced in his head. Fainting occurs at the slightest provocation; he faints after sleep, after rising or while yet in bed. Head feels heavy like lead. His gums are spongy and scorbutic. **The** teeth are decayed. Aphthæ or thrush are plentiful. His very breath is cold showing that the fire of life is about to be extinguished.

His breathing is short and labored, as if he has not enough energy left in him to draw in the necessary current of air. To minimise the exertion of respiration he wants to be constantly fanned. This difficulty of respiration causes cyanosis. His pulse is thread-like, weak and small, sometimes intermittent and almost imperceptible. To add to his distress, his abdomen becomes tympanitic, tense and inflated, which makes him feel very uneasy. Frequent involuntary cadaverous-smelling stools make his condition, already grave, more and more desperate.

It thus becomes an invaluable remedy in the final stage of many critical complaints.

From the above description of this valuable remedy, we must not be led to believe, that its application is totally confined to extreme conditions alone. We find in **Carbo veg**. an unrivalled remedial agent in lesser complaints such as dyspepsia or indigestion. In fact, it vies with some of the most important of our remedies applicable in disturbed digestion. The principal symptom is tympanitis, in consequence of which the epigastric region becomes tender and sensitive. With this tenderness there is also a sensation of rawness of the stomach extending all the way along the œsophagus to the middle of the chest. Great acidity of the stomach is complained of, and with this goes frequent eructation of wind. Tension is felt in the region of the liver which too is sensitive and painful. Colic attended with gurgling, the result of flatulence, is equally troublesome. The flatus passed, feels hot and is extremely offensive. Fatty food disagrees. Milk cannot be taken as it produces flatulence. These are symptoms of what we call chronic dyspepsia, and are the result of debauchery and excessive indulgence in rich and indigestible foods. **Carbo veg.** is particularly useful in such low adynamic form of dyspepsia, specially when it comes on after some exhausting and serious illness. They are frequently victims to hemorrhoids, the natural consequence of high living that clogs the liver. The hæmorrhoidal knobs are blue, and they frequently suppurate. The piles become more active each time they go on a spree. The temperament too, is peevish and irritable. The above symptoms also suggest **Lachesis, Nux vomica, Pulsatilla, Sulphur** and **Sulphuric acid.** Great deliberation is necessary to be able to arrive at the indicated remedy and to avoid confusion with many a similar ones.

Lachesis too, is a remedy for weak digestion due to vicious habits. Milk disagrees in both the remedies, but in **Lachesis** inspite of this intolerance of milk, there is a strong craving for it. **Carbo veg.** has fullness, heaviness and sleepiness after eating due mostly to flatulence, whereas in **Lachesis,** it is more a sensation of pressure than of fullness. It feels like a load, as if a stone was suspended in the intestinal region. The sensation of constriction, so characteristic of **Lachesis,** is wanting in **Carbo veg.** Then again in **Lach.,** the weakness is due to cardiac debility, whereas in **Carbo veg.,** it is due to profuse loss of some important fluid of the system. The craving for intoxicating liquor is very strong in **Lachesis.** In **Carbo veg.,** on the other hand the longing is wanting and it is generally used after bad effects of previous indulgence.

In **Nux vomica,** the condition is so similar to that of **Carbo veg.,** that at times, it becomes difficult to decide, as to which one of the two remedies, to resort to. The same fullness and sensitiveness to pressure are to be found. Pyrosis, acid eructations, borborygmi and nausea are same in two remedies, although in the latter remedy the intensity of the distention is more marked than in the former. The tympanitis in **Nux** is troublesome enough, but it has not got that bursting sensation that we have in **Carbo veg.** The **Nux** patient suffers from violent retching, more or less ineffectual, with a similar ineffectual urging for stool. The excessive irritability that marks the debauch of **Nux,** is far more to be dreaded than the cool distemper of the **Carbo veg.** patient.

Pulsatilla resembles **Carbo veg.** inasmuch as the etiology is same in both the remedies. The trouble originates in both the remedies without doubt, from indulgence in fat, rich and greasy foods. Flatulence, bitter or sour eructations are common in both the remedies but **Carbo veg.** lacks the sensation of lump in the mid-sternum. Neither has **Carbo veg.** aggravation at the peculiar time, when everything in **Pulsatilla** gets upset. It is more or less a case of slow digestion in **Pulsatilla,** as is evidenced by the bringing up of food, partaken several days ahead of the vomiting. The temperament and the thirstlessness in **Pulsatilla** are always guiding.

Sulphur has eructation, sour taste, fullness after eating, and strong craving for beer and brandy, and so far the similarity between **Sulphur** and **Carbo veg.** holds good. But the latter remedy lacks the abdominal plethora, the congested liver, the eternal piles, the constipation and above all the great hunger of **Sulphur** described usually as an empty all-gone feeling felt at about 11 A.M.

Sulphuric acid resembles **Carbo veg.** strongly in its sensitive epigastrium and in sour risings from the stomach. In both, the patient suffers from the bad effects of drinking, and in both have we got to deal with cachectic persons. But the main difference consists in the acidity of the former and the putridity of the latter remedy.

We will now discuss the action of **Carbo veg.** on the skin. Due to bad oxygenation of blood we have various forms of ailment arising from venous stasis. Ulcers, bed-sores are to be abundantly found in **Carbo vegetabilis.** They are flat with a tendency to spread in circumference. An intense burning, which becomes worse at night time, prevents him from sleeping. It is equally useful in carbuncles when the surrounding parts look livid and blue and the discharge is ichorous and fetid.

Charcoal from which this remedy is prepared, is as has been mentioned previously a great deodorant and disinfectant. In cases of carbuncles, ulcers and gangrenous degenerations we may use it externally as a sort of a poultice made up of a fine charcoal powder.

Carbo veg. is very useful in the collapse stage of cholera, but this collapse as has been mentioned before, is caused by the great drain on the vitality due to profuseness of its discharge. In **Camphor** the collapse is more or less due to a shock to the nervous system.

Carbo veg. is indicated in the more severe forms of dysentery where the stools show signs of putrid disintegration. Sopor. cramps, and symptoms of collapse, rarely found at the onset of a complaint, are its main indications.

Case 1.—I was called to a family (always allopathic, but wished to try Homœopathy as a dernier resort), and was brought before a child two months old, and apparently dying. The patient presented a hippocratic countenance, the eyes half open, nose pinched and cold, lips blue, pupils insensible; no complaining or crying from the child. The pulse I found small and quick, difficult to count, but beyond 130; the body thin, lean and marbled; feet and hands blue and cold, although constant application of hot cloths is made; abdomen distended with gas; respiration frequent, but not full. Auscultation revealed only tracheal sounds, and no vesicular murmur. The breath is cold. The previous history of the cause, although not very clear, was not more encouraging. The child had, during the last two months, three nurses ; since three or four days she had fever and a cough, and since noon has ceased to cough and to nurse; no stool or urine. Although preparing the parents for the speedy death of the child, I ordered a more frequent application of warm cloths, and in the meantime dissolved four globules of **Carbo veg.** 30, in seven or eight tea-spoonfuls of water. A few doses of this were given every ten minutes. The child improved from this time.—Dr. Gounard.

Case 2. Typhus.—Boy, aged fourteen. Third week, symptoms were: Unconsciousness; profuse, involuntary diarrhœa; abdomen distended; spleen enlarged; urine passed involuntarily; tongue dry, black, cracked; complete exhaustion; mucous rales in the lungs; dull sound on percussion, and respiratory murmur almost inaudible in posterior portion of tnorax; frequent, rough, hollow cough. Next day found him under the table, where he had fallen, in the midst of his excretions, cold, unconscious, almost moribund. After a few respiratory acts there would be an intermission of several respirations. At each respiration, the patient, with distorted features, snapped at the air, and gasped exactly like a dying fish; pulse small, frequent; skin cold. *Carbo Veg,* 200, every two hours and on the second day he was incomparably better. *Mur. acid* finished the cure.—Dr. Battman.

CARBOLIC ACID.

Carbolic acid is a powerful irritant poison and a great antiseptic. It acts primarily on the nervous system and produces deathly paralysis of respiratory centers. It is a coal-tar product and is an essential remedy in certain varieties of enteritis. The first time I ever used this remedy was in a case of this kind. A child of ten or eleven was suffering from mucus dysentery. The stools were full of big mucus shreds which looked like the scrapings of the intestines. Prostration was marked. A pale face covered with cold sweat, naturally reminded me of **Camphor, Carbo veg.** and **Veratrum album. Aloes, Cantharis** and **Colchicum** were tried but to no effect; **Carbolic acid** covered the totality of the case and cured it in a very short time. All the discharges of this patient were putrid.

Carbolic acid is a first-rate remedy in the adynamic type of diphtheria. It is characterised by absence of pain. The accumulation of the deposits in the fauces emits a very offensive stench. Excessive prostration and violent fever are also present. Great burning is particularly characteristic of **Carbolic acid.** The fauces look fiery red and are covered with diphtheric patches and exudations from the neighbouring glands, which are extremely swollen. The fever is high and the pulse extremely fast. Thirst is excessive but the liquids on being swallowed, are returned by nose due to blockage and constriction.

The pain of **Carbolic acid** is very characteristic. It is very much like that of **Belladonna** and **Magnesia phos.** It comes suddenly, lasts a short time, and disappears just as suddenly.

In headache **Carbolic acid** excels, when the patient complains of a sensation of a band tied tightly over the forehead from temple to temple. In this it is also similar to **Gelsemium, Cactus, Mercurius, Platinum, Sulphur, Nitric acid,** and **Spigelia.**

The urine in **Carbolic acid** is generally dark, smoky and greenish; and urination is accompanied by involuntary discharge of mucus from the anus. The smell is offensive. With regard to green urine we may also think of **Camphor, Arsenicum, Aurum** and **Colchicum.**

Nervous dyspepsia, of extremely painful character and in drunkards, has been cured by **Carbolic acid.** There is intense distress in stomach with deathly faintness and great sensitiveness to smells. The transverse colon suffers particularly from soreness. Diarrhœa and constipation come in alternation. There is also heavy flatulence. Breath is markedly offensive. We also notice a strong desire for stimulants and tobacco.

It has been often used with success in cancer, both of the stomach and of the uterus. We have strong menorrhagia in Carbolic acid. During hæmorrhage the patient looks almost bloodless and gets cold, clammy sweat. We also have profuse discharge of fœtid greenish, acrid matter from the vagina. The cervix uteri is indurated, ulcerated and corroded.

CARDUUS MARIANUS.

Carduus marianus is the holy thistle sometimes called St. Mary's Thistle. It is a native of Southern Europe and it grows plentifully in waste places. It was originally proved by Dr. Reil of Germany.

The tincture is prepared from the ripe seeds in the following manner. The seeds are covered with twice their weight of dilute alcohol and left in an well-stoppered bottle for a few days, the contents being regularly shaken. This is filtered and strained and we have the mother tincture of **Carduus marianus**.

Carduus mar. is pre-eminently a liver remedy. The whole range of its symptomatology proves its action over that organ.

Tenderness is felt in the left hepatic lobe where pressure causes oppression and cough. The other symptoms to follow are depression of mind, vertigo, dull heavy pain in forehead, eyes and temples, bitter taste. nausea and sour green vomiting. These symptoms remind us of **Nux vom.,** and they clearly show the great similarity that exists between these two sister remedies. At times the resemblance is so great that it needs the exercise of the greatest discretion to prevent confusion and mistake. **Nux vom.** as we all know, is a great remedy for affections arising out of alcoholic excesses, and so is **Carduus mar.** It remedies to a great extent the evil effects of alcoholic drinks, especially beer. I have used this remedy with great satisfaction in cirrhosis of the liver arising out of the same cause. Prœll relates two cases of cirrhosis of liver from over-indulgence in intoxicating liquors, in which **Carduus** helped. One was a cook and the other a brewery man, and they were so bad that they both developed dropsy. The indicated symptoms were flatulence, diarrhœa with clay-colored stools, fatigue and yawning after eating, chilliness, cramps, radiating stitching pains, and a peculiar sensation of band around the region of the liver.

I have used **Carduus** in jaundice in a lady aged about 55, who developed symptoms of icterus after an attack of gall-stone colic. **Carduus mar. Q** relieved the jaundice but not the irritation of the skin. Her symptoms were a dull headache, nausea, sour vomiting, heaviness in the region of the liver and a bitter taste in the mouth.

This remedy has been used with some success in gall-stone, and there are two cases on record by Dr. Liedbeck, who with half an ounce of the tincture in a pint of water, a table spoonful every two hours, cured two such cases in an admirably short time. I am also of opinion that **Carduus** not only expels the stones already formed, but if continued sufficiently long, also stops the formation of new ones. Dr. Nash reports of a case of gall-stone colic that he helped with the same remedy. He has not given us much of a symptom and his indications for this remedy are mainly negative. He says—"When other remedies fail for pain in the region of the liver, with dizziness, bad-tasting mouth, jaundiced skin and the usual symptoms called 'bilious,' if I have no especial indications for other remedies, I have given **Carduus,** and several times with very good results."

This remedy has also been used for ailments of the climacteric period such as megrim, metrorrhagia, leucorrhœa, asthma etc., with consequential disorder of the liver. In this way it is greatly similar to **Lachesis** and **Sulphur,** but in none of these two latter remedies do we find liver so afflicted as in **Carduus mar.**

CASTOR EQUIRUM.

This remedy was proved and introduced into Homœopathic Materia Medica by Constantine Hering. It is prepared from the rudimentary thumbnail of the horse. It is a small, flat, oblong, oval horn growing on the inner side of the leg above the fetlock of horses.

Hering recommends it in very high terms in cataract and ulcerated nipples of the worst kind in nursing women, and I feel, that we should all know something about it. Any remedy carrying such recommendation from such high authority should not be neglected. Times without number, during the course of your busy practice, you will come across cases, where the nipples, due to prolonged sucking by the infant, have turned extremely raw and sore. Fomentations, ointments and other measures as adopted by the attending physician having failed, knife the last help usually restored to in such instances is being contemplated. If you remember your master's eulogy about this remedy and do not fail to administer it, you will be rendering the most marvellous service and save her from the bright, shiny, sharp blade of the surgeon. Hering assures us, that even in neglected cases, where the nipple is nearly ulcerated off, and only hangs by small strings, where the reddened areola spreads for some distance around the nipple as in erysipelas, and where even axillary glands have become affected, this remedy will prove successful. It should therefore be compared and studied with **Asterias, Causticum, Graph.,** and **Phytolacca.**

CASTOREUM.

The medicine is prepared from a secretion contained in the preputial sac of the beaver. It resembles **Mosch.** and **Valerian** very closely. We find mention of this remedy in Galen, Hippocrates and Pliny. Most of our clinical symptoms of this remedy are derived from Trouseau and Pideux.

This remedy is mostly suited to nervous women and hysterical individuals. Dr. Farrington recommends it very highly in cases of weakness and prostration felt after a case of typhoid or any other exhausting illness.

Personally speaking my experience about **Castor.** is almost nil. What little I have gleaned from Hering, Allen and others will be given here. Dr. Hering speaks of using it with great success in a case of swelling of the tongue with a rounded elevation in the centre, the size of a pea surrounded by an angry, suspicious-looking base. It was extremely sensitive, and the patient felt a drawing sensation, as if a string was pulling the centre of the tongue towards the hyoid-bone. This looks like an important symptom. Cases of this kind, unless attended to immediately and successfully, may turn into a malignant sore.

Yawning seems to be an important symptom in this remedy. He yawns while suffering from abdominal colic. In diarrhœa, this symptom of yawning is present throughout the day. Even when he is sleeping, he is yawning constantly. We must, therefore, make an important note of this symptom.

Teste recommends it highly in amenorrhœa of nervous women. The abdomen is distended with wind and the pain starting in the middle of thighs, extends over to other limbs; blood leaves the uterus in drops, with tenesmus like pain.

We also use it in colic when confined to the small intestine. It is associated with paleness, coldness and sudden sinking of strength.

CAULOPHYLLUM

Caulophyllum is ' the blue cohosh.' It is one more of what we term the ' lady's remedy.' It acts specially on the uterus, and is very useful to women in the different stages of pregnancy, parturition and lactation.

We use it in congestive dysmenorrhœa with severe spasmodic pains in the first two days of menses. The intermittent nature of the pain is very characteristic of **Caulophyllum**. This is due to intermittent contraction of the womb. In this **Caulophyllum** differs from **Secale,** which produces continuous contraction.

The pains of **Caulophyllum** are spasmodic and they fly in all direction and during pain the patient experinces a sort of tremulous weakness over the whole body.

We use it also in leucorrhœa of little girls with moth-spots on their forehead and ptosis of the upper eyelids. This leucorrhœa is due to congestion of uterus, and is associated with a strong bearing down pain. The secretion of mucus from vagina is quite profuse, and it is accompanied by drawing pains in the lower extremities. The leucorrhœal discharge is sharp, acrid and weakening. The menstrual discharge in **Caulophyllum** is very scanty, and is preceded by pain in the small of back. Great aching and soreness of the lower limbs, bad breath, bitter taste, vertigo and chilliness are also present during menses.

The most important action of **Caulophyllum** however is seen in its application during pregnancy. It checks hemorrhage during pregnancy and prevents miscarriage. It is one of our best remedies to arrest the abortive process. Strange to say that its use in delayed and difficult labor is no less important. When the os becomes extremely rigid as in **Belladonna, Gelse., and Verat. vir.,** its use relaxes the rigidity of the os and hastens labor. Sometimes, as is very often the case, labor does not progress satisfactorily due to inharmonious action of the fundus and os uteri. When with the contraction of the fundus there is also constriction of the os, the result is exhaustion without the desired action; **Caulophyllum** establishes harmony of action between fundus and os and smooths labor.

Caulophyllum is an important remedy in rheumatism, but it has a special affinity for the small joints. Dr. Nash used it in the lower potency, in severe pain and swelling of the finger joints, in a pregnant woman. **Caulophyllum** removed the finger pains but brought on severe labor pains till its use had to be discontinued for fear of bringing about a miscarriage. With the stoppage or **Caulophyllum** the finger pain again returned. A sose of **Caulo.** high, rapidly cleared up the whole case. The internal trembling mentioned beforehand is a strong characteristic of **Caulophyllum.**

CAUSTICUM.

Causticum, a weak solution of Potassium hydrate, is a preparation peculiar to homœopathy. It is a polychrest. It is antisycotic, anti-psoric and anti-syphilitic combined in one. It is specially suited to patients who are melancholy, low-spirited and anxious most of the time, but particularly at that dread hour of evening, we call twi-light when shadows grow larger and the vanishing light of the day mingles with the darkness of the night. They are extremely timid, anxious and sensorious. The equilibrium of the mind is so disturbed that peace is nowhere to be found. They are apprehensive of some impending calamity; they are conscious-stricken, melancholy and despondent with a feeling as though they have committed some great crime. The anxiety referred to just now is associated with a frequent desire to pass stool. Redness of the face during anxiety with a frequent desire to pass stool is most characteristic of **Causticum.** They are sickly looking and yellow in complexion. In addition to the peevishness and irritability of temperament they are extremely suspicious and fault-finding. Another strange and contradictory feature of **Causticum** is that with this peevishness and irritability they combine an intensely sympathetic nature.

It is particularly useful in mental disorders, arising from long lasting grief, sorrow, and sustained night watching, and should therefore be compared with **Aur. met., Ignatia, Cocculus, Lachesis, Natrum. mur., Phos. acid,** and **Staphisagria.** Their complaints are always worse when thinking about them. **Causticum** patient is extremely chilly.

Causticum is a valuable remedy in chronic rheumatic arthritis and paralytic affections with contraction of flexors and stiffness of joints. In consequence of this contraction there is shortness of muscles which lead to various forms of deformity of the limbs.

The most important feature of **Causticum** is to be found in its tendency to cause paralysis of single parts. This is seen through-out the length and breadth of this remedy. We have ptosis of the upper eye-lids, which cause a sensation of heaviness. Paralysis of larynx causing aphonia, that of the muscles of throat causing difficult deglutition, and principally of the sphincter muscles of the bladder, causing either involuntary urination or retention are matters of every day occurrence in **Causticum.**

Another important feature is a sensation of rawness and soreness felt in different parts of the body. While coughing he feels it in the chest. A similar sensation of rawness and tenderness is to be found in many of its throat affections. In gastritis, sensation of soreness is felt at the pit of the stomach. In diarrhœa and other affections of the alimentary canal this sensitiveness causes him to loosen his clothing in the region of the loins; a similar sore feeling is also complained of, in the anus. It is thus almost an universal symptom in **Causticum,** and we must give due recognition to it.

Thirdly we must not overlook the paralytic weakness exhibit-ed by this drug. A faint-like sinking of strength is a constant complaint. The patient lolls about showing great disinclination to move or do anything. This is particularly the reason of his apathy and indifference. He is a great subject to vertigo which may be the precursor of oncoming paralysis. There is a tendency to fall either forward or sideways, on rising in the morning and sometimes even in bed at night. The sensation of weakness on which so much stress has been laid, accompanies this giddiness.

It is as well to discuss in this connection its use in spasmodic diseases such as hysteria, chorea, epilepsy and convulsions. Twitchings and clonic spasms are frequent. It is particularly useful in epilepsy occurring at the age of puberty, when connected with menstrual irregularities. Sometimes these attacks may be traced to a previous history of suppression of eruptions or to some fright The attacks are particularly worse during new moon, and is associated with involuntary micturition. Great uneasiness and fidgetiness are felt in the hands and the legs which are constanly on the go. However much they try, they cannot control these motions. During convulsions we have screams, gnashing of teeth and violent movement of limbs. These convulsive movements are often followed by real attack of paralysis.

In chorea we have constant twitchings of the muscles of the face. During sleep legs and arm are constantly jerked out. Speech is indistinct and the delivery is peculiar inasmuch as sentences are thrown out in spasmodic fashion with intervals between them. It principally affects the right side in preference to the left. The patient lies on stomach and keeps on making spasmodic jerks. The muscles of the face look distorted.

Causticum has been highly spoken of in deafness and in many affections of the ear. The principal symptom is a peculiar roaring buzzing noise in the ears which renders hearing defective. It is more of a sort of over-sensitiveness of the auditory nerve, that makes the slightest noise, resemble the roar of a distant cannon and this so over-powers, that other sounds fail to get an entrance. Even the patient's own voice reverberates; he speaks low for his own voice appears to him very loud. There is also a great accumulation of ear-wax of offensive odor in this remedy.

In the eye it produces symptoms which are of equally great importance. Intense photophobia is a troublesome symptom. It is so prominent that the patient is obliged to wink constantly. Flickering sparks and black spots before eyes are important indications of **Causticum.** They are constant. Sometimes they resemble swarms of insects before the field of vision. It is an excellent remedy for cataract. The patient feels a sort of obscuration of sight as though he was looking through guaze or a mist or as if a veil is drawn before his eyes. This dimness of vision becomes particularly objectionable, when he blows his nose. Also

we should think of **Causticum** in perpendicular half sight in cataract. Then again, there is the ptosis of the eye-lids referred to
beforehand. The sensation is one of heaviness in the upper lid as
if he could not raise it easily or as if it were agglutinated to the
lower lid and could not be easily loosened. He constantly rubs
his eyes to relieve this symptom of pressure and aggultination.
Being a scrofulous remedy, we find it indicated in scrofulous
ophthalmia, with corrosive lachrymation and shooting pains extending up to the head. Aggultination of lids with existence of warts
on eye-brows is a common feature.

    Causticum is a noted remedy in aphonia or failure of the voice.
This hoarseness may either be the result of paralysis of the laryngeal muscles, or it may be simply catarrhal. It is worse in the
morning, and is accompanied with a scraping sensation in the
throat. The whole canal down the chest feels as if it is raw and
denuded of its mucous lining. He has a sense of utter weakness
located in the region of the larynx. It is particularly thought of
in sudden loss of voice. The hoarseness may be accompanied by
a peculiar cough—a cough so characteristic of **Causticum** that a
mistake can hardly be permissible. It is violent and hollow, and
the patient is hardly able to expectorate. The patient feels as if he
cannot cough deep enough for relief or for expectoration of phlegm.
The sensation of soreness and rawness, spoken of previously, is
strikingly present. The cough is induced by a crawling sensation
in the larynx, and it is always worse after talking. Like the cough
of **Arsenic** we find that it is always worse on lying down. Another
peculiarity of this cough is that it causes pain in the hip joint,
and that it is followed by the involuntary passage of drops of
urine. Drinking cold water always relieves this cough. A sensation, as if lime were being slaked in stomach is a characteristic
sensation. The patient may not express his symptoms exactly
in these lines, but he will give you distinctly to understand, that
due to a putrid decomposition of food in the stomach, there is
a constant sensation of an acrid gaseous taste as if something
bitterly nauseous, is effervescing in the stomach.

    The action of **Causticum** on the urinary organs is of utmost
importance. It is indicated in involuntary urination, particularly
in children. This may take place either at night when they are
asleep or in the day while awake. In nocturnal enuresis, the emission of urine takes place during the first part of the night, after
they have hardly fallen asleep. At times this takes place, even be-

fore they have slept and it comes on so easily that they are hardly conscious of it. All sensations are wanting, and they only make certain of it, by feeling with their hands and finding themselves in a pool of urine. Then again, due to paralysis of the sphincter muscles, we have involuntary urination while coughing, sneezing and blowing the nose.

Causticum has a brilliant record of cure of constipation of the most inveterate type. The stools are tough and shiny and are covered with a shiny coating of mucus; sometimes they are passed in very thin pieces, scarcely larger than a goose-quill. The desire for stool is there, but it is rarely attended with success. The exertion needed is so great, that the patient becomes anxious and red in the face while defecating. It is the spasm of the rectum, that is responsible for this difficulty in passing stools, and evacuation is mostly attended with prolapsus recti. Then again we must not forget the opposite condition of involuntary escape of fæces with flatus. This is due to paralysis of the sphincter muscles of the rectum. The anus and the rectum are also the seat of great irritation. We notice large painful pustules near anus, discharging pus, blood and serum. There is also a sort of oozing of moisture from the anus. This constipation is frequently associated with hemorrhoids. The hæmorrhoidal knobs are hard, extremely painful and sensitive to touch. They particularly obstruct the passage and impede stools. They are particularly worse after standing. It will be an unpardonable omission not to mention that they are better able to pass stools standing. This reminds us of **Alumina,** where too, the patient prefers the standing posture, to any other, while passing stool. In **Medorrhinum** on the other hand the patient likes to lean backward to be able to pass stool. These symptoms are worth remembering, as they may prove of immense benefit at a critical moment.

On the skin its action is very characteristic. It cures itch, specially when it occurs on tips or wings of nose. Ill effects of burns and scalds come within its jurisdiction. Large pedunculated warts, exuding moisture, occurring in various parts of the body, have been removed with **Causticum.** These warts bleed easily.

In rheumatism we think of **Causticum** when the joints and the limbs get out of shape due to contractions of muscles and tendons. It affects principally the articulation of the jaw. The symptoms are invariably worse from cold, and better from heat and warmth.

Causticum may be called for in colic, when we have pains o a griping cutting character—a pain that is relieved by bending double similar to what we find in **Colocynth**. It is generally use ful after failure of that remedy, specially in menstrual colic. The menses come too early, and are too profuse with rarely any dis charge at night time. The pain is mostly felt in the back which feels as if torn and bruised. The yellowness of face, dizziness soreness in vulva and between legs, profuse leucorrhœa flowing lik menses and smelling same and smarting in pudendum as if from salt, are some more of the characteristic indications of **Causticum**

It is one more of Grauvogal's hydrogenoid remedies. Aggra vation is seen from washing, bathing, and relief comes from getting warm in bed.

Case 1.—Mrs. S., aged forty-six, full habit, dark complexion, phlegmatic deaf in both ears, worse in the right; no noises in the ear; ears dry in side, a little dark brown wax in the meatus externus. The tympani are covered with a similar shining mass. My voice appears muzzled to her. My cylin der watch was heard equally distinct on both sides, in the mouth and out side, half an inch before the right ear, and not at all on the left. She speak low, because her own words appear to her very loud. On turning he head, cracking and snapping in the ears. She is worse in the mornin Turn of life, her menses omitted one month, and then came on wors **Caust**. 80m, one dose cured.—Dr. B. Fincke.

Case 2.—Miss R., aged twenty, attended a meeting exposed to a sno storm, and indulged in vocal exercise. On returning home, experienc slight tickling and pricking in larynx accompanied by cough and no expe toration. During the night dryness and soreness of throat and fever, hoars ness and a deep cough set in, having a croupy sound. Articulation becam difficult as the hoarseness increased. The voice became extinct, and th patient could not speak above a whisper. All the while she had complain of soreness in the throat and pricking in the larynx. **Aconite** 6 was fir administered for an entire day, after which there was less fever: **Hep Sulph.** 6 was given, and before another twenty-four hours the charact of the cough was changed, whitish mucus expectoration in which the were no streaks of blood. During the next twenty-four hours the sor ness and pricking in larynx nearly disappeared and the cough was le severe; remained much the same for one or two days, expectorating co siderable tough, greenish mucus. Cough worse at night . **Hyoscyamus** two or three doses; expectoration increased in quantity, and quite a numb of lumps of thick, heavy mucus were thrown off, and yet there was restoration of the voice. **Causticum** 30 and 200 were given with good effe and hoarseness gave way and the patient was able to speak aloud.—Dr. A. Small.

CEANOTHUS AMERICANUS.

This remedy of recent date, has been prepared from the chopped and pounded leaves and pulp of the New Gersey Tea.

Though this is one of our new remedies, its claim as a great antidote to malaria, has been established without dispute. Drs. Hale, Burnett, and Majumder have cited numerous instances of its efficacy in the above complaints. The symptoms are enlargement of spleen with dull pain and fullness in the left hypochondria, chilliness and shivering principally down back, and dyspnœa and palpitation on exertion. All symptoms are aggravated while lying on the left side. In many instances it completes the cure where **Natrum mur, Cedron, Eupatorium** and **Arsenic** have left the work partly finished.

CEDRON.

We are indebted to Teste for the introduction of **Cedron** into the Homœopathic Materia Medica. The trituration is prepared from the seeds, and also a tincture is made from the entire fruit. It is a South American tree, also growing in the West Indies. Teste's attention was first drawn to this remedy by its tradional reputation in intermittent fevers. He also wanted to find out if it was indeed a specific for bites of venomous serpents, and stings of poisonous insects, for which it had a great reputation amongst the natives of Panama. We have the testimony of Mallert that it is so, who was bitten by a coral snake. The violent aching pains at the heart and in throat, that came on within a few seconds of the snake-bite, was immediately relieved by the chewing of its leaves and swallowing a small portion of **Cedron.** He also applied it locally over the sore; other after-effects were also removed, as if by a magic, by his partaking of a little more of the same fruit.

We have numerous proofs of **Cedron** being a first class remedy in malaria, specially of the quotidian type. We will come to a proper discussion of this later on. It is specially adapted to women and to persons of nervous, excitable temperament and of volup-uous disposition. Choreic attacks, epileptiform convulsions and trembling, are to be constantly seen in these patients. We also notice a great aggravation after coitus. She complains frequently of pain over her eyes, of languor, debility and lassitude after each act. I may as well mention in this connection that **Cedron** is a valuable remedy in menstrual epilepsy. Precursory symptoms, such as vertigo, tinnitus aurium, palpitation, irregularity of heart's action commence precisely on the same day, as catamenia starts. Then with aura epileptica the patient loses consciousness. We notice a distressing cry now and then, alternated with risus sardonicus and foaming at the mouth.

Lastly we come to the most important feature of **Cedron**—a characteristic that will enable us to recognise it, amongst thousand other remedies—I mean the clock-like periodicity in the recurrence of its symptoms. All symptoms come at regularly stated times, precisely at the same moment, and on the same day. This feature makes **Cedron** such a valuable adjunct in the treatment of marsh fevers. The fever which lasts from 15 to 17 hours recurs precisely at the same hour of the next day, week or month. The time of the attack may be either morning or the evening. But whatever time it starts on the first day, it is sure to recur at the same hour in all its successive attacks. This unerring periodicity, is the most important thing to remember always and everywhere in **Cedron.** The prodromal stage is marked by great mental excitement and exaltation of vital energy. The face gets red and hot. The stage of chill is marked by a general coldness, renewed by every movement as in **Nux** and **Cinch.** In the stage of heat he gets a strange craving for warm drink as in **Cas., Chel.,** and **Sab..** He would not touch any thing that is not warm during this stage of fever. This dry heat is soon followed by a state of profuse perspiration. In this respect, too, it is similar to **China.** The differentiating point, however, between these two remedies consists in the fact, that in **Cedron** the three stages are not so well marked and clear cut as in **Cinchona.** With the chill are intermixed heat, and hot fiush, felt in the hands, face, and particularly in the brain. Heat likewise is intermingled with shivering, shaking and cold limbs. Sweat though profuse in both remedies is not so debilitating as in **Cinchona.**

CHAMOMILLA.

Chamomilla is a plant which is also called Corn-Fever-Few. It grows in uncultivated fields, among wheat and corn, especially in sandy regions all over Europe. The plant grows to the height of one to two feet. It was first proved by Hahnemann.

The juice is extracted from the whole plant when in flower. The extracted juice is then mixed with an equal part by weight of alcohol.

Here we have to deal with the ugliest remedy in our Materia Medica—ugliest in the sense that nobody likes the company of our **Chamomilla** patient. If it is the husband, the wife soon gets tired of him; if it is the father, the child is afraid to approach him— he is so snappish; and if it is the child everybody else in the house except the parents, would rather have him dead. These patients do not know what they want; they are unhappy and they make everybody else around them so. It is very difficult to please the **Chamomilla** babies. Various things are wanted that are not to be had, and which when procured and offered, are refused with disdain and discourtesy. In this **Chamomilla** resembles such remedies as **Antim. tart., Cina, Antim. crud.,** and **Iod.** They are all peevish and irritable, but it is not at all hard to find out the lines of demarcation between them.

In **Antim. tart.** there is often the complication of rattling cough, the cold blue pale face, the irresistible sleepiness, and the tendency to vomit.

In **Cina** the symptoms of worms are very prominent—the canine hunger, the sickly white and bluish appearance around mouth, the pitiful weeping and whining, the screams and starts during sleep, the ever present digging and boring at the nose speak strongly against any other remedy.

In **Antim. crud.** the red strand of thick milky white tongue, indicative of gastric derangement, the longing for acids and pickles, the cracks at the labial commissures and the crusty nostrils, should easily disperse the prescriber's doubt and confusion of mind. Unlike the Chamomilla patient, he is quite unwilling to be touched or looked at, far less to be carried about. He is happy when he is neglected.

In **Silicea** we have a scrofulous rachitic child with open fontanelles and sutures, much sweating about the head, and a distended abdomen.

There is a remedy in our Materia Medica with just the reverse symptoms. Exceedingly affectionate, laughing, dancing, and whistling like a ray of bright sun-light, **Croc. sat.** kisses everybody around them—this mood very often alternating with the reverse symptom of crankiness.

It is also a remedy for the bad effects of violent emotions. When headache or colic or jaundice or some such like affection takes place due to extreme mental disturbance, we should think of **Chamomilla.**

It is a great remedy for dentition in children, and as such it bears a certain amount of resemblance to **Belladonna.** The baby starts during sleep, and is quite restless. Twitchings of the muscles of face and hands are also prominent. These symptoms though suggesting Belladonna should be looked into more minutely, and then it will be found that the face lacks the uniform congestion of **Belladonna.** It is true that one cheek is flushed and that the head is covered with hot sweat and that there is certain amount of fever, but still the intense erythism of **Belladonna** will be found lacking everywhere.

Moaning is quite characteristic of this remedy. We find this both in children and grown-up people. When the child is refused anything, it moans most piteously. The same is noticed in grown-up people who moan continuously on account of some trifling displeasure which arose out of mere triviality quite a long time ago. **Chamomilla** patients are quite averse to talking. They are short tempered, snappish and disinclined to talk. This snappishness is so pronounced in babies that they become quite stiff, bend backward, kick and scream in season and out of season, with reason and without reason, and nothing in the world would pacify them except being carried about. We find a similar impatience and irritability in women also. This is most pronounced during menstruation when they get extremely quarrelsome and headstrong. This impatience under pain means great excitability of the senses.

Chamomilla is one of our best pain-killing remedies, but not in the sense, in which our friends of the other school use morphia and other benumbing drugs. It simply cures the pain. Many a time and oft, have I seen the most distracting pain, leave under the influence of a single dose of **Chamomilla.** The pain is simply unendurable. It drives the patient to despair. Hahnemann says: "It is their peculiarity that they are worse at night, when they often drive one to the border of distraction, not infrequently accompanied by unquenchable thirst and heat and redness of the cheeks; also with hot sweat on the head and scalp." This is a general statement that holds good in Chamomilla pain, wherever it may be—tooth, ear, abdomen and heart. There is one other distinguishing feature about the pain of **Cham.** and that is numbness accompanying the pain. A few other remedies where pain is associated with numbness are **Aconite, Rhus tox, Platina, Kalmia,** and **Gnaphalium.** It is not at all difficult to discriminate between them.

In **Aconite** the pain may be just as intense, but with the pain and numbness, we notice tingling and formication. The constant fear, anxiety, restlessness and thirst make it impossible even for the variest tyro to make any mistake about its identity.

In **Rhus tox,** numbness is the most characteristic feature. The patient tosses about but not in agony as in **Aconite.** There is temporary relief from movement and it is in expectation of this that he tosses about.

In **Platinum** the pain increases gradually and decreases just as gradually. The irritability of **Chamomilla** gives place to the haughtiness of **Platina,** and the sexual symptoms come more in prominence.

The pains of **Kalmia** are stitching, darting and shooting. They move in a downward direction and are attended with or succeeded by numbness of the affected part. It is particularly useful, when as a sequelæ of gout and rheumatism, we notice a secondary derangement of the heart.

Chamomilla is very rich in gastric symptoms. We find it indicated in gastralgia, the effect of anger, brought about by the slighest contradiction. A pressive pain in stomach, as from a stone, is particularly characteristic of this remedy. A sensation of fullness and distention in hypochondria, nausea, eructation of putrid gas smelling like bad eggs, heat and sweat of face, bitter taste of mouth in the morning, a yellowish white coating on tongue, and collection of saliva of a sweetish metallic taste in the mouth, are a few more of its symptoms worthy of remembrance.

Chamomilla produces a peculiar green diarrhœa, and it is in the treatment of this complaint, that homœopathy easily proves its excellence and vindicates its principle. Regulation of diet, the use of purgatives and cathartics and the employment of many scientific methods, the outcome of much deliberation even fail in checking these abnormal-looking evacuations of the bowels. The hot, foul-smelling, corroding stools, looking almost like chopped eggs, changing frequently to a yellowish greenish color with all the accompanying symptoms of fever, crankiness, twitching of muscles and colic indeed show a desperate condition. It is impossible to estimate, how many such cases, after the failure of the dominant system of treatment, have been helped with **Chamomilla.** I feel certain every homœopath can vouch for the truth of this assertion.

Chamomilla is our great stand-by in some of those trying labor cases where there is great rigidity of the os uteri—cases that try to the utmost the skill of the most expert obstetrician. Labour pains press upward and is most spasmodic and distressing. The os is rigid preventing parturition. The patient is extremely hysterical, snappish, and fault-finding. There is also a great desire for fresh air. These long continued labor cases respond immediately to **Chamomilla.** Great trouble can thus be avoided, and a lot of unnecessary troubles saved, for the poor women, if only homœopaths would take pains and prescribe the proper remedy at the proper moment in the proper potency.

Chamomilla is also an invaluable remedy in threatened abortion. The discharge of dark blood, frequent urination, restlessness, yawning and shuddering with pregnancy predict serious trouble. **Chamomilla** prescribed on these indications will stop miscarriage. It is used in puerperal convulsions as well, specially those coming after a fit of anger.

Chamomilla is rarely thought of in fevers, although it makes admirable cures when indicated. There is chill without thirst. He shivers when uncovering or undressing. Another great characteristic is the intermingling of chill and heat at the same time. Certain parts of the body are extremely cold and chilly, whereas other parts feel hot like fire and this condition alternates. The whole body feels cold, but the face burns intensely—the breath feels hot. The posterior part of the body feels chilly, whereas the anterior part of the body is hot to touch. This state of alternation of symptoms with redness of one cheek and paleness of the other during febrile excitement is most guiding. The stage of heat is long lasting, and is characterized by violent thirst. He starts frequently in sleep. The same intermingling of heat and shivering is also to be seen in this stage. Great agitation, anxiety and the intense irritability of temperament seem to be more pronounced at this stage. The patient sweats most profusely over the face and the head, and the perspiration is hot,

Case 1.—W., aged forty, after exposure to a draught, got tearing in teeth and cheek. The pains continued in spite of leeches, creosote, clove oil, opium, etc., with aggravations and ameliorations for nearly a month; along with them were ptyalism and swelling, first of the cheek, then of the chin; the pains did not arise from any one tooth; they were worse in the night; he could not then lie in bed, he had to walk about his room for hours. The teeth are not loose nor decayed; they are hardly painful to touch, the gums are at present not affected. The pain seems to be owing to chronic irrita· tion of the nerve of the teeth and jaw. The pains yielded to **Cham.** 1, every three hours, in twenty-four hours.—Dr. Watzke.

Case 2.—A maid, aged twenty-four, has been suffering, at every monthly period, intense agony, partly from headaches but chiefly from painful menstruation. Her sufferings have lasted from puberty. A lady physician in New York, diagnosed retroversion of the womb. The headaches and a burning, drawing pain in the middle of the back, which was constant; with canine hunger, worst at 11 A.M.; great thirst; hot flushes of the face at times, and weakness of the knees, as if she would sink, were removed in about a month by **Sulph.** 3d. once a day. **The agonizing pain during menstruation** remained unmitigated, and resisted, **Bell., Coff., Puls., Sepia** and **Sulph.,** all in the thirtieth potency. Once only in three months was it relieved by **Nux vomica** 200. I was first consulted on the 7th of December, 1874, and, although her general health was greatly improved, it was not until April, 1875, when her headaches returned, that I observed **she was very irritable when spoken to, both before and during the flow of the menses. Chamomilla.** One week before menses, when her irritability begins, she has pains like those of labor, always in the morning before breakfast, with sickness and vomiting of her meals. Headaches, with throbbing in both temples, with a bursting feeling in vertex, relieved by pressure and cold; aggravated by reading, by bright light, and by looking at an object fixedly. Her sufferings ceased off generally on the second day after the flow was established. Eight years of the most intense suffering, as above described, was brought to a close; cured by **Cham.** 10m, in three doses of globules during the period, having been preceded by **Cham.** 3d, one globule every night during the interval.— Dr. Thos. Skinner.

CHELIDONIUM MAJUS.

The tincture is prepared from the extracted juice of calendine, a perennial plant growing in Germany, France and other adjacent countries.

The most striking action of this remedy is confined to the liver, and many of its symptoms are traceable to affections of that organ. The symptom that is considered most guiding is a constant pain, under the lower and the inner angle of the right scapula This brings to mind the name of a few other remedies such as **Kali carb, Mercurius, Chenopod, Rananculus, Angustura, Lobelia-s, Sanguinaria** and **Bryonia.**

Both in **Kali carb** and **Mercurius** we find sharp pains, through right lungs to back.   In **Chenopod.** the pain is found a little lower, on the right side, somewhat near the spinal column.   In **Rananculus** the pain extends from the inner angle of the left scapula to chest.

The other characteristic symptoms of **Chelidonium,** all indicative of deranged action of the liver, are a bitter taste in the mouth, a broad and flabby tongue that takes the imprint of teeth, thick yellow coated tongue, dirty yellow color of complexion, yellowness of the whites of eyes, grey white and clay-colored stools, high colored urine staining the linen yellow, nausea, disgust for food soreness and tenderness of the region of the liver, and a great desire for hot drinks.   Prescribed on these indications **Chelidonium** cures all sorts of complaints, such as gallstone, constipation, pneumonia, dyspepsia, diarrhœa and a host of other ailments.

I am grateful to **Chelidonium** for the service it rendered me in a case of hepatic fever.   It was in an octogenarian, ailing with a fever, he could not shake off inspite of the most scrupulous care and treatment.   The patient complained of constant stitches in the region of liver, that made breathing painful, specially while moving, taking deep breath, eating and drinking.   Bilious vomiting, sense of fullness and tenderness in the right hypochondrium, an extremely yellow watery diarrhœa, relief of pain and other complaints after eating, a great intolerance of cold drinks, a fetid odor of the mouth and a greyish yellow shallow sunken countenance, were symptoms that suggested the remedy.

A great craving for hot drinks, that bring untold relief, is a very prominent symptom of **Chelidonium;** unless boiling hot, their stomach will not retain them.   In this respect it is similar to **Arsenicum** and **Cascarilla.**

These patients are very lethargic mentally and bodily.   A great distaste is noticed for mental exertion of any description.   A state of weariness and fatigue is constantly on them.   They are sleepy and they yawn frequently, but when they try to sleep they find sleep unattainable.

A great heaviness, stiffness and lameness of limbs are quite charactertistic of **Chelidonium,** and so it becomes an important remedy in the treatment of rheumatism.   It may affect the arms, shoulders, hands, tips of fingers, hips, thighs and heels.   The affected limbs feel as if they are paralysed or as if heavy weights are hung on them.   The pains in the shoulder may extend to the deltoid muscle.   Ankles and wrist feel stiff.   The heels feel, as if they have been pinched by too narrow a shoe. The coldness of the tips of fingers is an important indication for **Chelidonium.** The pains of **Chelidonium** are always worse from the least touch and are definitely helped by bathing the part with hot water.

Chelidonium has been recommended in pneumonia, where bilious symptoms preponderate. Pronounced stitches are felt in the right side of the chest which render breathing difficult. Cough is persistent and the expectoration is bloody. Dyspnœa, yellow watery diarrhœa, prostration, loose rattling cough, violent motion of the alæ nasi, and hæmoptysis are indications of **Chelidonium** in pneumonia. The characteristic cough of **Chelidonium** is caused by a sensation of dust in the air passages.

We use **Chelidonium** in supra-orbital neuralgia, of the right side of the face, specially when associated with excessive lachrymation and gushing out of tears. The pains go from right cheek bone into teeth or into eyes. It must not however be forgotten that it is a neuralgia dependent on disorders of the liver.

It is invaluable both in constipation and diarrhœa of liverish subjects. When constipated, the stools become extremely hard and are difficult to pass. This difficulty again is augmented by a sensation of constriction and contraction of the anus. The stools are hard, bright-yellow, shiny, and clay-colored like sheep's dung. In diarrhœa they are brown, watery and involuntary. It may be either very yellow or clayish. The urine too, is high colored like beer, and it stains napkin yellow should it happen to soil it.

CHENOPODIUM ANTHELMINTICUM.

This is a rank odorous plant, commonly called the Wormseed, the Stinking Weed, and Jerusalem Oak. The seeds of this plant are in common use as a vermifuge.

The symptom that has been spoken of, as being highly characteristic of **Chenopodium** is pain beneath the joint of the right shoulder blade, with a sensation of giddiness in the forehead and ringing in the ears. This is very similar to our **Chelid.** This symptom, which has in late years been verified by many practitioners, was originally given to the profession by Dr. Jacob Gins.

This remedy should not be confused with Chenopodium vulvaria, which has been recommended by Cullen and Jahr in uterine complaints and hysteria.

I would also draw my readers' attention to another **Chenopodium** known as **Chenopodium glauci,** in which remedy we have severe pain under the left shoulder blade. Dr. Nash has great confidence in this remedy, and has spoken of it very highly. With this remedy he has relieved pain at the abovementioned locality, not once, not twice, but often. It was originally proved by Dr. Mayer.

Before closing, I must give its indication in toothache, where it has been of great service. The characteristic feature of this toothache, where Chenop glauci is helpful, is that it is relieved only after the patient breaks out in a general sweat. Dr. Raue effected a beautiful cure, in a very painful case of toothache, with this remedy, where many other remedies had failed, on the characteristic relief of all toothache from a general sweat.

CHIMAPHILA.

The plant known as the Ground Holly grows in all parts of the United State, Europe, and Asia. It belongs to the natural order of Pyroleæ. It was a favourite remedy with the aboriginal Indians and the early European settlers, in various complaints, principally scrofula, rheumatism, and kidney affections. It acts principally on kidneys and genito-urinary tracts, and increases renal secretions. Its influence on the bladder too, is very great as we will see presently. It is generally indicated in cachectic and scrofulous individuals and in constitutions broken down with intemperate habits. It is also a great remedy in plethoric and hysterical women suffering from dysuria.

It is one of our principal remedies in obstinate vesicle irritation due to catarrh of the bladder. The patient experiences great pain both in the region of the kidneys and the bladder. This pain induces a constant desire to void urine. The urine discharged, is dark-colored, thick and full of copious sediment. It is also ropy, bloody and full of pus. It scalds and smarts during and after the passage of urine. This painful irritation is felt along the whole length of the urethra and from the bladder to the meatus. It is so similar to **Cantharis** that at times it becomes extremely difficult to distinguish between them. The straining is as great as in **Cantharis,** but difficulty in evacuating the bladder, is more prominently present in Chimaphila than in the other remedy. He is unable to pass even a drop of urine without standing, with his feet wide apart and body inclined forward. All these symptoms are generally found in enlargement of the prostate and in acute prostatitis and hence its application in those complaints is a common affair. We must not also forget the peculiar sensation of swelling, felt in perineum which, on sitting down, appears like a ball pressing against perineum. The prostatitis referred to above, may be the result of sitting on a cold wet stone as it sometimes happens.

It is also efficacious in tumors of mammæ, benign or malignant. We use it, both in rapid atrophy of breast or in hypertrophy, hence we should think of it in women with large breasts as well as in women with no breast at all. It has been recommended in ordinary tumors as well as in cancers of the breasts.

CHINA OFFICINALIS.

Cinchona is of great interest to us, as being the first remedy with which Hahnemann experimented and that it is the drug that led to the gradual unfolding of the great principle of **Similia Similibus Curantur.**

The plant grows on the heights of the Andes and in India. It is so named after Countess Ellcinchon, wife of the Vice-King of Peru.

It is a great febrifuge. Huge quantities of this drug are consumed yearly. Administered as it is, without any true principle to guide us, it does more harm than good. I cannot do better than cite the opinion of our master about the abuse of quinine. " True, he can no longer complain that the paroxysms of his original disease occur any more on regular days and at regular hours; but behold his livid earthy complexion, his bloated countenance, his languishing looks. Behold how difficult it is for him to breathe, see his hard and distended abdomen, the swelling of the hypochondria; see how his stomach is oppressed and pained by everything he eats, how his appetite is diminished, how his taste is altered; how loose his bowels are, and how unnatural and contrary to what they should be; how his sleep is restless, unrefreshing, and full of dreams. Behold him weak, out of humour, and prostrated, his sensibility morbidly excited, his intellectual faculties weakened; how much more does he suffer than when he was a prey to his fever."

It cures certain varieties of intermittent fevers, I mean only those that simulate the pathogenesis of **Cinchona.** We will make a special study of the **Cinchona** fever, from a homœopath's stand point after we have finished discussing the few guiding charac- teristics of our remedy.

The first and the foremost point about **Cinchona** is its periodi- city. The ailments are worse every other day.

The second point is the great debility and prostration due to excessive loss of vital fluid. It is frequently the result of excessive lactation, long continued diarrhœa, chronic suppuration and profuse hemorrhage.

Great sensitiveness to pain and to drafts of air constitute the third feature of importance.

Lastly we must remember that **Cinchona** is second to none in respect of tympanitis and excess of flatulence. Of all my cures, the one that ranks best, is the case of a middle-aged lady, who in the opinion of our friends of the other school, was said to be suffering from peritonitis. When all available means failed, operation was advocated. Love of life and instinct of self-pre- servation prompted them, to give a trial to Homœopathy, before having recourse to that extreme measure. **Carbo veg** and **Rapha- nus** were tried, without much benefit, till the extreme sensitiveness of the abdomen and the feature of amelioration from hard pressure suggested **China.** To me it seemed to be a simple case of incar- cerated flatus with entire suspension of the action of the bowels. On administration of **China** 200 she moved 4 or 5 times and all that flatulence oozed away like gas from an exploded balloon.

The appearance of the patient is in keeping with his condi- tion. The face is pale and hippocratic, the eyes are sunken and surrounded by blue margins. We notice also a great dislike to all mental and physical exertions. Indifference, apathy and taci- turnity are well marked. He is lowspirited and gloomy.

He also suffers from fixed ideas. It is difficult to eradicate from his mind, the idea that has taken possession of him. These fixed ideas generally take the form of persecution by enemies. Wherever he goes or whatever he does, he feels that his enemies are at his heels trying to thwart him in every way. Such ideas get so strong a hold of his mind that we find him, jumping out of bed and even attempting to destroy himself to be able to escape from his implacable but imaginary enemy. In delirium and in insanity, he displays a great dread of dogs and other animals, particularly at night time. It is recommended in coma with complete uncon sciousness. On being called loudly, the consciousness revives and

the patient may even answer questions, but soon his consciousness ebbs away.

There is a great tendency to congestion of head. This is
evident from the flushing of face and the throbbing of the carotids.
The head feels as if the skull would burst.   These headaches,
strange to say, are frequently common after exhausting hemorrhages and sexual excesses. They are worse from draft of air,
touch and exposure to the sun. They are better by hard pressure.
Brain feels bruised. The pain is throbbing, hammering and tearing in nature. It extends from occiput to the whole head and
is worse by the slightest motion. He must stand or walk.

We notice great excitability of all the senses in **China.**
Intense photophobia, intolerance of noise, and acuteness of the
sense of smell are predominantly present in our remedy.   Voracious appetite, great longing for dainties, spirits, cooling things,
and highly seasoned food, and a violent thirst for cold water are
equally characteristic of **China.**

It is an important remedy in dyspepsia. Great aversion to
foods of all kinds is noticed.   He feels satiated all the time.
Slightest food taken into the stomach causes pain. Bread tastes
bitter. The patient's condition becomes a great deal worse after
drinking wine and other liquors. Sometimes the opposite condition of voracious appetite and canine hunger is noticed. He longs
for dainties. Belching, sour eructations, vomiting, pulsation in
pit of stomach, rumbling and gurgling in abdomen, sensation of
emptiness, qualmishness, pain and pressure, are all important indications for **Cinchona.**

We think of it in diarrhœa, when the stools are yellow, watery,
profuse, frothy, involuntary, putrid, painless and contains particles
of undigested food. It is always worse after meals and at night
times.

Tympanitis is particularly marked in **China.** This accumulation
of flatus passes neither up nor down. The abdomen looks like a
pyramid almost ready to burst.   The diarrhœa in China comes on
insidiously and gradually. The first stool perhaps is quite formed
and natural, but loose ones are sure to follow, each one becoming
more and more watery as the diarrhœa persists. It helps in hydrocephalus following an attack of persistent diarrhœa.

China finds its usefulness in the ailments of the male sexual
organs, specially in impotence from over indulgence, and in other
consequences of excessive or long continued seminal losses.

It is curative in its own type of intermittent fevers, which are generally antiponing in nature. It may be tertian, double tertian, quotidian or double quotidian. The time of the paroxysm is not of much importance. It may begin at any time of the day, but it rarely happens at night-time. The prodromal stage is prominent by reason of its thirst, canine hunger, nausea, anguish, headache, debility and palpitation of the heart. The patient suffers from a feeling of general illness at this period. He is unhappy because of an undefined feeling of languor, melancholy and want of ease. He does not appreciate that these symptoms are merely the precursors of an attack of ague. We must not forget, that this restlessness and uneasiness, coming before the paroxysm are the determining feature of our remedy. The ague starts with general shaking over the entire body, beginning in the legs below the knees and is accompanied by terrible shivering and chilliness. We notice real goose-flesh after every swallow of drink. In this respect we should take particular care, not to confuse **China** with **Eup. perf., Arsenic, Capsicum** and **Cimex.** In each one of these remedies we find aggravation after drinking, specially during the stage of chill. They all abstain from drinking water at this stage but each one from a different point of view. **Eupatorium** declines drink of water, though tempted with great thirst, because each swallow increases his chill. **Arsenic** would rather avoid drinks, because drinking aggravates his vomiting but, still he drinks as the thirst is too great. **Capsicum** is very similar to **China,** inasmuch as drink brings on fresh shuddering and chill each time. In **Cimex** on the other hand, drinking of water causes a general aggravation of all the symptoms such as headache, cough, oppressed breathing etc. The point that should be particularly remembered, is the cessation of thirst with the oncoming of the chill. It is very marked in the prodromal stage, long before the chill is on. It is absent during chill, but towards the latter part of the second stage, that is when the fever starts declining, the thirst commences again. It is also quite prominent during the stage of sweat. The presence of thirst in the stage of chill and heat is a contra-indication for **China.**

The stage of heat is characterised by the distention of veins which become quite prominent and noticeable. The congestion of head at this period is very marked. The patient uncovers frequently, but has to cover again due to a sensation of chill. In this **China** is somewhat similar to **Nux** where too we find frequent

covering and uncovering. The stage of heat is quite long lasting, and the patient avoids walking and prefers rest, as the least
movement aggravates the sensation of heat. With the sweat which
is very profuse, debilitating, and extensive, the thirst returns. The
thirst at this stage is intense. The sleep that we first noticed
during the stage of heat, deepens and becomes more profound, and
he becomes quite somnolent all throughout the stage of sweat. The
more he is covered, the worse he sweats. The tongue is yellow
and coated and the taste in the mouth is bitter. The pulse is quick,
hard and irregular during chill and heat, but slow during the other
stage. Ringing in the ears, a saffron yellowish tinge of the skin,
anemia, cachectic appearence, swelling and tenderness of the region
or hypochondria, loss of appetite, sinking sensation in the stomach,
and tympanitis are a few more of its characteristic indications.

Case 1.—A delicate girl, three years old, had an exhausting diarrhœa
three weeks. It is now painless, consisting of brownish-yellow fluid with
much undigested food. She had ten or twelve operations in twenty-four
hours, and is much debilitated. **China** 200, every two hours, produced decided improvement in thirty-six hours, and complete convalescence in two
days more.—Dr. Jas. B. Bell.

Case 2. Intermittent.—M. has had tertian fever five or six weeks
Puls 200 was given, which seemed to aggravate, changing the fever to a
quotidian type. Symptoms; Paroxysm commenced at 8 A.M. Hard and
shaking chills, lasting one hour, after which great thirst, followed by fever
with no thirst; headache; flushed face; dry, red eyes, and after the fever,
sweating, with thirst; but very profuse perspiration at night, particularly
upon the parts on which he lies. Great debility after perspiration. **China**
200, ten powders, one every three hours. Speedy recovery followed.—Dr.
T.D. Stow.

CHININUM SULPHURICUM.

Chininum sulph. is the sulphate of quinine. In the allopathic
system of treatment, this has practically taken the place of the
crude bark. The symptoms of **Chininum sulph.** and **China** are
similar to a great extent, the points of difference between them,
though not many, are striking, and it will be our object to differentiate between the two remedies as closely as possible during
the course of this lecture.

It is needless to enunciate once again the symptoms of quinine
poisoning. We all know, especially those of us inhabiting the
plains of Bengal, how emaciated, lean, pale and cachectic the poor

quinine-laden patient invariably looks.   Enlarged spleen, a cir-
rhosed liver, a constant ringing in the ears with deafness are
definite concomitants of the quinine cachexia.

Chininum sulph. is generally adapted to persons of dark complexion and to persons in a state of prostration, due to excessive
loss of blood.   They are naturally of a bilious temperament; with
the prostration just mentioned, is to be seen a great hyperesthesia.
The pulse force in these patients is diminished, due to a weakness
in propelling power of the arterial system.   This weakness, therefore, is universal and absolute, and hence should be considered an
important characteristic of **Chininum sulph.** Next to this weakness is the periodicity of the drug; everything happens at a stated
time.   The attack returns punctually at the same hour.   The skin
generally is flaccid and sensitive to touch.   We also find great
sensitiveness of the last cervical and first dorsal vertebræ to pressure.   During fever the entire length of the spinal column becomes
painful.

Chininum sulph. is particularly subject to neuralgia, which is
intermittent and occurs at regular hours.   These neuralgic pains
generally occur in supra-orbital and infra-orbital regions.   The
pains are lancinating in character and they are very regular in their
onset.   Dimness of vision, black spots before the eyes, extreme
sensitiveness of the eye to light, lachrymation, ringing and buzzing
in the ears, a jaundiced hue of the face and conjunctiva, a peculiar
whirling sensation in head are some of the other prominent symptoms of the remedy.

Another important symptom in **Chininum sulph.** is a sinking
sensation.   The patient is faint and feels as though she would die
and sink through the bed. **Ant. crud., Cina, Cocc., Dig., Hydrast.,
Ign., Merc., Nux vom., Phos., Podo., Puls., Sepia., Stannum, Sulph.,
Taba., Verat. album,** and **Zinc.,** also have a similar symptom.

In **Phosphorus, Sulphur** and **Zincum** the sinking sensation is
felt at 11 P.M. and is relieved after eating.   In **Sepia,** on the
other hand, the sinking sensation comes after the patient has partaken of food.   In **Cina, Lachesis, Muriatic acid,** and **Veratrum**
the sinking feeling is more persistent, and is not relieved by eating.   In **Mercury** the sinking sensation is not continuous, but
comes on after application of pressure on stomach.   In **Ignatia**
we have sinking, more especially, when the patient takes a deep
sighing breath.

We must not omit to discuss that particular chapter of **Chininum sulph.** considered the most important—I mean its application

in marsh malarial fevers or acute intermittents of supposed malarial origin. The type is generally tertian, rarely quotidian. As has been mentioned before, a perfect regularity is observed both in the invasion and in the progress of the disease. Before proceeding further I would like to quote from the famous lines of Adalphus Lippe as I believe, they will go a great way, in dispelling, a false belief entertained largely by the profession and the laity, that Homœopathy is unequal to meet malarial case.

"I lived for ten years in the country, where ague prevailed, and never resorted to quinine. I cured my cases. I have always been of the opinion that a physician who professes to be a homœopath must cure all his cases of intermittent fevers with homœopathic potentized remedies, under the law of the similars." I am fully convinced that it is possible to cure every case of malarial fever with speed and safety with homœopathic remedies, provided, of course, the homœopath takes pains.

The time of the paroxysm is generally 10 or 11 A.M. or 3 and 10 P.M. All the different stages are very distinctly marked and we have perfect apyrexia in **Chininum sulph.** The paroxysm anticipates about two hours each time. It starts with a decided strong shaking chill at 3 P.M. During chill the patient's lips and nails turn blue with ringing noise in the ears. The chill is very violent and it causes such trembling in the limbs as to prevent the patient from walking. Thirst is present during chill. This is a strong point of difference between **China** and **Chininum sulph.** In the former remedy the thirst is altogether absent during chill, whereas it is pre-eminently present in the prodromal stage. The heat, as it comes after the chill, is very violent and is frequently associated with yawning and sneezing. Thirst is also present in this stage. In fact it is present in all the stages of chill, heat and sweat, whereas in **China** the thirst which is absent in the stage of heat is markedly present in the stage of sweat. Another characteristic symptom is the presence of pain in the middle dorsal vertebra. Sweat which is either profuse during movement, or which comes on from time to time during sleep, is exhausting. We may consider regular paroxysm, clear intermissions, clean tongue, profuse sweat and thirst in all stages of chill, heat, sweat, and apyrexia as keynote indications of this remedy. Want of thirst during cold and hot stages and the absence of perspiration after heat, may be regarded as contra-indications.

A study of the relationship of thirst to the different stages of chill, heat, and sweat, will, in my opinion be very instructive.

Arn., Bryo., China, Eupat. perf. and **Sulph.** have thirst in the prodromal stage. For thirst during stage of chill, we may think
of **Apis., Arn., Ars., Bryo., Caps., Carbo veg., Chininum Sulph.,
Eupat. purp., Eupat perf., Ignatia., Nat. mur.**, and **Veratrum.** We
have thirst during heat under the following remedies: **Aco.,
Arn., Ars., Bryo., Chamo., Cina., Chininum sulph., Canth., Colchi.,
Casc., Eupat. purp., Elata.** and **Nat. mur.** Thirst during sweat
is marked under the following remedies: **Ars., China., Chininum
Sulph., Cactus, Nat. mur.,** and **Stram.**

CHIONANTHUS VIRGINICA.

Chionanthus is also called the Fringe tree. It acts powerfully
on the liver and is indicated in hypertrophy of that organ. Hence
it should be studied in conjunction with remedies like **Chelidonium,
Carduus, Podophyllum** and **Leptandra.** The liver is enormously
enlarged. Clay-colored stools, jaundice and high-coloured urine,
the natural sequences of a deranged liver, are to be found under
Chionanthus. Soreness in the region of the liver is a characteristic
indication. Emaciation is quite marked. Sometimes the urine
looks almost black. The stools are undigested, and show utter
absence of bile. It is particularly useful in jaundice that recurs
annually, and which refuses to get better inspite of all treatment.
Long residence in malarial districts, is very often the cause of this
obstinate jaundice. The cases calling for **Chionanthus** are so
similar to **Chelidonium** that at times it becomes very difficult to
differentiate between the two. The only distinguishing feature is
to be found in the absence of the intrascapular pain.

CHLORUM.

It is prepared from the element chlorin, and was introduced
and first proved by C. Hering in 1846. Its action is particularly
marked on the respiratory organs and is, therefore, indicated in
many affections of the respiratory tracts, such as spasmus glot-
tidis, coryza, aphonia, spasmodic cough, and asthma. It is in
these affections that I have used **Chlorum,** and had invariably
satisfactory results. It has been proved mostly in the form of
chlorine water. The symptoms of **Chlorum** poisoning are sudden
seizure of croupy symptoms, such as loss of voice, prolonged expiration, incessant dry cough, fever and profuse sweating.

The chief indication of **Chlorum** is the difficulty in exhaling. Air is admitted well enough, but its exit is prevented. A sensation of constriction is very well marked, and due to this constriction, tightness and suffocation seem imminent. Sometimes these attacks are very sudden; without warning the child makes a long crowing inspiration, but while attempting to exhale finds exhalation impossible. Inspiration after inspiration follows, but exhalation each time is found to be ineffectual, till at last the child sinks into a partial unconsciousness when free inspiration would take place and the child, almost turgid and livid, would sink into sleep. These symptoms are very marked and are invariably relieved with **Chlorum.**

CICUTA VIROSA.

It is our Water Hemlock. In common it is called Cow-bane. It belongs to the natural order of Umbelliferæ. It grows on the banks of rivers and rivulets, swamps, meadows, ponds, lakes, and all over the European continent, especially in Germany and in France. It is possible to confound it with **Conium maculatum,** as the two plants resemble each other very strongly. **Cicuta virosa** the Water Hemlock, should not also be confounded with **Phellandrium aquaticum,** which grows right in the water and not on the banks and borders. We have another variety of Water Hemlock, the American variety, which is called **Cicuta maculata.**

It produces congestion at the base of the brain and in the medulla oblongata. It is one of our convulsion remedies; we think of it especially, when the convulsions are of a violent character. Opisthotonos is a leading feature of this remedy. The whole body becomes rigid; we notice spasms in the muscles of neck and chest. The rigidity is so great that neither the curved limbs can be straightened nor the straight ones curved. The whole body in fact becomes hard as wood. Another leading indication that should not be lightly passed over, is that the head is turned or twisted to one side. The breathing becomes difficult. Foaming at the mouth, violent tremors, twitchings, strange contortions of the body and limbs, and bluish appearance of the face are important symptoms to remember.

It has also been recommended in the chronic effects of concussion of the brain after **Arnica** has failed. With indications mentioned before, we may use it also in chorea, meningitis, epilepsy, eclampsia, and other complaints involving muscular spasms and distortions.

The mind of **Cicuta vir** is characterised by a similar abnormality. He is violent in all his actions. He weeps, moans and howls. Mistrust, apprehension concerning future, indifference and sadness are marked features.

It has been recommended in periodical ecstasy. The patient gets into a state of temporary delirium. He cries, sings and speaks with open eyes without knowing any one. When consciousness returns he does not remember what had passed.

This remedy is rich in skin symptoms. We use it in eczema, impetigo and in pustular eruptions. The eruptions are, as a general rule, thick and honey-coloured. They appear at corners of mouth, spreading over face and in the scalp. It is an antipsoric like **Sulphur.** It has a long record of cures at its credit. I have used this remedy with great success in a case of eczema caput in a boy of eight summers. The pustules which had commenced on his face had spread to his scalp; they had run together and had formed into a solid cap-like mass, practically covering his entire head. A few doses of **Cicuta vir.** 200 cured the child completely in a very short time. It is used for eczema on the hairy part of the face like **Mezereum** and **Nat mur.** The eruption, though it appears mostly on the face and scalp, may come in other parts of the body. The characteristic feature to remember is that the exudation generally dries into a hard lemon-yellow scab.

CIMEX LECTULARIUS.

In **Cimex** we stumble across a remedy with the source of which most of us are unfortunately too familiar. Even those homœopaths that have never heard about **Cimex,** have to get up from their sleep at times suffering from the distressing effects of the bed-bug bites, for verily from the bed-bug, of the natural order of Hemiptera, our **Cimex** is prepared.

My experience with this remedy is very limited. It is considered a great remedy for intermittent fever. In the prodromal stage the thirst becomes intensified, and he complains of a feeling of heaviness in his legs. All his limbs, joints and tendons ache most violently during the stage of chill. The tendons feel as if they are contracted and they constantly yawn and stretch, as if to loosen the shortened tendons. The chill is violent indeed, and it becomes great deal worse on lying down. He feels better

sitting huddled up. Thirst is not very prominent. It is slightly
present during the stage of chill, scarcely any during the stage of
heat, and almost none during the stage of sweat. But the characteristic point about this thirst is that, when satisfied it aggravates
cough and brings on a violent headache.

CIMICIFUGA.

(See Actea Racemosa.)

CINA (SANTONINE).

Cina, also known as the worm-seed, belongs to the family of
Artemesia, or the natural order of Compositæ. The acitve principle of this drug is santoninum which affects powerfully the abdominal ganglia as a reflex of which we have convulsive twitching
and jerking of the limbs, and spasms. It is a powerful remedy for
the elimination of round worms alone. Those tiny little worms
known as oxyures which trouble children and babies, which come
in and out of the anus, and set up irritation of those parts do not
come under the influence of this remedy.

Cina is very useful in diseases of children and has
become a household remedy with us. Two very characteristic symptoms of this remedy, are ravenous hunger
and constant picking and boring at the nose. They want
to eat all the time. They are hungry immediately after the meal
is over. It is simply insatiable. In this respect **Cina** is like
Iodium, Phosphorus, Lycopodium, Natrum mur, Petroleum, and
Psorinum. Grinding and gnashing of teeth, rolling of eyes during
sleep, dark rings round the eyes, intense circumscribed redness of
the cheeks alternating with paleness and coldness, make **Cina** an
admirable remedy for helminthiasis.

The **Cina** temperament is exactly what is to be expected in
such patients. It is exceedingly ugly. We cannot imagine anything worse. The child cries and frets and strikes at everybody
around him. He is obstinate, wilful and head-strong. His sensitiveness is almost as great as that of **Staphisagria** and
Colocynth. Slightest thing offends him. Further what makes him
still more uncongenial, is uncertainty of mood. He wants things
difficult to procure, which when offered goad him to further fury
and irritability. Thus **Cina** resembles **Chamomilla, Ferrum**.

Manganum, Antim. crud., Antim. tart., Bryonia, and Staphisagria.
Hering thus describes a **Cina** child " Child is whining and complaining; very restless even during sleep; it will not lie awake even five minutes without crying; it must be rocked, carried, or dangled upon the knee constantly, day and night; does not want to be touched; cannot bear you to come near it; desires many things which it refuses when offered; it is not pleased or satisfied at anything; uneasy and distressed all the time."

We also use this remedy for night terrors of children. The child wakes up all on a sudden during night with hallucinations of sight, trembles and screams with anxiety.

We use **Cina** in affections of the eyes, specially in strabismus dependent upon helminthiasis. It also has optical illusions in bright colors. Blue, violet, yellow, or green color in all their optic grandeur dangle before the eyes and the patient has a real panoramic display in colors.

The urinary symptoms of **Cina** are very important and are in conformity with symptoms of helminthiasis. The child frequently wets the bed at night. The urine is strongly ammoniacal and profuse. This urine sometimes turns turbid and semi-solid on standing. Other remedies for milky urine are **Aurum mur, Lycopodium** and **Acid phos.**

We use this remedy for a certain variety of diarrhœa, specially in children during dentition. The stools are white mucus, like little pieces of popped corn. It may be also reddish or greenish mucus. Frequently the stools are full of ascarides.

Cina is an invaluable remedy in spasmodic periodical whooping cough. The cough is rendered worse by speaking and movement. Before the onset of the spasm the child behaves in such a way, as to lead the onlookers to think that it is going to get an attack of epileptic spasm. She raises herself suddenly, looks about in all directions in a bewildered fashion, then stiffens and loses consciousness. Duing paroxysms the child looks anxious, catches at her breath and gags. Towards the end of the paroxysm it throws its body backwards and a peculiar gargling sound is heard to go down the throat (**Cuprum met, Lauro., Hydrocyanic acid**). The sleep of the **Cina** patient is a disturbed sleep. The child tosses about during sleep and on awakening looks frightened and trembles. Sometimes it would not sleep unless rocked or kept in constant motion. The attitude of sleep is also very fantastic. The child loves to sleep on his belly. Sometimes we find him assuming a still stranger posture and sleeping on his hands and knees.

Case 1.—H. K., three and a half years old, suffered from a bronchial catarrh after catching cold, degenerating into bronchitis. Child pale and weak; respiration accelerated, short, rattling when coughing, which was done at short intervals; the chest seemed to be full of mucus, which could not be brought up, so that the child nearly suffocated; was very cross notwithstanding the great debility; obstinate, and crying, when his will was not carried out. Restless sleep, constantly broken by the cough; hardly any appetite; wants to drink water constantly; constipation; urine copious and involuntary; pulse 120; auscultation showed coarse, rattling murmur; spasmodic twitchings set in on the third morning, with threatening collapse; the child coughed decidedly weaker, still the rattling murmur could be heard from afar; twitching of extremities; pupils dilated, gnashing of teeth; deathly paleness; pulse 140. **Cina** 200. Suddenly severe convulsions of the whole body, with opisthotonos set in, which passed off as suddenly as they came; respiration quieted down; the twitching ceased, and the little boy fell into a quiet sleep; his eyelids perfectly closed as in natural sleep. Fully recovered.—Dr. M. Deschere.

Case 2.—Boy, aged fourteen (nine weeks sick); standing impossible constant muscular spasms in limbs and face; his arms and legs were in a continuous swinging movement; face so distorted by the spasm that speaking was impossible, and at each attempt the tongue and larynx became rigid; nourishing was only possible when one held the head firmly, while another put a spoonful of food in the mouth, which was swallowed with great difficulty; constant flow of saliva from mouth; staring eyes; spasms did not cease at night; no history of onanism or worms. **Cupr.** 6 did not benefit him. **Cina** 12, and in a few days the spasms ceased; in twelve days a great mass of ascarides was discharged.—Dr. Mossa.

CINERARIA MARITIMA.

This drug has been highly spoken of as a great agent in removing cataract and corneal opacities when applied externally in drops into the affected eye. Personally I have very little experience with it. It should be more widely used and its successes and failures published.

CINNABARIS.

Cinnabaris is the red sulphide of mercury and is a remedy of a very ancient status. It was handed down by the Orients to the Greeks and by the Greeks down through the Middle Ages, to the modern medicine. It is a remedy of great repute with us, in as much as it corresponds to the combination of the two vile poisons of syphilis and sycosis. Cases crop up in our practice, which inspite of great care on the part of the physician, always thwart and baffle him. It always pays to study the constitution of the patient.

When careful observation reveals the grafting of a sycotic history on a syphilitic base **Cinnabaris** comes our remedy. There is under **Cinnabaris** a great abundance of warty growths on the skin. These excrescences are especially fan-shaped and they are very common indeed on the prepuce. The ulcers in **Cinnabaris,** as well as other eruptions that may appear, are all characterized by an intense redness after the colour of this drug. Guernsey considers this to be a magnificient indication of **Cinnabaris.** It has been used in badly honey-combed fistulous ulcerations on the indication of this fiery redness of appearance. Violent itching of corona glandis with profuse secretion of pus, redness and swelling of prepuce, warts on prepuce and frænum, syphilitic phimosis with fetid gangrenous odor, induration of testicles and warty excres-cences in various parts of the body, clearly testify to the underlying malignancy of poison, find in **Cinnabaris** a ready help.

Long-standing cases of gonorrhœa with much pain, soreness and a great profusion of yellow-green discharge, when complicated with the above-mentioned syphilitic symptoms, come clearly under the influence of **Cinnabaris.**

A great sensitiveness is particularly characteristic of the remedy. The bones of the skull, and even the hair are painfully sensitive to touch. A sensation of congestion over whole head, but principally over forehead, is constantly present. But the most red strand symptom is an uneasy creeping and pressive sensation on bridge of nose, as if he has been putting on a pair of very heavy spectacles. This sensation of weight and pressure over the root of the nose oftentimes extends to the zygoma and the temples.

Like mercury there is a metallic taste in the mouth. Increas-ed flow of saliva is also present.

Cinnabaris is not often thought of in catarrhal troubles. It is an excellent remedy in those persistent forms of chronic rhinitis where the above mentioned symptoms are found compli-cating the case. The throat is swollen and the tonsils are enlarged. A great dryness in the throat annoys the patient, more especially at night, waking him up from sleep. It does yeomen's service in diphtheria, in sycotic and syphilitic constitution, when there is quiet, an accumulation of stringy mucus in the posterior nares. A tendency to hæmorrhage from the nose, is marked all along. The dryness of the throat and mouth is a capital indication. Syphilitic laryngeal ulcers, even when associated with tuberculosis have often responded to **Cinnabaris.**

The leucorrhœa of **Cinnabaris** also needs careful handling. The discharge causes a sort of a pressure in vagina, which is more akin to a sort of labor-like pain. Nodes on shin bones, tearing pains in legs below knees, pain in back of neck shooting to occiput with stiffness and hard swelling of glands at back of neck, and wandering rheumatic pains in various parts of the body, ought to leave very little doubt in our mind regarding constitution of these patients.

CISTUS CANADENSIS.

It is also called Rock-rose, Ice-plant and Forst-weed. It belongs to the natural order of Cistaceæ. It grows on low, dry, mica slate hills. It has been recommended highly in gangrene, ulcers, bites of mad animals, and poisoned wounds. As a local wash, it is said to arrest fœtid discharges from the ear, throat and other passages of the body. The ulcers for which it is recommended, are mercuro-syphilitic ulcers, surrounded by hardness and accompanied with swellings of neighbouring tissues. It is also used in ungainly cracks, on the hard and thickened surfaces on the hands of workmen or men used to hard manual labor.

This remedy though rarely used, is considered very useful in scrofula. We notice swelling of the glandular structures in different parts of the body. These patients as a rule are very sensitive to cold. Every draft of cold air seems to run right through them. Every exposure ushers in new complaints.

They also complain of cold feelings in various parts of the body, such as larynx, chest, and abdomen. A spongy feeling in the throat is very characteristic of **Cistus.** This last named symptom led Dr. Clarke to prescribe this with success, in a case of chronic sorethroat that baffled physicians for years. A continuous feeling of dryness and heat in the throat is complained of. The patient swallows constantly to relieve this unbearable dryness. The patient hawks up tough, gum-like mucus which are thick and tasteless. The least inhalation of air removes all sensations of heat in larynx and trachea, and produces a sensation of coldness in those regions.

It is useful in cancer of mammæ. But like all the homœopathic remedies it must be selected on proper indications.

COBALTUM.

It is a metal, and is mostly adapted to neurasthenic patients with sexual disturbances. The most characteristic symptom of **Cobalt.** is a backache—a kind of stiff pain in the lumbar region generally following seminal emissions. This backache is particularly worse from sitting as in **Agar., Berb., Can ind., Rhus tox, Sepia., Valerian.,** and **Zincum.** Distinct relief is experienced by walking, lying down and rising up. We have frequent nocturnal seminal emissions with dreams waking him up from sleep. Headache is constant, and it is worse bending forward. Weakness, trembling in limbs, footsweat and impotence are a few more of the indications of **Cobaltum.**

COCA (ERYTHROXYLON COCA).

Coca belongs to the natural order of Lineæ. The tincture is prepared from the leaves which are about two and a half inches in length and about half an inch in width. It is a bushy plant growing to a height of six to eight feet with white flowers and bright green leaves. It is a plant of very ancient lineage in use, since the time of the great Incas of Peru. Hence it is also known as the divine plant of the Incas. It contains an alkaloid called cocaine, which is very widely known all over the world. It is being abused so greatly that Cocaine has practically become a great manace to human health and happiness.

It is a great remedy for mountain sickness. It is useful in a variety of complaints incidental to mountain climbing such as painful shortness of breath, oppression, dyspnœa, hæmoptysis, anxiety, insomnia, and exhaustion. It is cultivated largely in Bolivia for the sake of its leaves, and it forms an important item of revenue for that Government. People there chew it same as an inhabitant of India chews ' pan,' for its exhilarating effect. It increases the frequency of the pulse and imparts courage and strength. It produces a constant desire to do something and generates a sort of excitability that tends to good people on to enterprises demanding strength and a rich fund of courage. It therefore acts as a beverage same as tea and coffee. Dr. J. W. Springthrope's delineation of the impressions of a cocainist is worthy of attention and which gives us a real insight into the feelings and sensations of a cocaine-fined. " You imagine," he says. " that in your skin are worms, or similar things moving along. If you touch them with wool, and especially with absorbent wool, they run away and disappear, only to peep cautiously out of some corner to see if there is any danger. These worms are projected not only on the Cocainist's own person but on his clothing as well. He sees them on his linen, in his skin, creeping along his penholder, but not on other people or things, and not on clothes brought clean from the laundry."

This sensation as if small foreign bodies or worms creeping over and under the skin is an important landmark of **Coca. Coca** patients are extremely bashful and timid. They are always ill at ease in society. These people get extremely shabby and negligent of personal appearance. We also notice a great blunting of the moral sense. They lose all sense of right and wrong.

It is a splendid remedy for angina pectoris with violent and audible palpitation,—angina particularly brought on by hill-climbing or over exertion.

On the males, we find it indicated in impotence with great relaxation of the external parts. A sensation, as if penis is absent, is a guiding symptom of **Coca.**

COCCINELLA.

It is prepared from an insect, generally known as the Lady-bird, belonging to the order of Coleoptera. It ought to be particularly remembered in neuralgia of teeth, gums, and mouth. The patient's sleep is disturbed at night time with bad toothache or an attack of neuralgia. One important symptom is, accumulation of profuse saliva in the mouth. We also notice an aggravation of all symptoms at sight of bright objects. Hence it comes in as an useful remedy in hydrophobia, and its action appears to be analogous to that of **Cantharis.**

The neuralgia of **Coccinella** is worse at night time. It also affects the right side of the face in preference to the left. The pains are accompanied by an icy coldness of the extremities. There is also a cold sensation in the teeth and the mouth as in **Cistus can.** The pains of **Coccinella,** be it on the face or teeth or gums are throbbing in character. Its attacks recur periodically. But when it comes it is of a brief duration.

COCCULUS INDICUS.

Cocculus indicus occupies a very high place in my estimation. The regard with which I hold it, is particularly due to its great usefulness, as we will see presently. In the days of my hardship when cases were few and far between, and when cures were rarer, **Cocculus** came to me as a God-send, in the treatment of a lady in the last throes of agony of climaxis. It was a case, where every hope was given up, after the best of treatments having failed, but still the patient could not resign herself to the inevitable. We will go into its detail while discussing its relation to the female sexual system; suffices to say that this cure procured for me a life-long friend, who has been ever since acting in the best of my interest, and to whom a big portion of my prosperity of later years is due.

Cocculus indicus, ordinarily called the Indian Cockle, is a native of the Levant and the East Indies. It belongs to the natural order of Menispermaceæ. In ancient time it was used to stupefy fish and thus render them an easy prey. It is used extensively at the present time, in adulterating Malt Liquors. It was first introduced into our Materia Medica by Sammuel Hahnemann who first proved it on himself and his disciples.

The active principle of **Cocculus,** to which most of its properties are due, is called Picrotoxine, a word meaning bitter poison. The principal action of this drug, is over the cerebrospinal system where it produces a kind of paralysis, depending on disorders of the spinal column. It has a special affinity for the lumber region of the spine. It also acts upon those portions of nervous system which control muscular movements. Hence we come across many symptoms indicating weakness of the legs. things, and the back. The **Cocculus** patient is constantly complaining of his back as if paralyzed. We notice unwieldiness of lower extremities; they cannot lift their legs while walking but drag them along. Knees sink down from weakness and they practically totter while walking, as if about to fall. Soles of feet go to sleep. Symptoms like these are particularly characteristic of **Cocculus** and should direct our attention to this remedy. Such symptoms of weakness and prostration are not confined to the lower limbs alone. We notice trembling in all the limbs. Lassitude permeates the **Cocculus** patient in his entirety. It is quite an exertion for him to stand; even talking is a taxation. A constant tendency to faint associated with a feeling of sickness and nausea, great hyperesthesia of all the senses and exalted susceptibility to impressions, startings and shudderings, migratory numbness which comes and goes inexplicably, and melancholia characterize **Cocculus** in a remarkable way.

Mentally, they are distracted; they experience great difficulty in reading and thinking; slowness of comprehension is apparent from their speech and behaviours. They take a long time where they have to deliberate, as mental process is deficient. They can not find right word while answering, partly due to forgetfulness and partly to difficulty in understanding what is heard. At times this becomes so pronounced as to border on imbecility.

Cocculus, like **Ignatia, Staphi., Hyos.** and **Platina** is a great remedy for the ill-effect of anger and grief. Dr. Adalphus Lippe cured a case of enlargement of the liver, on the indication of the pain in the liver being aggravated after a fit of anger, on the part of the patient. He is very easily affronted; every trifle makes him angry. In appearance he is pale and pinched—his features betraying a very low state of vitality, sometimes his countenance is almost stolid and expressionless, indicating entire cessation of all mental activities.

A very characteristic symptom of **Cocculus** is a sensation of hollowness and emptiness. This is complained of almost everywhere—head, chest and abdomen. It is a feeling as if the cavities of the body have been deprived of all their contents and that there is merely a sensation of emptiness, goneness and nothingness left inside. Allied to this is a sensation of lightness of the body.

It is in the sensorium that we find the most important indication of **Cocculus.** Great giddiness prevails. The patient feels as if he is intoxicated; nausea intervenes when he rises from a recumbent posture. During the attack, speech becomes difficult, and reading and thinking become an impossibility. This vertigo is brought on by the motion of a cariage. This leads to its application in sea-sickness.

Cocculus, like **Gelsemium** has a headache especially located in the occiput and nape of the neck. This headache is mostly of nervous and gastric origin—nervous, inasmuch as it is brought on by mental effort, and gastric disorder, because the headache is associated with nausea, vomiting and a great many other symptoms indicating a disturbed state of digestion. The strangest part of the headache is to be seen in the peculiar sensation of opening and shutting of the scalp in the region of the back portion of the head.

It is more like a dull and an undulating sensation in the brain. The patient is quite unable to lie on the back of the head and has to turn to the sides.

The headache is brought on by working or from riding in a carriage, boat, train or a car. The head feels as if it is tightly bound by a cord or as if nerves in the head are drawn up tightly. Brain feels as if it was compressed into a small bulk.

Cocculus has been very highly recommended in chronic dyspepsia, either from the abuse of stimulants or from long studies. The symptoms are a confused feeling in the head after eating or drinking, nausea, vertigo, salivation, and an absolute loss of appetite. There is a metallic taste in the mouth with a great afflux of saliva. Burning in œsophagus, extending to fauces with taste of sulphur in mouth, is more or less present. It is not so much the want of appetite that troubles the **Cocculus** patient, but an eternal aversion to food brought on even by the smell of food. Violent attacks of gastralgia, with cramping pain in stomach, is not an infrequent occurrence. Sensation of emptiness and hollowness, referred to previously, is particularly felt in the abdomen. There is great accumulation of flatulence, but this flatulence is not due to, defects in decomposition of food as it is in **Carbo veg.,** but mostly to retention of flatus, which when incarcerated, causes extreme distention of abdomen and great uneasiness. Diarrhœa, with sensation in abdomen as of sharp stones are being rubbed together, brought on by riding a short distance in an omnibus or car, lends peculiar interest to our remedy. This diarrhœa in **Cocculus** is also peculiar inasmuch as it occurs mostly in daytime. Throughout the night there is absolutely no disturbance, but it comes on directly after rising from bed. Certain amount of urgency is noticeable as he has scarcely any time to dress; stools are soft, yellow, and fæcal; prolapsus recti after stool is as much a feature of **Cocculus** as of **Podophyllum.**

Cocculus indicus is sometimes of great help to us in typhoid. The cases calling for it are rather cerebral than abdominal. The cerebrospinal system is more at fault than the abdomen. The symptoms indicating it are vertigo at the slightest movement, confusion of mind—a sort of a bewildered heavy state or wrapped state of mind, heaviness of eyelids, a strong sensation of tightness in the brain, white or yellow coated tongue and a great tympanitic distention of abdomen.

We have not yet discussed its relation with regard to the female genital organs. The menses are either premature, coming always ahead of time in profuse gushes, or they are tardy and are associated with violent abdominal spasms, extracting painful moanings and howlings from the patient. It thus, becomes an admirable remedy in dysmenorrhœa, and it was in such a case as this that I had occasion to prescribe **Cocculus**, as has been referred to previously. The patient, almost at her critical period of life, was very irregular with her menses. The taint of hysteria with alienation of mental faculties, the great and prominent weakness, paralytic sensation in back and lower limbs, trembling over entire body, excessive hysterical distention of abdomen and a peculiar serum-like purulent ichorous leucorrhœa, gushing out on bending or kneeling down, rendered her almost an object of pity. Pale, weak, cachectic and worn-out she was declared to be beyond redemption. **Cocculus** has removed all these undesirable symptoms, has put in a nice healthy flush of the rose on both of her cheeks, and a nicer healthier and a happier soul there does not exist all throughout this city!

Case 1.—Encephalitis. My youngest son, aged twelve, was taken with pains in the head, March 11. March 15. Face pale or flushed with eyes half veiled; cannot open eyes though insensible to light; unconsciousness; delirium with fear and fright or visions of wild beasts biting, and demons; great agitation, incessant talking, with paroxysms of shrill cries at short intervals, with great muscular strength; has to be kept in bed. Pulse 120 to 130, small and thread-like; difficulty of passing water which is abundant; pap-like diarrhœa; tossing about the bed. **Hyos.** 200. Some improvement up to 18th, when the symptoms changed. Short intervals of consciousness, during which he complained of great sensitiveness of the back of the neck and whole spine; light did not affect the eyes, the sight being gone; lips parched and dry, but slight thirst; angry and indignant form of delirium; when roused he complained of dizziness and cephalgia, as if the head were tightly compressed; soon falls again into a murmuring stupor, with tossing of the head and incessant trembling of the hands; has not slept an instant since the eleventh. **Cocc.** 200 instead of **Hyos.** Improvement followed on the third day and a recovery soon took place.—Dr. Malan.

Case 2.—Mrs. W. had been pregnant a few months before, but had miscarried at the third month, in consequence of vomiting and irritability of the uterus. Called on me in the fourth week of pregnancy, on account of morning sickness. **Puls.** 30, and **Bry.** 30, without relief. She then told me of her former miscariage, and that she was suffering from great pain and tenderness over the uterus; constipation, sour stomach, deadly nausea, etc. **Nux.** 3 regularly cleared the bowels, and improved the condition of the stomach. **Hell.** 3 cured the irritability of the uterus; the nausea and vomiting continued; very faint on rising up, with nausea and vomiting. **Cocc.** 30 soon arrested this trouble, and the case went on to full term with no further difficulty in this direction.—Dr. A. C. Rickey.

COCCUS CACTI.

My experience of this remedy is very limited. I have used **Coc. cact.** occasionally in whooping cough. It belongs to the natural order of Hemiptera. This medicine is prepared from a variety of female insects, found largely in Mexico and Central America, inhabiting different species of Cactus and allied plants. These insects after fecundation, deposit themselves on leaves of Cactus plant and increase rapidly in size and lose all shapes, till at last they look like mere excrescences on the plant.

The symptom that I consider very characteristic in **Coc. cact.** is the sensation of tickling in the larynx. This tickling sensation wakes him up at about 2-30 P.M., and makes him cough incessantly ending in the vomiting of profuse stringy, tenacious mucus. **Glonoine, Natr. mur, Sprum s., Phos, Rumex, Sarsaparilla, Sillic.,** and **Sanguinaria** are very similar to **Coc. cact.** in respect of this symptom of tickling in the throat.

In **Glonoine** the patient rather coughs in the fore-noon from tickling in the throat as if by a feather. The tickling sensation is first felt in the throat, gradually seeming to come from low down in throat and finally from the chest.

In **Sangunaria** the tickling sensation and cough start when the patient lies down.

Another important symptom is the peculiar nature of the expectoration. It is tough, white, viscid, gelatinous and gluey, like the white of an egg as in **Cann. sat, Kali bi, Paris, Phos, Stan.** and **Staph.** This cough is worse in the morning at about 6 or 7. It brings in its train severe paroxysms and it does not cease until a quantity of tenacious mucus is raised. The cough also gets violent after dinner and causes vomiting.

Now a short discourse on whooping cough for which it is such a splendid remedy, would not be out of place in this connection. **Ambra, Anacardium, Antim. tart., Arnica, Cina, Cuprum, Hepar, Hyosc, Ipecac, Lycop, Mephitis, Natrum mur, San, Spong.,** and **Sulp.** are much in demand in the treatment of whooping cough and a close examination will prove of real value to us in the determination of their relative importance.

We think of **Ambra** when the true nature of the disease becomes apparent, and the patient gets hollow paroxysmal coughs with expectoration of tough mucus after awaking in the morning same as in **Coccus cact.**

The most remarkable feature in **Anacard.** is the belching after each fit of coughing. **Anarcard.** is indicated in children, given to fits of uncontrollable temper, and in cough brought on by anger and vexation.

Ant. tart. is indicated when the accumulation of phlegm leads to a coarse rattling sound in the throat as well as in the chest, and the patient sinks into a sort of slumber after the paroxysms are over.

Arnica comes in painful paroxysms in young children with a tendency to hemorrhage, especially in the eyes.

Cina is very useful in whooping cough; it comes in violent, periodical attacks, caused by a titillating, tickling sensation as from a feather in the throat, accompanied with sneezing.

Cuprum is used, when there are excessive spasms not only of the muscles of the throat but of the entire body. The patient shows great anxiety before the attack. The child gets stiff and unconscious; breathing apparently ceases. Blueness of the lips, great prostration, complete exhaustion of breath, and expectoration of mucus with dark blood are true symptoms of this remedy.

In **Drosera** paroxysms get worse after mid-night and gagging and vomiting predominate. There is hemorrhage from the mouth and nose with excessive anguish.

Hepar is indicated in whooping cough with rattling sound, and choking as from mucus, in the larynx; it is always worse in the morning.

In **Hyoscyamus** the cough is more incessant than violent and is worse lying down but relieved by sitting up.

Ipecac is a remarkable remedy in whooping cough. There are spasms of the glottis before paroxysms. The child stiffens out during cough and becomes rigid, and turns blue in the face. There are also nose-bleed, bleeding from the mouth and vomiting.

In **Lycop.** the whooping cough is excited by irritation in trachea as from sulphur vapour (**Brom.**).

Mephitis is an important remedy to be thought of where during the spell of coughing, the child passes both urine and stool and turns so blue and seems so asphyxiated that it has got to be taken up immediately to be very much used.

Natrum mur. is indicated where the patient experiences violent pain in the forehead, which feels like bursting with each attack and is accompanied with involuntary micturition and stitches in the region of the liver.

Sanguinaria has the peculiar constricted sensation. It is always worse at night and is accompanied with diarrhœa.

The whooping cough in **Spongia** has a deep hollow burking sound which is excited by an irritation up in the larynx.

We will close this chapter on whooping cough with a few important indications of **Sulphur,** a remedy of first rate importance, not only in whooping cough but in almost all complaints. Under this remedy we notice the peculiar symptom of two paroxysms occurring in quick succession followed by a long respite.

We have gone through the whole gamut of whooping-cough remedies, and it will not be out of place to mention a few hints of hygienic importance. The patient should be kept in warm atmosphere, and should carefully avoid undue exposure to cool air. Relapses frequently occur in whooping cough from injudicious exposure to cold air.

A second important point is that the patient should not be given a full meal. Overloading the stomach frequently brings on fresh paroxysms of cough.

COFFEA CRUDA.

The Coffea plant is a small tree growing to the height of 20 to 30 feet. It abounds in the hilly tracts of southern India and Ceylon. It is characterized by extreme sensitiveness, nervous agitation and restlessness. A great and unusual activity of the mind and body is an important point with **Coffea cruda.**

This remedy is admirably suited to the sanguine temperament and the sensitive patient. This extreme sensitiveness is the most marked feature of **Coffea.** All the organs and the senses are overactive.

Mentally the patient is over-bright and too full of ideas. They flow in such quick succession as to prevent sleep. One idea leads on to another, one thought is linked with other thoughts, one memory conjures up a host of other memories. Such mental exaltation is the real cause of his sleeplessness. The acuteness and sensitiveness of the organ of hearing are just as great. The senses of smell, taste, touch and sight are equally acute. It is on account of this, that he feels his pains and aches to such an extent. What seems trifling and negligible to others is to him almost insupportable. It drives him to despair. He tosses about in extreme agony,

He is a great subject to ailments arising from sudden emotion and pleasureable surprises. This reminds me of a case of hysteria in a young girl, that was given to alternate laughing and crying and other variable phases of hysterical demonstrations. It was due to the news of recovery of her father, suffering from a very critical ailment and whose life was despaired of. **Coffea** brought about great amelioration of her condition.

The ailment for which **Coffea** is often used is headache brought on by over-exertion of mind, excessive joy, contradiction, vexation, noise and music. It feels as if the brain were torn or dashed to pieces. Sometimes it is onesided, and feels like a nail driven into the brain as in **Igatia, Thuja,** and **Nitric acid.** The headache of **Coffea** may be either congestive or neuralgic.

It is also used for toothache. The pain is excessive and causes weeping, trembling, nausea and tossing about. It is relieved by holding ice-water in the mouth, but the toothache returns when the water becomes warm. In this respect **Coffea** is similar to **Bismuth, Bryonia, Pulsatilla, Causticum, Sepia and Natrum sulph.**

Case 1.—On the 28th of November, 1875, I attended Mrs. S., a healthy woman in her first confinement, when she gave birth to a plump and healthy child. In a few days she arose from her confinement in a good condition. Nine days after, the child began moaning and crying with very little intermission, continuing for two days and nights. At noon of the second day I was called to treat the child for crying. After one hour of close examination of both child and mother, I reached the cause by asking the following singular question. Speaking to the mother I asked: "What do you desire most?" She replied: "I want a cup of coffee." "Have you been drinking coffee during the past few months?" "Yes, until the other morning, when mother said I must not drink it longer as it would dry my milk and oblige me to wean my child. Since then I have not taken coffee." I then requested her to take at once a cup of coffee, another of tea, and continue the use of coffee as she had previously done until further orders. At 7 P.M. of the same day, the child fell into a twelve-hour sleep, with after freedom of the crying. I gave no other advice or remedy.—Dr. T. L. Brown.

Case 2.—George W., æt. thirty-two, has had toothache for the past few nights, coming on about midnight, and keeping him awake until morning. Cold water, he says, relieves the pain. **Coff.** 200 was given, and he had no more trouble.—Hoyne.

COLCHICUM AUTUMNALE.

I want to make amends for my omission of this remedy in the first edition of my Materia Medica. by writing a full discourse on it in the second edition of the book. It is a biennial plant of the natural order of Liliaceæ. It is commonly called the Meadow Saffron; the active principle is an extremely bitter poisonous alkaloid known as Colchicine. It is a white or yellowish amorphous powder, soluble in water, acids, spirits, ether and chloroform. It is frequently used as an ingredient in many quack medicines sold in the market for the cure of gout or rheumatic affections. 25 to 30 minims usually make a lethal dose. We have various instances of poisoning with Colchicum. It is a very slow acting poison. Death comes on gradually after six or seven days.

If recovery happens, the convalescence, too, is a long protracted and a tedious process. It produces violent inflammation of the gastro-intestinal tracts, and a serious depression of the heart, and a great lowering of the temperature. The usual symptoms are abdominal pain, griping, severe nausea, vomiting, diarrhœa, great muscular weakness, severe cramps in the feet and calves. stupor, collapse and death. The kidneys are inflamed as well, and we notice the urine to be almost black. Bearing this description in mind, it will be easier for us to remember the homœopathic symptoms, on which alone the therapeutic value of this remedy lies.

The first important landmark of **Colch.** to be remembered, is the extreme relaxation of the entire muscular system, the same as we notice in **Gels.** This is manifested by the constant disinclination, on the part of the patient, to move or to work. He complains of sickness in the morning, at noon time, in the evening and at night. The slightest exertion, such as entailed by climbing a few steps, straining for a stool and talking, elicits complaints from the patient. Sometimes this exhaustion is so marked that as he sits up, his head falls either forward on his chest or on his back, as if he has not the strength to keep it up. This prostration is almost like the prostration of **Arsen.** only without the arsenic restlessness.

The second important point, is the general aggravation of all symptoms, mental and physical, from movement and from exposure to damp or cold, from getting wet, from bathing and living in damp dwelling or from the changes of the weather.

This leads to its application in diarrhœa, dysentery and rheumatism, and other complaints arising from change of weather.

The third characteristic feature is the great susceptibility of these patients, to all external impressions such as light, noise, and strong odours.

But the symptom that stands out most prominently in **Colch.** and practically eclipses all others, is the great nausea and faintness from the odor of cooked food, specially of fish, eggs and fatty meat. I can do no better than cite the testimony of Dr. Nash in a case that baffled him much. It was the case of an old dame of 75 who was suddenly seized with violent sickness, pain in the stomach, vomiting containing large quantities of blood and severe purging equally remarkable by the presence of blood. Tenesmus was great. **Acon., Nux., Ipecac., Ham.,** and **Sulph.** were all tried but in vain; no relief came and even the doctor felt that the patient was dying. Now during all this sickness this patient had been so nauseated and faint at this smell of cooking food, that they had been obliged to keep the doors closed, between her bed-room and the kitchen, which were two large rooms away. Baffled but still determined to succeed, the doctor referred to his Materia Medica, and was ultimately directed, by this symptom, to the selection of **Colch.** The result was most marvellous. I have another object in citing this particular case, from the annals of one of our great luminaries, and that is, to impress on all medical practitioners the importance of strong determination, perseverance and patience. Dr. Nash failed, not once, not twice, but many times but he was determined to fight it out—fight it out **" on that line if it took all summer ";** these are the doctor's own words. The genius of the man, shows out in this strong determination to fight. The repeated failures served only as a fuel, and showed out the real personality of the great doctor.

The fourth noticeable feature is the aggravation of all symptoms from sun-down to sunrise. In this respect, **Colch.** bears a strong resemblance to **Leuticum.**

Finally I must mention another important point in **Colch.** and that is the sensation of icy coldness over the stomach. I value this symptom greatly as it has guided me to the selection of **Colch.** in many instances of Asiatic cholera, which though obdurate, had responded well to our remedy on this symptom.

Now we will have a look at the constitution of our **Colch.** patient. He is generally an emaciated, sensitive individual and greatly disposed to rheumatic and gouty troubles. He is of a leuco-phlegmatic . melancholy temperament; memory is weak; confusion marks many of his ideas; intellect is clouded and dim. He reads, but he does not comprehend what he reads. He is surly, ill-humoured and his sufferings seem intolerable to him. There is lack of desire for exertion, mental as well as physical. His countenance betokens anxiety. He is sad, doleful and almost cadaverous-looking. There is circumscribed redness of cheek with marked paleness of nose and mouth, a symptom similar to that of **Ferrum met.**

A symptom that has already been touched on but which needs a little more explanation is the extreme nausea and qualmishness of the **Colch.** patient. He suffers from constant salivation and even the swallowing of this saliva causes nausea. Water he cannot drink, for that also produces sickish feeling. The slightest movement incites him to vomit. He is obliged to double up and he lies absolutely quiet the whole day, without the slightest movement for fear of this nausea. He vomits the water drunk; he vomits glairy mucus and even vomits stercoraceous matter. There is great burning and uneasiness at epigastrium. The whole abdomen is distended with gas as if he has eaten a great deal too much. With these symptoms, are associated painful urgings to stools. In this connection it will not be out of place to mention that **Colch.** is one of our grandest remedies for Asiatic cholera in its primary stage. Time without number have I used this remedy in that fell disease and checked it in its incipiency. The symptoms of **Colch.** in cholera are very clear-cut and precise and no one need make any mistake over it. The evacuations are very profuse and watery with a great abundance of jelly-like mucus floating on the surface. This denuding of the internal lining of the intestinal canal, is the most important point to remember. These attacks generally come on in the autumn. Tenesmus in rectum, long lasting agonising pain in the anus, severe cutting pain about the umbilicus, deathly nausea and prostration, constant vomiting, cramps and collapse are important landmarks, for us to be guided by, in its selection. It is also a valuable remedy in autumnal dysentery, where the bloody stools are full with scrapings from the intestines. The urging in each case is very great, leading sometimes to the protrusion of the rectum; sometimes the stools are only full of glairy jelly-like mucus. Tingling, itching, burning, tearing in anus, oozing of copious mucus, spasms of sphincter causing shuddering, long lasting pain in the rectum after stools, deathly nausea, and changeability of stools are symptoms ever to be trusted in **Colch.** for dysentery. Mention should be made in this connection that the relief after stools is so great that the patient falls asleep on the vessel as soon as tenesmus ceases.

Colch. is an important medicine in nephritis, especially with dropsy and after scarlatina. Urine is scanty, bloody, ink-like and albuminous.

We must not lose sight of **Colch.** in nausea of pregnancy. This is not a symptom to be trifled at. At times this symptom becomes so worrisome, constant, and trying that it baffles the best medical effort, and leads to fatal results. She feels a faint aching sensation about the navel as if she must eat, but the very thought and sight of food produce such loathing and disgust that eating becomes an impossibility. Sometimes this may go on for months, the mother almost dying from inanition. Allopathy, in these cases, advocates the bringing on of miscarriage to save the mother's life. But our Materia Medica is replete with remedies like **Colch., Cocculus, Ipecac, Kali carb., Kreosote, Nux, Petrol, Pulsat., Tabacum,** and **Verat. alb.** where a careful study and a judicious selection will stop the nausea and save the lives of both the mother and the child.

In **Colch.** the nausea is felt in the head and is worse while riding a carriage or sailing.

Ipec. is very much like **Colch.** The nausea is incessant and there is not a moment's relief.

In **Kali carb** we have nausea without vomiting, coming on only during a walk. She feels like lying down anywhere and prefers even dying to such nausea. Great sleepiness while eating is also a marked symptom of **Kali carb.**

In **Kreosote** the patient vomits sweetish water before breakfast. She retains her breakfast and dinner, but vomits out her supper.

We have nausea and vomiting in **Lobelia** with profuse running of water from the mouth. She is invariably worse after sleeping, and is relieved by taking a little food; after vomiting she breaks out into profuse sweat.

Nux vom. has ineffectual desire for vomiting. She feels she would be better if she could only vomit.

Pulsat. can be very easily distinguished from other remedies by the excessive bad taste in the mouth in the morning.

Tabacum should not be forgotten where we notice deathly faintness and pallor of the face relieved by going out into the open air.

Finally **Veratrum** is to be distinguished by the presence of cold sweat on forehead while vomiting and a great desire for fruits, juicy things, and for acid and salty food.

Colch. is a valuable remedy in asthma, caused by hydrothorax or hydropericardium with great dropsical swelling of the lower limbs extending up to the knees. Respiration is difficult and the breathing is oppressed. She is hardly able to lie down, and is greatly relieved by bending forward. Due to the hydropericardium already mentioned, the heart's impulse sounds muffled and indistinct.

Colchicum is an important remedy for rheumatic pains. We have pains in clavicle, shoulders, loins, hips, and especially in the right trapezius. It is used with great success in torticollis with severe pressing pain and tension in cervical muscles. The pain is so intense that even swallowing is difficult. It is especially applicable in rheumatism of the superior extremities. The pain in the arms is almost paralytic in character, and it is so violent that he can hardly hold even light objects. In the lower extremities we have pain in forepart of tibia accompanied with cramps in the legs and in the feet. In **Colch.** the pains are shooting tearing in character and are very changeable. They break out suddenly in certain limbs and disappear just as suddenly from others. We use it also in arthritic rheumatism. The joints affected are very painful, but they are not often accompanied with swelling or redness.

An important point to remember in **Colch.** rheumatism is the sensation of lameness in the limbs. The parts seem almost paralysed. The patient is very sensitive to the slightest touch. The least vibration renders the pain unbearable. The rheumatic pains are generally aggravated by exposure to damp and cold. They increase towards the evening and diminish by day-break.

H. C. Allen gives **Colch.** an important place in the therapeutics of the intermittent occurrings in late autumn with great preponderance of gastric and abdominal symptoms. The tongue is covered with a thick white downy fur; chill is felt in the extremities, and is relieved by the patient remaining quiet. The case cited by Allen in his therapeutics of fevers from the record of Dr.

Hawley is very instructive, inasmuch as, it shows the importance of fixing on the peculiar, strange and the characteristic indications in preference to the habit of prescribing on the routine basis. Here is a case of ague of the quotidian type, the fever coming on punctually at 10 A.M. with violent thirst, intense headache and great chill. **Nat. mur.** 200 was tried with scant success and great disappointment. The doctor floundered from remedy to remedy with no more success till at last he fixed on the important gastric symptom of nausea and disgust at sight or smell of food. After one dose of **Colch.** 2m, neither the fever nor the chill ever appeared. From my own experience I have had this fact repeatedly proved in more instances than one, that success responds quickly and undeniably, where prescription is based on characteristic indications rather than on the dry, usual and common-place method, of prescribing on the totality of unimportant, unnecessary, useless symptomatology, some real and others faked up.

Case 1.—Dropsy in a scrofulous young man of twenty-seven years of age. Fluctuation in the belly; œdema of the scrotum and feet. Urine scanty, albuminous, with epithelium or cylindrical casts, but containing phosphates and some sugar. Pressing headache; hot forehead; tongue coated whitish; violent thirst, no appetite; great palpitation of the heart, dyspnœa at night. In pit of stomach now and then burning; gulping up of water, afterward nausea, finally vomiting of food, or acrid, sour slime, with subsequent weakness, and sometimes ravenous hunger. Stool mostly diarrhœic and badly smelling; the mind is depressed; sleep disturbed at night by dyspnœa from 11 to 3 o'clock; pulse about 100 per minute; the skin is dry, pale; on the swollen parts it is cool, glistening. Auscultation and percussion reveal no abnormal condition of the heart or lungs. Liver and spleen seem unaffected, as there was no abnormal feeling in either of them, and the patient could lie on either side. **Arsenic** 30 for ten or twelve days, and then **Apis** 3 for a week did no good. **Colchicum** 6 in water, a teaspoonful every two hours, relieved in a short time.—Dr. Ign. Pollack.

Case 2. Hæmatemesis.—Mrs. M., æt. seventy-four. Vomiting of large quantities of bright red blood. After **Ipec.** 3 the vomiting gradually ceased, and she began to pass blood by the bowels, in considerable quantities at first, but afterward in small quantities, though very often, and with great tenesmus and pain in the bowels. The blood passed per anus was at first bright red, but afterward, when in connection with the tenesmus, became very dark colored and putrid. **Nux vom., Mercur., Ipec., Coloc., Hamam.,** with an occasional dose of **Sulphur** did not improve the case; it continued to grow steadily worse for two weeks, until sixty-five of the putrid, dark colored blood and mucous passages occurred in twenty-four hours, and the following symptoms presented: Extreme weakness, cannot move her head from pillow without help; great thirst; aversion to food on looking at it, and particularly when smelling it. The smell of broth cooking, two rooms away nauseates even to faintness (when doors are open between).

Irresistible sleepiness, drowsiness (when not too much pain). The pains increase toward evening, and did not diminish before daybreak. It was autumnal cold and damp weather. **Colchic** 2c, in solution, a dose once in two hours. During the following twenty-four hours she had but two passages, the pain had vanished, there was no nausea. The patient made a perfect recovery in a few days.—Dr. E. B. Nash.

Case 3.—Nov. 11, 1879, I was called in haste to see Nellie C., aged three years and a half. I found her delirious and inclined to stupor; pulse 140, temperature 103°; head very hot; hands and feet cool; face deeply flushed, with violent throbbing of temporal and carotid arteries; sleep restless and disturbed by starts and cries; frequent dysenteric stools of bloody, greenish mucus, preceded and followed by considerable tenesmus. The attack had been caused by errors in diet. Gave **Bell.** 200, which rapidly relieved the cerebral symptoms, but failed to control the dysentery. For the next four days the case steadily grew worse, in spite of the most careful medication. The stools occurred every half-hour during the day, and every twenty minutes during the night; were usually scanty, and consisted of greenish or white, jelly-like mucus with spots and streaks of blood. They were preceded by griping colic, causing the child to scream and bend double with pain; were accompanied by tenesmus and prolapsus ani, and followed by severe tenesmus, with desire to sit a long time, and such complete exhaustion that she would fall asleep on the vessel as soon as the tenesmus ceased. The urine was scanty; thirst well marked, but entire loss of appetite: patient exceedingly cross and peevish. The pulse varied from 100 to 120, and the temperature from 99° to 101°. Of course, there were rapid emaciation and loss of strength. **Merc., Pod.,** and **Sulph.** had already been given without effect. During these four days the child had not taken more than two teacupfuls of food. On the morning of the fifth day, I insisted that she must have more nourishment, and her mother replied: "Well, Doctor, i will try it, but every time we bring her food, the sight of it makes her gag, and have not been able to cook anything since she was sick, for the smell of the cooking turns her stomach." On this "keynote" **Colch.** 3 was prescribed, a few pellets in half a glass of water, a teaspoonful every two hours. During the twenty-four hours preceding its administration, there had been, by actual count, more than fifty stools. In the next twenty-four hours there was only five, and on the following day, two—the last one a perfectly natural evacuation. The patient was dismissed cured, and has remained well up to date of this report.—Dr. W. T. Laird.

COLLINSONIA CANADENSIS.

It is also called the Stone-root. It is a native of North America. It has a very tough hard knotted root. It was first proved by Dr. Burt. He experienced strong headaches with abdominal and rectal symptoms. It also produced rheumatic symptoms in many provers. F. S. Smith mentions having cured a case of subacute rheumatism in a wood-man with the mother tincture. Heart is markedly affected in this remedy.

Most of the symptoms of **Collin.** are due to portal congestion and hence it is such an important hæmorrhoidal remedy. The patient complains of great uneasiness, weight, pressure and pain in the rectum. It feels as if full of sticks and sand. It is thus very similar to **Æsculus hipp.** Symptoms that enable us to differentiate between these two similar remedies are hæmorrhage and the association of rectal irritation with heart and head symptoms. In **Æscul.** there is hardly any bleeding although there is always a sensation of fulness in the rectum. Constipation is obstinate. Stools are hard, sluggish and painful. In **Collin.** hæmorrhage is incessant, though not profuse. We think of this remedy, especially in the chronic variety of piles with heavy ache in the pelvis and a great itching and burning in the anus with a certain amount of prolapsus. This prolapsus ani reminds us of **Podo.**; but in **Podo.** it is associated with diarrhœa and not with hæmorrhoids as is the case with this remedy. The patient is prostrated due to great and continuous loss of blood.

Dull pain in the head with constipation, and the association of headache with hæmorrhoidal conditions are, in my opinion, two very characteristic features of **Collins.** to be always borne in mind by the homœopath.

Collins. is an admirable remedy for constipation. Dr. Nash has given us a very instructive case of constipation that he cured with this remedy. The patient who averaged only two stools a week for years, and who had taken any amount of cathartics without any lasting benefit, was cured perfectly within a month and the trouble never recurred. He was led to this remedy by the association of hæmorrhoids with the constipation and flatulence.

It relieves pruritus in pregnancy. The genitals are considerably swollen and inflamed. The soreness is so great that the patients can neither work, lie down, nor sit. Relief given during such distress will be always highly appreciated by the patient and is within the power of the homœopath to attain such results, provided he is well posted in his Materia Medica.

Before closing I will add a few more symptoms of **Collin.** with regard to its action on the heart. It is a cardiac irritant and hence this remedy should not be used in low potency in organic affections of the heart. It has relieved periodical spells of faintness, oppression, difficult breathing and attacks of syncope. But the indication to guide us, as I have repeated several times, is the association of hæmorrhoidal affections with heart complications. Dewey cured with **Collins.** severe constrictive pain in the heart, in a man who habitually passed blood in the stools—the heart symptoms coming on when the bleeding ceased and disappeared when it was re-established. This alteration is an important feature of **Collin.,** and should it be present, **Collin.** would be very strongly indicated. There are numerous instances of cures mentioned throughout our homœopathic literature, based on this grand characteristic.

COLOCYNTHIS.

In this remedy we have a real boon to humanity. Under the present-day life of stress and strain, no complaint is more common than indigestion and colic, and very few remedies come as handy as **Colocy.** towards the amelioration of this complaint. In common every-day language it is called Squirting Cucumber. It is an annual, that resembles the common watermelon. The fruit is globular, of the size of a small orange, with a thin leathery mottled green rind and a fleshy bitter pulp. The plant is widely distributed over most deserted places in India, Arabia, Syria, the Levant, and the Mediterranean islands. In the Arabian desert, a resinus extract from the fruit is painted upon the water bags, to protect them against the attacks of thirsty camels. The variety used in medicine is mostly obtained from Turkey.

Colocy. is a harsh and irritating drastic. In the allopathic pharmacopœia it is used in small doses in combination with other cathartics as an excellent laxative and after dinner pills, in chronic constipation.

This drug was originally proved by Hahnemann. It is a splendid monument, to last till eternity, of his glory and fine acumen as a student of science.

Colocy. causes violent intestinal irritation with profuse watery diarrhœa. An important concomitant of this diarrhœa is the colicky pain. It consists of griping in the abdomen, forcing the patient to bend double for relief. This doubling up is the chief characteristic of this remedy. He bends double or presses some thing hard against his abdomen. He leans over chairs, tables, bed-posts or anything handy and near about. The epigastrium is distended and tympanitic. There is constant rumbling and croaking of the bowels as from frogs. This is due to incarcerated flatus. The pain is felt more in the umbilicus. It is contracting, cutting, griping and pinching in nature; from umbilicus it spreads upwards over the whole abdomen. Relief is immediate, but temporary from evacaution; sharp pains soon return, and last till another stool. This goes on interminably, till the indicated remedy brings lasting relief. The bowels feel as if they were pressed inward, with cutting extended towards the pubic region and upwards, causing him to draw his legs up to the abdomen. He is restless from pain, and he moans and shrieks. This pain has been frequently described as a neuralgic pain. It is so distressing that the intestines feel as if they were being squeezed between stones and would burst. He is hardly able to stand straight; he walks bent with his hands pressed on his abdomen; a more vivid picture of colic cannot be drawn. Excruciating and unbearable though the colic is, the relief given by **Colocy.** is nothing short of marvellous. I have seen this verified time and again. Patients, suffering intensely and long, despairing of recovery, having had no relief from any treatment, have been restored to normal almost instantaneously, as if by magic. A gentleman, who was addicted to drinking, aged about 46, was suffering from intense pain,—pain that was almost distracting. He was under the treatment of the regular school, who had practically finished every available means at their command. There was a distinct area of hardness in the region of the liver, which led many of them to believe, that it was a case of abscess of the liver. They were not certain as to whether suppuration was complete, and if the case was ready for the surgeon's knife. To make certain, they were thinking of aspirating the liver. At this stage according to the suggestion of a near relative the homœopath was called in. As is usually the case with them, he prescribed **Colocynth,** according to the symptoms presented by the patient, irrespective of any pathological change in any of the organs. The pain that was dragging on from day to day for over a month, the hardness of the liver, the fever and all other abnormal symptoms disappeared, no one knew how, almost within 24 hours. This happened in the beginning of my practice, and it led the foundation of a sincere conviction in the efficacy of homœopathic treatment—a conviction never to be shaken any more, till the last spark of life burns out.

Of course, **Colocynth** is not the only remedy for colic. We have a host of other remedies such as **Aloes, Bell, Carbolic acid, Cham, China, Cocoul, Colch, Cupr, Dios,** and **Mag. phos.**

In **Aloes** the pain is just as intense and griping just as severe as in **Colocynth.** It is mostly caused by incarcerated flatus. After stool all pains cease, leaving the patient bathed in sweat and extremely prostrated.

In **Bell.** the pain is sharp and shooting in character. It comes on suddenly and disappears just as suddenly. There is tenderness to slight pressure, but a marked relief is obtained from hard pressure across the abdomen.

Carbolic acid should not be lost sight of in colicky pains of infants, and of old people. It is mostly indicated in colic of nursing infants.

Cham. has colic just as well marked as **Colocynth.** In both of these remedies we have colic as from after effects of anger. **Cham.** is to be preferred in the colic of children if there is much distention of the abdomen, and the child tosses about much in agony; but it is wanting in the doubling up of **Colocynth.** Irritability of temperament, dentition, hot face, red cheek, hot sweat, constant shrieking and screaming will help us to differentiate **Cham.** from other remedies.

In **China** the colic is relieved by doubling up, as in **Colocynth,** but here we have nausea, tympanitic distention of the abdomen and the etiological factor of indulgence in fruits causing the attack to come on. It is also used with success, in colic from gallstones.

In **Cocculus** the sensation, as if sharp stones were being rubbed together at every movement, is greatly similar to the cutting and twisting pain of **Colocynth.** The pain is in the epigastric or umbilical region. The abdomen feels drawn spasmodically towards the vertebral column.

In **Colch.** there is distention of abdomen with colic, but the differentiating features are extreme sensitiveness to touch or pressure, and a sensation of icy coldness in the region of the stomach.

In **Cup.,** as in **Cocculus,** the pain is crampy in nature, and the abdomen feels drawn in towards the spinal cord. It is specially used for colic in intussusception of the bowels with singultus. There is marked relief of the colic by a drink of cold water.

Dios. is just as noted for flatulent colic as any remedy we know of but unlike **Colocy.** there is relief by stretching the body out or by walking about. The pain, beginning in the abdomen suddenly shifts and appears in different localities such as fingers, toes, etc. It begins at the umbilicus and radiates all over the abdomen.

The remedy that comes next to **Colocy.** for colic is **Mag. phos.** It has violent cutting pains, so violent that he screams out. It is lessoned by bending double or by pressure with the hand, and it is mostly relieved by hot applications.

Finally we will discuss the colic of **Stannum.** The pain is stitching in character, and is aggravated by the slightest motion or touch, and is worse lying on the right-hand side. We notice a similar relief by bending double against a chair or table. If the colic happens to be in a little baby, there is signal relief by carrying the child, his abdomen pressed hard against the mother's shoulder.

In **Colocy.** the stools are saffron-yellow, frothy, liquid, sometimes greenish and slimy. Aggravations are always marked after eating or drinking, after vexation, indignation or grief.

We also think of **Colocy.** in sciatica, when the pains, in the affected part, are of a sharp and shooting character and extend down the course of the sciatic nerve to the feet. There is numbness and anæsthesia accompanying this pain.

Last of all, we will go through the indications of **Colocynth** in diabetes: The urine is milky. It coagulates on standing. When voided the urine is white, but it gets turbid on standing.

On the female sexual system, we must not lose sight of its indications in dysmenorrhœa. The pain is cramping, and the patient bends double with it. For several days before each period she experiences sharp, gnawing, darting pains in the stomach, which necessitate doubling up with extreme nausea and vomiting. All these symptoms are relieved at the appearance of the menses.

We must not forget **Colocynth** in suppression of the menses caused by chagrin.

Case 1.—A gentleman residing in Indiana, a banker by occupation and bitter opponent of homœopathy, said he would believe if it could cure him. An enthusiastic and intelligent layman promised him a cure and gave me his symptoms. In walking or riding in a carriage, could not turn his head to the left without producing vertigo, and he would fall if he did not take hold of something Could turn it every other direction with impunity. In other respects health was perfect. This had troubled him for years, and was increasing in severity; allopathy treated it in vain. **Colocynth** has vertigo on suddenly turning the head; it seems as if he would fall; vertigo when walking rapidly, and **Colocynth,** has a special affinity for the left side of the head. He was sent a drachm vial of **Coloc.** 200, which promptly relieved him.—Dr. H. C. Allen.

Case 2. Ovarian Tumor.—October 10, 1864. Was requested to visit Mrs. C. E. H., aged about thirty-eight years. She gave me the following history:. Had been always in good health; married ten years, but never pregnant. While travelling in France in 1854, she was attacked with what was then called acute peritonitis. She was confined to her bed several years. Partially recovering, she consulted Trousseau, who discovered the right ovary inflamed and somewhat enlarged. From this time she was more or less unable to walk, and suffered much from a tumor, which gradually developed in the pelvis, between the uterus and the rectum, and which was pronounced by Trousseau to be an enlarged and prolapsed ovary. In 1863, she came to New York and placed herself under one of our most experienced gynecologists, who confirmed Trousseau's diagnosis, pronounced the case incurable, and advised a sparing resort to anodynes to mitigate severe suffering. I found Mrs. H. confined to her sofa; she had not left her room for a year. A firm, elastic tumor occupied the space between the uterus and vagina anteriorly, and the rectum posteriorly, completely occluding the vagina and rendering defecation very difficult. It seemed not to be adherent to the walls of either passage. Attempts at walking induced paroxysms of acute pain across the hypogastrium in the sacral region and around the right hip-joint; from here the pains extended down the groin and along the femoral nerve. The pain was relieved by flexing the thigh upon the pelvis, and always induced or aggravated by extending the thigh. Even without the provocation of motion, there were frequent and severe paroxysms of pain, as above described. The appetite was not good and digestion feeble but the general condition of the patient was good. Nervous sensibility was very great. The pains had been ascribed to pressure of the tumor upon the sacral nerves. The patient had a dread of taking opiates, and had used them sparingly. I was requested to mitigate the pains if possible; no hope being entertained of a cure. With no definite expectations of accomplishing a radical cure, I prescribed **Colocynth** 200, a few pellets to be taken whenever a paroxysm of pain came on, and to be repeated every hour during the paroxysms. November 1. I learned that the paroxysms had been less frequent, much shorter and milder. March 2, 1865. The patient walked a half-mile to my office and reported that she had had no pain for a month, she could walk a half-mile daily, without fatigue or pain and had resumed the charge of her household after an interval of nine years. She thought the tumor had become smaller. Being about to sail for Europe, she desired some more **Colocynth,** that she might be provided in case the pain should return. June, 1869. Mrs. H. has returned from Europe; I find her perfectly well. There has been no return of the pain since 1865. The tumor disappeared from its position between the vagina and rectum, in the autumn of 1865, and was plainly perceptible in the abdomen, about as large as a Sicily orange. It has since disappeared entirely.—Dr. C. Dunham.

COMMOCLADIA.

The tincture is prepared from the fresh leaves and the bark of a very poisonous plant growing luxuriantly in Cuba and the southern parts of the U. S. A.   It is called "Guao" by the natives of the West Indies.   It belongs to the natural order of Anacardiacæ and is very akin to **Rhus tox.** with which remedy it has many symptoms in common.   The plant is so very poisonous that sleeping beneath its shade causes fatal illness, especially when the sun is shining on it.

It produces and therefore cures vesicular eruptions, malignant pustules and ulcers.   The ulcers are deep with hard edges, the surrounding skins being covered with small shining scales.   They discharge a thick, purulent, fetid matter.

Like **Rhus tox.** it is a good remedy for erysipelas, but of a much severer type and malignant nature.   Great swelling, intense itching, and much sloughing are some of the characteristics of this remedy.   We use it in erysipelas involving the tissues around the eyes.   The face gets most dreadfully swollen, and the eyes seem to project far out of their sockets.   They feel enormously enlarged, as if they are too big for the sockets.   This sensation of enlargement leads to its application even in glaucoma.   On similar symptoms it has been prescribed in ciliary neuralgia, the result of asthenopia and chronic iritis.   There is profuse lachrymation and aggravation of pain from movement.   Another symptom worth remembering, is that the pain is always worse when near a warm stove; open air relieves.

Its miraculous antidotal functions in malignant pustules and ulcerations have been proved repeatedly.   Dr. Navarro reports of having cured an indolent ulcer of six years' standing on the lower third of right leg, near external maleolas with **Commocladia.** He also used it successfully in a case of sloughing of the right breast.   The leading symptoms were, the hardness along the edges of the ulcer, discharge of thick purulent fœtid greenish yellow matter, the peculiar decayed-meat appearance, and the presence of shining scales covering the integument in the neighbourhood of the ulcers.

Commocladia is always better from motion as in **Rhus tox.**

CONDURANGO.

The **Condurango** tincture is prepared from a climbing shrub of Equador by adding five parts by weight of alcohol to the coarsely powdered bark; after the usual process of saturation and shaking, the tincture is poured off, strained and filtered. This drug was proved by J. P. Dinsmore.

When first brought to notice a few years ago, it was regarded by our allopathic brethren as a great panacea for all kinds of cancerous growths, but very soon **Condurango** lost its popularity. The reason is not far to seek. In medicine there cannot be such a thing as an absolute specific. **Condurango** may not cure every case of cancer, but for its own kind of malignant growths it is absolutely curative. To find out its curative sphere, according to the teachings of Hahnemann, Dr. Burnett proved this drug on himself. He regards rhagades at muco-cutaneous orifices and warty excrescenses, to be most leading indications for it. He has reported a case of cancer of the left breast in a middle-aged woman whom he cured with **Condurango,** the symptom to draw his attention to it being deep cracks in the angles of her mouth. Dudgeon has also recorded a cure with **Condurango** of a case of cancer of the left breast in a woman of 60. The nipple was retracted and a hard tumor of the size of an egg, the seat of much lancinating pain, had sprung up on the side of the retracted nipple. **Condurango** not only relieved the pain but took the tumor entirely away. Flat epithelial cancer on lower eyelid, the same on nose lip and chin, superficial ulceration of the cornea—have all been reported to have been cured when accompanied by sores or cracks at corners of the mouth.

Condurango has also cured cancer of the stomach with vomiting of coffea-ground masses, loss of appetite, and emaciation.

CONIUM MACULATUM.

In **Conium** we have stumbled on a very important remedy. It is the Poison Hemlock. It is a common old world plant, occurring in the temperate portions of Europe and Asia. All parts of this plant are active. The active principle is called Conine, a yellowish, oily transparent fluid of an acrid, nauseous, tobacco-like taste. We find mention of this remedy in the writings of Dioscorides, Pliny and Avicenna It is notorious as an ingredient of the State poison of the ancient Greeks. It was by means of this poison that Socrates was killed. It causes paralysis of the motor nerve filaments of the cerebro-spinal system. It produces depression of the temperature and the lessening of the arterial pressure.

Its use in the allopathic pharmacopœia dates from the time of Stoark. It was introduced first into our homœopathic pharmacopœia by Samuel Hahnemann It is generally indicated in persons of lively, quick, sanguinous disposition with a marked development of the glandular system. It is mostly adapted to the debility of old people, to diseases caused by a blow or fall, and to scrofulous people with tight rigid liver. It is also indicated in that peculiarly deplorable condition of young men addicted to masturbation. In the treatment of the bad effects caused by sexual excesses, **Conium** finds a ready use. Mentally these people are at very low ebb. Enfeeblement of memory leading to difficulty of apprehension, dulness and inability to sustained mental efforts, distaste for society, disinclination to business, complete indifference, great depression of spirit and anxiety and irritability of temper, are some of the symptoms to follow in the train of sexual excesses, and are quite well remedied by **Conium.**

The indication that stands out most prominent in **Conium** is dizziness. It is brought on and aggravated by turning the head sidewise. There is good bit of dispute as to whether this giddiness is worse lying down. Dr. Nash is of opinion that it is not so much the lying down as it is the turning of the head sidewise, whether in an upright or horizontal posture that causes vertigo. Dr. Guernsy writes: This remedy is characterised by great dizziness, brought on when lying down, and moving the head ever so slightly, or even eyes—all the contents of the room appear to be whirling around; the patient wishes to keep the head perfectly still." In my opinion too, as I have verified several times, the vertigo is distinctly worse, when the patient turns his head, however slightly. There is aggravation when lying down, but this aggravation is more the effect of movement nesessary in the act of lying down. Dr. Nash on this indication of aggravation of giddiness from the turning of the head sidewise used **Conium** in a case of locomotor ataxia with great success. This patient was gradually losing the use of his lower limbs. When he walked he would make his wife walk ahead of him or behind to obviate the necessity of turning his head which would be necessary, had she walked by his side. Other similar remedies are **Bryo, Calc. carb, Phos., Gels.,** and **Staphis.** Not only locomotor ataxia but other complaints have been cured on this golden indication. A case of lumbago is reported to have been cured with **Conium** in six days after a protracted suffering of seven months on the indication of her feeling dizzy by turning in bed.

Acting, as **Conium** does, upon the glandular system, we naturally expect it to be a great anti-scrofulous and anti-cancerous remedy. We use it for swelling and induration of glands after contusions and bruises; tumours of various kinds, especially scirrhus, coming on after injury, are also helped by this remedy Instances of such cures are numerous; the thing to remember everywhere is that the glands wherever affected are of stony hardness. These indurations are quite common in the mammæ, in the testicles, and in the uterus.

It is indicated in scrofulous ophthalmia—a characteristic symptom being intense photophobia, disproportionate to the degree of inflammation. It is so marked that there is profuse flow of tears, whenever eyes are forcibly opened; borders of eyelids are red and swollen; conjunctival vessels are highly injected.

Conium affects the wax in the ear. Under its use, accumulation of ear wax looking blood-red or like decayed paper, has been removed.

Now let us peep into the most important domain of **Conium**—I mean its use and efficacy in all complaints pertaining to the male and female sexual system. On the sexual sphere its action is profound. It is generally indicated in weakness of the sexual organs due to bad effects from suppressed sexual desire or from excessive indulgence. Hence we are called on to use this remedy in old bachelors, in old maids and in widows, who suffer from ill effect of suppressed sexual instinct and non-gratification of sexual appetite. It is useful in impotency due to constant nightly emissions. There is great sexual desire with partial or complete incapacity. The erection is insufficient, only lasting for a short time. There is discharge of prostatic fluid on every change of emotion, on the voluptuous line or even while expelling fæces. In this connection we may well compare **Conium** with **Agnas., Graph., Lycop., Nux vom., Sepia. Sulph., Phos.** and **Gelsemium.** In **Graph., Lycop.** and **Nux vom.** the sexual organ. all of a sudden loses strength during coition. In **Lycop.** and **Sulph.** the penis is always small and shrivelled.

I have used this remedy with signal success, in numberless cases, in sexual weakness of young men, from masturbation. The slightest stimulus, such as looking at women or being in their company, bringing on emission. is a very typical symptom, and it has been removed with **Conium.** Indurations and enlargements of ovaries and womb, prolapsus uteri complicated with induration and ulceration of the cervix, with profuse leucorrhæa, have been repeatedly cured with **Conium** on the indication of these complaints having been the result of suppressed sexual desire. In this connection I would like to impress on the mind of every homœopath another strong indication of **Conium,** *viz.,* the starting of the pain in the breast immediately.

We find it an admirable remedy for constipation and diarrhœa provided the characteristic symptom of coldness in the rectum is present. Dr. Mahendra Lal Sarkar of Calcutta effected a wonderful cure on the basis of this symptom. The patient had severe diarrhœa; some of the symptoms pointed to **Sulph.;** to make doubly sure he enquired whether the stools felt hot while passing. Being told that he had a cold sensation instead of hot during the passage of stool, the doctor prescribed **Conium** with brilliant effect.

Before closing, I must touch on another characteristic symptom of this remedy, I mean the sweat of **Conium.** The peculiarity of this sweat is, that it comes on as soon as the patient sleeps or even when he closes his eyes. Insignificant though this symptom may seem, it has helped to bring about many marvellous cures. On this indication Dr. Lippe cured an old man of hemiplegia. I am also indebted to this symptom for a cure of the most obstinate case of marsh fever. The patient was of a scrofulous diathesis. His fever started with great trembling, and there was a strong inclination to sit outside in the burning sun. The heat, when it started was great, and it was both internal and external. Various remedies were tried but none helped till my attention was drawn to **Conium** by the peculiarity of the sweat. Every time he fell asleep, he was almost drenched with sweat—dry he returning as soon as he woke up.   **Conium** stopped the next paroxysm, and since then he has had no more attacks.

It has a peculiar spasmodic cough; it is excited by itching and tickling in chest and it annoys him mostly at night time. It starts as soon as the patient lies down, and he is obliged to sit up for a respite.

Case 1.—Among the curiosities of practice I would mention the cure of a case of cataract following an injury to the right eye, which had caused total loss of sight. The patient was taking **Conium** 3 for a fetid ulcer on the leg, and after a course of about a fortnight, she, to her surprise, found sight returning to the eye in which for eighteen years she was totally blind. When I left Cambridge the sight was not fully restored, but the patient could distinguish colors and could tell whether the dress was striped, and whether a piece of paper was plain or printed upon.—Dr. Wm. Bayes.

Case 2.—The courses were scanty, offensive, and of a very drak clotty consistence and color. There were also, in each of the two cases, catarrh of the nasal and pharyngeal fossæ. One of the two cases was offensive in all her secretions, which compelled her to make free use of perfumes, in order to render herself barely presentable in society. The chief source of the fetid odor was the axilla. Soap and water were of little avail. The odor was aggravated in warm weatner, and also when the unhappy subjects of it were fatigued or became unduly excited or anxious upon any matter. In spite of the most vigorous attempts at disinfection, the presence of either of these cases could be readily detected by the peculiar tetor which they incessantly but insensibly, exalted. **Conium**, given at variable intervals, beginning with the 1st cent. potency, and ending with the 30th cent. was followed, in the course of three months, with a very gratifying amelioration of the distressing complaint, in each case. The defects of the catamenia were also partly removed, and the condition of the secretions and excretions generally improved by the medicament.—Dr. D. A. Gorton.

CONVALLARIA MAJALIS.

It is called the Lily of the Valley and it belongs to the natural order or Liliaceæ.   It is an important heart remedy with us.   It adds fresh stimulus and energy to an exhausted heart, and renders it more regular.   Even light exercise brings on a sort of fluttering at the heart, causing a sensation, as though the heart would stop beating.   This palpitation is usually worse on lying down.   But what renders the symptom important is its association with the soreness of the uterus.   The palpitation complained of, is sympathetic to the soreness in the uterus.   There is also pain in sacro iliac joint running down the legs.   Itching at urinary meatus and vaginal orifice is also quite prominen

It is serviceable in endocarditis with extreme orthopnœa. Heart-beat permeates the whole chest. It is used also in tobacco heart and in angina pectoris, with extremely rapid and irregular pulse. It should be studied side by side with **Dig., Cratæg., Lili. tigrinum,** and **Adonis.**

COPAIVA.

The tincture is prepared from the Balsam of **Copaiva,** and it belongs to the natural order of Leguminosæ. Its action is particularly to be seen on the mucous membranes, especially those of the urinary tracts and the respiratory organs.

Copaiva causes an urethritis with burning in the neck of the bladder and in the urethra. There is also a discharge of a milky, corrosive nature. The meatus of the urethra looks extremely inflamed and angry. These are symptoms of gleet and on these indications we prescribe this remedy for those persistent types of gonorrhœa which have taken on a chronic form after the subsidence of the acute symptoms. It may also be used in mild cases where the discharge is moderate and although certain amount of irritation in the urinary passage is present, no particular difficulty is felt. The allopath abuses this drug, by using it indiscriminately, in huge doses, in every case of gonorrhœa whether the symptoms call for it or not. Our procedure, as has been repeatedly hinted at, should be strictly based on the totality of indications.

The urine passed is high-colored with a thick deposit of abundant reddish sediment. Urine can only be discharged after great effort and even then it is emitted in drops, due very probably to induration of the prostate. Sometimes the smell of urine has the odor of violence as in **Cantharis, Osmium** and **Selenium.**

It is particularly suitable to urinary difficulties in women, especially when, due to chronic cystitis, there is suspicion of the thickening of the walls of bladder with frequent hæmaturia.

We will now look into its application on the diseases of the skin. Isolated patches of nettle rash with intolerable itching, due probably to gastric irritation with fever, are common. **Copaiva** in this respect is of equal importance to **Apis., Ars., Calc., Chloral, Mezereum, Rhus tox.,** and **Salic. acid.**

In **Apis** the urticarial rash is somewhat conical in appearance, and it occurs usually in the lower extremeties below the knees, sometimes on the arms, but rarely on any other parts of the body. Heat, redness, burning, smarting and stinging pains, dyspnœa, with the nettle rash are the important characteristics of the remedy.

In **Arsenicum** the wheals are caused by the eating of shellfish.

Calc. carb. is oftentimes indicated in a nettle rash of a chronic type which invariably disappears on slightest exposure or fresh air

In **Chloral,** the uriticarial rash is large in size and raised in appearance due chiefly to œdematous swelling of the base of the rash. It is caused by sudden exposure to chill.

In **Rhus tox.** the nettle rash is vesicular, and it appears after getting wet and in hairy parts.

CORALLIUM RUBRUM.

Corallium rubrum, the red coral, belongs to the natural order of Gorgoniaceæ. It contains carbonate of lime, oxide of iron, gelatin and various other elements. It suits constitutions tainted with a combination of syphilis and psora.

Its action is mainly located in the respiratory tract. **Corallium** has quite a lot of symptoms that simulate coryza; even epistaxis and ulceration within the nostrils arc not rare. The cough of **Corallium**—and it is pre-eminently the remedy for cough of a certain type—is a violent spasmodic cough. It has been described as the "minute-gun" cough by Dr. Guernsey. In my opinion no better suitable term for this cough can be given. It is like the booms of the maxim gun following so closely each on the heel of the other as to make it almost a continuous affair. The cough is so violent that children lose their breath, and become purple and black in their face. It commences with gasping for breath and continues with repeated crowing inspiration until the patient, purple and black in the face, is quite exhausted. Sometimes it is followed by vomiting of quantities of tough, ropy strings of mucus. A peculiar sensation is that of icy coldness of the air passing through the larynx.

At times the paroxysm is so great as to bring on bleeding from mouth and nose. Now, as regards this sensation of coldness in the air passage, we may compare it with **Bromium, Carbo animalis** and **Coccinella,** in all of which remedies we find this symptom present to a certain extent.

As has been said before, we have a profuse secretion of mucus in the nasal passage in **Corallium.** The mucus is generally fluent and odorless, looking like melted tallow. It is also quite a first-rate remedy in post-nasal dropping, obliging the patient to hawk frequently and clear the throat. Dr. Nash considers **Corallium** as the premier remedy in this affection.

Corallium should not be forgotten in syphilitic erosions exuding badly smelling ichor; the eruptions generally are, in the first place, slightly reddish like the colour of red coral, laterly these coral-colured spots change to a coppery hue. Flat ulcers which are extremely sensitive to touch, and which bleed on the slightest provocation, appear on the penis and scrotum. The whole of the inner surface of prepuce secrete a yellowish green offensive matter which causes great irritation, redness, and swelling. Smooth copper-coloured spots appear on palms of hands and fingers.

With just one more important landmark of **Corallium** we will close our chapter on this remedy. It consists of a peculiar sensation as that of wind blowing through skull on turning the head quickly or shaking it. Another sensation, as if the head had become very large, is also to be seen in **Corallium** same as in **Argentum nit., Bella., Bov., Nux vom.** and **Rananculus.**

Case.—E., æt., thirteen, nervous temperament; last November had a troublesome cough, which resisted all allopathic treatment; change of air was prescribed and the cough ceased. At Christmas it gradually reappeared, and now (Feb., 1,) had resumed its former intensity. I found her firing minute guns of short, barking cough; in the evening increased to a violent spasmodic paroxysm; health fair; cough gave no pain; had not yet menstruated. **Coral.** 30, three times a day, cured in a few days.—Dr. R. Hughes.

CRATÆGUS OXYACANTHA.

Here we have a remedy that is not very well known and consequently not often used; but I am sure, a better understanding of this drug will lead to a more universal use and greater advancement of the cause of Homœopathy. **Cratægus** is nothing but our English Hawthorn, a genus of plants of the natural order of Rosaceæ. It is used mainly for hedging purpose. There is a tradition that Hawthorn was the source of Christ's crown of thorns.

The preparation of the tincture is very simple. The fresh berries are pounded to a pulp and macerated in two times their weight of alcohol.

The history of this remedy is very interesting. It owes its origin to Dr. Greene of Ennis, Ireland, who made quite a name for curing diseases of the heart, and to whom people use to flock, from all parts of the United Kingdom, for his really wonderful cures. After his death it transpired that it was the common Hawthorn tincture, in 5 drop doses that procured for him the reputation of a medical necromancer. We owe much of our knowledge of this remedy to Dr. Jennings who proved it and rendered a scientific statement of its symptomatology. In those desperate cases of heart affections, such as valvular deficiencies or hypertrophy, where dyspnœa and dropsy have supervened, and the pulse is gradually growing weak and rapid, where physicians have lost heart, and the patient himself is gradually getting resigned to the inevitable end fast approaching, we can think of no better remedy than **Cratægus**. I have used this remedy scores of times with very great satisfaction. Sometime ago a man was brought into my office suffering from valvular disease. His lower eyelids were œdematous, his breathing short and difficult and his lower extremities showed signs of dropsy. Least movement aggravated his fits of dyspnœa; his skin was pale and waxy and his pulse 120 a minute. **Arsen, Digitalis** and a few other apparently indicated remedies failed till the idea of **Cratægus** dawned over me. I gave him the tincture in drop doses twice daily. He came back in seven days. The swelling of the eye-lids, the dropsy, the dyspnœa were gone. I advised him to continue the medicine for a month more, which as I learnt later on, made him perfectly well.

Dr. Halbert reports the following interesting and instructive case.

"Mr. S, a young man, sixteen years of age, had worked hard at manual labor since his twelfth year to support a widowed mother. He had, in fact, done a man's work before his physical maturity would permit it. For sometime he had shown signs of cardiac hypertrophy, and had been cautioned by physicians to take good care as to his heart. About a year ago during some gymnastic exercise in the nature of sport, he was suddenly admonished that something had ' given way,' and for relief was obliged to take to his bed. When I first saw him he was obliged to lie down, respiration was laboured and irregular and the heart's action was greatly exaggerated and erratic. There was decided precordial bulging; the apex beat was considerably displaced, downward and to the left, and the whole cardiac dullness was greatly extended; the impulse was heaving in character, with considerable mitral systolic blowing and the corresponding diastolic intensification;

there were also signs of considerable pulmonary engorgement and some pain in the chest region. The patient was put into a warm bath for twenty minutes and then carefully returned to bed. **Aconite 3x** was administered every half hour, and continued hourly for a day or two afterwards until he was somewhat relieved. **Cratægus**, five drop doses of the tincture, was then administered five times daily for a long time.

The effects of this remedy were most remarkable; the cardiac irritation gradually lessened, the area of dullness decreased and the rhythm improved; at the same time all the general symptoms improved rapidly. He has now been using the remedy several months and the result is most satisfactory. I have every reason to expect a cure of the extreme symptoms, and believe the heart will be reduced to a safe hypertrophy, which will virtually be a cure."

Dr. Hale advocates **Cratægus** in angina pectoris; he cites a case in which Dr. T. C. Duncan, relieved the terrible agonies of a woman, who suffered from this foul disease, with Cratægus.

CROCUS SATIVA.

Crocus sativa is the Saffron used frequently as a condiment. It belongs to the natural order of Iridaceæ. It has a few characteristic indications, which make it almost a sure cure, wherever such indications are found. The first of these consists in the hæmorrhage of **Crocus** where the blood becomes exceedingly stringy, tenacious, thick and black. It may be from uterus, nose, lungs, or bowels but the blood discharged is black, viscid and clotted, forming into long black strings and hanging from the orifice from which it is discharged.

The next keynote symptom is found in its mental sphere. We notice a great change of temperament. It is the uncertainty of temperament that lends importance to the remedy. This changeability of disposition, this depression and hilarity coming in alteration, the sudden moments of happiness, and affectionate tenderness giving place to insane hatred bordering almost on a frenzy, impart to **Crocus** an importance second to no other remedy in the Materia Medica. Dr. Clarke records a cure of a case of insanity, with this remedy, of a young artist, who had become subject to violent outburst of rage, in which he would take up a knife to throw at his mother and almost immediately after, would be abjectly repentant responded quickly to the action of **Crocus.**

Uncontrollable laughter is another peculiarity of **Crocus.** The fourth important characteristic is to be seen in a peculiar sensation as if something alive were moving in the abdomen, or in the chest. It may be either a real sensation or a hallucination. On this symptom it has been used with success in violent movement of fœtus during pregnancy. It is equally serviceable in phantom pregnancy where the sensation of movement in the pelvis, real or imaginary, leads on to a definite conviction of pregnancy.

Crocus patients are extremely sensitive to music, involuntarily joining in music on hearing a single note sung. A sixth characteristic of **Crocus** is to be seen in a peculiar feeling in the eyes as if he had been violently weeping. A constant desire to wink and wipe the eyes with a feeling as though a film of mucus were over them is noticeable. The vision seems dim as though the whole room were full of smoke. At times it feels as if he is looking through two sharp spectacles. On these indications it has been used with success in conjunctivitis, ophthalmia, and various other forms of eye troubles.

We have used **Crocus** with success in gastritis and gastric ulceration. The symptoms are fullness and bloatedness of stomach, rancid eductation, nausea, vomiting of decomposed fluids, cutting pain in stomach and that peculiar sensation of a living something jumping about in the pit of the stomach.

Its indications on the female sexual organs have been touched upon, but I have not yet mentioned the menstrual disturbances of **Crocus.** The menses appear too early, and are too profuse. It is a kind of metrorrhagia of dark, viscid, stringy blood due probably to overheating, straining, lifting or abortion. It is worse from the slightest motion.

In dysmenorrhœa too, it is equally applicable when the patient complains of a sensation of commotion in the stomach and the blood discharged is of the type mentioned before.

Case 1.—A few months since, I was called to a lady who had aborted at the fourth month, a week before, and who was in a very critical condition from uterine hæmorrhage with retained placenta. The celebrated "tampon" had been applied by the attending physician, according to the nicest rules of common sense; but however nicely applied, it would be invariably pushed out of the vagina. I proceeded to the examination. Whilst the woman lay quietly in bed, but very little blood would escape from the vulva, what did escape, came away in the shape of black strings. After a time she would feel that she must rise to the chamber, whereupon a large quantity of dark blood would escape. On making a particular examination of this blood it was found not to form a congealing mass, as ordinarily;

but the resemblance of an aggregation of black strings, or long, black angle-worms, with some of their heads and tails matted together. Here, then was the well-known characteristic of **Crocus sativus**. And it was found that the other symptoms of the patient corresponded with the pathogenesis of that drug. **Crocus 200** was given, in water, every half hour at first, and subsequently at longer intervals. She lost no more blood and rapidly improved.—Dr. H. N. Guernsey in "Transactions of Am. Inst. of Homœopathy," 1870.

Case 2.—A lady, who had just passed her climacteric period, consulted Dr. Smith with reference to her eyes. She had used glasses for some time, but of late they had failed to give satisfaction. The only symptom of which she complained was the one last stated viz., the eyes feel as if she had been looking through too sharp spectacles. One dose of **Crocus 200** relieved the trouble, enabling her to sew and to read as usual.—"Am. Jour. Hom. Mat. Med.," May, 1873.

Case 3.—Mrs. M., æt, forty-eight, medium size, fair skin, blue eyes, light hair, mild and sensitive disposition. Five days ago she awoke in the morning, about 3 o'clock, and coughed up blood in considerable quantity, at intervals, until about 7 or 8 o'clock, from which time it gradually diminished in quantity, there still being traces of blood in the sputa late in the afternoon. This had been repeated each day since, commencing at the same time in the morning. The blood was very dark and stringy. I put up three powders of **Croc. sat.** 6. The blood-spitting was as bad the next morning after, but ceased entirely after the second dose, and has never returned. The cough soon ceased.—Dr. H. Ring.

CROTALUS HORRIDUS.

Crotalus horridus is prepared from the venom of the deadly rattle snake of North America. Trituration is prepared by saturating sugar of milk with the venom; also a solution of the venom may be made in glycerine. This snake poison corresponds to low septic states and a general disorganization of the blood caused by septic toxæmia or zymotic and miasmatic diseases. The poison produces a rapid and direct depressing influence on sensorium and medulla oblongata deranging both circulation and nutrition. It acts primarily upon cerebro-spinal nerve centers, and secondarily, on the blood fibrin, causing decomposition of blood and hæmorrhages from all orifices of the body such as eyes, ears, nose, mouth, throat and urethra. It causes œdematous swelling of the body, and profoundly affects the organs of vision, even to the extent of annihilating their functions. After death the cerebrum, cerebellum and medulla are found to be in a state of engorgement with dark, fluid, decomposed blood. The cortical substance of the brain and the membranes as well look highly congested. The arachnoid mater gets thickened, tough and adheres to the pia mater, the meshes of which also show decomposition and engorgement.

Dr. J. S. M. Chaffee describes a case of rattle snake poisoning which he cured with **Crotalus** on Isopathic principle. The case is interesting, inasmuch as it gives us a vivid picture of **Crotalus**. We are not going to discuss the merit of Isopathy in this connection, but will quote the case for reason of utility, as it will help us to master, to understand and to appreciate the pathogenesis of our remedy. "I was to see James Wright, aged 54 years, who, while binding wheat, was bitten on third finger of right hand by a rattle snake. I found him bleeding from the bitten finger, and from eyes, nose, ears, mouth, rectum and urethra, pulse 110, small, wiry; respiration 40; temperature 105; haggard expression; whole body bathed in hot perspiration; delirium. This patient had had the regular routine treatment of whisky, quinine, and carbonate of ammonia for ninety-six hours, when the attendants withdrew and pronounced the case beyond the reach of medical aid. A marked characteristic symptom was a mouldy smell of breath, with scarlet red tongue, and difficult swallowing. Great sensitiveness of the skin of right half of the body, so much so that the slightest touch would produce twitching of muscles of that side. I prescribed **Crotalus hor.,** 30th trituration, 30 gr. in four ounces of water, a teaspoonful every hour until my return visit, twenty-four hours later, when I found marked improvement. Temperature normal; pulse full, soft and regular, delirium gone; saliva and urine slightly tinged with blood; appetite returning, he having asked for food for the first time since the accident."

Crotalus patients are mentally very snappish and irritable. They are so ugly in their temperament that they greatly resemble **Nux;** only in **Nux** the same degraded state of vitality as in **Crotalus** is wanting. They get almost furious at the slightest annoyance. Sometimes this irritability gives place to timidity, fear, anxiety and melancholia. Fear of death or rather thoughts constantly dwelling on death, oppress the patient. The **Crotalus** patient may be as apathetic and indifferent, as any remedy we know of, in our Materia Medica. It is an utter apathy almost simulating suspension of life that is to be seen in **Crotalus**. It is also applicable in the insipient stage of senile dementia characterised by mental delusion and forgetfulness.

As has been said before, we have a great tendency to hœmorrhage in **Crotalus.** The blood discharged is a dark fluid decomposed blood, that has lost all power of coagulation. Hence clots are not usually detected in the hæmorrhage of **Crotalus.** We have hæmorrhage in retina and ecchymotic spots in different parts of the body. There is oozing of blood from ears and nose. It stops epistaxis occurring at the onset of zymotic and septic diseases or in broken down constitutions. There is gastric hæmorrhage in which the patient brings up large quantities of almost black, watery, sanious blood. We have bleeding from the anus where the patient passes black, thin, coffee-ground stools. It is indicated in hematuria due to cancer of the bladder or the prostate gland. Menorrhagia, due to a toxic condition calls for **Crotalus.** In fact there is bleeding from every organ and orifice of the body. What really happens is a general state of disorganiation of the arterial walls and the veins. So that they lose the capacity to retain within them the circulatory fluid. The blood percolates through the walls of the channel, and mixes with the tissue products and contents of the different organs.

In this respect of hemorrhage we may aptly compare it with **Lachesis, Naja,** and **Elaps;** only in **Lachesis** the hæmorrhage is characterized by a charred-straw like sediment; in **Naja** a great preponderance of nervous phenomena accompanying the hæmorrhage and in **Elaps** the hæmorrhage is not a general hæmorrhage it occurs particularly in affections of the ears and the right lungs.

In eyes, its use extends over a variety of complaints such as ablyopia, momentary disappearance of vision, retinitis, ophthalmia, conjunctivitis and iritis occurring in eruptive diseases such variola, morbilli and syphilis. One very important feature of **Crotalus** is a deep yellow color of the whites of the eyes. This indication helped me in a case of cirrhosis of the liver in a constitution that showed signs of absolute dilapidation, and where almost all the stereotyped remedies had failed. The strong yellow color of the sclerotic coat of the eye reminds one more frequently of **Chelidonium** than **Crotalus.** The tongue is so swollen that it leaves very little room in the mouth, and snake-like it is frequently protruded from the mouth. The breath is offensive, and the saliva tion which is frothy and fetid is tinged with a show of blood. these indications it can be used in cancrum oris.

The sensation of constriction in throat, so characteristic of other snake poisons, is prominently present in **Crotalus.** We have used it with success in spasm of the œsophagus where deglutition was rendered impossible, and the patient swallowing liquid food only.

It is used in diphtheria of a very low type. The whole fauces look swollen, dark and red. Pulse is exceedingly fast. Much œdema and gangrene of the fauces, great prostration, much tremulousness, are its indications in malignant diphtheria.

In stomach we have frequent faint, empty, and hungry sensation. Great craving for stimulants, hæmatemesis, a very fast pulse, and other symptoms mentioned above lead to its indication both in cancer and ulceration of the stomach.

It is an excellent remedy in dysentery of septic origin as from foul drinking water and putrid food. Intense debility, tremulousness, fainting and sanious, bloody stools are characteristic indications. It is also applicable in diarrhœa brought about by absorption of septic matters in food and drink, and indulgence in "high game." Like **Pyrogen** it should be remembered in diarrhœa from obnoxious effluvia. In cholera it is indicated in the last stage with sudden and extreme coldness and blueness of the body. Suppression of urine, embarrassed respiration, and collapse lend further importance to its application.

Its application in febrile ailments is potent with great possibilities. It is indicated in ordinary bilious remittent, scarlet yellow, hectic, typhoid and cerebro-spinal fevers. In whatever fever it is applicable, it is applicable by reason of its symptomatology. The same low state of vitality, the septic condition, the history of septic absorption, the tremulous weakness, and the same tendency to syncope, hæmorrhage, petechial eruption and putrescence are to be observed everywhere. The tongue is always dry and cracked with a dark brown streak running down the centre. The edges are of a deep red color. The skin is yellow, and the sweat stains linen red, due to presence of blood even in sweat. It is also used in pyemic fevers, cellulitis dissection and lacerated wounds, malignant pustules and carbuncles, but on self same indication. It is thought of in burns and scalds, when threatening erysipelas or gangrene. Insect-stings call for **Crotalus** when they manifest the same symptoms indicating basic deterioration of tissues. Felon, pemphigus, and abscess also respond to **Crotalus,** when attended with low adynamic fever and bluish discoloration of the skin around the affected area.

CROTON TIGLIUM.

The tincture is prepared from the seeds of a species of Croton, which is a small slender branched tree. Although it was originally a native of China, it is now largely cultivated in India and other surrounding countries. The fruit is a three-shelled, three-seeded capsule. The seeds are largely used in Java for poisoning fish. A big quantity of seeds and oil are exported from Bombay and Cochin every year. The oil is a pale yellow, somewhat viscid, and slightly florescent liquid with a slight fatty odour, and a mild acrid burning taste. When applied to the skin, it produces rubefaction or a pustular eruption.

It is a drastic purgative. The allopaths generally use it as a quick purgative where the most rapid and complete emptying of the bowels is required. The rapidity of its action and the smallness of the dose required to bring it on are its two great advantages. The purging action of this drug is essentially an irritative one. There is increase of watery secretion. It also irritates the uterus and is abortifacient. The allopathic dose is one minim to one dram. It is a medicine that should be repeated with great caution.

In the hand of the homœopath (thanks to the genius of Samuel Hahnemann) this strong purgative has been turned into one of his principal curatives in persistent diarrhœa and purging of the worst variety. This ought to convince all unbelievers in the dictum of "Similia Similibus Curantur." To condemn a science, as being false without proper enquiry into and verification of its principle is unscientific, to say the least of it. Believe in nothing, till you are thoroughly convinced of its sangunity and truth. Disbelieve in nothing and pronounce no premature judgment, till the utter worthlessness of the thing is made evident to you. This, in my opinion, is the most sane attitude to take, for every student of science, that **Croton tig.** produces strong diarrhœa is undeniable. The diarrhœa thus produced has three important characteristics. Firstly, the stool is yellow and watery; secondly, it is expelled suddenly—the stool coming out as if shot out all at once; thirdly, the diarrhœa is aggravated by the least food or drink taken and movement.

Now, administer **Crot. tig.** in any potency for the kind of diarrhœa pictured above, and see whether your strongest bias against or disbelief in homœopathy is conquered. This is a challenge thrown out to all allopaths. Prove it to the contrary.

and get all homœopaths back into the folds of allopathy. If, on the other hand, the test succeeds, do not say any more that you do not believe in this most stupendous of natural laws, enunciated by Hahnemann for the benefit of mankind.

Now, in addition to the three principal characteristics of the **Crot. tig.** diarrhœa just mentioned, I like to add, that there is oftentimes a lot of flatus associated with this diarrhœa. The stool, though mostly yellow and watery, may be at times slightly greenish. As it has been said before, it comes on in a single gush each stool almost draining the patient dry. Stools are preceded by colic and borborygmus. There is quite a lot of gurgling in the intestines, as though nothing but water was in them. There is pressure on the umbilicus; a painful sensation of pressure is also complained of in the anus. This sensation of pressure in anus is as if a plug were forcing outwards.

With respect to the symptom of aggravation after eating and drinking, we should compare **Crot. tig.** with **Aloes, Argent. nit, Arsen., China, Ferrum, Podo., Nux vom., Pulsat.** and **Trom.**

In **Aloes** we have the involuntary stools associated with a sensation of heaviness in anus to guide us.

In **Argent. nit.,** though there is aggravation after eating and drinking the same as in **Crot. tig.,** we notice the causative factor to be excessive indulgence in sweets and sugars and nervous excitement.

Arsen. is very easily differentiated by the constantly increasing prostration, great restlessness, violent unquenchable thirst nausea and vomiting.

In **China,** we have nocturnal aggravation, distention of the abdomen, fermentation, rapid exhaustion, emaciation, drowsiness gradual deepening of the hydrocephaloid condition and the lienter stools; these make it easy for us to distinguish it from other similar remedies.

In **Ferrum met.** the desire for stool is almost instantaneous with eating and drinking. Here also the aggravation is at the night time and the stools are undigested, but the easy flushing of the face on the slightest exertion or excitement, painlessness prolapsus recti, and the chronicity of the disease are distinguishing features.

Nux vom. is of first importance in diarrhœa or dysentery from abuse of intoxicating drinks, high living, debauchery and drastic drugging. Backache, ineffectual urging for stools, over sensitiveness to external impressions, drowsiness after mea intolerance of pressure of clothing about the hypochondria, un-refreshing sleep at night, heat in the head with redness of the face, are such remarkable symptoms that a confusion is hardly possible.

In **Podo.** although, we have gushing, profuse diarrhœa and aggravation after eating or drinking, the same as in **Croton,** there is no reason for us to forget the other distinguishing features, such as the offensiveness of the stools, the time of the aggravation (from 6 A.M. to 12 noon), prolapsus ani during and after stool, exhaustion, gagging or empty retching, violent cramps in the feet, calves and thighs with yawning and stretching.

In **Pulsat.** we have great changeability in the stools; no two stools are alike. Irresistible desire for fresh air, chilliness, constant spitting of frothy cotton-like mucus, bitter taste in the mouth, thirstlessness, loss of taste, peculiarity of the temperament, and white coated tongue are guiding indications.

In **Trombid.** the thin brown (sometimes yellow) stools, con-taining particles of undigested food are expelled with force. We also notice stools after dinner and supper. But we must not forget that even after stools the pain in the abdomen continues, and that with the tenesmus there is chill in the back. We have also burning in the anus after stool.

Croton tig. is very rich in skin symptoms as has been men-tioned before. It cures eczema, specially of the scrotum. The peculiarity of this eczema of **Crot. tig.** is, that although the desire to scratch is very great, the patient cannot bear to scratch, due to extreme sensitiveness. The eruptions are generally vesicular. The scrotum looks raw and swollen, and the great itching disturbs the sleep. We have also intense itching of the genitalia or pruri-tus vulva in the females. It is recommended very highly in urticaria. The eruptions are large and copper-coloured.

There is another symptom which I would like to point out before closing. It is a symptom that has been spoken of very highly by many eminent homœopaths. This symptom is to be seen in the nipple of women, especially during pregnancy, par-turition and lactation. The nipple gets inflamed, hard, swollen, threatening a mammary abscess. Every time the child takes to the breast, excruciating pain runs from nipple through to the scapula of the same side. Many cases of cures of mastitis are reported on this indication.

Case.—A young lady had a severe neuralgia, which did not yield promptly to several medicines which seemed to be indicated. Suddenly its character changes, and the pains, as described by her, seemed to extend from the pupil of the left eye to the back part of the head. This symptom was so similar to the one which so frequently distressed nursing women, *viz.*, "a pain extending from the nipple through to the back," that I gave her **Croton tig.** In a few hours she was well and has no return since, now ten days.—Dr. H. N. Martin.

CUBEBA.

This medicine is prepared from the unripe berries of Piper Cubeba, a climbing shrub growing plentifully in Java, and other neighbouring islands. Its action is confined to the mucous membranes of the different orifices of the body, particularly to that of the genito-urinary tract. It is, therefore, that **Cubeba** becomes an important remedy for gonorrhœa, especially after the violent inflammatory stage of the disease is over. The violent strangury, and tenesmus as seen in **Cantharis** and **Mercury** are over, but there still remains a thick yellowish green discharge which is by no means scanty. There is a certain amount of scalding pain whilst urinating but it is nothing compared to the violent symptoms of **Aco., Arg. nit., Can. sat., Canth., Merc.,** and **Thuja.** It is also indicated in gleet when most of the violent symptoms have altogether subsided, and there still remains a pale, copious, slimy discharge causing soiled linen to become stiff, particularly after coitus or indulgence in spirituous liquors. Sometimes prostatitis and a chronic inflammation of the testicle are seen to respond to **Cubeba** while accompanying the abovementioned symptoms.

In women this is usefully employed in leucorrhœa where the discharge is profuse, yellow, greenish, acrid, and offensive spreading a sort of erythema at the inner surface of the thighs and causing pruritus vulva. We use it also in acrid leucorrhœa of children.

CUCURBITA PEPO.

This remedy, prepared either from the seeds or from the fresh stem of the plant, belonging to the natural order of Cucurbitaceæ, is a remedy well worth knowing, though we have not, so far, got any reliable provings of the same. It is an excellent remedy for tapeworm, and may be used with safety even in children. Its most important indication, however, is intense nausea immediately after eating; on this solitary indication it has been used with good deal of success in sea sickness, nausea, vomiting and salivation during pregnancy. Dr. L. E. Griste's recommendation, to use it in the above complaint is supported by the case of a woman who was almost starved to death during four months of pregnancy on account of this intense sickness preventing her from retaining a single meal. A tincture prepared locally by the doctor from the stem of a fresh pumpkin, when administered, a teaspoonful every two hours, effectively removed this nausea and stopped all further vomiting. The seeds give us a valuable remedy in tapeworm as has been mentioned before. The seeds are scalded and the outer covering peeled off, giving us the karnel which is mixed with cream and taken like porridge at night time before retiring. In the morning on waking, a tablespoonful of castor oil is recommended which will thoroughly wash out the intestines, and expel any worm that might have made the intestine its habitat.

CUPRUM ARSENICUM.

It is Arsenite of Copper. Its two metallic components are arsenic and copper. It is a great remedy with us in certain conditions and complications attendant on cholera, as for example, neuralgia of the abdominal viscera and uremic, convulsions resulting from œdema of the brain, nephritis etc. All these are serious developments, and **Cuprum ars.** by reason of its curative effects in such conditions, becomes an invaluable remedy. Abdominal symptoms are very marked in **Cuprum ars.** We would rarely think of prescribing this in cholera, unless there is violent colic, associated with frequent vomiting, purging, and cold sweat. The pains are spasmodic and intense, accompanied by extreme vesical and rectal tensions. The patient in his agony, squeezes his abdomen with both hands. The late Dr. B. L. Bhaduri mentions " icy coldness of the whole body with cramps and obstinate hiccough " to be the most characteristic of **Cup. ars.**

Dr. Salzer on the other hand lays special stress on the intermit tent nature of its sweat. These symptoms need further verifications; in a country like India where cholera is such an everyday affair, homœopaths should take particular pains, to ascertain and to announce to the world the curative value of these indications.

It is indicated even in diabetes when the urine becomes dark red and emits a peculiar garlicky odor. The high specific gravity and the presence of acetone and diacetic acid are further indications of **Cuprum ars.** in diabetes.

It is not to be forgotten in vomiting of pregnancy. The nausea is so constant and persistent, that the patient rejects everything, and thorough inanition renders the patient incapable of assuming the sitting posture. In conditions like these when even **Nux** and other remedies had failed, **Cuprum ars.** has been known to have given great relief.

CUPRUM METALLICUM.

It is the ordinary copper that is found plentifully in nature. It is a metal of a reddish color. The precipitated metal is triturated. This medicine was first introduced by Samuel Hahnemann.

Cuprum when taken in big doses, sets up an inflammatory colic. Abdomen becomes stony hard, diarrhœa either bloody, greenish or watery soon ensues, vomiting becomes intense, and pain in abdomen almost terrific. Gradually this gives way to a state of collapse with profuse cold sweat, great prostration, deathl anxiety, restlessness, tossing about, hiccough and difficult breathing This is very much like what we see in a case of cholera, an hence **Cuprum** becomes one of our great remedies in the treat ment of that dreaded disease. In India the home of Asiatic cholera it has become a custom from time immemorial, to hang a copper pice on the umbilicus. by means of a string, as a sort of prophyla tic against cholera. This theory of **Cuprum** being a prophylact agent is further supported by the fact that the workers in copp mines rarely fall a victim to this terrible disease. We in Ind owe to **Cuprum** an immeasurable gratitude, as it has saved inn merable human lives from this dreadful scourge.

The symptom that may be regarded as the most characteris point of **Cuprum met.** is spasm. Whatever may be the ailme calling for **Cuprum,** we expect to find some element of this spas

Thus in Asiatic cholera just mentioned, this remedy finds its application in the spasmodic stage, I mean the stage characterised by violent cramps. There is spasm of the stomach, of the abdomen, of the upper and lower limbs, and of the throat—a spasm so violent as to extort shrieks and cries from the poor patient. The particular feature to be remembered about this cramp is that it begins in the fingers and toes, and thence spreads over the rest of the body.

In whooping cough, for which **Cuprum** is a favourite remedy, the attacks are spasmodic in their nature. It is so long-lasting and suffocating that the patient turns entirely breathless, blue, and rigid. At the end of the cough he vomits out all the food taken and a little of tough gelatinous mucus. Before I run on to another item let me mention one or two other peculiarities of the **Cuprum** cough. It is a cough with a gargling sound in the throat, as if water were being poured out of a bottle. Another strange thing about this cough is amelioration from a drink of cold water.

In epilepsy, eclampsia, epileptiform convulsions, puerperal convulsions and other nervous affections, **Cuprum** becomes indicated by the same severity of its muscular spasms. There is generally great restlessness between the attacks either filling up the entire interval or only a part of the time. In epilepsy the aura begins in the knees and ascends; the first attack generally coming on during night. During epileptic spasm the face grows red, respiration becomes hurried and noisy, and arms and legs jerk; especially the left arm is convulsively jerked as if by electric shock. Urine flows involuntarily. The patient wakes up from the fit with dullness of the head, slow remembrance and excessive prostration. Frequently the thumbs are clenched across the palms of the hands during the paroxysm.

Cuprum is a capital remedy for the bad effects of repercussed eruptions, and as such it should stand side by side with **Agaricus, Bryonia, Calc. carb, Causticum, Sulph.,** and **Zincum.**

The mental symptoms of **Cuprum metallicum** are important and should be carefully studied. Maliciousness is the predominant feature of the mental state. They gloat over other people's misfortunes. and they feel happy when they find them in distress. The feature is manifest even in mania and delirium. They bite and strike and do everything to annoy their nurse or companion. In delirium they manifest great fear and become afraid of anybody approaching them. They shrink away and

try to escape from everybody.   Sometimes we find them be
lowing like a calf, and at other times they are seen to be
convulsive laughter.   The **Cuprum** mania is characterised by fier
rage, wild look and fear.   They try to bite and beat everybo
near them and tear things to pieces. They constantly protrude a
retract their tongue in the mouth like that of a snake, same
in **Lachesis** and **Crotalus.**   Marked loss of memory, unco
querable sadness. constant restlessness alternation of gaiety a
depression. are a few more of the mental indications of **Cupr**
metallicum.   It should also be thought of in bodily and men
exhaustion brought on by loss of sleep.

It is one of our remedies for the ill effects of fright.   Ca
of chorea in girls after fright are cured with **Cuprum.**   A case
epilepsy in a boy, after being locked up in the school, is also
ported to have been cured with **Cuprum met.**

Cuprum has congestion of brain as well marked as in I
ladonna. It is applicable in headache with convulsive moti
of the extremities and of the muscles of the face.   We think
it also in apoplexy when the above symptoms are present al
with half closed eyelids, heavy inspiration, and fixed stare of
eyes.   It is particularly useful in brain diseases due to me
tasis from other organs.   Tossing about of head, immovabilit
pupils, quick rotation of eye-balls under close lids, spasmodic
tortion of face, and frothing from mouth are a few more inc
tions worth remembering.

Cuprum metallicum has important gastric symptoms.   In
first place we will speak of the great nausea of **Cuprum**
It is almost as intense as in **Ipecac**.   The patient bring
gushes of whey-like fluid, and frothy bilious matter, and is
relieved by a drink of cold water.   Great burning is complaine
in epigastrium.   A deathly feeling of constriction beneath
sternum is characteristic of **Cuprum.**   Intense cutting pai
umbilical region as from a knife, associated with tenesmus or
traction of abdominal muscles should call for the remedy.

As has already been mentioned, it is an invaluable reme
cholera asiatica.   Its application is generally confined to the
part of the second stage, and the earlier part of the third sta
the disease—when the cramps start and collapse puts in an ap
ance, when lips, nails and the whole face turn bluish.   The ey
sunken and features go through a distinct change.   When
pass down with an audible gargling noise in throa, and
vomiting is preceded by a peculiar sense of constriction i

hest, we should seriously think of **Cuprum metallicum.** Deathly
nxiety, painful twitching of muscles, cramps of calves, aphonia,
ifficult breathing, blue colours and elasticity of skin and dis-
aarge of whitish fluid are valuable indications of **Cuprum metal-
cum.**

Case 1.—Asthma Millari. A delicate girl, nine months old, had for
veral days suffered with a cough, spasmodic and more violent during the
ght; peevishness, no fever; quick, difficult breathing; drawing in of the
uscles in the right and left hypochondrial region during inspiration; per-
ission normal; rattling of mucus far down; little appetite, tongue with
hitish coating; daily, one to two, thin, sometimes watery, sometimes
eenish stools. **Ip.** 9, every two hours.   While asleep the child suddenly
gan to breathe more quickly, and with greater difficulty; grew restless and
ssed about in bed; face bluish; eyes wide open; larynx drawn upward;
e braced herself against the bed with her hands; perceptible cramp in the
spiratory muscles; predominant abdominal respiration; the cough, which
is very exhausting, was attended by a very peculiar, hollow, somewhat
arse sound; at times, also, metallic-sounding piping, short coughs; hands
ld; cold sweat on forehead; spasmodic, small, very frequent pulse.
ie attack lasted five to six minutes; afterward, the child sank back exhaust-
, coughed a few times loosely and easily, and fell into a stupefied sleep. She
id five to six of these attacks for several consecutive nights,
t of longer duration.   **Ip.** every two hours.   The next day
ly one attack, which lasted only three to four minutes. During the day
eat debility, little appetite; cough easy and loose, and even none at all
r four or five hours at a time; respiration normal; two somewhat slimy but
herwise healthy stools. The next night, two rather lighter attacks, but
xt day still great debility. **Cuprum.** 9 in **Sacch. lact.,** one powder; if
cessary, another during the night. At midnight a very light attack, lasting
ly two to three minutes. The next day general health and appetite better.
ie dose **Cupr.**   No more attacks and soon restored to perfect health.
r. Hirsch.

Case 2. Paralysis of the Left Leg.—Mr. K., forty years old, found that
thin the last months the front part of the sole of his left boot was much
oner worn cft than any other part of his boots. After a while he became
nscious that he had to drag his left foot in a walking, and now he felt a
mbness and lameness in the sole of the left foot, which gradually extended
to the left knee. Finally, walking and standing became very difficult.
lopathic treatment was of no avail. Foot and leg were not noticeably
ophied, but skin, subcutaneous tissues, muscles and ligaments considerably
laxed; the sense of feeling was much decreased, so that the application of
t bricks to the constantly cold foot scarcely changed the sense of continual
ldness in it. At times, there was a dull pain from the hip down to the
ee.   His general health was not materially changed.   His apparent
sturbance of innervation (function and nutrition) of the **left** side, com-
ncing at the periphery and progressing toward the center, led me to choose
pr., which, according to physiological provings, has a special relation to
ch disturbances.   **Tinct. Cupr. acet. 3,** five drops, three times a day.
gns of improvement after eight days; cured in three months.—Dr. Heinigke.

CURARE.

This medicine is prepared from a powerful poison used by the South American Indians upon their arrows.   Authorities differ as to the composition of this poison.   Probably several totally different kinds of poisons are designated by the same name, According to Mr. Goudot, who learned the mode of preparation from an Indian tribe, it is made by adding to the concentrated juice of a creeping plant called Curari, the poison obtained from the virus bags of some of the most venomous serpents.   Another author and traveller, M. de Castellnau, who witnessed the preparation of the poison by another tribe, says that it is composed of the inspissated juice of the Cocculus toxiferos, and of a new species of Strychnos.   Further observation will doubtless show that there is great difference in the effects of the different specimens of Curara poison. M. Roulin says that the poison is obtained from a species of toad by half roasting the animal over a slow fire, when the venom exudes from the pores of its skin and is carefully collected on small wooden knives and preserved in small earthenware vessels.

" The Curara poison, which has found its way to Europe, is usually a brownish black, resinous-looking substance, something like the extract of liquorice.   It seems to keep well for an indefinite length of time. A heat of 212° does not seem to destroy its power. The active principle is soluble in all animal fluids whether acid or alkaline.   The aqueous and alcoholic solution are of a fine red color, the former looking great deal the darker A peculiar substance called Curarine has been obtained from it "- Bernard, B. J. H., Vol. 16.

It is a great remedy for paralysis of various kinds and various parts of our body. We have ptosis, facial and bucc paralysis, paralytic failure of power to swallow, paralysis of the deltoid muscles and the general paralysis of the motor system How it is caused is only conjecture, but there is hardly any dou as to the efficacy of **Curare** in combating such failures of the muscular system of the human body. A tired pain all ove weakness and heaviness of arm, weakness of hands and fingers ar trembling of limbs which frequently give way while walking a very prominent symptoms of this remedy.

The **Curare** patients are haggard-looking, pale, and nervor The eyes are sunken and they complain of dark spots before the vision. Noises in ears as of whistling, deep red cracked bleedi tongue, constant dryness of mouth are indications of a grave condition. Dr. Farrington considers **Curare** to be of great importance in vertigo when it is associated with weakness of the legs. At times this giddiness is most instantaneous. The patient falls down in a swoon or fainting fit while standing or walking.

We must not forget the distressing dyspnœa of **Curare.** This dyspnœa is most marked while falling asleep. On such occasions he is frequently threatened with paralysis of respiration.

It is very similar to **Nat. carb.** and **Crotalus.**

Case.—"Sometime ago I treated a man with cirrhotic liver. Every morning, at ten or eleven o'clock, he had an attack of bilious vomiting, followed by a chill. The vomiting continued for three or four weeks, and nothing seemed to stop it. But as he had the dizzy feeling just mentioned, I finally gave him **Curare** 500th, and it stopped the vomiting very promptly The man lived two or three months after that."

CYCLAMEN.

Cyclamen is the Sow-bread, a plant indigenous to the south of Europe. It was extensively used for medicinal purpose by the ancients. "It used to be considered that the root of **Cyclamen** applied externally, hastened difficult labor, and assuaged the pains : also that to touch **Cyclamen,** or to take it internally, would produce abortion and bring on premature labor."

It is very similar to **Pulsatilla** particularly in its relation to the female sexual system. Like Pulsatilla it is suited to plegmatic temperament. There is the same aversion and disinclination to work, the same ill-humoured moroseness and the same tendency to take offence at trifles. It differs from **Pulsatilla** in not having the amelioration from open air and the thirstlessness of that remedy. Mentally, these patients suffer from terrors of conscience. They grieve over duty neglected. There is also a great craving for solitude, and weeping affords them decided relief. They also suffer from a peculiar illusion of being deserted or persecuted by everybody. It has been used with success in mental derangement during climaxis, when the patient becomes extremely indifferent. This indifference gradually deepens and leads the patient finally to a state of total extinction of consciousness, when even questions are not answered, and stools and urine are passed involuntarily and unconsciously.

Its action on the female sexual system is as profound as in **Pulsatilla;** the menstruation comes too early and it brings a certain amount of relief to her melancholy. The menses are profuse, black, membraneous, and clotted. Like **Pulsatilla** again we find intense laborlike pains commencing in small of back and running down each side of abdomen to pubis. It is, therefore, as great a remedy for dysmenorrhœa as our **Pulsatilla.** The only difference is, as has been hinted at before, dread of fresh air. We think of it, also in menstrual irregularities with megrim and blindness. Leucorrhœa in blonde leuco-phlegmatic subjects with retarded or scanty mens turation need not always be given **Pulsatilla. Cyclamen** is just as often indicated in these conditions as that remedy, and lik **Pulsatilla** under similar conditions, it meets chlorosis and anæmia Buzzing in the region of the heart, tumultuous action of the heart, great lassitude, and a sensation of something alive running in the heart are symptoms that meet in **Cyclamen** a ready help. **Cyclamen** also relieves hiccough during pregnancy. Before finishing we must not omit to mention that Cyclamen relieves burning sore pain in heels, and that it has a peculiar sensation about anus and perinæum as if a spot were suppurating.

Case 1.—Mrs.—, æt. forty-four, of large frame. Has in former years had good health and has always worked hard. May, 1872, applied for medicine, stating that her menses had been troublesome for two months. The flow had continued all through each month; discharge pale and watery, at first dark and clotted. General appearance somewhat exsanguined; mouth, tongue and lips pale. She always felt best when moving about. The flow almost ceased as long as she was moving about at work, but as soon as she sat down quietly in the evening, the flow reappeared and continued after she went to bed. **Cyclam.** 2 relieved her promptly, and she improved in general health, and continued so, the menses returning monthly until March, when the troubles of last year reappeared. After two doses of same remedy she remained well.—Dr. H. Ring.

Case 2.—R., aged fifty-one years, has suffered greatly during twenty years from prurigo vulvæ. Her case had been considered incurable. She got along very well during the day so long as she kept moving about; but in the evening, as soon as she sat down, and especially after she had gone to bed, she was greatly annoyed by a troublesome itching of the vulva, compelling rubbing, and a bearing down sensation, necessitating counter pressure with the hand. The mucous surface felt raw, and there was said to be an eruption of some kind inside of the vulva. Cured by 12 powders of **Cyclamen** 30.—Dr. H. Ring.

CYPRIPEDIUM.

This remedy is very little known, and hence very little used. The tincture is prepared from the root of the 'Lady's Slipper.' It belongs to the same category as **Coca, Coffea** and **Thea,**—remedies in use as common beverages for temporary exhilaration. It acts on the cerebro-spinal system, and is useful in bad effects of mental exertion or reflex nervous excitement. It is supposed to be a good remedy for sleeplessness when due to the over-crowding of the brain with all kinds of pleasant ideas.

Little babies are often seen to wake up in the middle of the night and laugh and gambol in the bright light; if this continues night after night, the parents should take warning, as often such functional irritability and cerebral hyperæsthesia end in convulsions. A few doses of **Cypripedium** will avert the impending danger. In respect of sleeplessness it compares well with **Coffea** and **Scutellaria.**

In **Coffea** the insomnia is due to an over-excitement of body or mind, the result of excessive joy or agreeable surprise.

In **Scutellaria** the sleeplessness is due to neurasthenia. The patient wakes up suddenly with some disturbing disagreeable dream, and finds it hard to fall asleep again.

DAPHNE ODORA.

It is also called Daphne Indica or the sweet scented Spruce Laurel. It belongs to the natural order of Thymelaceæ. It particularly attacks muscles, bones, and skins, and thus bears strong resemblance to our anti-syphilitic remedies such as **Aur., Merc., Mezer.,** and **Staphisagria.**

This remedy, though not of great importance, has its own field of action where it becomes indispensable. I remember such a case. A common labourer, a great victim to rheumatism had a peculiar symptom. He felt that hands were detached from his body although he could control them at will. Various remedies were tried but to no effect, till **Daphne** removed this peculiar sensation together with the other annoying symptoms. This symptom, of a part of the body being separated from the rest of the limbs, is a characteristic point in **Daphne.**

Fetidity of breath, urine and sweat is another noteworthy feature of **Daphne.**

The tongue of **Daphne** is peculiar in that it is coated on one side only as in **Rhus tox.**

The pains of **Daphne** are erratic and eletric-like.

He has a great craving for tobacco, as in **Gambog.**

These patients suffer from great sleeplessness due to bone-pains; when they do sleep, it is disturbed by horrid dreams of black cats and of fire.

DIGITALIS.

Digitalis is the ordinary fox-glove. It is indigenous to the western parts of southern and central Europe. The Medicine is prepared from the leaves of uncultivated plants in their second season. The leaves are chopped and pounded and the juice extracted from them by means of pressure. The expressed juice is then mingled with an equal part by weight of alcohol. The mixture is then filtered after the usual process as in the preparation of other drugs. **Digitalis** was first introduced in medical practice by Withering. Samuel Hahnemann was the first to put it on a scientific basis by giving it a scientific proving.

Let us first study the action of **Digitalis** over the heart. It is a cardiac regulator. Its action upon the heart is dual in nature. By its effect upon the cardiac ganglia and muscles it induces contraction and strengthens the systole; by its action on the vagi it prolongs the diastole. As a result of this the diastole of the heart is lengthened and more blood allowed to enter the ventricles and the systole too is made stronger imparting more vigour to the flow of the blood in the arterial system. Thus a rapid and an irregular action of the heart is slowed and steadied, the arterial tension is raised.

In this connection it will not be out of place to cite from Beaumont Small regarding the applicability of **Digitalis** in defective heart conditions according to the theory advocated by our brethren of the other school. "In organic diseases of the heart, the guide for its use is the state of the compensatory action of that organ. It is not given as a remedy for the defective valves, nor with the expectation of benefitting any diseased condition of the organ; it is simply a stimulant and tonic to the muscular tissue. So long as the heart is able to overcome, the impediment to the circulation, and maintain a free flow of blood, nothing is to be gained by the use of the drug, but, with the earliest symptoms of failing power, its administration must be commenced. The system responds quickly to the first indication of this loss of compensation, the heart beats more feebly and quicker, the pulse becomes irregular, a slight degree of dyspnœa is noticed, and œdema of the feet and ankles begins. In such conditions the beneficial action of **Digitalis** is most marked. The heart beats more slowly and forcibly and propels the blood onward, the arteries become filled, the engorged veins relieved, and the equilibrium of the circulation is re-established. This slower action of the heart allows a prolonged period of diastole, during which it is at rest and recuperating; the succeeding contraction is rapid and strong, due to the renewed strength and stimulating action of the remedy.

" No form of organic disease contraindicates the use of **Digitalis** when the compensatory action is failing. Its typical action is produced in mitral disease, in which it acts rapidly and for a pro-longed period. In mitral stenosis it has been thought to produce a peculiarly important effect, as the prolonged dilatation of the ventricle permits a greater flow of blood from the auricle through the narrowed channel. In aortic disease it may also be given with confidence. The one condition in which **Digitalis** is contraindi-cated is fatty degeneration of the heart. In advanced stages of this disease, where the walls are thin and cavities are much dilated, it must be used with extreme caution as its action may be too violent for the feeble organ, and paralysis or rupture may follow. In the lesser degrees of degeneration, where the evidences of such a condition are indistinct, a want of action on the part of the remedy is a sign that must not be disregarded."

But we homœopaths have a surer principle to guide us. We do not depend on vague and abstract ideas, but on definite symptoms brought about by proving over healthy organism. The first symptom thus arrived at, is deathly nausea and vomiting with a faint sinking sensation at the pit of the stomach as in **Antim. tart, Tabacum,** and **Lobelia.** The symptom next to appear but not any the less important, is a peculiar feeling as though the heart stands still with great anxiety, especially through exertion or movement of any kind. There is a sort of indescribable uneasiness vaguely located in the region of the heart which can better be described as a sort of an oppresion. The pulse is very slow and weak, intermitting every third, fifth or seventh beat. Sometimes there is choking when trying to swallow, due to reflex spasms of the glottis. In extreme cases we notice cyanosis. The patient turns blue and sinks into a stupor which may verge on syncope. The breathing is deep, slow and sighing, at times approaching orthopnœa with short, dry tickling cough. Dropsy is very often present, oftener seen in legs penis and scrotum. The legs and thighs pit deeply on pressure. Urine is scanty, dark, sometimes highly albuminous.

Apocynum is another great remedy for dropsy from heart disease. In this remedy too, we find a great sinking feeling, a weak irregular, intermittent slow pulse; but the urine unlike that of **Digitalis** is copious and nearly involuntary from the relaxed sphincter; the skin is unusually dry.

Let us not forget that the dropsy of **Digitalis** is of cardiac origin, and is generally accompanied with a bluish colour of the skin unlike the alabaster hue of the renal dropsies. When the dropsy is of hepatic origin the remedies mostly thought of are **Aurum met., Chimaphila, China, Fluoric acid,** and **Lycopodium.** We will take up this discussion later on in connection with some of these remedies. Local dropsies too, like hydrothorax, hydro-pericardium, hydrocephalus, hydrocele, find in **Digitalis** a good remedy when of cardiac origin.

Digitalis acts on the liver but in an indirect way. That organ becomes sluggish secondarily to the affection of the heart. It becomes hard, tender, sore and slightly enlarged. Jaundice is very frequently noticed in such patients but this is not due to either retention of bile or catarrh of duodenum, but to a certain functional imperfection of the organ due primarily to some organic affection of the heart. Dr. Nash has reported a cure of a case of jaundice of the worst type with **Digitalis,** the sole indication for which was a too slow action of the heart, the pulse only giving thirty beats per minute. As a result of such hepatic disturbance stools turn white, ash-coloured or chalky. The taste in the mouth is bitter, but the tongue is clean, and there is great nausea at the sight of food. In this respect **Digitalis** resembles **Bryonia** and **Colchicum.**

On the mental side we notice great despondence, anxiety and melancholia. Sleep is very uneasy and unrefreshing. They wake up frequently during the night with anxious dreams, and a sort of a distresed feeling vaguely located at the cardiac region. The patient is constantly apprehensive of some evil coming to him.

We will now speak of the action of **Digitalis** on the urethra and genital organs. It brings about a condition simulating inflammation of the neck of the bladder. The patient makes many fruitless efforts to urinate. Hardly any urine comes out, and there is a feeling as if urethra were constricted. On the male genital organs it causes great irritability as a result of which we have frequent debilitating seminal emissions, weakness of memory, oppressed respiration and pain in præcordial region. Noctural emissions are frequent and are attended with great weakness of the genitals. It is a great remedy with us for the abuse of sexual functions, and is therefore called for, in the treatment of extreme debility in debauchees. Great debility, impaired digestion, foul taste in the mouth, palpitation of the heart, transient flushes of heat, fainting, ringing and roaring in the ears, and excessive loss of semen in consequence of onanism, are some of the indications of **Digitalis** in perverted function of the sexual economy. Similarly it finds application in nymphomania when excited by constant lascivious fancies with remarkably slow pulse and stools of a very light colour.

It is, like **Bryonia,** a splendid remedy for vicarious mensturation from lungs after suppression of menses. It has also a kind of uterine hæmorrhage of a low persistent nature, in weak emaciated women of pale waxy complexion suffering from quick respiration, lassitude, and icy coldness of the limbs. Cases such as these remind one of **China** and **Laurocerasus** which are oftentimes prescribed wrongly in place of **Digitalis.** A symptom that ought to be regarded as a guiding symptom and one that helps differentiation, is the peculiar, irregular respiration of **Digit.** Further more these respirations in **Digitalis** are always accompanied by frequent deep sighs.

Digitalis should be thought of in passive congestion of the lungs, when such congestion is due to a weakened dilated heart. Hæmoptysis from obstruction of pulmonary circulation when associated with engorged veins about the head, a pale waxy complexion, and coldness of the skin should immediately call for the application of **Digitalis.** It has been known to relieve the acute distress of asthma when it is secondary to heart affections. Frequent retching, laborious breathing, almost imperceptible pulse, tumultuous action of the heart, cough with hæmoptysis, scanty albuminous urine, œdematous swelling of the legs and ascites are symptoms that speak of a very grave situation; but even such conditions alter and a more methodical action of the heart established by the timely administration of **Digitalis.**

Case 1.—Mrs. B., a young married lady, had always enjoyed good health to within a year of my acquaintance with her, during which period she had been subject to frequent attacks of palpitation of heart. About September 1, 1853, having been exposed to cold and wet, she was taken with an acute pain in the hip-joint, which lasted about twelve hours, and then, as she expressed herself, "went to her heart," and for the following six or eight hours, and then, as she was afflicted with **angina pectoris,** and the following wer her symptoms; Constant pain or anguish in the region of the heart, with more or less palpitation, at times the pain and palpitation were greatly aggravated, exercise of the body and emotion of the mind caused an aggravation of her sufferings, but at times they were greatly increased without any apparent cause, while sitting perfectly at rest—such paroxysms were accompanied by sinking sensations; her face becoming purple, and ending in syncope, she would assert that she was dying. She had constant dizziness of the head and ringing in the arm and fingers; creeping all over her skin. Sometimes such paroxysms come on in the night, when it seems as if she were suffocating, wakes up in great anguish; has also terrifying dreams. Bowels and menstruation regular; appetite good. After the use of **Spigelia,** she received **Digitalis 24** with immediate benefit and perfect relief in two weeks. Physical examination of the heart gave no evidence of organic disease or of functionary disturbance, except excessive action.—Dr. A. S. Ball in the N. A. Jour of Hom. Feb., 1857.

Case 2.—A gentleman had had for eighteen months a curious and annoying symptom. Every night on going to sleep, he is suddenly awakened with a start by loud metallic crash in his head. This would frequently occur three times before he could fall into quiet sleep. It was very troublesome, and he had been treated for it some time without benefit. **Dig. 1** cured.—Dr. Dudgeon.

Case 3.—June, 1867, was called to visit Robert, a lad of sixteen, had been sick a year. Three or four physicians in turn had treated him, but without benefit. He was slender and very much emaciated, though able to dress himself and walk about. The case presented the following symptoms; Some appetite for food, but as soon as he ate, no matter what, it soured and regurgitations commenced. He spit it up by mouthfuls, as he expressed it, "sourer than any vinegar." After his stomach was emptied he had a terrible pain and uneasiness, which lasted one or two hours. Every time he ate there was the same repetition of symptoms. Bowels moved some, not costive. Gave **Calc., Carbo veg., Sulph., Acid sulph.** and other remedies in succession for four or five weeks, with no benefit. The boy was growing weaker, and I began to despair of curing him. I now observed his pulse was very slow, and he had a cold and blue look, and the surface and extremeties were cold. This led me to think of **Dig.,** and on comparing the stomach symptoms, I found it just the thing. Gave it to him, and the **effect** was like magic. In a week he was nearly well.—Dr. J. L. Gage.

DIOSCOREA VILLOSA.

It is also called the Wild Yam. It belongs to the natural order of Dioscoreaceæ. It is a perennial creeper growing wild in the Southern states of North America. It was introduced and proved by Cushing and Burt. The tincture is prepared from the root.

It is a great anodyne. A careful study of **Dioscorea** will amply repay us. Its actions far excel those of **Opium** and morphine as we will see presently. The pains of **Dioscorea** are neuralgic in character. It is difficult to explain the why and wherefore of this pain; all that is possible is to arrive at a problematic factor. **Dioscorea** probably acts upon the solar plexus and upon spinal nerves, and thereby causes pain over the body and in the viscera. It affects the ganglionic nervous system, particularly of the umbilical region, thereby producing symptoms simulating an attack of bilious colic. The statement of Burt is particularly illuminating and should be very convincing. "The grand sphere for the use of **Dioscorea** is among neuroses of the bowels and stomach; where the cœliac and umbilical plexus are in a state of great hyperæsthesia, the pain and spasm being unbearable." It is not a matter of much importance, as to what really happens; what we are concerned with most as homœopaths, is the proper application of our remedies on proper indications. The distress, as complained of in umbilical and hypogastric regions, is very severe. The pain is intense, cutting, twisting, and agonising, and it radiates all over the abdomen. The guts feel like being twisted most mercilessly. Another feature of this pain in **Dioscorea** is the sudden shifting from the original area of affection and the reappearance of the pains in distant localities, such as the fingers and toes. Great rumbling of bowels and discharge of large quantities of flatulence are not infrequent. It must be fully a year ago that I was called in to see a case of abdominal colic. The impression that the patient created on my mind will, I am afraid, never, be effaced till death brings oblivion. He was writhing in excruciating agony. The pains were neuralgic and paroxysmal. He felt as if his entrails were clutched by a powerful hand and twisted mercilessly. The intensity would increase with every second of pain till at last it seemed almost to tear asunder his string of existence, then all on a sudden, the remission would come bringing with it a few minutes of ease and quiet. This pain would begin in the region of the bowels and thence radiate upward and downward until his whole body would be involved eliciting shrill cries from him. A few doses of **Dioscorea** soothed it like oil on the surface of troubled water. Such then is the power and efficacy of **Dioscorea** in colic.

We must not however feel that these pains are only confined to the intestine alone. **Dioscorea** is equally applicable in renal colic and in other pains of spasmodic nature in urethra. The pain which is always agonising, writhing and crampy in nature, radiates from a small spot over the crest of the right ilium to the renal region and down the right leg and into the right testicle. Similarly it is applicable in angina pectoris where sharp, cutting pain, starting from the region of the heart, extends down the middle of the sternum into both the arms and hands. The same feature is to be observed everywhere.

DOLICHOS PRURIENS.

It is an West Indian climbing plant, from the fruit-pod of which the tincture is prepared. It is also called Cow-hage or Cow-itch. It belongs to the natural order of Leguminosæ.

I have used this remedy more than once with great satisfaction. Its symptoms, though not many, are very distinct and reliable.

The most striking symtom that I can think of, is a sensation of splinter felt in the throat below the angle of the right lower jaw. In this it resembles **Argentum nit., Hepar sulph.** and **Nitric acid.**

Another symptom worth noticing is violent itching all over the body without any visible eruption, and it is rendered worse by scratching.

It has been used with success in jaundice associated with irritation of the skin. Kraft has recorded the cure of a case of jaundice with **Dolichos** in a woman who also had with desperate itching an enormous distention of abdomen with flatulence. The symptoms of **Dolichos** are always worse at night.

Case.—A lady, æt forty-five, felt pain under left scapula, which continued three days, when an eruption made its appearance on the affected side, and assumed the herpetic form, spreading in rings forward to the sternum, and backward to the spine and attended with much burning and smarting Dolichos pruriens 30 was used successfully after **Rhus,** etc., had failed.—Dr Baikie.

DORYPHORA.

The tincture is prepared from the black Potato Bug, an insect greatly similar to **Cantharis,** to which it bears a strong resemblance. The tincture is prepared by crushing the live beetles and covering it with alcohol.

It produces an intense burning sensation in different parts of the body, such as mouth, throat, œsophagus, stomach, abdomen, rectum and the urinary passage. Hence comes its usefulness in gastric derangements, gonorrhœa and gleet.

It is also applicable in morning diarrhœa with intense pain in the abdomen and burning in the rectum. In gonorrhœa it is indicated by intense itching and burning in glans penis which looks swollen and bluish, and urination is associated with excruciating pain as in **Cantharis.**

Great trembling in extremities is another symptom to be remembered in **Doryphora.**.

It has been successfully used in urethritis in children caused by local irritation.

DROSERA.

It is also called Round-leaved Sundew and moor grass. This plant grows in Europe, Northern Asia, and America. The juice is extracted from the fresh plant before flowering, and is then mixed with an equal part by its weight of alcohol to make the tincture.

The plant grows in damp prairies, and is avoided by animals : when eaten by sheep it produces a cough which becomes fatal to them. On the system too, its effect is similar.

This remedy acts powerfully upon the system through its influence upon the pneumo-gastric nerve. The attacks of cough are of a spasmodic character frequently bringing on hæmorrhages from different orifices of the body.

It is one of our leading remedies for coughs of spasmodic nature. The cough is deep-sounding, hoarse, barking in nature and the paroxysms follow each other so closely that the patient gets out of breath and vomits large quantity of tenacious mucus.

The violence of such paroxysms can be easily guessed from the fact that hemorrhage takes place from the various outlets of the body during such fits of coughing. There is constant titillating and tickling in the throat as if from a feather, specially when the head touches the pillow, and at night. The cough is attended with a sense of constriction in the chest with pain in hypochondria, and the patient supports these parts with his hands during coughing. The cough is aggravated after midnight, from laughing, singing, drinking, talking and especially from lying down.

Whooping cough is such a distressing ailment, and the treatment is so difficult, that I think it will not be out of place to discuss a few other pertussis remedies in this connection:

Ambra grisea is a remedy of equal fame in whooping cough, but the cough here is always worse in a crowded place. The urine smells sour. This is one of the few remedies that have cough with eructations.

In **Antim. tart.** the whooping cough is provoked by anger, eating, and culminates in vomiting of mucus.

In **Bromium** the patient gets a sensation of coldness in the throat during the rough, barking, and whistling cough. Chilliness, shuddering and accumulation of frothy mucus in mouth are prominent concomitants.

The racking paroxysmal cough of **Coccus cacti** is very similar to that of **Drosera.** It differs only in the nature of the mucus that is vomited out. The tough, ropy and viscid mucus, very difficult to expel nearly causes strangulation and vomiting of food. The child on awakening in the morning is immediately seized with the paroxysmal cough.

Coral. rub. is another whooping cough remedy that bears great semblance to **Drosera.** I have found it more effective than many other remedies advocated in whooping cough. Under **Coral** the spasmodic nature of the cough is more marked. The cough starts with gasping for breath, and the patient turns purple and black in the face. It is worse at the later part of the night and morning. The cough in this remedy has been styled the 'minute gun' cough from the rapid succession of paroxysm after paroxysm that leaves of no breathing space between them.

Cuprum met. cough, though greatly similar to that of **Droser** has been so amply dealt with in that remedy that differentiation will be very easy.

Under **Dirc.** the gagging cough is accompanied by hoarseness and rawness of the larynx. The patient takes cold easily.

With **Senega** we will close this list of whooping cough remedies. This remedy is frequently indicated in chubby children. Mucus like that of **Coccus cacti** is very tough, transparent and albuminous consistency. Unlike **Coccus** the aggravation is toward the evening. The patient complains of a crushing weight on the chest.

Drosera has been highly recommended by many physicians in tuberculosis both of the lungs and larynx. Chronic persistent hoarseness, the effect of repeated catarrhal attacks, rapid emaciation, a sense of constriction of the larynx when talking, constant motion to and fro of the epiglottis, a rough scraping feeling of dryness deep in the fauces, severe sitches in the chest felt when sneezing and coughing, purulent expectoration and foul pus-like taste in the mouth are symptoms that warrant its application in the last named complaint.

In Laryngeal phthisis the indications calling for its application are anemia and pallor of the larynx, redness and swelling of the mucous membrane covering the arytenoid cartilages, weakness, loss of appetite and a dry, tickling, persistent cough.

We also use it in harassing titillating cough in children that commences troubling as soon as head touches the pillow at night. During cough the fingers are spasmodically contracted.

Case 1.—A boy, three years old, had whooping cough for three weaks. Symptoms: The cough appears at times during the day, but is worst during the night. It is excited by laughing, weeping and mental excitement and usually terminates with vomiting of the ingesta and a large amount of tough mucus. For several days profuse epistaxis with the attacks; also, protrusion of the eyes, purplish hue of the face, suffocative spasms. Emaciation, exhaustion. Cured by **Drosera 30**.—(Tietze in Annalen der Hom. Klinik, iii., 188.)

Case 2.—Lady twenty-five years old; came under my treatment suffering from what she termed asthma; about two years ago, while residing in London, she was with a number of children exposed to the whooping-cough; the children all contracted the whooping-cough, while this lady also suffered from cough which was treated by a learned specialist in London, who pronounced it "bronchitis." The lady was sent to Brighton, and there became asthmatic; returned to London, and the learned pathologist tortured her for six weeks; at last a diarrhœa ended the attack, and she was ordered **Ars.** for six months only three times; besides other tonics; she was reduced to a skeleton. This summer she returned to Philadelphia, and was again attacked as before with violent asthma, for which she took first **Lobel.** in large doses, each dose for a moment palliating the asthma; but finding no permanent benefit, and growing worse under that palliative treatment, she desired homœopathic treatment. The first remedy administered for the nightly return of the asthma, which did not permit her to lie down, but made her very restless, was a solution of **Ars.** cm. (Fk.); the great restlessness ceased; she began cough, and expectorated great quantities of white, ropy phlegm; cannot lie down; **Coc. cac.** cm. (Fk.) very much relieved her for a fortnight. Now came another exhibition of the disorder; the cough is much worse, shaking her over; worse from 9 P.M. till 1 and 2 A.M.; diarrhœa also appeared; very frequent, dark, almost black, loose painful evacuations with much mucus violent palpitation of the heart in the evening; **Phosphor.** cm. (Fk.) ever: two hours, for twelve hours relieved the palpitation of the heart, the diar rhœa and wheezing breathing. She could now-lie down, but in another wee the cough came on in paroxysms, coughed more at night; the irritation wa described as coming from the diaphragm, causing a catching of her breath and a real whoop. A single dose of **Dros. cm.** (Fk.) very soon relieved he and she has since then been free of any complaints.—Dr. Ad. Lippe.

DUBOISINUM.

It is prepared from the Corkwood tree of Queensland, belong ing to the natural order of Solanaceæ. It, therefore, belongs the same order as **Belladonna.** The tincture is prepared from extract of the leaves. It dilates the pupil and is, therefore a go substitute for atropine. It also dries the mucous lining, chec perspiration and causes hyperæmia of retina. Its most impo tant symptom consists of a vision of red spots floating before eye In the lower limbs it causes loss of power, hence we find the patients staggering as if stepping on empty space. We find indicated in pharyngitis with a varicose condition of the thro There is hardly any secretion of any kind in consequence of whi the throat feels excessively dry. Hyperæmia of the epiglott engorgement of the laryngeal cavity, frequent hawking up viscid semi-transparent mucus, and a frequent desire to clear throat are important indications calling for **Duboisinum.**

DULCAMARA.

Dulcamara commonly known as the "Bitter-sweet" i climbing shrub, belonging to the natural order of Solanaceæ. grows to a height of 6 to 8 feet, and it flowers in clusters. tincture is prepared from the fresh stems and leaves gathe before flowering. It is generally adapted to scrofulous const tions with a marked susceptibility to weather changes. It principally on the mucous membranes and muscular tissues, gives rise to symptoms like those resulting from exposure to d: and rain. It also acts on lymphatic tissues producing gland enlargement and cellular effusions. The Dulcamara constitu therefore, is a phlegmatic one. It takes cold easily, and su from all changes of weather.

Mentally the **Dulcamara** patient is very depressed, an solicitous about the future. A great deal of mental confu prevails, and it manifests itself in his want of power of concentration.

Paralysis is a common feature in **Dulcamara**. Any portion of the body or any organ such as the lungs, the heart, and the vocal cords, may be affected. The paralysed part feels icy cold. The outstanding feature in all these affections, where **Dulcamara** is indicated, is seen to consist in its modality. The complaints of **Dulcamara** are brought about by exposure to cold and damp, getting wet and working in water. Hence it is generally called for in ailments of persons accustomed to live in basements or damp cellars.

Dr. Clarke brought complete relief with a single dose of **Dulcamara** 30 in a case of sarcoma of the bones at the base of the skull in which there were stabbing pains in the front of the head, and partial paralysis of the tongue. It was the latter symptom that drew his attention to **Dulcamara.**

Like all scrofulous remedies, it is very rich in skin symptoms. We notice various kind of eruptions, some of them dry, some moist, some vesicular and some papular. Eczema, nettlerash itch, and warts are plentiful. They may come on scalp, cheek and elsewhere. The warts are large, fleshy and smooth, and are seen in hands and back of fingers. It is a great remedy for crusta lactea. Thick brown yellow crusts cover sores on cheek, scalp, and other parts of the body. It is also a great remedy for retrocession of eruptions due to exposure to damp cold air.

Dulcamara vies with **Bryonia** and **Rhus tox** in the treatment of rheumatic affections. It is generally the chronic form of rheumatism, where the affection occurs after exposure, that demands **Dulcamara.** Sometimes this rheumatism is the effect of suppression of cutaneous eruptions, and it frequently alternates with diarrhœa as in **Abrotanum.** The pains are sticking, drawing, and tearing in character, and the affected parts feel as if they have gone to sleep. The pain becomes very severe when they remain in one position, and it subsides a bit when they move about, reminding one of **Rhus tox.** We should also think of **Dulcamara** in that intolerable pain in the shin bone at night time, that compels the patient to get up and walk about. It is not the syphilitic bone pain that we find in **Aurum met.** and **Asafœtida.** It has been recommended in lumbago when the back feels lame and cold, and the patient complains of a drawing pain from the small of the back down the thighs, as if he has been stooping for a long time.

Dulcamara has a characteristic diarrhœa inasmuch as the stools are simultaneous with vomiting, and are associated with prolapsus recti. The stools are changeable, white, yellow or greenish and are always aggravated at night time and in wet weather. We use it also in a certain form of chronic diarrhœa where the patient shows constant drowsiness, aversion to food, and lies quietly in an apathetic condition—the stools being thin, yellowish, greenish, watery and involuntary. It is a condition that strongly resembles **China,** and shows an equal amount of drained vitality.

The urine generally is scanty, fetid, and turbid; sometimes it contains a tough, jellylike white mucus giving a milky appearance to the urine. Dr. Clarke recommends it in cystitis and other ailments of the bladder, particularly when a muco-purulent urine is associated with one-sided sensitiveness of the abdomen.

Dulcamara strongly resembles **Antim. tart.** in catarrhal troubles. There is increased secretion of the mucous membranes and glands, although usually the elimination from the skin is much decreased. Like **Antim. tart.** it is useful in the cough of children and of old people. We think of it particularly in threatened paralysis of the vagus.

Case 1.—Mr C., labourer, worked in water for three hours, ten day previous to my visit. The next morning awoke with pain in left kidney and could not urinate, but since then has passed a few drops ten or twelve times per day. Urine bloody, with white sediment; also has severe pain in abdomen, and urging to stool without effect; appetite poor; tongue coated a dark, dirty color; nausea; kidneys very sensitive to pressure; pain extending along the ureters. **Dulcamara** 1 cured.—Dr. N. C. Ricardo.

Case 2.—M., aged fifty. For three years suffered with intolerable pain in the tibiæ. During the day was comparatively free from pain, but "wa obliged to walk the floor half the night." The pains were aggravated b rest and wet weather, and ameliorated by the opposite conditions. Well i every other respect. Suspecting a syphilitic taint, I questioned him closel but he denied strenuously ever having been infected. **Rhus tox.** in varyin potencies, **Merc. viv.** and **Merc. sol.; Rhod.** 30 and 200, **Ruta grav.** 20 **Thuja** 200, and several other remedies failed to relieve, and I was on the poi of giving him up as a "bad job," when the last prescription of **Dulc.** 200, s doses did the business. He is not cured yet, but reports himself very muc better.—Dr. W. F. Shepard.

ECHINACEA ANGUSTIFOLIA.

It is also called the purple cone-flower, and it belongs to the natural order of Compositæ. In **Echinacea** we have a grand remedy for all conditions tending towards malignancy. It promotes suppuration, but checks the spread of the infection through lymph channel. Hence it should be thought of in snake-bites insect stings, boils, carbuncles, and gangrene when there is profuse slouging discharge and progressive emaciation and debility. It is, therefore, as good a remedy in blood poisoning and septic conditions as **Baptisia**. We think of it in puerperal septicemia, when the discharge turns extremely offensive, and tympanites and abdominal sensitiveness indicate serious complications. Chilliness with nausea is a cardinal indication.

ELAPS CORALLINUS.

This medicine is prepared from the venom of the Brazilian coral snake. It was proved by Mure and Lippe, who extracted the poison from the living snake, and triturated it with sugar of milk. We notice that this remedy seriously affects the auditory, nasal, and the throat passages, and is consequently curative in many affections of those regions. Thus for example, we use it in chronic otorrhœa when accompanied with deafness. The patient complains of constant buzzing in the ear as if a fly were imprisoned in the auditory meatus. He is also subject to epistaxis and eruptions about the nose and the face.

This is a grand remedy for ozœna. The nose feels stopped up and occasionally emits a foul smell. This is accompanied with chronic pharyngitis. The posterior wall of the throat is found to be covered with a dry greenish-yellow membrane, wrinkled and fissured, extending to the nares. Occasionally portions of this membrane are expelled through nose of throat leaving an angry, raw surface. Deglutition is extremely painful.

All the discharges of this remedy are black, and this is so prominent that we can call this a characteristic symptom. Thus in the epistaxis the blood is black. The blood from the uterus too is dark coloured. Even the wax from the ear is dark.

Lastly before we close let us add that **Elaps** is a capital remedy for uterine cancer. The flow of dark-coloured blood, in these cases, is so very free that the patient becomes severely prostrated. She feels as if something had burst in the womb, and there follows a continuous stream of dark fluid blood.   This extreme hemorrhage gives them a pale, haggard, cachectic look.

About the skin symptoms of **Elaps** we know very little, but we have read about Dr. Clark curing a case of long standing irritating rash in axilla, which frequently used to give rise to suppuration of the axillary glands.

ELATERIUM.

This is also called the Squirting Cucumber. The fruit is cucumber-like in appearance, but it is only about one and a half inches in length. It is three-celled, and contains numerous seeds in a very bitter pulp. When the ripe fruit drops from the stem, the seeds and the pulp spurt out of the aperture left by the stem. This feature supplies an important characteristic of the drug, namely that of any discharge spurting out of an orifice particularly the stool from the rectum.

The preparation of this drug is a bit different from the other remedies we have gone through so far.   The juice is extracted from the fruit before it is quite ripe by means of pressure. The expressed juice is then mixed with equal parts by its weight of alcohol, and allowed to stand 8 days in a well-stoppered bottle and then strained and filtered.

This is one of our main remedies for cholera and choleric diarrhœa. As I have mentioned before, the dark olive-green frothy stool is expelled with great force from the anus. It is thus like **Croton tig., Gratiola, Jatrop, Podo, Thuja, Aloes, Calc-phos, Gambogia** and **Phos.** The difference consists in the nature of the expulsion.   Here the stool squirts out like water as from a small aperture at the bottom of a vessel. There is very often violent colic recurring at short intervals. Sometimes, this is accompanied with nausea and vomiting of a watery substance, or of a greenish bilious matter.

Dr. H. C. Allen recommends it very highly in cases of quotidian, double-quotidian, tertian, double-tertian and quartan types of fevers when suppressed by quinine, as a result of which urticaria breaks out, all over the body, with intense pain and a peculiar disordered state of the mind. When as a result of such drugging, we find them suffering from a strong propensity, to wander from home even in the night time, **Elaterium** will be a capital remedy.

At the onset of the fever, great chilliness is noticed with constant gaping and yawning. Sometimes, this yawning is so loud and of so peculiar a nature as to resemble the neighing of a horse. This is followed by intense heat with violent thirst. The pains shoot to the very tips of the fingers and toes. Very often a diarrhœic condition is noticed during the stage of heat. There is profuse purging, nausea, vomiting, and violent pains in the abdomen.

Elaterium is very useful for jaundice of new-born infants.

EPIGEA REPENS.

This is an æsthetic-looking plant also known as the Trailing Arbutus and Ground Laurel.   It is an analogue of **Uva ursi., Mitchella, Chimaphila, Cannabis, Copaiva, Cubeba, Ipomea nil.,** and **Osimum.**

This drug has not been properly proved, but we have had various proofs of its usefulness in many complaints of the urinary system, especially dysuria and strangury attending renal calculi. It is especially adapted to the Uric acid calculi. Dr. Hale used it, in a case of strangury where the urine was full of blood and a large quantity of muco-purulent sediment, in 10 drop doses of the tincture. The patient passed a copious deposit of fine brown sand, and was relieved of all his troubles.

Uva ursi is another capital remedy for dysuria, due to stone in the bladder. The flow of urine stops suddenly as if a stone had rolled into the internal orifice of the urethra. The little urine that comes out after great straining is hot, scalding, bloody, slimy, and ropy. In cases where operation is deemed absolutely necessary, it relieves the inflammatory thickness of the wall and ameliorates to a great extent the suffering of the patient.

In **Chimaphila** the urine is full of mucus sediment, due to cystitis, the result of stone in the bladder. The patient has to stand with his legs wide apart, and a slight forward inclination of the body when he wants to pass urine.

Osimum is indicated when, like **Cantharis,** we notice a great quantity of blood in the urine passed with intense strangury and trial. The urine smells intolerable like the smell of musk. It is a right-sided remedy.

Ipomea nil, a rare remedy, is very useful in cases of cutting pain in the renal region extending down the ureter to the bladder. The distinguishing features are the nausea and vomiting that accompany the pain.

The other remedies, that we have mentioned, need not be touched on, as they are very common and their indications have been given elsewhere.

EPIPHEGUS.

The other names for this remedy are Cancer-root and Clap-root. It is comparatively little known, but as homœopaths we can not neglect it; occasions may arise when **Epiphegus** and nothing but **Epiphegus** will help.

The only use that I ever made of this remedy was in cases of headaches of a very peculiar nature. These headaches are neurasthenic in type, brought on by strenuous exertion, such as going on a visit, doing a day's shopping, etc. The patient suffers from a constant desire to spit a ropy, viscid salivation. Vision too gets a bit blurred. It is always worse on rising from supine position and in the open air. There is a decided relief after a sound sleep.

The pains of **Epiphegus** are pressing in character and they are generally referred to, in the temples, travelling inwards; they are worse from working in open air. The headaches are, as has been pointed out before, nervous headaches caused by mental and physical exhaustion, and they are preceded by hunger.

EQUISETUM HYEMALE.

It is called the Scouring Rush, a plant growing in damp soils of Europe and North America. It is a very popular remedy for gonorrhœa, gleet, hematuria, gravel and dropsy. Its principal action is over the bladder; it is a great urinary remedy with us. The most important symptom is a constant desire to urinate with severe or dull pain in the bladder. This pain is not relieved after the patient has pased urine. The entire region of the bladder is tender to pressure. A pain extends, at times, to the testicle and the spermatic cord. The urine passed is scanty, inspite of the great desire to urinate.

We must not forget it in incontinence in old women. **Equisetum** has been known to restore full control over stools and urine.

ERECHTHITES.

It is called the Fire weed, and it belongs to the natural order of Compositæ. It is a grand hæmorrhagic remedy, and is therefore allied to **Erigeron, Millefolium, Hamamelis,** and other hæmorrhagic remedies of our Materia Medica. The hæmorrhage may be from any part of the body such as the lungs, throat, ear, nose, mouth, bowels, kidneys, and uterus. The hæmorrhage is attended with excitement of the circulatory system.

ERIGERON CANADENSIS.

This is an annual plant that grows plentifully all over the world in fields, commons, and glades. It grows in such profusion that it is regarded as a very trublesome weed by the farmers. It flowers in July and August. The medicine is prepared from the whole plant when in bloom. It was first proved by Dr. W. H. Burt of the Uuited States. It is known by various names such as fleabane, daisy, field-weed, mare's-tail, etc.

Times without number I have used this remedy and it was mostly in cases of bad hemorrhages, and I must say I was rarely disappointed. It is a remedy good for hemorrhages of all kinds, but like all our homœopathic remedies it must be used with discretion and the discretion consists in prescribing on totality of symptoms with due deference to the singular and the peculiar ones amongst them. The hemorrhage of this remedy, it is immaterial from what orifice it may take place, is character- ized by the bright redness of the discharge.

Hematemesis due to ulceration or rupture of blood vessels in the stomach may be helped by **Erigeron.** In epistaxis and hemor- rhage from the bowels we have used it with as great advantage. Even local application of the tincture is advocated. Not very long while ago a gentleman came to me for hemorrhage from the anus. Examination revealed bad fissures in the rectum. The hemorrhage was very profuse. I tried various remedies but not with much satisfaction till I had to resort to **Erigeron** which had to be applied locally by means of gauze soaked in the drug and than inserted into the rectum.

Such local application of the tincture though advocated by many is unhomœopathic, for the principle of Similia does not countenance local medication. Pure homœopathy, as taught by Hahnemann, is meant simply to help the diseased vitality—vitality that ought in every case, to solve all its own problems, fight its own battles, and make its own destiny. By interfering with the spontaneous working of vitality which, local medication really amounts to, we not only interfere with the proper working of nature but endanger and upset a plan which physicians, however skilful, may never really understand, and the method of which might never come within the limit of his intelligence.

Erigeron is good for bright red hemorrhage from the uterus. But this is still putting it very vaguely for there are innumerable remedies with bright red uterine hemorrhage; the indication that we deem very important is the association of this hemorrhage with dysuria and irritation of the rectum. There are a few other remedies which require consideration here.

One of them is **Mitchella repens.** The bright red hemorrhage from the engorged uterus is associated with dysuria, but unlike **Erigeron** the flow is in a continuous stream.

Yet another is **Phosphorus.** This is one more of our great hemorrhagic remedies. The menses are almost always preceded by leucorrhœa and a sad melancholy mood. The patient feels like weeping, and is troubled with frequent desire to urinate.

A third is **Sarsaparilla.** In this remedy too, we meet with frequent desire to urinate which ceases as soon as the flow is established. Another important feature of this remedy is that micturition is followed by almost unbearable pain. The menses are ushered in by a few itching eruptions on the forehead.

Senecio is another remedy that claims the association of dysuria with menses. The patient complains of a burning pain in the neck of the bladder before menses, giving rise to much tenesmus. This remedy is indicated mostly in nervous women who suffer from sleeplessness due to prolapsus or flexion of the uterus. She is a great subject to catarrh of the nose, throat, and lungs, and we have hæmoptysis in place of menses.

We must not suppose that **Arnica** and **Sulphur** are only remedies for ecchymoses; **Erigeron** has this symptom quite well marked.

Sometimes during dentition, children suffer from great difficulty in passing urine. They want to urinate very frequently, and they cry as often as they pass urine. Whatever may be our explanation of this symptom. it is true that **Erigeron** cures it.

Lycopodium is another remedy where the child cries during micturition and the napkin is stained red.

It has been recommended in placenta prævia by Dr. Moore who reports of having saved numerous cases, through the medium of **Erigeron.** We can very easily put our trust in Dr. Moore's assertions considering it is a powerful hemostatic. Its indications in such a condition are, profuse flow of bright red blood, pallor, weakness, and an aggravation of the flow from the slightest movement on the part of the patient.

ERYNGIUM.

It is also called the Button Snake-root, and it belongs to the natural order of Umbelliferæ. It grows in low, wet places and is an excellent remedy in urinary disorders. Its action is mainly confined to the mucous membranes lining the eyes, ears, nose, mouth, urethra, and vagina. It sets up a sort of irritation in those places and produces a thick yellow mucus discharge. It is, therefore, somewhat similar in action to **Pulsatilla.**

Its main action, however, is located in the bladder and the urethra. Tenesmus of the bladder with difficult and frequent micturition is an important indication. On this indication, it has been known to cure renal colic. Dr. W. K. Leonard reports of having cured a young methodist minister who was having repeated attacks of renal colic every three days. After Morphia and other remedies had failed, **Eryngium** in five drop doses, three times a day, put an end to the trouble.

ERYTHROXYLON.

(*See* **COCA**)

EUCALYPTUS.

It is also called the Fever or the Blue Gum tree. It belongs to the natural order of Myrtaceæ. It is a tree of great height, and is a native of Australia. It has a capacity for absorbing water. It is also supposed to destroy malarial poison. The tincture is prepared from the fresh leaves. It has a marked catarrhal effect; hence it makes an important remedial agent in influenza and other ailments affecting the mucous surfaces of the human body. It is also a powerful diaphoretic; it has been used with very fine result in exhausting nightsweats. Fistulous ulcers discharging offensive, ichorous matter and other varieties of putrid sore, also respond to its influence. It has been recommended as a wash, in distilled water, in foul smelling, ill-conditioned ulcers and wounds. It is also a great antidote against strychnine. It has been found, that a decoction prepared from **Eucalyptus** not only alleviates, but also modifies convulsions caused by strychnine.

It has been strongly advocated in chronic catarrh of the nasal passage discharging purulent and fetid matter. A stuffed up feeling in the nose, with thin watery coryza and a sensation of an acute catarrhal condition respond equally to the influence of **Eucalyptus.**

In the mouth we have an aphthous condition and an excessive secretion of saliva. Enlarged ulcerated tonsils and inflamed throat also improve under its influence. As a catarrhal remedy it comes in after **Aconite** and **Belladonna** had partially relieved the virulence of the acute stage, but failed to arrest the progress of the disease.

The most important symptom of **Eucalyptus,** however, is a peculiar vascular condition of the region near about the abdominal aorta. A distinct pulsation, due to increased vascularity, is referred to in the above-named region. Sometimes it is described as an uncomfortable feeling of weight and fullness in the epigastrium. This feeling is associated with a sensation of goneness as in **Phosphorus, Sepia,** and **Sulphur.** It has been recommended in dysentery when found in conjunction with the above-mentioned symptoms. Heat in the rectum, tenesmus, prostration and hemorrhage from the bowels are some of its indications.

On the kidneys, however, its actions are still more marked. The urine becomes loaded with pus. Burning and tenesmus, suppression of urine, and hæmaturia call for its application in acute and chronic nephritis. We have records of **Eucalyptus,** curing vascular tumors of female urethra. Ulcers around the orifice of the urethra have also been cured by **Eucalyptus.**

Thus it makes quite an important remedy for us, not to relegate it to the forgotten shelf of useless remedies.

EUGENIA JAMBOS.

This tree, commonly known as the Malabar Plum-tree and Rose-apple tree, is a native of the tropics. It belongs to the natural order of Myrtaceæ.

It produces a kind of inaction and talkativeness. This talkativeness is due to a sense of exhilaration. It is also marked by great indolence. The patient evidences a strong desire for rest and inaction. He avoids exercise of all descriptions.

It has one peculiar symptom that deserves mention. We notice a great change of the mental atmosphere after micturition. Every sign of gloom vanishes and things seem clothed in beauty and grandeur after every action of the bladder, but this is only shortlived for the gloom comes back again.

The modality should be carefully studied. There is a general aggravation on exposure to sun and by closing the eyes. The eyes fill with water on going out into the sun. Tears run out on exposure.

We have a peculiar nausea in this remedy inasmuch as it is better by smoking. The pains in **Eugenia** are wandering in nature.

EUPATORIUM PERFOLIATUM.

Eupatorium perf., commonly known as the Bone-set or Ague Weed, is a remedy with which every homœopath is more or less familiar. It was first proved by Drs. Williamson and Neidhard. The preparation, of course, is same as in other remedies— two parts by weight of alcohol being added to the chopped and finely pounded pulp. It acts upon the gastrohepatic system, fibrous tissues and bronchial mucous membranes giving rise to symptoms of serious bilious derangement, engrafted on a malarial cachexia.

The leading characteristic for its use is to be found in the distressing and universal bone pain, it causes throughout the system. Soreness is everywhere to be found. The scalp, the parietal protuberances, the eye-balls, the chest, the trachea, and the rest of the limbs become one mass of soreness, as if terribly bruised, struck, and hammered. The name bone-set is very apt inasmuch as it conveys to the mind this supreme characteristic of the drug. So important is this symptom that its absence may be regarded as a contraindication for **Eupatorium.**

I have used **Eupatorium** on various occasions in cases of
influenza. The patient complains of a severe bruised feeling all
over his body. His back, limbs, head, chest and all his joints
ache most fearfully and even the eye-balls become painful; severe
lachrymation and photophobia are present; the nose too runs
freely; great prostration is felt, partly because of the pains and
partly of the lassitude, that naturally accompanies 'La grippe.'

The troubles for which it is especially indicated are fevers of
various types. It is used in tertian, double tertian, anticipating,
remittent and bilious fevers. The time of the paroxysm is generally 7 to 9 a.m. The patient knows of the approaching fever
from the insatiable thirst and the bone pains that come on long
before the chill sets in. In this respect it is similar to **Capsicum,**
China, and **Natrum mur.;** for in all three of them we notice
violent thirst before the chill, but they are wanting in the bone
pains of **Eupatorium.** The thirst is also present during the stage
of chill, but vomiting is particularly apt to result from drinking,
and this fact is an important feature of this drug. The chill
begins especially in the back and runs up the spine. Nausea and
vomiting of bitter fluid and bile towards the close of the stage of
chill, and their aggravation from drinking, are in my opinion
the most important charactertistics of this drug. There is not
much thirst during the stage of heat. The cheeks become mahog-
any-red, the head throbs violently, and the soreness of the
body continues. Sweat may be scanty or absent; if present it
relieves all the other symptoms excepting cephalalgia, which it
aggravates. The sluggish action of the liver is responsible for
the slight attack of jaundice so often to be met with in the
Eupatorium patient.

The chill, let me mention again, is exceedingly severe. The
patient shivers inspite of all the warm clothing and blankets,
heaped upon him. We find him almost crouched up even under
a whole mountain of blankets. Extreme tenderness of the
epigastrium, fullness and hardness in the hepatic region with
stitches and soreness on movement and coughing, remind one of
Bryonia. We also notice a sort of a hectic cough during the
paroxysm. Yawning and stretching are the precursors of an
attack of ague. The trembling, referred to above, is a kind of
nervous trembling. Great weakness is complained of during the
attack which also is of nervous origin. The tongue is coated
white or yellow. The taste in the mouth is at times insipid, but

it is mostly bitter. Like **Nat. mur.** we have also fever blisters on the lips.

Dr. Allen considers **Eupatorium** as important as **Arsenic, Cinchona** and **Naturm mur.** in the treatment of malarial fevers of the miasmatic districts, marshy places, and river banks.

Let me add in this connection that the **Eupatorium** fever does not always come at the aforesaid period. It alternates between the hours of 9 a.m., one day and 12 noon the other day. The noon attack is always a milder one than the earlier paroxysm.

Before closing I must not forget the cough of this remedy. The universal feature of soreness is also to be found here. The chest is so painful that the patient holds it tightly with his hands before he coughs. This is very much like **Phosphorus, Bryonia,** and **Natrum carb.** Dr. Clarke has mentioned of another peculiar characteristic of the **Eupatorium** cough which I have not found elsewhere. According to him the **Eupatorium** cough is greatly ameliorated by getting on hands and knees, and in support of this statement he has cited a case from Dr. W. P. Defriez who with **Eupatorium** cured a hacking cough, always relieved by getting on hands and knees. This will be an important symptom after further verifications.

Lastly let me add that **Eupatorium** bears a strong semblance to **Arnica, Bryonia, Bellis., Ruta, Pyrogen, Baptisia, Medorrhinum** and **Nux mosch.,** in respect of the bruised feeling, to which so much importance has been attached.

EUPATORIUM PURPUREUM.

The common name of this plant is Gravel root. It is also called the Queen of the Meadow, It belongs to the natural order of Compositæ.

Eupatorium purp. is very rich in urinary and sexual symptoms as we will see presently. It is a powerful diuretic producing a great increase in the quantity of urinary secretion. Vesicular irritation is also set up leading on to urgent and painful urination. The opposite condition of suppression of urine, too, comes under its domain, hence we have œdematous swelling and dropsy in **Eupatorium purp.** It has been recommended in albuminuria and diabetes, its leading indication being an excessive irritation of the bladder. The smarting and burning in bladder is so excessive that the patient does not know what to do, and finds ease nowhere. The desire to pass urine is almost constant, but he passes only a few drops at a time, and is obliged to renew his efforts every few minutes; with each passage of urine the smarting increases. These are certainly symptoms of chronic cystitis, and like **Cantharis, Eupatorium purp.** has been known to soothe and relieve after the failure of the first named remedy. On the sexual system, it produces impotence in the males and sterility and uterine atony in the females.

Like **Perfoliatum, Purpureum** is equally serviceable in the treatment of malarial fevers. We have bone pains in **Purpureum,** only not as severe as in **Perfoliatum.** The chill begins between scapulæ and then spreads over the entire body like so many waves. In **Purpureum** the chill is not preceded by thirst. There is hardly any thirst even during the stage of chill; if there is any thirst at all, it is in the form of a longing for lemonade and other cold drinks. The shaking is just as violent as in **Perfoliatum** or it may be worse, but there is comparatively little coldness of the limbs. The heat is long lasting and is accompanied with thirst and at this stage the longing is more for hot drinks. The stage of sweat is without thirst. The sweat is mostly to be seen in the upper part of the body, and it is hardly profuse. The chilliness drags on even in the stage of sweat. Any movement, however slight, brings on a sensation of creeping chill. Towards the latter part of the stage of chill, there is only nausea with hardly any vomiting.

EUPHORBIUM.

Euphorbium is prepared from the resinous exudation of a plant growing in Morocco. It belongs to the natural order of Euphorbiaceæ. It is an irritant to the skin and mucous membranes. It produces gastro-intestinal as well as cutaneous irritation. It is also an important remedy in caries and other diseased condition of the bones. It has also been recommended in torpid ulcers and cold gangrene of old persons. It renders excellent service, particularly in gangrene of internal parts consequent on inflammation of stomach and bowels.

A great indication for this remedy is burning pains in the bones and this symptom alone will help us, in differentiating it from **Fluoric acid, Silicea,** and other remedies having degenerative influence on bones. I have used it with success in caries of the hip-joint, being guided to it by the burning pain at night time, that made rest almost impossible for the patient. It also relieves painfulness of coccyx, worse from rising from a sitting posture and on beginning to move.

It acts as a great anodyne in pains of cancer. Dr. Clarke speaks very highly of **Euphorbium,** for with it, he relieved the excruciating pain in a desperate case of sarcoma of the pelvic bones after other remedies had failed.

It has been used with success in cataract. Lenses become milkywhite, and the patient sees better in dim light.

The ailment, where it has done the best work, is erysipelatous inflammation of the cheek. The affected area becomes covered with vesicles, full of yellow liquid. The burning pain is simply excruciating.

EUPHRASIA OFFICINALIS.

Euphrasia, in common languge, is called the Eyebright. This significant name is very appropriate as we will see presently. It acts particularly on the mucous lining of the eyelids where it produces a state of inflammation. The conjunctiva is reddened. The vessels on the conjunctiva are enlarged, secretions mostly mucous in the beginning but turning purulent later on, are increased. Photophobia, lachrymation and burning, fluent running of nose are accompanying symptoms. The eyes become puffed. Blurring of the eyes, distressing sensation of dryness, and itching are also present.

Euphrasia is also indicated in conjunctivitis of a traumatic origin. Little blisters also form on or near the cornea. It is also indicated in rheumatic iritis. The pupils do not react to light, and if they react at all, they react tardily. The aqueous humour too, gets cloudy due to the inflamed products getting mixed up with the fluid. All the symptoms can be relieved effectually by the timely administration of **Euphrasia.**

I shall add a few other characteristic symptoms of **Euphrasia** before closing. We have a characteristic cough in this remedy—a cough that appears after the disappearance of hæmorrhoids. This cough is usually accompanied with severe coryza. Profuse expectoration of mucus while coughing and sometimes vomiting while attempting to cough out phlegm are strong indications for **Euphrasia.** Another noteworthv symptom is frequent yawning while walking in the open air.

Case 1.—Staphyloma. Staphyloma of the cornea in a man fortytwo years old. After enucleation of the left eye, he lost completely the sight of the right cne. The lids could hardly be closed; the cornea was thickened and all at once opaque; he had ant. synechia as a result of rheumatic ophthal. mia; violent surrounding pains; a great congestion of the conjunctiva and lachrymation. Patient could hardly distinguish day from night, and every oculist had pronounced it incurable. **Rhus.** at first, then **Euphrasia;** this latter in low dilution and mother tincture as instillation into the eye. The cornea has become almost clear; there remains only a little opacity above and below. Pupil has the dimension and form of horse's pupil, and remains motionless; meanwhile patient sees enough to guide him and reads well the names of streets and numbers of houses.—Dr. Deventer.

FAGOPYRUM.

Fagopyrum is nothing but Buckwheat, belonging to the natural order of Polygonaceæ. This remedy is comparatively little known, and it cannot boast a big record of verif-l symptoms although authentic and extensive provings have been made.

It has a marked action over the skin where it produces pruritis, erythema, blind boils, phlegmonous dermatitis, and eruptions both vesicular and pustular. Itching is general, and we find it in the scalp, eyes, margins of lids, ears, and nose. There is even soreness in the inside of the nose with heavy crusts covering the sore parts. The lips are dry and cracked. All the excretions are characterised by offensiveness. All these symptoms remind us of **Sulphur** to which it bears great resemblance. There is another symptom which brings it still closer to **Sulphur,** and that is a sinking feeling in the stomach at about 6 or 7 p.m.

FEL TAURI.

This medicine, originally introduced into our Materia Medica by Buchner, is prepared from Impissated gall of Ox triturated with sugar of milk. It is, as a remedy, very little used and very few of us can submit much from clinical experience to substantiate the pathogenetic properties of **Fel tauri.** Our friends of the other school use it occasionally for combating disintegrating influences in the intestines. We, on the other hand, acting on principles of Similia Similibus Curantur, use it for disorders of digestion, biliary calculi and pain in the nape of neck etc. Of the symptoms on which our prescription of **Fel tauri** is based the following may be mentioned .

1. A great tendency to sleep after eating.
2. Violent peristaltic movements causing great deal of gurgling and rumbling motions in abdomen.
3. Odorless and tasteless eructations.
4. Tension in nape.

FERRUM ARSENICUM.

It is the Arseniate of Iron. We are greatly indebted to Late Dr. P. C. Mozumdar of Calcutta for our knowledge of this remedy. He had ample opportunity to verify most of its symptoms, and has left us quite a legacy in his splendid date of the symptoms of this remedy. Its most characteristic indications, as defined by the Great Doctor, are enlargement of the spleen with continued high fever, disinclination for work, constipation, sometimes colliquative diarrhœa, emaciation, debility and want of thirst in any stage of the fever. It is, therefore, useful and curative in that type of pernicious malarial fevers that now-a-days easily acquire the designation of Kala-Azar. **Ferrum ars.** is no way inferior to the modern arsenic and antimony treatment of this malignant disease, as advocated by our friends of the other school. Here is a cure effected by the same doctor with **Ferrum ars.** worthy of close attention and thought. A robust healthy young man of 25, had occasion to go to a district ridden with malaria, with the result that his health gradually declined, strength failed, and there came on occasional attacks of fevers that insidiously destroyed the red blood corpuscles, till at last he returned home—a changed man with pale cachectic look and abdomen enormously distended, with an enlarged spleen that hardly left any space in his abdomen for anything else but an indurated liver, almost as enlarged as the spleen. Large doses of quinine, instead of checking the former, made it more persistent and his health dwindled till almost every hope was given up. **Ferrum ars.** 6, administered twice daily by Dr. Mozumdar, showed improvement in three days and after a treatment, extending over a month and a half with occasional doses of the same medicine completely restored him to health.

FERRUM IODATUM.

It is the iodide of Iron. This preparation is mostly adapted to scrofulous patients with glandular enlargements, tumors and tendency for crops of boils, while such a condition is associated with very distinct anæmia. Rachitis, exostosis, periostitis, and various forms of spinal curvatures with deformity, in constitutions betraying turgescence of the capillary system, generally call for **Ferrum iodatum** in preference to the pure metal. The Great Doctor P. C. Mozumder of Calcutta recommends it very highly in enlarged spleen and liver while unaccompanied with any rise of temperature.

My experience with this remedy, however, is more limited to the female sexual system. I have derived great benefit from its application in prolapsus uteri with amenorrhœa, associated with great itching of vulva and vagina. The sensation is one, of a constant bearing down, as if everything was coming away. I have used it both in anti-version and retroversion, and the symptom that has mostly guided me in its selection is the peculiar starchy leucorrhœa.

Ferrum iodatum has been used with success in albuminuria and diabetes. It relieves and sometimes radically cures œdematous swelling of the lower extremities in albuminuria. The urine is sweet smelling. At times it is dark-coloured depositing a thick white sediment.

We should also think of this in hæmoptysis in phthisical patients. Great debility with emaciation, evening chilliness followed by heat and sweat all night, greenish, purulent expectoration containing small cheesy particles, and oppression of chest and presence of rales under clavicle lead to its indication in the tuberculosis of the lungs.

FERRUM METALLICUM.

Ferrum metallicum is the pure metallic iron. It is a medicine of very ancient lineage. Our friends of the other school prescribe it extensively in anæmia and chlorosis.

Iron, being a component part of the human blood, is supposed to be a good supplement for deficiency of blood wherever found. This theory, based on a fallacious conception of the working of the human system, is utterly materialistic, and as such unworthy of serious attention. Verily, the want of proper proportion of iron in the blood can not be rectified by the addition of extra iron in the shape of food or medicine. The source of the trouble lies in the defective assimilation—in other words, to the incompatibility of the vital force in adopting itself to the changing environments. Homœopathy takes a fuller view of the situation and aims at putting things right at the source, rather than interfere or meddle, in a process known only to the force within the individual concerned.

This is done by strict adherence to the principle of Similia Similibus Curantur. Our method, therefore, of the study of **Ferum metallicum,** must be the same as in other remedies. The strange, the uncommon and the keynote symptoms, supplemented as usual by the totality, will invariably lead us to exactly where **Ferrum metallicum** becomes a necessity.

The first amongst these is the peculiar modality of our remedy. There is always and invariably an aggravation after eating and drinking, and while at rest. Everything in **Ferrum met.** is ameliorated by gently walking about. Sudden motions aggravate.

We must not hesitate to give anæmia, the next place in the chart of importance. It is either a cachectic state, due to faulty nutrition and assimilation or simple poverty of blood induced by hæmorrhages, deficience of air, light, and suitable food. To prescribe **Ferrum met.** in such conditions alone would be unhomœopathic to the extreme, unless in addition to this symptom mentioned above, we have a great irregularity in the distribution of the blood. The cheeks are flushed with a rosy hue as if in the best of health; but in spite of this marked local plethora, this bloom in appearance, there is an universal pallor of the lips and mucous membranes. The face which is ordinarily of a pale, waxy complexion, belying a low state of vitality, flares up on the slightest excitement, such as the meeting of a friend, entering a warm room, meeting with a slight rebuff or a disturbance in the mind caused by the slightest variation of her physical or mental environments. Veins as seen in **Ferrum met.** are generally full and prominent. The blood vessels all over the body throb violently. Sometimes the anæmia is so profound as to lead to a swelling of the feet.

The appetite, desires, and aversions supply us with the next charactertistic indication of **Ferrum met.** Both the opposite conditions of extreme hunger and total anorexia are found under this remedy. At times there is voracious appetite, the patient eating double the amount of ordinary meal and still feeling hungry, and then there is the extreme dislike to all kinds of food. The stomach is always out of order; regurgitation of food without nausea and inclination to vomiting are two grand characteristics.

On these symptoms, it has been used with success in extreme cases of diarrhœa and dyspepsia attended with a good deal of swelling and painfulness of the liver. Eructations are almost constant. They may be sour, foul, and burning. Every particle of food, taken during the day, is vomited out, especially towards the hours of midnight. There is generally a steady flow of water from the mouth after vomiting. At times the nausea is so great that the patient rolls and staggers as if intoxicated. In this respect, it is so similar to **Ipecac.** that a confusion may be very easily made, but then again, we must remember that the regurgitation, so characteristic of **Ferrum,** is wanting in **Ipecac.** A great soreness of the walls of abdomen is always present.

It is a great hæmorrhagic remedy. We have hæmorrhages from almost all the orifices of the body. The blood is light, and it coagulates easily. The characteristic point is the association of this hæmorrhage with anæmia. The bleeding is explained by sudden ebullitions due, as has been said before, to irregular circulation, and sudden rush of blood to single parts. We prescribe it for epistaxis in anæmic children with frequent changing of colour of the face. We prescribe it in hæmoptysis, in metorrhagia and menorrhagia, and in hæmorrhages from other parts of the body affected with temporary congestion caused by a disruption in the equilibrium of circulation.

It is best adapted to young anæmic persons with oversensitiveness, weakness, and great pallor of the skin and mucous membranes. Mentally they are very gloomy and despondent. Irritability, peevishness, quarrelsomeness, and intolerance of contradiction are prominent mental features. Giddiness is a constant feature; they feel as if they are balancing themselves most of the time. On rising suddenly, everything around them grows black, and they reel and stagger, and have to lean against something.

Headache—yes, they are martyrs to it. It is a congestive, hammering, pulsating headache. During these headaches the feet get cold and the face turns fiery red. It is so violent that the patient has to take to bed. Rush of blood to head is so great that the veins of head swell, and the patient experiences roaring, buzzing, and prickling sound in the brain. During these attacks though anæmic, they simulate a false plethoric appearance. The headaches are generally worse after midnight and are relieved by getting out of bed and slowly walking about. Although during headache the patient, due to ebullition of blood, looks very full-blooded like **Belladonna,** we must not be misled; the two remedies are characteristically different. One has, merely the semblance of plethora, and the other is really plethoric.

We use this metal in diarrhœa. The stools are generally watery with much flatulence, and are more frequent after food or drink. They are acrid and excoriating making the passage extremely sore. As a rule they are painless, and they are full of undigested particles of food. It has been used very successfully in chronic diarrhœa and in colliquative diarrhœa in phthisical subjects. The pale miserable complexion, emaciation, hardness and distention of the abdomen, bulimia alternating with anorexia, involuntary and the peculiar regularity of afternoon evacuation, give us indubitable right to prescribe **Ferrum met.**

On the female sexual system its indications are numerous. The menses appear too soon and are too profuse and too long lasting and all throughout this time the face looks fiery red with great deal of ringing in the ears. The copiousness of the discharge forbids all movements, as the least movement aggravates the flow. The flow of blood is partly watery and partly coagulated though at times we have a profuse discharge of a grumous character. The menses intermit and then reappear. It is extremely debilitating. During menses the varices in legs are worse; the face, red at times, betrays a great pallor and bloatedness. Skin is cold and pits upon pressure especially about ankles.

It is extremely useful in vomiting in pregnancy, especially when it is of a spasmodic nature. The patient suddenly leaves the table and with one effort vomits all the food taken and then returns and eats another complete dinner.

Let us now study the action of **Ferrum** on the respiratory system. It is recommended in asthma, with great deal of oppression of the chest and a feeling as if someone is pressing on it with his hands. It is generally worse about midnight, when he must sit up or better still walk about for relief. The cough is spasmodic, worse after meals, making him vomit all his food. We use **Ferrum** in incipient stage of phthisis florida. Hæmoptysis morning and night, intrascapular pain, heavy breathing, great prostration, and a tickling teasing cough associated with a sore bruised feeling in the chest in young florid subjects with a remarkable erethism of vascular system, generally call for **Ferrum met.**

We have some very clear-cut indications for **Ferrum** in rheumatism. It is mostly in omodynia of a constant drawing tearing nature that we think of this remedy. The pain is worse in bed, and he must get up and walk about. Dr. Nash cured a patient on this indication after having failed with other remedies, in a case of chronic rheumatism of the shoulder joint. Aggravation is also seen from warmth of bed, uncovering for any length of time and folding of arms.

Lastly **Ferrum met.** is indicated in intermittent fever particularly after abuse of quinine. The important symptoms, indicating it, are the following: (1) Chill at 4 a.m. (2) Distention of the blood vessels during heat particularly of the temples and face; (3) Red face during chill; (4) Throbbing pulsating headache during fever.

Case 1.—B., aged thirty-nine. Is able to talk only in toneless whisper, and only that which is absolutely required from him; pain in the larynx and trachea; after talking, burning; frequently a sensation as if something were in the larynx which he wished to remove by hawking and coughing; a sensation externally as if the throat were being pressed together. By day, as well as by night, there occurs, from a sensitive tickling in the larynx, such violent attacks of cough that he loses his breath, the blood mounts to the head, tears run from his eyes and he sinks down exhausted; very easily vexed; the least thing excites him; pulse accelerated toward evening, and after he does fall asleep, sweat breaks out, which awakens him, and he has to lie a long time before he can go to sleep again, and so on until morning. Some nights, congestion to the chest; palpitation of the heart; pulsation in all the arteries, and anxiousness. Mind in the highest degree oppressed; despondent; great solicitude about those belonging to him, with constant thoughts of death; pale, earthy color of the face. **Chel. 6, Nux vom. 30,**

Sulph, 30, Lach. 30, had but slight effect. **Ferr.** one dose daily for six days, cured.—Dr. Th. Ruckert.

Case 2.—A young lady had omodynia last spring affecting both deltoid muscles, for which she had taken **Bry., Rhus tox.** and various remedies without effect. I prescribed a single dose of **Fer. 200.,** which very soon entirely relieved the pain, and she felt no more of it until this fall, when there was a recurrence of the rheumatism, but this time only in the left deltoid. When moving the arm, the pain was violent and lancinating, causing her to cry out. Two doses of the same remedy completely relieved the omodynia, and there has been no return for nearly three weeks.—Dr. H. V. Miller.

FERRUM PHOSPHORICUM.

It is the Phosphate of Iron, and constitutes one of the organic tissue salts of Schussler. Its function is to lend colour or pigment to the blood corpuscles. It also carries oxygen to all parts of the body. The deficiency in this cell salt leads to disturbance of circulation. Disturbed circulation again in its train causes other disturbances in the normal equilibrium of the human system. Hence, according to Von Schussler this remedy is of great economic importance in setting things right through the supplying of the deficiencies of the cell salts.

This remedy has not been fully proved. Most of our symptoms are derived from the writings of Schussler and from stray clinical experiences of homœopathic practitioners.

It is a great hæmorrhagic remedy; the hæmorrhages are of bright red blood and may come from any outlet or orifice of the body. It is generally indicated in the pale and anæmic subjects, who, in spite of want of blood and exhaustion, are subject to sudden gushes of bleeding. It is generally useful in the first stage of such attacks, before exudation, usually a follower of strong inflammatory processes, has taken place. It is indicated in hæmoptysis after concussion or a fall. It relieves expectoration of blood in pneumonia.

We will do well to give this remedy a thorough Hahnemannian proving. Most of the symptoms, as have been recorded previously, are not authentic, as they are not the result of a thorough scientific proving.

FERRUM PICRICUM.

Ferrum picricum is a trituration from the Picrate of Iron. We are indebted to Dr. Cooper for this remedy who made extensive provings and who is our chief authority on this subject.

It is particularly suited to bilious patients with dark hair and eyes.   A kind of dirty discoloration, due probably to bile pigments about the joints, is another leading indication of this remedy.   It has a few more indications of equal value, and we would do well to go thoroughly into its symptomatology.   One such indication and a very rare one, is a sensation as if warts were growing on the thumb. This symptom has come out repeatedly in many provers. A third indication refers to its use in excessive fatigue and bad effects thereof. Whenever any organ or any function of any organ gives out under strain of excessive use and fatigue, we should at once think of **Ferrum picricum.** Failure of voice in public speakers, deafness arising from living in very noisy quarters, and rheumatic attacks after very strenuous bodily labour, call for **Ferrum picricum.**

Like **Picric acid, Nitric acid,** and **Thuja,** it is one of our noted remedies for warts and lupoid growths.   These warts of **Ferrum picricum** appear mostly on the hands. and they are multiple and pedunculated. The co-existence of warts with deafness is a sure indication for our remedy. and this symptom carries with it the seal of repeated verifications. It is regarded as almost a specific in epistaxis. We must not forget another specification of **Ferrum picricum,** and it is seen in its action on the prostate gland. There is generally hypertrophy of that organ in consequence of which the patient experiences a frequent desire for micturition at night and a feeling of fullness and pressure on the rectum. Senile hypertrophy of the prostate gland, a very common complaint of the old age is thus amenable to the influence of **Ferrum picricum.**

FILIX MAS.

Like **Cina, Areca,** and **Granat,** it is one more of our vermifuge remedies. In common language it is called the Male Fern and it belongs to the natural order of Filices. According to Hering, the tincture must be prepared from the fresh root, and the best time for its application in tapeworm is summer, as the root can be obtained fresh at that time. If an ounce of this powdered-root is given in the forenoon, the tape-worm will come in the after-noon. Pale face, blue rings around the eyes, gnawing, boring pains in bowels worse from eating sweet things, loss of appetite and furred tongue are some of the symptoms indicative of worms, and are invariably relieved by the application of **Male fern.** A woman, who had repeatedly passed segments of tape-worms, was seized with severe colic which quickly disappeared under **Filix mas,** and was followed 8 days later, by the discharge of tapeworms, fifty inches in length. It also causes atrophy of the optic nerve, leading on to blindness, and hence it should be used with great caution.

FLUORIC ACID.

Fluoric acid is a highly excoriating acid, prepared by treating Calcium fluoride with Sulphuric acid. It even corrodes or eats into the glass.

It is to be particularly remembered for its action on bones and skin. It is a kindred remedy to **Sil., Cal. fluor., Hepar sulph.,** and the like. There is usually a syphilitic and mercurial dys-crasia. In **Fluoric acid** old cicatrices become red around edges and threaten to become open ulcers as in **Graph.** Varicose veins, obstinate ulcerations, caries and necrosis, especially of the long bones such as the femur, humerus, radius, etc are greatly amenable to the influence of **Fluoric acid.** The discharges of this remedy are thin and excoriating. The symptoms are frequently relieved by cold applications. In inflamation of osseous tissue and in exos-toses, in threatened gangrene, especially of the scrotum and penis, and in bed sores (especially where there is a syphilitic history), we cannot do better than to administer a few doses of **Fluo. acid.**

Fluoric Acid increases muscular ability. It adds a stimulus to the free coursing of blood to the affected area, and thus helps in the healing of a sore. Homœopathy admits of no half-way process and allows no patch-work. All its cures are permanent.

natural and spontaneous. I have noticed some remarkable change in the nails of patients after they have been given a course of **Fluoric acid** treatment. Nails that were crumbling assumed their normal complexion and gloss. Whitlow and panaritium which are signs of a rundown state of health, disappear permanently under the influence of **Fluoric acid.** Altogether it ensures a better state of health in the patient.

One characteristic feature, we should always keep in mind regarding **Fluoric acid** is, that the ulcers etc. are relieved by cold dressing. This is an important point of distinction between **Fluoric acid** and **Silicea.** Under the latter remedy relief is obained by dressing with hot water alone.

Fluoric acid and **Silicea** are complementary, and that the ill-effects form the over-use of **Silicea,** can be rectified by the exhibition of **Flouric acid.**

Case 1.— Mr. D——, musician, aged fifty-nine, medium height, weakly constitution, sallow skin, emaciated; so weak he can scarcely walk, and greatly depressed in mind; had the diseases of childhood; remained well til' his thirtieth year, when he came under allopathic treatment for a fever Twelve years ago he had tertian intermittent, which was successfully treated since then his health had remained tolerably good, but he commenced to drink during the last months; his present symptoms have made their appearance, which, no doubt, are due to drinking. He complains principally of mental weakness; loss of appetite; whitish, dry tongue; feeling of fullness and pressure in the epigastrium; great tension and dropsical swelling of the abdomen; tardy, infrequent and hard stool; scanty, dark-red urine, painful in passing. He has hydrocele, the size of an infant's head; the penis i curved in the shape of an S, at least four inches in circumference, swollen the prepuce œdematous to such a degree as to hide the orifice. Short frequent cough, mostly dry, occasionally whitish, frothy mucus; grea dyspnœa: has to be propped up in bed. Anxiety; sleeps little and seldom great and unquenchable thirst; craves refreshing drinks; legs œdematous a far up as the abdomen; very ill-humored; small, frequent pulse; dry skin an weak voice. Physical examination revealed enlargement and induration o the liver particularly of the left lobe. Prescribed **Arsenicum, Carb. veg., an Zincum,** without the slightest benefit. The disease made rapid progress; th ascites and hydrocele increased, the latter to a degree which threatene gangrene. There was now suppression of stool and urine; one night th patient suddenly and involuntarily passed a large quantity of urine, and wa attacked by fear of death, with great prostration. **Tart. emet.** was prescribe in alterantion with **Acon.** Two days later, his condition was as bad as eve **Fluoric acid 6,** in water, a teaspoonful, every four hours. This remed worked such a rapid and remarkable change as I have never before witnesse in similar chronic cases. His forces rallied, the swellings decreased, an entirely disappeared within eight days; stool became regular, urine pass copiously and without pain; appetite, sleep, and pulse in a short time became normal. In two weeks he was well enough to work; continued his medicine for two weeks more, and he had no relapse during the next year.—Dr. Carl Haubold.

FORMALIN.

Formalin is the saturated cold aqueous solution of Formaldehyde. It contains 35 to 40 per cent of the gas by weight, and is colorless. It has a sharp taste. It is a powerful disinfectant, deodorant and a strong poison. It is largely used as a hardening and a fixing agent and as a preservative for anatomical and biological specimens. It is also used as a preservative of food and medicines. It is a powerful irritant to the eyes and mucous membranes of the respiratory notch. Applied to the skin, it causes severe urticaria and taken in strong solution, it may cause vomiting, weakening of the pulse and respiration. Our friends of the other school used it as a prophlyactic and curative in influenza and pertussis and in allaying the cough and the night sweat of tuberculosis. Surgically it is, an antiseptic of great value, and is used for sterilising the hands, dressing sutures, and instruments. Our use, as has been mentioned repeatedly, is based on the symptomatology of the drug. Dyspnœa, anuria, albuminous urine, forgetfulness, coryza, and ptyalism are some of the symptoms of **Formalin.** With further proving we will come to a better understanding of this remedy which has, up to now, been very sparingly used by homœopaths.

FORMICA.

This remedy is prepared from the common ant. It belongs to the natural order of Hymenoptera. Only that variety of ants are used in the preparation, which would attack and defend themselves by biting with their mandibulæ or jaws, and bend their abdomen outward and forward, at the same time ejecting from the anus a sharp sour fluid into the wound.

My experience of this remedy is very meagre. Most of the symptoms mentioned here are taken from "Hering's Guiding Symptoms." The provings of this remedy were principally made by Dr. Lippe and Hering. They both recommended it very highly in the apoplectic diseases as it strengthens the brain.

It has been praised highly in rheumatic affections, especially in rheumatic inflammations of the eyes and in affections of the spinal cord. The rheumatism for which it is particularly efficacious is said to appear mostly in the joints, and causes great restlessness. The patient desires motion, although it makes the pain more acute.

GALLICUM ACIDUM

Gallic acid is obtained from ordinary Tannic acid by boiling it with dilute acids. It occurs free in Nut-galls, Oak-apples, Tea, and in fruits of various other plants. It is an astringent substance, and is a great disinfectant. It dissolves slowly in water, but readily in alcohol and ether, and has a faintly acid taste.

In **Gallic acid** we have a splendid remedy for phthisis, especially of hæmorrhagic variety, and for asthma. The old school uses it in night-sweats, diabetes, and chronic diarrhœa.

Dr. Mercy of New York records a wonderful cure of a case ot phthisis in a young lady with a cavity in her left lung. It was a far-gone case. Purulent expectoration, night-sweats, evening fever, rapid pulse, and a rapid loss of flesh pointed to the inevitable end; but under the prolonged use of **Gallic acid 1x** she recovered her normal health with the exception of a slight dullness in the region affected. We have also authentic reports of various cases where an application of ointment containing Gallic acid brought on attacks resembling " Hay-Asthma."

Its principal symptoms, however, are great weakness with irritability, excessive dryness of mouth and throat, and a sensation of contraction of the anus. A distinct pain is felt in the lungs. The other symptoms are wild delirium, photophobia, epistaxis, increased secretion of phlegm in the throat, and hæmorrhages.

GAMBOGIA.

This remedy is prepared from the gum resin of a tree, native of Cambogia, Siam, Cochin and China. It was first proved by Nenning and Hering. It is a tropical evergreen tree with yellow juice. **Gambogia** is collected by cutting or wounding the trunks, whence the bright yellow juice flows slowly out and collects into the vessels tightened at the lowest part of the incision. This juice slowly hardens. It is used in India and China as a pigment of high excellence. The taste is very acrid. It is soluble in alcohol and in ether, but not in water. It has strong purgative properties. It is one of the most violent cathartics. It produces abundant watery stools with considerable griping. The allopaths use it as an ingredient in many of their cathartic pills. Although the full dose is five grains, it is risky to use it in such large quantity owing to its violent cathartic properties.

The chief reputation of **Gambogia** amongst homœopaths is for its usefulness in diarrhœa. In this complaint they have utilized it to the best advantage. As we do not prescribe our remedies for diseases by name, (for that would throw us into great confusion, there being so many hundreds of remedies for diarrhœa), we must find out the characteristic features of **Gambog,** pointing to its application. The first and the foremost is the way in which the stools are expelled. They come out all at once with a single and somewhat prolonged effort. The second point is the suddenness of the urging; the third and final point consists of the feeling, obtained immediately after the stool, of great relief in the abdomen, as if some irritating substances were removed from the intestines. There is great burning in the anus.

It is used both in the acute and chronic cases of diarrhœa and dysentery. It closely remembles **Aloes, Croton tig., Gratiola,** and **leander.** We have also great rumbling and gurgling and inflammation of the abdomen. The stools are profuse, watery, sometimes yellow, sometimes greenish and lienteric.

It has some important symptoms of the eyes and the throat. Violent itching of the canthi and eyelids, pain in the small of the back as if sprained, pain in the sacrum, and gnawing pain in the coccyx are important landmarks of **Gambogia.**

The pain in this remedy, wherever it may be, is of a burning character.

GAULTHERIA.

In ordinary language it is called the Winter-green; it is an ever-green trailing vine, found growing in cool, damp woods. It belongs to the natural order of Ericaceæ. The tincture is prepared from the fresh leaves. It is a great remedy for neuralgic and other inflammatory pains. Hence inflammatory rheumatism, pleurodynia and sciatica come under its jurisdiction. Cystic and other prostatic irritation too, come within its sphere. The symptom that stands out most prominently in **Gaultheria** is acute prolonged vomiting associated with severe pain in the epigastrium and uncontrollable appetite, notwithstanding the irritability of the stomach. With time and years and with further verifications, **Gaultheria** also may climb the ladder of importance.

GELSEMIUM.

Gelsemium is our common jasmine. It is a climbing plant indigenous to the southern parts of Europe. Medicine is prepared from the fresh root which is chopped and pounded, and then mixed with alcohol in proportion of one to two. It is highly poisonous and is one of our valuable vegetable polychrests. The remedy has been proved by Dr. Hale. It causes active or passive congestion of brain, spinal cord, lungs, liver, and other organs, and leads to general paralysis of the voluntary and involuntary nerves, although its principal action is centered upon the motor side of the spinal cord. We will consider a case of **Gelsemium** poisoning as mentioned by Dr. Clarke in his dictionary. " J. H. Nankiva drank two ounces of the tincture of **Gelsemium** instead of sherry. He walked a few feet with assistance and in another minute his legs were paralysed. He dragged himself to the bed-side with his arms, but they were unable to help him to bed into which he had to be lifted. As long as he lay quiet there was not trouble, but on the least exertion there was excessive tremor. Vomiting occurred during the next twenty-four hours. Temperature rose to 101.5°F. Heart's action became very violent and intermittent. All the muscles of the eyes were affected but of the voluntary muscles those on the right side suffered most. There was somnolence and absence of mental excitement."

In this case of **Gelsemium** poisoning we find paralysis to the most prominent feature. The best indication that I know **Gelsemium** is prostration, and excessive languor. When this is little more pronounced we call it paresis, and in extreme cases this paresis assumes the form of real paralysis. This feature runs throughout the length and breadth of this remedy, as will be amply proved before we have finished discussing it.   We have paralysis of various groups of muscles about the eyes, throat, chest, larynx, sphincter, and extremeties. This loss of power of the entire muscular system gives to the patient a played out feeling. The muscles lose power to contract at will of the patient, but he has all his sensibilities left in tact.

The next important characteristic of **Gelsemium** is tremor. On this symptom, numerous varieties of ailments such as fevers, convulsions, hysteria, epilepsy, apoplexy, and various other types of nervous disorders have been helped.

Dr. Eriskine White has reported of a case of a baby born in convulsions, that he cured with **Gelsemium.**   The symptoms to guide him were a history of fright in the mother a few weeks before the baby was born, and the incessant quivering of the child's chin.   Within thirty seconds of the administration of **Gelsemium** the quivering ceased, and in three minutes' time the convulsions were at an end.   What else can add to a practitioner's fame than cures like these! Patient study, diligent discrimination, and above all thorough fidelity to the principles of Similia Similibus Curantur are objects that we should all aim at.

The mental condition of these patients is characterised by the ever-present phenomena of lassitude. We find them in a very depressed mood. They would like to be left alone without any desire to speak or be spoken to. They lack the capacity to think or fix their attention on anything. In extreme cases we notice a sort of cataleptic immobility. These patients are great cowards, and are fearful of death.

Gelsemium is a grand remedy for troubles brought on by fear and dread. We have occasion to use this frequently in singers and orators in troubles like diarrhœa, headache, etc. when brought on by this fear of going before the public. **Gelsemium** is also a remedy for complaints that arise from exciting news, sudden emotions, fear, anger, etc. In this respect it is similar to **Coffea, Colocynth, Staphisagria,** and **Opium.**

Gelsemium is a reliable remedy for occipital headache. Here too, the characteristic feature is the languor, the drowsiness and the lassitude. The simply want to lie down and rest.   There is passive congestion of the brain as a result of which the face looks suffused. The headache begins at the nape of the neck, passes up and settles down over the eyes. The neck feels stiff. The headache is almost always preceded by dimness of vision, and is better by copious urination. It is a good remedy for the sun-headache—meaning thereby the headache that starts early in the morning, continues all throughout the day, and becomes better when the sun goes down. A sensation of sickness accompanies this headache. They stagger as if drunk when they move about. It is also a good remedy for headaches from astigmatism diplopia, and paralysis of ocular muscles. In respect of headache **Gelsemium** compares very well with **Kali bich., Natrum mur., Iris** and **Sepia**; in all of these remedies we find a certain amount of blurred vision or blindness before headache. It is also similar to **Aconite, Ignatia, Kalmia, Mellilotus,** and a few others in respect of amelioration of the headache after profuse urination.

As there is intense congestion in **Gelsemium,** it becomes splendid remedy for threatened and actual apoplectic seizure. The symptoms are stupor, general paralysis, headache, nausea, giddiness, dilatation of the pupils and twitching of the single muscle It has been used in cerebro-spinal meningitis, but its use is confined to the first stage of the disease and at its onset. Livi cheeks, dilated pupils, loss of strength, icy coldness of hands, wea and a hardly perceptible pulse, and involuntary closing of eyelie are symptoms calling for **Gelsemium** in meningitis.

Gelsemium is also frequently needed in the treatment of inte mittents. The patient suffers from nervous chills running from sa rum to the nape of the neck. This chill is so very severe that wishes to be held tightly, so that he may not shake so much. this it is like **Lachesis,** where also we find severe shaking and t desire to be held. Another peculiarity of the **Gelsemium** chill the want of thirst and profuse urination all throughout the sta of chill. The stage of heat too is without thirst, and it is inter and burning. He simply wants to lie still and sleep, as he feels tired and exhausted. Sometimes we find him in a semi-stuporo condition. In children during this stage there is frequent starti and twitching, and a desire to grasp the bed or the attenda they frequently get the sensation of falling and it is merely save themselves from such imaginary catastrophy that we f them grasping at everybody or everything around them.

Gelsemium is also a good remedy for fevers with typh tendencies, especially when we notice great prostration in initial stage, and constant trembling of muscles, sleeplessness, a great sore and bruised feeling all over the body, slow pulse, extreme lassitude and somnolence. The sweat is slight or partial, but if relieves all the pains.

It is invaluable in eruptive fevers of children with a tendency to convulsions at the time of the eruptions. The fever is almost as intense, the heat as great, and the erethism as marked as in **Aconite**, but the restlessness of that remedy is wanting. There is no need for a confusion with **Belladonna**, as **Gelsemium** is wanting in the violence and suddenness of **Belladonna**. The stupor, the somnolence, and the twitching may suggest **Belladonna** but **Gelsemium** lacks the fiery intensity, and the great arterial excitement of the latter remedy. The chilliness in **Gelsemium** is very great indeed, and the patient can not move away from fire without feeling chilly. During fever torpidity and heaviness are felt. The pulse is full and quick, but not hard and throbbing as in **Belladonna**. The sleep is interrupted by muttering delirium, whereas in **Belladonna** we have either fierce delirium or moaning accompanying coma and stupor.

Now let us turn to another important feature of **Gelsemium**—I. mean the inco-ordination of the muscular system. We have functional paralysis of the motor nerves, but the sensory ones are unaffected. Thus we find it indicated in all kinds of paralytic affections—starting from a mere weakness or heaviness of limbs to absolute paralysis of the entire muscular system. Dr. Farrington has cited a case of post-diphtheritic paralysis in a child where **Gelsemium** effected an absolute cure. The child's spine was bent and one side of the body was paralysed. He would more stagger than walk. Strabismus was marked.

We use **Gelsemium** in aphonia, but only when it is due to paretic state of the laryngeal muscles.

Gelsemium is also good for dysphagia when the difficulty in swallowing is due to weakness of the muscles of deglutition. Similarly it is a good remedy for ptosis, but the ptosis in **Gelsemium** is different from that of **Causticum, Rhus tox, Sepia** and **Kalmia**.

In **Rhus tox** the ptosis is due to paralysis from getting wet.

In **Sepia** it is almost always associated with menstrual irregularities.

Kalmia is indicated in ptosis of rheumatic subjects with an attendant feeling of stiffness in the lids. It is also a great remedy for locomotor ataxia.

The male and the female sexual system needs a certain amount of consideration. The weakness which has been spoken of as being the backbone of **Gelsemium,** finds ample play in the physiology of the males. Involuntary emission of semen without an erection, spermatorrhea from relaxation and debility, flaccidity and coldness of genitals and complete exhaustion of the sexual parts are phenomena to be encounterd daily in **Gelsemium.** The sexual power is so completely exhausted that even the most powerful stimuli fail to excite the patient and bring an efflux of blood into his sexual organs. He presents a complete picture of impotence, and his features are those of a man broken down morally, mentally and physically. Pale face, dark circle around the eyes, weakness of mind and memory, emaciation, and constant thoughts of suicide speak of an unenviable state of affairs. In this respect **Gelsemium** should be compared to **Dioscorea, Caladium, Selenium, Conium, Nux vom.** and **Agnus castus,** remedies noted for great sexual debility.

Gelsemium is equally invaluable in the diseases of the females We think of it particularly in reflex headaches due to ovarian irritation. The head feels enormously enlarged, with an accompanying sensation of heaviness in the uterine region. White leucorrhœal discharge, nervousness, excitability, and backache while accompanying headache with temporary blurred vision should remind us particularly of **Gelsemium.** There is undoubtedly a strong congestion of the uterus giving rise to sharp, labor-like pains in the uterine region extending to back and hips. Like **Caulop.,** it is excellent in congestive dysmenorrhœa. The symptoms indicating it are a suffused countenance due to congestion to the head, bearing down sensation in the abdomen, cramps in the uterus and legs, general hysterical condition, and partial suppression of menses.

Its efficacy, however, is most marked in pregnancy and parturition. It is not only applicable in the normal healthy state but also in many abnormalities of pregnancy. We think of it in threatened abortion from sudden depressing emotions, as is cause by fright, anger, hatred, and jealousy. **Gelsemium** re-instates the normal state of mind. Mind has great deal to do in the easy sailing of the events that are of the utmost importance to us. Coolness of temper soothes matters, and renders easy, the complicate and the intricate affairs of our life. Hysterical women have always a difficult time of it in the lying-in period. They tremble, the shiver, and allow themselves to be dominated by many nervous excitement, with the result that the progress of labor becomes retarded. If **Gelsemium** is to be the remedy for such a condition, a kind of paretic condition of the uterus becomes manifest. The womb becomes inert and loses all its tone and elasticity, as a result of which, even at the proper period, it becomes incapable of expelling the fœtus. **Gelsemium** is a wonderful remedy in the rigidity of the os as well. In this respect **Gelsemium** should be differentiated from **Belladonna,** a remedy noted for spasmodic contraction of the os uteri. **Gelsemium** is thought of in tardy dilatation of the os, a condition often to be met with, in labor that has lasted several hours. Also the os in **Gelsemium,** though rigid does not feel so thin to the examining finger as in **Belladonna.** A great indication is, however, nervous chills in the first stage of labor. It ushers in real substantial labor pains and thereby renders labor a matter of comparative ease and safety.

The most important condition to remember in **Gelsemium** however, is the uterine inertia. Everything seems relaxed. The neck of the uterus feels flabby, the os looks open, the bag of water keeps bulging out through the open os, but the labor does not progress; the patient grows more and more drowsy, speech thicker, till at last there is the whirlwind of terrible eclamptic fits. It is for the accoucheur to take note of things in time, and prescribe **Gelsemium** before the utmost has happened. When the patient gradually sinks into a semi-stupid state, when her speech becomes thick as of one intoxicated, and when face looks flushed, it ought to be time enough for us to prescribe **Gelsemium** which usually puts a stop to the downward progress and ushers in fresh labor pains and finishes the case without allowing any thing untoward happening.

Gelsemium affects the heart in its own peculiar way. The patient feels that he must be constantly on the move if he wants his heart to continue beating. As soon as he rests, he feels that his heart will cease to beat. These sensations come on more during sleep from which he wakes up in distress. In this respect it is very similar to **Grindelia** where too the patient is afraid to fall asleep, on account of the smothered feeling which wakes him up.

The pulse of **Gelsemium** is, as a rule, large, full, and quick, but not hard.

Gelsemium is antidoted by **Atropin, Cinchona, Coffea, Digitalis,** and **Nux mosch.**

Case 1.—Mrs. M., thirty-five years old, has had two children and with her last child had a tedious confinement, owing to rigidity of the os uteri. I was called to attend her in confinement, found the os uteri somewhat dilated, with the edge hard as a stout copper wire, and great rigidity of the perineum. The uterine action was strong but irregular. I immediately gave her twenty drops of **Gelsemium** in half a wine glass of tepid water. In about ten minutes the uterus began to yield, and the resistance of the perineum subsided. Previously to this, she was in an intensely nervous state, calling aloud to her husband and declaring she should die. The skin was hot and dry, lips parched and haggard, wild look of the eyes. She was delivered of a boy within two hours.—Dr. E. W. Alabone, Hom. World, Oct., 1874.

Case 2.—I have cured with **Gelsemium** a case of tertian ague in a single lady of twenty years. The case was one of two years standing. After exhausting a long list of homœopathic remedies, I gave the woman in all half a drachm of quinine in forty-eight hours without making any impression upon the chill and fever. In perfect despair I finally insisted upon the lady's reconsidering her case, reviewing all of its histroy and symptoms with the utmost care, hoping to find some symptoms which she had failed to communicate to me and which might suggest some remedy not yet tried. Upon thinking the matter over, my patient was discouraged at her inability to assist me in my search for "something new." She had told all she knew, unless she had forgotten to mention the fact, that, while the paroxysm was on, she "had no control over the lower limbs." Following this hint, as a last resort, I gave **Gelsemium** 1st decimal, ten drops in a gobletful of water, two teaspoonful every two hours. The lady never had another chill, but regained her health perfectly.—Dr. I. N. Eldridge.

Case 3.—Fever. Man, aged sixty-nine, dull heavy headache; complains that he feels drowsy and stupid, and that when he attempts to move, is so weak that he can hardly control his movements; feeling of great prostration; tongue slightly coated, can hardly put it out, it trembles so; mouth sticky; no thirst; no appetite; skin hot and dry; pulse 120 and full; the eyes look dull, eyelids drooping; hands tremble violently when trying to lift or move them; legs tremble very much when trying to walk. Patient came near dying three months before with typhoid fever, but had been in good health since. Had been exposed a few days before to a cold snow storm. Acon 30, **Bry.** 30, **Rhus.** 30, did no good. **Gels.** 30, every hour, cured.—Dr. E. B Nash.

GINSENG.

This name is applied to the root of every species of Panax quinquefolium L. It is a highly priced article in China, as according to the Chinese system of therapeutics it is supposed to be a remedy of high medicinal repute.

It contains a considerable amount of gum and starch and a little volatile oil.

In America it is a domestic remedy for the after pains of labor, but the complaint for which it is supposed to be a valuable remedy is sciatica, its indication being a bruised pain in the small of the back and thighs on rising from bed and a great languor. The pain extends as far as the big toe. The patient complains of a nightly digging pain in the right lower limb from the hip to the big toe The pain is lancinating and tearing in its character. With this is noticed a frequent desire to urinate.

It is a right-sided remedy.

GLONOINUM.

This is commonly known as Nitro-glycerine. This was discovered by Sobrero. It is a highly explosive light yellow oily liquid. It is prepared by slowly adding one part of glycerine to a mixture of two parts of concentrated Sulphuric acid with one part of Nitric acid.

This is one more of the many monuments of Constantine Hering's patient, persistent labour, great genius, and devotion to the cause of Homœopathy. It produces great and sudden irregularity of circulation with sensation of expansion, bursting and throbbing. The whole symptomatology of **Glonoinum** is based on this keynote of the remedy.

It is pre-eminently a remedy for congestive headaches, in which every throb of the arteries of the brain seems to be synchronous with the beat of the heart. The patient complains of a crushing weight across the forehead. His skull seems too small for the brain. The brain seems like expanding and bursting through the confinement of the skull. He holds his head with both hands. Sensitiveness to jar is very great. He cannot lie down. The intensity of the throbbing makes even the pillow pulsate. These attacks in **Glonoinum** are, as has been mentioned before, due to irregularities of circulation. These circulatory disturbances are very sudden, and that is what forms the keynote of the remedy. The patient, who was feeling absolutely well a moment ago, all on a sudden, gets unnerved with such upheavals of his circulatory system. His whole head, seems crowded with a great onrush of blood. This sensation of fullness in the vertex keeps increasing all the time from the constant pumping of an accelerated heart. All the arteries seem to be on the breaking point and as a sort of a protection he is obliged to hold on to his head, during every movement, to prevent a threatened rupture of his cranium. Sometimes these sensations in the brain are described as the rising and the falling of the waves of a turbulent sea. The cutaneous veins of the head and face show obvious signs of enlargement. In consequence of this congestion the most obvious happens. We have purple face, hot vertex, and blood-shot eyes. It sometimes gives rise to a sensation of ice-cold sweat on the forehead which however is not there. It also causes a sort of choking sensation, as if legatures were tied round the neck preventing the returning of the blood from the head. He is even afraid to shake his head as it feels that the slightest movement would break the head to pieces. The eye-balls protrude during headache, and the capillaries look as if injected. There is almost deathly sickness with the headache. This sickness, it must be remembered, is of cerebral origin. In consequence of this congestion, we have ringing in the ears. The patient's own pulsation is audible and prevents him from falling asleep. There is also deafness accompanying the throbbing fullness in and around the ears.

Another effect of this cerebral congestion is to be seen in its symptoms of convulsions. The patient froths at the mouth, and is unconscious. The hands are clenched; the thumbs overturned being in the palms of the hands. The pulse is full and hard, and the face looks bright red and puffed.

It is good for what we call the season headache—a headache that begins with the warm weather and lasts all summer. The **Glonoin.** headache increases and decreases with the sun. It is specially suited to headaches of people that work under the sun or gas light when the heat falls straight on the head.

Glonoin. patient is very susceptible to the rays of the sun. He always walks on the shady side of the street, and carries an umbrella all the time as a precaution. It thus bears certain amount of semblance to **Belladonna,** but the characteristic difference consists in the modality of the two remedies.

Belladonna patient likes the head covered whereas **Glonoinum** is better from uncovering.

Glonoinum has a few mental peculiarities. He suffers from loss of the sense of location. He does not know where he is. Well known streets seem strange to him.

Case 1.—B., a methodist clergyman, aged forty-four years, large and fleshy, and in the enjoyment of perfect health, with the following exception, came to see me, saying that he was troubled with loss of location, several times daily, each attack lasting from fifteen to thirty minutes, and that it began about ten years ago, at long intervals at first, but has increased in frequency from an attack of once a month to several times a day, and now, even when walking in streets that he has travelled in for years, when this feeling comes on him he cannot tell where he is, and is obliged to inquire. When coming to my office, he was obliged to inquire where it was, although standing directly in front and in plain sight of it. When in this peculiar mental condition, he says he is "all right" in regard to everything else, and can converse upon any topic and think accurately, and to test himself upon this point, he has sat down and added up long columns of figure, and left the work to be reviewed "when Richard was himself again," and invariably found it correct. Says he feels perfectly well every way, eats well, sleeps well, and this is all the trouble or annoyance of any kind that he has. In looking over the Materia Medica for a similimum, I found, under **Glonoine,** this symptom, "loses his way in the known streets," and gave him some powders of the 20th potency, with instructions to take a powder, dry, on his tongue, whenever he felt this sensation coming on. He returned to my office some ten days after, saying that the first powder had cured him entirely, and he had had no occasion to use the other powders.—Dr. C. A. Cochran.

Case 2.—A lady, æt. twenty-eight, of extremely nervous temperament, complains of severe headache, pulsation in the temples, fullness, and heavy aching on the vertex; she had her hair cut off to within two inches of the scalp, because the heaviness and heat of it almost distracted her; the least motion makes the pain much worse; she has not slept for three nights; keeps her eyes closed, because the light is disagreeable, though not painful; tongue coated heavily on the back part; moderate thirst; putrid taste; perspiration alternately, with chilliness, which causes her to cover herself up very heavily, till perspiration breaks out again; oppressed breathing, caused by a sense of weight in the chest, and occasional light cough; pulse 106, small and empty; hands hot; aversion to food; on attempting to rise, such weakness of the limbs she could not stand. **Glon.** cm, in water, every two hours, gave quick and permanent relief.—Dr. Ad. Lippe.

Case 3.—R. S., æt. three, had been sick several days. At midnight of the third day, the child presented the following symptoms. Severe diarrhœa; stools frequent and copious; very watery and yellow containing undigested particles of food that had been eaten the previous day. Had also nausea and vomiting. Gave **Ant. crud.** 6, with only partial relief of diarrhœa and vomiting: otherwise, no change for the better. On the day following, cerebral symptoms were manifested; twitching of limbs, particularly when asleep; would start suddenly out of a sound sleep and sit up in bed, looking about as if to inquire the case, would then lie down and fall into another dose, and thus on, alternately waking and sleeping with startings; tendency to drawing backward of head. Dark red spots, of various size, appeared on child's face and neck, chest and arms. Opisthotonic spasms now set in, gradually; teeth were clinched, jaws firmly locked; limbs extremely cold, the latter as far up as the knees, the former up to the elbows; at times the patient would cry out as if in sharp pain; eyes rolled about in their sockets, followed by intervals of comparative freedom of pain. Patient made vain efforts to sleep; after a night or two were thus passed, the breathing became more labored; insomnia ensued, subsequently coma set in; discharges from bowels continued more or less watery, and became involuntary; eyelids relaxed and dropped, eyeballs turned up; strabismus convergens was present; skin harsh, dry; gradually insensibility set in; eyes became insensible to light, and the mind to all that transpired around the child; all efforts failed to attract any attention from the child; the Chapman spinal ice-bag was applied at this stage, embracing within its limits the spine from occipital protuberance above to fifth lumbar vertebra below. The rigidity of body gave way in five minutes, and patient passed into a state of quiet repose. Skin became soft and moist; stools, both urine and fæces, were evacuated at regular intervals during the same night, requiring some effort on the patient's part, indicating return of vigor and tone to sphincters; no more involuntary stools; **Glonoin** 10 was administered every two hours, and the patient passed on to complete convalescence in a few days.—Dr. C. H. Von Tagen.

GNAPHALIUM.

Gnaph. is a fragrant bitter aromatic annual, growing in fields and woods. Though not so well known, we can hardly do without it, as it is one of our great standby in the treatment of sciatica and lumbago. The pain along the course of the sciatic nerve and its larger ramifications is intense. Numbness is generally associated with this pain. In this connection it is better to mention that it is very similar to **Colocynth,** not only with regard to neuralgic affections but in respect of many of its abdominal symptoms.

A short comparison between these two remedies will be to our advantage. In **Colocy.** the pain extends from the hip, down the posterior portion of the thigh into the popliteal space. The pains are sharp and shooting in character, and the patient must keep perfectly quiet, as every motion aggravates. In **Gnaph.** the pain commences from the hip, and rushes downward posteriorly to the feet. The leg feels cramped, and has got to be drawn up. The pain is worse in cold and damp weather.

Dr. George Shelton has recorded the case of a clergyman who had been persistently suffering from sciatica of the right side. This pain starting from the inner side of the thigh used to travel downward along the course of the anterior crural nerve. During cold and damp weather it used to extend along the right cord into the testicle, and caused him to draw up his leg and flex the thigh on the abdomen. A few doses of **Gnaph.** cured him completely.

We will now compare **Gnaphalium** with the following remedies with regard to their application in sciatica.

Ammon mur.—Here the pain is severe and long continued. It is most often left-sided, and the tendons of that side feel as if they were too short, making him lean sideways while walking. The pains are altogether better by rubbing and while he lies down.

Calc. carb.—It is a great remedy for sciatic pain, caused by working under water. The pain is aggravated when the limb is kept hanging down, and hence he has to elevate his knees constantly.

Euphorbium.—The tearing and tingling pain of this remedy is relieved by motion. In this respect it is somewhat similar to **Rhus tox**.

Ferr met.—The pain in the hip-joint is violent, and it is more so from the evening till midnight. There is a distinct lessening of the pain from walking slowly. The patient, although he can hardly put his feet on the ground, walks about for relief.

Kali iod. is good for sciatica in patient with a syphilitic and mercurial history. The pain, is apt to be worse at the night time, and as in the former remedy, is better by motion.

Kali phos. is almost a specific for neuralgia when the patient feels most of the pain in the sole of the foot. He is very restless.

Ledum.—In this the pain runs from the feet upward, and the affected limb is cooler than the remainder of the body. The left side is more affected than the right side.

Menyanthes as a remedy for sciatica has a very peculiar indication. The pain throws the affected thigh and leg spasmodically upward in a jerking fashion at every attempt to assume a sitting posture.

Nat. mur. has tensive pain in right hip and knee of a remittent character as in **Ammon mur.** Feeling of contraction of the hamstrings, emaciation of the affected limb, and relief by heat, are marked features.

Plumbum is used in chronic sciatica with muscular atrophy.

Ruta is indicated in sciatica where pain is very deep-seated, and feels as if it is in the marrow of the bone. There is generally a history of injury and contusion.

In the stomach its action is similar to that of **Colocy.** Like the latter remedy there are rumbling in the bowels, copious watery stool at night, much colicky pain, vomiting and purging.

GOSSYPIUM HERBACEUM.

This remedy is prepared from the root of our everyday Cotton Plant. It is cultivated in Asia and the southern parts of the United States of America. The fresh inner root is chopped and pounded and mixed with two parts by its weight of alcohol, and then after a few days strained and filtered. It belongs to the natural order of Malvaceæ.

This remedy is rich in sympathetic symptoms of the stomach, heart, bowels, and the nervous system arising from disturbance of uterine function. It is generally indicated in tall women who are comparatively anemic, and who are extremely nervous. In big doses, it acts as a powerful emmenagogue, but in homœopathy it should be used only on the principle of similia. It relieves a tardy flow of menses, specially when accompanied with a sensation as though the flow is about to start but yet does not do so. It removes a state of granulation in the mucous covering of both labias which seem studded with innumerable reddish eruptions.

I have used this remedy once or twice in my practice and with great satisfaction. It produces and hence cures morning sickness of pregnancy. We notice great nausea from least motion in the morning soon after waking; as soon as she raises her head from pillow, the retching starts. At first very little comes up, and then a little saliva, and lastly some bilious matter, but rarely any ingesta.

Intermittent pain in the ovaries is another characteristic feature of this remedy. It has scarcely disappointed me in after pains. Very excruciating and agonising pain, so frequently met with after labor in nervous females, has been repeatedly helped with this remedy. This is not much, but it will pay us immensely to remember these symptoms.

GRANATUM

It is prepared from Pomegranate, a very beautiful shrub or small tree producing a dense crown of dark green foliage. It is a native of Asia. The homœopathic tincture is prepared from the bark of the root of this plant. The important constituents of pomegranate bark is an alkaloid called Pelletierine. There is also a large amount of tannin, and some mannite.

This remedy is an important vermifuge. I have successfully used the decoction made from the bark of the root of this tree, forgetting rid of tape-worm.

GRAPHITES.

Graphites is called Plumbago. It is our common black lead. It is a mineral carbon. Its preparation is a bit difficult. In the first place graphite has got to be purified, which is done by boiling it in a sufficient quantity of distilled water and then digesting it in a solution of equal parts of Sulphuric acid and Hydrochloric acid, diluted with twice their volume of water. The purified graphite is then triturated coarsely with powdered sugar of milk and water. The drug was first proved by Hahnemann.

Graphites is an anti-psoric of great power. We will do well to bestow proper attention to the study of a remedy of such high repute. The first point for us to take note of in **Graphites**, is its constitution. These patients are rather stout and anemic with a tendency to skin affection and constipation. The terms. that vary aptly sum up the whole essence of this remedy, are to be found in the three words—fat, chilly and costive. This tendency towards obesity is distinctly marked. It is not the healthy flesh of the strong, healthy and the solid constitution but an unwieldy accumulation of adipose tissues, the result of mal-nutrition and imperfect assimilation. It may, therefore, be likened to **Calcarea carb.**, which remedy it resembles in its great sensitiveness to draughts of air and constant chilliness. There is distinctly a scrofulous basis as is manifested by its tendency to lymphatic œdema. The hair is blond, the face pale, and the spirit is low. In women this obesity is associated with habitual constipation and a proneness to delaying menstruation. Although the face shows occasional patches of color, due mostly to rush of blood, the

Graphites patient looks haggard, bloated, and yellow. The eyes are sunken betraying a low state of vitality. We must not also forget that **Graphites** is characterized by a great tendency to falling off of hair and whiskers. In consequence of this there are many nude spots on the scalp which look bold and shiny at places.

The next great trait is to be found in the unhealthy nature of the skin and nails in **Graphites.** The skin is found to be dry and absolutely deviod of moisture and is parchment-like. Every injury suppurates. Like other remedies, it has got its favourite sites. Most of the eruptions of **Graphites** are to be seen between the toes and fingers and on the scalp and behind the ears. The eruptions, in whichever part of the body they may be, are papular; —they contain a glairy, tenacious, honey-like fluid. Cracks, fissures, and rhagades are innumerable. They appear on the skin between the fingers and toes, on the nipples, labial commissures, and in and around the anus. These eruptions are not very sensitive. The nails are brittle, and they crumble on the slightest excuse. Further more. they are deformed and painful. In this respect **Graphites** bears great resemblance to **Calcarea carb., Petroleum, Mezereum, Psorinum, Oleander, Vinca minor,** and **Nitric acid**.

Calcarea carb is a great remedy for eczema scrofulosum. There is eczema on the scalp and face, same as in **Graphites,** but crusts that form are white unlike the crusts of **Graphites** which are yellowish.

Petroleum is very similar to **Graph**;—the skin is dry, harsh and parchment-like; the locations are about the same; fissures and cracks too are just as prominent. We notice thick scabs of yellowish green colour discharging an amber-colored fluid; the aggravation is specially in winter.

In **Mezereum** the vesicles are very itchy, but the point is that the secretion dries quickly, from under which an acrid, thick pus oozes on pressure. The itching is worse when the patient gets warm in bed or is wrapped up. These eruptions generally come on in parts normally deficient in fat.

Psorinum is a great antipsoric. The eruptions, dirty and greasy in appearance, disappear during summer but reappear when the cold weather comes on.

In **Oleander** we have crusta lactea on the scalp and the back of the ears as in **Graphites.** The vesicular eruptions about the head are smooth and shiny with drops of serum standing out here and there, but the scabs when they dry look brown. It is a remedy specially indicated in skin troubles complicated with gastro-enteric affections.

Vinca minor so rarely used and so little known, is good for humid eruptions on head, face, and behind ears.

In **Nitric acid** the humid, stinging eruptions appear on vertex and temples; they bleed easily when scratched. Profuse granulations, proud flesh, and splinter-like pains are some of the guiding characteristics of **Nit. acid.**

Graph. is no less a remedy for the bad effects of repelled eruptions of any kind. Suppression of an eruption as well as of a habitual secretion or excretion sets up a great turmoil and disturbance in the human constitution. It is very often the cause of many misfortunes. Failure to take cognizance of such facts leads to many catastrophies—catastrophies that might have been easily averted, had it been for a little more discretion and intelligence on the part of the attending physician. Dr. Nash records the case of a child that had been relieved of an eczema on the head by means of local applications with the result that severe entero-colitis had set in. Symptoms gradually assumed alarming proportions, till at last it was disposed of as an incurable case of consumption of the bowels. Nash found the child greatly emaciated; restless and passing frequent stools of brown fluid, mixed with undigested particles of food partaken. They were also extremely offensive. **Graphites** 6m promptly cured the case.

The **Graphites** patients are not over-cheerful. Sadness and despondence are their ever-present companion. They weep and are constantly miserable and unhappy. This sadness is characterized by a taint of apprehensiveness. A kind of a fearful foreboding is constantly on them. A particular point that should be carefully remembered, is that this sadness is particularly worse during music. This is indeed an abnormal trait as usually human nature is susceptible to music on the pleasing side. In the case of **Graphites**, however, the opposite is true; instead of making her happy and forgetful, music tends to deepen the inherent trait of sadness that lurks in her system. In this respect **Graphites** may be compared to **Aco., Dig., Kreo., Nat carb., Natrum sulph.,** and **Sabina.** In this connection we may also think of **Manganum** as being the opposite of **Graphites.** The sadness of **Manganum** is distinctly ameliorated by sad music. Another characteristic of **Graphites**, that I have omitted to mention, is fidgetiness while at work. They cannot sit in one place long, but must rove about being impelled by anxiety, solicitude, and fear. It has been recommended in impudence and idiocy, when the patient laughs all the time and laughs even when reprimanded.

Graphites has been aptly termed the **Pulsatilla** of the climacteric age because of the great semblance, in the uterine symptoms of the two remedies. The menses are too late and scanty, and are generally preceded by severe menstrual colic Eruptions make their appearance at this time. As a result of such scanty and irregular menstruation, patients turn chlorotic Sometimes leucorrhœa appears in the place of menses, and thi is fetid and excoriating. It gushes out night and day, and i oftener seen before than after the menses.

It has been recommended highly in dysmenorrhœa. Th patient complains of great weakness, lassitude and tiredness i lower extremities. Sick headache, with pain over the eyes, numbness and pain in the sacrum and down the legs, great emaciatio with paleness of the face, acne solaris in the face, bearing dow pain in the womb and swelling and hardness of the ovaries are ind cations to lead us to **Graphites**. It has been prescribed in cance of the uterus. I dare say if prescribed properly, it may ameliora and alleviate and in certain cases cure where cure is possibl Great heat and painfulness in the vagina, swelling of the lymphat vessels and mucus follicles near about, hardness and swelling of t neck of the uterus with tuberculous nodes and cauliflower excre cences, discharge of black, lumpy, fetid blood, inveterate constip tion, florid complexion, obesity, and the peculiar parchment-li skin, covered over with its characteristic rash are sure indicatio for **Graphites**.

On the male sexual side its application is confined to sexu weakness due to great abuse leading on to a total aversion coition. Involuntary seminal emission, flaccidity of the pe herpetic eruptions on genitals and scrotum indicate **Graphites**

In some cases of dyspepsia where **Graphites** would help, otl remedies are oftentimes prescribed. Such mistakes can easily avoided by careful study of the remedy. Great flatulence is notic and the abdomen is so full from accumulation of old fæces : incarcerated flatus that they cannot stand anything tight about tl waist. The taste of the mouth is bad as of rotten eggs. T suffer from excessive canine hunger. Sometimes eat becomes a necessity as it relieves pain in the stom: **Graphites** should be particularly remembered in all cases wl there is amelioration from eating. On this indication, it has been used in gastro-dynia, gastralgia, chronic gastric catarrh, chronic gastritis, and even in asthma with marvellous success. I have known a patient who had to keep bread or some other articles of diet handy, to be able to eat quickly as soon as suffocative paroxysm of asthma was about to start. I have also cured impending cases of gastric ulceration with **Graphites** on the same characteristic feature of amelioration from eating. In this respect it resembles **Petroleum, Chelidonium,** and **Anacardium.** They have great disgust for sweet things and to all animal foods, the very thought produces **nausea** and loss of appetite as in **Angustura, Calcarea carb, Carbo veg., Cocculus,** and **Colchicum.** We give below a brief discussion of the above remedies as it will be to our advantage.

In **Angustura** we find particular aversion to meat, but there is a great longing for coffee.

Calcarea carb, we all know, is a great remedy for chronic dyspepsia, or rather of dyspepsia in strumous subject. The same disgust and repugnance to meat and to warm cooked food is noticeable; they crave cold victuals. Palpitation of heart, constant tendency towards diarrhœa, sour smell, sour vomiting, sour stool, and excessive sweat of the head are all prominent symptoms.

In **Carbo veg.** the same excessive flatulence, the same repugnance to meat, especially to fat, fish, and oysters are present; but a confusion with **Graphites** is not likely as the other symptoms are so distinct and clear-cut. It is a dyspepsia of a chronic form, mostly seen in the old people, and it is brought about by over-indulgence in strong spirituous liquors, debauchery, late suppers and rich food.

In **Cocculus** great nausea and extreme aversion to food, inspite of great hunger, are more marked than in any other remedy. The very sight or the smell of food sickens and brings on vertigo and an efflux of saliva into the mouth.

Lastly, we come to **Colchicum.** Appetite for different things is present, but as soon as he sees them or still more smells them, he shudders with nausea and is unable to eat. It may even bring on fainting.

Whenever diarrhœa is present, although such a thing is not very common in **Graph.** the stools are brown, fluid, mixed with indigested substance and of an intolerable fetor. But constipation is of more frequent occurrence—the stools are large, hard knotted, and are joined together by mucus shreds. As a result of such passage of large, hardened, fæcal matter, although lubricated with mucus, the anus becomes fissured and varices make their appearance. These hemorrhoids are very painful, especially on taking wide steps. They are itchy and sensitive.

In troubles of the eye, very few remedies can excel **Graphites** We use it in scrofulous ophthalmia with intense photophobia and profuse lachrymation. The mucopurulent discharge from the eye is thin and excoriating. We also use it for ulcers, pustules and herpes on cornea with sore and fissured eyelids. In chronic ciliary blepharitis, especially in blepharitis angularis with cracked bleeding and ulcerated margins, full of scabs and eczematous eruptions, no other remedy can approach **Graphites.** This is very much like **Sulphur,** but the margins of the eyelids in **Sulphur** are red, whereas in **Graphites** they are paler than usual.

Graphites also affects the vision. Letters appear double when writing and run together when reading. He also sees fiery zigzags around his field of vision. Hyperæsthesia of eyes intense photophobia, great sensitiveness to sun light, vanishing of sight during menstruation, thickening of the cartilage of the lids, and finally the wild condition of eye lashes are a few of its symptoms worth remembering.

It is used in tinnitus aurium with lots of humming, hissing ringing, rushing, and crackling sound in the ears, specially far during the full-moon. Sometimes there is complete deafness. H suffers from a sensation as if a skin were before the ear obstructing sounds. Strange as it may seem, these patients hear better in noise, as when riding in a carriage or in a crowd. The sense of smell is abnormally acute in these patients. They can not tolerate any smell especially that of flowers.

The headache of **Graphites** is very peculiar. When fat anemic women, with disordered menstruation, complain of a numb and heavy feeling in the head, specially in the occiput, we can think of no other remedy that will suit them better than **Graphites.** The sensation of a heavy weight in the occiput is very strong that they frequently rest their head on some support.

We will mention a few peculiar sensations of **Graphites** before we close. One is a sensation of a cob-web over the face This symptom led me to prescribe **Graphites** in a protracted ca of low delirium in a young gentleman of about 23 summers. As I entered the sick room, I found the patient constantly wiping his face. On enquiry I learnt that he was trying to get rid of some tangled thread on his face which he could not accomplish inspite of the constant manipulation of his hand. **Graphites** was greatly instrumental in curing that case. Another peculiar symptom is a sensation as if the skin of the forehead was drawn into folds.

Case 1.—Miss H. N., aged thirty years, living in comfortable circumstances and obliged to exert herself, had always been delicate since her menses commenced, at the age of twelve or thirteen years. About ten years ago she experienced "bearing down"; her menses became too profuse and protracted. Under routine treatment the menstrual flow at last disappeared. Since then, she began to suffer excessively from unilateral headache of periodical character. These headaches at first appeared about once a week. On awaking in the morning a numbness in the left side of the head would be the forerunner of a day of nameless misery. The numbness gradually concentrated near the supra-orbital region of the left eye, where it seemed to expend all its force. At noon violent nausea set in, but without ability to vomit; the patient was tormented by retching and straining. There was obstinate constipation, backache, and sensitiveness of the spine, with great prostration on the least exertion. During the intervals, she was able to be out-of-doors and to do light work. She had also a continuous headache of a dull aching kind, every day, especially mornings. **Nux vomica** and **Lachesis** relieved the constipation, but did not the headache. Under the action of two doses of **Graphites** in the 200th dilution, she gradually improved, and the headache ceased permanently. She now enjoys good health, but the menstrual function was never re-established.—Dr. C. Wesslhoeft in the New Eng. Med. Gazette, October, 1876.

Case 2.—Two months after confinement Mrs. T. applied to me for relief from a trouble which her physician pronounced fissure of the anus (which diagnosis I confirmed), and for which he recommended forcible dilatation. Pain during evacuation, severe, sharp, cutting, followed by constriction and aching for several hours, and especially severe at night. By her physician's advice she had been using small enemata of water, retaining them as long as possible, and then voiding them without effort, I recommended a continuance of the enemata; and gave **Graph. 200** in solution, a teaspoonful every four hours. Within three days the pains had ceased—an evacuation after enema was painless. The enemata were continued for a fortnight, and could then be dispensed with. There has been no return of this trouble.—Dr. C. Dunham.

GRATIOLA.

This is also called Hedge Hyssop. It grows on the borders of rivers, lakes, and ditches in central and southern Europe. It was proved by Nenning of Germany. The whole plant is used in the preparation of the tincture. It belongs to the natural order of Scrophulariaceæ. It acts specially on the gastro-intestinal tract.

Gratiola is a remedy of wide renown, especially for its efficacy in cholera and choleric diarrhœa. The most important point in this diarrhœa is the characteristic rush and force with which the fæces are expelled from the anus. It thus resembles **Aloes, Calc-phos, Croton tig., Gambogia, Phosphorus, Podophyllum,** and **Sulphur.**

The stools consist of a yellow-greenish watery substance and are very frothy. Often do we find great rumbling and gurgling in the abdomen with violent colic. Vomiting is particularly severe, and is accompanied by pain in the head, severe cramp in the solar plexus, intense nausea, and a great rectal and anal irritation in the shape of burning. A peculiar cold feeling in the abdomen is considered a very important symptom of **Gratiola.** C. W. Sonnenschmidt has recorded a cure of a case of diarrhœa of which the stools were yellow, watery, frothy and urgent. **Colocynth** and **Ipecac** failed, till at last enquiry revealed the cold feeling in the abdomen. **Gratiola** was then prescribed and effected a speedy cure.

Mentally the patient is very peevish, irresolute, hysterical and ill-humoured. Teste considers **Gratiola** the **Chamomilla** of chronic diseases. The patient is almost always worse during and after eating; this is especially noticed in vertigo.

The head and the eye symptoms of **Gratiola** are important. There is a frequent rush of blood to the head and a consequent vanishing of sight. This is another of Gratiola's important characteristics.

GRINDELIA ROBUSTA.

Grindelia is also called the gum plant, because of a viscid balsamic secretion. The tincture is made from the whole plant when in flowers. The proportion is one part of the chopped plant to two parts by its weight of alcohol.

Grindelia is noted for its efficacy in the treatment of asthma. It is mostly indicated in mucus asthma. There is an abnormal accumulation of tenacious, viscid mucus in the smaller bronchi, but the most important peculiarity of the drug consists in an aggravation during sleep. On falling asleep his respiratory movement ceases and is not resumed until awakened by the ensuing suffocation. The patient has to keep up in a sitting posture in the bed and sleep is entirely out of question due to interruption of breathing during sleep. It is also used in asthma from heart troubles. This asthma is secondary to heart affections. This difficulty of respiration during sleep is due to its paretic action on the pneumogastric nerve.

In the head, we have a peculiar sensation of heaviness as if the patient had taken too much quinine. Pain in eyeballs, running back to the brain and worse from movement of eyes, pain in thet region of spleen, cough and dyspnœa are symptoms that should be clearly remembered.

It has quite a lot of symptoms on the skin. Eruption, vesicular and popular, herpes zoster, roseolar rash, insects and beebites are materially helped by **Grindelia.** Gatchell recommends external application of a lotion of **Grindelia robusta** one in ten of water as a sovereign remedy in itches and painful erythematous eruptions.

GUAIACUM

The tinture is prepared from the gum-resin of Lignum sanctum or Lignum vitæ, a large tree growing in West Indies. It belongs to the natural order of Zygophyllaceæ. This remedy was introduced into our Materia Medica by Hahnemann, and proved by himself. It is one of Hahnemann's anti-psorics and is a noted remedy in gout and rheumatism, engrafted on a syphilitic constitution. It acts principally on muscular and fibrous tissues, causing contraction of limbs and a consequent deformity. Caries, spongious affection of bones, especially of tibia and tarsal bones, acute inflammation with all the redness, heat and swelling of **Belladonna,** are some of its principal actions and it will be our business in this chapter to go into it thoroughly and differentiate it from remedies of like nature with similar dyscrasia and predilection. It also promotes suppuration and spontaneous evacuation of gouty abscesses, greatly relieving the sufferings of the patient. Another characteristic of **Guaiacum,** that should be clearly remembered, is that all its excretions are intolerably offensive. The pains are pressive, drawing, and tearing in nature, often ending in a stitch. The tendency of this pain is to travel backwards or from below upwards.

It is, as has been hinted at before, a remarkable remedy in syphilis, mostly in its secondary stage. It helped to cure a harassing case of secondary syphilis, recorded by Proell, after the failure of **Mercurius, Nitric acid, Aurum mur.,** and **Mezereum.** It was in the case of a gentleman who had an inflammation of the palate, threatening perforation. Confusion of thoughts, melancholia and weakness of memory were additional symptoms. Inflammation of the palate grew deeper, till at last perforation of the palate was threatened. **Guaiacum 3x** was administered, and within the course of two weeks the whole trouble vanished; mind became clear and cheerfulness was established and memory had returned. This is indeed a wonderful cure and brings **Guaiacum** nearer to **Fluoric acid, Kali bich., Mercurius,** and **Nitric acid.**

In **Fluoric acid** we have extensive ulceration of the mouth and throat. Syphilitic caries and necrosis, boring bone pains, and the offensiveness of the acrid ichor, are common in both remedies but **Guaiacum** wants the peculiar pungent strong urine of **Fluoric acid.**

Kali Bich., a noted remedy in syphilis, has a tendency for per-forated ulcers in nose, mouth, throat but it differs from **Guaiacum** in its stringy, jelly-like discharge.

In **Mercurius** we have ptyalism, flabby, broad tongue and the peculiar lardaceous appearance of the base of ulcers—symp-toms entirely wanting in **Guaiacum.**

Nitric acid has splinter-like pains and the ulcers are inclined to spread more in circumference than in depth.

We should think of it, particularly in syphilitic sore throat and the keynote symptom here is a great burning in the throat, œsophagus, larynx, and the whole of buccal cavity. In this respect it is greatly similar to **Phytolacca** where too, the pain is a burning pain and each time patient swallows, he feels like swallowing hot liquids.

GUAREA TRICHILIOIDES.

It is also called the Red-wood and the Ball-wood. It belongs to the natural order of Meliaceæ. We are indebted to Petroz for our knowledge of this drug which is of great impor-tance in many affections of the eyes. Although it needs further verification and proving, we may safely depend upon some of its eye symptoms. Numerous cases are on record, of cures of chemosis of an extreme type. It substantially helped in a case of chemosis, after extraction of cataract, where the pad was so extended and thick that nothing of the eye could be seen but the pupil at the bottom of a veritable tunnel.

GYMNOCLADUS CANADENSIS.

Gymnocladus is also called the American Coffee-tree and it belongs to the natural order of Leguminosæ. One symptom, which is supposed to be of paramount importance, and which has been the basis of numerous cures with **Gymnocladus,** is the peculiar, bluish-white coating of the tongue. Dr. C. T. Bingham cured a case of persistent headache, located in the front part of the head, specially under eye-brows and upper part of the nose with **Gymnocladus,** being guided by the peculiar tongue of the patient which was distinctly bluish-white in colour.

It is also a good remedy for sore throat which is charac-terised by the dark livid redness of the fauces and tonsils.

Over the eyes the patient experiences a peculiar sensation as of flies crawling over it.

HAMAMELIS VIRGINICA.

Hamamelis is our common witch-hazel.   This plant grows extensively in the United States.   Having first learnt of its efficacy from Mr. Pond of 'Pond's Extract Fame' Dr. H. C. Preston had it thoroughly proved and its symptoms systematically arranged. The tincture is prepared from the fresh bark of the twigs and roots.

Hamamelis stands at the top of the list of all our hæmorrhagic remedies, but its action is confined altogether to the venous system of the blood vessels. It may thus be called the **Aconite** of the veins; that is, it acts upon the veins in the same way as **Aconite** acts on the arteries, but the grand characteristic of this remedy, a characteristic that pervades the length and breadth of **Hamamelis,** is found in the sensation of universal soreness. It is found in the wounds either incised or lacerated, rheumatic affections, phlebitis, ulcers, orchitis and the various other affections for which **Hamamelis** is homœopathic. The parts feel bruised.

Coming back to its hemorrhagic properties we must lay special stress on its power of causing passive congestion or venous stagnation of the skin and mucous membranes.   The blood in **Hamamelis** is dark and clotted, as is to be expected in all venous hæmorrhages.   This hæmorrhage may take place from any orifice or outlet of the body.   It may be from eyes, ears, nose, throat, lungs, stomach, abdomen, urinary organs and the sexual channels.   In the eyes we have extravasations due to rupture of small vessels, due either to a strain, as is caused by whooping cough or violent concussion and other external injuries.

In epistaxis the blood is non-coagulable and dark-colored; it is associated with a feeling of tightness across the bridge of the nose and a considerable pressure in the forehead. Dr. Preston cites of a case of epistaxis in a hemophiliac, where he had to insert a piece of linen soaked with **Hamamelis,** through the nostrils, to check the hermorrhage.

In varicosis of the throat, the parts look bluish from distended veins and there is more or less discomfort and pain on swallowing, with frequent hawking up of mucus tinged with dark, grumous blood. In hematemesis the same characteristic is to be found. In dysentery where **Hamamelis** is our remedy, the quantity of blood passed is unusual, amounting almost to an actual hemorrhage. We should think of it particularly in that variety of dysentery, where the patient passes huge quantities of blood with the stools which are usually accompanied by crampy pain around the umbilicus. The blood discharged may be either bright red or of a tarry consistency. It is an excellent remedy in melæna when the abovementioned characteristics are present. Hemorrhoids, when attended with profuse bleeding at regular intervals and without much expulsive effort, stand in equal need of **Hamamelis.** Varices protrude through the anus and the hemorrhoidal veins, look distinctly bluish and distended to fullness, with their contents of venous blood. Hæmaturia and hæmorrhoids of the bladder, when characterized by dull pain in the renal and vesical region and associated with constant urging to urination, can be easily checked with **Hamamelis.**

With regard to the uterus it checks both active and passive hæmorrhage. Numerous lives have been saved, through its agency in various ages and climes, where death seemed imminent from the constant escape of blood, which nothing would stop, and the patient looked shrivelled and blue as in the collapse stage of cholera. It also checks hemorrhage of the lying-in-women and prevents threatened abortion as is heralded by a persistent oozing of blood and brought about either idiopathically or by injury. Its power to regulate and restore equilibrium of the venous and arterial side of the circulatory system, is further manifested by its capacity to relieve varicose enlargements of veins of the lower limbs in pregnant women. I have used it more than once and with ample satisfaction, in varicose veins on legs during pregnancy, in women, who could hardly move or stand, due to swelling and painfulness. Once I had occasion to prescribe **Hamamelis,** in a case of huge hæmorrhoidal tumor as large as the head of a small baby, that came on, a few days after the birth of her child. Milk-leg, swelling of the labium, congestion inflammation and neuralgia of the ovaries, chronic parenchymatous metritis, sub-involution and hypertrophy of the uterus and prolapsus of both vagina and uterus have been helped by **Hamamelis,** when the universal symptom of soreness was present along with the other indications mentioned above.

The action of **Hamamelis** on the male sexual organ is great. I have used it frequently in orchitis following gonorrhœa. The indications are soreness and severe neuralgic pain in testicles shifting to bowels and causing nausea and fainting. The enlargement of the spermatic veins, the result of violent exercise, horseback riding, etc., also comes under the influence of this remedy when associated with a feeling of soreness.

Hamamelis is similar to **Arnica, Calendula** in injuries; and to **China, Phosphorus, Crocus, Erigeron** and **Trillium** in hemorrhage.

HECLA LAVA.

This medicine is prepared by triturating the lava thrown out from the crater of mount Hecla in Iceland. The remedy was first proved by Dr. Garth Wilkinson of London. While on a visit to Hecla he noticed that the cows and sheep, grazing on the pastures on the slopes of the volcano, generally suffered from exostoses of the jaws. On post-mortem of some of these animals, it was found that their tissues had become calcareous and friable. Further experiments and provings were made and its efficacy in the treatments of tumors, indurations, exostoses, nodosities, caries, and other syphilitic destructions of nasal bones, were established without doubt.

HELLEBORUS NIGER.

This is also called the Christmas Rose because the flower blooms in mid-winter. The tincture is prepared from the dry root coarsely powdered and mixed with five parts by its weight of alcohol. It belongs to the natural order of Ranunculaceæ.

This is another of our master's immortal monuments. It is not a remedy that we are called on to use every day, but that does not make it in any way less important. It is generally needed in the more serious forms of ailments where its marvellous effects will often astound and startle the disbelievers. Its effects are specially felt over the sensorium, where it produces a state of stupefaction and insensibility. It acts principally upon the kidneys and serous membranes giving rise to dropsical effusions as will be seen in many of its applications in typhoids, nephritis and meningitis. These effusions may be in the brain, thorax, peritoneum and cellular tissues. It thus makes an excellent remedy in many dropsical diseases.

It produces " a condition where with sight unimpaired nothing is seen very fully and the patient does not pay attention to anything ; with the hearing perfectly sound nothing is heard distinctly; with perfectly constituted gustatory organs everything seems to have lost its taste; where the mind is often or always without ideas; where the past is forgotten or little remembered." Such a condition is often met with in typhoid states. The expression of his face is stupid. His look is vacant and the pupils are dilated. Constant somnolence is an important feature of this drug, out of which the patient may be roused with difficulty, but he rarely gains full consciousness. He has no desire of his own and when left alone, he sinks back into slumber. He lies upon his back with his limbs drawn up. There is occasional sliding down in bed. Of all these symptoms the most important one is the boring of the head into the pillow; this is intermixed with occasional screams that possibly indicate sharp shooting pain felt somewhere in the cranium. He is thirsty and drinks water greedily and in so doing he bites the spoon. The water drunk descends audibly into the stomach, the same as we find in **Cina, Hydrocyanic acid** and **Phosphorus.** There is a sort of a wrinkle on the forehead with cold sweat on it. Another symptom, that helped me on many occasions and which I consider the most important in **Helleborus,** is the continual motion of one arm and one leg, the other lying perfectly still as if paralysed. The urine is generally suppressed or scanty with dark specks floating in it. In the urine we very often notice a sort of a coffee ground sediment. Dr. Nash is of opinion that the first sign of improvement after the administration of **Helleborus** is an increase in the quantity of the urine; it is worth our while to remember this, so that we may not run on to a new remedy to seek speedier relief. Another symptom that should be mentioned is a sort of a chewing motion of the mouth. His jaws are constantly moving as if he is chewing something. In this respect **Helleborus** is like **Belladonna, Bryonia, Calcarea carb.** and **Natrum mur.**

In **Belladonna** the symptoms are more violent indicating a higher degree of inflammation and deeper cerebral erethism at the bottom of the trouble.

In **Bryonia** there is a certain amount of depression in the sensorium, but there is no perversion of the senses. We also notice a great want of secretion of the mucous surfaces of the body,

The chewing motion in **Natrum mur.** is mostly noticed during the stage of chill. It is only when he is covered up during chill that we find him performing this act.

In **Calcarea carb.** the chewing motion is noticed during sleep and in the prodromal stage of epilepsy.

From what has already been said, it becomes evident that **Helleborus** is an important remedy in the therapy of typhoid fever. It is towards the later stages, when continued high fever has given rise to symptoms of effusion in the brain with a corresponding state of depression in the sensorium, that we think of **Helleborus**. It is true we have sensorial depression in **Rhus tox, Baptisia, Pyrogen** and **Acid phos,** but in none of these do we find the same amount of sensorial depression as in **Helleborus**. In **Rhus tox** the sensations are eminently present though bedimmed to a certain extent by the light delirium of the remedy. In **Baptisia** and **Pyrogen** it is a bit more profound than in **Rhus tox** and the condition of the patient somewhat more desperate, considering the tissue changes that are rapidly taking place under these two latter remedies. **Phosphoric acid** has the apathy and the indifference of **Helleborus,** but this state is nothing compared to the deep-seated lack of sensibility of our remedy. The expression of the face is stupid, the look in the eyes vacant and the patient is utterly indifferent to everything that is happening around him. It is more a state of somnolence than indifference from which the patient cannot be roused or if roused at all, it is done with great difficulty. He stares at his physician without the slightest look of recognition. All his perceptions and senses have grown extremely dull. He utters no desires, expresses no wish and slowly sinks back into a slumber from which there is hardly any awakening. He lies upon his back with limbs drawn up and even then slides down in bed. The action of his heart is slow and his respiration is laboured and behindhand of the normal. Inspite of the great heat, he is covered with cold sweat and his limbs, specially hands and feet, are icy cold. Automatic motion of one arm and leg, involuntary throwing about of the limbs, weak unintelligible voice, unconscious discharge of urine which is scanty, high-coloured and albuminous, sooty appearance of the nose which is cold and looks as if about to tumble down, white blisters on swollen lips and a wrinkled appearance of the forehead are symptoms that point clearly to **Helleborus.** This apathy and sensorial depression is more akin to the stupor of **Opium,** but then in the latter remedy cerebral congestion is more profound, the breathing loud and stertorous and the face dark and purplish. In **Helleborus** the face is pale, often cold or at least cooler than what is found in **Opium**. The pulse of **Helleborus** is weak, small and perceptible, whereas that of **Opium** is slow.

The mental side of **Helleborus** is characterized by total unconsciousness and a diminished power. Frequent involuntary sighing, much lamenting and moaning and a state of woefulness are particularly present in **Helleborus**.

Helleborus is frequently needed in meningitis, hydrocephalus, convulsions. epilepsy, apoplexy and other affections of the brain, when many of the above-symptoms, are present. The nearest remedies to **Helleborus** in these affections are **Apis, Zincum, Bell., Bryonia,** and **Cuprum**.

Helleborus finds its scope in post-scarlatinal dropsy when the patient breathes easier lying down than sitting up. In this it is similar to **Digitalis** and **Terebinth.**

It is a good remedy for mucus dysentery where the stools are white, jelly-like and tenacious. These attacks come on in children frequently during dentition, also while suffering from hydrocephalus. There is quite a good bit of smarting and burning at the anus after the stool. In this, **Helleborus,** is similar to **Aloes, Colchicum** and **Rhus tox.**

The time of aggravation in **Helleborus** is 4 to 8 p.m.

Case 1—Geo,.B., æt. sixteen months, after two week's allopathic treatment for diarrhœa, had soporous sleep, with screaming and starting; lower jaw sinking down; constant motion of the jaws, as if chewing something; face pale and puffed; scanty, dark-colored urine; forehead drawn in folds, and covered with cold perspiration. After **Nux** 30, one dose **Hell.** 200 was given, and soon relieved. Child was well on the third day.—Hoyne.

Case 2.—Feb. 25, 1871. A. K., a girl twelve years of age, black hair and eyes, dark complexion. has had dropsy for three days, following an attack of scarlatina. No thirst, face flushed, pulse 96, upper eyelids bag out; cheeks, body and legs œdematous; urine scanty and highly albuminous, color dark, with floating dark motes, no sediment. **Apis** and **Ars.** have failed to arrest the disease. Two years since I remembered having promptly cured with *Helleborus* a similar case with coffee-ground sediment. In that case the urine was likewise dark, with floating dark motes, hence I gave the same remedy this time; 200th potency, in water, every three hours. In five hours, the pulse stood at 80, skin moist, bloating diminished, urine copious. Same remedy was continued three days; urine greatly increased in quantity, but the albumen undiminished. February 27. Great orthopnœa from midnight to about 1 o'clock· **Ars.** 200, two doses. March 1. Copious urine, with dark sediment; **Hell.** 200, March 2. Bloating increased, but urine more profuse; orthopnœa at 1 o'clock A.M. **Ars.** 30. March 3. Bloating diminished, urine still copious and clearer—less albumen; some pink sediment, like hematin; no more orthopnœa; **Ars.** 30. March 7. Pulse 72; non-synchronous with respiration; calves of legs only dropsical; urine copious—Placebo. March 9. Slight dropsical swelling of calves of legs only. Patient feels quite well—discharged, May, 1871. Has been well ever since. —Dr. H. V. Miller.

Case 3.—An old lady of fourscore, who was threatened with a low form of nervous fever, but under treatment developed only an intermittent. On close study of the case, I could find but one symptom wherein her case differed naturally from that of the ordinary type of ague, and it belonged solely to her. This symptom was rheumatic pains in the knees during the chill, and **Helleborus** was the only remedy which we know has that symptom, under these conditions, and one dose of Fincke's preparation cured her. This happened four years ago, and to this date there has been no relapse.

HELODERMA.

This is a medicine of recent origin and is prepared by triturating sugar of milk saturated with the venom of Gila Monster, a serpent of the lizard type found in Arizona. It is an ugly looking object, the entire body being encased in a thinly-coated armour of fixed skin, marked over with yellow and black spots. In dark, it becomes excessively languid and slow of movement, but assumes great activity and liveliness when brought into the reviving rays of the sun light. This is true mostly of every species of the serpent class. They all assume great energy in the hotter part of the season and go comparatively low during the cold months of the winter and the snow. Its bite produces symptoms of locomotor ataxia and paralysis agitans. The poison is a slow lingering poison and when it does kill, it kills after months of suffering, pain and torture. Death takes place rather from failure of heart than from respiratory failures. Dr. Robbert Boocock made bold provings of this remedy and brought it to a scientific basis. He took 3 or 4 drops of tincture prepared by mixing one dram of 6x trituration to 4 ounces of alcohol. He was seized with an internal coldness in the region of the heart as if being frozen to death. It was a coldness that came from within outward and was so intense as to be described as an " arctic coldness." Other provers had this symptom just as prominently as Dr. Boocock. Hence we can consider this symptom to be the cardinal symptom of the remedy. It also has a sensation of constriction and aggravation from sleep as in other snake remedies. Other indications are tremor, spongy feeling of feet on walking, numbness, staggering gate and great thirst with dryness

of the mouth.   The sensation of coldness, referred to above,
is felt everywhere.   In the head we have a sensation of
a cold hand.   In the mouth the tongue feels cold, dry and tender.
In the chest, even the lungs and the heart feel cold. Coldness
is felt along scapula and along spine.   On these indications, Dr.
E. E. Case effected great improvement in a case of locomotor
ataxia in a woman who had all the classical symptoms of the
disease.   Under the application of **Heloderma** she recovered a fair
control of her muscles and usefulness.   Dr. Boocock used it
successfully in a case of impending failure of the heart with all
the symptoms of death gradually making their appearance, such
as blueness of the hands, coldness of tongue and breath, and sudden
loss of strength and energy.

In fever we have excessive internal coldness and sensations
of cold waves ascending from feet or going down from base of
the brain.   **Helo.** thus becomes akin to—**Abies can.,** and **Camphor**
in the treatment of marsh fevers.

HELONIAS DIOICA.

This is also called the Blazing Star.   The plant is indigenous
to the United States of America.   Medicine is prepared from the
fresh root, gathered before flowering.

Helonias has a specific action over the uterine organ, and is,
therefore, regarded as a great uterine tonic.   The one key-note
indication of this remedy is a 'consciousness of the womb.'   In
the normal condition, due to the autonomous action of the vitality
and a perfect co-ordination of the different parts of this complex
machinery we are never conscious of the different organs of the
system; when such a consciousness dawns, it means a deviated
vitality and a disordered condition.   Such then is the import of
his ' consciousness of the womb.'   The ligaments become loose
and flaccid due to a general exhaustion of the system, as a result
of which we have uterine displacement.   The uterus moves when
she moves; when she stands the organ dangles about; the result
is a sore and a tender feeling.   This is reflected in the sacrum as
dragging and an undefined feeling of weakness.   This is not
about all.   The cervix of the prolapsed uterus is full of ulceration;
constant dark offensive discharge, more pronounced on the least
exertion, lends further pathos to the shallow, sad, suffering ex-
ression of the face.   Menorrhagia due to ulcerated os or cervix

is a common occurrence. It lasts longer at every period and drains her already exhausted vitality to its very bottom. She loses more blood than is made in the intermenstrual period. To add to her discomfort. there is that intense pruritus of the vulva and vagina. The labia and the pudendum are hot, red and swollen. They itch and burn terribly; even the mucous surface of the labia becomes red, swollen and covered with curdy deposits. Dr. L. L. Danforth reports of a case that he cured with **Helonias.** The pruritus was so intense that " she could tear the flesh out." The cause of this was a thin albuminous leucorrhœa from a congested cervix coagulating on the surrounding parts giving rise to further irritation.

When the affection of the kindey is secondary to uterine trouble, we may think of **Helonias.** Thus when in albuminuria, the result of amenorrhœa, we notice weariness, languor, emaciation, debility, loss of appetite, paleness, chlorosis, constant aching and an extreme tenderness in the region of kidney, especially the right, with profuse, clear, light-colored urine, **Helonias** will do yeoman's service.

On the chest, **Helonias** has got a peculiar symptom. There is a sensation as though the chest were gripped in a vice. Dr. Farrington reports, of a case of blood spitting accompanying prolapsus uteri and a long-lasting lochial discharge that he cured with **Helonias.**

There is another peculiarity we must not overlook. These patients feel better when they are forgetful of their ailments; the moment the consciousness of their sickness comes to them, their distress becomes unbearable. In this **Helonias** is similar to **Calc. phos** and **Oxalic acid.**

These patients, as a rule, are very lethergic and dull when they start on any work, but very soon the lethargy gives in to a fulness. of energy and action. Mentally they are very melancholy, irritable and fault-finding. We notice great intolerance of contradiction.

HEPAR SULPHURIS.

Till very recently the prevalent belief that obtained amongst laymen and even physicians of this country, was that homœopathy was not efficacious in cuts, bruises, boils, abscesses, carbuncles, gangrenes, and the like ailments. They were supposed to belong to the domain of the surgeons. Fortunately for suffering humanity such notions no longer exist; experience having resulted in knowledge and knowledge in the inculcation of wisdom, there has been a thorough disillusionment of all such false conceptions and the Materia Medica of the homœopath has, to a great extent, superseded the scalpel of the surgeon. It has happened time and again that when the regulars were contemplating an amputation, the distracted patient escaped and saved himself from mutilation by the administration of a timely and appropriate dose of homœopathic medicine. **Hepar sulphuris** has helped much in the transformation of the erroneous belief. It is the surgeon amongst our homœopathic remedies.

We will come to this aspect of the remedy later on. Now let us begin with a few words about its preparation. The common oyster shell is first cleaned, then it is finely powdered and mixed with an equal part of pure flours of sulphur. The mixture is then kept for about ten minutes heated to a white heat in a crucible hermetically closed. The potencies are then made by trituration. This drug was first proved by Hahnemann.

It is a compound of two of our great remedies, **Calcarea** and **Sulphur**; hence we meet with a lot of symptoms common to both of them. Allen says "It simulates mercury in its action on the liver and kidneys, **Sulphur** in its action on the skin and mucous membranes of the intestinal tract, **Calcarea** in affecting the respiratory tract and all the foregoing in its action on the connective tissue." But we must not let ourselves be misled by this statement, for though there are many symptoms in common with the two remedies, **Hepar sulphuris** presents a train of symptoms peculiar and characteristic of **Hepar sulphuris** alone. The most important feature of this remedy is to be found in its sensitiveness. It runs through the entire rubric of **Hepar sulphuris.** The pain which another will not mind at all will drive this patient to the border of despair.

He can hardly bear the slightest touch. When by accident somebody touches the affected part, which the patient is ever careful to guard against, he may even faint. I have repeatedly prescribed **Hep. sulph.** with excellent results in boils and abscesses when this over-sensitiveness was present. We meet with a similar sensitiveness to touch in **Cinch off, Arnica, Ruta, Kali carb., Spig.** and a few other remedies. In every one of these remedies we notice great fear of being hurt.

In **Cinch off,** we have a patient with agonising pain, holding up his hands in appeal, to any one approaching him.

The **Ruta** patient starts from sleep with a scream when touched, ever so lightly. So also is **Kali carb.**

Spigelia is afraid of pointed things. While in **Asaf.** and **Sanguinaria** we have pain that vanishes on touch to reappear elsewhere.

Hand in hand with this sensitiveness to touch we have the sensitiveness to cold. He is so accustomed to get it that he does not know how or where he got it. He seems to know by instinct whether the doors or windows are open in the next room. This is like **Nux vom., Psor., Sil.,** and **Tuberculinum.** These remedies are all alike susceptible to the least draught of cold air.

This susceptibility and sensitiveness are alike characteristic of the moral sphere of this remedy. Teste speaks of his mental condition in the following admirable sentences:—

" Dissatisfaction with one's self and others; dreamy, atrabilious mood, a sort of ferocious spleen as though one could murder a man in cold blood (even in persons who are generally of a merry and benevolent disposition)."

Sometimes he is melancholy and low-spirited, brooding on suicide. Generally he is very irritable, which makes itself manifest by his hasty speech and actions. He finishes long sentences in one breath. This last symptom reminds us ot **Bell., Dulc., Lach.** and **Sulph.**

Hahnemann spoke of this as a great antidote to mercury. He at first used it in big quantities to neutralize the effects of mercury chemically, but later on he discovered a dynamic antidotal virtue in it which has been verified time and again. The secret of this statement is that many of the symptoms of **Hep. sulph.** become manifest in patients of mercurial infection.

For instance in ophthalmia or inflammation of the eyes of mercurial origin we use **Hep. sulph.** when we meet with great sensitiveness to touch and to air, a zone of pimples surrounding the inflamed eye, ulceration of the cornea, intense photophobia, profuse lachrymation, great redness of the cornea and even chemosis.

We must not overlook the action of **Hep. sulph.** in suppurative inflammations. A great difference of opinion prevails amongst several authorities on this point. Dr. Farrington says:—

"If you give it in high potency when the throbbing, stabbing pains in the affected part and the general rigor show the onset of inflammation, it may abort the whole trouble. In other cases if you see that suppuration is necessary, and wish to hasten the process, then you give **Hepar** low."

Drs. Allen and Norton seem to think in the same way. There are others again like Drs. Clarke and Nash that differ. We are also inclined to believe that the " indicated medicine " works with nature and promotes either absorption or suppuration as the vitality demands. Dr. Nash makes mention of a case in which the cm. potency of this remedy brought about " the most rapid pointing, opening and perfect healing." Dr. Clarke mentions another case of " an axillary abscess with a large collection of pus " in which **Hepar** 6 induced the most striking absorption. We could add to these instances by citing numerous cases from our own practice.

There are two other remedies with marked influence over the suppurative process, such as **Sil.** and **Merc.** and we want to discuss their applications.

In **Silicea** the pus is thin, bloody, ichorous and sanious whereas in **Hepar** it is rich, thick and creamy; both have aggravation from cold and relief from warmth and hot applications.

In **Merc.** the aggravation is pre-eminently a nocturnal affair.

Hep. sulph. acts especially on the skin, lymphatic and glanddular systems and the respiratory mucous membrane. I think we will do well to cite the nice differentiation that Dr. L. P. Foster makes between this remedy, **Kali sulph.** and **Calc sulph.** " **Kali sulph.,**" he says, " acts on the epidermis, while **Calc sulph.** acts very much the same as **Hep. sulph.** only more deeply. **Hepar** acts on abscesses before they open, **Calc sulph.** after." Foster mentions a case of multiple ulcers in the gluteal region of a lady about 3 inches in diameter and three-fourth of an inch deep that he cured with **Calc sulph.**

Now we come to the skin symptoms of **Hepar sulph.** The skin is very unhealthy; little injuries suppurate. like what we see in **Merc., Sil., Cham., Lycop., Graph.,** and **Acid flour.** We also notice vesicular and papular eruption in flexures of joints. According to Dr. Guernsey the flexures of the elbow and knee are the especial seats of those eruptions.

He also recommends it in eczema, crusta lactea, and inter- trigo which spread by means of new pimples appearing just beyond the old parts. We also use it in humid soreness on the genitals, scrotum, and the folds between the scrotum and the thighs. But we must not forget the chief characteristics of all these skin affections, namely the great sensitiveness and the mercurial origin of the trouble. Dr. Hughe's experience with it in "grocer's itch" and "psoriasis palmaris" is worth noticing.

It will be an unpardonable omission if we do not mention the lung affections of this remedy. In the stage in which exudation becomes purulent, especially in the chronic form of this trouble, this remedy is called for oftener than other remedy. The symp- toms to indicate it are a loose and choking cough and a lentescent fever. The aggravation is from cold air and towards morning. Bæhr in his 'Science of Therapeutics' mentions a brilliant cure of pneumonia in a boy of six summers with this remedy. "The poor child was exceedingly emaciated, had a slight hectic fever, was constantly troubled by a spasmodic cough, with a purulent and a fetid expectoration, diarrhœa and loss of appetite. The right side of the thorax had caved in quite considerably, the left was abnormally bulging........The child was put on **Hepar** 3rd tritu- ration, with such excellent success that in eight days the caving of the chest was considerably less. In about four weeks the right lung had almost been restored to its normal condition and the curvature of the thorax had entirely disappeared, so that the child now looks thoroughly sound and healthy."

The **Hepar** croup is brought on by a dry, cold wind. The cough is rattling and choking. It is worse towards the early hours of the morning. The breathing is short and suffocating and the distressed patient has to sit up and bend the head backwards to get relief. He complains of a sensation as if a fish-bone were lodged in his throat.

Aconite has got a somewhat similar croup brought about by an exposure to a dry, cold, northwest wind. Aggravation is espe- cially marked in respiration, for every respiration ends with a coarse, hacking cough. The febrile symptoms are well marked.

Hepar has been used with success in Tuberculosis before that dreadful disease has advanced very far and we have a harsh, croupy cough with production of tenacious mucus in the chest, aggravation in the morning and great sensitiveness of the system.

We must not forget the action of **Hepar** on the sexual organs There is a great congestion of blood to the uterus and we have a consequent hemorrhage in women with chapped and unhealthy skin. Very frequently with this we have uterine ulcers; they are superficial, serpiginous and indolent. The discharge is purulent and sometimes bloody and it smells like old cheese. The edge of the ulcer is very sensitive.

It is very rarely that we use **Hepar** in dyspepsia, but there are cases that only **Hepar** and nothing but **Hepar** will help. The symptoms calling for it are a great longing for acids, wines, sour and strong tasting things; a sort of heaviness and pressure in the stomach after eating, though after eating the patient feels strong and comfortable. Constant sensation is felt as of water rising in the œsophagus, as though the patient had eaten something very sour. Sometimes there is vomiting in the morning. A few hours after a meal he feels a sort of distention in the region of the stomach and he has to loosen his clothing. With this we may have either constipation or diarrhœa. The constipation is of an atonic form; that is, as if the intestines had become faulty in their expulsive powers. The stools are soft, but they are passed with great difficulty. It is not the kind of constipation that we have in **Bryonia**, for in that remedy the difficulty arises from the hard and burnt condition of the stools.

In **Sulphur**, too, we have constipation, but then it is due to the stools being hard and enormous in size.

The **Hepar** constipation resembles that of **Alumina, Anacardium, Caust., Plat., Sil.,** and **Verat alb.** In each one of these the difficulty arises from an atonic condition of the intestinal tract.

In diarrhœa the stools are undigested, thin, papescent, whitish and sour-smelling. We have sour-smelling stools also in **Calc ost, Magn. c., Rheum** and **Sulph., Bell., Benz. ac., Cina, Dulc., Hell., Phos.** and **Acid phos.** resemble **Hepar** in the lightness of the color of the stools.

In **Hell.** the stools are white and jelly-like.

In **Phos,** they are like little pieces of tallow or particles of sago constantly oozing from the open anus.

In **Acid phos.** it is white or yellow, watery diarrhœa characterized by painlessness and absence of any marked debility.

The white or the light-coloured diarrhœa of **Acid benz.** is copious and very offensive; it smells like burnt gun powder or like the very offensive and highly fetid urine of the patient.

Like the atonic state of the intestinal tract we have a semi-paralytic condition of the bladder. The urine is passed so tardily that it seems that there is scarcely any expulsive power in the bladder. The patient is unable to finish; it seems to him as if some urine always remains in the bladder. In this respect we should compare **Hepar** with **Alum, Sil.,** and **Sepia.** Also with the above symptoms there is occasionally wetting of the bed at night.

We should never forget **Hepar** in marasmus of children. There is great weakness of the digestive system and however well chosen may be his food, it disagrees. The child smells sour all over. The child is subject to catarrh from the least draft of cold air. He is sad, but it is nothing compared to the indifference and apathy of **Acid phos.** where the child wants nothing and craves for nothing.

Last of all we come to the fever symptoms of **Hepar sulph.** The time of the paroxysm is generally 6 or 7 p.m. (the 6 p.m. paroxysm is more marked under **Fer.** and **Ver.**). Over the already present susceptibility to cold, the patient begins with a fresh chill. It is so great as to make him shiver. His teeth chatter; sometimes the intensity of the chill is so great that he is compelled to seek shelter near a warm stove. This last symptom also reminds us of **Bovista** and **Lach.,** for in them too, we find that with the onset of the chill, the patient is compelled to seek the warmth of a stove or some such heating apparatus. The **Hepar sulph.** patient also complains of icy coldness of the face and feet.

Another very important symptom to guide us is the appearance of a sort of nettle rash during the chill. It burns and stings. There are also fever blisters around the mouth. These fever blisters are very misleading, for with many of us they mean only **Nat mur.** Hydroa or fever blisters as they are called, are indeed a great feature of **Nat mur.** but then we have **Ignat., Nux vom.** and **Rhus tox.** claiming the same symptom. The patient sweats profusely on the slightest locomotion and the perspiration smells terribly sour, sometimes offensive. There is no relief from sweating.

Case 1.—Girl, aged thirteen, cough for five months, with hoarseness. Since two months painful diarrhœa, alternating with constipation. Every evening, fever, chill, heat, and sweat till next morning. Cough dry, brought on by talking, laughing, moving, eating and always worse from evening; expectorates a little yellowish, blood-streaked mucus; during cough, burning pain in larynx which is painful to touch; soreness in larynx; burning pain in chest, changing localities; soreness in left side of chest. Dullness on percussion in left supra and infra clavicular region; bronichial breathing; wheezing sound in right apex. **Phos.** 20, every night for two months. Cough became less frequent and was attended with copious expectoration of gray-yellowish sputa; fever and nightsweat gone. **Hep.** 9 finished the cure.— Dr. Stens. Jr.

Case 2.—A farmer, had suffered from piles for a long time, and was becoming debilitated from the continual loss of blood. He was almost incapacitated from riding on horseback, and even driving in a gig would often bring on the hæmorrhage. Though a spare man, his liver was engorged and his abdomen swollen and somewhat tender. **Hep.** 6, three times a day. After the first week the bleeding ceased, and in a few weeks he was wholly cured. His family were prejudiced against Homœopathy and I saw no more of the patient for eighteen months or two years. He went to the seaside and got dysentery, was treated Allopathically then, and became so seriously ill as to raise apprehensions for his life. When he had rallied so much as to enable him to get home, he sent for his former Allopathic adviser. He was well treated Allopathically. But the system, not the man was at fault, and the patient continued to retrograde till he began to look death in the face as a more than possible contingency. Then he also looked medicine in the face as well as death, and said to himself, "when the old system couldn't cure my piles the new system did, why shouldn't I try if it couldn't cure my dysentery." So he bade old physic good-bye, in the shape of his former surgeon, and called me in. Again, Homœopathy triumphed, and this time finally, for he got well rapidly, and said with reason that he had escaped a double danger, for that if the disease had not killed him, he fully believed that the Allopathic physic would have done so. And realizing the double-headed danger of disease plus drugs, he determined that henceforth, his family as well as himself, should be placed under Homœopathic care, when ill.—Dr. Bayes.

HIPPOMANES.

It is a meconium deposit out of the amniotic fluid of the mare or the cow. Triturations are made from the soft gelatinous mucous substance of a urinous odor taken from the tongue of a newly born filly. This remedy has so far very little clinical standing but a few characteristic indications have been cited and we will do well to be conversant with them. The first and foremost is the sensation of coldness in the stomach. The next is a sensation of sprain in the wrist. The arm feels as if paralysed. A great pain in the wrist, accompanied with great weakness of hands and fingers, has frequently led to its application in chorea in young people growing too fast, with remarkable results.

HIPPOZAENIUM.

It is a powerful nosode, introduced into our Materia Medica by Dr. Drysdale. It clearly testifies to the assertion so often made, that what Homœopathy thinks of today, Allopathy thinks of on the morrow. Homœopathy has anticipated, in various instances, many of the modern, so-called discoveries and innovations of the scientific schools. This powerful nosode is prepared from Bacillus Malleni, the micro-organism of glanders. When injected into the circulation of a glanderous animal it causes an elevation of temperature. It has been, therefore, utilized for early diagnosis in suspected cases of glanders.

In the homœopathic system of therapeutics its unquestionable utility is derived, same as in other remedies, from a thorough scientific proving and its application is based on totality of symptoms. We notice great debility and emaciation and a great tendency for lymphatic swellings and inflammations everywhere under this remedy. The entire system presents a strong resemblance to pyemic condition of the body. The entire mucous membrane manifests symptoms of inflammation and ulcerative disease. Putrescence, destruction and decomposition of tissues are seen everywhere. Malignant erysipelas, carbuncle, plague, cancer, confluent small-pox, lupus exedens and other varieties of connective tissue destructions are not only checked, but are radically cured by the timely administration of this nosode.

This remedy has not so far received the same clinical verifications as many of our other nosodes, but it has been recommended highly in chronic ozena and bronchitis. The nasal affection particularly calling for this remedy is ozena of the most obstinate type, involving ulceration of the nasal cartilage and bones. The destruction at times is so great as to lead to an exposure of the necrosed septum-vomer and palate bone. It is indicated in bronchitis of elderly persons, threatening suffocation due to excessive secretion of mucus. Extensive rhonchi are heard all over the lungs.

It is also used in pulmonary abscesses and in phthisis where it tends to diminish expertoration and abate constantly recurring aggravation and inflammation.

HOANG-NAN.

This is a plant belonging to the strychnos family and is also called Strychnos Gaultheriana. It is a native of Tonquin and it belongs to the natural order of Loganiaceæ. The tincture is prepared from the dried bark. It has a great local reputation as being a remedy for leprosy, hydrophobia and snake bites. In animals poisoned with it, we notice tetanic convulsions beginning in the hind legs and thence spreading over the rest of the body. In homœopathy its use is confined to carbuncles, leprosy and syphilis, but it should be strictly remembered that its application is based on the universal principle of similia, the same as in other remedies. It should be studied in comparison with **Curare, Angustura** and **Hydrocotyle.**

HOMARUS.

Homarus is prepared from the digestive fluid of the Lobster. It is a thick reddish offensive liquid contained in a sack situated in the neighbourhood of the mouth. It is prepared by triturating sugar of milk saturated with this liquid. The remedy was extensively proved by Dr. Cushing and we are indebted to him for whatever knowledge we have of this remedy.

It makes an important remedy in digestive troubles. It is particularly useful in patients who are awakened at night time by an urgent desire to pass stools which, however, is relieved by the patient passing only a large amount of wind. Another important symptom is a peculiar languid tired feeling in the morning, which reminds us of **Nux vom.** This tired feeling however passes off shortly after he starts on his usual daily avocations.

A third symptom which may very well be considered the leading indication of this remedy is an aggravation from milk. In this respect it is like **Calc. carb., China, Conium, Nitric acid, Sepia, Sulphur, Mag. carb.** and **Æthusa.**

HYDRASTIS CANADENSIS.

The tincture is prepared from the root of Hydrastis, a perennial underground stem. It is also called the Golden Seal, and it
belongs to the natural order of Ranunculaceæ. The color of the
tincture is highly yellow. Here let me mention that an intense
yellow color characterises all its discharges. **Hydrastis** has a spe
cial affinity for all the mucous surfaces of the body. We use it in
nasal, pharyngeal, laryngeal, œsophageal, bronchial, duodenal, in
testinal, urethral and vaginal catarrh when the characteristi
yellow tough stringy discharge is present.

A second characteristic of **Hydrastis,** one that is not seen in
many remedies, is a peculiar gone feeling in the stomach, fel
particularly after meals. This symptom renders it an importan
remedy in dyspepsia. The other indications are a large flabb
coated tongue indented by teeth, eructation, putrid taste in th
mouth and debility. As a result of sluggishness of the liver consti
pation is prominent. The stools are lumpy, and are covered wit
tough yellow mucus.

Quite a few cases of cancer of the liver, uterus, breast an
other parts of the body have been cured with **Hydrastis.** Th
skin becomes adherent and looks mottled and puckered. Grea
emaciation, marked depression of mind, intense irritability of tem
perament and general anasarca are prominent symptoms. I
uterine cancer we have offensive, tough, stringy, pus-like discharg
from the vagina. Excessive bleeding attended with pain and anem
are also present. Tenacious, viscid leucorrhœa, either uterine o
vaginal, looking like long threads and causing a sort of pruritus
a prominent symptom.

It is reported to be efficacious in removing the tendenc
towards habitual adherence of placenta.

HYDROCOTYLE ASIATICA.

This is a small Indian plant, commonly called the Indian Pennywort. In Bengal it goes by the name of **Thankuni.** Its chief action is centered on the skin and the female generative organs. A great variety of skin affections such as acne, eczema, pemphigus, lupus, leprosy, copper-coloured eruptions, papular eruptions etc. have been cured with it. This remedy has been proved elaborately by Dr. Pramada Prasanna Biswas of Pabna. The complaint in which it has been found to be particularly efficacious is copper-coloured eruptions on the face. A tubercle covered over with a thick crust, on the right alæ nasi, as large as a four-anna bit, which was diagnosed as lupus exedens, was cured with **Hydrocotyle asia-ica.** Great thickening of the epidermoid layer and exfoliation of the scales have led to its use in scrotal tumors as well as elephantiasis. **Hydrocotyle** also has fungus growths and granular ulceration on the upper lip and neck of the uterus. Insupportable itching of the vagina is a characteristic indication.

HYDROCYANIC ACID.

Hydrocyanic acid is commonly known as Prussic Acid. It is also called Hydrogen cyanide. It is a colorless volatile liquid with a peculiar odor, resembling that of bitter almonds. It is a very powerful and deadly poison. A fraction of a grain is enough to kill an adult in ten to twenty minutes.

It acts powerfully on the medulla oblongata and the upper portion of the spinal cord and causes extreme dyspnœa, giddiness, dilated pupil, and tetanic and epileptiform spasms. Suddenness of the attack and great prostration are two important features of **Hydrocyanic acid.** Primarily, it acts upon the cerebral veins producing congestion and secondarily, upon the heart and nerves. It destroys life by causing disorders of respiration. It has the property of preventing proper appropriation of oxygen by the tissues and the elimination of carbon dioxide. The very odor of this strong poison causes one to fall unconscious and motionless. It brings on a sensation of constriction in chest that interferes with the respiration. Severe tetanic spasms are produced, to be followed ultimately by profound coma. An administration of a lethal, yet not overwhelming dose of **Hydrocyanic acid,** causes dyspnœa, hurried respiratory movements, powerful tetanic spasms, dilatations of pupils, protrusion of tongue and eye-balls, a glassy appearance of the eyes, involuntary evacuation of urine and fæces and a rapid diminishing in force and frequency of the pulse, till at last the tortures are ended by death. If, however, death does not occur, the condition of tetanus passes into one of general paralysis with total loss of reflex irritability.

It is thus a powerful agent as capable of destroying life as it is of curing any serious deviation of our vitality. Homœopathy utilises in full this latter property of the great poison but its application is based on the immutable principle of Similia Similibus Curantur. The suddenness of the attack, referred to above, is the guiding keynote of its application according to the homœopathic principle. Whenever there is sudden loss of consciousness, sudden rigidity of limbs, sudden attack of convulsions, and sudden stoppage of the heart's action, **Hydrocyanic acid** should be thought of, before any other course is resorted to.

Epileptiform spasms and tetanic convulsion demand **Hydro cyanic acid** on the above indications being present.

In epilepsy we think of **Hydrocyanic acid** when the seizures come every three months or so and last for two or three weeks leaving the patient extremely prostrated. It is useful in those cases where the attack lasts for several days at a stretch, the patient vomiting green fluid and passing green motion all the time.

In traumatic tetanus **Hydrocyanic acid** is reported to have done an immense amount of good, specially when the paroxysms come on without any provocation and leave the patient in an extremely prostrated and exhausted condition. The patient is afraid to fall asleep or even close his eyes for fear of the attacks coming on. The appearance becomes cyanotic and cold.

The tetanic grin should always draw our attention to **Hydrocyanic acid.** The patient's jaws are firmly fixed. He lies on bed with head fixed and thrown backwards and legs fixed and rigid. The abdominal muscles are so firmly contracted as to resemble a piece of hard board.

Hydrocyanic acid like **Picric acid** is a great remedy for neuræsthenia and nervous dyspepsia due to over-work and anxiety. The most prominent symptom here is a great sinking sensation at the epigastrium. It is described more as an anguish felt at the pit of the stomach. Two or three hours after eating, the patient complains of a burning pain in the region of the navel, extending to œsophagus and throat . Vomiting of food or of a slimy bilious matter, emaciation, intense gastro-dynia and entero-dynia and above all, the peculiar noise while drinking, indisputably point to **Hydrocyanic acid** as the correct remedy.

It is a great help to us in the collapse stage of Asiatic cholera, specially when collapse follows the sudden cessation of all discharges. The stools cease and vomiting decreases, but the patient instead of reviving becomes remarkably cold, pulseless, cyanotic and full of anguish. **Hydrocyanic acid** eases the breathing, brings back the heat of life and slowly revives the patient.

It is also to be thought of in threatening paralysis of the lungs. I have used it often and with success in the fatal stage of many critical ailments on the indicaton of the respiration being laboured, co-existing with a feeling of suffocation and a torturing pain in the chest.

One more symptom faintly referred to already is, that when he drinks, the water rolls down audibly through his throat, as though it were being poured into through an empty barrel. On this symptom alone many remarkable cures have been effected.

HYDROPHOBINUM.

(*See* **Lyssin**)

HYOSCYAMUS NIGER.

Hyoscyamus is the Henbane. The plant grows both as an annual and biennial. The highly active second year's growth of the biennial plant is the only form which is used in the preparation of the drug. It is a native of Europe and Western Asia, where it is a very common and an abundant weed. It is also cultivated for medicinal purpose in several other countries. Its odor is heavy and narcotic while its taste is bitter and acrid. The plant is very similar to Tabacum, Stramonium and Belladonna From Tabacum it can be distinguished by its incised leaves, from Stramonium by its hairiness.

The alkaloidal percentage of Henbane is very much lower than that of **Bell.** Although it is very similar in its action to **Bell.**, there is considerable difference between the two remedies in our omœopathic Materia Medica.

This drug is poisonous to fowls, hence its name of Henbane is very appropriate. There is an interesting case of poisoning with **Hyoscyamus** which we will do well to examine. A patient of Dr. J. S. Mills objected to the taste of water to which he had added few drops of the mother tincture of **Hyoscyamus**. To encourage the patient the doctor himself took a few teaspoonfuls of the mixture with remarkable sequence of symptoms. Dr. Mills writes to say " A few moments later I found that it produced a queer feeling throughout the body. I felt as though without weight, as though I walked on the air My head felt light. I had an insane desire to laugh and shout. It was only by the utmost use of my will-power that I could keep myself from doing something ridiculous. Even when I forced myself to think of my position of responsibility as medical attendant on this very sick man, and the absolute necessity of keeping my wits about me, it was hard for me to restrain my hilarity. I can liken the condition only to one of mild hilarious intoxication ' funny drunk.' I knew I was silly, but I could not help it. To keep myself from losing my dignity before the nurses and the family, I locked myself in the bathroom for a few minutes and made faces at myself in the mirror "

From the above case it is very easy to see how rich is **Hyoscyamus** in mental symptoms. Although many of its mental symptoms are similar to those of **Belladonna,** they are not so violent as in the latter remedy. The mood is a reflective one. He makes no complaint. He answers questions mildly, but the answers are mostly irrelevant; he sees persons who are not and have not been present. Sometimes while left to himself he chatters unintelligibly. He smiles but it is a silly smile, the expressionless smile of an imbecile.

A very important characteristic of **Hyoscyamus** is jealousy and suspicion. He is constantly afraid of being poisoned, betrayed, sold or injured and naturally he wishes to run away from everybody. He is very reluctant to take any medicine offered him as he considers everybody, his medical attendant included, bent on taking his life. This distrust is manifested by all his actions and behavious. Such suspicion is also to be found under **Cench., Merc., Lach.,** and **Anacardium.**

Loquacity is another feature of **Hyoscyamus.** This loquacity is due to excessive animation. He jumps from subject to subject as in **Agaricus, Cimicifuga, Lachesis, Lachnanthes, Podophyllum, Selenium** and **Teucrium.**

In **Agaricus** the patient goes on talking, unmindful of all interruptions. He will hardly answer any question asked while he is in his talkative fit. In **Lachesis** the talkativeness is most marked in the evening. **Lachnanthes** is characterised by a peculiar fit of talkativeness that is most marked between the unusual hours of 1 to 2 A.M. **Podophyllum** and **Zincum** are to be particularly thought of in loquacity during the stage of chill and heat. **Selenium** is talkative far into the stage of perspiration.

Amativeness constitutes the third important landmark, but the peculiarity of this amativeness lies in its shamelessness. He goes about naked and will not be covered; he constantly throws off his bed clothes shamelessly, exposing his modesty. This desire to be nude, this lasciviousness are important factors in **Hyoscyamus**. In this respect it should be compared with **Bell., Camphor, Cantharis, Phos., Lil. tig., Stramonium,** and **Secale cor.**

Sometimes the **Hyoscyamus** patient goes into a stupor from which he can be readily roused. He will answer questions quite correctly but will relapse into the stupid state almost immediately. This is very similar to what we find in **Phos. acid, Bryonia,** and **Muriatic acid.** But in **Hyoscyamus** the stupor is not so pronounced as in the last three remedies. In **Phos. acid,** the patient can be roused but with great difficulty. In **Muriatic acid** the adynamic state is very prominent and the patient can hardly be roused from his stupor.

In **Hyoscyamus,** we have sordes appearing on the tongue and teeth. Associated with this, we have rattling during breathing. The mouth remains open; the lower jaw hangs down and the patient lies in a state of stupor. The muscles all over the body twitch intermittently. This is a clear picture of a typhoid state and hence **Hyoscyamus** oft comes handy in the treatment of typhoid and typhus. The brain is active but it wanders. The patient labours under a distinct hallucination, which is mostly centered in a desire to escape from the room or from those around. Sometimes he would lie on his back, his eyes quite open, staring and immovable. The urine is involuntary; it leaves streaks of red sand on the sheet. The sphincter muscles of both the anus and the bladder are in a state of paralysis. The delirium is of frequent occurrence. The patient attempts to jump out of bed and run away. He thinks he is at a wrong place. He constantly spits on his bed clothes. He puts his hands on his genitals and plays with same, being devoid of all sense of propriety and decency. The patient's tongue is red and cracked. He is disturbed with a dry nocturnal cough which prevents sleep. The head and face are hot and there may, comparatively speaking, be a general coldness of the body. These are very clear-cut indications on which numerous cases have been treated and cured and we shall do well to remember that, when allopathy fails and the prospect looks gloomy there is still a strong ray of hope for the patient should he be put under the principle of Similia which treats human system as an autonomous, self-sufficient organism capable of managing its own affair with only a slight help from remedial agencies in times of dire distress.

Hyoscyamus is also useful in convulsions, hysteria and epilepsy. Convulsions begin with twitchings of the mouth and face and especially of the muscles about eyes. The spasms are clonic in nature and this differentiates **Hyoscyamus** from **Belladonna,** where they are mostly tonic. Movements are mostly angular, face is dusk-red and bloated. We also use it in convulsions of children, especially after fright and from intestinal worms. It is used in epilepsy, when before the attack the patient complains of vertigo, sparks before eyes and ringing noise in the ears. The convulsions are so violent that it seems that the joints and the spine will be broken to pieces. After the attack the patient falls into a deep sleep which continues for several hours. It is also used for intense sleeplessness in excitable and irritable persons, who are much harassed by business embarrassments **(Phosphorus).**

We have quite a characteristic cough in **Hyoscyamus.** It is a dry, tickling and hacking cough. The tickling is caused by the elongated uvula or titillation by uvula on the dorsum of the tongue. The cough is worse while lying down, so much so, that the patient has to sit up in bed at night most of the time. I have used this remedy with signal success in cough of children while asleep. In my opinion, it is not the lying down alone but falling asleep that causes the aggravation.

I have already hinted at its action on the female generative organs. It excites sexual desire to such an extent as to make them inveterate nymphomaniacs.

Case 1.—(Typhus) Ninth day. Patient lying on back, eyes wide open staring and immovable; is unconscious; face red, lips black, tongue dry and black, lower jaw hangs down; urine involuntary; it leaves large streaks of red sand on the sheet; skin dry; pulse over 200. Dr. Hering was called in consultation; both he and Dr. Lippe feared paralysis of the brain. Before Dr. Lippe found the red sand he was deliberating between **Opium** and **Hyos** the sand pointed to **Hyos. Opium** has the symptom more often state of snoring with the eyes half colsed (**Lyc.** had red crystals in urine and falling of lower jaw; increase of urine only at night.) **Hyos.** 200 one drop in half tumblerful of water; several spoonfuls were given, and in six hours the patient perspired, the jaw closed, and he was out of danger. Reported by Dr. J. Heber Smith.

HYPERICUM PERFOLIATUM.

It is called St. John's wort and it belongs to the natural order of Hypericaceæ. This drug was proved principally by Muller. If any remedy can vie with **Arnica** in traumatism, it is **Hypericum.** But its usefulness is more confined to injuries of parts rich in sentient nerves. This is shown by the intolerable pain accompanying the injury. Piercing wounds from sharp instruments, gun-shot wounds, crushed wounds such as, mashed fingers, punctured wounds as those caused from trading on nails, needles, pins etc., come under the influence of **Hypericum.** Even rheumatism, bunions, corns etc., call for **Hypericum** when the pains are disproportionately severe, indicating involvement of the nervous structure. Excessive painfulness, therefore, should be considered an index of the remedy. Dr. Guernsey treated a case of rat-bite on the first finger in a boy, who was in a state of tetanic convulsions with locked jaws and stiffness of the head and neck. Although he thought of prescribing **Ledum,** he was induced to change to **Hypericum** by the symptom of intense tenderness about the region of the wound. This remedy in its 500th potency was administered every few minutes, till at last the child fell asleep, to wake up the next morning practically convalescent.

I also had an opportunity of testing its efficacy in a somewhat similar case. A man utterly incapacitated, said to be suffering from an injury, was carried into my office one day. Examination revealed a tiny spot on his heel caused by his inadvertently stepping on a rusty nail. The pain was out of proportion to the injury sustained. A few doses of **Hypericum** enabled him to resume his usual gait in a short while.

This remedy is also useful in incised or lacerated wounds, in injuries of the spinal cord and in bad effects of spinal concussions. **Hypericum** prescribed at proper time after such injuries, prevents lock-jaw. It is of great use in pains after a fall on the coccyx.

The headache of **Hypericum** is peculiar. The patient feels as if he is lifted high into the air. He is in great anxiety lest he should fall from this great height.

In vertigo the head feels elongated. It starts troubling at night time and is frequently associated with a strong desire to pass urine.

IGNATIA.

Ignatia is a climbing shrub found growing in the Philippine Islands and Cochin China. The tincture is prepared from the powdered seeds of this plant found growing within its fruit. These seeds are about an inch in length; they contain a big quantity of strychnia. It belongs to the natural order of Loganiaceæ.

It produces a distinct hyperæsthesia of all the senses and because of the presence of strychnia in its composition, it has a tendency to produce clonic spasms. It is specially adapted to the nervous temperament, particularly to sensitive women who are alert, nervous, rigid, and apprehensive.

In **Ignatia** we have to deal with the female counterpart of **Nux vom.** By this I simply mean, that it suits the nervous temperament, the sensitive easily excitable nature that is quick in perceiving, prompt in appreciation and rapid in execution. This is very different from the thin irritable quarrelsome spiteful and the nervous disposition of **Nux vomica.** The two remedies differ widely in their mental characteristics. **Nux vom.** is vehement, careful and zealous in disposition. It is an ardent character that we have to deal with in **Nux.** You displease him, which can be easily done, he will snap you right in the face; whereas our **Ignatia** patient, though equally intelligent and sensitive, is more of a forbearing nature. She takes things easily to heart and instead of retaliating then and there, broods over her supposed wrong and pines over it in solitude. She is taciturn, sad and fond of solitude. She weeps and she sighs in silence unperceived by her imaginary aggressor and her friends. It is a thing that furrows deep on her mental structure and leaves a permanent evil-bearing effect. We thus find **Ignatia** resembling another sister of her tribe, **Pulsatilla.** The latter remedy as we all know, is equally sad. tearful and melancholy. She too weeps but she lacks that introspective mood of **Ignatia.** She makes her grief known to everybody around her and finds consolation in their sympathy. This tearful weeping disposition of **Ignatia,** also reminds us of **Natrum mur,** another tearful weeping damsel. This last-named remedy resembles **Ignatia** in its irritability, which **Pulsatilla** very characteristically lacks. **Natrum mur** is inconsolable. She weeps bitterly. Naturally people sympathises with her troubles, but this sympathy and consolation aggravate her complaints and elicit a fearful rebuff. We must be on our guard, even when we want to do such a charitable thing as offering consolation to the grieved soul of **Natrum mur.**

A further trait of **Ignatia,** is a great dislike to contradiction. They are fault-finding in the extreme. They must have things just as they want them. A little disappointment, a little delay cause untold misery and bring on an endless train of ailments in their wake. They are too sensitive to be repremanded or scolded. I have seen children get into convulsions from such suppressed mental phenomena. In this **Ignatia** resembles **Staphisagria** and **Colocynth.**

I have forgotten to mention one other peculiarity of **Ignatia.** It is found in the paradoxical nature of many of its symptoms. For illustration we may cite a few peculiar conditions, such as an empty feeling in the stomach not getting better after eating, cough getting worse on coughing, noise in the ears getting better by noise, piles feeling better while walking, sore throat feeling relieved on swallowing, fever with thirst during chill only and so on. Such absurd uncommon and unexpected occurrences are very characteristic of our remedy.

This remedy is also characterised by a great changeability of mental conditions. In an incredibly short time, joy changes into sorrow, laughing into weeping, a mental calm to a furious rage and so on. This uncertain state of mind and changeability of temper make association with these patients a matter of great risk. We feel uncertain as to where we stand, and do not know how to proceed. In this respect **Ignatia** compares with **Aconite, Nux moschata, Pulsatilla, Lycopodium, Sarsaparilla, Platinum** and **Zincum.**

Ignatia is particularly useful after the bad effects of grief specially when it is of recent origin. For the chronic or long-lasting effects of grief, that happened long while ago, we should think of **Acid phos.** and **Nat. mur.** It is also a great remedy for suppressed mental sufferings, due to shame and disappointed love. They are inconstant, impatient, irresolute and quarrelsome. Sometimes we find them suffering from an extra-delicacy of mood and a super-conscientiousness.

Ignatia resembles **Sepia** and **Lilium** in its indifference of mood. This indifference becomes more marked during menstrual period when she feels particularly melancholy. Anxiety and disquietude always lend a sort of unhappiness which, as it blends with the peculiar sensitive temperament of **Ignatia,** renders her a strange conglomeration of contradictions and impossibilities.

Another trait of this patient is a great intolerance of tobacco. They cannot smoke.   Even the smell of other people smoking brings on a terrible headache. With these peculiarities in mind we will go into a detailed study of **Ignatia.**

Ignatia is considered to be a great remedy for hysteria.   Dunham's remark in this respect "Of all our remedies none so completely corresponds to hysteria and so often cures it as **Ignatia**" is worth noticing.   Great melancholy, changeability of mental state, despondency, a sensation as if stomach were hanging on a thread, nausea, are all characteristic indications. We have globus hystericus very well marked. . The patient falls into a state of semi-unconsciousness, clenches her thumbs, froths and foams at her mouth and at last returns to consciousness with a long drawn sigh.   The causative factor is found in long concentrated grief, suppressed anger, disappointed love and indignation.   In this respect we should compare **Ignatia** with **Asaf., Moschus, Valeriana, Cocculus** and **Nux mos.**

Ignatia is a great remedy for headaches of nervous, hysterical subjects. The pain is felt over a small spot that can be covered with the tip of a finger. It feels as if a nail were driven through the skull and she feels better by lying on it. The characteristic feature of changeability is also noticeable here.   The pain is erratic in its nature. Sometimes it comes gradually and abates suddenly; at other times it comes on suddenly and goes away in a similar way. This headache is brought on by mental labour, strong disgusting odors, disturbing emotions and indulgence in coffee, alcohol or tobacco. It is often periodical in its nature. Another point about the **Ignatia** headache is relief of the pain from a flow of profuse colorless urine. In this respect **Ignatia** is similar to **Aconite, Gelsemium, Kalmia, Sanguinaria, Silicea,** and **Veratrum alb.**

I have used this remedy very successfully in dyspepsia of hysterical women. The symptoms are, a flat taste in the mouth, copious salivation, aversion to tobacco, warm food, spirituous liquor and frequent regurgitation of food.

This aversion is nothing but a fanciful, groundless aversion. There is hardly any reason underlying her likes and dislikes. She is so inconstant even in her fancies that there is hardly any depending on it. There is also an empty gone-feeling at the epigastrium and the most strange part about it all is that it is not relieved by eating. There is also an excess of flatulence which leads to protrusions on various parts of the abdominal wall. The bowels are inclined to be loose, with a tendency towards hemorrhoidal knobs, in the rectum. Sometimes the patient feels an urgent desire for stool which, however, is caused mostly by an accumulation of flatus and is followed simply by a mere expulsion of wind with a certain amount of protrusion of the rectum.

Ignatia has a constipation of its own. The desire for stool is felt more in the upper intestines. After severe straining he passes either a hard or a soft stool with certain amount of procidentia recti. Most of this straining is to be accounted for by a certain amount of constriction in the rectum. In consequence of this straining, he becomes an easy victim to hemorrhoids. This gives rise to a sharp stitching pain that shoots up the rectum and causes quite a little annoyance and distress. Another feature, an illustration of the paradoxical nature of Ignatia, is that the prolapsus becomes worse when the stools are soft.

Toothache of Ignatia, is another illustration of the same dominant feature of contradiction. It is worse, not so much during the acts of eating, as in the intervals. It is also rendered more acute by smoking tobacco and lying down.

The action of Ignatia on the genital organs of the female deserves our attention. It is indicated in dysmenorrhoea· when associated with hysterical symptoms. Constant sighing and sobbing, a faint feeling at the pit of the stomach, despondence and intense labour like pains are characteristic symptoms. The blood may be either profuse or scanty and dark black or bright red. Frequent desire to take deep breath, which temporarily relieves some of her sufferings, should be considered a guiding indicaton of Ignatia.

The place of Ignatia in the therapeutics of fever is not an unimportant one. It cures quotidian, tertian, quartan types of malarial fever. The paroxysms are generally irregular, more postponing than anticipating. We notice violent gaping and stretching in the prodromal stage. The chill is ushered in with great thirst for large quantities of water. In Capsicum., Carbo veg. and Eupat., we have thirst before and during chill, whereas in Ignatia the thirst is present only during chill. This chill commences in upper arms and then spreads to back and chest. The patient shakes with chill and the face shows great deal of redness due to congestion. The chill is relieved by the patient repairing to a warm room or hot stove. Hahnemann considers this symptom of "febrile coldness relieved by external warmth" particularly characteristic of Ignatia. The heat is only external and is characterised by the absence of thirst. During this stage a great dislike is evinced by the patient towards external warmth. As soon as heat begins, he throws away all coverings as they are simply intolerable. Like **Chamomilla** it also has redness and burning of one ear, one cheek, and one side of the face. He falls asleep at this stage and like **Apis** and **Opium** snores heavily. A very characteristic feature here, as elsewhere, is frequent sighing. Another symptom worth remembering is the breaking out of urticaria over the whole body at this stage, disappearing with the next stage of sweat.

Case 1.—Intense pain over right eye and seemingly through the supra-orbital foramen; pains as though a needle were pushed through into the brain, pressure from without inward; appetite disordered; sometimes mad delirium, nausea and vomiting. Eyes red, swollen and protruding. Comes on in the morning at or near nine o'clock, generally stopping at 2 P.M. Aggravated by noise, washing hands in cold water, dropping the head forward, stepping heavily. Amelioration by soft pressure, lying on back and heat. **Ignatia 200** one dose, relieved in two hours, and cured permanently. —Dr. T. D Stow.

Case 2.—Since birth of first child, eleven years before, Mrs. D. has suffered with piles, bleeding but slightly, and protruding at stool, which is followed by severe contractive pain in the anus and stitches up the rectum, lasting until exactly 5 P.M. each day, when the pain suddenly ceased. There was prompt relief from **Ignatia 6.**—Raue's Record.

Case 3.—Spasmodic affection in a boy, after "fright," in spells, from six to ten times daily. He suddenly feels sleepy, and lies down or he goes to sleep while standing, and falls; he then lies quietly and unconscious for half an hour, or for several hours, when at once, with still closed eyes, he forms his hands into fists, hides under the bed-cover, and peeps timidly from under it; his extremities commence jerking upward; even his body is thrown upward, and his lower jaw thrusts forward. He then awakens suddenly, with a jerk of respiration, and complains of hunger. **Ignatia 12** one dose every night; well in two weeks.—Dr. Ruckert.

INDIGO 361

INDIGO.

Indigo is the blue dye made from a herbaceous plant of the natural order of Leguminosæ. The commercial indigo is of a dark blue hue and is sold in the form of cakes. It is tasteless and odorless. It was first proved by Drs. Martin and Schuler of Germany.

It has a profound action over the sensorium. They feel melancholy, sad and down-hearted. We may say they are very subject to the blues, a condition quite in conformity with the appearance of the crude material. **Indigo** used to be plentifully cultiavted in this country. It was a popular home remedy with people for worms and ascarides. Its usefulness in worm troubles has been amply vindicated by homœopathy which strongly advocates its application in children that are roused at night with horrible itching of the anus; but it is rarely indicated unless the melancholy temperament is present.

The trouble for which it is frequently used is epilepsy, specially when associated with worms. A peculiarity about this epilepsy is that they become vehement and furious before the attack is over. These attacks apparently originate in the solar plexus and give **rise** to a sensation of heat over the whole head. Another **sensation**, particularly complained of at this time, is an undulating wave-like sensation in the brain.

Indigo affects the muscles in a way similar to **Rhus tox**. We find aggravation from rest and also at the commencement of every movement. A decided amelioration from movement and pressure is noticeable. Another peculiarity about this **Indigo** pain, one that will help us to differentiate between this remedy and **Rhus tox,** is the aggravation after meals.

The **Indigo** has a characteristic cough inasmuch as, it is almost always associated with epistaxis. It is mostly of the form of whooping cough where the great violence and the long duration of the attack bring about hemorrhage from the nose.

INDIUM METALLICUM.

It is a rare metal, looking very much like lead in color and softness, and is so named from the Indigo blue line in the spectrum by which its presence was discovered by Reich and Richter in the Zinc-blende. I rarely had occasion to use this remedy except once in a case of obstinate constipation, which nothing would relieve except **Indium.** The stools which were mostly pasty, had to be evacuated with an extreme degree of straining which caused the face to look purple, as if full to bursting. **Sulphur** and other similar remedies were tried in vain, till the patient in the course of conversation happened to mention of a severe lightning pain in the head, each time he strained at his stools. This reminded me of a case reported by Berridge who had marvellous effects in a case similar to mine and which **Indium** cured.

It is somewhat like **Selenium** in its action over the male sexual organ, where it causes a diminution in sexual desire and power. It is also used in nocturnal emissions when such emissions become very frequent and debilitating and as such should be compared with **Acid phos.** The urine smells highly offensive after it is allowed to stand for a little while.

IODOFORMUM.

It is prepared by the essential reaction of alcohol on free Iodine. It occurs as yellow lustrous crystals having a peculiar penetrating persistent objectionable odor. Applied locally, it tends to benumb and repress suppuration by virtue of absorbing the juices of the exposed parts and by the action of free Iodine liberated through decomposition of the **Iodoform.** It is a good anodyne and is supposed to be particularly curative in syphilitic and tubercular lesions. Grave symptoms, however, may supervene from a careless use of the drug. The smallest fatal dose probably is 45 grains. A frequent symptom, however, in a case of **Iodoform** poisoning is somnolence followed by stupor with other symptoms, resembling meningitis such as contracted motionless pupils, restlessness, exceedingly rapid pulse, muscular twitchings and delusion of persecutions and suicidal tendency. Death occurs generally from paralysis of the heart. From this it can be easily judged that it should be an important remedy in the treatment of tubercular meningitis and other tubercular conditions. The symptoms are sharp neuralgic pain in the head, a sensation of heaviness in the head as if it could not be lifted from pillow, sleep interrupted by sighs and cries, drowsiness, distention of abdomen, swelling of the mesenteric glands, chronic diarrhœa with greenish watery undigested stools and weakness of the knees and the legs.

IODIUM.

Iodium is a nonmetallic element found plentifully in sea water, mineral springs, in certain land plants such as tobacco, and in various sea animals. It is bluish black in colour, its odour is pungent, and its taste is caustic and acrid. The homœopathic preparation of Iodium consists in taking one part by weight of Iodium and dissolving it in ninetynine parts by weight of alcohol. It was first introduced into our Materia Medica by Samuel Hahnemann.

It is specially suited to persons with dark hair and complexion and thus it differs from **Bromium** which is a remedy for fair people with light complexion and golden flaxy hair.

Iodium is an anti-scrofulous remedy. The tissues that specially come under its influence are glands. Here as in other remedies our procedure is the same; we do not prescribe for troubles by names but on symptoms. The symptom that impresses itself as the most striking is the great emaciation and absorption of the tissues of our body. The allopaths take advantage of this phenomena when they make local applications of **Iodium** for swellings and other hypertrophied conditions of different tissues of our body. The emaciation that I have mentioned is a progressive emaciation and it continues in spite of all attempts made to stop it. What makes it more striking is the ravenous appetite that goes along with this. He eats often and much but loses flesh all the same and finds a sort of a relief from eating. Emaciation is also seen under **Abrot., Natrum mur., Sarsaparilla, Tuberculinum** and **Kreosotum;** but they all have their points of difference and can be easily discriminated. Regarding the hunger of **Iodium, I** must say that it is the most remarkable feature of the remedy. This hunger is constant and continuous. He must eat every few hours or else all his symptoms are aggravated. It is a hunger that finds satisfaction nowhere He feels almost like fainting and the hunger is not satisfied. Dr. Clarke used **Iodium** with remarkble success in the opposite condition of anorexia in a young woman who, owing to a nervous shock, had lost all appetite and had made up her mind to strave herself to death. Five drops of **odium 3x** in a wine-glass of water, half an hour before meal times produced such marvellous appetite that she had to give up the idea of suicide from starvation.

Another feature of great importance is a remarkable and unaccountable sense of weakness coming on the patient. He trembles and is unable to move; even the exhaustion of talking brings on profuse sweating and nervous excitability. He is not fit for any violent exercise. This weakness is particularly felt when the patient makes an attempt to go up-stairs. He loses his breath and has to rest several times before he gets to his destination. The debility is more marked during menses.

A third characteristic is excessive flatulence. Every particle of food that he takes seems to turn into gas and we find him eructating most violently from morning till night.

Iodium has a remarkable aggravation of all his symptoms from warmth and heat. He cannot bear any hat on his head as it tends to increase his warmth. Washing in cold water, and cold air always ameliorate. Even the warm air in a warm room causes aggravation and brings on a throbbing of the head. In this way it is like **Pulsatilla** where too, we find a great craving for fresh air and a longing to open all the doors and windows.

Lastly there is another characteristic that should be clearly noted—a characteristic which is almost universal in **Iodium**. This characteristic consists of great torpidity and sluggishness. No haste is to be found anywhere in this remedy. Everything is slow and lingering; even diseases are not speedy in their termination. This indolence of the disease should be particularly suggestive of **Iodium**.

To look at him, one would hardly believe that there is much life left in him. His face is dark, yellow and tawny with many yellow spots—a complexion, indicating a cachectic and debilitated condition. The skin is rough, dry and dirty with a marked tendency to papules, boils and abscesses. In this connection it will not be out of place to mention that **Hepar** is one of the best antidotes to **Iodium**.

Mentally he is dejected and lachrymose and is disposed to be very impatient. He runs about all the time and hardly sits not knowing where to go or what to do. He is in a state almost bordering on mania. It has been recommended in mania with irresistible impulses, such as to commit a murder or run or to be engaged in some laborious occupation. It is this tendency to keep in motion day and night that should be particularly associated with **Iodium** and be made an important landmark of the remedy.

Iodium is indicated in enlargement of the heart. Great precordial anxiety, necessitating constant change of position, sensation as if the heart were squeezed together and grasped by an iron hand and severe palpitation of the heart brought on by the least exertion are important indications of **Iodium**. It is also helpful in mitral insufficiency when associated with great weakness, referred to in the region of the chest. A feeling of vibration over the heart like that caused by the purring of a cat, is also noticeable. In this respect **Iodium** is similar to **Spigelia** which remedy too, has a similar symptom referred to in the same region.

By reason of its power to cause induration of glands, **Iodium** becomes helpful in scrofula. We find hypertrophy of the cervical glands, mesenteric glands, thyreoid glands and numerous other glands imbedded in other parts of the system. When young men and women grow fast and due to falling off of appetite emaciates, it is time that we should be careful. A slight tickling cough, gradual but steady enlargement of the glands and at last a little spitting of blood showing bronchial and pulmonary congestion, unless taken in hand at once, may develop into tuberculosis of the lungs. **Iodium** would form an admirable remedy and check the onward progress of the fatal malady if it is prescribed on such well-marked symptoms as emaciation, weakness, profuse night sweats, tickling cough, expectoration of transparent mucus streaked with blood, diarrhœa and even strong hemorrhage from the lungs. Cough, membranous croup, larynigitis and bronchitis all find in **Iodium** an excellent remedy. The cough is dry and croupy in nature and is excited by the sensation of feather tickling in the trachea and under the sternum. On account of great soreness in the larynx the patient grasps it at every attempt on coughing. Sometimes we notice a shrill whistling and rattling in the chest with great soreness and oppression and a sawing hissing respiration. This tickling is the most important part of the **Iodium** cough. It is constant and unendurable and it annoys the patient immensely. It at times extends to the lungs.

Iodium finds application in pneumonia, specially when the lower lobe of the right lung is affected and the disease takes on an indolent form. Violent chill followed by great pressure on the chest, interruption and impediment of respiration, expectoration of tenacious yellowish matter occasionally tinged with blood, and a sensation of weakness in the chest with anxiety and oppression, are important indications for **Iodium.** But we must remember that in **Iodium** the suppurative process is slow and unless handled with tact and caution, it will slowly progress on to a hectic condition, ending ultimately in tuberculosis of the lungs.

Iodium is helpful in many of the complaints affecting the sexual organs of the males as well as the females. In the former, we may have atrophy of the testicles with complete loss of sexual power as well as hypertrophy with sexual excitement. It meets both the condition and is, therefore, curative in both. On the female sexual side an exactly similar condition prevails. There may be either atrophy of the ovaries and mammary glands with sterility or induration with extreme sensitiveness. It also produces and hence cures, swelling and induration of the uterus. It is even indicated in cancerous degeneration at the neck of the uterus. Usually such a condition is associated with profuse metrorrhagia with chronic leucorrhœa. Such condition, if found in conjunction with symptoms like progressive anæmia with emaciation, great debility and constant hunger, **Iodine** will be almost sure to ameliorate, if not cure.

It causes a peculiar diarrhœa and when found in chronic cachectic subjects, it will have the most marvellous effect. The stools are white, watery and foamy and are of a chronic exhausting character. They may be even whey-like and fatty—a stool generally indicative of pancreatic insufficiency. Similar stools, if associated with inflammation and swelling of the mesenteric glands indicate tuberculosis mesenterica. Bloatedness and distention of the abdomen, itching and burning in the anus, ptyalism, ulcers in the mouth with putridity of breath and a canine hunger that is hard to satisfy are all symptoms of tabes mesenterica and are fully covered by **Iodium.** Hence **Iodium** should have a special claim to our attention as being curative in a complaint that has long been pronounced incurable.

IPECACUANHA.

Ipecacuanha is a small shrub that abounds in the moist shady woods of Brazil. It is bitter, acrid, and nauseous. It was first introduced into our Materia Medica by Hahnemann. The tincture is prepared by adding five parts by weight of alcohol to the coarsely powdered root of this plant. It belongs to the natural order of Rubiaceæ. The name of this drug which is adapted into most European language, is borrowed from the South American Indians. The roots are long, tortuous, white and filiform when young but at maturity thickens to 3 or 4 times the diameters of their woody columns by the accumulation of starch-bearing tissue in the bark.

It is a moderate local irritant producing smarting redness and pustulation on the skin. Its systemic effects consist of severe inflammation of the lining of the stomach and intestines. The emetic action of the drug is characterised by nausea and salivaiton. It is also a cholagogue. Its chief action is centered on the pneumo-gastric nerve, producing spasmodic irritation in the chest and stomach. It also causes extreme prostration and exhaustion.

It is almost an everyday remedy. Its symptoms are very clear-cut and definite. The most important trait of this remedy is a constant, distressing and a continual nausea. **Ipecac** is rarely indicated when this symptom is absent. It is a sort of qualmishness with profuse salivation; it is an ineffectual desire to vomit. Even when he is able to vomit, his qualmishness instead of subsiding becomes aggravated hundredfolds. This qualmishness is accompanied with a peculiar sensation in the stomach as if it is hanging down relaxed. **Ignatia, Staphisagria, Thein, Lobelia** and **Tabacum** are a few others that can boast of a similar sensation. The substance vomited is glairy jelly-like mucus, sometimes bile. Other remedies with such deathly nausea are **Arsenicum, Cadmium, Crotalus hor., Tabacum, Antim. crud., Pulsatilla, Zincum, Apomorphin** and **Cocculus,** but each one of these remedies has its own differentiating marks.

Another symptom of **Ipecac** almost equally important is a general sore feeling all throughout the body. The bones feel as if they are all broken to pieces. This pain makes him quite restless. Here we should compare **Ipecac** with **Arnica, Medorrhinum, Ruta, Baptisia, Pyrogen, Nux mosch, Eupatorium** and **Rhus tox.**

Ipecac is a great hemorrhagic remedy. We find hemorrhage from almost every organ of our system such as lungs, bowels,

consists in a steady flow of bright red foamy blood associated with nausea. The appearance of this patient is in keeping with his internal condition. His face is deathly pale with blue margins round his sunken eyes. Mentally he is very irritable, taciturn, and uncertain. He is full of desires but he does not know what he wants.

The gastric symptoms of **Ipecac** are many and important. It is brought about by indulgence in rich food, such as pastry, pork, fruits and ice-cream. The tongue of **Ipecac,** inspite of all this gastric disturbance, is quite clean. The vomiting, as has been repeatedly said, is almost incessant. At first he brings up quantities of ingesta to be followed by huge masses of bile and then mucus of grass green colour. The presence of blood either bright red or pitch-like in colour is not infrequent. This retching and the unavailing desire to vomit are also associated with intense cutting pain in the belly. Loss of appetite, a great disgust for food, emaciation, acute distress in epigastric region, coldness of extremities, hippocratic countenance, imperceptible pulse and a profuse discharge of cold, clammy sweat are symptoms that are invariably present and should be carefully remembered. In this respect **Ipecac** should be compared with **Pulsatilla, Arsenicum** and **Antim. crud.** in all of which we find the causative factor to be the same.

In **Pulsatilla** the distinguishing features are a thick white-coated tongue, absence of thirst and a peculiar bland taste in the mouth.

Arsenicum is more deep-acting in action. It rather follows or supplants **Ipecac,** when as a result of indulgence in these rich articles of food catarrh of the stomach has set in with irresistible burning, nausea and intolerance of food. There is always relief from hot drinks.

Antim. crud. is the remedy when gastric derangement follows the overloading of the stomach. The symptoms are a peculiarly white coating on the tongue, fetid eructations, slow digestion, anorexia and a diarrhœa alternating with constipation.

It is an invaluable remedy both in diarrhœa and dysentery. The stools have the appearance of fermented yeast and it spurts out with much flatus as in **China, Elaterium** and **Croton.** In color it may be lemon-yellow or green as grass. This **Ipecac** diarrhœa is mostly seen in children during teething. The pain in the stomach causes the child to scream unceasingly. It tosses about in bed with all the discomfort of an over-loading of the stomach with sweets, fats and pastries. If with the above symptoms we have a clean tongue and an incessant tendency to vomiting we could not be far wrong in prescribing **Ipecacuanha.** In dysentery the stools which are frequent are tinged with the presence of blood or they may be quite dark, resembling frothy molasses. This latter stool is particularly characteristic of **Ipecac.**

In choleraic affections it may be needed in the first stage, when nausea and vomiting predominate. The face looks pale, indicative of great suffering. Blue rings around the eyes, vomiting immediately after a drink of water, the anguish and the uneasiness, the frequent long drawn sighs, a peculiar distressed feeling in the abdomen as if the stomach were empty and were hanging down relaxed and constant griping and colic lead to the indication of **Ipecac.** In teething children all the above-mentioned symptoms may be found in conjunction with convulsions.

Affecting, as it does, the pneumo-gastric nerve we find it useful in asthma specially of the spasmodic type where the patient complains of great constriction in the throat and the chest. There is usually a great accumulation of mucus in the bronchial passage which gives rise to a peculiar wheezing sound. At times this collection is so great as to threaten suffocation. Due to presence of emphysema the patient finds it difficult to throw off the accumulated mucus in sufficient quantity. In this respect it is so similar to **Lobelia inflata** that at times it becomes difficult to distinguish between the two. Another remedy to which it bears a great resemblance is **Antim. tart.**, the difference consisting only in the quantity of accumulated phlegm in the bronchial passage. Although **Ipecac** finds it difficult to expectorate, still the patient manages to get rid of a portion of accumulated phlegm either by means of coughing or vomiting, whereas in **Antim. tart.** the patient fails in every attempt to over-throw the phelgm, which weighs heavier and heavier, the cough getting less and less frequent, till at last the patient chokes and succumbs from paralysis of the lungs due to failure of expectoration. It is equally useful in capillary bronchitis of infants. The cough is spasmodic and is caused by tickling in the larynx. Nausea and vomiting usually follow an attack of coughing. Very frequently the cough is so suffocative that the child turns blue, faint and stiff. All these symptoms make it an admirable remedy in whooping cough. The paroxysm is usually so strong as to bring about an attack of epistaxis as well as bleeding from the mouth.

We should think of it even in hæmoptysis, generally the precursor of phthisical affection of the lungs. The blood is usually bright red and is expelled without much effort. It is provoked by a dry tickling cough and is preceded by a sense of bubbling in the chest. The blood discharged is usually frothy and is associated with gasping for breath.

Ipecac is indiscriminately used in the treatment of ague and intermittent fever. Its use, like those of other remedies, is based on the same immutable law of Similars. We use it in every case where that prominent characteristic of persistent nausea is present. The chills are short and free from thirst. A strange part of this chill is that it is always worse in a warm room and from external heat. The patient feels ever so much better in the open air and by drinking. This is one of our remedies where during this stage. we find redness of one cheek and paleness of the other. The heat is long lasting and is accompanied with thirst, nausea and vomiting. Oppression of breathing and a dry hacking cough are present at this stage. A symptom, that escaped my mind and one that is worth our while to remember, is that the patient complains of great prostration during the stage of chill. Nausea and vomiting, the two most characteristic features of **Ipecac** extend even into the stage of sweat. In fact they are worse at this stage and are distinctly better after the stage of sweat is over. The sweat is usually sour and the urine turns turbid at this stage. **Ipecac** is particularly useful in those cases of malarial fevers which have been tempered with by the mal-administration of quinine.

Case 1.—During a cold day, a gentleman was taken down with a severe, painless diarrhœa. He took **Dulc.** which produced only undigested stools, without any improvement; then **China,** then **Phos.,** then **Bry.,** but without any benefit. Thinking he saw the best effects from **Phos.,** as it removed the undigested food from the stools, he concluded to take it in larger doses; but undigested stools returned, now worse than ever. He took **China** again, in repeated doses; but aggravation, with flatulence, was the consequence. I found him at stool, expelling the fæces promptly, with great violence and with copious flatulence; the stool had a foul smell, and in color and consistency looked like fermented yeast. **Ipec. 30,** one dose, cured.—Jahr.

Case 2.—Miss Alice B., æt. eleven, black hair and eyes; had long been subject to attacks of ague, for which **Quin,** had been successfully given, without, however, preventing the recurrence of the paroxysm with every new provocation; chill every other day, about 11 A.M.; she shivers a while, then shakes for twenty minutes; headache; hands first cold; nausea as the chill goes off; nausea all the time; no thirst with the chill; chill followed by fever; thirst with the heat; perspiration when the fever passes off. Found her covered up on the sofa, shaking with the chill, when I visited her in

July 26. Blank powders to take during the afternoon, and one powder of **Ipec. 1m.** (Fincke) to take at bed time. Was sent for before bearkfast in the morning; found her still in bed; she had passed a comfortable night but had just been vomiting. Satisfied that this was the effect of the **Ipec. 1m.,** I gave her only a blank powder in water, to take a teaspoonful every hour, and promised to call in the evening. After tea, I found her out at play. Nearly a year has now elapsed, and she has had no chill since; but once in a while, when her sister (**in loco parentis**) finds her complaining of headache etc., as formerly, before the chill, she sends for a few powders, and the danger is avoided.—Dr. J. H. P. Frost.

IRIDIUM.

It is a metal of very high specific gravity and is found in combination with Platinum in platinum ore. It is one of the heaviest of substances known.

This metal which has not yet received a substantial proving, is supposed to be a good specific for anæmia by reason of its capacity to increase red blood corpuscles. It has also been recommended in exhaustion after any serious disease and as such it is similar to **China** and **Laurocerasus.** The symptoms which are not too many and too reliable and on which **Iridium** may be prescribed are the following: a feeling of self-confidence and equanimity, a feeling of numbness in the ears and throughout the body and a sensation as if the mind were void and difficulty of concentration of thought.

IRIS VERSICOLOR.

This is commonly called the Blue flag and Flower-de-luce. The tincture is prepared from the fresh root, gathered in late autumn or early spring. It belongs to the natural order of Iridaceæ. The most important action of this remedy is found over the gastro-intestinal mucous membrane and its numerous glands. When taken in big quantity, it brings on profuse ropy salivation, lachrymation, and intense burning of the mouth, œsophagus and the stomach; profuse purging that excoriates the anus and vomiting of extremely sour fluid with a consequent burning of the passage are also found.

This is one more of our sour remedies. We can call hyperacidity the most marked feature of **Iris.** It is noticed everywhere. Thus **Iris** becomes an important remedy in dyspepsia, gastric ulceration, gastric catarrh, duodenitis and diarrhœa when this symptom is present. Dr. Kitchen relieved a case of gastro dynia with **Iris** when this important symptom of vomiting of sour foods after meals was present. This vomiting is the red strand of the remedy. There is first of all vomiting of ingesta, then sour fluid and last of all yellow and green bile. The substance vomited out is thick and ropy mucus hanging from the mouth to the receptacle. Great burning, distress and violent pains are felt in the epigastrium. It has been used very successfully in colic with pains coming in successive shocks in the umbilical region. Nausea, with straining and belching of wind, great commotion and rumbling in the bowels in the affected area, much mental depression and great anguish of the mind and constant expulsion of enormous discharge of wind are symptoms indicating **Iris.** Dr. Nash cites a case of chronic gastritis, which from its persistent nature was feared to be cancer of the stomach that he cured with **Iris.** It was in a middle aged lady who had frequent attacks of vomiting of ropy mucus, which after a lapse of a little time, turned dark and coffee colored. Judging from the growing weakness and the color of the vomited substance together with the persistence of the trouble, the supposition arrived at was endorsed by many physicians who were in attendance on the çase. After the failure of **Kali bi., Iris** was prescribed and it cured in a short time and permanently.

It is used with benefit in diarrhœa and cholera morbus when such troubles start between 2 and 3 A.M. with violent vomiting of extremely sour bile and mucus and purging of profuse corrosive watery stools.

But the ailment, that has brought **Iris** its greatest renown, is sick headache. Generally speaking this headache in **Iris** is of gastric origin. It is due to acid stomach or irritation of that organ through excessive acid secretions. It is a headache that affects the right side principally as in **Sanguinaria.** It is aggravated by rest and on first moving the head but relieved by continual motion. The headache is associated with lowness of spirit, nausea and acid vomiting. I have forgotten to mention that **Iris** headache is periodical in its nature. The attack comes on a certain day every week. The pain is intense, and throbbing and it ushers in a blurred state of the vision or temporary blindness with vomiting at the height of the attack. Dr. Kitchen considers **Iris** the most prompt and effectual remedy for headache of this type. He also recommends it in neuralgia of the head and eyes.

Everything considered, **Iris** bears a strong semblance to **Mercury.** It affects the mouth, and the glandular systems in the same way as **Mercury.** The difference between the two consists in the fact that it is comparatively powerless on the osseous tissues.

JABORANDI.

It is a Brazilian plant that often grows to a height of twenty feet. It contains an alkaloid jabourandin or pilocarpin that is used by the old school as a diaphoretic and sialogog. The tincture is prepared from the powdered dried leaves and stems saturated with alcohol. It belongs to the natural order of Rutaceæ. Dr. Robbin's summing up of the effects of **Jaborandi** in heroic doses is interesting and we quote below the jist of his statement: Very soon face becomes red; temporal arteries throb more strongly; then there is a peculiar feeling of heat in the mouth and on the face and the flow of saliva begins. Soon the forehead becomes moist and the face more red; then beads of perspiration appear on forehead, cheeks, and temples. The flow of saliva increases, all the salivary glands contributing. The mouth is filled with immense quantities of fluid and expectoration is incessant. At same time perspiration covers the face and neck; then the whole body becomes red and moist, and a pleasant warmth is experienced; in a few minutes perspiration breaks out over entire surface and soon runs down on all the sides. Meantime other symptoms have supervened. The eyelids first become moist, then tears increase, collect in the canthi, then roll down the cheeks; at the same time there is increased secretion of the Schneiderian membrane, and increased activity of the mucous glands of the pharynx, the trachea, and the bronchi. These effects reach the maximum intensity forty five minutes after taking the drug and last thirty or forty minutes more. Salivary glands enlarge. Thirst is intense. Pupils get slightly contracted. When perspiration and salivation have ceased the subject becomes prostrated and drowsy, and the parts that secreted excessively become abnormally dry.

This establishes beyond doubt the red strand of the remedy to be hyper-secretion of all the glands of the human system. We have profuse and copious sweating, starting on forehead and face and thence spreading all over the body. Profuse salivation, free flow of tears and nose and then watery copious diarrhœa are all characteristics of **Jaborandi.** It is used with great benefit in uremia, nephritis, renal dropsy, hydro-thorax, ascites, pleurisy, bronchitis, coryza, glycosuria and diabetes, when the abovementioned symptoms are present.

Jaborandi is credited with marvellous curative power in various complaints of the eye, such as hyperopia, choroiditis, asthenopia, hypermetropia, cataract &c. Vision becomes dim; objects at distance look hazy. The eyes tire soon. Sometimes nausea is brought on by looking at a moving object.

I remember using **Jaborandi** in a case of climacteric flushing of the face. It was in a lady of about 47 years. She was ashamed to go before other people lest they thought she had painted her face. The flushes used to be succeeded by beads of perspiration over her forehead. **Jaborandi** removed the feeling of heat and lessened the perspiration.

Jaborandi is contra-indicated in adynamic patients, also in cases of pronounced cardiac embarrassment and pulmonary congestion or œdema.

JACEA.

(*See* **Viola Odorata.**)

JALAPA.

It is a tuberous rooted plant that grows in Mexico. The tincture is prepared from pulvarised dried root. It belongs to the natural order of Convolvulaceæ.

I know just one or two symptoms of this remedy which I will make it a point to discuss just now. Firstly, it is a remedy generally called for, in the ailments of infants—infants, who laugh and play all day but scream and kick all night; all their troubles are worse at night and that is why they scream and toss about at that hour.

The **Jalapa** baby is a frequent subject of diarrhœa—a diarrhœa that is watery, sour-smelling and associated with colic.

Jalapa helped me in a case of entero-colitis in a little baby of about seven summers. The baby came to me from allopathic hands after three months of prolonged diarrhœa. The baby was so emaciated and feeble that it was a piteous object to look at and the poor thing was constantly undergoing contortions of the body, due most probably to a colic to which it was a constant subject. **Jalapa** cured the child's diarrhœa, relieved the colic and the last that I knew of him, he was a healthy nice chubby child.

JATROPHA CURCAS.

This medicine is prepared from a shrub indigenous to West Indies and South America. The tincture is prepared from the coarsely powdered seeds of this plant by saturating the same with alcohol. It was introduced into our Materia Medica by Hering. The common name of this plant is Physic Nut, a name that amply illustrates the use that is generally made of this drug. It belongs to the natural order of Euphorbiaceæ.

It is one of our chief remedies for choleraic diarrhœa and cholera, when the main characteristic of the remedy, I mean the marked and peculiar gurgling in the abdomen, is present. The noise is very loud as if caused by the emptying of a full bottle inside the abdomen. We may also liken it to the ' bhug-bhug ' sound caused by the sudden immersion of an empty vessel into water.

The second characteristic of the **Jatropha** diarrhœa is the sudden expulsion of abundant alvine evacuations, sometimes containing a large number of lumbrici and ascarides. They come out like a gushing torrent. The onset of the diarrhœa in **Jat.** is quite sudden.

The third important point consists in the nature of the staff that is vomited out. It is a thick albuminous glairy sort of a fluid. The thirst is unquenchable. Anxiety and anguish, indifference, prostration and occasional cramps, make it a splendid remedy in the first stage of cholera. Judicially used and oft repeated, for it is a remedy that needs repetition, it will avert the fatal end in a large number of cases.

JUGLANS CINEREA.

It is also called Juglans Cathartica. It is our common Butternut or the Black Wal-nut. This remedy like its sister juglans regia is an important hæmorrhagic remedy. The characteristic feature about this hæmorrhage is that the blood is dark, inky and clotted. We shall go into finer differentiation between these two sister remedies a bit later on. It is sufficient to say just now that the blood in both these remedies is fluid, dark and pitch-like in colour.

The headache of **Juglans cinerea** is very characteristic. The pain is sharp and shooting in character and it is mostly an occipital headache. It is a headache associated with frequent micturition and it comes in the morning, same as in **Nux., Bry., Chel.** and **Iris.**

Another feature of **Juglans** is a sinking sensation felt in the epigastric region. In this respect it compares well with **Sulph., Phos., Phos. acid,** etc. With this sinking sensation is felt a sharp stitching pain in the region of the liver which extends to the right scapula as in **Chel.** and **Bryo.** Thus it is as important a liver remedy as our **Nux.** We also have the morning aggravation as in **Nux.;** but in **Juglans** it is an occipital headache more than anything else that disturbs the patient and frequently wakes him up at about 3 o'clock in the morning preventing him from falling asleep again, to be followed in the morning by a bilious yellowish greenish jaundiced stool.

JUGLANS REGIA.

It is our famous Walnut. The word Juglans really means Jovis Glans or Joves' Nuts. In classical literature it was supposed to form the staple food of the great JUPITER, hence this lofty appellation. We are indebted to Dr. Muller for many of our informations regarding this remedy. As I have mentioned in connection with our previous remedy, the hæmorrhage is black, pitchy and clotted. In **Juglans regia** the hæmorrhage is from the uterus, whereas in **Juglans cinerea** it is mostly from the lungs. I give preference to **Regia** where skin symptoms predominate, especially in scrofulous subjects. We have eruptions and scabs on the scalp behind the ear, on the arms and in the axillæ. The itching is so intense at night that he is hardly able to sleep. Many of the skin eruptions of this remedy closely resemble syphilis. The symptoms are generally worse by motion, after fat food, at night and from undressing.

JUSTICIA ADHATODA BASAK.

This Indian shrub is highly efficacious in the affections of the respiratory tract, especially of the catarrhal type. It has been in use in this country for hundreds of years and its reputation in many bronchial affections is established beyond question. In ordinary bronchitis, in asthma, in whooping cough, in laryngismus stridulous, in influenza, in pneumonia and even in phthisis it has been extolled as a remedy of high curative value. The Ayurvedic pharmacœpia is very loud in its praise in all the above-mentioned complaints. This medicine in its new roll, as a homœopathic drug, deserves more extensive proving.

The guiding symptom of **Justicia** is a constant and an eternal flow of mucus discharge accompanying any one of the complaints mentioned above. The head feels full, hot and heavy. The mucous membrane of the nose and eyes is violently congested, leading to a continuous flow of profuse coryza. There is entire loss of smell and taste. The entire sternal region feels heavy, narrow and impacted. The larynx feels painful, showing congestion of the laryngeal mucous membrane with the attendant symptom of hoarseness. Paroxysmal cough associated with sneezing and severe dyspnœa due to a sensation of tightness across the chest are some of its symptoms. In whooping cough, it is greatly similar to **Ipecac** and **Drosera.** The child turns blue and looks, as if it is going to be suffocated. It has been used in asthma and it has been known to relieve the intense tightness accompanying a fit of this disease. Like **Ipecac** it has been found to be efficacious in the first stage of tuberculosis with the spitting up of blood which it checks immediately. Like **Ipecac** again, we have great wheezing and rattling of mucus in the chest and throat.

KALI BICHROMICUM.

This is commonly known as Bichromate of Potash. It was first proved by Dr. Drysdale of England. This is an anti-syphilitic remedy of great repute and wide application.

Its principal action is centred over the mucous membrane. It causes a secretion of a tough stringy mucus,—mucus that adheres to the part and weaves into a long string when pulled. This symptom is the result of an inflammatory process which leads to the formation of plastic exudation. This exudation again, in its turn, tends to the formation of false membranes. We use it in ophthalmia, ozena, sorethroat, laryngitis, gastritis, ulceration of stomach, gonorrhœa, leucorrhœa and in various other ailments when this characteristic symptom is present.

The next important feature of **Kali bich** is found in the nature of its pain. This pain shifts rapidly from one part to another as in **Kali sulph, Lac can, Pulsat, Magn. phos, Lilium tig** and **Kalmia.** It is a pain that often comes in small spots as in **Ignatia;** it can be covered with the point of the finger. The pain of **Kali bich** resembles that of **Belladonna** in its onset. It appears and disappears suddenly. We use it also in neuralgia when it occurs at the same hour every day.

Kali bichromicum is applicable in a certain type of headache—a headache that begins with blurred vision or blindness. The sight returns as soon as the headache increases. Often it is due to suppression of the discharge from nose. Great aversion to light and noise during headache is common. It commences in the morning and lasts practically all day and is accompanied by persistent retching and vomiting of food and bile which does not bring any relief. The pain is situated in the forehead, round about the eye and on the malar bone. At other times again, we have periodical attacks of semilateral headache on small spots that could be covered with the point of a finger. These headaches are mostly ameliorated by pressure, in open air and by eating.

It has been used in trachoma with pannus and in syphilitic iritis. One other condition of the eye for which this remedy is very valuable is ulceration of the cornea. It is just the right place to mention that the ulcers of **Kali bich.**, in whichever part of the body they may be located, are perforating in their nature. The part looks, as if it has been punched out. This tendency to cause deep eating ulceration is also found in other preparations of Potassium. This feature is almost as prominent in **Kali iodatus** as in **Kali bich.** The inflammatory process in **Kali bich,** is generally slow and indolent, with a tendency to get into chronicity. The symptoms are never very violent, but they are troublesome enough. A great lack of reactive power is always manifested by these patients. It is applicable in conjunctivitis either scrofulous or sycotic; but here too, the same tendency towards chronicity is to be observed. True enough, the lids are swollen and the eyes get agglutinated in the morning but then the other violent symptoms, such as photophobia and intense pain are wanting. It is also indicated in iritis which may or may not be of syphilitic origin. Certain amount of conjunctival injection and lachrymation on exposure, are to be observed. But the most important point, for the prescriber to remember, is that this remedy should not be prescribed until exudation has taken place posteriorly between the iris and the lens. **Kali bichromicum** helps in the absorption of the exuded matter.

The organ that comes most under its influence is the nose. Many cases of chronic ozena, some of them of the very worst type, have been helped with **Kali bich.** It has healed vast ulceration in the nose when destruction of the entire cartilaginous septum has happened. The mucus discharge from the nose is tough ropy, green and bloody. Oftentimes it is like plugs and clinkers. Little pieces of caried bones sometimes come out with these discharges. The nose feels unnaturally dry due to obstruction, caused by these hardened masses of fetid clinkers. Loss of smell is an early symptom. The frontal sinus is often affected. A very important symptom is a pressive pain felt at the root of the nose. Violent pains shoot from root of nose to external angle of eye and are accompanied with dimness of sight. Due to this feeling of pressure at the root of the nose and a sensation, as if nose were swollen, he keeps on blowing at his nose with hardly any discharge. The dryness of nose is so great that he has a sensation as if his nostrils were made of parchment. The air that is expelled from the nose feels hot. The plugs and clinkers already referred to, cause a sensation of stuffiness and blockage. The discharge, as has been already mentioned before, is green but they are often tinged with a little show of blood. Unless the discharge continues freely, he experiences a sort of pain from occiput to forehead. The smell that emanates from the nose is extremely objectionable.

Kali bichromicum very strongly affects the mucous membrane of the throat. This takes the form of an inflammation but we must not lose sight of the fact that this inflammation, unlike the inflammation of **Aconite** and **Bell,** is of a highly indolent nature and there is a great tendency towards formation of exudation. The tonsils look large but there is hardly any inflammation, and fever; there is a marked tendency to formation of ulcers on tonsils and the velum. The ulcers are covered with an ash-colored slough and the patient hawks up large quantities of tenacious mucus which is so viscid that it draws out like a long thread from the gullet and the throat. The membrane when it forms, is quite thick and leathery. The tongue is coated yellow and is dry and glossy. In diphtheria we notice the formation of a membranous deposit of a pearly white fibrinous consistency extending downward into the larynx and trachea. The uvula becomes œdematous and bladder-like. The cough is violent, rattling, hoarse, and metallic. He expectorates tough fibro-elastic casts. Another peculiarity of this cough is that it is caused by eating.

The tongue is broad and flat like that of **Mercurius** and takes the imprint of teeth. A thick yellow fur, more towards the base of the tongue, is also noticed. Very often large insular patches, are visible on the tongue. In typhoid, typhus, malignant dysentery and other varieties of serious ailments, the tongue becomes glassy, smooth, red and cracked.

Like the mucous membrane covering the other orifices of the body, it affects alike the mucous lining of the stomach and produces gastric symptoms, varying in intensity from simple indigestion to malignant affection of the stomach. It is prescribed in common dyspepsia with vomiting of food which has turned sour in stomach. This dyspepsia, though wanting in the severity of an acute disease, becomes, if not taken in hand at once, a forerunner of chronic catarrh of stomach which may ultimately turn into ulceration of stomach and duodenum. It is the effect of over-indulgence in beer or other malt liquors. After food the patient complains of a great weight in the pit of the stomach. Loss of appetite, nausea, a flabby sordid looking tongue and dull pain in hyponchondrium are symptoms which lead to **Kali Bichromicum.** The stools are brown, watery, and frothy and they gush out in the morning as in **Sulphur, Rumex** and **Natrum sulph.**

KALI BROMATUM.

Potassium Bromide occurs as a colorless or white cubical crystals or granules. It is odorless and has a pungent saline taste. It abates all forms of nervousness, fidgetiness or even spasms and creates a tendency to mental calm and indifference Used in large and repeated doses, it may even create idiocy and imbecility with total destruction of the mental faculties There is a certain amount of aphasia and physical weakness amounting to paresis, with impotence in **Kali bromatum.** Fetidit of breath, hoarseness, acne on face, and œdematous swelling o the faucial arch are some of the symptoms of **Kali bromatu** poisoning. This gives us food for reflexion. According our principle of Similia Similibus Curantur it becomes effic cious in relieving certain variety of symptoms that accompani physical and mental weakness. In overwhelming doses paralys of sense and motion becomes absolute and death ensues quiet by failure of respiration or cardiac action. It is used medicina by allopaths to quiet a qualmish stomach or to calm a restle subject and to invite sleep. It is also used in epilepsy and tetar in heroic doses but with doubtful benefit.

The procedures, followed by homœopaths, are howe altogether different. Here, as in other remedies, the totality symptoms produced by Bromide of Potassium on healthy bei is our main guide. In the first place it causes a great depression of the mind. The patient is very fretful, crying at trifles and constantly brooding. These fits of crying sometimes become almost uncontrollable. The melancholy is so profound that the patient weeps constantly and nothing relieves the remarkable depression of mind. This depression partly owes its origin to a great despondence—a despondence that almost drives him mad and makes him very apathetic. Another trait of his character is a great suspicion of mind. He imagines that he will be poisoned; that he is pursued by some evil spirits; that he is hated by every body or that his honor is at stake. Ideas such as these actually drive him mad. I fully believe that this is how he gradually gets into a state of acute mania. Forgetfulness of mind is almost complete. He forgets how to talk and has to be told the word before he could speak it. Horrid illusions, hallucinations of sight and sound and actual delirium take possession of him. On these indications it has been repeatedly employed in puerperal mania, melancholia and delirium tremens. We have used this remedy for spasms and convulsions due to fear, anger and other mental disturbances.

It is a splendid remedy for night terror of children. They wake up at night with some horrible dream and scream, moan and cry. To soothe them into silence is a hard job. These night terrors of children in **Kali bromatum** are due to over-excitement of the brain. Not only is this remedy efficacious in such disturbances in children, but they are useful in grown-up men as well, who have worked hard and worked long and have practically exhausted themselves. It relieves giddiness and a benumbed feeling in the brain due to merciless applications over hard, difficult and intricate problems.

A second characteristic of **Kali bromatum** is extreme nervous restlessness of hands and fingers. They are in constant motion. The fingers are twitched without any cessation and that without any reason whatsoever. This is different from fidgetiness of **Zincum** where only the lower limbs are involved. Sometimes this nervousness spreads all over the body and we find the patient moving about constantly. They shake all over with anxiety. This trembling is often accompanied by unsteadiness rolling and traggering, as if drunk. Inco-ordination of muscles, amnesic phasia, anæsthesia, particularly of gums, pharynx and genitals, are frequent complications with these patients. It is on account of this that **Kali bromatum** occupies an important place in the treatment of ataxia.

Kali bromatum has important indications in the male and female sexual spheres. It causes sexual and lascivious fancies and dreams, leading on to satyriasis. The opposite condition of impotence, the effect of sexual excesses is also to be found under **Kali bromatum.** But everywhere, whatever may be the condition, symptoms of great melancholia are always guiding. They may be also accompanied by staggering gait, weakness and great forgetfulness. On the female sexual side it is a great remedy for indurated uterus due very probably to fibroid growths. Ovarian cystic tumors, neuralgia of ovaries, sub-involution of uterus have been helped with **Kali bromatum** on indications suggested before. It is equally applicable in menstrual epilepsy when associated with great irritation and nymphomania, the result of much ovarian irritation.

It is needless to say that **Kali bromatum** is a great remedy for both acne simplex and indurata. They generally appear in young, fleshy persons and lymphatic constitutions and leave unsightly marks, thereby causing great mental depression. It also removes the tendency for small boils that come in successive crops over the face and the tongue and are the source of much troublesome itching.

KALI CARBONICUM.

Carbonate of Potash is a white granular substance of alkaline taste. In nature it exists in large quantities in plants of all varieties and descriptions and was originally obtained from the ashes of plants and vegetable tissues. It is a polychrest of very high repute and is applicable to elderly people with lax fibre and dark hair. A great tendency towards obesity is noticed in these patients. They are usually fleshy and flabby, but they differ from the **Calcarea carb** patients in respect of profound anæmia to which they are frequent subjects. Their skin is almost milky-white with tendency to dropsical effusions. It is on account of this anæmia that we find them to be very susceptible to cold and chilliness. They prefer to remain indoors, as the least draught of air makes them shiver. Inspite of this anemia, we find the patient, at times looking very flushed and crimson. This does not really mean full bloodedness, but only a temporary influx of blood into certain localised areas. The peculiarity about this flushing, is that it is most one-sided and partial. We find one cheek to be red and hot, the other pale and cold. The patient usually very pale, looks flushed during a fit of coughing. All these do not betoken a healthy state, but only a localised hectic condition. Yet another characteristic of these patients is to be seen in their debility. It is more an exhaustion than a debility. The patient seems almost worn out and that inspite of doing nothing, there is a constant tendency to lie down. Walking, talking or indulging in any other activity, however slight, are irksome. This weakness and this exhaustion gradually grow in intensity, till at last they amount almost to a state of paralysis. This is how weakness in **Kali carb.** slowly and insidiously develops into real paralysis. The patient yawns continuously and complains of great sleepiness all throughout the day and even in the early hours of the evening, when every body around him is happy, cheerful and enjoying themselves. This sleepiness, however, grows very intense, specially after eating when they can hardly keep awake. It has been said that they fall asleep even while they are having their food. But this, after all, is not the restful sleep of the healthy. During sleep they start, twitch, grind their teeth, talk and cry. The sleep is further disturbed by dreams of thieves, ghosts, diseases, dead people and various other erotic sentimental fantacies. Still another peculiarity of these patients is to be found in their touchiness. By this is meant a great dislike to be touched. They cannot bear anybody to touch them. It makes them start. This touchiness is praticularly prominent about feet.

The greatest characteristic of **Kali carb,** however, is to be seen in the nature of its pains. They are stitching and lancinating in character and are worse from rest and lying on the affected side. They are aggravated at the early hours of the morning at bout 3 a.m. This pain is present everywhere in **Kali carb** and we will have ample opportunity to verify it before we ave progressed far. Mentally they are peevish, nervous and ritable. Noise is disagreeable and even human voice is intolerae. Due partly to touchiness mentioned above, and to intense ervousness, we find them getting startled easily. They are most as easily frightened. Apart from this and inspite of much elancholia to which they are easy victims, we find them to be rticularly fond of company. This desire for company is not account of any social instinct, but it owes its origin to a ead of being left alone. They suffer from hallucinations. They agine, as if there are people in the room where really there are none. They are being tantalised by imaginary figures and fancies which cannot really be substantiated by facts. The **Kali carb** patient is also found to be very indifferent to his surroundings. In this way he is like **Acid phos.,** the only difference being that in **Acid phos** it is of nervous origin whereas in **Kali carb,** it is the effect of physical exhaustion.

A characteristic, that has not yet been touched though of outstanding importance, is the occurrence of bag-like swelling between the upper eye-lids and the eye-balls. It is more of the type of puffiness which gives a sac-like appearance to the above-mentioned region.

We must not forget the backache of **Kali carb,** a symptom worth its weight in gold. This backache is accompanied by great weakness and profuse sweating. Farrington considers this combination a great indication for **Kali carb.** The patient constantly speaks of his back as giving out. This is so bad while walking that he feels like lying down in street to obtain relief. It is pressing in character and is relieved by rubbing. It feels like a heavy weight in the pelvis. The pain shoots down the glutei muscles into the buttocks and thence through the thigh into knee and even downwards. On this symptom Dr. Clarke made a remarkable cure in an aged lady that used to suffer from 'Rheumatic pains' in the back accompanied with a foul vaginal discharge that was diagnosed as cancer by an allopathic practitioner of repute. Under the influence of **Kali carb.** the pain disappeared, the discharge stopped and the patient lived many long years to die from another ailment altogether. On this symptom of backache, so important is **Kali carb,** insufficient labor pains have been rendered efficient, abortions stopped, confinement made easy, severe hemorrhage from uterus stopped and lumbago cured. Speaking about this backache Farrington mentions about a case of dyspepsia in a nervous female which he cured on the strange indication of aggravation of the backache from eating. This odd symptom led him to **Kali carb** which not only cured the backache but removed the dyspepsia as well.

Its indications in dyspepsia need close attention. It characterized by great repugnance to food. Sour eructation, acid up-risings of food, great sensitiveness of the epigastric region, a strange feeling of emptiness and gone-feeling in the pit of the stomach and above all, a painful distention of the abdomen due great accumulation of flatus are some of the symptoms to lead **Kali carb.**

Lastly we shall discuss the action of **Kali carb.** on the respiratory system. It is indicated in bronchitis, pneumonia and phthisis pulmonalis. The most characteristic symptom in all these affections, however, is a stitching pain referred to, in the walls of the chest. The cough is dry and paroxysmal. One peculiarity, about this cough, is that the viscid mucus or pus, whatever he happens to bring up, is swallowed. The expectoration usually consists of hard, white mucus which practically flies out of the throat while coughing or else the patient swallows them without being able, in the least, to throw it away. Great dyspnœa, purulent expectoration, great bubbling and rattling noise in the chest, the 3 a.m. aggravation, vomiting of ingesta while coughing are some of the symptoms worth remembering. The cough is usually worse after eating and drinking and the patient complains of a feeling of weakness and faintness in chest specially when walking. It has been recommended very highly by Hahnemann as a great remedial agency to counteract the disorganising effect of tuberculosis. According to him, almost every case of ulcerated lungs should have this anti-psoric as a starting remedy. It affects frequently the base of the right side of the lung in preference to the left. The cough is worse from any exertion and when lying down.

Kali carb has a tendency to produce fatty degeneration of the heart and has a great salutary influence in insufficiency of mitral valves. The pulse is intermittent, slow and weak. A sensation, frequently complained of by these patients, is as if, the heart were suspended by a thread. Another feature is easy choking. Food easily gets into the wind pipe and is followed by severe paroxysm of coughing. It is even useful in angina pectoris with the following symptoms: Stitching pain worse on strong inspiration and on coughing; burning in the region of the heart; arms go to sleep after violent exercise; chocking in the throat; difficulty of breathing; tumultuous action of the heart.

Case 1.—H. R., a lad of eleven years, was taken with neuralgia of the heart, complicated with pneumonia of the left lung. I found the patient in a half-recumbent position, inclined to the left side, and he could lay in no cough. Pulse 145 per minute and respiration about fifty. Gave **Aconite** for other posture, owing to the aggravation of the severe stitching pains in the chest by the slightest movement, and the increase of the distressing dry 4 hours without any relief, followed by **Arsenic** for an equal length of time with no benefit. **Bryonia** followed by **Phosphorous** were given for the next 8 hours, at the end of which time I think the patient was less comfortable than when I first saw him, being unable to recline the head, or turn the body to either side, not having slept more than ten minutes at a time for four days, and such naps far between. At this juncture I gave **Kali Carbonicum 200.** The effect was immediate. The stitching pains were relieved, and the cough softened, and the night following the first dose, the patient was able to lay comfortably, with the body reclined at an angle of forty-five degrees, and slept several hours. From this moment convalescence commenced. While other remedies were given at the commencement of these cases, no permanent improvement took place until **Kali Carbonicum** was given, and after it had been given, improvement was permanent.—(Dr. Preston)

Case 2.—Anna Custer, of delicate constitution, aged twenty years, was attacked by asthma and severe pains of the joints and was treated at the hospital. Since her dismissal from there, more than a year ago, she suffers from gastric and other troubles; everything she eats produces continual pressure; tension in the stomach; small portions of coffee or weak soup fill her up, with eructations, nausea and vomiting; she complains also of frequent headache and toothache; hot flashes with abdominal pulsations; vertigo; continual chilliness; cold feet; internal chilliness, with constant inclination to micturate, but the urine flows slowly and causes a burning sensation; stool dry, retarded; pit of stomach hard and painful to the least touch; respiration heavy, oppppressed especially when walking; when stooping, the pain at the pit of the stomach increases and the respiration becomes more oppressed; the pain frequently moves over the ribs to the back; feet cold; features pale, œdematous around the eye; sleep restless and dreamy; skin dry. The patient suffered on as long as she was able to work, but as the sufferings increased, she felt obliged to take to her bed, Dec. 2, 1869. Cured by three doses of **Kali carbonicum 200.**—(Dr. Schelling in "**Am. Jour. of Hom. Mat. Med., vol iv.**")

KALI CHLORICUM.

It is the chlorate of potash and is used in the old school as an antiseptic wash in aphthous mouth and foul ulcers. It is a strong poison and it produces destructive degeneration in the kidneys; hence it is used in nephritis and hæmoglobinuria with albumen and blood in the urine. It is usually indicated when secretion of urine decreases in quantity and becomes highly albuminous with a great percentage of hæmatin and casts. The urine either looks black or greenish black and has got to be frequently drawn off by catheter.

Its greatest application, however, is to be found in ulcerative and follicular stomatitis. The whole mucous lining of the mouth becomes red and tumid. Even the tongue becomes full of ulcerations. These ulcers have a sort of a grayish base. Salivation becomes profuse and acid. Submaxillary glands become swollen red and œdematous. The effluvia from the mouth becomes highly offensive. The secretions are excessively tough and stringy. Epistaxis, difficult swallowing, incessant cough and difficu respiration are a few indications of **Kali chloricum.** All these symptoms make it an admirable remedy for the worst type of stomatitis and diphtheria. This remedy too, has not been proved satisfactorily and hence its use is somewhat limited.

KALI CYANATUM.

This is the Cyanide of Potash. Most of our symptoms are derived from toxicological reports. The first proving was made by Dr. Lembke. This ingredient is used to a great extent in photography and cases of poisoning are not infrequent.

Kali cyan. is not an everyday remedy, but still I would like to give this remedy an important place in my Materia Medica. My indebtedness to this remedy is very great. It was about some five years ago that an elderly lady came to me with an ugly looking ulceration on her tongue. The pale worn out appearance, anæmia, exhaustion and the chronicity of the complaint had led many physicians to declare it to be a case of epithelioma of the tongue. Several preparations of Mercurius were tried, but none proved effective. At last I was led to prescribe **Kali cyan.** after coming across a cure of similar case by Petroz. The improvement was not only rapid but permanent. Within the course of a fortnight, the ulcer with all its abominable symptoms, such as dribbling from the mouth, offensive odour, occasional hæmorrhage, sharp shooting neuralgic pains in the cheek and temple of the affected side, disappeared. The lady is alive and it has not reappeared. I am sure other practitioners will be able to verify my statement. Dr. E. T. Adams has reported a similar case in an inveterate drunkard, who had a swelling on the right side of the tongue, excavated by a surgeon that left a huge ugly looking ulceration that would not heal and was pronounced cancerous. He gave her 1100 part of a grain of **Kali cyan,** once in every four days. In a fortnight the suffering was diminished and the tongue practically looked healed up. Even the pernicious cachexia disappeared and she made a complete and permanent recovery.

But the symptom that ought to have been mentioned first, as being of the greatest interest, is neuralgic pain for which it is almost a specific. This pain is particularly felt in the temporal region, sometimes between the temporal region and the ciliary arch. It may be also felt in the orbital and supramaxillary region. It is almost maddening and unbearable. Aggravation is seen after a full meal and a relief is distinctly felt by motion in the open air.

Before closing I must touch on another important characteristic and that is slow breathing. This symptom came out in almost every case of poisoning. They breathe so slowly that at times we feel that they are hardly breathing. These indications though not many are effective and useful.

KALI IODATUM.

The Iodide of Potassium or Kali hydriodicum, particularly affects the periosteum, connective tissues, the lymphatic glands, and the central substance of the nervous tissues. I have used it repeatedly in syphilitic nodes, condylomata and in tumours of the breast and the uterus. It has a tendency to bring on atrophy of the glands. It also produces infiltration and that is why we usually find œdematous swelling wherever this remedy is indicated.

Iodide of Potassium, if used continuously and long, brings on progressive wasting with voracious appetite. It is an anti-syphilitic and anti-scrofulous remedy combined in one. Rilliete carried on many interesting experiments with this drug on the healthy. A man, who was given 40 centigrammes of **Kali iod.** mixed with table salt, slowly extended over a period of two years, developed the following symptoms:—" Palpitation, melancholia with fixed ideas, great indefinable weakness, progressive atrophy and wasting." Dr. Clarke has reported a case of a gentleman of 74 who was suffering from psoriasis. This gentleman's health was in excellent condition. He consulted a homœopath, who did not do him any good, neither did he do him any damage. In desperation he went to an allopath, who gave him massive doses of **Kali iod** with the result, that within a fortnight, he lost over a stone in weight. Appetite disappeared and palpitation set in; pulse became irregular, intermittent and frequent. Although the psoriasis disappeared, the patient died shortly after. Such disastrous consequences from injudicious application of poisonous drugs are not uncommon in the opposite school of treatment. I know of another instance where after suppression of a similar skin disease by some external medication, the patient lost appetite so completely, that he dwindled to almost nothing, till at last the release came in the shape of death.

Now about a few characteristic indications of **Kali iod.** The symptom, that in my opinion ought to be given the first place, is extreme sensitiveness of the parts affected. It is not a localized sensitiveness as is seen in boils and ulcerations. The whole surface is tender; slightest touch and pressure cause pain, which is more or less diffused over the whole area. Dr. Clarke in his Dictionary reports of a case of supra-orbital neuralgia that he cured with **Kali iod,** simply on the indication of a diffused soreness over the whole head that accompanied the paroxysm of the neuralgic pain.

Secondly the constitution for which **Kali iod.** is especially effective has a mercurio-syphilitic taint. It works marvellously in patients who after an attack of syphilis had been over-dosed with mercury. Buboes, chancres, deep-seating ulcerations, bone swellings, nocturnal bone pains, falling out of hair, enlarged glands, gout, rheumatism, and emaciation all point to a mercurial history superadded to syphilitic constitution. Such cases, therefore, come well under the influence of **Kali iod.**

Aggravations and ameliorations are very well marked and peculiar and should be carefully considered as they constitute the third differentiating feature of our remedy. Like all syphilitic patients we see a nocturnal aggravation from sun-set to sun-rise. This we find in all affections where **Kali iod.** will be needed. Aggravation from touch has already been mentioned. Another prominent aggravation is to be seen by a drink of cold milk. Like all other Kali preparations we also notice a marked aggravation after coitus. Needless to say that these patients are as sensitive to atmospheric changes as **Hep. sulph., Bell, Merc.** etc.

Fourthly, discharges from all the mucous surfaces are ichorous, corrosive and green. We find this symptom in ozena, otorrhœa, ophthalmia, and in various other complaints, where there is a discharge from any of the orifices of the human body.

Now as to the constitution of the **Kali iod.** patient; it is generally suited to pale, delicate subjects with a tendency to flatulent distention, depression of spirit and a pronounced emaciation with progressive weakness. We also think of it in children. with big heads, emaciated limbs and big teeth. These youngsters generally cannot bear any jerk or jolting, not because of any definite lesion in any of the limbs, but on account of a general sense of tenderness which has been previously described as a diffused sensitiveness, not confined to any particular limb or organ. A few doses of **Kali iod,** which is a great constitutional remedy with us, will very often rectify the constitutional dyscrasia and lead to a general amelioration of all his ailments.

Mentally these patients are very irritable and harsh. They are very passionate and spiteful with an inclination towards sadness and weeping. They suffer from very strong lancinating hammering headache, due to the congestion of the brain, the result generally of a suppression of a long-standing nasal discharge. Sometimes lachrymation is associated with this headache. As has been mentioned before, these headaches are mostly syphilitic or mercurial in their origin. Very often **Kali iodatum** headaches are more external than internal, due probably to the action of the drug on the aponeuroses of the occipito-frontalis muscles. Sometimes it is a periosteal headache, with great deal of heat in the skull. In this connection I should mention that **Kali iod.** is a splendid remedy for acute and chronic hydrocephalus, especially when there is a history of hereditary syphilis and mercurial infection. As I have mentioned before, it is a great remedy for effusion and infiltration. This may happen not only in the cellular tissues but in brain substances as well. In acute hydrocephalus, it should be prescribed where there are strabismus, elaborate respiration, convulsions, paralysis and dilatation of the pupils with automatic movements of the limbs.

Iodide of Potassium causes great coryza or catarrh with great tendency to catch cold on the slightest exposure. We notice repeated attacks of a violent acrid coryza from least exposure with violent sneezing, bloated eyelids and profuse lachrymation. This catarrhal inflammation gradually spreads to the Schneiderian membrane which thus becomes a potent factor in the chronicity of the complaint. Red swollen nose with continual secretion of a watery colourless acrid fluid, violent and painful sneezing, swelling of the eyelids, injected conjunctiva, hammering pain in the head with sensation, as if it has become enormous in size and coated tongue are symptoms that will naturally follow. This discharge, instead of subsiding, as it does in an ordinary cold, gradually becomes purulent and the watery colourless fluid gradually turns into yellowish greenish matter of foul disgusting smell. In such cases, it is the taint that we have got to combat, rather than the acute symptoms of the trouble and this can be best done by the administration of a constitutional remedy like **Kali iod.**

In affections of the eyes, **Kali iod.** is called for principally in syphilitic iritis with a history of abuse of mercury. We think of this remedy, especially where the inflammation is very severe and due to the violence of the inflammatory process, the pupils inspite of repeated administration of atropine, contract to a pi point. Chemosis, œdema of the lids with lachrymation, purulent secretion and injection of the conjunctivæ and periosteal pain of the orbit, are symptoms generally found accompanying iritis.

Dr. Farrington speaks of Iodide of Potassium very highly in pneumonia but the indications given by him are far from satisfactory. He advised us to prescribe this remedy where the symptoms do not call for **Bryo., Phos.** and **Sulph.** This is indeed not a very sure principle to go by. The other indication, given by him, that of extensive hepatization, leading to cerebral congestion with effusion, is more to be depended on. Red face, dilated pupils, drowsiness, heavy breathing and want of reaction of light on the pupils, though pointing to **Bell.,** when secondary to extensive hepatization and due to serious serous effusion into the brain, will be better met by **Kali iod.** The homœopath that prescribes on symptoms without a proper understanding of their real import, is likely to fall into blind pit holes. It will always pay us to think, contemplate and to try to understand, patients as well as symptoms, rather than rush blindly and prescribe on the first bunch of symptoms that we encounter on our first inspection of the patient.

After most of the pneumonic symptoms have disappeared, we sometimes have a peculiar harassing cough to deal with——a cough that is sometimes dry but oftentimes accompanied with profuse expectoration of copious green sputum. This mucus or purulent matter, whatever it may be, is frothy and has the appearance of soapsuds. It keeps on coming in endless quantity from deep down the chest and is accompanied by a sharp stitching pain through the sternum to the back, same as in **Kali carb.** With this we have exhausting nightsweats and a general prostration. Unless things are rectified soon, there is every danger of our patient running into phthisis. A few doses of **Kali iod.** at this stage are invaluable. **Stann.** and **Sang.** are two other remedies that may be needed in similar a condition. In all these three remedies, the expectoration is copious; with **Stann.** and **Kali iod.,** it is greenish. In **Sang.** on the other hand, it is frothy, sanguinous and fluid. The taste of the sputum too, differs in all these remedies. In **Sang.** it is fetid; in **Stannum** it is sweetish and in **Kali iod.** it is salty.

Kali iod. is marvellously successful in removing tinnitus aurium. There is a sharp, shrill, hissing sound. Some little while ago a gentleman, holding a very high place in the diplomatic service of our Government, came to me almost distracted, with continual singing and hissing in his ears. Various remedies such as

Bell., Caust., China, Graph., were tried but with no appreciable result. **Kali iod.** finally gave him great relief and it was prescribed on basis of the patient's mercurio syphilitic constitution and a lot of bone pains to which he was a constant subject. We have **Kali sulph.** and **Nit. acid** for noises in the ear when chewing. We think of **Kreos.** for noises before menses; of **Ferr., Petr.,** and **Verat.** during menses; of **Dulc.** when the noises, which are mostly of buzzing character, come on at night time. **Caust., Lycop., Phos.,** and **Sepia** are remedies for echoes and re-echoes. They hear their own voice echoing and re-echoing.

Let us now discuss the indications of **Kali iod** in diseases of the sexual system of the males and the females. As has been repeated so often, it is used with great success in syphilis. It abounds in gummatous tumours involving the nervous tissues Chancres are deep and hard edged. There is a curdy cheesy deposit at the bottom of these deep-eating ulcers. The discharges are offensive, corrosive, ichorous and greenish. Sometimes, if long neglected, these chancres become almost gangrenous. **Kali iod** also has obstinate vegetative growths on glans penis same as in **Thuja.**

Great confusion generally prevails as to the indications of **Aurum met., Cinnab., Hep. sulph., Merc., Nit. acid** and **Kali. iod.** in syphilis. Hence a short summary of the indications of all these remedies will be useful. It unfortunately is a complaint so prevalent now-a-days that it will be advisable for every homœopath to be well posted on this subject.

Aurum met. is generally applicable in secondary syphilis where there has been a great abuse of Mercury. The most prominent and characteristic symptom of this remedy, is boring pain in the mastoid process. The nasal bones and some of the bones near about are the ones mostly affected. Nodes on the bones and the skull, cerebral or meningeal tumours of syphilitic nature with excruciating headaches, caries of the palate and other flat bones, offensive and putrid smell in the mouth and great melancholia are the characteristic indications of **Aurum met.**

Cinnab. our next remedy, is very valuable in syphilis when complicated with gonorrhœa. The chancres are hard with elevated edges, same as in **Kali iod.,** but it lacks the sensitiveness of the latter remedy. Still, however, the patient is just as uneasy and unhappy due to his having a free discharge of pus from the urinary passage with great redness and swelling of prepuce, and violent itchiness of corona glandis.

Help. sulp. is called for, sometimes, but not as often as some of these remedies. I generally find it useful in growths and ulcerations where profuse suppuration is the predominant feature and where the constitution is a mercurio-syphilitic one.

Mercurius and many of the preparations of Merc. have been, from time immemorial, regarded as a great antidote for syphilis. They are needed only when the indications are present. We do not, like our brethren of the other school, use our remedies as buckshorts. Each has got to be individually selected on proper indications.

Merc. dulc. is used mostly in the syphilis of the females where there are many condylomatous growths in and around the external genitals, perineum and anus.

Merc. cor. becomes useful in phagedenic chancers with lardaceous bottoms. Extensive ulceration in the mouth, gums and throat, fetid breath, profuse salivation, enlarged tonsils, tendency towards the swelling of other glands, and broad indented tongue call for the above remedy.

Merc. sol. is a remedy that I have used oftener than any other remedy, with great success, in cases where chancers are red and which spread inward, with a great tendency for bleeding. Inverted edges and yellowish fetid discharge are guiding.

Merc. iod. rub. has been found useful in syphilis, with a soreness of the bones of the face and a great unhealthiness of the glandular and cerebral tissues of the body.

Nit. acid is a great standby with the homœopath, for those types of syphilitic ulcerations that spread more in circumference than in depth. The pain is of the stinging character; it feels like so many splinters hurting him all the time. Great tendency for bleeding, exuberant granulations, irregular edges, condylomatous and cauliflower-like growths on thin pedicles and the peculiar sites of its affections (the junction of the skin and mucous membrane) are all characteristic of **Nit. acid.**

On the female sexual organs, it has been used both in tumours of the breast as well as in atrophy of the mammæ. Scabby eruption on labia, corrosive leuchorrhœa, severe burning and tearing pain in the ovarian region, and dysmenorrhœa with constant urging to urinate, are symptoms to be carefully remembered.

Even fibroid tumours of the uterus have been known to be cured with **Kali iod.** This sounds almost absurd to our allopathic friends. They cannot conceive how a growth, sometimes as big as the head of a small child, can disappear with the infinte small

dose of the homœopathic medicine that neither tastes nor smells
and that, when wrongly applied, does not, like their poisonous
drugs cause death, torture and suffering.   I have cured several
cases of fibroid tumors of the uterus with the minimum doses of
the indicated remedy. Here is another case reported by Dr.
Cooper, of a fibroid tumour cured with **Kali iod.** " Mrs.—æt 30.—
womb packed with fibroids, pain in the right inguinal
region on exertion, spirit depressed, tinnitus, like buzzing of flies, constantly tired, sleepy feeling down the limbs, hot
burning feet, though sometimes intense shivering all over, pains
in the breasts, which are tender, unable to go long without food,
constant distension as from flatus, sinking at scrobiculus cordis
at 11 a.m., sleep dreamy—all these symptoms moved away under
Kali iod. 30 leaving the patient in absolute comfort."

KALI MURIATICUM.

Kali muriaticum is Chloride of Potassium as distinguished
from **Kali chloricum** which is chlorate of potassium. Its application is confined to catarrhal affections and subacute inflammatory
stages giving rise to fibrinous exudations. These exudations are
sticky and they cause swelling of the interstitial connective tissues, due to resulting infiltrations. It is simply on account of
this property of **Kali mur.** that we use it in dysentery, diphtheria,
laryngeal croup and croupous pneumonia, when acute infiltrations
are suspected.   It causes diminution of secretion and hence a
gradual going down of the swelling. It is particularly useful in
acute and chronic rheumatism, with deformities, due to hard
scorbutic infiltrations of subcutaneous tissues. It may even be
thought of in peritonitis, pleuritis and præcorditis, while present
ing the same features.   The great keynote of **Kali mur.** is there
fore whiteness, as these secretions, referred to before, are
generally of a white color. The tongue is coated white. Even the
eruptions, pustules, and pimples discharge a whitish mattery substance. We should think of **Kali mur.** in vesicular complaints
when the contents of these vesicles are of a white fibrinous nature
     The conditions and symptoms, most frequently marked in
Kali mur., arise from its peculiar affinity for the middle ear and
Eustachian tube, where it sets up chronic catarrhal inflammation
We have noise in the ears. It is particularly useful in deaf
ness due to swelling of the internal ear and Eustachian tube an
the tympanic cavity. It is equally applicable in earache when

such is found to be associated with white furred tongue, swelling of glands and cracking noise in the ears when swallowing.

Kali mur. is also a remedy for indigestion, due to portal congestion and enlargement of the liver. There is always aggravation from fatty food and pastries. The presence of the white or grayish coated tongue, frequent diarrhœa from rich food and the light-coloured evacuations remind one of **Pulsatilla** but the similarity does not carry very far.

KALI NITRICUM.

It is Nitrate of Potassium. In common language it is called saltpetre. This is a permanent salt occurring in colorless, transparent, six-sided rhombic crystals or in crystalline powder. It is odorless with a cooling, pungent taste. It is a gentle diuretic and diaphoretic. A special therapeutic application of saltpetre in the old school is the inhalation, for the relief of spasmodic asthma, of the fumes arising from its combustion. It is also used as a preservative of meat and other articles.

Extensive provings have been made by homœopaths and we have a nice lot of symptoms to go by. In the first place, the pains of this remedy are stitching in character, of the type found in **Bryonia** and **Kali carb.** Such pains may be felt anywhere, and wherever found, they generally tend to impede respiration. On this indication it may be used in pleurisy, as well as pneumonia. Its indications in the above complaints are severe cough with shortness of breath, expectoration of blood, red or turbid urine and great and constant thirst. A very great symptom here, as well as in asthma, is a peculiar dyspnœa that prevents the patient from drinking, as drinking brings on suffocation. If he is at all able to drink, he takes in small sips, so as not to bring on an interruption in breathing. This oppression of chest is considered an important landmark of the remedy.

Another symptom particularly characteristic of **Kali nitricum** is the ink black flow of menses. A third symptom worth remembering is the aggravation of all his symptoms from eating veal, wine and beer.

KALI PHOSPHORICUM.

The phosphate of potash is one of the most important amongst the twelve tissue remedies introduced by Schussler. It has been used very extensively and has been lauded universally It is generally adaptable to cases, showing a great want of nerve power. All the nerve cells are in a state of depletion. This total bankruptcy of vitality belies a true state of adynamia. It may be the result of exhaustion of the nerve cells or a general anæmia or leukæmia caused by long lasting mental depression. Extreme sensitiveness is particularly characteristic of **Kali phos.** He starts on being touched ever so lightly or at some sudden noise as from banging of the doors.

KALI SULPHURICUM.

It is the sulphate of potash and is one of Schussler's famous twelve tissue remedies. It is found in the cells of the human body and its action is to transfer inhaled oxygen to all the cells. A lack of this substance gives rise to extensive disquamation of the cells of the epidermis and epithelium and a catarrh with a secretion of yellow mucus. These two symptoms have come out very prominent in our proving and we may consider them two principal indications of **Kali sulph.** The tongue furnishes the third characteristic point of our remedy. It is always coated with yellow mucus and is covered with yellow slimy secretion. The pain of **Kali sulph,** which is migratory, supplies the fourth keynote symptom. The modality which is particularly striking should be carefully remembered. Everywhere under this remedy, we find a general aggravation from warmth and amelioration from open air. It has been very aptly described as **Schussler's Pulsatilla** as all the symptoms mentioned above are to be seen in **Pulsatilla** as well.

KALMIA LATIFOLIA.

This is the mountain laurel, an ever-green shrub found on rocky hills. It belongs to the natural order of Ericaceæ. It is specially adapted to people of rheumatic and gouty diathesis with tendency to metastasis to the heart.

The pains of **Kalmia** are intense. They are sticking, darting and pressing in nature. They change place suddenly as in **Lac caninum, Pulsatilla, Magnesia phos., Kali sulph.** and **Phytolacca.** The pain shoots in a downward direction; a further characteristic is a sensation of numbness felt in the affected part. It thus simulates **Aconite, Chamomilla** and **Platinum.**

We use this remedy in hypertrophy of the heart and valvular insufficiency. The heart's action is tumultuous, rapid and feeble. Dyspnœa and anguish are extreme. The patient is propped up in bed. He complains of a very sharp pain in the heart, a pain that pretty nearly takes his breath away and shoots down into the abdomen and the stomach.

Kalmia is particularly useful in heart disease, following an attack of rheumatism or sometimes alternating with it. As in **Digitalis** and **Apocynum,** there is also a remarkable slowness of pulse—sometimes coming as low as 40 beats per minute. Great palpitation is complained of and it is felt even in the throat. It gets worse leaning forward. The patient trembles all over. With the palpitation there is constriction of the throat as well.

Kalmia is a great remedy for neuralgia in general. We find it almost everywhere. It is useful in prosopalgia, especially when affecting the right side. This pain, starting after an exposure to cold, extends over the head, ear and face and then goes down to the arm. The pain is either accompanied with or succeeded by numbness in the affected parts. It occurs at irregular times and then shoots in a downward direction.

It is particularly serviceable in neuralgic and rheumatic pains in the eyes and the eye-balls. The pain is so severe that it becomes almost an agony to turn the eye-ball. There is a stiff, drawing sensation everytime he moves his eyes.

We think of **Kalmia** in rheumatic fevers. Almost all the muscles of the body are affected. The fever is high. Every attempt to move is attended by excruciating pain. Urine when analysed shows presence of albumen.

KAVA-KAVA.

(*See* **Piper methysticum**)

KRAMERIA.

(*See* **Ratanhia**)

KREOSOTUM.

Kreosotum another indispensable remedy is a product of distillation of wood tar. It affects the mucous membrane very powerfully, specially that of the sexual system of the females, as we shall find presently. Its keynote feature is corrosiveness. This is seen in the various discharge of the body. Leucorrhœa is putrid, acrid and corrosive. Menstrual blood has also a similar characteristic. It produces corrosive itching in vulva. The urine smarts and burns the pudenda. Similarly the discharges from the ear, nose, eye and throat are excoriating in their nature.

The fluids and secretion of the human body, undergo rapid decomposition in **Kreosote,** and that is why all the discharges of this remedy become extremely offensive and fetid. The otorrhœal discharge from the ear, the catarrhal discharge from the nose, the stools, the urine and the leucorrhœal discharge are not only corrosive but putrid as well. It is on account of this tendency to decomposition that **Kreosote** becomes such an excellent remedy in carbuncles, carcinoma and other forms and varieties of gangrenous, cancerous and putrefying ulcers. This destructive tendency is also substantiated by carious decay of the tooth—a feature most common in **Kreosote.** The teeth show dark specks and begin to decay as soon as they appear. The gums show an equally bad condition. They are spongy, soft, bluish, ulcerated and scorbutic. They bleed very easily and are generally infiltrated with dark, watery fluid. After extraction of teeth, we notice persistent oozing of dark, slightly coagulated blood. The taste in the mouth, as can be easily imagined, is putrid.

Its action on the kidney is well-marked. It is one of our grand remedies for incontinence of urine. The urging is so great that the patient cannot get out of bed at night quick enough. The urine is chestnut brown, fetid, alkaline and deposits a white sediment. It is a first class remedy for nocturnal enuresis of children. They wet the bed during the first sleep from which they are roused with difficulty. They frequently dream that they are passing urine in the proper place but they wake up, alas, to find out that it has been done in the most incompatible manner and in the most improper place.

The organ where its action is most marked is the uterus. We use it in chronic ovarian affection, in ulcers on the neck of the uterus, in cauliflower excrescences around and on the uterus, in menorrhagia and in leucorrhœa. It is particularly efficacious in uterine affection of middle-aged women who have passed clim,xis. It has cured inveterate cases of ulceration of the neck of the uterus with long-lasting-fetid leucorrhœa or frequently occurring uterine hemorrhage, causing much burning and eruption on the parts. On such symptoms **Kreosote** has been beneficially used in cases of cancer of the uterus. In fatal cases where cure is not possible, its administration brings great relief to suffering and ease to the patient. The patient complains of a sensation of pressure towards genitals. Constant burning pain in small of back; leucorrhœa, bland to start with but finally becoming acrid, ichorous, bloody and pungent; severe pain during coition; dwindling and falling away of mammæ; general aggravation during menstruation; heat and puffiness in the vagina are infallible indications of **Kreosotum.** The putrid, acrid, corrosive leucorrhœa stains clothing yellow and stiffens them like starch. The smell of this vaginal discharge is peculiar inasmuch as it has the odor of green corn. This discharge sets up a kind of voluptuous itching deep in vagina; even external genitals look swollen, hot and hard.

It is one of our hemorrhagic remedies. Small wounds bleed freely and easily, but the flow is passive. We use it for the persistent oozing of dark slightly coagulated blood after extraction of the teeth. We use it in metrorrhagia when the blood is dark, offensive, clotted, and the flow continues for weeks causing fainting and collapse.

It is an important remedy in gastromalacia, gastritis and cancer of the stomach. The patient vomits large quantities of undigested food taken throughout the day of a sweetish taste. There is a sensation of a painful hard spot in the stomach. Other symptoms are rapid emaciation of the neck and the face, intense thirst, bloated sensation in the region of the stomach, offensive whitish grey or chopped stools, hiccough, belching, sunken eyes, coldness of hands and feet and drowsiness. The appetite is keen but drinking brings on vomiting.

Case 1.—Mrs. L., aged thirty-five, feeble, prosopalgia, mostly confined to right side; at times extending to left side and whole of chest and to all parts of the body and extremities; pains of burning or smarting character. sometimes twitching or lancinating or pricking, as if pins were being thrust into the parts; feeling, at times, as if wind were blowing on affected side of the head, sometimes as if cold water were dropping; trembling of extremities; feeling of coldness of entire body from the least exposure, as from lifting the bed clothes; feet and legs cold to the knees; short and quick breathing on the least muscular exertion; much of the time a cold perspiration on the body; twitching, starting and moaning in sleep; very tired and languid, can scarcely stand alone; sunken, dark appearance about the right eye; no appetite; pains aggravated at night during motion, by bathing affected parts; by application of heat and taking either warm or cold things in the mouth. **Kreos. 200** cured.—Dr. F. W. Payne.

Case 2.—Patient a ruddy blonde, tall, full habit, æt. twenty-two, un-married. Has always suffered much at the menstrual period, and for many years, has been troubled with profuse leucorrhœa. Menses too early, profuse and long-lasting, color dark, with very fetid odor: marked nausea and prostra-tion during first two days, with heavy pains through the uterus and coccyx; leucorrhœa of a yellow white color; quite thick, very foul odor, and just before menses. **Cal. carb,** was given with benefit; after more thorough study of the case, **Kreos.** 30th was prescribed on January 4. Patient reported on the 30th of the month. Menses still early and profuse, but some decrease of nausea and bad odor. Ordered no medicine to be taken, until within ten days of next menstrual period, the same drug to be then resumed. Report-ed February 21. Menses three days early, decrease of quantity of pain and odor. Prescribed **Kreos.** 200, to be taken every other day through the month. Patient reported again in March. Menses one day early, little pain, no nausea, bad odor almost gone. **Kreos. 500,** one per week. Reported May 1. Menses normal, but still no change in leucorrhœa, which troubled her very much. For this condition **Aralia rac.** was given, with most grati-fying results; the patient having now been perfectly free from all menstrual and uterine disorder for many months.—Dr. May Howells.

LAC CANINUM.

Here is one more of the homœopath's indispensable remedies. It is prepared from the dog's milk. It has a few very characteristic symptoms that should be carefully studied. The grand keynote of this remedy is found in its mental symptoms. The patient is very forgetful. Sometimes his mind becomes a total blank; he buys things in the market and walks away without them. He omits letter or letters of a word when writing. While speak-ing, he unconsciously and inadvertently substitutes objects seen instead of objects thought of. This is due to absent-mindedness. With him concentration of mind is difficult. In this respect it can be compared favourably with **Acid phos, Anacardium, Baryta carb,**

Can. indica, Glon., Lycopodium, Medor. and Thuja. Of course all these remedies have peculiarities of their own and differentiation should be mainly based on individual characteristic.

Acid phos. like Nat. phos. and Caladium has marked forgetfulness after sexual excesses.

In Anacardium the forgetfulness is to be accounted for by excessive mental exertions; also in this remedy the forgetfulness is most marked in the morning hours.

Baryta carb. is indicated in forgetfulness of old people where age has taken the keenness of all mental faculties.

Can. ind. is so utterly forgetful that he has to stop while speaking because of his forgetfulness.

In Glonoine, forgetfulness renders the patient ludicrous. He forgets the name of well-known streets, the number and the location of his own house, although he has been living in same for years.

Medor. forgets even his own name. Symptoms like these may seem ludicrous to an allopath who prescribes on generalisations, but to a homœopath, taking detail of each minute occurrence, these symptoms will be of immense benefit. In Thuja as in Kali bich., the patient becomes very forgetful, specially after waking up from sleep As time elapses, his memory gradually dawns on him.

We also find him suffering from a chronic blue condition He loses interest in everything. World seems to him too dark and cheerless a place to live in. Destitute of hope and ambition, he becomes very irritable and cross. Very often he fears as if he is becoming insane.

Another peculiar mental condition of Lac caninum is found in a strange delusion about snakes. He imagines as if he is surrounded by snakes. He falls asleep thinking of snakes; during sleep dreams of snakes and wakes up from sleep in fright as if about to be beaten by snakes. Another symptom that this remedy is credited with, consists of a peculiar state of mind in which he thinks that he is wearing someone else's nose. This is not all. We find him possessed of a few other absurd notions. He feels as if he is too light and as though walking through the air without his feet touching the ground. While lying down his body does not seem to be touching the bed.

The next characteristic of Lac caninum, is to be found in its changeability. In rheumatism the pain and the swelling keep on changing the location every few hours or days. In diarrhœa the stools are not the same every time. In sore throat, tonsillitis, diphtheria, the same changing of sides is noticeable. I remember having cured with **Lac caninum** scrofulous swellings of the axillary glands that used to alternate sides very frequently.

Its chief sphere of action is found in affections of the throat. In diphtheria the membranes leave one side and go to the other side alternately. Pains too repeatedly shift from side to side and shoot into the ear on each attempt at swallowing. Inspite of this difficulty he feels like swallowing all the time. The breath smells horribly. Profuse salivation, external sensitiveness of the throat as in **Lachesis**, a shining glazed appearance of the fauces and of the diphtheritic deposits, are all additional indications. One nostril feels quite stopped up, while the other keeps free and discharging. Dr. Nash cites two cases of tonsillitis in one house that were put under the two opposite systems of treatment, allopathic and homœopathic. He cured one case with **Lac caninum** on this great symptom of constant changeability of sides, in such a short time, that on the same evening of the prescription, when he visited the patient, he found her taking oyster broth. The other case under expert allopathic treatment progressed on to suppuration and took a week longer in getting round.

The other important indications of this remedy are the following :—

Great sinking feeling in the epigastrium and faintness in the stomach. Inflammation of the breast worse from the least jar and movement, so she holds it fast and firmly while moving, to prevent the jar from reaching them. Intense, unbearable backache felt more in the supersacral region. Like **Rhus tox** this backache is worse from rest and on first moving. In fact, the whole spine becomes painful from coccyx to the base of the brain and is very sensitive to touch and pressure.

Violent palpitation while lying on the left side, better lying on the right side. While lying down, she feels as if her breath would leave her and she has to get up and walk about.

———

LAC VACCINUM DEFLORATUM.

This remedy owes its origin to Dr. Swan who in his turn got the idea of potentizing skimmed milk upon reading "Donkin's Skimmed Milk Treatment of Diabetes and Bright's Disease." The patient feels completely tired and worn out. Great fatigue is felt from the slightest exertion; hence there is a marked disinclination to exertion of any kind. It also has a marked effect over the secretion of the milk which it diminishes to a great extent; hence it is used in cases of deficient milk secretion in young mothers which it restores in an incredibly short period by virtue of the principle of Similia Similibus Curantur.

It is a noted remedy for sick headache. The pain is first felt in the forehead from which place it extends to the occiput. The pain is most excruciating and unbearable and is associated with intense photophobia, nausea and vomiting. It is aggravated by movement and is relieved by frequent and profuse urination. The pain is also periodical in its nature and it frequently occurs in patients who have a tendency to constipation. Menstrual time is also a critical time with these patients inasmuch as that this headache occurs mostly at that time. Due to great anæmia, these patients are constantly chilly even when near the fire. Nausea is almost as characteristic of **Lac deflo.** as it is of **Ipecac.** It is intense and can be aptly described as a deathly nausea. The patient first brings up undigested food of intense acid taste and then a brownish fluid which looks very much like coffee ground. The constipation, already referred to, is an inveterate constipation. It is intensely chronic and is associated with headache, as has been said before. We use it in cases where the most powerful purgative fails. The fæces are dry and hard and large and it lacerates anus extracting cries as well as a considerable amount of blood. In this way it is greatly alike **Sulphur.**

It has a certain amount of influence on the female sexual system. It is useful in restoring the menstrual flow after it has stopped, due to the patient having put her hand in cold water. It relieves the consequent congestion of blood to head and the pressing, bearing pain in the ovaries.

LAC FELINUM.

There is no limit to the great possibility of expansion of the Homœopathic Materia Medica. The entire organic and inorganic kingdom, all conceivable objects, must have in them great potentialities which, when properly utilized, may develop into great remedial agencies. We have one such instance in **Lac felinum.** Like milk from many other animal, the cat's milk too has been brought into prominence by Dr. Swan who conducted elaborate provings with it. Personally speaking, I have had no opportunity to verify his experiences about **Lac felinum** but then that should be no reason why this remedy should be left out of this Materia Medica.

Most of its symptoms, at least important ones, are located in the head and the eyes. The headache is terrible and it penetrates the left eye-ball to the centre of the brain. The pain is acutely felt on the vertex as well. A sensation of constriction along the bridge of the nose is prominent. One of the provers felt her head drawn down so that the chin pressed heavily on the chest and in her agony which was great, she rushed from room to room screaming and holding her head firmly in her hands. We also have pain in the eyes and a sensation, as if the eyes were drawn back. It thus makes an important remedy in ciliary neuralgia. The indications are sharp lancinating pains in the centre of the left eye-ball, extending externally to the temple and frontal region over the eye, with intense photophobia, redness of the conjunctiva, and lachrymation. The symptom on which most stress is laid, is that the pain appears to be in the interior of the eye-ball and thence extends backwards as well as to the temple and forehead. Dr. Berridge used it with great success in a case of keratitis, where the pain was so excessive for three nights and days, that the patient did not have a wink of sleep, and the pain felt like a knife running from the affected left eye to the left occiput. **Lac felinm** 40m potency every hour not only relieved the pain but brought on a steady recovery. In this respect it may very well be compared with **Mercurius, Ruta** and **Spigelia.**

LACHESIS.

This medicine is prepared from the virus of surukuke, the deadly bushmaster of South America. It grows to a length of about seven feet and more; the fangs are nearly an inch in length. The skin is reddish brown, marked along the back with large rhomboidal spots of a blackish color. The poison is inodorous, tasteless and somewhat greenish white in color. This medicine was first proved by Dr. Constantine Hering at great risk to his life. It has some very grand characteristics and I will discuss them in order of their importance.

The first and the foremost key-note of **Lachesis** is the aggravation of all troubles from sleep. We find this in headache, diphtheria, heart affections, laryngitis, peritonitis, pyemia and many other affections where **Lachesis** is indicated.

Selenium, Spongia, Stramonium and **Sulphur** are a few more with a similar modality. I remember the case of a young gentleman who wanted to be treated for a severe pain in his heart, that always used to bother him while falling asleep. He told me the pain was so severe and the fright so great that he used to sit up night after night, to be free from this pain. A dose of **Lachesis** 200 cured him permanently.

It is difficult to explain this aggravation of **Lachesis.** It may be partly due to its action on the pneumo-gastric nerve or partly to its influence on the centres of respiration. Whatever may be the true reason, the fact remains. As we are concerned with facts alone, we leave it to the students of science to speculate, investigate and verify deductions arrived at by themselves as to the real essence of these symptoms. We are glad to be satisfied with symptoms that are always our guide, our sole guide and the only guide.

Next in importance, is the great sensitiveness of the surface of the body with intolerance of touch and light pressure. They cannot stand hard and tight collars on the neck. They dislike tight bandage on their waist. Dr. Hering, who first proved this drug and as a result of which, he became delirious and unconscious, could never tolerate hard and tight collars about his neck all throughout his life. So great is this sensitiveness that **Lachesis** patients even dislike the weight of bedclothes on them; hard pressure and rubbing they do not mind so much.

The third point is, that it is a left-sided remedy. It principally affects the left side of the body. We cannot advance any explanation for this phenomenon but it is a fact just the same and we have to accept it.

The fourth point about **Lachesis** is the amelioration of all its symptoms from the onset of a discharge. The suppression or non-appearance of discharge always makes **Lachesis** patients worse. This is what makes **Lachesis** such an admirable remedy in climacteric ailments. When the period stops, all kinds and sorts of troubles make their appearance such as hot flushes, headache, mania, etc.

Lachesis, although it may be indicated anywhere and when indicated should be prescribed for all types of conditions and constitutions, is adapted to thin emaciated persons or to those who have changed physically and mentally through their illness. These patients are generally choleric in their temperament and have a vivid imagination. Their complexion is generally of a sickly hue. This remedy is particularly suited to drunkards, who suffer from bad head and hemorrhoids and are prone to erysipelatoid inflammations.

The mental side of the **Lachesis** patient is no less striking. His mind is so full of ideas that he jumps from subject to subject. Ideas flow very rapidly in his head and he goes chatting about them. In this it is similar to **Agaricus, Mephitis, Actea, Paris, Hyoscyamus, Caladium, Teucrium, Cannabis indica, Lachnanthes** and **Podophyllum.** This excess of imagination prevents sleep at night.

The **Lachesis** mentality as has been mentioned before, is characterized by a spirit of suspiciousness. He suspects everyone around him—servants, wife and children are no exceptions. Even the poor doctor attending on him, is looked upon with dread. He will not take medicine from anybody thinking that they would poison him. He is afraid to taste even his food as he believes that to be merely a bet for his destruction. At times, this suspicion takes the form of fear and he imagines as being followed by enemies. He would run in desperate anxiety, to escape them. There is, indeed, no limit to which he would not go and unless good precautions are taken, he would throw himself out of the window. He gets the most absurd ideas into his head. He imagines himself to be dead and believes everybody about him making preparations for his funeral. Like **Nat mur.,** we find him, at times, believing in robbers being in the house whom he would try to avoid by jumping out of his window.

Lachesis patient is subject to insane jealously. He suspects the fidelity of his wife. I remember treating a case of puerperal insanity in a lady whose entire mental phenomena revolved round one idea of her husband being faithless to her. **Lachesis** cured the case. In this respect it resembles **Apis, Hyoscyamus** and **Pulsatilla.** Another peculiarity of the mental state consists in the derangement of the time-sense. They confound morning with evening, night with day and so on.

The delirium of **Lachesis** is mostly of a muttering type like that of **Rhus tox.** The face is red and the patient is drowsy to a certain extent. Either we notice a great talkativeness with frequent changing of subjects or a slow difficult speech accompanied with the dropping of the jaw. He sings, whistles and makes odd motions with his arms.

The patient is tormented with a morbid state of conscientiousness. It takes the form of religious mania. He dreads society and is quite solicitous about his future. At times he feels as if he is in the hand of a superior power and has been charmed into doing things which he would hate to do and is anxious to break away from this spell.

These symptoms show that **Lachesis** may be an invaluable remedy in the severer forms of typhoid fever and other diseases of a typhoid type. The facial expression is one of anxiety and confusion. It looks red, swollen and puffy as after a debauch; there are blue rings around the eyes; cutaneous hyperesthesia is very prominent inspite of great depression of the vital force. The least touch, even when the patient is unconscious, startles him. The pressure of bedcloth on his abdomen is intolerable; inspite of his unconsciousness he manifests his dislike for the covering by constantly lifting it up with his trembling hands. Delirium is slow and muttering. Loquacity is marked from the beginning, though at times we find him in stupor with coldness of the extremities and trembling of hands. He sleeps with his mouth open; his lower jaw drops down showing great drain in his vital force. When asked to protrude the tongue it comes out trembling or catches at the teeth. The tongue is dry black and stiff like leather. Teeth are covered with sordes. Often this condition is associated with a debilitating offensive diarrhœa. The blood that he passes shows signs of decomposition; it is black and looks like charred straw. It thus compares with **Opium, Hyoscyamus, Arnica, Apis, Mur. acid, Baptisia** and **Pyrogen.**

Opium, which indicates a condition in no way less morribund than that of **Lachesis,** should be prescribed when the reactive power is very deficient.   It is indicated by stertorous breathing and a threatened paralysis of brain due to violent, engorgement of blood in arteries, arterioles and veins of cerebellun and cerebrum. In **Lachesis** the complexion of the patient is bluish and in **Opium** it is dark red.

Hyoscyamus betrays great sensorial depression as is evidenced by trembling of limbs and twitching of muscles.   The great differentiating feature consists in the involuntary placing of the hands on the genitals.

In **Arnica** we have the dropping of the lower jaw, the stupor and the involuntary passage of stool and urine.   The condition, perhaps, is just as grave as that of **Lachesis.** The stupor may be just as profound and it may be really a difficult problem to differentiate between the two. It may be a great help to remember that ecchymotic spots are to be found specially in the latter remedy.

Apis shows more of meningeal inflammation than **Lachesis.** The sudden screams, the constant movement of the head and the constant oozing of fetid substance from the open anus are symptoms not to be found in **Lachesis.**

Muriatic acid shows a condition more desperate than that to be found in **Lachesis.** The involvement of the whole of the alimentary canal, from the mouth to the anus, as manifested by numerous ulcerations in both the orifices, the great sensitiveness to touch of the rectum, the constant sliding down from bed, the presence of numerous hæmorrhoidal knobs in the anus and the smooth, glossy tongue are conditions to be found in **Muriatic acid** alone.

Baptisia means a sensorial involvement and a toxic condition. The besotted appearance and the drowsiness, not so complete and deep as in **Lachesis,** call for **Baptisia** but generally in a condition, less precarius than what is found in **Lachesis.**

Pyrogen precedes **Lachesis** in respect of the decomposing and the disorganising process. Under both the remedies disintegration has commenced but in **Lachesis** we find the completion of what was originally started in **Pyrogen.** The tendency for hæmorrhage and the over-whelming activity of the poison are more marked in the latter remedy than in the former.

Lachesis is also very important in the treatment of malarial fevers. The chill starting from the small of the back, assumes such voilent form as to make the teeth chatter. Another peculiarity with these patients during chill, is that they want to be held tightly and pressed. "A lady wanted her daughter to lie with her full weight across her during chill: A boy wanted a sack of flour put on him to keep him from shaking." This desire for weight is not so much to keep him warm as to keep him still. In this respect it compares well with **Gelsemium.** The sweat is profuse and smells like garlic. Trembling, a mapped tongue, intolerance of pressure on the throat and chest, burning in palms and soles, internal sensation of heat with cold feet, restlessness, icy cold- ness of ears, lip and nose, shrivelling and lividity of the skin, rapid yawning and incessant sighing are some of the other symptoms to be found in conjunction with those mentioned above.

Lachesis affects circulation in a remarkable way. It causes flushing of the face due to an abnormal rush of blood to the head, coldness of the feet, palpitation of the heart and a sense of constric- tion in that organ. This sense of constriction in the heart compels him to sit up. The feeling of constriction frequently ends in a cramplike pain in the præcordial region causing palpitation and anxiety. The pain is accompanied with a choking sensation and is aggravated by the slightest exertion. He feels sick and faint and his face becomes white, till he is compelled to lie down, which restores normal action of the heart. Great dyspnœa, a sense of suffoca- tion and weight in the chest, a very fast and rapid pulse and trembl- ing are symptoms of **Lachesis** that should be carefully borne in mind. It will help us in the treatment of many varieties of aliments of that most vital of organs of the human system. **Lachesis** also helps in the atheromatous condition of arteries in old people and in induration of veins accompanying cellular inflammations. Sometimes he feels as if his heart is hanging by a thread and every beat of heart would tear it off. In this respect it is similar to **Kali carb.**

Lachesis has important urinary symptoms. It is indicated when the urine becomes dark, I may say almost black; this is due to presence of decomposed particles of blood in the urine. The urine also contains albumen. Sometimes we notice black specks or flakes floating in the urine. Other remedies presenting **black urine are Colchicum, Carbolic acid, Digitalis, Helleborus and Tere- binth.** Another peculiar symptom worth remembering is a sensation of a ball rolling loose in the bladder, specially when he turns over. This sensation of ball may occur elsewhere as throat, abdomen and other organs or cavities of the body.

Lachesis is not often required in the treatment of diarrhœa, but when indicated it becomes essential. So it would not do to neglect this aspect of the drug. We need it specially for chronic cases and for diarrhœa of drunkards and for diarrhœa during climaxis. The stools are watery, chocolate-colored and cadaverous smelling. The decomposed blood mostly looks like charred straw. The tongue too is quite peculiar. It is smooth, red and shiny. They suffer from a tormenting urging, but cannot pass anything as the anus feels closed. There is quite a bit of constriction in the rectum which makes defecation extremely painful and they have to desist in consequence. Protruding piles complicate this constriction. Each attempt at stool is followed by terrible pain in the rectum as from the beating of little hammers.

Lachesis stands very high in many complaints of the throat. We may use it for simple sorethroat, tonsillitis and diphtheria. The indications are elongation of uvula, swelling and purplish color of the fauces, sensation of a lump in throat which descends on swallowing but returns soon, excessive tenderness of throat to external pressure and constriction of throat. As a rule, the left side is affected. A peculiar indication is the difficulty of swallowing liquids specially saliva; solids can be swallowed more easily— they even relieve. Sometimes when swallowing fluids, they escape through the nose. We must not forget or overlook that in all these affections, the patient has a sensation of a foreign substance in his throat. He feels as if a crumb of bread or a morsel of food or even a piece of bone is sticking into his throat and he is relieved to a certain extent by hawking, though the feeling does not go away entirely. The pain in throat extends even to ear and is aggravated on deglutition. **Lachesis** is used in phlegmonous inflammation of throat in children or in women during climacteric years. The pain is further aggravated by hot drinks. In diphtheria we have excessive swelling of throat, internal as well as external. The unbearable fetor, the besotted appearance, the rapid pulse, the high temperature, the muttering delirium, the purplish appearance of the membrane as also of the lips, buccal cavity and throat and the affection of the submaxillary gland, indicate a serious state of affairs, but not too serious when placed under the certain curative influence of **Lachesis**. **Lachesis** also is helpful in syphilitic phagedæna of soft palate and fauces and gangrenous sore throat

Lachesis is curative in aphonia caused by paralysis or œdema of vocal chords. It is relieves the hoarseness of phthisis. The same symptoms of constriction, dryness, rawness, sensitiveness to touch and aggravation from sleep, spoken of previously, will be our guide here as well as elsewhere.

Lachesis has a dry hacking cough caused by the touching of the throat. This cough is always aggravated after sleep and is associated with a sensation as if some fluid had gone into the wrong passage. The cough is mostly dry and is raised with great difficulty. It is sympathetic to cardiac affections.

Lachesis is very useful in ulcers, carbuncles, abscesses, malignant pustules, etc. They are generally very sensitive to touch. The affected parts look bluish. Discharges are ichorous and often sive. I have used this remedy in carbuncles of the worst type. The symptom that I consider the most important in this complaint is the intense burning. They must rise at night and bathe it with water to relieve the burning. The surrounding parts are always covered with numerous small boils. Suppuration is generally tardy. **Lachesis** increases the quantity and improves the quality of matter and brings about a speedy cure.

Lachesis affects the head in a material way, causing heaviness with nausea and dizziness. The **Lachesis** headache, as has been mentioned before, is due to the stopping of some natural discharge of the body such as menses, coryza, perspiration, nose-bleed, etc. With the headache the patient wants to close the eyes. It is pressing and bursting in nature and is worse from motion, pressure, stooping and sleeping. There is pressure on the vertex as from lead. Sometimes we find this headache ushered in by debauch and excessive drinking.

Lachesis may be indicated in severer forms of brain troubles such as meningitis. It is particularly useful after suppression of exanthema. The patient experiences sharp pain in head and screams out in distress. Drowsiness, trembling palpitation of the heart and stupor gradually supervene. In the above symptoms partly resembles **Belladonna** from which it should be carefully differentiated. Though drowsiness and stupor are common to both the remedies **Belladonna** is only indicated in the initial stage of the trouble before dangerous and fatal transformations have the opportunities to take place and the vitality had not been drained to its last.

These patients are very sensitive to the heat of the sun. It makes them languid, dizzy and faint and produces congestion. In this respect **Lachesis** compares well with **Glonoin, Camphor, Belladonna, Nitric acid** and **Theridion.**

Case 1.—R. H. S., aged forty-two years. Sanguine temperament. Mother of two children, usually in good health, is subject to attacks of asthma which is somewhat hereditary. Was taken, November 2nd, with a most violent attack of spasmodic asthma; characterized by the following symptoms, viz., sharp pain through the lungs, with great dyspnœa; both pain and dyspnœa are aggravated sitting erect or by lying down, alleviated by bending forward and throwing the head back. There was a feeling of intense constriction in all parts of the chest, as if the lungs were being pressed up into the throat, causing such extreme agony that she despaired of life. These symptoms were accompained by a feeling of constriction about the neck, as though a cord was tightly tied around it. The sensation of constriction necessitated loosening the clothes at the neck and waist. At times during the paroxysms, she suffered from a sensation as though the heart turned over and ceased beating for a moment, then commenced again with increased force. Auscultation revealed numerous cracking, whistling sounds, induced by the passage of air through a tenacious, glairy mucus in the smaller bronchiæ, as was evident when the paroxysm was relieved and the mucus began to be expectorated. The lung seemed full of mucus, yet none coul be raised. The paroxysms are sometimes induced by rapid walking or by laughing. When the paroxysm was most severe, the face was so congested as to be almost purple. After administering **Ipecacuanha**, **Arsenicum**, **Cuprum** and **Hyoscyamus** with no effect, I selected **Lachesis** as the similimum to the case, and gave one dose of **Lachesis** 3000. The remedy was given about 5 p.m. of a cold cloudy, damp evening of November, in the increasing stage of a most violent paroxysm, with a fearful foreboding in the mind of the patient that she would suffer intensely through the night. In less than ten minutes I saw an evident amelioration of the symptoms. The wheezing, whistling sounds in the chest and throat began to yield. The patient gradually improved and was able to sit erect with comfort when I left. The dose was repeated after an interval of three or four hours, when the remedy was discontinued with the exception of an occasional dose for two or three weeks and no paroxysm has since appeared, though nearly ten months have elapsed.—(Dr. C. L. Hart., **Med. Investigator, April, 1874.)**

Case 2.—Young man, aged twenty-two; ankle badly injured by being caught under a large grindstone; tibia and fibula both broken, about three inches above the ankle joint; severe contusions of parts, which were also much lacerated, leaving openings to the tibia (compound fracture). Adjusted the parts, dressed and applied **Arnica**, as usual in such cases; gave **Arnica** internally. All things went well, seemingly, until the seventh day, when on entering the room, my attention was arrested by an exceedingly offensive fetor; I recognized it as an indication of gangrene, and exposure of the parts confirmed my suspicion. For some distance around the borders of the flesh, appeared bluish-purple vesicles, covering a dirty looking ash-gray ground; and it really appeared as if amputation would be forced upon me as the only rule of practice. An experienced physician, who saw it at the time with me, said as much; but I determined upon trying **Lachesis**, and gave one dose of the 6th, which acted as if by magic. In six hours, the nature of the case was entirely changed; in twenty-four, the blisters had disappeared and the swelling gone down, and two days later the dead portions sloughed off, bringing to view a healthy granulating surface

The wounds henceforth healed kindly, and in due time the cure was complete and a foot saved which, but for **Lachesis**, would, in all probability, have been sacrificed.

LACHNANTHES.

Lachnanthes is a herb that grows on the coast lands of the United States. It belongs to the natural order of Hæmodoraceæ. The tincture is prepared from the whole plant. Several nice cures are attributed to **Lachnanthes,** so it behoves us to know something about this remedy.

Head, chest and circulation are profoundly affected by **Lachnanthes.** It has headache of great intensity extending down to jaw. The pain is a splitting, bursting pain aggravated on movement of head and is associated with a disposition to keep eyes closed. Slightest noise, even that of a person walking over a carpet, terribly disturbs the patient. Its effect on circulation of blood is great indeed. In no remedy do we have such constant chilliness as in **Lachnanthes.** The patient has a sensation of a piece of ice, lying on back between shoulders, which causes him to shiver and gives him goose flesh. His whole body is icy cold, and even getting under a warm feather quilt, would not appease his chill. A hot flat-iron is the only thing that relieves the chilliness.

The occasion that first brought me into contact with this remedy was a case of intermittent fever in a young girl of about seventeen summers. The most characteristic feature about the case was icy coldness. She wanted her mother to rub her back with hot iron. This was associated with stiff neck. During the height of fever her cheeks were highly flushed and her eyes were glossy and bright. As these were sound indications of **Lachnanthes,** the remedy was prescribed and the result was a further verification of Samuel Hahnemann's principle, ' **Similia similibus curantur.'**

It is a great remedy for torticollis. The neck becomes stiff and the head gets drawn to one side. The pain in the nape of the neck is so great as to give him a sensation of dislocation. When this occurs with sore throat, it is a very strong indication for **Lachnanthes.** Another important symptom that I have omitted to mention, is a circumscribed redness of the face with an abnormal brilliance of the eyes. Loquacity of **Lachnanthes** is remarkable and in this it resembles **Lachesis** to a certain extent.

LACTIC ACID.

This corrosive acid was first discovered by Scheele in sour milk the result of spontaneous fermentation of sugar of milk under the influence of casein. It is also met with in many vegitable products which have turned sour. It was introduced into our Materia Medica by Reisig.

Lactic acid is so corrosive that it eats into every tissue of the body, not excepting the enamel of teeth. It is generally suited to thin, pale, anemic women who lose much blood at each menstrual nisus. It is a great remedy with us for diabetes mellitus, morning sickness during pregnancy and chronic osteitis. A grand characteristic of **Lactic acid** is nausea and sickness, so constant as to lead us to think of prescribing **Ipecacuanha** with which remedy it is often confused. With this nausea is associated a constant water brash with continued discharge of profuse saliva. The saliva brought up feels hot and is exceedingly sour and corrosive, so much so, that it leaves an acute burning all along the passage, from stomach to mouth, in its progress upward. On this indication I have repeatedly used it in morning sickness and with great success. A lady aged about twenty-three, primipara, was vomiting so continuously, from the time of her conception, as to be reduced to skin and bone. The only food she lived on was given per rectum. Faintness, from want of food, was a marked feature. The spitting from the mouth was continuous, lasting from the time she got up in the morning till late at night when she dozed into a faintlike sleep. Her medical attendant—an allopath was thinking of bringing on miscarriage, every available means having been exhausted. The extreme acidity of saliva, constant eructations of hot acrid fluid and canker sores in her mouth induced me to prescribe **Lactic acid.** The result was more than what the fondest hope could dream of. The vomiting stopped and it stopped so suddenly that even the patient could not believe that she was ever the subject of such serious ailment.

In diabetes its indications are evacuation of large quantities of foamy strong smelling dark urine, voracious appetite, great thirst, dry parched stickly tongue, chilliness of extremities, weariness and debility, a feeling of emptiness and sinking in stomach and distress and pain in renal region. Dr. Nash considers the concomitant of rheumatic pain with diabetes, a guiding indication

profuse sweat, rheumatic inflammation of elbows, knees and small joints of upper and lower extremities, profuse and offensive sweating of feet, nocturnal aggravation, thick white coating on the tongue, fetid metallic sour taste with nausea and epistaxis in the morning.

LACTUCA VIROSA.

Lactuca virosa is the poisonous lettuce, a plant that has a strong disagreeable smell, like that of opium and a bitterish acrid taste. There are two varieties of lactuca—the sativa and the virosa, former being the garden lettuce. The juice contains an active principle called Lactucin and is somewhat like **Opium** in its action. We notice in this remedy great sleepiness and lethargy. This irresistible drowsiness is a close bond of resemblance between **Lactuca** and **Opium.** A similar sleepiness, though not quite as pronounced as in **Lactuca virosa,** is also to be seen in **Lactuca sativa.** People after a good feed on garden lettuce are seen to be very drowsy.

The most characteristic symptom of **Lactuca,** consists in a sensation of constriction and tightness, affecting the whole body but more especially the chest. It is experienced in pit of stomach, in abdomen, in the neighbourhood of heart and also in rectum and anus. This symptom makes it an admirable remedy in angina pectoris, asthma, whooping cough, hydrothorax and in dyspepsia where such symptoms are characteristically present. Crampy stitching pain in the left chest, extending to left scapula, an indescribable tightness of the whole chest at night, obliging him to sit up with anxious suddenness and causing a feeling of terrible suffocation, lead to its indication in angina. A similar sensation, causing him to awake suddenly with pain and cough lead to its indication in asthma. The cough is most incessant and spasmodic, threatening almost to burst his chest. It feels as if his chest would fly to pieces. The cough is caused by a peculiar sensation of tickling in the fauces.

Another keynote symptom of **Lactuca virosa** is a sensation of lightness. The whole body feels light as if swimming in the air. We should think strongly of **Lactuca** in dreams of swimming in the air and of walking above the ground.

In its action over the female sexual system, we notice it to be a powerful galac-togogue. It promotes the increase of milk in the female breast. Dr. Hering recommends it in gonorrhœa of females.

On the male urethra we have a " sensation as of a drop were continually passing along the urethra when seated."

LAPIS ALBUS.

The " Lapis albus " means white stone. This medicine is prepared by triturating a species of gneiss, which Dr. V. Grauvogl found in suspension in the mineral springs of Gastein, Germany. He was led to the proving of this drug by the fact that critinism and goitre abounded among people accustomed to drink from these springs flowing over formations of gneiss. It has since been proved and verified and is credited to be very useful in various forms of new growths. It is reported to have cured cases of carcinoma and scrofulous growths of various descriptions. Its leading indication is burning, shooting pain in the cardiac muscles, pilorus, uterus and mammæ. On this indication, Dewey cured a swelling, of the size of a goose egg, in the right sterno-clavicular region of a patient. Dr. Nash reports of having done excellent work with Lapis albus in a woman suffering from a fibroid tumor with profuse debilitating hemorrhage. The black horribly offensive discharge, the burning pain in the diseased parts, the rough serrated edge of the cervix and the profound anemia made the prognosis very gloomy, till he had recourse to Lapis albus. The doctor writes:—" I had no hope that she could live more than two weeks at the longest. Under the action of this remedy she began to improve immediately and from the half dead wreck, that could not turn in bed without help, a skeleton, white as a ghost, she steadily improved. She is now doing her house work, the discharge having all ceased except her natural menses at her regular periods." This speaks lots about it.

LAUROCERASUS.

This medicine is prepared from the chopped matured leaves of the common laurel of our garden. It belongs to the natural order of Rosaceæ. It contains a certain amount of Hydrocyanic acid and many of its symptoms are to be attributed to this. It is a handsome evergreen shrub growing in the Caucasus, Asia minor, and Persia. From those countries it has been introduced into Europe for ornamental gardening.

It is a great remedy to be frequently thought of, in debilitating affections, showing a great want of reactionary force of the vitality. This lack of reactive power is the greatest keynote of this remedy and is particularly so when occurring in chest affections. The patient's appearance is particularly striking. The eyes are sunken and the complexion is blue. There is a great obstruction of vision; everything looked at, seems shrouded with veil. The muscles of face keep on twitching and titillating. The tongue is cold and numb. We notice much gasping for breath; in fact, everything points to a very low ebb of life. Life seems like a little flame in constant danger of being over-powered and extinguished by any passing breeze. In many respects, therefore, it resembles **China,** another remedy showing an equal amount of depletion of the vital force; only **Laurocerasus** is applicable in a more desperate condition than that represented by the former remedy.

The **Laurocerasus** patient gets out of breath from slight exercise, such as running, climbing steps, walking etc. Least exercise brings on gasping. This in my opinion is the most important symptom of this remedy.

It is particularly useful in long faint. The patient suddenly loses consciousness from which he does not recover for a long time. His lower jaw drops, his arms sink to side, respiration becomes suspended and the pulse weak and scarcely perceptible. The eyes remain wide open and staring. There is hardly any foaming from mouth. The patient takes deep breaths at long intervals.

Laurocerasus has a dry, harassing cough. It is particularly useful in the spasmodic cough to be seen in the later stages of whooping cough when the patient becomes much prostrated. It is also useful in cough with valvular diseases of the heart.

Laurocerasus has a kind of green diarrhœa. Drinks roll audibly through œsophagus and intestines. Coldness of body, pulselessness, cloudiness of brain, fainting, suppression and retention of urine, sensation of constriction of throat when swallowing and a complete paralysis of sphincter make it almost a specific in certain condition of cholera and choleric diarrhœa.

Case 1.—Boy, aged thirteen, had rheumatism during the past winter which was mostly confined to the lower extremities. He was treated with internal applications. We now find him with disease of the heart, as the result of such treatment. He says he has cough mostly after midnight; can scarcely sleep, because of difficulty of breathing. Sitting posture causes gasping for breath, great fluttering and beating at the heart. We might, from these symptoms, reasonably suspect a disease of the heart; and, upon physical exploration of the chest, we find, by percussion, considerable enlargement of the organ, and by ausculation, we find the murmur most prominent near the apex of the heart, with sound of regurgitation, and insufficiency of the mitral valves. There is a very sharp beat of the second sound of the pulmonary artery. Our diagnosis in this case is, insufficiency of the mitral valves, with hypertrophy of the heart. His legs are largely swollen; his face also shows signs of dropsical effusion. He also has that peculiar look of the eye common in this disease. The eyeball seems prominent and full staring. **Laur.** September, 21. Feels much better. Can sleep now with more ease. The gasping has disappeared, and the œdematous swelling of the legs has very much improved. This boy did not return, but, on the 19th of November, I sought him out, and found him hard at work in a grocery. He was entirely relieved of all his sufferings, and felt well. Auscultation revealed the same abnormal sounds of the heart, although somewhat modified in degree.—Dr. H. M. Nartin.

Case 2.—A lady was suddenly taken with violent uterine hæmorrhage. Dr. H. was called for, who prescribed **Ip., Hamamelis. Nux., Crocus** etc., but without effect. Finally, the doctor advised to send for the German brother. At 11 P.M. eight or ten hours have elapsed; we greeted our brother at the door, and learned that we had probably arrived too late. The patient was almost gone—was cold, clammy and white, like the sheet that covered her. She had been vomiting, but that was all over, and only constant, faint efforts to vomit were made three or four times every minute; there was no strength left to vomit. The eyes were closed; she was unconscious; pulse and breath scarcely perceptible. We gave at once a dose of **Cuprum** 2 (not because we preferred this attention, but because we had just that and no other). She immediately made a few violent efforts to vomit, after which that trouble subsided at once. On making a local examination, we found the vagina stuffed with cotton. The anxious doctor, who was urged and had to do something, had restored to this kind of tampon because nothing else would answer. Prescribed **Prunus laurocerasus, 10 drop-doses** in water every fifteen minutes; removed all the stuffings, and the flowing ceased within a few minutes. The patient insisted upon being henceforth treated by the consulting physician; but this was refused. The "counsel" justified his young neighbour, and vouched for him that he would do well, and so he did.—Dr. J. L. Arndt.

LEDUM PALUSTRE.

It is also called the Wild Rose-merry, Marsh Tea and Labrador Tea. It belongs to the natural order of Ericaceæ. Hahnemann says, "It is suitable for the most part, only for the chronic maladies in which there is a predominance of coldness and deficiency of animal heat."

This is one of our rheumatic remedies. It is specially adapted to people of rheumatic diathesis and to constitutions abused by alcohol.

The most characteristic feature of this drug is an extremely cold feeling of the surface of the body, specially of the affected part, to touch. This is due to lack of vital heat of the system. It is generally used in complaints of people who are cold all the time. In spite of this cold and chilly sensation warmth aggravates.

What makes it very striking, is that in spite of this extreme cold sensation he is relieved by application of cold. Dr. Clarke reports (Medical Dictionary vol. II. p. 268) of having cured with **Ledum,** rheumatism in the left arm of an octogenarian. This patient used to take cold baths at night to be rid of the pain and this alone enabled him to sleep. I can remember a similar case of gout in the ankle joint, that found relief from immersion in ice-water. **Ledum** relieved most of the symptoms.

Ledum is used both in the acute and chronic forms of this complaint. It has a special tendency towards affecting the smaller joints such as the ankles, the heels and the finger joints. It commences in the lower limbs and gradually ascends. It relieves rheumatic swelling of feet and legs extending above calf to knees. It is also useful in gouty nodosities on joint and in pain in ankles, ball of great toe and in heels and soles of feet. The pain is sticking, tearing and throbbing in character and the affected parts feel as if bruised or beaten.

It is one of our remedies for punctured wounds. It is equally great for bites of animals and insect. We think of **Ledum** in injuries that leave long lasting discoloration behind them.

Ledum is an excellent remedy in arthritic fevers brought on by exposure to cold. The chills are very violent. He shivers with chilliness. He feels as if cold water were poured over the whole body. In this it compares well with **Lachnanthes,** a remedy where the patient has a sensation of a lump of ice between the shoulders that gives him horripilation. Heat of the body becomes excessive but it is characterised by an intolerance of the warmth of bed and a distended condition of the veins of the hands.

Case 1.—(Hæmoptœ, alternating with Rheumatism). A young man was attacked with a violent stitch-pain in right hip. The pain gradually grew continuous, and was especially at night in bed so violent that he had to leave the bed and lay upon the floor; sometimes it was relieved by washing the whole leg with cold water. After a while the joints of the knees, then of the feet, and at last those of the hands commenced swelling. Some months later, when this inflammation had all subsided, he was suddenly attacked by a violent cough and spitting blood. The spitting of blood was subdued, but the cough continued for several weeks, until again in violent attack of hemorrhage set in with profuse expectoration of thick, greenish, foul and fetid masses. Examination revealed a cavern in the left subclavicular region. **Acon.** 2, a teaspoonful every hour. Great improvement. Four days later, the cough still continues, the expectoration is difficult and consists of thick, tough mucus. **Tart. em.** 3, every four hours. In about eight to ten days the patient seemed well, but all at once, without any apparent cause, he was attacked again with inflammatory rheumatism of the hands. **Bry.** 1, every two hours, relieved within four days; but ten days after another sudden attack of cough and hæmoptysis set in, and an examination of the chest revealed another vomica. **Acon.** and **Tart. em.**, administered, as before, did no good. The patient sank rapidly, with all the signs of a galloping phthisis. In this critical moment, I thought of a case which Rau had reported in his "Homœopathischen Heilverfahren," of a young man with coxalgia alternating with hæmoptysis, whom he had cured with **Led.** I at once gave to my patient **Led.** 30, four globules upon the tongue. The change was wonderful, and improvement continued for four days, when it ceased. **Led.** 30, another dose, was not followed by improvement in the next four or five days. **Led.** 200, one dose, again set nature to work, and in four weeks the patient was completely restored without another dose of medicine.—Dr. Stens, Sr.

Case 2.—Mme. Borel, thirty-three years of age; changed at fourteen; married at fifteen; had two children before she was twenty, and an abortion at twenty-five. The present disease appeared as consequent to this abortion. Present condition: menses profuse; constant sanguinous flow between the periods; pain in the kidneys and in the left iliac fossa; enormous fibrous tumor occupying the anterior wall of the uterus, and perceptible through the abdominal wall. **Led.** 12, at first, very much diminished the flow; but the menses having returned profusely and prematurely, with violent pains. I substituted **Calc.** 30, for the **Led.**, which produced a happy effect. After this improvement, which continued two or three weeks, the usual hemorrhage returned, in spite of the **Calc. Led.** 12 and 30, continued for several months, with intervals of repose, finally checked the flow and reduced the menses to their physiological measure. This partial cure held good for some months; but it was necessary to recur, from time to time, to the **Led.** This patient is subject to rheumatismal pains.—Dr. Jousset.

LEPTANDRA VIRGINICA.

It is also called the Black-Root or Culver's Root. The drug was introduced into homœopathy by Dr. Hale and was first proved by Dr. Burt. It acts very prominently upon the liver and causes congestion and catharsis of the intestinal mucous membrane. Dr. Burt's experience after taking a tincture of the fresh root of Leptandra which I am quoting below is very interesting and it fairly epitomises the action of the drug:—"For the last two hours I have been in awful pain and distress in the umbilical and hypogastric region; drinking cold water aggravates the pain very much; there is dull, aching, burning distress in the region of the gall bladder, with frequent chilliness along the spine; there is great distress in the hypogastrium with great desire for stool. A very profuse black stool, about the consistence of cream, with undigested potatoes in it, gave amelioration, but was followed by great distress in the region of the liver extending to the spine; for the last four hours there has been constant distress, with pains in the whole abdomen, but for the last half-hour the pains in the umbilicus and hypogastrium have been awful to endure, with rumbling and great desire for stool; a very profuse black, fœtid stool, that ran like a stream from my bowels, and could not be retained for a moment, gave great amelioration, but did not stop the pain altogether."

This proves beyond doubt the grand characteristic of **Lept.** to be black tarry stools. We also notice dull aching in the right hypochondrium and over the region of the gall bladder. This pain extends into back and over the spine. A colicky pain in the abdomen with great deal of rumbling is also present. The gastric disorder for which **Lept.** is used is generally of a chronic type and is caused by derangement of the portal system. Dr. Hering reports of a chronic case of camp diarrhœa of three months' standing. The patient was emaciated beyond measure. His features were haggard and jaundiced. Prostration was so great that he was hardly able to stand. The stools were muco-purulent and bloody. **Lept.** removed all his symptoms.

Amongst other remedies with black stools we may mention **Arsen., Merc., Opium, Platina, Plumb.,** and **Verat.**

In **Arsen.** the diarrhœa is generally the effect of chilling of the stomach with cold drinks. The stools, though black like **Lept.,** are generally samll in quantity. The prostration is much more prominent and out of all proportion to the amount and the number of the stools.

Merc. is very closely allied to **Lept.** The main distinction rests with the pressing pain and tenesmus of **Merc.** **Lept.** lacks the tenesmus though it may have griping colicky pain after stools.

Opium is a remedy for diarrhœa of a very chronic type. It is also used for acute diarrhœa after fright or sudden joy or any other sudden abnormal, disturbance of the mental equilibrium. The patient's condition in **Opium** is more serious than in **Lept.** Comatose sleep, apathy, bloated dusk red face, heat of the head, suppression of urine point more or less to a typhoid condition not observed in **Lept.**

Plumbum is applicable in diarrhœa with black stools when we have actual retraction of the umbilicus, a sensation of pulling at the navel, severe cutting colicky pain in the abdomen and a pain that radiates to the brain, lungs and other parts of the body extorting violent screams from the patient.

In **Verat,** together with the severe pinching colic, violent thirst, and big evacuation, we have a frigid state of the entire body with great abundance of cold sweat.

LILIUM TIGRINUM.

This plant is a native of China and Japan, but it is cultivated widely in other countries as well. It was introduced into homœopathy by Dr. W. E. Payne. Drs. Dunham, Lilienthal and others have proved it very carefully and it has since become a first-rate remedy with us for various complaints of women, specially of the uterus and its appendages.

It has three principal spheres of action:—(1) It causes congestion and hyperæsthesia of the female sexual organs. (2) It causes extreme sensitiveness of the posterior spinal cord. (3) It increases the reflex excitability of the heart. However, as homœopaths are not much concerned with pathology, symptoms being our main guide, we shall confine ourselves to the symptoms.

The symptom that shows itself most prominently in all its provings is a downward dragging sensation. This downward dragging sensation involves the rectum, the bladder, the uterus and the loin. There is a distinct consciousness of the uterus, the ovaries, the bladder and the tubes—all weighing down like lead and trying to force their way through the vagina. The patient frequently has to put her hands on the vagina or to sit down to prevent these organs from coming out. This bearing down sensation is unfortunately a very common complaint with women. A very big majority of patients, that we come across, complains of a similar sensation. They, therefore, come within the scope of remedies like **Lili. tig., Sepia, Bell., Kreo., Murex.,** etc. We shall go through a thorough differentiation a bit later on, but it will just suffice to say here, that it is not the knife that is always necessary to put such things right. I have done it and others before me have done it and many of you will do it later on and verify things for yourselves.

Lili. tig. has been used in retroversion, anteversion, subacute and chronic ovaritis, subacute endo-cervicitis, metritis and other varieties of uterine troubles. The patient complains of a bearing down pain particularly while walking, as though menstruation would come on or as if the bowels would move; there is distress in the pelvic region, and pressure upon both retum and bladder; she has often to wear a " T " bandage to hold herself together.

Lili. tig. has a peculiar pain. It is sharp, burning, stinging in character. It extends across hypogastrium to groin and then travels downwards. The menses come early. It is scanty, dark and offensive; it flows only when she moves about and ceases when she stops walking. The continuous pressure in the region of bladder brings on a constant desire to urinate with scanty discharge. Smarting in the urethra and a certain amount of tenesmus are also present.

The mental condition of the **Lil. tig.** patient like that of **Sepia** is characterised by a profound depression of spirits. She can hardly keep herself from crying. She does not know what she cries about, but she must. This melancholy attitude, practically speaking, marks all patients suffering from uterine disorders. They are all very timid, down-hearted and forlorn. Another great feature of **Lil. tig.** is to be seen in its indifference and apathy. Like **Phos., Phosphric acid, Opium, Platina, Pulsat., Nat. mur.,** and **Apis** the **Lil. tig.** patients take no interest whatsoever in the usual avocation of their lives. Their household affairs are neglected; they take no interest in their personal appearance, and their loved ones are not hankered after as before; sometimes again this depression takes on a religious aspect. They doubt about their salvation; they think that they are doomed to expiate for their sins or for those of their family. Sometimes this doubt becomes so intensified that they walk the floor day and night in a disconsolate mood, and would neither rest, nor partake of any refreshment. An important symptom that has escaped my mind and which I must not forget to mention, is a desire to do everything in a hurried manner. This hurry is particularly to drown and suppress strong sexual desire. They are afraid to be left alone; they fear they have heart disease, which they believe, is incurable.

As I have mentioned before **Lil. tig.** has some important heart symptoms. They have a sensation as if their heart was grasped and squeezed in a vise. In this respect it is greatly similar to **Cact. grand.**

LITHIUM CARBONICUM.

Carbonate of Lithium is a white light powder.   It is found in solution in the mineral springs of Carlsbad and other places. It has an alkaline taste. It was proved by Dr. Hering.

This is an invaluable remedy in chronic rheumatism, specially when accompanied with valvular troubles. Any little excitement causes fluttering of the heart. Pain in the heart is very frequent; it is specially felt when the patient bends forward. This pain is relieved when he passes water. These symptoms are very import-ant as well as characteristic and should, therefore, be carefully borne in mind. Another peculiarity of this rheumatism, consists in the appearance of an eruption on the affected part. The small joints are specially involved. We notice great tenderness, swel-ling and redness of the last joints of fingers. The skin of these patients are dry, harsh and rough.

Another great charactertistic of **Lithium** is soreness. Like **Hamamelis,** bones, joints and muscles feel bruised as from fall or blows. Even the eye-balls feel sore. Symptoms which indi-cate this drug are, rheumatic soreness in cardiac region, a trembl-ing and fluttering sensation of heart after mental agitation and induration of aortic valves.

As is generally the case, we find certain amount of urinary complications. It is turbid, strong, scanty flocculent and full of uric acid deposits. While passing urine, flashes of pain are felt in the region of the bladder, extending into spermatic cord.

Lithium is useful in headache of females brought on by sud-den cessation of menses. It is felt in the vertex, head and eyes. The eyes feel very sore and they find it difficult to keep the eye-lids open. This headache is rendered peculiar by the fact that it is always better when the patient eats something, but it returns and remains till food is taken again.

Lithium has some important eye symptoms that need careful attention. It has entire vanishing of right half of whatever the patient looks at. It may be the result of excessive use of eyes with insufficient light or direct exposure to the blinding effects of strong sunlight. Also, we find chronic hardening of the meibomian glands.

I will mention one more symptom of this remedy before closing. As a rule, the nose is swollen red and a bit puffy. It is dry when inside the house, and moist when he goes into the open air. Very often, patients come to us to get rid of this excessive congestion of their olfactory organs; when the totality is there **Lithium carb.** will invariably help to restore the lost beauty of the sensitive patients and earn for us their life-long gratitude.

LOBELIA INFLATA.

Other names for this plant are Asthma-root and Indian tobacco. It belongs to the natural order of Lobeliaceæ. Its chief action is centered in the pneumo-gastric nerve. This medicine was introduced into our Materia Medica by Dr. Jeanes of the United States.

Taken in a big quantity, it produces intense nausea, vomiting, profuse perspiration and great prostration. These are the keynotes of this drug. Prescribed on such indications, **Lobelia** will be useful in various complaints. We think of it particularly in periodical headache that comes on in afternoon and continues increasing till midnight, every third attack being more violent than the two previous ones. The other accompanying symptoms are profuse salivation, cold sweat on the head, faintness and an indescribable weak feeling in the epigastrium. It is also used in neuralgia of the left side of the face and temples when such neuralgia is the effect of retarded menses. These patients exhibit a great distaste for tobacco. They cannot bear the smell of tobacco or tobacco smoke.

Lobelia has been recommended highly in gastralgia and dyspepsia. There is hiccough with profuse flow of saliva. Frequent gulping of a burning sour fluid, due to acidity of stomach, a faint or weak feeling at pit of stomach—a feeling that is a mixture of pain, heat, oppression, and excessive uneasiness and which he finds very hard to describe,—worry him constantly.

It is an excellent remedy in asthma. Dyspnœa, due to constriction of the chest is most incessant. It is usually described as a pressure or weight in chest and is relieved by rapid walking. A distinguishing mark of the **Lobelia** asthma is a pricking sensation felt all over the body, previous to an attack of asthma. During these attacks he gets a peculiar sensation about his heart as if it would stand still. Vertigo, a threatened loss of consciousness and an extreme tenderness over sacrum are three guiding characteristics of **Lobelia.** It resembles **Digitalis** and **Tabacum** in heart affection, **Arsenic** and **Veratrum** in gastric troubles and **Ipecac** in spasmodic asthma.

LYCOPERSICUM.

Lycopersicum belongs to the natural order of Solanaceæ. In common language it is called the Tomato or the Love-Apple. It is used extensively all over the world as an edible vegetable. Its use is confined mostly to coryza, rheumatism of the Deltoid muscle and diabetes. This remedy has been proved by Cooper, Gross and Roberts. It develops a decided pain in the right Deltoid muscle and in this respect it is similar to **Sanguinaria.**

On the nose, it produces a strong coryza which is always worse out of doors and is greatly similar to **Cepa** which has a similar coryza with the difference that in **Cepa** the patients are always better while in open air. It causes polyuria and therefore has been recommended in diabetes.

LYCOPODIUM CLAVATUM

Commonly this is known as clubmoss or Wolfs-claw, a low creeping perennial plant that grows almost everywhere but specially in the northern countries. The medicinal part is the powder, a fine mobile light yellow dust. Put into the fire it burns with a mild roaring hissing sound, hence it is utilized in stage lightening and in pyrotechnic displays. It belongs to the natural order of Lycopodiaceæ.

Lycopodium is the premier remedy of our Materia Medica. From the time it has been introduced into our Materia Medica by Samuel Hahnemann, it has effected innumerable cures, some of which are simply marvellous. Almost every practitioner can cite some such instance and confirm the wonderful efficacy of this remedy. We find it particularly indicated in persons of keen intellect but feeble muscular development. Like **Nux** they are highly intelligent, precautious and their physical condition is not in keeping with their mental state. Lean and puny, thin and emaciated, they rarely leave any strong impression at first sight. It is only after a certain amount of intercourse with them that we find out the inherent superiority of their mental calibre. They are far from being self-possessed. Extremely sensitive, they take offence at trifles and are easily excited to anger. They are discontented, impatient and misanthropic. All these traits may easily lead one to prescribe **Nux vomica.** If not for certain strong points of difference which we will discuss later on, it may be permissible to substitute one remedy for the other. The mental traits are indeed similar; the difference, however, between the two remedies is not negligible. It is true that they are both ugly in their build and mentality but there is this difference that **Nux** is snappish only when you go near them. **Lycopodium** patient on the other hand will go a long distance out of his way to pick quarrel with his neighbour. They are fault-finding, domineering, vehement and intolerant of contradiction. I distinctly remember Dr. H. C. Allen comparing the **Lycopodium** patient to a man with a club going about, seeking whom he could thrush. They are both dyspeptic and bilious but **Nux** is a bitter remedy whereas **Lycopodium** is sour. In **Nux vom.,** the aggravation is in the morning hours whereas in **Lycopodium** it is in the afternoon. **Nux vom.,** eats heartily and his troubles start after eating whereas **Lycopodium** is characterised by a strong satiety which prevents him from having a hearty meal. **Lycopodium** patients are greedy, avaricious, malicious and parsimonous and as is always true with such temperament, they are generally pusillanimous. We notice a great predisposition to lung and hepatic affections in **Lycopodium** constitutions. They are, as has been mentioned before, very emaciated and this emaciation is generally due to loss of fluids. Dropsical swellings, consequent upon disease of liver, is of frequent occurrence. The face is rather pale and sallow with dark rings round the eyes. Furrows and wrinkles on the brow are plentiful. These give him the appearance of an old man over-burdened with thought, anxiety and worry.

Lycopodium is pre-eminently a remedy for lithic acid diathesis; hence we find much red sediment in urine. Gravel, small calculi either in kidney or in bladder frequently occur in **Lycopodium,** as a result of the lithic acid diathesis. We will have ample opportunity to study this thoroughly when we come to discuss its application in diseases of the urinary organs.

A symptom that has been sadly omitted is the lachrymal mood of **Lycopodium.** The patient weeps all day and cannot calm herself by any means. She cries even when she is thanked. This is different from **Natrum mur.,** where sympathy elicits tears. With this lachrymal mood, however, there is a sort of imperiousness in **Lycopodium.** We find him always assuming an air of command. She is stiff and pretentious. She does not hesitate even to strike her attendant when thwarted. Such is the type of patient we have to deal with in **Lycopodium.**

We shall now discuss a few red strand keynotes of **Lycopodium.** A very good one is the excessive accumulation of flatulence. Fermentation is constant. This is confined more to the lower part of the abdomen. In this it differs from **China** and **Carbo veg.** In the former the flatulence spreads over the whole abdomen; in the latter, in the upper part only. This accumulation of flatus in **Lycopodium** is so excessive and the distention of the abdomen so great, that they feel bloated and full all the time.

The next characteristic is the peculiar 4 to 8 p.m., aggravation. These patients, whatever may be their trouble, are better in the morning hours and in the afternoon till about 4 p.m., when the exacerbation commences and lasts till about 8 o'clock and then gradually subsides. In this respect we should also think of **Sabadilla, Nux moschata** and **Helleborus**, although in none of them it is as prominently marked as in **Lycopodium.**

The next point that I would ask every practitioner to bear in mind, is the direction that the affections of **Lycopodium** generally take. They begin from the right side and go to the left side. In headache, sore-throat, ovarian complaints and in various other ailments this peculiar feature of the disease spreading from the right to the left is noticeable.

Another peculiarity of **Lycopodium** is amelioration from uncovering and warm drinks. We will have ample illustration of this while dealing with its application in diphtheria and other varieties of throat affections.

Lycopodium is a first-rate remedy for dyspepsia. It is difficult to tell, how many cases of this kind I have helped with this remedy. I can boldly say that **Lycopodium** covers at least fifty per cent. of all cases of dyspepsia of this world. The tongue is coated white. The patient complains of a bland putrid taste in the mouth that sometimes changes to sour. The tongue is covered with numerous small blisters that burn and scald. This dyspepsia is atonic in type and is found in persons of weak health, who are constantly sleepy and irritable. They also suffer from canine hunger. They want to eat all the time, but their appetite is very uncertain. Inspite of such appetite a few mouthfuls bring them satiety and a sense of fulsomeness. They feel as if they have eaten clear up to their throat and there is no space for any more. In this matter of distress after eating it bears a great semblance to **Nux vomica,** but unlike **Nux** the distress commences immediately after eating. The worry and trouble in **Nux** commence some little while after eating, when the process of digestion has partly commenced. Nausea, hiccough and vomiting are very frequent in these patients. **Lycopodium** has cured many cases of dyspepsia with heart-burn that commences a⁺

about 3 p.m., and ends with the vomiting of intensely sour food and bile at about 7 p.m.

The epigastric region is extremely sensitive to touch and tight clothing. Rumbling or more correctly, a sensation of churning in stomach, tension in hypochondria as from a chord, sensitiveness of the liver to contact, icterus entrailgia due to an accumulation of gas in intestines and great depression of mind are symptoms that are frequently encountered in **Lycopodium.**

Lycopodium patients are generally costive. They suffer from frequent ineffectual desire for stool. This is not due to irregular peristalsis as in **Nux vom.,** but to the presence of constriction in rectum. Each evacuation causes terrible amount of pain and urging that leaves the patients in a very prostrated condition. In some bad cases we may notice syncope after the stool. The mucous membrane of rectum is very much injected, excoriated and is full of numerous hemorrhoidal knobs. The examining finger encounters spasmodic constriction of the sphincter. There is also narrowing of rectum due to the same cause. The most striking symptom to remember is the persistence of pain after evacuation. It is so severe as to arrest breathing. The pain is cutting, tearing, stitching and cramping in nature.

From what has already been stated and by reason of its action on the liver, we may easily guess the importance of **Lycopodium** in swelling or enlargement of veins. Everywhere we come across distended varices showing great stagnation of circulation. There are big, tortuous varices in the legs that bring on fatigue, weariness after slight walking. The labia, too, are swollen with varices particularly during pregnancy showing great impediment in the circulatory system. The piles of **Lycopodium** are generally bleeding piles. The flow of blood from them is almost like hemorrhage. The discharge of blood is immense, not at all warranted by the small size of the vein from which they exude.

Lycopodium is also serviceable in constipation of young men, who are tormented with night pollutions or addicted to masturbation.

It is also useful in diarrhœa and the keynote symptom is chilliness in rectum before stools.

The action of **Lycopodium** on the urinary organ is very striking. It has been recommended in diabetes insipidus where the thirst is very great, the patient drinking an enormous quantity of water and passing an equally large quantity of pale, watery urine,

It is useful in chronic cystitis. The urine becomes turbid, milky, purulent and offensive. Urging to urinate is very great but he has to wait long before it passes. Sometimes he finds it impossible to void urine. The bearing down pain becomes so great that he has to support his abdomen with his hands.

He is constitutionally inclined towards gravel and calculi. We notice in his urine a large deposit of red sand. Dr. Nash urges practitioners to differentiate this gritty sandy substance from the brick dust sediment of other remedies. Unless this condition is rectified by the timely administration of **Lycopodium** the patient will sooner or later run into a regular attack of renal colic; this sandy substance imperceptibly leads to the formation of regular crystals. This sandy sediment is often seen in the urine of young children and babies. When such is the case we find them shrieking before every attempt at urination.

The importance of **Lycopodium** on the sexual organs should not be overlooked. It is one of our best remedies for impotence. The sexual desire, as well as power, is greatly diminished. The penis becomes small, cold and relaxed; erections are feeble and he falls asleep during an embrace. Such conditions are specially seen in old men after excessive sexual indulgence and in young men suffering from exhausting pollutions. **Lycopodium** has helped many such cases.

On the female sexual system its importance is equally great. We notice discharge of blood from genitals during every passage of hard or soft stool. There is great dryness of vagina and the patient complains of great burning during and after coition.

In the more serious forms of uterine affections such as, inflammation of the uterus, **Lycopodium** finds plenty to do. The inflammation which **Lycopodium** disperses is generally of a chronic character. Profuse milky bloody corroding leucorrhœa, neuralgic pains referred to internal genitalia, chronic dryness of vagina, physometra, varices of genitals, presence of polypi, erectile tumors and other painless pedunculated condylomatous growths are symptoms that should lead in the selection of **Lycopodium.**

Its use is not only confined to the pathological conditions of the generative organs but to the physiological phases of pregnancy, parturition and lactation. It is a great medicine for morning sickness. We think of it in neusea, vomiting, anorexia and swelling of veins in the first month of pregnancy. In some cases the movement of the fœtus in the womb becomes a regular source of annoyance and distress to the mother. It seems to be turning somersault within the womb. **Lycopodium** will not only check this excessive movement but will help in the ultimate expulsion of the child at the proper time. Its application during labour is based on the spasmodic contraction of the cervix, preventing parturition. The pain though unbearable is ineffectual and is accompanied with jactitatory movements of the body. The patient dances up and down during pain. She must keep constantly in motion. Labor-pains run upwards and are temporarily relieved by placing feet against a support.

We use it in phlegmasia alba dolens. The saphenous view becomes enormously swollen and tender and can be distinctly traced all its way.

We will now study the indications of **Lycopodium** on the respiratory tract. There is a decided catarrhal inflammation of the nasal mucous membrane. Violent coryza with acrid discharge from a nose, swollen with the effects of inflammation and profuse lachrymation from red and burning eyes, indicate a real onset of a bad cold. The other symptoms are snuffles, discharge of crusts and elastic plugs from nose, great dryness and stoppage of nose causing frequent starting and choking during sleep and great soreness of the upper lid. This cold may travel downwards and we may have serious involvement of the lungs. **Lycopodium** becomes serviceable in that condition of pneumonia where the area of hepatization is extensive and in consequence, the breathing becomes diaphragmatic. The patient is bolstered up in bed and presents a bluish white appearance with pinched nostrils. The eyes look staring due to great dyspnœa. The temperature, respiration and pulse are very high. The nostrils are in rapid fan-like motion. His mind wanders and his voice is anxious and tremulous. Fine crepitations, later on giving place to coarse rattling render existence unbearable. His mouth and throat very often get filled with ropy mucous, having a distinct streak of blood in them. Much pain is complained of in lungs. The right is more affected than the left side. Cough is hacking and more troublesome from 4 to 8 p.m. **Lycopodium** serves to tide over the case on to the next stage and ultimately helps to restore the normal equilibrium of the patient. We also use it in impending suppuration of the lungs when the patient brings up mouthfuls of purulent rust-colored stringy mucus.

The action of **Lycopodium** on throat is very important and it deserves our special attention. It is applicable in tonsillitis, ulcerated throat and even in diphtheria. Great dryness is particularly characteristic of **Lycopodium.** Even the saliva dries on the palate and lips and becomes stuff. Gums and the palate get a lardaceous coating and stink very badly. **Lycopodium** is an important remedy in diphtheria. The most important indication is a feeling of contraction in throat. It prevents food and water from going down. They regurgitate through nose and cause a sensation of choking. There is a constant desire to swallow but swallowing is accompanied with violent stinging pains. The patient is worse from swallowing drinks, especially cold drinks. The tonsils are enlarged, swollen and congested, over the surface of which are noticed numerous ulcers covered with coatings of pus. In diphtheria, in conjunction with the abovementioned symptoms, we also have great prostration, swelling of glands of the neck, diminished secretion of urine, heavy stupor and aggravation from sleep. The membrane which is generally of a dirty grayish color, starts from the right side and gradually goes towards the left. In this connection we should compare **Lycopodium** with **Mercurius protoiodide,** where also the same side is involved but the peculiar tongue of the latter is wanting in **Lycopodium.**

Lycopodium occupies a prominent place in the therapeutics of fever. It may be needed in all types of fevers. Firstly we will discuss the usefulness of **Lycopodium** in the intermittent type of fevers. The paroxysm may come on between 8 and 9 a.m. or in the evening between 6 and 7 p.m. It is ushered in with shaking chill and incessant yawning and nausea. The patient feels as if lying on a piece of ice. Between chill and **heat** he vomits an extremely sour fluid. This is different from the bitter vomiting of **Eupatorium** and **Ipecac.** During the stage of heat he complains of great thirst and wants to uncover. In this place, let me mention, that in **Lycopodium** perspiration often follows the chill, stage of heat being totally absent.

It is an excellent remedy in typhoid and typhus; but generally its application comes in, at the end of the second week or the beginning of the third week, when due to suppression of the rash, we find the patient sinking into a state of unconsciousness with many other alarming symptoms. The patient becomes stupid and lies with dropped jaws and half opened eyes. Muttering delirium, picking at the bed clothes, materialism, involuntary micturition or retention of urine, snoring rattling breathing, a swollen blistered tongue and distention of abdomen are symptoms that do not impart a very favourable impression of the case. A timely administration of **Lycopodium** even at this stage, will react on the sinking vitality and turn the course of the disease curewards. The tongue just mentioned is particularly characteristic of **Lycopodium.** It is so swollen that it cannot be protruded when you ask him to do so. It only rolls from side to side like a pendulum, in his attempt to talk, which at most is indistinct, stammering and heavy. The eyes do not react to light. They have lost their bright lusture of health and have a sort of a fishy look. Hands and feet are cold and there is a general want of bodily heat; a symptom on which particular stress has been laid by Dr. Farrington, is the coldness of one foot and the warmth and heat of the other.

Case 1.—Mr. H., aged forty years, has been exposed to the night air for years. He was suddenly roused from his afternoon nap by copious spitting of blood. By the use of powerful astringents the hæmorrhage was checked after he had lost about half a pint of blood. On July 20th I was called and found him feverish, restless and weak. Prescribed **Aconite** 2 every two hours. In the evening I was called again; he had then raised about one pint of bright-red blood. The fever was much more severe and he was quite weak. **Millefolium** 3 soon arrested the hæmorrhage. **Aconite** and **Millefolium** were then given in alternation. When the fever had abated and danger from hæmorrhage had passed, he was to take one dose of **China** 3 every two hours. July 21st.—On examination, the upper of both lungs disclosed dullness, on percussion, with some bronchial respiration and mucus rale. The dullness was mainly on the left side, while the soreness was principally in the right side. There was constant hacking cough with bloody sputa. Prescribed **Ipecacuanha** 3 every two hours. The condition of the patient demanded frequent change of remedies; the symptoms improved until August 5th, when they grew more violent and alarming. During the month of September, **Lycopodium 200, Arnica, Kali carbonicum,** and **Arsenicum** were given, but without relief. October 1st.—He has had **Calcarea phosphorica** by advice of counsel. The prognosis both from myself and my medical adviser was very unfavourable. He is now daily losing flesh; appetite very poor; much pain in the lungs, severe hacking cough; eyes bright and glassy; sunken cheeks; paroxysms of fever, with bright, red spots on the cheeks; very restless at night; profuse night-sweats · dull sound on percussions of the upper lobes of both lungs. At 4 P.M. each day, he has a fever and is much worse generally; prescribed **Lycopodium 200** every two hours. October 2nd.—He had a better night; perspirationless; feels much better every way. From this date the improvement was so rapid, that at the sixth day I suspended all medicine. Now five months have passed and he has been able to be out in all weather; but, by advice, takes care to guard against the influence of sudden changes.—(Dr. A. M. Cushing, **New Eng. Med. Gazette, May, 1873.)**

Case 2.—Mr. D. had suffered day and night, with short intervals, for six weeks, severe colic. The pain was constant most of the time, with paroxysms of great severity, when it seemed as if the intestines were grasped with two hands and drawn into a knot in the umbilical region, and then slowly torn asunder. During these paroxysms he was drawn forward and would lie across the end of a **lounge** with his arm between it and his abdomen, as it seemed to relieve the pain. Alternate diarrhœa and constipation. Constant feeling of fulness, which was increased to repletion after eating a few mouthfuls. Loud rumbling in the left side of the abdomen. Emission of flatus was followed by relief. Pain and feeling of fulness were always worse about supper-time. Prescribed **Lycopodium 200,** one dose. The pain began to lessen soon after the dose was taken and disappeared within a few hours. A relapse was cured by one dose of **Lycopodium 5000.** He has been well since. The relief of pain from pressure seemed to call for **Colocynth,** but the feeling of repletion, the loud rumbling in the left iliac region and the time of aggravation made the selection of the proper remedy an easy matter.—(Dr. E. A. Ballard, **Med. Investigator, December, 1872.)**

Case 3.—Several years ago I had a very severe case of diphtheria, affecting both the throat and nare. Counsel was called. We found the symptoms to correspond to the following symptoms under **Lycopodium** in Raue on "Pathology and Therapeutics," page 119: Worse on the right side; the nose is stopped up, and the patient cannot breathe with her mouth shut; she keeps her mouth constantly open, slightly projecting her tongue, which gives her a silly expression. **Lycopodium 30** acted like magic. I had cured three or four other, nearly similiar cases. More recently I have tried it in several cases of diphtheria in the nose, that did not have "Projecting tongue and silly expression," as only one nostril was stopped up at a time, and it failed to act.—Dr. E. C. Price.

LYCOPUS VIRGINICUS.

In common parlance this herb is known as the Bugle-weed or the Virginia horehound. It grows plentifully all round the year in the bogs and swampy lands of the United States of America. Tincture is made from the fresh plant when it flowers by adding two parts by weight of alcohol to the chopped and pounded plant. This remedy was first proved by Drs. Chandler and Morrison.

Lycopus virginicus is a remedy for which I will always have a grateful regard in consideration of the useful service it rendered to me sometime ago, in a case of valvular disease of the heart. The luckless patient was in a very wretched condition. His heart-beats generally slow and weak, was tumultuous and forcible when he attempted to do any hard work, such as climbing steps or the like. At such times he would almost feel faint and his heart-beats could be heard even from a distance. Various remedies were tried, such as **Digit., Cactus, Spig.,** but they all proved failures till **Lycopus** was administered. It gave him so much relief that he thought himself practically cured and went back to his work.

These patients generally show signs of exophthalmus. Their thyroid glands become enlarged and they suffer from pain, tachycardia and tremor. Their eye-balls protrude; this protrusion is at times so excessive as to amount to a practical dislocation of the eve-balls from their sockets.

Lycopus is a great remedy for erratic pains. Generally the pain begins on the left side, jumps from place to place and at last returns to its original site. It is better from warmth but worse from cold air and movement. We will do well to compare this remedy with **Kali bich., Lac. can., Led.,** and **Puls.,** because the resemblance between them is indeed very great.

In **Kali bich.,** the pain shifts like that of **Lycopus,** but it is a pain that is generally in small spots and can be covered up with the tips of the fingers.

Lac. can. stands unrivalled with regard to changeability and erratic nature of its pains. Like **Lycopus** it begins on the left side but it changes its locations much more frequently than **Lycopus.**

In **Ledum** too the pain shifts but it shifts down-wards.

Last of all we come to **Pulsatilla.** Here the pain, which is erratic in nature, is accompanied by chill and shivering, the intensity of which is determined by the intensity of the pain.

Another peculiarity about this **Lycopus** pain, is that the patient is more sensitive to it when he concentrates his thought upon it. Thus it forms a valuable trio with **Oxalic ac.,** and **Helon.**

Sometimes this pain becomes located in the heart and then it is something which we must be cautious about. It is more of a sort of an ache in the precordial region and at the apex; but the peculiarity about it, which will help us to distinguish it from other remedies, is that the pain shifts to the left wrist and inner side of right calf, and then comes back to its original location. Many of the important symptoms of this remedy are similarly characterized. Thus for example the pain in the testicle shifts to the supra-orbital region and sometimes from one teste to the other.

Hamamelis is very similar to **Lycopus** in this respect. The patient gets a sort of a dull, ache in the testes. It is more a bruised sensation, a sore feeling than a real pain which distinguishes this remedy from its other sister remedies.

Lycopus has some very important symptoms in the urinary sphere. It has been recommended very highly in diabetes mellitus. The patient passes huge quantity of urine daily. Thirst is exceedingly great—the patient drinking large quantities of water. It is a thirst that nothing but the coldest water would satisfy. The specific gravity is much diminished and the urine shows deposits of mucus, epithelial cells, abundance of spermatozoa and oxalate of lime crystals. Sometimes the urine gets very thick and scanty and is accompanied by œdema of the feet. Another peculiarity that we must not omit to mention, is that, so long as the bladder is full, it does not trouble the patient at all; but as soon as he passes urine and the bladder becomes empty, he feels a great distended sensation in that organ.

Now we come to the symptoms of the remedy as manifested in the female sexual organs. The menses are very scanty lasting from half an hour to about six or seven hours, and generally, intermitting for ten or twelve days. We have a similar menstruation in **Euphrasia** where it lasts about an hour and is very painful.

Lycopus has been used with great success in consumption. It is useful in the tickling cough of phthisis when accompanied by hæmoptysis and tumultuous action of the heart. Hale recommends it highly and regards it as a great palliative in those advanced cases where cure is not possible.

LYSSIN (Hydrophobinum.)

It is a Nosode. The medicine is prepared from the saliva of a mad dog. The first saliva was obtained by Dr. Hering in 1833; that is about 50 years before Dr. Pasteur commenced his experiments with the serum. Dr. Pasteur's experiments led him to produce the rabic poison in extreme form on the spinal cord of rabbits. Therefrom he produced different degrees of modifications of the poison. He inoculated his patients, suffering from dog-bite, with the rabic poison prepared by him, commencing with the one of the lowest intensity, and gradually going up the gamut. Lots of mishaps have happened to several patients through this treatment, although it cannot be denied that Dr. Pasteur has added a very valuable item of information to the medical science, which has been greatly improved upon, since his death and is doing endless good to millions. But our point here is, that the idea germinated in the brain of a homœopath in the first instance which has gradually blossomed into a fine science. The homœopathic application of **Lyssin** is free from all dangers. Its method is accurate, scientific, safe and efficacious. The most characteristic symptom of this remedy, consists of an aggravation of all the symptoms and of all the ailments, by the noise of running water or at the sight of bright light. All symptoms centre round this peculiarity. In mania, headaches, dizziness, toothache, diarrhœa, diphtheria, sorethroat and in almost every complaint, where **Lyssin** is indicated, this symptom forms the most vital point round which the whole case revolves.

Other characteristic indications are the following:—

Memory for single words much improved.

Strange notions and apprehensions during pregnancy.

Inclination to be rude and abusive, to bite and strike.

Not afraid of dogs, but dislikes to see them because their sight renews her fear.

When he hears water poured out, or if he hears it run, or if he sees it, he becomes very irritable, nervous; it causes desire for stool and other ailments.

Frequent gaping without being sleepy, most when he has to listen to others.

Pain as if head would burst during pregnancy.

Headaches from bite of dogs, rabid or not.

Sight of water renews idea of pain and causes convulsions. (Pregnancy).

Hearing water poured out in next room makes him very irritable and nervous.

If during the night, or in the morning before rising, he heard pouring out of water in next room, he was immediately obliged to rise and have an evacuation.

Hearing water poured out brought on convulsions during pregnancy. Toothache and other complaints during pregnancy. with internal ebullition of blood from chest to head; head feels as if filled with air to bursting.

Large quantities of tough saliva in mouth, with constant spitting in diarrhœa.

Spits all the time small quantities of a frothy saliva; with pain in limbs.

Periodical spasm of œsophagus, continual painful inclination to swallow without being able to swallow anything; constriction is most severe when taking water into the mouth, if he tried to swallow it forcibly, he had burning and stinging pain in the throat, cough and retching which forced fluid from his mouth; difficult speech.

Difficulty in swallowing; particularly fluids.

When taking water into the mouth, constriction was greatest.

Periodical spasm of œsophagus.

Gagging when he forcibly attempts to swallow water, forces it out of his mouth.

Dysenteric stools with tenesmus; renewed as soon as he hears or sees water run.

Straining to evacuate, causing a violent pain in the small of back and in the rectum, afterwards compelling him to walk about, although weak, in dysentery.

Constant desire to urinate on seeing running water; urinates a little at a time.

Complaints resulting from abnormal sexual desire.

Menstruation, with hæmorrhoids, pulsations in the anus and weakness of back.

Sensitiveness of vagina rendering coition quite painful.

During pregnancy: strange notions, desires or cravings; rush of blood from chest upward; toothache, backache and other complaints; great sense of bearing down.

Spasms excited whenever she attempts to drink water, or if she hears it poured from one vessel into another; sight or sound of water affects unpleasantly, even though desiring water.

Sighing, with pain in the heart.

He could neither lie down nor stand up for any length of time, in dysentery.

Unbearableness of heat of the sun.

MAGNESIA CARBONICA.

Magnesia carb. is a salt. It is a light white friable mass obtained as a white precipitate, on mixing solutions of Magnesium Sulphate (Epsom Salt) and Sodium Carbonate. It is odourless and tasteless, insoluble in alcohol but soluble in dilute acids, where it causes copious effervescence.

It is a great gastro-intestinal remedy, as its action mostly centres on that portion of the human anatomy. We shall discuss this in full after we have taken an account of the constitution of our **Mag. carb.** patient. It is used in all ages and sexes, but everywhere we find great constitutional debility brought about by the excesses of cares, anxieties and worries of life. Muscles are lax and flaccid; the normal tone is gone. The sprightliness, the agility and the normal outburst of vitality are wanting. How often in our practice do we see such derelicts of humanity—worn out in tatters, barely sustaining a burdened and careworn existence. **Mag. carb.,** if symptoms indicate, is a great tonic to such individuals. If the patient is a child, it is puny, sickly and of defective nutrition. If it is a woman, she is nervous, sad, despondent and morose. Trembling of hands, constant absence of mind and vertigo indicate the low ebb at which her vitality is flowing.

These patients are extremely sensitive both bodily and mentally. The slightest touch causes startling; the slightest noise irritates; the slightest pressure aggravates almost all symptoms and the slightest exposure to draughts of cold air brings on untold miseries.

Another great characteristic of **Mag. carb.** is the extreme acidity. This sourness runs throughout the length and breadth of **Mag. carb.** The stools, the vomited materials and the sweat, have an acid taint in them. In fact I would consider the absence of this symptom a great contra-indication for **Mag. carb.**

Our **Mag. carb.** patient is a great martyr to neuralgia. The pain is lightning-like, sharp and unbearable. This pain is usually worse at night. The slightest touch, draught, and change of temperature would bring on and aggravate the pain. An important peculiarity of **Mag. carb.,** is an aggravation of all the symptoms, specially pains from rest and amelioration from walking about. The patient is obliged to run from room to room all night on account of the pain. As soon as the patient stops, the pain returns. It is also a great remedy for tearing, digging, boring pain in the malar bone (prosopalgia). This pain, too, becomes insupportable during rest and keeps on driving him from place to place.

Tumors and bony growths also have yielded to **Mag. carb.** Dr. Clarke cured with it a tumor of the right malar bone in an aged sea-captain on whom he tried various other remedies but without much avail. How amidst confusion Dr. Clarke came to the selection of **Mag. carb.,** is an interesting study and I am citing below his own statement.

"His face was quite distorted; right cheek bulging out, nose pushed over to the left side, right nostril stretched out. The malar bone was especially prominent near the wing of the nose. This was the only part that was tender. The tumor was soft as if cystic. There was no discharge. Inside the mouth, the right side of the hard palate bulged into the mouth and was slightly tender to pressure. The tumor was the seat of a constant gnawing pain; but the thing that troubled him most was sensitiveness to cold winds and cold weather. This was so great that he was afraid he would have to give up his calling. This led me to give **Silic.** 30 in the first instance (on February 27, 1895); but **Sil.** only increased the pain. One night he awoke feeling all his back aching. I worked up the case more carefully and found this under **Mag. c.:** 'Throbbing pain in antrum of Highmore with swelling of right malar bone'; and 'facial neuralgia, left side, shooting like lightning, aggravation from touch, draught, change of temperature; cannot stay in bed, must walk the floor.' Putting those together I prescribed (on March 13th) **Mag. c.** 30, giving four doses a day. March 28th: 'Much less pain. Face much reduced, swelling softer, fluctuating. Swelling inside mouth softer.' April 10th: 'Very much beter. Tumor smaller and softer.' August 14th: 'Face almost normal in appearance. Swelling inside mouth quite gone. Has no pain whatever, no sensitiveness to cold air.''

Magnesia carb. is equally well-indicated in toothache. This tooth-ache comes on while riding a carriage and is aggravated at night time and by exposure to cold. It compels him to rise and walk about, the pain being insupportable while at rest. It is a great remedy for toothache during pregnancy. In this respect it should be compared with **Ratanhia** which has exactly the similar symptom.

Now we come to the important action of **Mag. carb.** on the gastro-intestinal tract. Cutting pain about the navel, distension of abdomen, audible rumbling and gurgling followed by loose diarrhœic stools are present. The stools are green, watery, frothy with green scum like that of a frog-pond. Sometimes we notice large masses of white tallow like substance floating in the green watery stool. The green colour, the sourness and the froth are the three distinctive characteristics of the stool of this remedy. Milk is mostly intolerable and it is passed out in the stools in the form of curds. It causes great distention, nausea and uneasiness. Hence it is an object of great aversion to the patient. Talking about aversion I must mention that it has also an inordinate craving for meat.

The menses under this remedy are usually late and scanty and they have this peculiarity, that they flow more at the night time while the patient is at rest, becoming scanty while the patient is up and moving about in the morning, ceasing altogether later on in the afternoon. Before menses we have coryza, headache and obstructed nostrils, sorethroat and labor-like pains. We must also remember that in all preparations of Magnesia the menses are always dark, black and pitch-like.

I shall just mention one symptom before closing, as I consider it to be very important. It is a peculiar sensation in the face as if it has been smeared over with the white of an egg.

The patient's sleep is very much disturbed and unrefreshing. They get up more tired in the morning than when they go to bed. It is full of dreams of dead persons, of fire and of thieves.

MAGNESIA MURIATICA.

It is the chloride of Magnesia. This preparation of **Magnesia**, though greatly similar to **Mag. carb.**, has some peculiar characteristic symptoms of its own. Hence the need of a separate chapter on this remedy. It is particularly a woman's remedy; I mean woman who suffers from hysterical paroxysms, complicated with uterine disorders. Indigestion with all its symptoms is also a characteristic feature of **Mag. carb.** A coated flabby large yellow tongue, accumulation of water in the mouth, continual rising of frothy saliva, severe hiccough after dinner causing vomiting, regurgitation of food while walking, rotten rancid eructation, "waterbrash, oppression in the pit of the stomach, intolerence of milk, pressing pain in the liver, a sensation of weight in hypochondriac region, biliousness, constipation and colic" are some of the symptoms that indicate it as a cardinal remedy in gastrohepatic affections of the hysterical woman. Aggravation from mental exercise, rest, meals and coition are as characteristic as its amelioration, from movement, hard pressure and open air.

They suffer from congestive headache. The head feels as if it would burst. It is relieved by strong pressure and wrapping up of the head. The pains are referred to the temples.

The complaint in which, however, it is mostly indicated is a peculiar obstinate constipation. The characteristic stool is knotty like sheep's dung, crumbling at the verge of the anus. This constipation is mostly common in children during dentition. The stools are sometimes covered with mucus and blood. They are so hard and dry that they seem as if they are burnt. After stools the rectum feels sore and painful. Such constipation is very common in poor, puny, rachitic children with enlarged abdomen. Quite a lot of urging is necessary before defæcation.

We have a peculiar palpitation in **Mag. mur.** It is rendered worse by sitting. Every time the patient rests, the pulse gets accelerated and he feels a peculiar sensation of ebullition in the region of the heart. This necessitates constant motion.

On the female sexual organs, as has been mentioned before it produces quite a lot of characteristic symptoms. The flow is black and clotted, and it is accompanied with violent pains in the back when walking and in the thighs when sitting. The flow is profuse at night, in bed and it causes hysterical symptoms. The menstrual pain is generally relieved by having back pressed. There is frequent desire to pass urine and it can only be passed by bearing down with abdominal muscles, showing an atonic condition of the bladder. They sleep a lot during the day with great deal of sleeplessness at night.

MAGNESIA PHOSPHORICA.

Phosphate of Magnesia is one of the most important of the twelve tissue remedies of Dr. Schussler, the propounder of the Biochemic System of Medicine. It has proved itself to be an important remedial agent. It is found in blood corpuscles, muscles, brain, spinal marrow and in various other tissues of the human body.

Magnesia phos. occupies an important place amongst some of our best neuralgic remedies. It has been said and very truly, that homœopathic prescribing is no easy matter. A careful study of **Mag. phos.** will convince every student of homœopathy, the utter need of discrimination, careful cool judgment, and a constant burning of incense before the Goddess of Materia Medica. There is no Balm of Gilead, nor a general anodyne in our system of Therapeutics.—There are infinite varieties, types and gradations of pain, each calling for different remedies. We have boring pains, digging pains, griping pains, dragging pains, crampy spasmodic pains, benumbing pains, bruised pains, cutting stitching pains, gnawing pains, stinging pains and thousand other varieties of pains that need careful balancing and the finest powers of penetration and discrimination. This explains the scarcity of physicians of the type of Hahnemann, Hering, Lippe, Allen, Majumdar, Roy, Bhaduri and Salzer. Then again, the pains vary in their way of coming and going. In **Kalmia, Nat. mur., Phos., Platina, Spigelia, Stann.** and **Sulp. acid,** the pain appears gradually and disappears gradually. In **Bell., Kali bich., Pulsatilla, Magnesia phos.,** and **Nitric acid,** it comes on suddenly and disappears just as suddenly. We shall therefore make a special study of the symptoms of pain of some of these remedies.

The pain of **Mag. phos.** is mostly neuralgic. It is sharp, shooting, cutting and is almost unendurable. The pain darts along the course of a nerve like lightning flash and extorts scream from our patient. It rapidly changes its place. It is felt now in the head then all on a sudden it radiates to every part of the body. The patient hardly knows where it is going to come on next. This is what has been described as wandering pain and in this respect our remedy is similar to **Kali bi., Kali sulp., Lac can., Led.** and **Pulsat.** The pain of **Mag. phos.** has also been described as a crampy pain. It comes on spasmodically and bends our patient double with colic. It is mostly a nocturnal pain. It comes on almost every night and leaves him with the light of the dawn. Periodicity is a further characteristic of this pain. The **Mag. phos.** pains are invariably better by heat, warmth, pressure and bending double (**Colocynth**). They are aggravated by motion and draught of air. We will next compare **Mag. phos.** with a few other great pain remedies and note points of similarity and difference.

Acon.—In this remedy the pain is almost as excruciating as in **Mag. phos.** In fact it is more so. It drives our patient almost mad. The neuralgia in **Acon.** is caused by exposure to dry cold winds. It is particularly indicated when there is violent congestion of the affected part. In **Acon.** the pain is worse at night time ; it is burning, lancinating, pulsating, tingling and benumbing, with great hyperæsthesia of the affected part. There is also much apprehension and anxiety.

Ammon. mur. has an important place in the therapeutics of neuralgia. It is worse while sitting, better while walking (**Rhus tox**) and entirely relieved while lying down. It is particularly indicated in sciatica. The patient limps when walking and there is a sensation as if the tendons were too short.

Actea racemosa has neuralgia of any part of the body as a reflex symptom from uterine and ovarian diseases. The pain is sharp, lancinating and neuralgic in character. It is felt around eyes and supra-orbital region, whence it shoots up to the top of the head.

Apis has migrating pains same as in **Mag. phos.,** but the pains in **Apis** are stinging and burning in character and there is a great deal of soreness connected with **Apis.** The pains are ameliorated by cold application and open air.

Arsen. is as great a neuralgic remedy. The pain in this remedy is of a burning character occurring mostly in patients of malarial habit, who had their system ruined by heroic over-medication. The pains are worse especially after midnight and from cold.

Cactus grand. is a great heart remedy and enjoys an equal reputation in the treatment of neuralgia—but only in those cases which are characterised by the onset of pain at the missing of an accustomed meal. Periodicity is even more marked here than in **Mag. phos.**

Capsicum resembles **Mag. phos.,** in that the neuralgia of the face, is aggravated by the slightest draught of air whether warm or cold. These patients are generally of a lax fibre. The pain is a burning pungent pain like that caused by taking red pepper.

Cedron is very efficacious in malarial neuralgia of the supra-orbital region. The pain is of a burning type and the affected part feels as if on fire. Periodicity here, as elsewhere in this remedy, is the guiding feature. There is marked aggravation after coition, during menses and lying on the left hand side.

Cham. is not inferior to any remedy in the treatment of neuralgia. The pain is shooting, tearing and pulsating in character. Although there is extreme impressionability, the part affected feels numb. Excessive irritability, hot sweat on the head, redness of one cheek and paleness of the other and aggravation from anger are important points on this remedy. Hot perspiration breaks out on the face and forehead.

China is another important remedy in neuralgia and is characterised by great periodicity. It is generally indicated in anæmic patients and it usually involves the infra-orbital region on either side. **China,** too, is indicated in neuralgia of malarial origin and is aggravated at the slightest touch or draught of cold air.

Chininum ars. is indicated in violent neuralgic pain in the left mammary region.

Ignatia should be thought of in neuralgia of the nervous and sensitive individuals. The pains are exetremely severe and are often associated with globus hystericus.

Kali bich. has a strong resemblance to **Mag. phos.,** with respect to the wandering nature of the pain.

Natrum mur. should not be forgotten in neuralgia. In this we have another remedy for neuralgia due to suppression of the malaria poison. It is chiefly a ciliary neuralgia from sun-rise to sun-set. The pain is of a darting, shooting, throbbing character and almost drives the patient mad. It is accompanied with flow of saliva or involuntary tears. It is generally better at the sea-side.

Plumb. met. is used in neuralgia of the rectum,

Pulsat. should not be forgotten as it has many points of resemblance to **Mag. phos.** The pain in **Pulsat.** is erratic and paroxysmal. In this remedy we have neuralgia mostly on one side of the body and is accompanied with great chilliness; the greater the pain, the worse being the chilliness.

Rododen. should be remembered with **Ham.** in scrotal neuralgia.

Spigelia is a great rival of **Mag. phos.,** in neuralgia. It is generally associated with the sun; that is beginning early in the morning with sun-rise and gradually getting worse towards the noon and eventually subsiding with the sun-set in the evening. It generally begins in the occiput, then coming forward, it settles over the left eye. It may also involve the cheek, specially the left. At the height of the pain, there is always bilious vomiting. The sensation is as if the eye-balls are enormously enlarged. It is an important remedy for glaucoma. We notice aggravation from noise, motion, jarring of the body and stormy weather.

Staph. should be thought of in neuralgia, of shoulder-joint and arms.

Thuja may also be used in neuralgia. The pains are intense, stabbing and well-nigh unbearable. If the patient sits up, these pains almost drive him to distraction. He has got to sit up to get relief. Frequently these patients display sycotic history. The pains are apt to be worse in the damp atmosphere.

Mag. phos. is a splendid remedy for headache of school children, suffering from optical defects. It is mostly neuralgic in character and is, as has been said before, ameliorated by external application of warmth. It is also of particular interest in headache of young mothers after child-birth. Sudden flushes of pain in the back part of the head and neck, thence spreading all over the head, and involving the eyes, are of frequent occurrence necessitating rest, darkness and tight bandaging.

It is also used for spasms or cramps in the stomach. Nipping, griping, pinching pains are felt at the pit of stomach. These pains are also accompanied by a sensation of tight lacing around the body. Similar cramps are also felt in the abdomen, often accompanied by watery diarrhœa. It is sometimes not at all easy to distinguish **Mag. phos.** from **Colocynth.** Like **Colocynth** we have flatulent colic in **Mag. phos.,** forcing the patient to bend double. It is particularly of interest in flatulent colic of children and new born babies, who like **Colocynth,** double up with crampy pain between the hours of 3 and 4 p.m. The flatus neither passes upward nor downward. The stools in **Colocynth,** are fluid, copious, fecal, papescent, or slimy and bloody. The evacuations and the pains are provoked by the slightest food or drink. It has been used with great success in spasmodic hiccough and persistent vomiting. The patient spits up what he had eaten even while at table with little or no nausea.

MAGNESIA SULPHURICA.

Magnesia sulph., otherwise known as Epsom salt, is an ingredient of sea-water and of the water of some saline springs. It occurs in small colourless, rhombic prisms. It is odourless but has a cooling saline, bitter, disagreeable taste. It is a typical saline purge. In excessive dose it induces nausea, vomiting and profuse purging. It is by far the most commonly used saline purgative. It is a diuretic as well.

The homœopathic provings have brought us real good results. Its field of action, though narrow, is quite important. My experience with **Mag. sulph.,** is very limited. I have used it occasionally with certain amount of success in diarrhœa. The great cardinal indication, that frequently led me to this prescription, has been copiousness of the stools. Cases requiring **Mag. sulph.,** very often simulates a case of cholera. Vomiting of food. copious, yellowish, slimy, stinking stools and the presence of a large quantity of watery serous fluid demand **Mag. sulph.**

It has got a peculiar toothache. It comes on as the patient enters warm room after being in the fresh cold air for some time. It is aggravated by the least contact of food either warm or cold.

It has been extolled as a remedy for warts. Dr. H. T. Webster recommends it highly in such affections on the emperical ground of having cured many such cases.

Lastly it has been recommended in diabetes. Personally speaking I have had no experience to support this assertion, but as it is a strong diuretic and as it causes great thirst it may possibly prove a valuable adjunct in the treatment of that obstinate malady. The urine is clear, green and profuse. Often we have involuntary nocturnal micturition.

MALANDRINUM.

Malandrinum is another nosode prepared from the virus of the disease in the horses called Grease. Dr. Boskowitz of Brooklyn was the first to introduce **Malandrinum** into our therapeutics.

It is a great prophylactic against small-pox and like **Silicea**, it rectifies the bad effects of vaccination. Dr. Allen advises us not to use this remedy oftener than once a fortnight, as it is a deep and long-acting remedy. My experience is that it should be used oftener specially when the epidemic is violent. Living in a country where small-pox is not uncommon, I have had occasion to use this remedy often, both as a prophylactic and as a therapeutic agent in small-pox and also in chicken-pox. The result has been uniformly satisfactory. During the last 16 years, I have used this remedy in thousands of cases as a prophylactic and I have not known one single case of failure. Every year before the epidemic commences, hundreds of patients come for the internal vaccination as they call it. I have hope that with further verification we shall be able to substitute vaccination altogether with **Malandrinum.** How far this hope will be realised is for our posterity to judge. Dr. A. L. Marcy relates his experience with **Malandrinum** and it is in full accord with what I have said:— " During a small-pox epidemic he vaccinated himself, taking at the same time **Malandrinum** 30 night and morning. The vaccination did not take. It was twice repeated and still did not take; nor was small-pox contracted." He was called to vaccinate four children in a family whose parents had small-pox; he vaccinated all and gave **Malandrinum** 30 to three of them at the same time; the remaining child was the only one whose vaccination " took." This was so severe that **Malandrinum** had to be given to modify its intensity, which it did effectually. The other three were re vaccinated but none " took." In another instance out of a group of four children, from six to seventeen years of age, only the eldest had been vaccinated, and he had a good scar. All except the eldest were given **Malandrinum** and were vaccinated and none of the three " took." The eldest took small-pox. **Malandrinum** was then given, and in a few days he was convalescent. In another case of small-pox, **Malandrinum** was given, and the disease only lasted a few days, the eruption drying up."

I have had exactly similar experience with **Malandrinum**. It has been prescribed in very severe types of small-pox and I find that in nine cases out of ten it invariably cuts the disease short.

Now as regards the symptomatology of **Malandrinum**. Dr. Burnett considers the following symptoms very characteristic of our remedy—Lower half of the body affected; greasy skin and greasy eruption, slow pustulation never ending, as one heals another appears. The following symptoms are worth noting:—

Diarrhœa: acrid, yellow, offensive, discharge followed by burning in the anus and rectum.

Dark brown, foul-smelling stools, almost involuntary diarrhœa; pains in abdomen may supervene.

Black, foul-smelling diarrhœa, with malaise and weariness.

Child constantly handles the penis.

Pain along the back as if beaten.

Soles of feet bathed in sweat, scald and burn when covered or warm. Deep rhagades, sore and bleeding, on soles of feet ameliorated in the cold weather and after bathing.

Restless sleep; dreams of trouble, of quarrels.

Malandrinum 30, while being used as a prophylactic of variola cured a stubborn case of aphthæ, which had resisted many well selected remedies.

Each member, in a family of six, had been vaccinated; three receiving **Malandrinum,** and their arms were only slightly affected by the vaccination and ran a short course of a few days; the other three, who did not receive **Malandrinum,** were very ill, arms sore for weeks and required treatment.

A lady had an ulcer as large as a silver dollar and three-fourths of an inch deep, which continued to suppurate and would not heal; but under the curative effect of **Malandrinum,** recovered promptly.

"In a family of eight persons, none of whom had been vaccinated, the eldest boy took small-pox. One of his brothers slept with him after it had broken out all over; the mother expecting to be confined in a few days, we sent her away, and I at once put the rest of the family on **Malandrinum** 200, with the result that none of them took small-pox. The boy that slept with his brother, had a light fever the twelfth day, but that passed off without any further trouble."—Dr. Bryant.

MANCINELLA.

Hippomane Mancinella, a species of the Euphorbiaceæ, is a poisonous tree of the West Indies, bearing poisonous fruits somewhat resembling apples. The plant is extremely irritating; even water dropping on the skin from Mancinella leaves causes blisters and intense erythema of the skin. It was introduced and proved by Dr. Bute.

Its chief action is centered on the skin and throat. We notice intense redness of the skin with numerous small vesicles containing yellow serum which desquamate on the following day. The redness resembles the deep blush of scarlatina and has been used with great success in that disease. Large vesicles appear all over the body and specially on the soles. In respect of erythema and vesiculation it should be compared with **Canth., Croton tig., Yucca fian, Euphorb.,** and **Rhus tox.**

It is particularly useful in affections of the throat after scarlatina and also in post-diphtheretic ailments. The uvula is greatly elongated; even the tonsils are badly swollen and they are about to suppurate. The passage is rendered so narrow that there is constant danger of suffocation. The breathing is of a whistling character. There are numerous burning ulcers on the tonsils and in the throat. But the most important symptom is a constant sensation of choking, particularly when the patient tries to speak. A great thirst for cold water with inability to swallow, on account of the choking sensation, is of no less importance. This aggravation from the drinking of cold water may be considered the leading symptom of this remedy. The following are a few other importan indications of **Mancinella:—**

Sudden vanishing of thought, forgets from one moment t next what she wishes to do.

Fear of getting crazy; of evil spirits; of being taken away b the devil.

Tongue coated white as in aphthæ.

After drinking water: colic; pain in the abdomen.

Pains in abdomen after drinking water.

Colic; after drinking water; with diarrhœa (at midnight); wi fainting; constipation, alternating with diarrhœa.

Choking sensation rising up into the throat, hindering speec

Nasal tone of the voice.

Cough; aggravated at night; after drinking.

Constriction of the chest.

Hands as if too thick, "asleep," heavy and clumsy.
Hands feel icy cold.
Icy coldness of hands and feet.
When awaking, hands go to "sleep" and feel as if too thick.

MANGANUM.

There are two preparations——Acetate of Manganese and Carbonate of Manganese; but the symptoms are so very similar in both, that no distinctions have been made. It is found in nature in combination with iron to which it is a close ally. After the general manner of heavy metals, in small dosage, it tends to improve blood quality and quicken general assimilation, and in large dosage, to derange the nutritive process leading to emaciation and nerve poisoning. Our homœopathic proving has brought out a whole series of important indications to which we will refer just now. It was proved and introduced into our Materia Medica by Hahnemann himself.

I have had occasions to use **Manganum** in rheumatism and in affections of the ears, and I have been highly pleased with the results. I am sure, used on proper indications, it will give similar satisfaction to other homœopaths. There are a few characteristic indications in **Manganum** same as in other remedies. The first and the foremost amongst these is soreness of almost every part of the body when touched. Limbs are very tender and they feel lame, pretty much the same as in **Arnica**, but in **Manganum** the pain is deep-seated. It feels that the very bones are affected and that the soreness extends down to them.

The next important feature consists in its modality. Nearly all symptoms are aggravated at night time, from cold, in cold rainy weather and by change of weather. Ameliorations are found from lying down, in open air, by eating and by swallowing.

The third point for us to remember, is that it has particular affinity for the ankles and the ankle-joints. We use it in inflamation and swelling of malleoli with stitches in the leg running upwards. Many of the complaints in this remedy begin in the lower limbs and generally run upwards.

Mang. has been used with great success in catarrhal deafness of the ears. It is also used in catarrh of the Eustachian tube with stitching pains and wheezing noise in ears. The dulness of hearing is always relieved by blowing nose and is aggravated in cold damp rainy weather. It is also associated with a cracking noise every time he swallows.

Mang. is as important a remedy in climacteric ailments as **Sulph., Lach.** and **Sang.** We have sudden flushes of heat same as in the other remedies; also we have discharges of blood between periods, with pressing in genitals.

Mang. has a special claim on us homœopaths, for its great usefulness in a certain variety of cough——a deep cough with expectoration, ceasing on lying down. An irritation is felt about the middle of the sternum. This is a strange peculiar and an unusual symptom. Generally speaking, cough is usually aggravated on lying down; whereas under this remedy the opposite condition prevails. A symptom like this is rarely met with and when we do come across such a symptom, we should never foget **Mang.** The few other remedies that I know of, having a similar symptom are **Acon., Ammon. mur., Euphra., Sepia** and **Zinc.** It is not difficult however, to differentiate **Mang.** from any of these remedies.

In **Acon.** the cough is ringing or whistling in character. It is a violent, hollow, high-sounding cough but croupy in nature. The aggravation in **Acon.** is mostly in night time whereas in **Mang.,** is always an afternoon cough. In **Acon.** the sound is a barking sound and is accompanied with suffocation.

The **Ammon. mur.** cough is caused by tickling in the throat whereas in **Mang.** the tickling is felt deep down, behind the sternum. The secretion of a quantity of thick yellow matter present with stitches in the chest. Although the cough ameliorated by lying on the back as in **Mang.,** it is always aggravated on turning on the side and is always marked with a strange coldness between scapulæ.

In **Euphrasia** the aggravation is marked more in the morning hours when the patient gets out of bed; sometimes it is so harassing that he has to lie down again for relief. This cough also better from eating. The most peculiar part of the **Euphras** cough is that it always comes on in the day-time, never at night.

The **Sepia** cough is very easy to differentiate as it is found mostly in women suffering from uterine derangement. This cough is also rendered worse by walking fast.

The **Zinc.** cough is spasmodic in nature and is caused by a sensation of tickling in the larynx. This cough is always worse after eating and drinking of milk. We think of **Zinc.** particularly in that spasmodic variety of cough in children when during a fit of coughing the infant automatically puts his hand on his genitals.

Before closing I would like to touch on one other indication of **Mang.** that has led many homœopaths to effect remarkable cures. It is a symptom on which Dr. Lippe amongst many others, placed great importance. It consists in unhealthiness of the skin around the joints. Very often we notice suppuration of the skin around the joints. This is a red strand symptom and should always draw our attention to **Mang.** The presence of other characteristic indications and also the totality will, as usual, help us in making the final selection.

MARUM VERUM.

(See **Teucrium**)

MEDORRHINUM.

Medorrhinum is prepared from the gonorrhœal virus. It was rst introduced by Dr. Swan. Most of the provings were made ith the fifth potency. It is an invaluable remedy. By this I do ot mean that it is more important than any other remedy when dicated, but simply that this remedy is oftener indicated than any others. It must however be borne in mind that the principle f its application is exactly the same as that of any other homœo- athic remedy. To prescribe **Medor.** on the simple basis of sycosis therefore a great mistake. Dr. Nash is very doubtful on this int. Numerous cases are reported throughout homœopathic terature, of marvellous cures, based simply on sycotic history, ther inherited or acquired. Instead of propounding a theory my own I would rather leave it to the better judgment of the dividual homœopath to form and evolve theories on the basis his own experience.

These patients are, as a rule, subject to enlargement of lymphatic glands all over the body. Their facial appearance is characteristic. Great pallor, yellowness of the face, particularly around eyes as if occurring from a bruise, yellow band across the forehead close to the hair, greenish shining appearance of skin: great tendency towards rheumatic affections, peculiar serrated teeth, offensive odour about the body, scaly scurfy margins of the eyelids and falling of eye lashes, are all characteristics of **Medor.** Many cases of stunted growth in children are due to some latent gonorrhœal factor in their constitution, and **Medor.** is said to have remedied such defects. After an administration of this remedy, children, who were defective in various ways and showed no sign of progress either mental, moral or physical, have blossomed forth into health and vigour. This theory has been verified time and again and we have numerous instances in hand to prove its correctness.

The time of aggravation in **Medor.** is particularly characteristic. It takes place from sun-rise to sun-set; this constitutes an important factor in differentiating it from **Syphilinum,** where the aggravation is seen to take place at night from sun-set to sunrise. In **Medor.** the patient is much ameliorated at seaside whereas in **Syphilinum** the amelioration takes place in high altitude and on mountain tops.

It is a great constitutional remedy. In our sojourn of thousands of years through various generations and centuries and due to pernicious influence of many of our antagonistic environments we, all of us, are born with various kinds of taints and dyscrasias These manifest themselves in various forms throughout our lives. The ebb and flow of health, the susceptibilities, the cravings, the aversions, the ailments to which we fall a ready victim are some of its phenomena. The span of life, the emotional peculiarities, the peculiar bends of character, and the physiognomy are moulded to a greater or to a lesser extent, by the latent poison and miasms of our system. Ovarian tumors, oophoritis, salpingitis, metritis, parametritis, endometritis, hydrocephalus, nasal polypi, epistaxis, psoriasis, albuminuria, cystitis, epididymitis prostatitis, and synovitis, are complaints that are particular manifestations of, and are traceable to the latent gonorrhœal poison communicated to the patient from some ancestor. Hence it is we find **Medor.** so marvellously efficacious in so many complaints where proper symptomatic indications are wanting, forming such a bulwark in many of our prescriptions. I am going to cite below a few instructive cases for the benefit of homœopathic practitioners who are to decide whether to prescribe on dyscrasia or to go by indications.

Case 1.—In summer, 1875, I had an obstinate case of acute articular rheumatism in a man æt. 6£, from June 11th to September 5th. He suffered excruciating agony from neuralgia. After a desperate battle for life the first week of September, he was relieved, and arose from his bed a wreck. It was expected that time and out-door life and the best hygienic measures would restore him. But weeks and months passed without a change; he walked the streets leaning on a cane, bent over, muffled in wraps to his ears, and looking like an old man about to fall into grave. Three months after my attendance I saw him pass my office, and considering his previous good health and robust frame the question arose: Why does he remain in this condition? Is there any miasm hereditary or acquired, to explain the obstinacy of the case? Could it be a gonorrhœal taint? For reasons unnecessary to mention I would not ask him.

Dr. Swan's suggestion now occurred to me:—

"An obstinate case of rheumatism might be due to latent gonorrhœa and **Medorrhinum** might well cure it; in many cases where improvement reaches a certain stage, and then stops, **Medorrhinum** has removed the obstruction and the case progressed to a cure; and this too in cases where gonorrhœa appeared to be most unlikely cause, teaching us, if anything, the universality of latent gonorrhœa and the curative power of the dynamic virus."

His wife consulted me on another matter, and said, "Her husband was as well as could be expected considering his age; she believed he would not do anything more, as he regarded his feeble state due to his age." However, he came next day, and I gave him three doses of **Medorrhinum**, to be taken every morning; within ten days he returned feeling well and looking better. I then gave him one dose to be taken after some time; this was the last prescription he had required. Within the month, after the **Medorrhinum**, he dropped his cane and muffler, walked the street erect with a firm step, a perfectly well man, having increased in weight from 140 to 212 pounds.—Dr. Allen.

Case 2.—A girl of eleven had been treated by many physicians with salves and ointments to the general impairment of her health. Face mottled with a profusion of red scurfy sores; eyelids involved and nearly denuded of lashes; hairy scalp and a diffuse mass of thick yellow scabs, from beneath which oozed a highly offensive mixture of ichor and serum. Passing down neck, back, perineum and involving genitals and pubes was a fiery red band as broad as a child's hand, oozing a pale yellow serum, which caused the clothing to stick to the body. I told the mother I could cure the case but it would certainly get worse the first three months. **Medorrhinum** CM was given one dose dry on the tongue. The external appearance grew rapidly worse, but appetite, sleep and general health steadily improved, and in nine months she was completely cured.—Dr. Wildes.

Case 3.—A child of six, since infancy was horribly disfigured with tinea capitis. The scalp was a mass of dense crusts exuding a fetid ichor and the only semblance of hair were a few distorted stumps ending in withered roots. One dose cured in a few months, and at the time of writing, the patient was a healthy and extremely talented young lady, and the possessor of a luxuriant head of chestnut hair.—Dr. Wildes.

Case 4.—During a manœuvre in the army in 1885, Dr. V. got wet by a heavy rain coming into the tent during a wet night. From this he got a hacking cough, on rising in the morning and in the open air. It sounded as if he would call some one, and people would turn and look at him with angry eyes. His throat was thoroughly examined by a specialist, but nothing was found. In 1901, after 16 years of coughing he consulted Dr. Ide, one of our greatest homœopathic physicians. He ordered the doctor to take **Medorrhinum** one dose, and wait the result. On reaching home, he took the dose, and next morning had no cough, nor did he cough afterwards, even in the open air. As an officer he had had a gonorrhœa, of which he could not get rid. From this he always had an unpleasant feeling and burning pain. All this vanished like a magic.

Case 5.—A girl of twenty years had a violent cough for many months, that nobody could (or did) cure, until I learned that her father had had gonorrhœa a year before her birth; then a few doses of **Medorrhinum** worked like magic.

Case 6.—Sycotic warts were cured by one dose, after nine months' careful treatment had failed. He contracted gonorrhœa during December, 1886 and was nearly cured. In May, 1887, he had another sycotic attack, with chancroids. The ulcers were all over the prepuce, and as they improved the warts began to grow all over the glans, back of the corona, inside of the prepuce, and frænum. The head of the penis was two three times of the natural size; the warts very moist, and secreted a yellowish, stinkling fluid, and bled very easily, and the odour was very perceptible in a room with him; but his general health was much improved. From the 26th May he had **Merc. sol., Nit. ac., Sulph., Corallium, Cinnab., Silic., Thuj., Phos. acid, Sabin, Staphis.**—all in high potencies, but got no better.   In March 7th, 1888, Dr. W. P. Wesselhœft advised **Medorrhinum**, CM.   In a week he was better while the discharge and the odour were gone. In two weeks more the warts were about one-third their size and in six weeks they were entirely gone.

Case 7.—Miss X. æt. 23, had chronic blepharitis since eleven. Her suffering was intense. Light, especially gas-light, was intolerable, and this prevented her from going into society. She could not read in the evening, and in the morning the lids would be closed, and she suffered much on getting them separated. There was much discharge. Before coming under me she had been under strict homœopa. .c treatment all the time. I remembered treating her father for gonorrhœa before his marriage, and I suspected the taint had reappeared in this form. **Medorrhinum** was given in a high potency, single doses repeated as the effect of each wore off, and she was entirely cured.—Dr. Deschere.

Case 8.—One case (a middle-aged lady) was n ' able to attend church, a few rods from her residence, for a long time, the trouble being in her feet and ankles and soles of the feet. The ankles were so sore and the soles so tender that she could not walk on them. **Antimonium crud.,** which had cured some bad cases with similar symptoms for me, was without any beneficial effect, but **Medorrhinum** CM one dose, so benefited her that she could walk wherever she pleased.

This remedy is very rich in mental symptoms. The most prominent of which are the following :—

Great weakness of memory.

Entirely forgets what she has read, even the previous line.

Forgetfulness of names, words and initial letters.

Cannot remember names ; has to ask name of her most intimate friend ; forgets her own.

Time moves too slowly.

Dazed feeling ; a far off sensation, as though things done to-day occurred a week ago.

Loses constantly the thread of her talk.

Great difficulty in stating her symptoms, loses herself and has to be asked over again.

Wild and desparate feeling, as of incipient insanity.

Cannot speak without crying.

Is in a great hurry ; when doing anything is in such a hurry that she gets fatigued.

Wakes at an early hour with a frightened sensation, as if something dreadful had happened ; feels a heavy weight and great heat in the head ; cannot rest in bed ; feels as if she must do something to rid her mind of torture.

Medorrhinum is very rich in symptoms of the throat. The patient is troubled with hoarseness, specially while reading with occasional loss of voice. It is very useful in choking caused by a weakness or spasm of the epiglottis. The larynx gets constricted so that no air could either escape or enter. Relief is obtained by lying on the face and protruding the tongue. This is a very curious amelioration and should be carefully borne in mind.

The cough under **Medorrhinum** is caused from a sensation of tickling under the sternum. It is incessant, dry and harassing. It is always worse at night and when the patient is about to fall asleep. It is worse on lying down and it is better by lying on the stomach. Indications like these are very strange, peculiar and uncommon, and hence they are of greater importance than those that are otherwise. A case cited by Dr. McLaren is very instructive and inspiring. It shows exactly what can be done and it also shows the other side of the picture that we have forgotten to draw, I mean the efficaciousnes of **Medorrhinum** as prescribed on indications. I am citing below a case for the edification of the homœopathic profession in general :—

"A young French Canadian of delicate constitution, after working in a factory all winter, began coughing in spring and running down in health. He returned home and came under my care in May. The cough persisted and prostration increased, in spite of carefully selected remedies, and the patient took to his bed. It was then observed by me that the cough and general condition was ameliorated from lying on the face. This, coupled with a knowledge of his having a sycotic taint suggested **Medorrhinum**, which was given. The next day a profuse gonorrhoeal discharge appeared, and the cough and all threatening symptoms promptly disappeared. Exposure to contagion had occurred several weeks before, but from lack of vitality the disease could not find its usual expression and was endangering the patient's life.—Dr. D. C. McLaren.

Before closing I will touch on the indications of **Medor.** on the male and the female sexual organs. It has been used with great success in impotence. Nocturnal emissions are very common; the discharge is watery and it hardly causes stiffness of the linen. It is transparent and is of the consistence of gum arabic mucilage. Gonorrhoea for which it is supposed to be such a great remedy is amenable to its influence, only when it has attained the chronic stage. We never think of using it in an acute case. The flow is thin and transparent and it drags on for months. Hardly any acute symptom is noticeable. Slight burning in the meatus during urination and a slight soreness in urethra are the only symptoms that we notice. So it is more gleet than gonorrhoea that comes under its influence. We also notice chancre-like ulcer on the prepuce.

On the female sexual system it is used for ulceration on the neck of the uterus. The menses are very dark and the stains are difficult to wash out. Generally speaking, it is attended with intense colic causing drawing up of the knees. The pain is terrible and is bearing down and labour-like in nature. Menses are sometimes followed by neuralgic pain in the head. I am citing below an interesting cure of membranous dysmenorrhoea by Dr. Close with **Medor.** It was prescribed not on any sycotic history nor on any supposition of latent sycosis but on the strict and clearcut symptomatology.

The menstruation was accompanied by terrible pains of a griping character. The flow was scanty, and on the second day there was a passage of a firmly organized membrane. The mental symptom was a constant feeling as if something was behind her. She could not get away from that sensation. It was of nothing definite, simply something terrible behind her, peering over her shoulder, causing her to look around anxiously. Under **Medorrhinum** I found many of her symptoms, including the peculiar mental symptom, and gave it to her. The next period was without membrane. Repeated the remedy and the third period was painless again.--Dr. Close.

MEL CUM SALE.

It means honey with salt. It is supposed to be a splendid remedy for prolapsus uteri when associated with chronic metritis. Symptoms of sub-involution and inflammation of the cervix are also associated with the above complaints. I have not used this remedy and hence am not in a position to pass any verdict on it. Its chief indications are (a) a feeling of soreness across hypogastrium from ilium to ilium, (b) sensation as if bladder were too full, (c) pain from sacrum towards pubis.

MELILOTUS.

It is also called the Sweet Clover and it belongs to the natural order of Leguminosæ. It was first proved by Bowen in 1852, since which time it has been re-proved by Dr. H. C. Allen in late years.

The most important keynote of this remedy is found in the engorgement of the blood vessels in any part or organ of the body. This is specially noticed in the head. The congestion is so great as to make the face distinctly livid and purple. This leads on to such violent headache as to make the patient bed-ridden for hours. Any trifling thing provokes this headache and it is almost always relieved by epistaxis. The congestion is so violent that the patient feels as if his brain would burst through the forehead. When talking, the headache leaves forehead and settles in occiput. It is relieved by the application of vinegar and cold water or lying down. The headache is accompanied with retching and vomiting. With regard to the congestion it may be compared to **Acon., Ailanth., Amyl. nit., Bell., Ferrum met., Gelsemium, Glonoine, Sanguinaria** and **Veratrum viride.**

In **Aconite** the headache is brought on by exposure to sun's rays. The congestion is just as violent and the feeling much about the same as in **Melilotus**. Also in this remedy we have relief from nose-bleed; but the livid appearance of **Melilotus** is wanting in **Aconite** where the face, though flushed, looks pale as compared with the engorged appearance of the other patient.

Ailanthus has passive congestion of the head and relief from nose-bleed; but the want of inclination to think and act is in striking contradiction to **Melilotus** where the mental faculties and the brain are left more active than ever.

Amyl nitrate has marked congestive headache and hemicrania but in this remedy the affected side looks paler than the other side.

Belladonna has marked congestion of blood to the head; the headache is relieved not by lying down but by sitting propped up.

Ferrum met. is characterized by marked congestion of the head of people who are debilitated and anæmic and is associated with sudden vertigo. The headache is momentarily relieved by pressure and entirely in the open air.

Gelsemium has marked passive congestion of the brain and is associated with dizziness and blurring of vision before headache.

The congestion of **Glonoine** is characterised by a crushing weight across the forehead. This is mainly a sun headache, increasing and decreasing with the sun.

Sanguinaria congestion is associated with dizziness in the head and is relieved by a quiet rest in a darkened room and from pushing head deep into the pillow.

Veratrum vir. is an excellent remedy when the congestion is most intense.

MENTHA PIPERITA.

It is our well-known peppermint. It has marked action over the respiratory organs and hence it is remarkably helpful in dry cough caused by irritation of the respiratory passage. The peppermint cough is a dry cough caused by the air going into the larnyx during an effort to talk and hence it is very similar to **Rumex.** The voice is husky and the tip of the nose is sore to touch. The throat feels dry and sore, as if pins were laid crosswise in it. The trachea is painful to touch. The case as related by Gibson Miller, of a teacher who used to suffer from a dry spasmodic cough, is quite interesting. The inhalation of the smallest quantity of smoke at once induced the most distressing paroxysm of cough. The least breath of air and the slightest attempt at singing or speaking aggravated the trouble. **Mentha piperita 30,** completely removed the cough and cured him so thoroughly as to enable him to smoke, talk and sing without the slightest return of the paroxysm.

MENTHOL.

It is the essential oil of Mentha. It has strong action over the mucous membrane of the naso pharynx; hence it is of great use in acute nasal catarrh, Eustachian catarrh, pharyngitis and laryngitis. In the head we have frontal headache and pain over the frontal sinus. Pain in the face above the zygoma and pain in the eyeballs are prominent symptoms of this remedy. It relieves tickling in the fauces, also short cough and asthmatic breathing. It has also been recommended in pruritus vulvæ.

MENYANTHES TRIFOLIATA.

Menyanthes is a perennial which grows in boggy places in America and in Europe. In common language it is called the Buck Bean. In Ireland where it grows profusely it is called the Bog Bean from its being a water plant. It was introduced into homœopathy by Hahnemann who proved it on himself.

Menyanthes is a great remedy with us for the treatment of ague and malarial fevers. We will go into this in detail after having picked out its prominent and characteristic indications. The symptom that stands out most prominently in this remedy is a general sensation of chilliness. This is felt in the head, ears, abdomen, feet, legs and fingers. There is a sensation of chilliness felt even in the œsophagus. I have seen **Menyanthes** prescribed in various ailments on the simple indication of extreme coldness of the tips of the nose. The next important indication is a sensation of tension. This tension is felt in the root of the nose, arms, hands, fingers and head, and in fact over the whole body. The skin feels tight everywhere. It is a feeling as if he has been cramped and crowded into the tight fitting of his own skin. This is a peculiar sensation and should be carefully borne in mind. It will help us out of many tight corners. The next and the third important feature is fidgetiness. Spasmodic jerkings and physical twitchings are found everywhere. These are always worse during rest. As soon as the patient lies down his legs jerk and twitch so that he has to sit up. In this respect it is very much like **Zinc. met.** This spasmodic jerking is usually seen in gouty persons with deposits of calcarious tissues in many of their joints. It has been used with great success in sciatica where stretching and contractive pains are felt in the region of the hip-joint, causing spasmodic jerkings of thighs and legs when in a sitting posture.

The aggravations in this remedy, are mostly seen during rest and in horizontal position. The headache found under this remedy is very characteristic. It is a sort of pressure on the vertex from above downwards and is invariably helped by hard pressure. It feels as if a heavy weight has been put on the top of the head, and the peculiar amelioration derived by still heavier pressure, is striking and characteristic. In this respect it may be compared with **Arg. nit., Bismuth, Cact., Cina, Hellebore., Nux vom., Puls., Spig.,** and **Thuja.**

Next we come to its most important sphere, I mean its usefulness in the treatment of malarial fevers. It is generally adapted to cases where there has been a great abuse of quinine. We should therefore think about it whenever a patient comes to us from the opposite school of treatment where quinine is such an universal favourite. To be honest and outspoken every medical man must admit that there are cases where quinine is absolutely of no avail and still how often we find such patients being given quinine repeatedly and in huge doses. Such maladministration not only complicates the case but produces a sort of a drug disease far more difficult to eradicate. All the enlarged spleens and livers that we come across are not the effect of marsh miasms alone. A little judgment, scrutiny and a little more unbiased thinking will make it plain to many of our fellow practitioners that poisonous ingredients and drugs may, if misapplied, produce a great many symptoms and far more potent damages than are caused by many of the dreaded bacteriæ. However, the maladministration of quinine should not constitute the sole reason for the prescribing of **Menyanthes.** A far more important indication is the predominance of the chilly stage. Chill, to which such a high place has been assigned in this remedy, is as well marked here as in other complaint where this remedy is indicated. Chilliness, though specially felt in the fingers and toes is practically present all over the body.

It is felt most severely on the back, and it is greatly relieved by warmth of heat of the stove. In this respect our remedy differs from **Verat. alb.** and **Ipec.** In the former remedy even the heat of the stove or for the matter of that, any other hot application does not bring any relief. In the latter remedy all such attempt produces the reverse effect. The **Menyanthes** patient feels the coldness in the abdomen and in his feet as far up as the knee on the slightest movement. As soon as he rises from his bed in the morning, he feels coldness creeping over abdomen, back and sides. His hands and his feet are icy cold as if they have been kept immersed in ice water. There is shivering with yawning. Horripilation is noticeable all over his back.

The stage of heat is not half as marked as the stage of chill. Indeed, there are flushes of heat with hot ears and cheeks, but this hot flush are nothing compared to the severity of his chill.

These patients are ravenously hungry and show a marked desire for meat. This is unlike **Arnica**, where we have the opposite condition of aversion to meat.

A feature that has not been sufficiently emphasised is the unequal distribution of chill and heat in **Menyanthes.** Fingers and toes are cold, although the rest of the body retains its animal heat. This is a great feature with **Meny.,** and it constitutes an important point in the differentiation with other similar remedies such as **Led., Mag., Sepia,** etc. Dr. A. L. Fisher gave **Menyanthes** a very high place in the therapeutic of fevers. "Quartan intermittents were the pest of my life until I struck **Menyanthes.** I feel sure, many of us would do well to study our homœopathic Materia Medica a bit more thoroughly and not despair as they often do, whenever they come face to face with a case of intermittent fever."

MEPHITIS.

This medicine is prepared by dissolving one part by weight of the liquid obtained from the anal glands of the skunk or the polecat to ninetynine parts by weight of alcohol. This substance, secreted in a pouch near the anus, from the follicular gland is highly pungent and disgusting in odor. It nearly stifles when smelt. The peculiarity of this medicine lies in the strange constitution of the patient. They seem to have a power of withstanding extreme cold. In fact they thrive in cold weather. Washing in ice water is very agreeable to them and relieves all their suffering.

Very lately, I helped an elderly lady suffering from asthma with **Mephitis.** The symptom, that led to the prescription, was the relief she had from bathing, which she did five or six times a day.

They frequently wake up at night time suffering from a peculiar congestion of the legs which gives them a sensation of heat in those parts. This brings on an uneasy feeling in the legs and makes them fidgety. This fidgetiness of the legs also reminds us of **Zinc. met.**

Like **Lachesis, Stramonium** and **Podophyllum** the **Mephitis** patients talk incessantly. They are led from subject to subject by the vividness of their fancy.

It is a valuable remedy in cough of a certain type. The cough is brought on by reading aloud, talking and drinking.

In this respect it is similar to **Rumex** and **Sticta.** Dr. Stewart cured with **Mephitis** a constant hacking cough in an elderly man, who could hardly talk because of the cough. **Ambra grisea, Rumex, Kali bi.** and **Phosphorus** were used without much success but **Mephitis** 1m cured him promptly. It has been recommended very highly in whooping cough when the catarrhal symptoms are more or less absent and spasmodic symptoms are most prominent. It is so violent and spasmodic that each spell would seem to terminate life. The cough is worse at night and after lying down and is attended with a suffo-cative feeling. To exhale is very difficult. Food taken hours before are vomited. **Mephitis** thus resembles **Drosera** and **Coral. rub.**

MERCURIUS.

There are various preparations of Mercury, but under the heading of **Mercurius** we will combine the study of **Mercurius solubilis** and **Mercurius vivus. Merc. sol.** was first introduced by Hahnemann but later on he abandoned this preparation preferring to it that of metallic mercury known as **Mercurius vivus.** Virtually the action of the two remedies appear to be the same.

Mercury is a brilliant silver-white metal. At ordinary tem-perature it is liquid. It is also called quicksilver. It is mostly obtained from **Cinnabar,** the red oxide of mercury, by heating the ore and condensing the mercurial vapours by an elaborate pro-cess of cooling.

Mercury has been long known to be a medicinal substance and amply abused by the Old School of practice. In their hands it has done more damage than good to humanity and as such it has been an object of dread to the layman. In the hands of the homœopath on the other hand, used as it is on a fixed law and prepared as it is on the harmless principle of attenuations, it has been a very potent therapeutic agent distributing health, happiness and life to the ailing multitude.

When used in poisonous quantity, Mercury produces general anæmia due to disintegration of the red blood corpuscles. Im-

mediately after taking the poisonous substance, there is experienced by the victim, an intensely disagreeable, acrid, metallic taste
followed almost at once by a burning pain in the mouth,
throat, and epigastrium; this pain rapidly extends with
increasing severity to the abdomen. There is excessive thirst.
Nausea sets in, followed by frequent retching and vomiting of
mucus often tinged with blood and sometimes containing shreds
of mucus.   There is diarrhœa with frequent serous, mucous, and
usually bloody stools. The pulse is small and frequent. The victim exhibits great anxiety. The mucosa of the mouth and throat
becomes white and shrivelled and in a short time there follows
severe swelling of the fauces. The swelling of the throat is often so
severe as to threaten asphyxia, and cases are known in which
tracheotomy became necessary to save life. Breathing becomes
difficult. A period of vertigo precedes insensibility, collapse
and death. Convulsions may sometimes occur before death.
The fatal period is from twenty-four to thirty-six hours.

The whole of the alimentary canal is more or less inflamed; the
mucosa of the mouth and throat is red or even ulcerated, especially
in the upper part, or in very acute cases it may be shrivelled and
whitened; that of the stomach is ecchymosed, even ulcerated; in
only one case has perforation been observed. The intestines are
more strongly affected than the stomach and may exhibit
greenish-yellow ulcerations, especially in the lower part of the
ileum; not infrequently the mucosa is œdematous, swollen, and the
submucosa infiltrated with serum. In such an event the intestines
are anæmic. These appearances follow the absorption of mercury
by no matter what channel; usually the large intestine exhibits
appearances identical with those seen in dysentery. The
liver and kidneys are anæmic, enlarged, and show fatty
degeneration unless death has been quite rapid. The liver
may be icteric and pasty. The kidneys exhibit a somewhat analogous appearance, which may sometimes be suggestive
of Bright's disease. The bladder is contracted and usually empty
The muscles of the heart are hemorrhagic and show some
fatty degeneration. The blood in acute cases is usually dark
thick, and coagulates with difficulty. In chronic cases it i
anæmic. The mouth may appear grayish in color; this appear
ance occasionally extends down the œsophagus. The wall
of the intestines are not infrequently grayish or blackish from
mercuric sulphide, the result of putrefactive changes. This clear
ly shows Mercury to be a potent agent for good or for evil.

is for us, homœopaths, to utilise the best that is in **Mercurius,** and this can only be done by following the sound principle handed to us by our great master.

In the next chapter we will discuss, from the homœopathic standpoint, the long train of symptoms produced by Mercury when taken in the healthy condition and evolve out of the confusing mass, a mode, a procedure that will be safe and easy for us to depend on.

In the first place the characteristic that seems most striking is the nocturnal aggravation of this remedy. It is a modality that is invariably present in every case of **Mercurius.** This aggravation is particularly noticed after the patient gets into the warmth of his bed. Be it toothache, rheumatic pain, mumps, diphtheria, tonsillitis or dysentery, this characteristic must always be present; that is why the **Mercurius** patient dreads his bed and the warmth thereof. There are other remedies like **Apis, Chamomilla, Drosera, Ledum, Pulsatilla, Sabina, Secale** and **Sulphur** that have similar modality, but then each one of these has its own individual peculiarity to help differentiation. This modality is so important that its absence may be regarded as a contraindication for **Mercurius.**

The second characteristic is to be found in the perspiration of the patient. He perspires very freely but this brings him no relief. This is debilitating and constant. This reminds us of **Hepar sulph.** and **Sambucus,** two other remedies similar to **Mercury.** The sweat of **Sambucus** differs from that of **Mercurius** in that it is not fetid. Talking about perspiration we are reminded of **Kali bich.** and **Causticum** two more remedies with certain amount of peculiarity attached to their sweat. In the former the perspiration is noticed while the patient sits quietly. In **Causticum** the patient perspires more in open area than in a closed confined place. In **Hyoscyamus, Graphites, Murex** and **Veratrum** the perspiration is more evident during menstrual period.

The other characteristic points of **Mercurius** are all confined to the mouth. The gums are invariably swollen and spongy with a tendency towards bleeding. In this **Mercury** is similar to **Kali mos, Kreosote** and **Lachesis.** The tongue is broad, swollen and flabby almost filling up the buccal cavity. Its broad edge is invariably dented with the imprints of teeth. There is no mistaking about the odor of his mouth. It is so offensive and disgusting that it annoys everybody around him. No remedy has this con-

cadaverous and putrid smell we should also think of **Arnica, Arsenic, Carbo veg., Chamomilla, Kali phos., Kreosote, Natrum mur., Nitric acid, Phytolacca, Spigelia** and **Tuberculinum,** but they do not cover all the other conditions of **Mercury.**

It is necessary to mention that there is a great and constant overflow of saliva from his mouth. We find him constantly spitting. The saliva is tenacious, soapy, stringy and profuse and it gives him a peculiar coppery metallic taste. Inspite of such profusion of saliva he is very thirsty and drinks tumblers of water at a time.

Mercury affects teeth in a very characteristic manner. We mostly find crowns of teeth decaying. The remaining roots look black, dirty and carious. Sometimes a bright red margin is noticeable on the gums which has a tendency to recede, thus exposing the roots of teeth and making them loose and painful. The teeth feel as if they are too long and loose. It is a capital remedy for toothache. The pain is tearing, lacerating and shoots into the face and ears. It is always worse in damp weather, evening warmth of bed and from taking cold things. He feels better by rubbing his cheek.

The taste of the mouth is, as has been said before, sweetish metallic and putrid. The speech is difficult on account of trembling of the mouth and tongue. The mucous membrane of mouth is full of burning, aphthous ulcers which keep on secreting the characteristic discharge. These ulcers are generally of syphilitic origin or they may at least have a substratum of syphilitic poison behind them. The ulcers spread rapidly till they practically involve larynx, pharynx, the tonsils and the surrounding parts. There is tendency also, on the part of these ulcers, to extend in depth. The uvula too, looks elongated, enlarged and greatly swollen.

Mercury is a great hemorrhagic remedy. We think of specially when the blood coagulates easily. Thus in epistaxis the blood gets congealed very soon and hangs from nostrils like icicle. The same condition is noticed in metrorrhagia, menorrhagia hemoptysis and hematemesis.

It affects the mucous membrane of the intestines in a remarkable manner, hence its great efficacy in dysentery and other similar ailments. Its symptoms are very clear-cut and definite. Violent tenesmus and continued urging, a never get-down feeling, prolapsus recti, slimy bloody stool are too charateristic to be mistaken. Sometimes the stools look greenish; even when watery we may notice a sort of a greenish scum floating on the surface. Naus chilliness, excoriation of the anus are also very prominent symptoms. It is the frightful pain that we must always keep in sight of, in **Mercurius.** The bowels feel as if they were cut into pieces. The pain gets most violent when at stool. He strains so hard that it feels as if the entire bowels would be forced out. The most peculiar portion of it all, however, is that the quantity of stool discharged is exceedingly small—not at all in proportion to the huge urging induced by **Mercurius.**

The mental condition of **Mercurius** is characterised by the same poverty as that found in other departments of the remedy. Weakness of memory, absent-mindedness, obtuseness of sense and imbecility are characteristics of **Mercurius.** There is also great uneasiness that causes a sort of restlessness preventing her to remain long, in one place or in one position. It is as if she has committed a great crime and that her conscience is making a coward of her. These conditions are usually aggravated at night time. Another peculiarity of **Mercurius** is a strong desire to commit murder. This desire is not the effect of a premeditated plan of vengeance but it is simply a desire to kill—sometimes directed against persons, she is particularly fond of. Something urges her to kill her husband of whom she is very fond and she implores him to hide his razor. Such abnormal state of mind should receive our special attention. At times, this desire to kill is directed towards her ownself. Whenever she sees an open window or a sharp instrument, she is seized with an uncontrollable desire to commit suicide either by jumping out of the window or by cutting her throat. These types of patients should be treated with great caution. Such mental phenomena, though abnormal, are often to be met with in hysteria, puerperal mania and melancholia. Other symptoms permitting, **Mercurius** becomes an admirable remedy for these complaints.

One great characteristic of **Mercurius** which I have so far omitted to mention is tremor. This symptom is so pronounced and prominent, as to render **Mercury** almost a specific for paralysis agitance. The patient trembles all over. There is tremor of the head, hands and tongue. These motions are mostly involuntary and can be momentarily suppressed by volition. Even the speech is stammering, showing signs of the general tremor. She is unable to lift anything or to write. These are partly paralytic in nature and partly due to great exhaustion to which our **Mercurius** patient is an eternal subject.

Hahnemann's preparation of **Solubilis** is preferred in syphilitic complaints to that of **Vivus**. I have cured innumerable cases of syphilitic sores on prepuce and glans penis with great deal of phimosis and paraphimosis with **Merc. sol.** The chancres are indurated with lardaceous cheesy base and inverted red edges. It spreads both in circumference and depth and secretes a yellow excoriating discharge. I remember a case in which the glans were practically eaten away and the patient had two huge buboes on both sides, that got totally and permanently cured with **Solubilis** in a very short time. That the cure has been a permanent one is evident from the fact that within the last six years not a single mark of syphilis, primary or secondary, has manifested itself.

· **Mercurius solubilis** is equally efficacious in treatment of gonorrhœa. The symptoms are burning pain, frequent painful erections. a purulent greenish discharge, pain in the testicles, phimosis. frequent urging to urination, offensive odor from the mouth, ptvalism. threatened bubo and great redness of the inner surface of the prepuce.

Merc. sol. is useful in ophthalmia specially of syphilitic and scrofulous origin. The symptoms are intolerance of light. discharge of muco-purulent matter, thickening of the tarsal edges of the lids, vesicular ulcers on cornea, pustules on cornea, photophobia, lachrymation, profuse watery excoriating coryza and spasmodic closing of the lids with hypopyon.

It is also helpful in syphilitic iritis. The aqueous humor becomes hazy and pains of a tearing boring character are experienced around the eyes, forehead and temples, especially at night time.

We find **Mercurius** indicated in offensive otorrhœa of either syphilitic or scrofulous nature. The discharge is bloody and purulent. Lots of furuncles are noticed in the meatus. Otalgia is equent and distressing. Cervical glands are seen to be enlarged The ears look inflamed internally and externally. The relationship between **Mercury** and inflammation should be studied very carefully. It is recommended in the later stage of inflammation when inflammation merges into suppuration. The more has pus formed, the more it is indicated. It, therefore, follows **Belladonna,** which is pre-eminently a remedy for the inflammatory stage. **Hepar sulphur** is also a remedy that comes between **Belladonna** and **Mercurius.** We think of it when inflammatory stage is just about over and suppuration is about to step in. It works both ways. It prevents suppuration when suppuration has not taken place and hence is a remedy to be used in doubtful cases of suppuration. **Mercurius** does not prevent formation of pus, but rather helps it and should, therefore, be used when you are convinced of formation of pus. **Silicea** follows **Mercurius** after **Mercurius** has done its work. It prevents further suppuration and tends to hasten the already long-drawn process of slow healing.

Case 1.—M. Kiernan, aged thirty-five years, of good constitution; violent pain in his throat, worse during deglutition, with much heat about head; throat inflammed, and tongue coated. **Bell 1.** Two days later, face flushed, vessels of eyes injected; lips bluish; his tongue twice its natural size, coated and red at tip, almost complete inability to move the same; interior of mouth much inflamed; constant profuse flow of saliva and fetor from the mouth; expression of face indicated much anguish; was unable to swallow a few drops of liquid, complaining of much pain in the head, tongue, and adjacent parts; stiffness of the jaws, and burning heat in the mouth, accompanied with much thirst. **Mercurius 3d**, four powders, every day. The effect was so surprisingly gratifying, that the patient was completely cured in nine days.—Dr. O. Fullgraf.

Case 2.—Mrs. McA., aged forty-seven, most excruciating pain, caused by two large ulcers on the left leg, on the anterior aspect, about midway between the knee and the ankle. Had been dosed with **calomel** seven years before, for disease of the liver. Some few months after she noticed a small pimple on the leg, which, on being broken, produced a foul ulcer, very painful; this was followed by several others. The present ulcers have been in existence for one year (about), and present the following symptoms and appearance; Deep, foul ulcers; gray-colored, though slough; thin, ichorous pus; edges raised, swollen, and inflamed; the viens in their vicinity are varicosed; pain rather worse on getting warm in bed, and on motion, or touching it, in fact, nothing seems to relieve it; both hot and cold applications produce aggravation; the pain on pressure is intolerable; pain sharp, shooting, or lancinating **Nit. ac. 30**, without benefit. **Merc. sol. 1000**, one powder dry on the tongue, and one powder of **Sach. alb.** daily. In addition, the limb was firmly strapped, and a bandage applied over all. One week after, the pains had nearly disappeared; and at the expiration of six months, the ulcers were entirely healed.. Only two doses of **Merc.** were given.—Dr. J. G. Gilchrist.

Case 3.—G., tailor, past sixty. Troublesome itching of the body and limbs. Skin covered with crusts and papulæ. Eruption first appeared over two years ago as very small elevated spots on back of wrists, gradually extending to the other parts of body. Itching so intolerable it almost sets him crazy if he gets a little warmer than usual while at work. When he first gets into bed the cool sheets feel so nice he goes right to sleep, but after sleeping about half an hour he is awakened by this awful itching and has to get out of bed and walk the floor until the sheets get cool again. **Merc. viv. 200** relieved very much, and **Merc. viv.** 30m completely cured all except a slightly troublesome itching in the daytime while at work. **Sulph.** 55m completed the cure.—Dr. H. N. Martin.

MERCURIUS CORROSIVUS.

This is called Mercuric Chloride. It is commonly called the corrosive sublimate. It is a salt and it occurs in the form of heavy colourless, transparent, glistening, rhombic prism. It has an acrid, disagreeable, metallic taste. It is soluble in water, the solubility increasing with temperature. When swallowed it produces a sense of constriction almost amounting to suffocation. A burning sensation in the throat, violent pain in the abdomen, nausea and suppression of urine, are important symptoms of its poisoning. In chronic poisoning the symptoms are gradual inflammation of the salivary glands, redness and swelling of the tongue, ulceration, fetid breath, ptyalism, etc. Quantity required to destroy life varies from three to five grains.

The keynote symptom of this preparation of *Mercury* is tenesmus. This occurs mostly in the rectum and in the bladder. This tenesmus is incessant and persistent. It is not relieved by passing of stool and voiding of urine. This symptom assumes double importance when we have rectal and vesical tenesmus going together.

It is a great remedy for various kinds of eye troubles such as cyclitis, chorioditis, iridocyclitis, irido-chorioditis, episcleritis, retinitis hæmorrhagica and albuminurica iritis and kerato-iritis. Most of these inflammatory troubles are syphilitic in their origin. The lids become œdematous, red and inflamed. The trouble starts with excessive photophobia and acrid lachrymation. The patient sits in some dark corner with his eyes closed and a dark bandage on, to occlude any strong light. Gradually the inflammation becomes purulent. Pustules, ulceration on the cornea, phlyctenulæ discharging ichorus acrid matter very soon make their appearance. The corrosive nature of the discharge from the inflamed area disfigures and excoriates the surrounding parts. We have a similar corrosive discharge from the nose and the ear. This corrosiveness is particularly characteristic of all the discharges of this preparation of *Mercury.* In diarrhœa and dysentery the anus gets raw and inflamed. In cystitis the corrosive urine scalds and burns. In gonorrhœa the discharge corrodes the urethral opening and all the surrounding parts. The leucorrhœal discharge makes the surrounding parts red and excoriated.

In **Mercurius cor.,** we find a powerful remedial agent in diseases of the intestinal tract. It occupies a very high place in the treatment of dysentery. The stools are frequent, hot, scanty bloody, slimy, offensive and they contain shreds of mucous membrane. Sometimes we find the patient passing pure blood in large quantity. The urging is great before, during and after stool. He feels a sort of pressure in sacral and hypogastric regions that excites desire for defecation. There is frequently cutting pain in the rectum and prolapsus. These symptoms are associated with tenesmus vesicæ. The straining is almost continuous. In dysentery, diarrhœa and enteritis, these are our sole indications for **Merc. cor.** The quantity of blood discharged in **Mercurius cor.,** is more than is to be found in many of its sister remedies. The number of stools is generally many. The constricting pain with prolapsus of the rectum, the constant urging to stool and the tenesmus of the bladder associated with suppression of urine are symptoms that will prove helpful.

I have used it frequently and with success in cystitis. The symptoms are intense tenesmus of the bladder, passing of hot burning bloody urine in drops with great pain and presence of flesh-like pieces of mucus and filaments in urine.

Three more characteristics of **Merc. cor.**—characteristics that are invariably present in complaints calling for this remedy are faintness, weakness and shuddering. The debility, prostration and lassitude are so great that their limbs tremble on standing and trying to move.

MERCURIUS CYANATUS.

Mercuric cyanide is a white transparent crystal turning dark on exposure to light. It is odorless but has a sharp metallic taste. In action this salt is highly irritant and intensely poisonous. One part by weight of this pure mercuric cyanide is dissolved in ninety-nine parts of distilled water. Trituration may also be made.

The symptoms of this remedy are mostly clinical and toxicological. This preparation of mercury is particularly suited to all sorts of buccal affections. I have used it with remarkable success in diphtheria, putrid sorethroat, follicular tonsilitis and chronic laryngitis. I give **Cyanatus** preference to other forms of mercury in malignant and gangrenous diphtheria. The symptoms are unmistakable. The entire cellular tissue of the neck becomes infiltrated and the odor of the mouth becomes excessively putrid. The salivation, as in other preparations of mercury, is incessant. The entire mucous membrane of the mouth and fauces presents a dark red appearance. The tonsils are greatly inflamed and enlarged; they soon show deep-seated ulcerations which are saturated with a peculiar putrid greenish-yellow pus. These obnoxious symptoms are very soon superseded by the formation of a tough whitish gray membrane which rapidly envelopes the whole of the buccal cavity, extending over the palate and descending even into the gullet and the laryngeal cavity. Green exudations of a thick leathery consistency are constantly ejected from the nasal cavities and are hawked up from the fauces, pharynx and larynx. The power of speech is soon lost and he finds it extremely difficult to swallow liquids which escape through the nose. Profuse debilitating epistaxis, high fever and extreme prostration are marked indications for **Merc. cyanatus.** The pulse becomes excessively weak and fast. Urine when it is not suppressed looks dark and scanty. The parotid glands are enormously swollen. Necrotic destruction of soft parts, of palate and fauces should invariably turn our attention to **Mercurius cyanatus.**

MERCURIUS DULCIS.

The common name for this is Calomel. It is a white impalpable powder, permanent in air, odorless tasteless and insoluble in water, alcohol and ether. Locally the action of Calomel is absolutely bland, but after swallowing, local and constitutional symptoms, such as nausea, griping, and passages of mucus and green stools, declare themselves. In homœopathic therapeutics, it is utilised principally in catarrhal affections of the mucous membranes of the eyes and the ears; hence it makes such a popular remedy in otitis media, otorrhœa of scrofulous children, catarrhal deafness in elderly people and in obstruction of the Eustachian tube.

It is especially suited to scrofulous children who are liable to bilious attacks and whose complexions are characterised by a peculiar corpse-like pallor. They are flabby, ill-nourished and are subject to chronic swelling of cervical and other glands of the body.

A great characteristic of **Merc. dulcis** consists of the peculiarity in the appearance of the interior of the buccal cavity. The tongue and palate look black. Salivation is constant, putrid and intolerable. The mouth is full of ulcerations. The gums are sore.

Its application in inflammatory complaint is based on the formation of plastic exudation; it is advocated in meningitis, peritonitis and other varieties of inflammatory ailments when symptoms denote the formation and secretion of a plastic substance, as a result of the inflammatory process.

It has been used with benefit in inflammation and hypertrophy of the prostate gland, the result of maltreated gonorrhœa. The symptoms are burning pressing pain while urinating, constant desire to urinate and scanty urine.

It has been recommended in condylomatous growth around external genitals, perineum and anus of the females emitting an extremely offensive smell. We also use it in copper-colored eruptions of syphilitic patients.

It takes precedence over all other preparations of mercury in green diarrhœa of children. The stools may have all shades of green in them. They may be grass green, coppery green or whitish green as is often seen in chopped-egg stool of scrofulous children. Over and above the green color of the stools, we have enlargement of the liver, bloatedness of the abdomen, excoriating soreness of the anus, aphthous mouth and enlargement of submaxillary, cervical and inguinal glands. These make such a complete picture of **Merc. dulcis** that there should be no chance of confusion between this and such other remedies with green stools as **Chamomilla, Ipecac, Argentum nitricum** and the different preparations of Magnesia.

MERCURIUS IODATUS FLAVAS (Mercurius Protoiodide).

This is commonly known as **protoiodide** or the yellow iodide of mercury. This preparation is highly useful in diphtheria but the distinguishing feature is a thick yellow coating at the base of the tongue. The lips and the edges are red. The tongue is broad and flabby and takes the imprint of teeth as in other preparations of mercury. We should also remember that this remedy has a special affinity for the right side of the throat. The diphtheritic membranes too look yellow. The nose is obstructed with thick yellow scabs and membranes. There is often a post nasal dropping. The taste of mouth is coppery. Other symptoms are great prostration, glandular engorgement, œdema of neck, scanty and high-colored urine, high fever, aphonia, difficult respiration and frequent spells of suffocation. There is aggravation from warm drinks and empty swallowing.

This is a great remedy for chronic catarrh in old people and children. They frequently expel thick plugs of nasal secretion and complain of severe frontal headache.

We think of **Mercurius protoiodide** in yellow leucorrhœa of young girls and children. It is also good for copious chronic muco-purulent leucorrhœa in females.

MERCURIUS IODATUS RUBER. (Mercurius Biniodide).

Another name for this is Bin Iodide of mercury or Red Iodide of mercury.

This preparation of mercury is also useful in diphtheria. It principally affects the left side. The symptoms are not quite as severe as those of the **Cyanatus**. We notice a certain amount of glandular swelling, but this is not quite so alarming. The exudations, are limited, transparent and easily detachable; salivation is profuse. There is quite an accumulation of phlegm in the throat and nose and the patient constantly hawks up hard tough greenish lumps of phlegm. The tongue feels scalded.

We use **Mercurius bin iodide** in syphilitic sores of the mouth; numerous mucous patches are on the lips and inner surface of the cheeks with their bases covered with a creamy exudation. It is specially recommended in hard Huntarian chancre. I have used it with great satisfaction in threatened gangrence of the glans in paraphimosis. It is specially useful in chronic open buboes that does not heal easily. It has been used in sarcocele with success.

In females, leucorrhœa of greenish color and in males, a whitish gonorrhœal discharge have been helped with **Mercurius bin iodide.**

I have had very gratifying results from **Mercurius bin iodide** in a case of chronic multiple ulceration of the legs that refused to heal for years; they were of syphilitic origin.

MERCURIUS SULPHURICUS.

Mercurious sulphuricus is the yellow precipitate of Mercury. We are indebted to Dr. Lippe for our knowledge of this remedy who gave it a thorough clinical proving and has left us quite a few dependable indications for **Mercurius sul.** It is particularly useful in hydro-thorax if occurring from heart or liver disease. Dyspnœa is so intense that the patient is compelled to sit up night after night and is thoroughly exhausted. The extremities are exceedingly swollen, stiff and numb. The hands are icycold and the nails blue. The above conditions which generally supervene in the latter part of an extremely dilated heart where compensation is gradually giving way and death seems imminent, **Mercurious sulphuricus** may yet stay the hand of fate by bringing in a sort of a loose watery diarrhœa which gradually leads to a distinct amelioration of the annoying symptoms and may yet bring a few years of ease, comfort and life to the dying man.

MERCURIUS SULPH. RUB.

(*See* **Cinnabaris**).

MERCURIUS VIVUS.

(*See* **Mercurius**).

METHYLENE BLUE.

Methylene blue is one of the aniline dyes and is used in old school practice in rheumatism of joints and muscles and in rheumatoid arthritis. In the homœopathic therapeutics, we use it in malaria and typhoid when associated with great tympanites. This remedy has not yet received good clinical verification and hence we are greatly handicapped with regard to its administration. The following are some of its symptoms: irritation of the bladder, greenish urine, tortuous breathing, dark bluish color of the skin and habitual

MEZEREUM.

Mezereum is a hardy shrub growing to a height of three to four feet with fragrant red flowers and is a native of Europe and Asiatic Russia. It belongs to the natural order of Thymelaceæ. It is a poisonous shrub. If applied locally, it produces intense burning and swelling, severe painful sneezing and erysipelatous eruptions. Fever, burning while passing urine, debility, mental depression, intense thirst, narcotism, coma, difficult swallowing, and itching all over the body are some of the symptoms to be noticed in a case of poisoning.

It was first proved by Hahnemann and associated with him as one of the provers was Constantine Hering, at that time a medical student at Leipzig. It is called the vegetable analogue of mercury and is also one of the most important antidotes to it. A careful study will reveal the close resemblance between the two remedies. The same unhealthiness of the skin, the same sensibility to damp cold and warmth, the same nightly aggravation, the same tendency towards affections of the bones and the same characteristic of the eruptions and ulcerations make differentiation a difficult problem. It is generally adapted to light-haired, phlegmatic persons of irresolute temperament. Hypochondriasis and despondence are two cardinal mental indications of this remedy. A great indifferance marks his behaviour everywhere. He takes no pleasure in anything. Everything seems to him dead and still and nothing leaves any lasting impression on his mind. Vanishing of ideas is another mental characteristic. He looks through the window for hours without being conscious of objects around. He knows not what he is about. He forgets what he is about to say.

I have already mentioned that it has important skin symptoms. A general unhealthiness is seen all over the body, although certain parts are more affected than others. The skin gets wrinkled and in folds. Intense itching is felt all over the body, as though thousands of insects were creeping The parts scratched get covered with innumerable red or reddish elevations, as if covered with nettlerash. A general roughness of the skin with scabbing is also to be noticed. Scurfs like fish scales are to be seen all over on the back, chest, thighs and scalp. It is also a first-rate remedy for the itch-like eruptions that appear after vaccination. Eczema finds in **Mezereum** a ready help.

They are characterised by intolerable itching and copious serous exudations. These eruptions are mostly moist and scabby. They bleed easily when touched. We prescribe it also in ulceration when characterised by extreme sensitiveness, thick yellowish scabs and a band of vesicles appearing around the ulceration. These vesicles itch violently and burn like fire. The itching is aggravated in the bed and by touch. The favourite site for many of the eruptions of **Mezereum** is the scalp. The head is covered with a thick leather-like crust under which white and honey coloured pus collects matting and gluing the hair and giving the general appearance of extreme uncleanliness and filth. Sometimes the scabs, growing over these eruptions, are white and chalk-like concealing underneath a heavy crop of vermin. It is sometimes so bad that it gives the appearance of a skull-cap. **Mezereum** is often of great service in herpes zoster.

Mezereum is one of Hahnemann's antipsorics Dr. Carroll Dunham has recorded a cure of deafness in a boy of 17 years, the result of suppression of eczema on the head. When 3 years old, he had an erruption of thick white, hard, almost horny scales over his head which were fissured in numerous places. Through these cracks, there oozed a copious discharge of thick, yellow foul smelling pus. The scabs were removed by means of a pitch plaster and the exposed surface painted with nitrate of silver. The eruptions disappeared but deafness intervened. **Mezereum 30** was given once a month for four months, finally, resulting in the complete restoration of hearing. It is very useful in blepharitis with tinea capitis and in eczema of lids. It is also used in ulcers of upper lids extending to nose. Red pustules on chin should also remind us of **Mezereum.** The symptoms, especially pointing to this remedy, are a sort of a scabby eruptions on hairy part of face, which on slight pressure exudes a sort of bloody lymph, producing intense itching and irritation. It is worth our while to remember that this greenish discharge constitutes a cardinal indication of **Mezereum.**

It has special action upon bones and periosteum and it constitutes a valuable remedy for ostitis, periostitis, cystic osteoma, abscesses of fibrous parts and tendons and in tumors of frontal and malar bones. It principally affects the shaft of cylindrical bones. Swelling and pain of cranial bones also call for **Mezereum,** especially when there are several elevated nodules on the skull, the result of suppressed syphilis. The pain, especially at night, is so severe as to cause fainting and this intensity leads us to a surmise of pressure on the brain substance by the bony growth. The sensations are as if the bones are distended. It is particularly indicated in periostitis and swelling of tibia with violent night pains.

We should make a special study of the pain symptoms of **Mezereum** as they are very characteristic. The pains are lightning-like; they come suddenly while talking or eating and disappear leaving the part numb. These pains starting in infraorbital foramen, sometimes in zygoma, travel to temples, corner of the mouth and down neck to the shoulder. Increased lachrymal secretion, injected conjunctiva and great sensibility to touch are sure indications for **Mezereum.** Dr. Nash has cited an obstinate case of facial neuralgia that he cured with **Mezereum** on the history of aggravation from eating and relief obtained by holding the face as near as possible to a hot stove. Application of heat of other descriptions was not of any value.

In toothache, the tooth feels elongated and excessively sensitive. It may be due to carious degeneration and the carious process in **Mezereum** affects principally the root, crown remaining intact.

It is also an admirable remedy for a certain type of constipation after confinement. It should be prescribed particularly when the stools are hard as stone and are immense in size. It feels as if they would split the anus open. They are so big that they cannot be expelled wholesale. They keep on coming in sections and exhaust the patient so that she trembles. The stools are preceded by chill and followed by long stitches in the rectum. In this respect it can be very conveniently compared to the following remedies:—

Ammon. mur.—The stools are hard and they crumble to pieces; they are covered with a glairy mucus but they are not so big in size as in **Mezereum.** They require great effort and force to expel them.

Antim. crud.—It is generally indicated in constipation of old people. The stools here are hard and the fæces too large, same as in **Mezereum.** Another point of resemblance is that it is serviceable in constipation during child-bed, but the suicidal despondency, white coated tongue, anorexia and the dyspeptic symptom such as gulping up of fluids, tasting of ingesta, nausea and vomiting are symptoms that render distinction quite easy.

Apis mellifica is an admirable remedy for chronic constipation. The stools are hard, large and difficult to pass and are evacuated only once or twice a week. The feeling in the anus is as if it were stuffed full with heat and throbbing.

Bryonia has very hard dark round or black stools, as if burnt dry. They are very large in size and passed with great difficulty. Great dryness of tongue, mouth and lips, intense thirst, irritable and angry mood and a strong rheumatic diathesis characterise **Bryonia.**

Graphites.—The stools, which are very large in size, are passed with great difficulty and are covered with mucus. Defæcation is rendered difficult by the fissured condition of the rectum and a great dryness of the part.

Lachesis should not be left out of the list of remedies with large stools. In fact the stools of **Lachesis** are simply enormous. While evacuation takes place the sphincters nearly become paralyzed and after evacuation they close very slowly. After evacuation the patient feels as if thousand hammers were beating inside the anus.

MILLEFOLIUM.

Another name for this plant is Nosebleed, a very appropriate term because of its great tendency to produce hemorrhage, not only from the nose but from every orifice and organ of the human system. Its medicinal properties were known to the ancients. It is mentioned in Homer's *Iliad* as being utilised by Achilles to heal the wounds of his soldiers and hence it is also called **Achillea millefolium.** It belongs to the natural order of Compositæ.

The characteristic point about the hemorrhage of **Millefolium** is that it is almost always painless and that the blood passed is bright red and fluid. These two characteristics being present we may use it in hemorrhage from the mouth, nose, lungs, stomach, bladder, rectum and uterus. It thus belongs to the same category as **Hamamelis, Ipecac, Ustilago, Aconite, Sabina, Arnica, Phosphorus, Secale, Trillium, China** and others of the same type.

It is a noted convulsant but this property too, is based on suppression of hæmorrhages or other secretions. It is indicated in convulsions of women due to suppression of menses or lochial discharge. It also finds application in pregnancy. It is an important remedy for painless or bleeding varices in pregnant women.

Millefolium should be thought of in hæmopysis of phthisical
patients. The expectorated blood is florid and comes out without
much coughing. This is preceded by a sensation of ebullition in
the chest. There is also a sensation of warmth as blood rises into
her throat and flows out of her mouth. Sometimes this spitting of
blood is associated with violent palpitation. Another great characteristic with the hæmorrhage of **Millefolium** is the want of
anxiety and in this it differs from **Aconite.**

MITCHELLA REPENS.

Mitchella is prepared from a small trailing evergreen commonly known as Partridge Berry, a plant very common in the
United States. It produces a small scarlet berry. My experience
with this remedy, though not very great, has been very satisfactory. I had occasion to use **Mitchella** in an elderly lady of about 49
who was suffering from prolonged and protracted uterine hæmorr-
age. On examination her uterus seemed hard, enlarged and heavy.
In the theory of climaxis various remedies—remedies that are
usually prescribed at this period—were tried but to no effect. The
hæmorrhage continued till at last it was brought to my notice
that this presistent hæmorrhage was associated with frequent
desire for urination, which was not very free and satisfactory.
This association of dysuria with hæmorrhage, the keynote symptom of **Mitchella** led to the prescription of this remedy with the desired effect.

This plant was in great use among the Red-Indians of the
United States. The Indian women on the eve of confinement used
to drink a decoction made from this plant as it had the reputation,
among them of bringing on safe labour. We also use it for false
labour pains in the last month of pregnancy; when the pains are
slow, feeble and inefficient, it stimulates and completes labour

MORPHINUM.

Morphinum is prepared from morphia, the alkaloid of **Opium.** The activity of **Opium** is principally due to this vegetable alkaloid and it is present to the extent of 8 to 17 per cent. Apart from morphia, the alkaloid, we use three other preparations, the acetate, the muriate and the sulphate. The properties vary so little that we will study them altogether.

Many of its symptoms are also to be found under **Opium** but there are a few very characteristic differentiating points, which a good homœopath should make it his business to understand. It is in vertigo principally that we find **Morphia** of great use. This vertigo is very intense and it is felt from the slightest movement of the head. All on a sudden, after movement of any kind, especially of the head, everything turns dark and the patient becomes unconscious.

The next important characteristic is excessive hyperesthesia. Extreme susceptibility to pain is, in my opinion, the most important symptom to remember. Either the pain is more than he can bear or his power of endurance is diminished. It has been successfully employed in cancer or in other complaints where the violence of the pain almost threatens convulsions. The pain causes twitching and jerking of the limbs.

It has a few important gastric symptoms, such as tympanites and vomiting of green substance. Delusion of vision on closing eyes is also to be found in **Morphia.** He sees a man standing at the foot of the head; he also finds the room full of white and coloured babies. Anxiety, restlessness delirium and terror make him cry out in alarm. Flow of ideas, rapid and pleasant, stupefaction and coma, make it very much like **Opium.**

MOSCHUS.

It is commonly known as musk. This is nothing but the dried preputial secretion of the musk-deer that abounds in the mountainous parts of Asia and Siberia. This glandular secretion is found in a sack between the umbilicus and the preputial orifice. It is a fatty, waxy, gelatinous, albuminous substance with a very strong smell. It was known to the physicians of India long before the birth of Christ. It was a favourite stimulant with them. Even the Kavirajes of the present day use it extensively in the stage of collapse. Samuel Hahnemann was the first to introduce it into the Homœopathic Materia Medica. It has a strong action over the circulation of blood. Under its influence, the icy surface of the body warms up and continues even far after the stage of death. Used on the principle of 'Similia Similibus Curantur' it becomes a sturdier medicinal agent than the Mriganavi of our Baidyas and the ordinary musk of Allopathy, as we shall see presently.

A great indication for **Moschus** is a frequent tendency to fainting even from the least excitement. The nervous hyperæsthesia is most intense as is manifested by extreme tremulousness and restlessness of the patient. She faints even when talking or eating. Their relatives and friends are at their wits end as to what to do about this distressing symptom. It is not painful incidents alone that cause fainting. She is so prone to it that the slightest disturbance of her mental equilibrium or the least emotional changes bring on a state of fainting. We have known cases where even the fragrance of a sweet flower has brought about this condition. Everything points to a hysterical temperament, as it indeed is one of our principal remedies for that disease. The most noted indication of **Moschus** for hysteria, as well as for epilepsy and hystero-epilepsy, is, however, a sensation of coldness and shivering. Before and during such attack, the patient shudders as from a great chilliness. Spasms of the larynx and spasms of the chest accompany these convulsive fits. They are so violent that everybody around the patient dreads, as if she would succumb during such an attack.

We must not feel that **Moschus** is the only remedy that has this symptom of fainting so prominently marked. There are others that can boast of this symptom, only we must, as homœopaths, use our proper function of minute discrimination. It is true, we hear of **Aconite** and **Opium** fainting, but they faint only when they are frightened. **Pulsatilla,** too, faints but she only does so when placed within the four walls of a closed room and where there is a palpable want of proper ventilation. **Sulphur** and **Phosphorus** faint from hunger at about 11 a.m., but they revive as soon as they partake of a hearty meal. We must not omit to notice that our **Sulphur** patient faints after a stool. It is quite strange that **Magnesia** exhibits the reverse symptom as she faints when she sits for her dinner. The **Alumina** patient behaves well and nicely so long as she is allowed to sit. A great aversion to standing is displayed by **Alumina,** and she faints when circumstances compel her to do so. The **Carbo veg.** patient, on the other hand, does not mind standing but she loses all consciousness and faints right off. We must associate **Conium** and **Podophyllum** with **Sulphur** for like **Sulphur** they too, faint after stool. **Murex, Lyco,** and **Thuja** are remedies noted for fainting before menses. Throughout the rest of the month they are happy, easy and quite but as the time for the period approaches, they lose their natural equilibrium of mind, become languid and faint every now and again without much of a cause. We must not lose sight of **Asafœtida** and **Agaricus,** two great remedies for fainting; in **Asafœtida** this happens after emission and in **Agaricus** after coition. The last remedy to discuss with regard to this symptom is **Sepia.** She faints during chill and on exertion.

The mental symptoms of **Moschus** are somewhat like those of **Palladium.** The hysterical temperament renders **Moschus** very fickle and changeable. She cries one moment and bursts out the next in an uncontrollable fit of laughter. She is very frightened and exhibits a great dread of death. Quarrelsomeness, malice and rage bring her to the same pedestal of ugliness as **Palladium.** Once angry she keeps up to it for a long time and in her rage keeps on scolding till her lips turn blue, eyes stare and she falls down in a long spell of fainting.

Under the action of **Moschus** we find sexual desire to be greatly excited in both sexes and even in aged persons. It is also very effective in a certain type of diabetes that is associated with impotence. The patient emaciates daily and suffers from an insatiable thirst. Large quantities of urine containing sugar are passed daily.

There is one other indication of **Moschus** that should be mentioned—an indication that brings it very close to **Carbo veg., Antin tart., Phosphorus, Ammon. carb.,** and **Ipecac.** It is indicated in threatened paralysis of the lungs. Loud rattling of mucus is hear in the chest but hardly any expectoration. The pulse grows weaker and weaker, till finally the patient goes into a syncope. The stools and the urine are passed involuntarily and when swallowing, fluids are heard to roll down the throat. Such symptoms make it an admirable remedy in that critical stage of typhoid where the most minute differentiation becomes necessary between **Moschus** and the abovementioned list of remedies, the one to which it bears the greatest amount of resemblance being **Carbo veg.**

Case 1.—A boy, five years old, of light complexion, pale but strong, had the whooping cough in September, 1859, which was treated at first with **Belladonna 3**, and afterward with **Veratrum 3**. On October 20th, new symptoms appeared. At the moment of inspiration, without anxiety, or cyanosis, or pain, the respiration became crowing and lengthened, as in laryngismus stridulus. Then followed some normal breathing, interrupted again by that crowing and lengthened inspiration. During play, eating, laughing, even during sleep, the laryngismus continued, and as the attacks got worse, without anxiety and restlessness, I gave him **Moschus** 12 every two hours. In three days the laryngismus was removed, and the whooping cough was cured by the end of October. —(Dr. T. S. Hoyne, **Med. Counselor,** April, 1879.)

MUREX PURPUREA.

This medicine is prepared from a sea snail found on the coast of the Mediterranean and Adriatic, called the purple fish. Like **Sepia,** the ink fish, this purple fish secretes a peculiar matter. This peculiar colouring is of a fine red hue. Like **Sepia** again, this remedy is particularly a woman's remedy. It is used in ovarian cyst, prolapsus uteri, dysmenorrhœa, carcinoma uteri and in bad effects of abortion. This remedy was first proved by Petroz.

Now as regards the guiding symptoms of **Murex purp.,** the first and the foremost is violent excitement in the sexual organs. She is afflicted with almost a frantic desire for sexual gratification. In this respect, she resembles our **Origanum** patient whom we will discuss later on. The desire is so violent that it outweighs all reasons and sense of propriety. This venereal desire is excited by the slightest touch. In this respect **Murex** is very similar to **Sepia;** the differentiating feature consists in its having profuse and excessive hæmorrhage, whereas in **Sepia** the flow is always scanty. Furthermore during this period of hæmorrhage she passes large clots and blood coagula. It therefore forms an important remedy for hæmorrhage during climaxis. The excessive sensitiveness about the genital reminds us also of **Coffea.** We have strong desire in this remedy for intercourse but there is a fear on account of the excessive pain it entails. On the above symptoms it has been used in a large ovarian cyst with very satisfactory result. This patient that was confined to her bed for over a year, not only got better on the administration of **Murex** but recouped her former strength in an incredibly short time.

Another symptom of importance is a distinct sensation of the womb as in **Helonias.** The patient is constantly aware of a heavy substance dangling about in the pelvic cavity. It is more a sensation of bearing down than anything else. It feels as if the internal organs were being pushed out.

The third characteristic indication is the sinking, all gone sensation. The patient feels a great emptiness and void. It thus resembles **Cocculus, Digit., Ignat., Phos., Sepia., Stann., Sulph., Tabac.,** and **Verat. alb.** In all these remedies we have the all gone sensation very well marked.

Murex is an admirable remedy for prolapsus uterus when the displacement is associated with sore pain of the uterus. The pain extends upwards from right side of uterus, and crossing the body goes to the left mamma. Sometimes the uterus feels as if it is cut by a sharp instrument. This myalgic pain in the uterus generally comes on when the patient is in bed, and is relieved by sitting up or walking about. This aggravation from lying down which necessitates sitting up and walking about tires her out completely. In this respect we must compare her with **Lil. tig.** In **Lil. tig.** also we notice a similar pain, but in it the pain originating from mamma traverses downward to the uterus. Greenish irritating leucorrhœal discharge, pain in the hip, loins and down thighs, hæmorrhage at the slightest touch of the examining finger, weakness in the stomach, sensation of pressure towards genitals, heavy weight pressing upon the rectum, discharges of pure blood by vulvæ at stools, painful weariness in the loins and sharp lancinating pain in the uterus are guiding indications of **Murex,** and on them we can safely depend to tide us over all troubles. The leucorrhæal discharge referred to just now has one peculiarity It generally comes on in daytime and disappears at night.

The mental state of **Murex** is one of great depression of spirits. This sadness is generally aggravated at the approach of menses. It seems to her that she is hopelessly ill and is never going to get well. We also notice constant desire to urinate in our **Murex** patient. She has to rise several times in the course of night to pass water. The specific gravity is often as low as 1000. Although no trace of sugar and albumen is found, the patient gradually loses weight. A peculiar pale cachectic appearance coming on her indicates a general break-up of her constitution. This last symptom together with those mentioned before hand has often led to a prescription of **Murex** in cancer of the uterus.

MURIATIC ACID.

It is a colorless gas with a peculiar pungent distressing odor and acid taste. It is manufactured from salt through the aid of Sulphuric acid, hence it is also called the " Spirit Of Salt ". Another name for this is Hydrochloric acid.

Most of the indications of this remedy point to a very desperate condition. It thus deserves careful study and close attention. The symptom that towers over others in importance is extreme debility. He is even wanting in that last tinge of vitality necessary to maintain his position in bed. We find him constantly sliding down. The lower jaw hangs down. His buccal cavity is studded with numerous ulcers. The mucous lining of the lips is inflamed, red and painful. The tongue is dry, shrunken, leather-like and paralysed. Unconsciousness with constant moaning is another prominent indication. Involuntary defection, unconscious urination, great sensitiveness of the genitals to touch, peevishness and irritability deserve an important place in the symptomatology of this drug. The ulcers have a black or a dark base, and a great tendency is noticed towards perforation. Such a desperate combination of symptoms represents a critical typhoid state. **Mur. acid.,** therefore, heads the list of our typhoid remedies.

Other ailments manifesting great prostration and exhibiting a similar typhoid state have an equal demand on **Muratic acid.** Thus in diphtheria, it should be given a very prominent place when we have much rattling of mucus, swelling of submaxillary glands, gangrenous condition of the entire throat, fetor oris, profuse epistaxis, sordes on teeth and lip and above all an over-whelming prostration.

It is one of Dr. Guernsey's "Big Four" in hemorrhoidal ailments. The hemorrhoids look swollen and blue and are intensely painful to touch. The sensitiveness is so excessive that he even dreads contact of bed sheet. There is amelioration from application of warm water and a decided aggravation by bathing the parts with cold water. This sensitiveness also leads to its indication in diarrhœa. Great smarting and cutting sensation in the anus is felt before, during and after stool. The stools are thin, watery and involuntary, discharged while urinating. There is also prolapsus ani during stool and while urinating. It is particularly useful in diarrhœa of infants, threatened with marasmus and muscular debility.

The urinary symptoms of **Muriatic acid** should not be passed unnoticed. We notice great difficulty in micturition. In many instances this is due to weakness of the bladder. He must press long and press hard before the urine passes. From such excessive straining the anus protrudes during the act of urination. Oftentimes there is pain at the close of urination.

Another peculiar symptom of **Muriatic acid** is pain in the stomach while talking.

MYGALE.

It is prepared from a large Black Cuban Spider. The tincture is prepared by putting the living insect into alcohol. It was first introduced and proved by Dr. Howard. It belongs to the natural order of Arachnida. It will not be out of place to mention in this connection that all remedies, belonging to this order, have choreaic symptoms well marked in them, and **Mygale** is no exception to this rule. It is one of our principal remedies for chorea. It mostly affects the muscles of the face. **(Cicuta).** Dr Howard has given the following indications for its use—"The muscles of the face twitch, the mouth and the eyes open and close in rapid succession; cannot put the hand to the face; it is arrested midway and jerked down. Gait unsteady; legs in motion while sitting and dragged while attempting to walk; constant motion of the whole body."

Other additional symptoms are tremulousness; constant contortions of the face; throwing his head backward and then forward with a jerk; frequent feeling of oppression and difficult breathing; convulsive movement of shoulders; jerking of the head to the right side; impossibility to keep hands in the same position for a single minute etc.

The remedies most similar to **Mygale** in chorea are **Agar., Actea racemosa, Tarent., Ignat., Stram.,** and **Zizia.**

Agaricus has angular choreaic movements, but the distinctive features are itching of the different parts of the body as if frostbeaten and extreme sensitiveness of the spine to touch.

Actea racemosa is useful when the left side is mostly affected and when chorea is associated with rheumatic ailments and **uterine** displacement.

Tarentula is a right-sided remedy.

Ignat. is useful in chorea due to emotional disturbance.

Zizia is indicated where the choreaic movements continue even during sleep.

Another symptom worth remembering is the association of nausea with strong palpitation. The presence of this symptom with those of choreaic movements make its usefulness doubly certain.

MYRICA CERIFERA.

Myrica is prepared from Bayberry, a shrub that grows to a height of about 10 ft. and is obtained in sandy soils, along sea-shores. This remedy is very akin to **Chel.**, **Dig.**, and **Kali bich.**, by reason of great similarity in their symptomatology.

It is one of our great liver remedies. There is constant aching pain in the liver immediately below the ribs. The tongue is thickly lined with yellowish white coating. Bitter taste, offensive breath, want of appetite, yellowness of the skin, dark-coloured urine, drowsiness, tenacious, thick and nauseaous secretion in the mouth, extreme lassitude, jaundice, pains under the scapulæ—are clear cut indications of **Myrica** and they further point to the liver to be the seat of trouble. Dr. Burnett, on such indications as these, used **Myrica** with excellent result in cancerous and other grave diseases of the liver.

Myrica produces abundant secretion of tough tenacious mucus from many of the mucous and serous surfaces of our body. We thus meet with profuse catarrhal discharges from the nose, throat and other mucous and serous surfaces. We use it in leucorrhœa, bronchorrhœa, laryngeal and pharyngeal catarrh, stomatitis etc., when the secretions are tough, tenacious and profuse; it is therefore similar to **Kali bich.**, **Hydrastis, Coccus cacti,** and such other remedies.

Its akinness to **Dig.**, is mostly through its jaundice, though there are a few other common symptoms such as sharp pain about the heart, increased and audible pulsation, and slowness of the pulse. With **Dig.**, the jaundice is to be traced from organic derangement of the heart, whereas in **Myrica** the affection is only functional. For some reasons, which it is not always possible to detect, the bile does not form properly and therefore its elements remain in the blood to be manifested later on in various symptoms of jaundice. It is more superficial in its action on the heart than **Dig.** These are about all the important symptoms of **Myrica** that we need remember.

MYRISTICA SEBIFERA.

It belongs to the same order as **Nux moschata** but unlike that remedy, its action is principally confined to suppurative inflammation of joints and in whitlows. For the latter complaint, it is almost regarded as a specific. The pain in the finger nail is excessive with intense swelling of the phalanges. Quite a few cures have been ascribed to it by doctors practising all over Europe. Dr. Cartier cured a case of suspected osteomyelitis and purulent arthritis in an old man of 87 after some of the eminent old school authorities of Paris had practically given him up. Dr. Cartier found the shoulder full of pus and the scapula exceedingly tender to touch. **Myr. seb. 3,** five drops, three times a day, was given with the result that in 10 days time all the suppurative process had stopped. The size of the joint had become normal and the tenderness of the scapula had vanished. It certainly has great power over suppurative process, especially when affecting the joints.

MYRTUS COMMUNIS.

It is prepared from the Myrtle. Flowering shoots and leaves are used in the preparation of the tincture. This plant was well-known to our ancestors. We find mention of this in writings of Hippocrates, *Galen,* Dioscorides and many ancient Arabian writers. We have no real provings of **Myrtus** but there are many important clinical symptoms which establish its claim as a great remedial agent. Its chief indication consists in the sharp stitching pains in the upper portion of the left lung, going right through from the front to the left scapula. This pain is always aggravated on taking a deep breath, on yawning and on coughing. On these indications it has been used with great success in phthisis and in pneumonic affections. The cough is dry and hollow and is caused by tickling in the upper and anterior aspect of the lobes of the lungs. The cough is always worse in the morning and is better in the evening. Great lassitude is felt towards the evening. This evening amelioration and pronounced evening lassitude and tickling in the lungs are very characteristic of **Myrtus.** Taken in hand in time and with proper care even complaints like phthisis may be arrested and **Myrtus communis** is one such implement in our hands to check the onrush of this fatal disease.

NAJA TRIPUDIANS.

This medicine is prepared from the poison of the deadly Cobra of India. Cobra poison has always found an important place in the therapeutics of ancient India. In the Ayurvedic system, even now, this drug is extensively used. It was introduced into homœopathy by Russell and Stokes. This drug has a strong affinity for the medulla oblongata and cerebellum. It strongly acts on the pneumo-gastric and glosso-pharyngeal nerve. Hence this drug is very rich in symptoms of the heart and the throat as we will find out very soon. Dr. Clarke in his Dictionary quotes the experiences of Frank Buckland from 'Curiosities of Natural History." He skinned a rat that was killed by cobra bite. He had a slight abrasion near his nails, through which in an indirect way the attenuated cobra virus affected him. " I had not walked a hundred yards, before all on a sudden, I felt just as if some body had come behind me and struck a severe blow on my head and at the same time I experienced a most acute pain and a sense of oppression at the chest, as though a hot iron had been run in and a hundredweight put on the top of it." His face turned blue. Almost staggering, he entered into a Chemist's shop and was given four glasses of brandy. This sensation of hot iron running through and the symptom of a heavy weight on the chest have been verified repeatedly by several other provers. We also find that these two symptoms are mentioned in the writings of many other homœopaths of note. In my opinion they constitute two important landmarks of **Naja**. Constriction and pressure of the throat, a sensation of choking, spasmodic stricture of the œsophagus, dyspnœa, fluttering of the heart, stitching pain in the region of the heart, are always to be remembered as symptoms constituting the essence of this remedy. On these indications it has been used with great success in the treatment of diphtheria, angina pectoris, plague, septic and other fatal complaints, affecting the throat and the heart. Chronic hypertrophy and valvular diseases of the heart, rheumatic carditis, threatening paralysis of the heart, œsophagismus find in **Naja** an important help.

Talking about diphtheria, we must not forget two other valuable remedies, namely—**Crotalus** and **Lach. Crotalus** is generally selected where there is persistent hæmorrhage from the nose and the mouth. **Lach.** is indicated when the left side is more affected than the right side, and when the site of action is more the larynx than the pharynx. Great swelling and involvement of the lymphatic glands, as well as a gangrenous state, are characteristics of **Lach.**

NAPHTHALINUM.

Naphthaline is a hydro-carbon of colorless, transparent, crystallised prism. In the old school, it is used as an intestinal antiseptic, vermifuge and an expectorant. People working in naphthaline factories are found to suffer from hay fever. It thus becomes a great remedy for acute coryza with fluent excoriating discharge and much sneezing. It has also a cough of spasmodic nature; the patient is unable to take his breath due to paroxysms of cough, following each other in quick succession. It thus makes a splendid remedy for whooping cough and as such should be compared with **Drosera.**

It has a marked affinity for the eye, where it produces detachment of the retina, papillo retinal infiltration and patches upon the retina. It also causes and therefore cures opacity of the cornea as well as the lens.

————————

NARCISSUS.

This remedy, prepared from the Daffodil, belongs to the natural order of Amaryllidaceæ. The tincture is prepared from unexpanded blossom-buds. It causes symptoms of nausea with violent vomiting and diarrhœa—a diarrhœa somewhat similar to that found in **Colchicum.** The stools are watery, relaxed and loose and they are accompanied by hiccough, sinking and a fainting feeling. Great drowsiness and faintness are two prominent characteristics that should remind us of Daffodil.

On the skin, it produces a sort of erythema of a papular, vesisular and pustular type. This rash is always aggravated in the damp wet weather.

NATRUM ARSENICUM.

This remedy, Sodium Arsenate, has been extensively proved by Gourbeyre. It is an important remedy for nasal catarrh with headache and pain at the root of the nose. There is a general feeling of stoppage of the nose with discharge of watery fluid and a postnasal dropping of a thick bland yellowish mucus. Dry crusts also form in the nose which, on removal, leave raw surface behind them. We also use this remedy in supra-orbital headache with a feeling of fullness in the head and in the face and heaviness and soreness of the eye-balls. In the throat, it causes a purplish appearance and a general œdematous condition and thickening of the uvula, tonsils and pharynx. There is also a great hawking out of thick yellowish green mucus. It vies with **Apis** in diphtheria inasmuch as under **Natrum ars.,** we find great swelling, much prostration and dark purplish hue of the throat same as in **Apis.** The uvula hangs down like a sack of water. Like **Apis** again, there is absence of pain. The symptom however, that should lead to the selection of **Natrum ars.,** is the pain at the root of the nose—a symptom greatly characteristic of this remedy. Another symptom that is particularly characteristic of this remedy is a general coolness of the surface of the body which is covered with a cold clammy sweat. These patients are extremely sensitive to cold and dust.

NATRUM CARBONICUM.

Natrum carbonicum, the Sodium Carbonate, is the common soda purified. It is one of Hahnemann's great antipsoric remedies and a polychrest of very great importance. In the old school, its use is confined to burns and eczema and as a douche in nasal and vaginal catarrh; in homœopathy, however, its application extends over an immense tract as will be seen presently.

It has a very marked irritating action over the skin and mucous surfaces of the human body. The skin of the whole body becomes dry, rough and cracked in places. Itching with a sensation of formication is constantly present. Eczema, herpes, warts, ulcerations are everywhere present.

On the mucous membranes the effects are equally marked. The whole of the alimentary canal from the mouth to the anus is in a state of irritation bordering on inflammation. Redness of the mucous membrane of the mouth and fauces with rawness and soreness, painful blisters, a constant desire to hawk and flat ulcers point to the presence of an irritating influence. A similar condition is evident in the nose and in the eyes. Humid herpetic eruptions, ulceration in the nose around the mouth and lips, coryza with copious thick yellowish greenish musty smelling discharge, corneal ulcerations with great photophobia, indicate the universal characteristic or irritation present everywhere.

Another great characteristic of our remedy—a characteristic that is particularly its own, is aggravation of many of its symptoms from mental exertions. He is unable to think or do any mental work without bringing on severe headache, giddiness or some such trouble. His head feels stupefied if he tries to exert himself in the least. His memory is weak. There is a marked inaptitude for meditation or mental labour. Difficulty of comprehension, inability to combine ideas while listening or reading, show clearly the gradual dwindling of the mental faculties. Such a state of the mind gradually leads to a sort of aversion to mankind and society. At times this aversion becomes so strong that even the proximity of his near and dear ones becomes intolerable. This symptom makes **Nat. carb.,** a close ally of **Sepia** where a similar aversion is noticeable. This is not all. Another feature, just as marked and as important, is sadness and depression of spirit. The mood is a typical hypochondriacal one. The patient constantly feels a intolerable melancholy and apprehension. This is specially marked after a meal, particularly after dinner. The anxiety, restlessness and apprehension are rendered worse by music. Hence music is detested.

Another characteristic worth noticing is a great susceptibility of the head to the rays of the sun. It is therefore a valuable remedy in acute and chronic effects of sun-stroke. In this respect it should be compared with **Glon.** and **Lach.**

Nat. carb. exhibits great debility after every exertion. His movement, becomes slow unsteady and tired. Any little obstruction causes him to fall. There is further evinced a pronounced weakness in his ankle joints. Easy dislocation and spraining of the ankle is therefore a matter of common occurrence with him. Ankles are so weak that they give way and bend every now and again, as he attempts to walk. Often it comes to our notice that people who are apparently healthy and well in almost every respect suffer from such defect of the ankle joints. They fall repeatedly and often without any apparent cause. Such defects may be easily rectified by the administration of a constitutional remedy such as **Nat. carb.** Other remedies having similar weakness in the ankles are **Caust., Nat. mur., Sulph.,** and **Sulph. acid.** We also use this remedy for ulcerations on or about the heels. It should not, however, be confused with **Lycop.,** which has ulcers on the insteps rather than on the heels.

We shall now look into the action of **Nat. carb.,** on the female sexual organs. The most important feature here is a strong bearing down feeling as if every thing would come out. This is partly due to the passive congestion of the uterus, noticed particularly during and after coitus, due to an extra influx of blood caused by sexual erethism. In this respect, too, it bears strong resemblance to **Sepia** which seems to have many symptoms in common with this remedy. This backache or rather this bearing down feeling is aggravated by sitting and is ameliorated by moving about.

Nat. carb. is an important remedy for sterility due to ejection of semen after coition. There is also to be seen profuse leucorrhoea of thick and yellow mucus with putrid odour.

Amelioration by rubbing is an important characteristic in **Nat. carb.** I have used this remedy with great success in weak and deficient labour pains, having been guided to it by a great desire on the part of the patient to be rubbed while in pain. It expels moles or the products of false conceptions.

Lastly with the mention of one more characteristic symptom, we shall close this chapter on **Nat. carb.** These patients are particularly susceptible to electrical changes in the atmosphere **(Phos., Rhod.).** The nervousness, sadness, headache, giddiness and all other ailments to which they are subject are distinctly worse during thunderstorm. We should therefore do well to compare this remedy with **Bryo., Nat. mur., Nitric acid, Petrol., Phos., Rod.,** and **Sili.**

The strong aversion to milk which causes diarrhœa and indigestion is specially marked after vegetable diet and starchy food. Great desire for cold water which produces a distinct aggravation, ravenous hunger from a sensation of emptiness in the stomach from 10 to 11 A.M., scrofulous enlargement of the glands specially cervical, blisters on the points of toes, cold feet, inflammation of the external nose with redness, are some of the other important indications to be borne in mind along with the symptoms mentioned before.

Case 1.—Man about twenty-six years of age; nervous temperament; had frequent headache; his occupation in a close room near the roof made it worse; also aggravated by being in the sun; pain mostly in the forehead, although occasionally in vertex; confusion and inability to think accompanied attack. **Nux vom.** somewhat ameliorated, and **Natrum carb.** 30 cured.— Dr. G. M. Ockford.

Case 2.—**Natrum carb.** 200, cured loss of hearing of right ear for seven or eight months; sounds seem to come from the left side when they really come from the right; at times, singing in the right ear, or a noise like a bubble bursting in the ear, or of fullness in the right ear when eating, or, on swallowing, feeling as if something moved in right ear.—Dr. E. W. Berridge.

Case 3.—L. aged forty-five, diarrhœa for ten days, but slightly benefited by **Sulph.** 200, and later **Phos.** Watery diarrhœa, gray, often during the day, worse after eating, the discharge passing with a gush; before stool, cutting pains in upper part of abdomen; the desire to stool very sudden; after stool, burning and soreness in the anus and rectum, which were worse in the evening and during the forepart of the night; great weakness, sensation of sinking in the lower part of the abdomen and frequent perspiration. **Natr. carb.** 200, one dose cured.—Dr. A. Lippe.

NATRUM MURIATICUM.

Natrum muriaticum, also called the Chloride of Sodium, is our common table salt. It is a polychrest amongst polychrests. In the human economy, it plays a very important part. It is found in almost all the tissues of our body, although it exists more largely in the aqueous humors of the eyes and the crystalline lens. It also stimulates digestion, firstly by increasing flavour of food and secondly by increasing the quantity and quality of gastric juice, secreted after food has reached the stomach. It, therefore, fills an important roll in the physiology and pathology of the digestive system. We will go into this more in detail later on. It is our object at present to get a thorough and a clear understanding of the action of the remedy on the human system in general.

It is one of the greatest of our remedies for emaciation and loss of flesh. They are very thin and inspite of every care, the emaciation progresses. At times, it becomes quite difficult to explain this loss of flesh—the patient eating well and partaking of every thing nutritious and fattening, but still losing flesh all the time. Anemia, weariness and complete prostration manifest themselves and our patient gradually becomes powerless, prostrated and bed-ridden. The skin becomes flaccid; anasarca, accumulation of serum in areolar tissues, puffiness amounting at times to complete dropsy and enlargement of varicose veins in different parts of the body are natural consequences that follow in the wake of the downward progress of our ill-fated patient. The loss of flesh, mentioned above, is most conspicuous about the neck. This gives our patient a ludicrous, unsymmetrical proportion, who indeed is an object of pity with his pendulous abdomen, suspended from a narrow strip of a throat on which is mounted a head, no way proportionate to the rest of the body.

Nat. mur. also leads to an impoverished condition of the blood People living on sea-shore or taking long voyage, are frequently seen to suffer from anæmia and a scorbutic state of the system Ulcers of the tongue, mouth and gums, swelling of the gums and a peculiar mapped appearance of the tongue are frequent occurrences with these people. It, therefore, is curative of these conditions, wherever found, provided other symptoms also point to this remedy.

The skin is rather harsh, dry and parchment-like and we have a great profusion of perspiration in **Natrum mur.** They sweat so much as to be thoroughly drenched with it.

Another peculiarity, equally great, is the thirst of **Natrum mur.** They drink an enormous quantity of water. If they are offered a glass of water, they will invariably drain it dry. It is a thirst that is constantly on **them** and no amount of drink quenches it.

As has been already mentioned, they are very pale, wan and anæmic. It is not at all difficult to recognise a **Natrum mur.** patient. The dirty leaden hue merging gradually into a earthy yellowish complexion bespattered with numerous brown spots, the greasy shiny appearance, the swollen upper and the lower lips with pearly blisters around the corners of the mouth and the baldness of the head with the falling off of whiskers, betokening a sycotic basis, are symptoms too clear-cut to be confused with those of any other remedy.

The mental condition of **Natrum mur.** is characterised by excessive irritability. They cry from the slightest cause and get into a passion about trifles. This lachrymal disposition and this hypochondriacal mood are two striking features of our remedy. They weep constantly but without knowing why they are doing so. You speak to them however gently, and it would simply bring on lachrymal depression. You console them, thinking it will be welcome but that aggravates matters. In this respect **Natrum mur.** differs from **Pulsatilla,** where consolation brings relief and soothes the troubled spirit. **Natrum mur.** finds a sort of happiness in indulging in sad and painful thoughts. They have a sort of fascination for them. They try to recollect past disagreeable occurrences, to be able to think over them, brood over them and then indulge in the grief they cause. It is very much like the fascination of sin. We try to fight with it, grapple with it, fly from it and then of our own accord fly back into the arms of its terrible embrace. This hypochondriacal mood is almost always associated with constipation and palpitation. They are disheartened, gloomy and apprehensive and they frequently seek solitude. Taciturnity, quarrelsomeness and vindictiveness render her the most disagreeable of companions. As has been mentioned before, we notice great impairment of mental faculty in these patients, rendering them quite disinclined to undertake mental work of any kind. When, however, they are forced to do so, they make many mistakes, show evident confusion and betray entire loss of memory.

Awkwardness characterises all their movements. Like **Apis** and **Bovista,** they feel nervous, drop things and break them. Intellectual ability is impaired. We find a great loss of memory and aggravation of many complaints from mental work.

It is an admirable remedy in headaches of anemic school girls. There is a great rush of blood to head and the arteries throb mercilessly. It feels like thousand hammers knocking against the brain. The headache of **Natrum mur.** is periodical and is rendered worse by moving the head and the eyes. Sometimes it starts in the morning and lasts till evening. It begins with blindness as in **Kali bich., Iris, Gelsemium,** and **Lac deflor.** I might as well remark here that **Natrum mur.** is inferior to no remedy when intensity of the headache is concerned; it is so violent that they become even maniacal. They speak in blasphemous language. During such paroxysms of maniacal headache the tongue becomes dry and clings to the roof of the mouth and the pulse becomes intermittent.

Natrum mur. produces manifest weakness in the muscles of the eyes, in consequence of which they suffer from asthenopia, amblyopia and amaurosis. Sight becomes obscure and objects look dim, as though seen through a gauze or veil. It is particularly indicated when the internal recti muscles are affected.

It is highly serviceable in scrofulous ophthalmia due to abuse of nitrate of silver. Lids are swollen and there is profuse discharge of mucopurulent matter. Swelling of conjunctiva, fissures at canthi, chemosis and intense lachrymation are important symptoms. We also have great sensitiveness, smarting, and a sensation of sand in eyes. The eye-lids are so excessively sore, as to look like raw beef; they close spasmodically and it becomes difficult to force them open. In this complaint, **Natrum mur.** can well be compared with **Argentum nitricum** and **Graphites.**

We should not overlook the action of **Natrum mur.** on the mucous membranes of our body. It causes a kind of catarrhal inflammation, leading on to hypersecretion of mucus; hence it becomes a good remedy in fluent coryza, alternating with attack of sneezing. Loss of smell, loss of taste, frequent hawking of mucus from throat, a sensation of plug in throat causing choking redness of tonsils, elongation of uvula are symptoms calling for it application in this complaint.

This is a splendid remedy to be thought of in delaying cata menia of young girls. Prescribed in proper time it stops thes chlorotic girls from running into consumption. The menstrua blood is dark and flows day and night. Sadness, anxiety, flutte ing of heart, headache, become very troublesome at this time.

Displacement of uterus is a common feature in **Natrum mur.** Every morning after getting up the bearing down feeling becomes so accentuated that they have to sit to prevent prolapsus. This is accompanied by backache. This backache is so troublesome that they have to lie down on their back or press a pillow against it to obtain relief.

A characteristic urinary symptom that generally accompanies this prolapsus is an increased desire to urinate. I may as well add here that they suffer from weakness of the bladder. In consequence of this they suffer from involuntary escape of urine every time they laugh, cough, sneeze, or in any other way exert themselves. When this weakness is exaggerated we have what is known as incontinence. Urine flows incessantly necessitating frequent change of clothes. This condition is somewhat similar to what we find in **Causticum, Pulsatilla** and **Rumex.**

The opposite condition of difficulty in the expulsion of urine is also to be met with in **Natrum mur.** They have to wait ever so long and press ever so hard to get the flow started. In this respect **Natrum mur.** should be compared with **Ambra grisea, Hepar sulph,** and **Mur. acid.**

It is a remedy *par excellence* in sexual debility of the males. We frequently notice impotence as a result of excess. Great physical weakness and even paralysis may follow such errors. Emissions are frequent. Great loss of hair from pubis is also noticed.

In consequence of these frequent losses, they suffer from backache, night-sweat, weakness of legs, constipation and palpitation.

It is very useful in chronic gonorrhœa when repeated injections of nitrate of silver change the thick yellow matter into a gleet-like clear discharge of transparent slimy mucus that stains the linen at intervals. It is therefore a remedy for the chronic type of gonorrhœa when all the acute symptoms of pain and tension have disappeared. The discharged matter is very thin and causes slight itching and burning. We must not forget the strong smell so characteristic, in the genitals of these patients.

On the female sexual system, **Natrum mur.** manifests a decided diminution in the sexual appetite of the patient. This loss of desire sometimes amounts to a regular aversion to coitus. This may be partly due to great dryness of the vagina which renders the act painful and causes smarting and burning after the act. The menses in **Natrum mur.** appears too early, is too profuse and

lasts too long. This renders them more anæmic and cachectic.
Before menses they are anxious, sad and irritable. During menses
they suffer from headache, colic and palpitation. After menses
they suffer from a sort of congestive headache and leucorrhoeal
discharge which may be either greenish or transparent.

It is particularly useful in what we call hydroa-labialis or in
other words fever blisters. In this respect it is similar to **Arsenic,
Hepar sulphur** and **Rhus tox.**

The effect of common salt in our food is, as has been already
hinted at, to increase our appetite and to help digestion of food
by inducing due secretion of the gastric juice; when potentized
a more powerful action of the drug is generated, of which the proof
lies in its efficacy in the treatment of the most difficult of ailments—
dyspepsia. Our use of this drug in that complaint is not based on
crude physiology but on symptoms, according to the principle laid
down by our master. We notice a great aversion to meat, bread
and coffee and a longing for bitter things. Hunger is excessive
and they do not stint themselves when it comes to good living; but
inspite of this emaciation progresses. A feeling of fatigue, weariness and lassitude is constantly on the patient. They are disinclined to move, walk or undertake work of any kind. There is
distress in the stomach after eating but it is relieved by the tight-
ening of the clothes. Heart-burn, acid eructation, singultus,
nausea and vomiting, are common.

They are great martyrs to the most obdurate variety of constipation. The stools are hard. They are absolutely devoid of
moisture in consequence of which they crumble when passed. The
dry stools and the utter want of secretion in the guts make defecation absolutely trying. It gives rise to fissures in the anus and
every act of defecation is followed by bleeding and intense smarting. This constipation is marked by a decided aggravation of all
their usual ill-humour.

The tongue of **Nat mur.** is mapped with red insular patches
and this characteristic tongue reminds us of **Taraxacum, Nitric
acid, Lachesis, Mercurius** and **Aresenicum.**

Their sleep is full of vivid dreams. It is a remedy of great
value in patients who constantly dream about robbers and feel so
terrified about it that they do not feel satisfied till a thorough
search is made.

Natrum mur. is very rich in skin sypmtoms. It helps in raw
inflamed eczema specially when it crops up near the edges of the
hair roots and on genitals and legs. Like **Graphites** we think of

it in tetters in bends of joints oozing an acrid fluid that dries up and forms crusts with deep fissures and cracks about them. Nettle-rash, shingles, and corns have also been helped by **Natrum mur.**

Finally we come to the most interesting part of **Natrum mur.**,—I mean its place in the therapeutics of intermittent fever. There is no denying the fact that it has cured more cases of inter-mittent fever, specially of the chronic variety, than any other known remedy. **Arsenicum** is the only remedy I can think of that can approach **Natrum mur.**, in respect of utility in the treatment of such fevers. Its indications are very definite and precise. The four chief points of importance are the intensity of chill, almost unbearable bursting hammering headache, great thirst and pro fuse perspiration. Of this the headache is found in all the stages. It is present in the prodromal stage. It is so violent in the stage of chill that it makes the patient unconscious. It lasts all through-out the stage of heat, when the intolerable hammering almost stupefies the patient. And lastly its presence in the stage of sweat announces its overwhelming importance.

About chill I may add that it is not possible to overrate its severity. So agonising is this chill that they dread it before it really sets in; it begins in the extremities such as fingers and toes and thence spreads to the small of the back. It is so severe that it turns the lips and the nails blue.

The thirst of **Natrum mur.**, is present in all the stages. He drinks large quantities of cold water.

The sweat as has been said before is profuse and relieves all pains except the headache.

It is well worth knowing that under **Naturm mur.**, we notice vomiting of bile between the stages of chill and heat as in **Eupato-rium perf.** Hydroa or fever-blisters over the lips as in **Ignatia, Nux vomica** and **Rhus tox,** are of frequent occurrence.

The time of the paroxysm is generally between 10 and 11 A.M., but it may come on any other time and still be within the domain of **Natrum mur.;** the absence of one important symptom, however prominent should never override the totality. The **Naturm mur.** fevers are more frequently to be met with in marshy malarial districts.

Lastly there is one other point that I feel like emphasising in our study of **Natrum muriaticum.** This remedy affords a clear proof of the superiority and the high curative value of dynamiz-ation. Its great efficacy in the treatment of many obsti-nate complaints is a living illustration of the value of potentization of drugs. We all consume a certain quantity of this inert substances without developing symptoms but on dynamization they become more' potent than the most powerful poisonous drug that our book on therapeutics can boast of. It may shock the credulity of our scientific objectors but there is no denying the fact that where crudest arsenic fails and when that universal panacea of quinine proves inert and ineffectual in coping with ailments like pernicious malaria, malarial cachexia, kala-azar, affections they deem incurable, **Natrum mur.** works like a charm.

We will discuss the significance of this remedy in those affections later on; for the present we will be satisfied with a glimpse at the **Nat. mur.** patient. Lean and emaciated she shows signs of great depletion of the vital fluid, which leaves her very anemic and cachectic. Irritability is very excessive. She cries from the slightest cause; gets into a passion about trifles; but the trait that draws our attention the most is a lachrymal disposition. She is constantly weeping but she does not know why she weeps. Unlike **Pulsatilla** where consolation brings relief and soothes the troubled mind, **Natrum mur.** is rendered worse by all such acts of grace. It brings on fluttering of the heart, intermittent pulse and renders the already ugly disposition almost insupportable.

This hypochondriacal mood which becomes more prominent when she suffers from constipation, is due to an undefined apprehension of some impending calamity. Sometimes she gets into fits of taciturnity and avoids company.

Case 1.—Mrs E., aged thirty-five years; nervo-billious temperament; tawny complexion and of rather spare habits. She has been much troubled for five years by attacks of sick-headache of a severe character, which comes on periodically, commencing a day or two before a catamenial period the menses being regular and somewhat copious. The attacks were generally first felt early in the morning, even before rising, increasing during the forenoon; the sensation being that of a tight pressing ache across the forehead and across the eyebrows, and extending outwardly to the temples A confused feeling of the brain and a confined, full, and compressed feeling over the whole frontal portion of the head, with a desire to lie down and be quiet, with occasional nausea and even vomiting, were symptoms which were usually developed and lasted during the catamenial period of four or five days. There was a marked desire to keep still and quiet during the entire course of the headache. I was called to her at the onset of one of these attacks, which came on two days before the menstrual flow, and with such regular procedure, that she predicted a severe attack. I gave her a single dose of **Natrum muriaticum 10,000** on the tongue, and requested her to note any effect that might occur and report the same to me. About ten days afterward she reported that the attack of headache had passed off during the afternoon and evening, the menses came on during the next day, and ran the usual course without being accompanied with headache, and with less general malaise than usual. I gave her a powder of **Natrum muriaticum 10,000,** to be used in case of a return of a similar attack, but not otherwise. Two years afterward she still had this, as she had no return of the headache.—(Dr. W. Gallupe, in **Trans. Am. Ins. of Hom.,** 1878.)

Case 2.—T., aged sixty-five. Six years ago, had ague for sixteen months in spite of **Quinine,** which temporarily suppressed paroxysms. On visiting the uplands of Tully, the disease became again developed, continuing five months under **Quinine.** In five months patient started on his well day for his former home; for four years after the ague ceased, general health was poor; he took **Quinine,** had dyspepsia, liver complaint, suppressed urine, **China** cachexia. He now visited Tully again, when the tertian ague returned. Tried salt water, **Oxalic acid,** with no effect. Present symptoms: chill, beginning every day at 10 A.M. continuing one-and-a-half hours, with severe shaking; heat all the afternoon; profuse and offensive sweat all the night, severe aching in the knees and legs during chill; during heat, much thirst, terrible headache, delirium; during sweat, relief of symptoms. **Nat. mur. 200.** one dose, cured.—Dr. H. V. Miller.

NATRUM PHOSPHORICUM.

This is also called Sodium Phosphate and is prepared from Calcined Bone. It acts upon the glandular organs of the intestinal tract and is a useful remedy in all complaints, arising from excess of lactic acid in the system. Acidity is the most important characteristic of **Natrum phos.,** and is seen to taint practically every organ under this remedy. On awaking in the morning the patient experiences an acid taste in the mouth which practically persists throughout the day. Sour eructation, sour vomiting are also frequent. The stools and the perspirations as well smell acid **(Mag. carb.).** Almost every complaint in **Nat. phos.,** has this symptom of acidity pre-eminently marked. Such an excess of acidity would always direct our attention to **Nat. phos.,** and place it in the same category as **Calc., Carbo veg., China, Lycop., Mag. carb., Nat. carb., Natrum sulph., Phos., Robinia** and **Sulph. acid.** From what we have seen, it stands to reason that it should be one of our principal remedies for chronic dyspepsia and as such ought to be carefully studied by every homœopath. Dyspepsia is such a hydra-headed trouble and is so frequently encountered that it should not dismissed with scant attention. Many of the so-called serious troubles of our life, if traced carefully, will be found to have their origin in some type of dyspepsia. Careful attention in the initial stage may curtail endless troubles. **Nat. phos.**, if judicially pres-cribed, would form a powerful instrument in our hand to fight a type of dyspepsia that sometimes proves most baffling. A yellow creamy coating at the back part of the roof of the mouth, a simi-lar thin moist creamy golden yellow coating at the back of the tongue, acid taste in the month, acid risings, flatulence, headaches, giddiness, and morning sickness with vomiting of sour fluid, are some of the important features of **Nat. phos.** These, however, are not all the symptoms. A diarrhœa specially in children with green, sour smelling stools, caused by an excess of acidity, is of frequent occurrence. Flatulent colic, vomiting of curdled masses much straining at stool, a constant urging to stool with passing of jelly-like masses of mucus, pricking of the nose, itching at the anus, inability to retain urine, sensation of hair at the tip of the tongue dropping of thick yellow mucus from the posterior nares at night and constant attacks of gastralgia and enteralgia accompanied by vomiting of sour fluid as vinegar are a few more characteristics of our remedy.

It is also recommended in consumption, characterised by an intense acidity of the expectoration, so much so, as to cause sore ness of the lips and rawness of the tongue and mouth.

A similar acidity also characterises the secretion from the uterus and the vagina. Such an extreme acidity is an important cause of sterility, and **Nat phos.** has been successfully used t combat this condition.

Leucorrhœa with watery creamy yellow acid discharge, caus ing itching, rawness and soreness of the part find in **Nat. phos.** speedy cure. The discharges smell sour and sickening.

Before closing I will also mention a few indications of **Na phos.**, in the ailment of the eye. It has been recommended an very rightly in inflammations of the eyes specially when there is secretion of golden yellow creamy matter. The eyes are glue together in the morning with a creamy discharge, In conjunct vitis, in scrofulous ophthalmia and for the matter of that, in an complaint or disease of the eye, **Nat. phos.** will make itself a sple did curative agent when prescribed on the characteristic creamy di charge. An interesting case from Dr. Schussler's own practice being cited below :—

" In May last a little girl of 'eight was brought to me who su fered from severe conjunctivitis, with great dread of light. Sł had been treated for some time by an ordinary practitioner, but without effect. I ascertained that her eye affection dated from the time, she had had measles some years previous. **Cal. carb.,** and other medicines proved ineffectual. The enlargements of the glands of the neck, and the creamy secretion of the eyelids, led me to try Sodium Phosphate, of which I administered a dose three times daily. A week later on, the child was brought to me, her eyes being perfectly cured."

Like **Cina, Nat. phos.** is highly efficacious in ailments arising from worms.

NATRUM SALICYLICUM.

It is the Salicylate of Sodium. Its chief chemical property is to prevent fermentation and hence it is utilised in the manufacture of beer. An excess of this substance in beer very often leads to painful symptoms of tenderness of feet and dark, discoloured, enlarged veins in beer drinkers. It also causes a great depression of spirit and bodily prostration. Great weakening of the pulse and a lowering of the body heat are two other symptoms of **Natrum salicylicum.** This remedy, though not so popular with us, is a curative agent for giddiness, particularly the type of giddiness associated with intense tinnitus aurium and deafness. Thus it becomes an important remedy in Meniers's disease. This giddiness is always better lying down and is worse raising the head or sitting up. The noises in the ears are constant and most distressing. In this respect it is similar to **Cocculus, Phosphorus** and **Pulsatilla** where due to great giddiness, the patient is almost compelled to spend most of the time lying down. There is one more symptom worth noticing is **Nat. salicylicum** and that is dyspnœa. It is so alarming as almost to stiffle the patient, who is compelled to assume a half-sitting posture and breathe with the greatest of difficulty. He gasps like fish out of water. This latter symptom also leads to its application in those types of chronic bronchitis where life becomes an agony due mostly to the intensity of the dyspnœa that practically chokes life out of him every second of his existence,

NATRUM SULPHURICUM.

It is also called Sodium Sulphate. It was discovered by Glauber in 1658. Hence it is also called **Glauber's Salt.** This is one of the most important of Schussler's 12 Tissue Remedies. This inorganic salt is found in the intercellular fluids of the human body and its function in the human economy is to regulate water in the human blood and other fluids of the body. It keeps blood, bile, pancreatic juice at normal consistency by eliminating excess of water in the system caused by malassimilation and want of harmony in the working of the various influences of life and health. The deficiency of this salt prevents the elimination of such water from the tissue as is produced by oxidation of the organic matter. This is the theory on which is based the biochemic prescribing of **Nat. sulph.** In homœopathy, on the other hand, the prescription is based on the surer foundation of the totality of the symptoms. As homœopaths, we are, therefore concerned with the symptomatology of **Nat. sulph.**

The first point to note in this remedy is the constitution of our patient. It is the famous hydrogenoid constitution of Von. Grauvogl, that attracts our attention. The patients, having this constitution, feel keenly every change of temperature. They cannot tolerate air or atmosphere surcharged with moisture, nor can they eat with impunity plants or vegetables that thrive in or near about water. They feel healthy and happy in dry weather. Their ailments worry much less when the weather is fine and prosperous. Furthermore symptoms are worse by touch, pressure, and in the morning hours.

Mentally these patients are depressed and tearful. There is also a great inclination to commit suicide specially by shooting. Another peculiarity about the sadness of **Nat. sulph** is that like **Acon., Dig., Graph., Kreo.,** and **Nat carb.,** it is aggravated by music. This disposition towards self-destruction is not confined to **Nat. sulph.** alone. We find it in **Aurum met., China, Cimici., Mercury, Nux vom., Arsenic, Psor.,** and **Silicea.**

These patients are just as prone to get sick headaches as **Gels., Sang., Nat. mur.,** and others. The top of the head feels hot. Brain feels loose when stooping as if it would fall forward. As in **Rhus tox** it is associated with giddiness, bitter taste in the mouth, vomiting of bile, bilious diarrhœa, and colicky pain. Very often it is like a basal headache. Violent pains are felt in the great depth of the brain and it feels as if the bones at the base of the brain were crushed. Great deal of congestion is felt in the brain and there is often bleeding of nose associated with great heaviness of the head (Bry., Rhus., Lach.). We must also note the colour of the patient's tongue; **Nat. sulph** invariably has a dirty greenish, greyish or greenish-brown coating. Another symptom is that it removes the salivation with the headache. Dr. Baltzer prescribed **Nat. sulph** with great effect, after **Puls.** and **Phos.** failed, in a case of periodical headache in a young girl. The symptoms were shooting pain in the right temple, beginning early in the morning and increasing till evening and only ceasig at about midnight when she was able to get asleep. It was relieved by cold compress, open air, dark room and vomiting. Noise, light, eating, stooping, menstruation, invariably aggravated the headache. During headache her mouth used to get full of saliva causing her to spit constantly. It is a symptom worth noting although it needs further verification.

A great characteristic of **Nat. sulph**, a characteristic that dominates it everywhere, is that its discharges are invariably thick, yellow or yellowish green (**Pulsat**). I consider this a valuable symptom. In ophthalmia, conjunctivitis granulosa, ozœna, diphtheria, gastritis, diarrhœa, dysentery, gonorrhœa, leucorrhœa, cough, asthma and for the matter of that in every other variety of complaint characterised by a thick yellow or yellowish-green discharge we should accord **Nat. sulph.** our first consideration.

It is a great remedy for acute and chronic diarrhœa. The diarrhœa is principally worse in the morning, hence resembling **Sulphur,** and **Thuja; Sulph.** drives the patient out of bed, long before it is time for him to get up. **Thuja** gets an urgent call as soon as he takes his first cup of tea in the morning; but **Nat. sulph.** like **Bryo.** starts getting his stools after he gets up and moves about. The urging is sudden and the gushing stool is accompanied with flatulence. There is quite a great deal of rumbling in the bowels due to flatulence and this rumbling is mostly located in the right side of the abdomen in the ilio-cæcal region. The stools are dark, bilious or of green bile. It may be also yellowish-green, slimy or bloody. The stools are occasionally, involuntary while passing flatus or urine or during sleep as in **Aloes.** Before stools we notice a contractive pain in the abdomen extending into the chest. Violent colic as if pinching and a good deal of rumbling characterise this stage. During stools there is a profuse emission of flatus associated with a voluptuous feeling and burning in the anus. But the most important part is that after stools there is immediate relief of colic and patient feels distinctly happy and cheerful. It is as great a remedy for chronic diarrhœa as it is for the acute. Torpidity of the liver is at the root of this diarrhœa. We also notice great sensitiveness and soreness in the right hypo-chondriac region. Inability of bearing tight clothing about the waist, soreness of the liver to touch, stitching pain in the liver while walking, and taking deep breath, vomiting of bitter fluids, greenish brown and greenish grey tongue, enlargement of the liver, dis-tention of the stomach, prevalence of acidity, constant taste of bile in the mouth, yellow complexion, loss of appetite, constant rising or gulping up of sour water in the mouth, qualmishness before eating, disgust for bread and a great desire for ice-cold water are the great indications of this remedy and should lead to its application not only in chronic diarrhœa but in dyspepsia and other hepatic diseases.

Let us now look into its action on the respiratory tract. The most important symptom here is great and constant dyspnœa. The patient has a strong inclination to take deep and long breath (**Bryonia, Phos.**). Slightest exertion brings on short breathing (**Calc. carb.**). Such difficulty of breathing is particularly notice-able on a damp, cloudy day. Hence, **Nat. sulph.** makes an admir-able remedy for asthma both acute and chronic. Copious green expectoration, offensive breath and harsh asthmatic breathing, audible even at some distance, lead to its application. One peculiar symptom which is of great value and which has frequently led to its application in asthma, is looseness of bowels with each attack. Dr. Guernsey has recorded the case of a woman of 36 who suffered from violent attacks of asthma, and where after many remedies had failed, he was led to prescribe **Nat. sulph.** on the indication of loose evacuations starting since the onset of the asthma. Heavy pressure on the chest as from a load, stitches in the chest when yawning and during inspiration, soreness of the chest when coughing relieved by pressure, cough attended with muco-purulent expectoration, loud rales in the chest and an empty all-gone feeling have led to its application in sycotic pneumonia and phthisis.

It is a very valuable remedy in panaritium. We also have inflammation and suppuration around the roots and nails. Œdema of the feet, ulcerative pain in the soles and heels, podagra are also to be found in **Nat. sulph.**

Numerous wart-like eruptions on the arms, thighs and anus betray the sycotic taint in **Nat. sulph.** Condylomata and soft fleshy excrescences on the male genital organs also belie the same constitutional taint.

It has been used successfully in remittent, bilious, malarial and intermittent fevers. Symptoms indicating it are icy coldness of the limbs, absence of thirst in all the stages, bilious vomiting and aggravation in wet weather. A curious symptom that led Dr. S. M. Pease to prescribe **Nat. sulph.** with signal success in a case of intermittent fever is that " when he took off his boots at night the ball of the right great toe invariably itched." Itching is therefore a very valuable symptom in **Nat. sulph.** that will lead to its application not only in intermittent fever but in various other deviations of the vital force from the normal condition.

Dreams of **Nat. sulph.** are remarkable. Soon after falling asleep he starts up in a fright. His dreams are mostly about fighting. Other remedies having similar dreams are **Allium cepa, Ferrum, Nat. mur., Ran.** and **Staph.**

Dreams, to a homœopath, are oftentimes quite guiding. They give us a far better insight into the deeper nature of our patient than many of the so-called symptoms that crop up and float on the surface to meet our superficial gaze. It is not for nothing that dreams differ. Some dream of accidents, other of amorous subjects, others again of topics of varied nature—each dream in its turn specifying a particular temperament, or more correctly a special deviation of the individual from the normal. Important cures have been recorded, based on dreams alone. Hence a special study of the dreams, together with their remedies, will not be out of place here.

Dreams of animals—**Arnica, Mercury, Nux vom., Phos.** and **Puls.**

Dreams of battles—**Allium cepa.**

Dreams of business—**Bryo., Chelid., Lach., Lycop., Nux vom.,** and **Rhus tox.**

Dreams of the dead—**Anacar., Argent. nit., Arnica., Arsen., Mag. carb., Phos., Sulph.,** and **Thuja.**

Dreams of falling—**Bell., Cact., Dig., Kreo., Puls., Sulph.,** and **Thuja.**

Dreams of fire—**Anacar., Hepar. sulph., Lauro., Mag. carb., Mag. mur.**

Dreams of flying—**Apis.**

Dreams of robbers—**Alum., Mag. carb.,** and **Nat. mur.**

Dreams of snake—**Argent. nit., Lac. can.**

The homœopathic system of treatment is thoroughly scientific. It encompasses the patient in his entirety. It does not, like the other schools of treatment, regard its patient as a conglomeration of various detached self-sufficient, autogenic units, each working out its own salvation, independent of the central vital force, that really stimulates, guides, protects and preserves all the different organs in a system of complete harmony and unision. Therefore, we take into account not only the workings and deviations of all the organs of our patient and their functions, both normal and abnormal, but look deeper even into the thoughts, ideas, sentiments, and even further into the unconscious and subconscious state of our patient.

NICOLUM METALLICUM.

It is a metallic substance found in conjunction with Cobalt. I have not had much experience with this remedy except that I have found it useful in a certain type of cough, associated with intense pain in the head and where during the paroxysm, the patient is compelled to sit up. It is a cough that, at first sight, would remind you of **Bryonia**. Everytime he coughs, he must sit up and hold the head with both the hands or else the shooting pain in the head becomes most agonising. This would very naturally suggest **Bryonia** but minuter analysis reveals that it is not holding of the head that relieves but the act of sitting up that is really the relieving factor. Another peculiarity of this cough which I have not had occasion to verify, is that the patient has to put arms on thighs when coughing.

NITRIC ACID.

Nitric acid is a colorless, highly corrosive, transparent liquid. It was introduced by Hahnemann.

This is one more of our polychrests. **Nitric acid** patients are as a rule lean, thin and of nervous temperament. They catch cold easily and are frequent subjects of diarrhœa. They are further characterised by excessive weakness of mind and body, trembling of limbs and great physical irritability. At times they are so prostrated that they have to keep to bed constantly. The least exertion tires them.

The main characteristic of this drug consists in extreme fetidity and corrosiveness of all its discharges. In coryza the wings of the nose seem to be highly inflamed. In otorrhœa the purulent ichorous discharge makes the part red and angry. The leuccorrhœal discharge is equally acrid; so are the urine, the menstrual and the alvine discharges.

The next important characteristic is found in the sticking pricking pain as from splinters in the affected part. In diphtheria, sore-throat, hemorrhoid, pneumonia, bronchitis, diarrhœa, dysentery, chancre, bubo and in numerous other ailments, this peculiar and characteristic sensation becomes our main indication for the remedy. Other remedies having a similar symptom are the following: **Æsculus, Alumina, Argentum nit., Baryta carb., Carbo veg., Dolichos, Hepar sulph.** and **Silicea.**

A further symptom of **Nitric acid** worth remembering is a sensation of a band. This may be felt in any part of the body and is always a characteristic indication of **Nitric acid.**

Mentally **Nitric acid** is characterised by great depression of spirit, indifference, irritability of disposition, hopelessness, despair and sadness. He is very self-willed, head-strong, and obstinate. Entreaty, apology, coaxing, love are equally incapable of moving him. He also suffers from a morbid fear of cholera. This shows an anxious state of the mind and anxiety indeed is a great characteristic of **Nitric acid.** He is constantly worried over various things. He is anxious about his health, about his future and about things that do not really concern him. This state of mind is, to a great extent, generated by continued loss of sleep or from a loss of a dear friend. Such anxiety, is to be met with in various other remedies but in **Nitric acid,** we have a deep-seated remedy to deal with. The constitution of the patient, which is tainted with poisons of syphilis, mercury and scrofula, should always be a para

mount feature in the selection of the remedy. **Weakness**
plays an important part. The patient is so **weak** and
exhausted that he is obliged to lie down every now and
again. The slightest exertion causes him loss of breath.
We frequently find him speechless. He trembles in all
his limbs and complains of great debility and heaviness, particularly in the hours of the morning. A great subject to constant
diarrhœa, we find him emaciated and thin almost to bone. Over
and above this, due to his tainted constitution, we find him suffering from inflammation of the bone and the periosteum. It is altogether a broken down cachectic constitution that we encounter
in **Nitric acid**—a constitution that is thoroughly sapped with
syphilis and mercury. The proofs are many and numerous. In
the first place, he is a chronic martyr to ozena———an ozena
of syphilitic origin. He expels yellow plugs and green casts from
the nose. Frequent epistaxis and disagreeable odor from the nose
are also present. Other useful remedies for syphilitic ozena are
**Asafœtida, Aurum met., Flouric acid, Kali bich., Merc. iod., Phytc
lacca,** and **Stillingia.** The gums are, as in all similar cases of
mercurial and syphilitic cachexia, scorbutic.

It is adapted both to primary and secondary syphilis, though
its application in the latter stage is oftener called for than in
the former. It is most useful after abuse of mercury. The
chancres are phagedenic. Nocturnal bone pains, particularly of the
ones of the head and the long bones, development of warts and
copper-coloured spots when associated with pronounced debility,
sweat and exhaustion render **Nitric acid** a sure remedy.

In the acute and primary stage we have flat suppurating
ulcerations which are of irregular shape and zigzag edges. They
discharge a thin copious bloody corroding ichorous fluid. They
are inclined to spread more in circumference than in depth and are
further full of exuberant granulations—the base looking like
raw flesh. The least touch or movement causes bleeding from
the ulcers. In some bad cases we notice sloughing of the entire
integument of the penis that leaves the organ entirely denuded.
In the females, similar destruction of tissues is also to be
seen. Instances are numerous where the entire integuments,
covering the pubic region, had sloughed away, leaving muscular
structure entirely bare. The chancres in **Nitric acid** increase very
fast, especially along the circumference where the edges are
raised. The pains are generally splinter-like. Buboes threaten to
suppurate.

Another characteristic point is a tendency towards fungus growths. As I have mentioned before, the pain in these sores are splinter-like in character; they also burn and smart. They are always worse from application of cold water. Condylomatous growths and warts that bleed pretty often and on the slightest touch, are of constant occurrence. Let me add here that the choicest locations for these **Nitric acid** chancres are the junctions of the mucous membranes and the skin and the edges of the orifices of the body, such as the mucous outlets of the mouth, nose rectum, anus, urethra and vagina.

Nitric acid is a great hemorrhagic remedy. We notice bleeding excrescences in the vagina and on the mouth of the uterus. The leucorrhœa, as has been already mentioned, is acrid, offensive, greenish yellow in character and is specially seen in subjects with venereal history. The menses in **Nitric acid** are too early and too profuse. The blood is dark colored like muddy water. During menses the patient complains of pain down thighs, labor-like pain in the abdomen and the back, palpitation, anxiety, trembling and tiredness.

It is as great a remedy for gonorrhœa as any we know of. The discharge is yellowish, bloody or greenish. Bubo, painful micturition, tenderness of testicles are a few additional symptoms. We use it also in strictures and prostatitis due to suppressed gonorrhœa.

The action of **Nitric acid** over the bladder and the kidneys is of surpassing importance. It is particularly useful in albuminuria of syphilitic patients. Excessive prostration, nausea, sour taste, bilious diarrhœa, fetid and turbid urine and œdema of the feet are strong indications for its application. The urine of **Nitric acid** is very characteristic. It is scanty, dark brown and strong smelling. The smell is that of horse's urine. It feels cold when passing. Another condition often met with is difficult micturition. He must stand and press a long while before urine appears, but once the stream starts, it comes on uninterruptedly. We have also hematuria in **Nitric acid.** This is accompanied with shuddering and followed by intense urging.

We will now study the action of **Nitric acid** on the digestive organs and its application in various disorders thereof. The liver is seriously affected, as a result of which we have obstinate jaundice. There is a strong longing for fat, chalk, lime and other absurd substances. Bread and meat cause strong aversion to food. Milk disagrees. With this, as has been hinted at before,

we have persistent diarrhœa.   The discharges from the bowels
are offensive, green and watery.   They frequently contain long
pieces of mucus resembling scrapings from the intestines.   The
patient experiences a constant pressure in the rectum, but this is
not always followed by an evacuation Sometimes after long straining he may pass a little mucus but the feeling remains as if the
rectum were full of fæces that could not be expelled.   The most
characteristic feature of all is violent cutting and drawing pain
in the rectum continuing for hours after defecation.   The patient
walks about the floor with this intense burning tearing splinter-
like spasmodic pain in anus.

It is of great use in dysentery of diphtheritic type.   Here also
a great and a constant pressing in the rectum is experienced without very much of an evacuation.   The sero-croupous discharge,
ineffectual urging to stool with sharp splinter-like cutting pains
in the rectum should be constantly borne in mind.

Hæmorrhoids are plentiful and annoying.   They come out
with each stool.   They are very often the source of the sensation
of weight and pressure in the rectum and are frequently the
cause of the agony that accompanies and follows evacuations.
Constriction of the anus is a very frequent feature.   Another important point is the discharge of a fetid watery substance from
the anus that keeps it constantly moist.   The constant urging
and tenesmus are very exhausting.

The constipation of **Nitric acid** is somewhat like that of
Alumina and **Graphites.**   The stools are hard and small like
sheep-dung and are accompanied by a mucus secretion.   With
every stool there is protrusion of hemorrhoidal tumors and profuse bleeding.   This remedy is specially useful in patients of bilious
habits, and of syphilitic and mercurial infection.   Fissures of the
anus are very often associated with this constipation.

Case 1.—I found the patient in the following deplorable condition:
Sloughing of the entire integument of the penis, and of the prepuce, leaving
that organ entirely denuded.   At one inch posterior to the corona glandis
on the left side of the corpus-spongiosum, was a fistulous ulcer extending
into the urethra, so that in micturition a portion of the urine escaped through
this orifice.   The integuments which cover the pubic region had likewise
sloughed away, leaving the muscular structure bare, and ulceration was
extending upward under the pubes.   The entire diseased surface was in a
very unhealthy, or phagedenic, ulcerated condition.   The urine emitted an
intolerably strong odor on being voided, and gave rise to considerable burning and smarting.   Sleep at night was much disturbed; appetite poor and
there was considerable emaciation.   Frequent painful erections occurred in

the latter part of the night. He had had chancres on the glans, and buboes were still in a condition of ulceration. I had the entire diseased surface dressed with sweet oil and raw cotton, and ordered **Nitric acid 200** in water, to be taken night and morning. This resulted, in a comparatively short period, in a perfect cure, the fistulous opening into the urethra even being closed. Of course, the true skin, prepuce and hair, which had been destroyed, were not reproduced.—Dr. H. N. Guernsey. **Hahn. Monthly, November, 1870.**

Case 2.—Mr. G., aged twenty, of good constitution, consulted me about numerous large warts, which disfigured the back of his hands. He had suffered, for four years, the most excruciating pains with them, and neither cauterization, ligatures, nor red-hot iron has ever done him any good. Since four or five months the disease is on the increase, and begins to tell more and more on his constitution. The backs of his hands are covered with mammilated warty excrescences, hard and horny in places, and so close together, that the least friction produces laceration of the skin. Deep rhagades, always bleeding, prevent him from any manual exertion; especially as hæmorrhages from them, which quite frequently set in, are stopped only with difficulty. He frequently suffers also from inflammatory affections of the lymphatics, and glands of the arms and axillæ. Prescribed **Nitric acid 30**, six globules, to take a dose in the morning, fasting; and to repeat it every four days, for twenty days. Then **Nitric acid 200**, six globules, once a week. The patient soon began to feel great relief; the rhagades healed up, the larger warts disappeared, and the others looked softer and less irritable. The remedy was continued for two months and the patient was perfectly well when the case was reported, three years later.—Dr. Gaillard. **Am. Jour. of Hom.**

Case 3.—Mrs.——, aged twenty-eight, aborted at second month in consequence of a rough sleigh ride. First few hours she experienced considerable pain. Contractions came on regularly, and the embryo was expelled. The post partum hæmorrhage was quite profuse and long continued. When the pains had ceased, the **Secale** which I had prescribed ceased to be of service. The flow then became passive, and the discharge dark-coloured and shreddy. As an effect of keeping her in proper position, and the use of appropriate diet and drinks, she convalesced, but relapsed several times. The usual remedies would cause the flow to cease for a little but on attempting to change her posture in the least, the discharge commenced again. Matters went on thus for four weeks, in all of which time she had really gained nothing, but lost much in strength, color and spirits. Tuesday, prescribed **Nitric acid 2x** in water, two spoonfuls every half hour. On Wednesday she had no flow since midnight. Medicine was continued every three hours. On Friday there was no return of it, and she sat up a little. Discontinued the **Nitric acid**. Sunday she came out into the parlor, and afterward convalesced rapidly.—Dr. R. Ludlam.

NITRO-MURIATIC ACID.

It is also called Aqua Regia. It is a mixture of Chloro-nitric acid, Chloronitrus acid, Chlorin and water. It is a remedy of comparatively recent origin and although our experience with it is meagre, it has been highly recommended in oxaluria in which complaint it is almost regarded as a specific. The urine generally is cloudy and is associated with urging in the penis and the bladder and aching in the hips, thighs and small of back. When such symptoms are associated with intense salivation, bleeding gums and ulceration of mouth and tongue, **Nitro-muriatic acid** becomes particularly useful. I have very rarely used this remedy.

NUPHAR LUTEUM.

Nuphar luteum is the Yellow Pond Lily, belonging to the natural order of Nymphæaceæ. This medicine was first proved by Dr. Pitet. Its field of action though very limited is not to be ignored. It produces important and marked symptoms of weakness in the sexual sphere. There is entire absence of erection and sexual desire **(Agnus)**. Voluptuous ideas fill imagination but do not cause excitement. The penis is retracted and the scrotum is relaxed. Involuntary seminal losses are frequent during sleep **(Phosp. acid)**. We also notice involuntary emissions during stool **(Nux v., Sel., Sulph.)** and when unrinating (Prostatic discharge during diarrhœic stool—**Arsenic**). In this respect our remedy compares well with **Agnus., Con., Graph., Lycop., Sepia** and **Sulph.**

It is also a great remedy in entero-colitis. The most marked feature of this diarrhœa is that the stools are extremely yellow like that of **Chelid.** It also has a morning diarrhœa like what we find in **Sulph.** Quite early, long before it is time for the patient to get up in the morning, he experiences intense urging which obliges him to go to the bath-room. He gets two or three passages of liquid light-yellow stools and no more till the next morning.

NUX MOSCHATA.

It is prepared from the powdered dried root of nutmeg. It belongs to the natural order of Myristicaceæ. The nutmeg tree is a native of the East and West Indies. It was introduced into our Materia Medica by Helbig.

It is at all times a great remedy with us. Although it suits all kinds and classes of people, it is particularly adaptable to children, old people and women during pregnancy. It has a particular action over the nervous system and hence we find it applicable in such nervous ailments, as hysteria, locomotor ataxia, chorea, epilepsy, catalepsy, fainting fits and various forms of convulsions. Jactitation of muscles, trembling, fatigue, lassitude and restlessness are prominent characteristics of **Nux moschata.** He suffers from great restlessness and must constantly move about. He staggers while walking; often we find him falling. The weakness so frequently complained of by him, is not anything like the weakness of **Arsenicum.** It is more or less a nervous state, brought about by abnormality in the economy of the nervous system. He complains of great fatigue and wishes to lie down after the slightest exertion. This condition, more a lassitude than anything else, is not the after-effect of a great loss of vitality but merely a nervous feeling that may be conquered by sheer force of will. Sometimes this languor assumes such proportions that we find our patient frequently going off into faints.

The mental aspect of the patient also betrays the same tendency. Frequent vanishing of thoughts while talking reading or writing, great weakness or loss of memory, listlessness and indifference also speak of real depletion of the nerve force. He has no will power of his own and is the plaything of whims and fancies. He accomplishes nothing; he undertakes no enterprise. He stands in one place for hours together and he does not know what to do and where to go. He does not know where he is and betrays great incoherence attempting to express his ideas. This shows total imbecility and **Nux moschata** frequently meets with, cures and rectifies all such mental disorders. Stupor, unconsciousness and insensibility are merely stages of his downward journey.

A leading keynote symptom of **Nux moschata** is drowsiness It is constant and irresistible. Most of the time he feels sleepy and muddled, as if intoxicated. The eyes are constantly closed and he lies perfectly silent. In this **Nux moschata** bears a great resemblance to **Opium,** but in the latter remedy the drowsiness is more akin to coma. The suffused countenance, the stertorous breathing, the involuntary defæcation and micturition, the thorough blunting of all the senses following intense acuteness, are keynote symptoms of **Opium** and are thoroughly absent in **Nux moschata,** where the lassitude and the lethargy, purely nervous, are nothing compared to the thorough intoxication of the whole system as in **Opium.** Furthermore, in **Nux moschata** it is associated with chilliness and thirstlessness. The patient is always worse in damp and in cold. Warmth always brings in amelioration.

The second keynote symptom is dryness. Everything in **Nux moschata** is dry. The tongue is so dry that it adheres to the roof of the mouth. The skin is dry; the eyes are dry Nose, lips and throat also betray dryness. Due to such dryness in the mouth, the saliva is lessened. It gets thick and it looks like cotton. Inspite of this dryness, there is hardly any thirst. This dryness in the mouth and throat is particularly troublesome after sleeping. In fact, it wakes him up from sleep. Nothing can be done to relieve this dryness. There is difficulty of deglutition due to the same cause. Food sticks in the throat due to want of lubrication from proper saliva. Speech is indistinct and articulation difficult, due partly to a sort of paralysis but mostly to this want of secretion of the glands imbedded in the mouth whose function is, in a secondary way, one of lubrication.

Finally, we must discuss its tendency to fainting, another keynote indication of **Nux moschata.** These patients faint on the slightest provocation. At times it becomes extremely difficult to discern its cause. The sight of blood, even standing for a long while, strong odor of flowers or scents and slight emotional disturbance will cause the patient to swoon away. This tendency to faint or swoon is more marked after a stool. Such characteristics always indicate a hysterical temperament and **Nux moschata** is indeed a great remedy for hysteria with us. The fickleness of temperament, already referred to above, is another illustration of such temperament. We also notice in these patients an inordinate inclination to laugh and make a jest of everything. The alternate changing of mood and symptoms of halucinations also speak of it as a priceless remedy in hysteria.

Nux moschata has always been highly spoken of as being a valuable remedy in dyspepsia. They suffer from a tormenting flatulence. Whatever they eat seems to turn into wind. The stomach becomes intensely bloated and pressure on the heart and the lungs bring on palpitation and dyspnœa. It is not, therefore, inferior to either **Nux vom.,** or **Lycopodium,** two remedies, generally thought of in such instances. Like either of these two remedies, **Nux moschata** too has hiccough, nausea, waterbrash and vomiting. Enlargement of the liver and the spleen, colicky pain, looseness of bowels with great sleepiness make the resemblance between these remedies still closer. But we must not forget that even the dyspepsia of **Nux moschata** is more or less of nervous origin and is generally to be found in nervous hysterical subjects. One important symptom of **Nux moschata,** absent in the other two remedies, is that this tympanites is brought on by unpleasant mental emotions. The stools may be profuse, watery, exhausting, thin and yellow. It is generally brought on by cold drinks in hot summer or after taking boiled milk. It is particularly useful in chronic diarrhœa during pregnancy.

We must not forget its efficacy in hæmorrhage from bowels in typhus. The putridity of the smell, the profound coma, rolling, rumbling and gurgling noise in the bowels, thirstlessness, the red or bloody sweat and the intense drowsiness, in conjunction with chilliness make **Nux moschata** as valuable a remedy in typhus as any we may think of.

From what has been already said, we may easily guess that **Nux moschata** is an excellent remedy in many affections of the females. In the first place, we should think of it in dysmenorrhœa of hysterical women. Menses are preceded by intense pain in small of back which feels almost like breaking as from the weight of a hard board placed on the back. During menses we have intense backache, a great bearing down sensation, lassitude and headache. The menses are generally irregular, both as to time and quantity. It may appear too early and too profuse or too late and scanty. The blood discharged is generally thick and dark.

It has been used very successfully in checking threatened abortion in hysterical females, disposed to fainting. Hering reports of a case of impending abortion in a female after six months of pregnancy due to a severe kick in the lower part of the abdomen from a child who was sleeping with her. **Nux moschata** stopped the semi-sanguinous, foul-smelling discharge from vagina which was accompanied with a strong bearing down pain, abortion looking almost imminent.

Case 1.—Mrs. B., aged twenty-nine years, mother of four children, of vigorous build; nervous constitution; sanguine temperament. When a child, he suffered from an eruption on the head; her menses appeared early, have always been copius and accompanied with much pain. She was married at twenty-one and soon became pregnant. At the time when the menses should have appeared she had violent congestion to the chest and neck; she felt as if her head would burst and her heart be squeezed off; she had violent stitches as if a knife were plunged into her chest and head; frequently, unconsciousness and epileptic convulsions; she was bled several times without any but temporary relief. Her confinement brought no change in her condition; at the time when her menses should have re-appeared, her symptoms were the same. She was bled about once a month. The effects became manifest. Her complexion became earthy and pale, she became emaciated, and so weak that she could hardly attend to her household duties. Great oversensitiveness of the nervous system; the least thing excited her very much.   Sometimes after mental excitement, especially if a short time before her catamenia, she was attacked, in the midst of her work, with slight vertigo, vanishing of thoughts and fainting, from which she recovered in a few moments, without, however, being fully conscious; she attended to her work automatically and on awakening from this condition, she had not the slightest recollection of what she had done. If forcibly aroused, she fell into violent convulsions.   If unmolested, she would usually, after finishing her work go to bed and fall into a quiet slumber, from which she awakened after forty-eight hours, invigorated and unconscious of what had happened. At times she was in a clairvoyant state and answered questions accurately on subjects entirely out of her sphere; but on returning to consciousness, she was perfectly ignorant of what she had said.   There was great debility and tendency to constipation.   The blood taken from her arm was thin and pale; the pulse, after the congestions, small and weak; in the carotid, a light murmur was audible At the time of her menstrual period, when the congestions were most frequent, there would, occasionally, appear an eruption on her face, which spread to her neck and consisted of irregular, slightly elevated, reddish patches, scaling off under violent itching, and gradually disappearing. A careful physical examination revealed no organic disease.   **Nux moschata** accomplished a complete cure in a year and a half.—(Dr. Lohrbacher, **Am Jour. Hom. Mat. Med.** vol. iv.)

   Case 2.—Mrs. H., thirty-five years old, pregnant six months, after violen blow on the abdomen, and next day getting feet wet; severe paroxysmal colicky pains all over the abdomen followed; could not keep her feet still on moment; was restless all over. **Coloc.** and **Rhus** gave no relief. At th same time a semi-sanguinous, foul-smelling discharge set in, per vagina with bearing-down pains; felt very drowsy, yet unable to sleep. **Nux mosch** 200. Slept all night and all pain gone. After few days took **Puls.** whic' discharged dead foetus.—Dr. S. Lilienthal.

NUX VOMICA.

This is the king of our polychrest remedies. This is commonly known as the poison nut, a plant indigenous to India and East Indies. It belongs to the natural order of Loganiaceæ. The tincture is prepared from the seed of this plant, deprived of their hard shells. They are disc-shaped, about an inch in diameter and a quarter of an inch in thickness. They are intensely bitter and poisonous. It contains strychnia and Brucia to which most of its properties are to be attributed.

The symptoms of poisoning are tetanic rigidity of the muscles of the body with occasional relaxations and renewal of the spasm from the slightest touch. The convulsions are accompanied with consciousness. Death is caused by the arrest of the respiratory movement. The smallest fatal dose is said to be three grains.

It is truly the king of our polychrest remedies and its dominion is vast. It extends from pole to pole and it encompasses a perplexity of character that is truly astounding. If the inhabitants of this big universe were to be grouped according to their characters, I truly believe that **Nux vomica** will fully cover three-fourths of this enormous mass of humanity. It is a remedy that suits ardent characters. It is never in the nature of the **Nux vomica** patients to be lukewarm in anything they undertake. They are always in the front rank of all enterprises and in consequence they generally occupy the topmost places in all occupations and all departments of life. They are the foremost scientists, the best doctors, the best lawyers, the commercial magnets and the sure leaders of every movement and enterprise. By this I do not mean that these people, occupying such high places in life, should be always and invariably given **Nux vomica** when they get ill, but most of them when ill may need this remedy, as it suits their temperament. We must not, however, be misled by this eulogy into believing that they are always as pleasant as they are great. They are thin, irritable, choleric persons with nervous, melancholic temperament. It is thus suited to careful and zealous persons, to people who are over-cautious, intellectual and irritable in their disposition. The irritability of **Nux** knows no bounds. **Chamomilla** seems pleasent and companionable when compared with the vile malicious and the quarrelsome nature of this thin ill-humoured dyspeptic. Do whatever you like, try however much you can, it is hard to please them. All their senses are over-sensitive. Noise, smell, light and music are equally unbearable. Even harmless words annoy them. It is an excellent remedy in ailment of literary and studious persons, who are constantly indoors and who stuff themselves with strong powerful drugs for little or no ailments, and suffer from sluggish liver and constipation. They lead too much of sedentary life. The only part of their system that is exercised is their brain and intellect. The inevitable happens and we find them pale, lean, worn out with high intellectual forehead and eyes staring out of their sockets in the true intensity of their zeal and fierceness of character. These are the people that are bidding high to buy the universe with their whole life, body and entity. They never waver, they never pause and they never think of the enormous price they are paying for their success. The health is ruined; the intellect at times seems to be almost giving in under the intense strain and stress of their activity but still they plod on and to what end? With a broken down constitution and tottering legs, they hurry fast to a premature grave and this is what I meant when I said that they are buying the universe with their soul.

Another aspect of these characters is to be found in their habit of taking drugs and intoxicating liquors. This is a necessary corollary to their way of life. When faculties get dim and blunt, when nature gives up in exhaustion, they still want to keep up the space and this can only be done by means of artificial stimulation and that is why we find them indulging in coffee, tobacco and alcoholic stimulants. Under the influence of these strong narcotics, they keep up but only to break down in a collapse, and then we have merely the skeletons of those masterminds that wanted to buy the universe. Such then is our **Nux vomica** patient.

Nux vomica patients may at times evince a homicidal tendency It is said to be useful in women who when alone get an insane desire to kill their husbands. This is not due to any lack of affection on their part. They want to commit suicide but they dare not They lack the courage. These patients are indisposed to mental exertion and to work of any kind.

Nux vomica patients are very subject to headache. It is the result of a certain amount of congestion to the head and is accompanied with heat and redness of the face. They feel as if their head would split or their skull would be pressed asunder. This headache is generally felt in the morning on waking, as if they did not sleep well at night. Sometimes it is described as a feeling of confusion or stupefaction. The **Nux vomica** headache is rendered worse by eating, exposure to open air, mental exertion anger, chagrin, masturbation, constipation and debauchery. It is better in a warm room and from pressure and wrapping up of the head.

Nux vomica is a favourite remedy for cold. We think of it in the first stage of coryza when the nose feels dry and obstructed inspite of an acrid watery discharge and frequent sneezing. The catarrh is fluent in the morning but becomes dry in the evening and at night time. It is worse in a warm room but better in the open air. This catarrh is frequently associated with headache, heat in the face and chilliness. The nostril feels sore as if ulcerated

Let us now study the action of **Nux** on the liver. That it acts on this organ very powerfully is evident from what little has been said about the remedy. It is our sheet anchor in induration and swelling of the liver caused by high living, debauchery and drunkenness. The region of the liver becomes so sore that they constantly loosen their clothes to relieve the oppression. This oppression is partly due to the distention of abdomen with flatulence. The accumulation of wind is great and it now presses on the heart causing palpitation, uneasiness and difficulty of breathing, and now downwards over the intestines and the bladder causing frequent desire for stool and constant urging for micturition. Frequent colic, periodical belching, violent griping and tearing in the abdomen, jaundice, aversion to food, constipation, bilious attacks, loss of appetite, yellow skin, high colored urine, backache, are symptoms too characteristic and violent to be overlooked.

Its influence over the digestive organs is no less marked. The stomach becomes distended and sensitive to pressure. After eating food seems to lie heavy like a stone in the stomach causing sensation of fullness, weight, pyrosis, acid eructation, lassitude, nausea and confusion of ideas. Qualmishness is felt immediately after eating with constant water brush. Nausea is constant in the morning but the most important symptom is ineffectual desire to vomit. He feels that he will be ever so much better if he can only vomit but that vomiting rarely comes. Sometimes however he succeeds in vomiting a kind of green bitter substance that leaves him more irritable, indisposed and ill-at-ease.

The opposite conditions of diarrhœa and constipation, though both illustrate the same detective assimilation are common in **Nux.** The diarrhœa generally comes on in the morning after rising from bed or immediately after eating some food. The urging is constant but it is more or less fruitless in that the stools are in small quantities and that they are accompanied by a longing to pass more. He constantly feels that there are more stools to be passed out. The stools are either papescent or watery, sometimes a bit frothy and sour. They are also brown, offensive and involuntary. Intense backache is felt before and during stool. This diarrhœa is the result of debauchery, abuse of alcoholic spirits, night watching and over-exertion of mind and body. In constipation the stools are large and hard but the characteristic point here, as elsewhere, is the same ineffectual desire for stool. It is not due, as in **Alumina,** to atony of the rectum but to the fitful action of the intestines. It is often seen in people who lead a sendentary life but does not like to forego the luxuries of the table.

As a result of this ineffectual urging hemorrhoids become plentiful in the **Nux vom.** patient. Prolapsus recti due to sereve pressing, tearing, smarting, itching, painful and spasmodic closing of the anus, are some of the accompanying symptoms.

Diabetes, renal colic, hematuria, cystitis, all find in **Nux vom.** a ready help. The symptoms are ineffectual urging to urination spasmodic strangury, paralysis of the bladder with dribbling of urine and involuntary urination.

Nux vomica is a powerful and oft-used remedy in sexual debility of males when due to excesses of all descriptions, such as onanism, high living, excessive venery and prolonged mental and physical exertion. It often meets the extreme condition of impotence when we have the same etiology. In gonorrhœa we think of **Nux vom** when the discharge drags on after the abuse of strong drugs like **Copaiva** and **Cubeba.**

The place of **Nux** in the therapeutics of intermittent fever is of supreme importance. It is useful for fevers of all types but specially for the tertian when the paroxysms occur in the morning hours. Here let me mention that constant chilliness, the most striking characteristic of **Nux,** forms an important indication of this remedy in the treatment of fevers. The patient is chilly in all the stages and at all times.

Even during the stage of heat when he is burning all over there is an internal sense of chill which manifests itself on the least exposure. He does not like to move or go into the open air. Cover too he cannot keep permanently for it brings on a wave of heat and an uneasy ebullition of warmth. So this stage of heat properly speaking is a combination of one and the other. It is thus a stage of alternate heat and chill.

The fever sets in towards the latter part of the night or the early hours of the morning such as 6 or 7 A.M. with violent rigor and coldness and blueness of the face and the hands.

A noteworthy feature about the onset of the **Nux** paroxysm is that it is anticipating in its nature, that is, the fever comes on a few hours earlier every day. The stage of chill is characterised by gaping, pain and numbness of the limbs and thirstlessness. The second stage or the stage of heat is the only period in which he is tormented with a great thirst. This thirst disappears during the stage of sweat but the sense of chilliness so often emphasized in **Nux** hangs on and plays hide and seek with the sweat. Gastric and bilious symptoms are almost always present.

His tongue is coated yellow or white; taste of his mouth is bitter, oftener it is so bitter that he feels like rinsing his mouth every now and then. Vertigo, headache, soreness of liver and spleen, obstinate and ineffectual constipation, loss of appetite, aversion to bread, water, coffee, tobacco, and debility are ever present.

Nux vomica is indicated in a variety of diseases of the female sexual system. If properly prescribed it meets with a whole lot of abnormalities beginning from simple nymphomania to regular prolapsus of the uterus. It causes and therefore cures a great excitement of the sexual organs leading on to sexual dreams and orgasms in irritable and headstrong women. They lead an idle life and partake of rich and highly seasoned food and drink large quantities of stimulating liquors which act as a sort of fan to the fire and stimulate excessive venery and exaggerated passion. The menses are generally too early and profuse. They occur too soon and last too long. A great tendency to fainting and oversensitiveness to nervous impressions, nausea in the morning, constant chilliness, frequent palpitation and last of all great irritability of temperament are symptoms that will make a false prescription impossible as there are not many remedies that can present such a strong combination of symptoms.

During pregnancy **Nux vomica** often becomes the remedy for morning sickness. We invariably run to it and are rarely disappointed. It stops the frequent rising up of bitter sour fluid at night and nausea in the early hours of the morning. Its strong point here is the ineffectual nature of the vomiting. There is certainly a strong predominance of retching over vomiting.

We must not, on any account, neglect the action of **Nux** on the respiratory organs. It is an excellent remedy in asthma of gastric origin. Dyspnœa is marked: the breathing is short, hard and oppressed. It is due to pressure upward of the diaphragm, in consequence of accumulation of gas. The attacks are always worse after a hearty meal. Belching relieves the difficulty of breathing. It is generally worse from cold air and exercise. It is applicable also in pneumonia of drunkards. Catarrhal symptoms find preponderance over inflammatory ones. Gastric and bilious symptoms are also pronounced. It is particularly useful in those slow types of pneumonia where hepatization occurs without fever cough or any other marked symptoms. indicating lung affections.

Lastly, we will discuss its applicability in typhoid fevers. It is a remedy generally called for in the early stage of the disease. Here too, gastric symptoms predominate over cerebral. Vertigo bitter taste in the mouth, pressure in the epigastrium, constipation, sometimes diarrhœa, disturbed restless sleep, chilliness on the slightest movement, a great and a strong desire to lie down, constant headache located generally in the occiput, great aversion to food and unintelligible muttering delirium are sure indications of **Nux vomica.**

The most important point to remember in this remedy is that the patients are always worse after a disturbed sleep. They generally wake up at about 3 A. M. in the morning and find it difficult to sleep again. Ideas keep on crowding upon them till at last out of sheer exhaustion, he falls asleep again, tired and irritable.

Case 1.—A young man, twenty years of age, the son of an oil manufacturer thin and weakly, had been from his childhood subject to a spasmodic asthma, which used always to increase from the commencement of autumn until the depth of winter, and gradually decline from that period until the mild weather in spring. Every year he had grown worse and this autumn he hoped might be his last. Already the attack commenced more violently than the last year at this time. The probable issue was evident Last year, and for years past, every fall of the barometer, every south-west and more particularly north wind, every approaching fall of snow, every gale of wind, had brought on an asthmatic paroxysm lasting hours and days he would not infrequently pass the night with both hands grasping the table, exerting all his strength to draw the smallest quantity of breath, and every moment in dread of suffocation. The intervals between such fits were occupied by slighter attacks, brought on by a draught of air, the vapor from the heated oil-cakes, dust, a cold room, or smoke. He told me of these symptoms with the utmost difficulty of utterance, elevating his shoulder to draw a scanty breath, and this at a season of the year when his condition was as yet pretty tolerable. This case occurred in Hahnemann's practice at the beginning of his professional career as a homœopathic reformer The remedies which are usually recommended for asthma in allopathic pra tice had been tried in vain, a medicine was procured which could produce anxiety and diminish the easy action of the bowels. The choice fell on Nux vomica. Four grains, given twice daily, removed gradually but perceptibly, the constriction of the chest; he remained free from the spasmodic asthmatic attacks, even in the worst autumn weather, even in winter, in all winds, all storms, all states of the barometer, all humidity of the atmosphere, during his now increased domestic, manufacturing and travelling business, in the midst of the oil vapor, and that without any important change in his diet, or any change in his place of abode. He now slept comfortably at night, whereas formerly he had passed the whole night in an arm-chair, bent forward, or leaning against the wall, or coughing without intermission During this season, which had threatened to be so dangerous to him, he gained strength, agility, cheerfulness, and capacity of resisting inclement weather. He was eventually cured.

Case 2—Mrs. T., always well except previous to her first confinement, when she suffered from neuralgia of the nipples. Miscarried four months ago and was treated by a "regular" with drastic purgatives, and had constant bearing-down pains in the uterus and the rectum, causing her to scream incessantly. During the past three months has been treated liberally to opium, wine, brandy, champagne, leeches; now suffers from constant violent thirst; obstinate constipation; drinking water causes return of uterine pain; nausea, occasional vomiting; extreme emaciation; hair, formerly abundant, was now white, thin and dry; her face bore the expression of great anguish; perfectly helpless; pulse 100; febrile excitement during paroxysms of pain at night and towards morning. Nux vom. 200 every four hours was ordered and after taking it twice had a spontaneous discharge from the bowels. Patient gradually recovered.—Dr. C. Wesselhoeft.

OCIMUM CANUM.

It is also called Ocimum Sanctum. In common English it is called the Holy Basil. It is the sacred ' Toolsi ' of the Hindus and is used extensively by the Kavirajas of this country. This plant which grows to the height of 2 to 3 feet, is an aromatic plant and is looked upon by the Hindus with great reverence. There is hardly a Hindu home that is without it and a home without this plant is supposed by them to be a doomed home. Its sacred leaves are indispensable in every offering and worship. The whole of Hindu life is intimately associated with this plant and it is given an important place even after that life is extinct.

This drug was originally proved by Dr. Mure of Brazil, but since then the provings of Dr. Mure have been verified repeatedly by many physicians of note in several countries, amongst whom we may mention the names of Dr. Clarke of England and Drs. P. C. Mojumdar and Promoda Prasanna Biswas of India.

Ocimum has a specific action in diseases of the kidney, bladder and urethra. It has proved itself of incalculable value in renal colic due to calculus. The symptoms are excruciating crampy pain in the region of the kidney with violent vomiting every few minutes; the patient twists and turns in agony and wrings her hands with the intensity of the colic; urine is thick and purulent with an intolerable smell of musk; oftener it is full of brick dust sediment indicating presence of blood. These are the symptoms of an acute attack. On these symptoms alone, several cures are reported. We will quote a few interesting experiences of the late Dr. P. C. Mojumdar. He was sent for at about 4 a.m. and he found the patient, who happened to be a medical man himself, in great agony the pain which commenced from the upper part of the right kidney extended down to the pubis. Bilious and acid vomiting was a marked feature of the case. After all the routine remedies had failed Ocimum canum gave immediate relief. The second case was that of a man of 50 who sent for Dr. Mojumdar on the sixth day of the attack—the Allopathic treatment with all its injections having failed. Here too the extreme vomiting of bile and the intensity of suffering drew the doctor's attention to Ocimum canum which was prescribed in the 3x potency. The relief was speedy, the patient having passed in a very short while some uric acid calculi.

It has been also recommended in bilious remittent fevers. Dr. Biswas of Pabna who experimented with it extensively, found it an admirable remedy in those types of bilious fevers that were accompanied by slight catarrh or congestion of the bronchial tubes and a certain disturbance of the gastric functions. According to him the redness of the tongue with a slight coating in the back aphthous sores in mouth, moist mucus rales in chest, slight pain while breathing, dyspnœa, worse from lying down, loose fetid stools and great irritability of spirits are some of its indications that place it in the same footing with Bryo., Gels., especially in the treatment of autumnal fevers and asthma.

My experience with this remedy is practically nil and does not warrant any opinion. A further proving and a more extensive application are necessary.

ŒNANTHE CROCATA.

Œnanthe Crocata is also called the Water Hemlock. It belongs to the natural order of Umbelliferæ and is one of the most rankest amongst poisonous plants. It grows in damp soil and produces a fascicle of fleshy roots. Its leaves bear a strong resemblance to those of celery for which it is frequently mistaken and such mistakes are the causes of numerous cases of poisoning with this plant. It is free from disagreeable or warning taste

The symptoms of poisoning develop very rapidly and death occurs within an hour or two due apparently to heart failure. The symptoms of poisoning are at first a sensation of great heat in throat, to be followed soon after by unconsciousness with terrible convulsions. These convulsions resemble epileptic fits. Other symptoms are livid face, dilated and fixed pupils, bloody foam from mouth, stertorous breathing, complete insensibility and severe clonic convulsions. Hence it is strongly homœopathic in epilepsy It is generally indicated in nocturnal epilepsy and in epilepsy arising from sexual disorders. The fit generally comes on at night time, although its occurrence in day time is not a contra-indication. Most of the cases in which I have used it with success are those occurring in women mostly about the menstrual time and where absence of menstruation at the allotted time leads to priapism and subsequently to epileptiform convulsions. Dr. Clarke reports of a case of a young woman who never menstruated and had become almost idiotic in consequence and a sufferer from epileptiform convulsions, especially at the time when menstruation should have appeared. After various treatments had failed, **Œnanthe crocata** was administered which effectively checked the epileptic symptoms. Dr. F. H. Fish also cured a girl of epilepsy with **Œnanthe crocata.** In this particular case however, the fits had nothing to do with the menstrual period. The spasms in this remedy come in quick succession and with entire unconsciousness. The eyes are half closed; alternate redness and paleness of face, involuntary urination and defæcation, want of aura, redness and swelling of face and neck, foaming from the mouth, and tight closing of jaws and hands are important symptoms. There is also a singular noise in throat, as if being chocked. Dr. Clarke considers vomiting, tympanites and semi-priapism during attack special indications of **Œnanthe crocata.** Time of occurrence is an important item of interest in these cases. Other remedies having nocturnal epilepsy are **Artem., Ars., Aurum, Calc. carb., Cuprum,** and **Nit. acid.**

In **Artemisia,** however, the fits are brought on by violent emotion. Several convulsions come close together and then there is a long interval of rest.

In **Arsenic** prostration and restlessness are very marked. The spasms are preceded by burning heat of the whole body; at times the patient complains of a sensation of warm air streaming up along the spine into head.

Aurum almost always has a hereditary syphilitic taint underlying the patient's constitution.

In **Calc. carb.** the fits are worse during solstice.

Cuprum met. has nocturnal epilepsy and the fits occur at regular intervals. The convulsions are very violent in this remedy. They occur during dentition or from retrocession of exanthema. Coldness of hands and feet precedes the attack.

In **Nit. acid.** the fits generally occur after midnight. There is also the syphilitic substrata to be considered in **Nitric acid.**

OLEANDER.

It will be short-sighted to leave out **Oleander** in a Materia Medica written out in India, the premier country in respect of gastric affections of various degrees of fatality. This plant commonly known as the rose-laurel is an ornamental plant growing to a height of 10 to 15 ft. in various parts of Southern Europe, Arabia and Northern Africa. The drug was first proved by Hahnemann. The tincture is prepared from the fresh leaves chopped and pounded and mixed with two-thirds by their weight of alcohol. The plant is highly poisonous. It causes prostration of the nervous system, weakness of memory and forgetfulness, slowness of perception, vertigo, inflammation of stomach, diarrhœa and certain kinds of painless paralysis; hence it is curative in all these affections and we will try and study its indications in proper order.

The keynote indication of **Oleander** is found in its gastric symptoms. We notice great rolling and rumbling in the abdomen with emission of foul-smelling flatus; the stools are yellow, undigested and involuntary. The presence of the undigested particles of food taken on the previous day is very characteristic of **Oleander**. With regard to the presence of undigested particles in stools it compares well with **Antim. crud., Calc. carb., Calc. phos., China, Ferrum, Graphites, Phosphorus** and **Sulphur**.

Another symptom calling for **Oleander** is the involuntary nature of its stools. The patient imagines he is only emitting flatulence. In this respect it is similar to **Aloes**. In children and babies, we have frequent soiling of diaper simultaneously with passing of urine. The stool is apt to occur during a meal as in **Ferrum, China** and **Argentum nitricum**.

Oleander resembles **Graphites, Cicuta, Mezereum, Petroleum** and **Viola tricolor** with regard to the unhealthiness of the scalp. The whole scalp looks like a seething mass of pimples, some of them papular, some pustular—the latter discharging a kind of mattery substance, which very soon form into hard crusts. Disquamation of the epidermis, violent gnawing and itching as from lice are symptoms that have been repeatedly verified. Great sensitiveness of the skin and a tendency towards chafing are also prominent features of **Oleander**. The headache of **Oleander** is very peculiar. It is pressive and stupefying. It feels, as if a heavy weight were crushing on the head. A curious feature of this headache is its amelioration by looking sideways and crossing eyes. This oft verified symptom is valuable inasmuch as it is a rare one. On this symptom, Dr. Farrington relieved a persistent case of headache in a young lady who tried various measures and remedies unsuccessfully, till at last he was led to it by this peculiar symptom of its amelioration.

OLEUM ANIMALE.

This is rectified animal oil. This colourless or slightly yellow oily liquid was discovered in 1711 by Johann Conrad **Dippel** of Prussian-blue fame in his process of preparation of bone-black. Hence it is also called Dippel's Oil. It acts principally on the nervous system and is a medicine of great repute in certain ailments which we will discuss in this chapter. **Oleum animale** like all our other remedies has a few characteristic indications to guide us in its selection—the most important of which is the peculiar nature of its pain. It is, as in **Kali carb., Carb. animals** and **Bryo.**, a stitching pain but the stitching is associated with a burning sensation. The part feels as if it is being stitched with red hot needles. Another characteristic of the **Oleum** pain is that it shoots from behind forward. Also we have a " pulled-upward " sensation connected with some of its pains. These indications are considered very important and they have led to important cures of neuralgia of the spermatic cord and scirrhus of the breast.

Its other characteristics are to be found in its modality. We notice amelioration from rubbing, in open air, and by pressure. The aggravations usually take place after eating.

It is a remedy for migraine and in this respect it is very similar to **Gels., Ignat., Sang., Nat. mur., Spig.** and **Kali bich.** There is polyuria of perfectly clear urine accompanying these attacks. **Oleum animale** is helpful in toothache of irritable patients. It is invariably relieved by pressing the teeth together.

The mucous membranes of the buccal cavity are very relaxed. Hence these patients are constantly biting them. They can hardly eat without biting their cheek. The following are a few other indications worth remembering: Profuse accumulation of snow-white saliva in mouth **(Nux moschata)**; eructations taste like urine **(Agnus cast)**; sensation as if water were in stomach; chronic asthma nervosum for which no organic basis could be detected but which was caused by repelled foot sweat **(Sili., Sulp.)**; sour taste in mouth; twitching in lips; slow pulse **(Dig., Apocy.)**.

OLEUM JECORIS ASELLI.

Oleum jecoris is the cod-liver oil. It is a nutrient as well as a hepatic and pancreatic remedy. It is prepared from the liver of the Gadus Morrhua. It belongs to the natural order of Gadidæ It was proved by Neidhard.

I have not so far had any occasion to use this remedy, although I have prescribed this on several occasions in crude form for various scrofulous affections. Homœopathic proving also emphasises its usefulness in weakness, emaciation, anæmia, defective nutrition, particularly in children. It has been found to be useful in atrophy of infants with hot hands and head and a great tendency to catarrhs, rickets, and bone affections. It has also been found to be useful in diseases of joints in pale, thin, cachectic subjects, that is people who are tubercular and scrofulous in their temperament. Scrofulous abscesses, ulceration of glands and old abscesses in similar subjects, hectic fever, night sweats, and chronic persistent diarrhœa with marked emaciation cough and hæmoptysis, have been helped with **Jecoris.** Tabes mesenterica in pale emaciated children has also given way under its persistent use. It is thus seen to be a tubercular remedy *par excellence.*

We will now discuss a few characteristic indications. One is a very decided pain in the liver. The second is a general soreness, not only in the liver, but all over the body, such as throat, chest, abdomen, kidneys, ovaries etc. The third keynote symptom is the occurrence of palpitation of heart in association with the other symptoms. The fourth and a very important one is a great burning in palms of hands. The last characteristic symptom is yellowness of expectoration, of the leucorrhœal discharge and other secretions of the body. Even the tongue has a coating of yellow on it. The remedy needs a more extensive proving and further verification of all of its symptoms.

ONONIS.

This remedy is very little known and is still less used. But still it is being given a place in this book on account of its usefulness in certain varieties of epilepsy where aura begins in the occiput and thence spreads all over the head. This plant is also called Rest-harrow. It is indigenous to Britain and it grows in waste lands and in the borders of cultivated fields. As epilepsy is such a formidable ailment, it behoves us not to neglect anything that may be helpful in its treatment. My personal experience with this remedy is almost negligible; but a cure recorded by Cooper is worth mentioning. A labourer aged about 45 after exposure to strong sun commenced making grimaces which ultimately resulted in unconsciousness with convulsions. A few doses of **Ononis** θ removed all such symptoms and produced a permanent cure.

ONOSMODIUM.

Onosmodium is also called false Gromwell and it belongs to the natural order of Boraginaceæ. It has proved itself of great use in locomotor ataxia and in Meniere's disease and hence should be placed in the same category as **Gels., Caust., Argent. nit.** and others. Its most important symptoms are want of power of concentration and co-ordination. Concentrated relevant thoughts, logical reasoning, sane judgment, in fact any process of the mind calling for diligent application are impossible to these patients. Hence their talks are disconnected and they are irresolute.

Co-ordination is just as much at fault here as in **Gels.** They stagger, as if drunk and are constantly afraid of falling. They also lack proper ideas of distance and height. Hence they are constantly inconvenienced. Inability to focus eyes is an important symptom with these people. They want objects held at distance to be able to look at them properly. It is also a first-rate remedy for headaches, brought on by eyestrain. The feeling of tension in the eyes due to inco-ordination of occular muscles, ushers in strong headache which gives way to **Onosmod.** pretty readily.

E. S. Norton used this remedy, in its lower attenuation, with signal success, in many cases of headaches due to myopia and also in catarrh of the middle-ear that led to a similar headache with constant roaring and hissing noise in the ears.

It is a remedy for sexual impotence both in the males and in the females. This impotence is more of a psychical nature. The sexual desire is entirely lost.

A great symptom of **Onosmodium** is dryness of the throat, nose and mouth. This symptom accompanies it almost everywhere. Guided by this symptom, Yingling prescribed **Onosmodium** in a woman whose breast was only partially developed. **Onosmodium** not only removed the dryness but restored breasts to their usual size and proportion. An important modality of **Onosmodium** is aggravation of headache in the dark and by lying on back.

OOPHORINUM.

This is a sarcode prepared by the trituration of the expressed juice of the ovary of the sheep or the cow. It has been highly advocated in ailments after excision of the ovaries and in climacteric sufferings, especially those characterised by skin disorders, such as acne, prurigo etc.

In this connection I may as well speak of another sarcode **Orchitinum** which is the testicular extract. This remedy properly speaking is the predecessor of the new endo-crine doctrine of inner secretions. **Orchitinum** too has been advocated in climacteric sufferings and in premature senile decay and other disorders of the sexual system.

OPIUM.

Opium is a blackish brown substance with a peculiar unpleasant odor. Its taste is bitter. It is simply the dried milky juice so abundant in the poppy plant, that exudes from the capsule when incised. The Homœopathic preparation is made by covering the powdered opium gum with five parts by their weight of alcohol. It belongs to the natural order of Papaveraceæ. It contains at least twenty different alkaloids, the chief of which are morphine, apo-morphine, codeine, apocodeine and narcotin. Among the less important constituents of **Opium,** we should mention resine, pectine, fixed oil, wax, glucose and some coloring matters. The poisonous nature of **Opium** was known to the ancients as early as 1853 B. C. Nicander gives us the toxic effect of a " Drink prepared from the tears which exude from poppy heads." Dioscorides and Pliny also speak about **Opium.**

It is a strong poison. The symptoms produced by **Opium** poisoning vary according to the quantity of **Opium** taken. In mild dose, it produces a sort of transient exilarating effect involving the emotional side of our nature more thoroughly than the intellectual sphere. There is also an increase in the nervous excitability of the system. The patient forgets all pains and troubles of life and seems to live for the time being in a heaven of peace, quiet and contentment. Imagination runs rampant, giving rise to all sorts of pleasurable emotions to be followed by a stage of easy drowsiness. This is why we find such a lot of men getting addicted to this strong narcotic and anodyne. Loquacity, increased imaginary power, amounting at times to hallucinations, and priapism are all symptoms that occur at this stage. The symptoms of increased dosage simulates an attack of apoplexy. The pleasant drowsiness, spoken of previously, passes into complete and absolute unconsciousness. Muscular relaxation, a very red bloated turgid face, rattling stertorous breathing, contraction of pupil to a pin-point, blood-shot eyes and hot sweat on the skin are important symptoms of this stage. The patient can no longer be roused even by the most violent means. He lies motionless and senseless with eye-lids closed or partially closed. The surface of the body is bathed in profuse perspiration. The face is pale, the lips are blue, the lower jaw is dropped and the muscles are completely relaxed. Retention of urine occurs early in the history. Gradually the skin becomes more cyanosed and covered with cold clammy sweat. The pulse becomes slower and feebler, till i vanishes. The agitations and twitchings of individual groups of muscles gradually subside, betokening the dawn of complete paralysis. Respiratory movements are made at longer intervals and then finally cease, death taking place from asphyxiation. Heart's action continues for a short while even after death. The treatment in case of acute **Opium** poisoning should be directed first, to removal of unabsorped poison from the stomach; and secondly to prevention of death by coma and cessation of respiration. Autopsy reveals the vessels of the brain and the meninges to be gorged with blood. The brain substance presents numerous dark spots. Serous effusions are frequently met with in the space between the meninges and the ventricles. The lungs show signs of intense congestion and turgescence.

With these symptoms of poisoning before us, it will be easier for us to understand and appreciate the symptomatology of the drug from the homœopathic standpoint. We, as homœopaths, individualise each remedy same as we individualise each patient. To do so it is necessary to find out the strange and the peculiar characteristic of each remedy so as to be able to differentiate, discriminate and individualise. One such strange characteristic of Opium is its painlessness. On this indication we use this in diphtheria, abscesses, boils, carbuncles, malignant growths, pneumonia, typhoid, typhus and in other ailments. A short while ago, I treated a case of bloodpoisoning of which the most important indication was painlessness. She was delirious. There were huge patches of inflamed areas in different parts of her body. The fever was high and the face was intensely red almost livid. But when questioned as to how she felt, her invariable answer was "Now I am feeling a bit better." She complained of nothing, she wanted nothing—and fell into dozes of stertorous sleep.

Sleepiness is the next important feature of **Opium.** The sleep is heavy and stupid. Once he falls asleep it becomes hard to wake him up. Sometimes however a different condition is noticed. He feels sleepy but he finds it hard to fall asleep as in **Bell., Cham., Caust.** and **Coca.** The opposite condition of sleeplessness is equally characteristic of **Opium.** But it is a sleeplessness that is associated with acuteness of hearing. They hear the clocks striking, the cocks crowing, the wagons rattling on the street, the doors closing and shutting, and they wake up in the morning unrefreshed and tired.

The stertorous rattling breathing should be given the next important place. On this symptom I cured a middle-aged gentleman who was unconscious for three days and was supposed to be **suffer-ing** from cerebral apoplexy—a case that was declared absolutely hopeless. After a few doses of **Opium** the breathing became normal and he fell into a sound sleep from which he woke up perfectly conscious.

Opium presents a variety of mental states, some of which seem apparently contradictory, whereas in reality they are merely differ-ent grades of the same process. In the first place, we have extreme sensibility of all the senses. They all become atuned to a degree of perfection not to be found in any other remedy. The functions of the eyes, ears and nose become extremely acute. The faintest sounds and the lightest odors that would escape others are percep-tible to him. The brain becomes more active and the eyes glisten with terrors of the most intense mental activity. The other aspect is dulness of mind giving way to complete imbecility; at times we notice total annihilation of the mind. These different states, instead of being confusing and contradictory, rather show the need of a broad scientific and psychological attitude of mind, necessary for the study of the various phases of a truly complex machinery— the human mind.

Opium is a very useful remedy in delirium tremens. It is particularly indicated in "old sinners," who have lived a life of excess and have burnt their candles from both ends. They wear a constant look of fright and terror. They imagine, they see all kinds of animals and frightful objects and are in a state of nervous dread. They believe themselves to be criminals, mur-derers and objects of suspicion and they constantly run away from people thinking everybody is after arresting them. It is also a remedy for dementia, the result of a long-continued habit of masturbation.

Opium checks all the secretions of the body except those of the skin which is generally covered with a peculiar hot sweat. This want of secretion renders **Opium** such an admirable remedy for constipation specially of children and of corpulent good-natured women. It is not merely dryness that accounts for this constipation. It is, to a very great extent, caused by inertia of the rectum and the entire intestinal tract. Such paresis also leads to want of peristaltic action and we have total want of evacuation for days at a time. But strange to say, due to great want of sensibility, they hardly experience any inconvenience from such accumulation of fæces. The stools are hard small round black balls, like sheep-dung. They make a sound as soon as they strike the vessel. In respect of constipation **Opium** reminds us of **Chelidonium, Plumbum, Thuja, Bryonia** and **Silicea.**

It is no less a remedy for diarrhœa—a diarrhœa brought about by fear, sudden joy or other emotional disturbances. The stools are generally involuntary, black and offensive. The abdomen becomes highly tympanitic, hard, swollen and sensitive to touch. It may also be used in cholera infantum, particularly when selected remedies fail to act due to lack of vitality and when patients show signs of advancing coma and other brain symptoms.

Opium is useful in retention of urine due to excessive use of tobacco, also in nursing children after a fit of passion in nurse. It is valuable in retention due to paralysis of bladder or the sphincter in women after parturition. This is different from **Stramonium** where the absence of urine is due to suppression.

Opium is a grand remedy for typhoid or typhus when the patient gets into a state of muttering delirium with glistening of the eyes, redness of face, dullness of senses and snoring. It is also useful in profound coma when the patient cannot be roused from the stupor and the face looks puffy and red. The pupils are greatly contracted or widely dilated.

Case 1.—A Woman, aged eighteen; very stout, primipara, after cathartics, had puerperal convulsions, not ceasing after child was born; pulse 120; pallor; sunken eyes, pupils much dilated; muttering; borborygmus; comatose; spasm; throws legs and arms about; stretching legs and arms at right angles with body; trembling; pulse working rapidly; eyes turned inward and upward; head bent back, over to left; left hand and foot turned to left side; tongue quivering, coated dirty yellow; the spasm would scarcely relax when it would run into another; more than thirty having occurred, finally stopping very suddenly for ten minutes. **Op.** was given. Only three light spasms followed.—Dr. O. P. Baer.

Case 2.—Have recently corroborated an old symptom of this drug in a case of typhus abdominalis. Many slight indications for **Op.,** and most prominent among them the peculiar sopor. Gave **Op. 23m,** in water, every hour. Found at next visit that the pulse and temperature had both been much reduced, and the symptoms for which I prescribed the medicine also better, but in their place a wellknown symptom, which I accepted as an aggravation of this drug, viz., a constant complaining that the *bed was so hard.* I at once stopped the medicine, and under **Sach. lac.** had a rapid recovery.—Dr. William Jefferson Guernsey.

ORIGANUM.

Origanum is prepared from Sweet Marjoram, a plant generally used for the seasoning of food in cookery.   This medicine was proved by Dr. Cessoles.   This plant ought to be distinguished from Wild Marjoram (*Origanum vulgaris*) from which oil of thyme is made.   This remedy has a particular affinity for the female sexual organs, where it sets up great irritation and excitement.   Erotomania, unconquerable lascivious impulses, and voluptuousness are symptoms that call for **Origanum.**   The irritation is so great that in spite of every attempts she makes, she is driven to onanism and selfabuse.   All her life, emotion and impulses are centered around the sexual system.   Everything around her is suggestive of sexual phenomena and she rushes on to its gratification on the slightest pretext.   In this respect it compares well with **Calc. phos., Camph., Canth., Conium, Hyos., Lach., Phos., Plat., Pulsat.,** and **Verat.**

In **Calc. phos., Phos.,** and **Verat.,** the excitement is greatly increased before the menstrual period.

In **Canth., Hyos., Lach., Plat.,** and **Pulsat.,** the aggravation of sexual impulses, is particularly noticeable during menstruation.

Another curious symptom of **Origanum** is an impulse to run a symptom also found under **Iod.**

ORNITHOGALUM.

This is also called the Star of Bethlehem.   It belongs to the natural order of Liliaceæ.

I have never so far used this remedy and I can only say I am sorry, as much on my own account as on the account of a patient that came to me, in almost the last throes of agony of cancer of the stomach.   It has a especial affinity for gastric and other abdomnal indurations and it has been spoken of most highly in ulceration and cancer of both pylorus and cæcum.   The symptoms are a great depression of spirit, intense prostration, constant nausea coated tongue, flatus rolling in balls in the abdominal cavity from side to side, increase of pain after meals particularly when food passes through the pyloric orifice, vomiting of coffeground substance, a sensation when turning in bed as if a bag of water were falling from side to side, distention of stomach and abdomen with frequent belching up of mouthfuls of offensive flatus, amelioration by warm food and aggravation from cold drinks, coldness of the limbs before the onset of pains and restlessness on account of the creepy feeling in feet which causes the patient to be fidgety and walk about.

Some of the cures effected by Cooper on these indications are nothing short of the miraculous. The one that I want to refer to in particular, in this connection, is that of a man of about 40 who was operated on for cancer; but the operation had to be abandoned on account of numerous adhesions and cancerous tissues that could not be removed. The man was in intense agony, writhing from side to side and unable to retain any food. The tongue was coated red and there was a visible protuberance near the region of the diaphragm. **Ornith.** was given in repeated doses at reasonable intervals and the patient after bringing up quantities of dark clotted blood became quite well. The swelling subsided, strength returned and he became as well as well could be.

Another case reported by the same author was that of an old maid who suffered from severe gastric pains and vomited blood. Her other symptoms were pain in stomach, sickish feeling, a great deal of wind and " sometimes a swollen feeling across the lower chest." Here too **Ornith.** effected wonders and the patient regained sound health. A third, just as interesting as the first two, was that of an old lady of 62 who was seized with profuse vomiting of blood and who since then had been living simply of slops. Her feet and legs were swollen and she had " fluid sack " that rolled from side to side as she usually turned in bed. Here as well as in the last two cases, the effect was more surprising than what the fondest hope could desire.

If I had only thought of this remedy, I might have helped an old gentleman that came to seek relief at my hands, quite recently and who on account of my ignorance and for no fault of the system of treatment I practise, had to seek help at the hand of the surgeon, which alas brought him relief—but a relief which every patient shuns and flies from.

OSMIUM.

Osmium is a metal found in association with Platinum. Its principal action is centred on the respiratory organs where it causes distinct pain and sensitiveness. This pain and tenderness in larynx, trachea and sternum are the keynote symptoms of our remedy. The whole of the respiratory tract is irritated from one end to the other. Mucus secretions are noticed from nose and throat. The cough which is hollow and convulsive is caused by an irritation low down in chest and is associated with tearing pain all along the passage. The cough sounds, as if it is coming from an empty tube or as if caused by resonance and it shakes the whole body as it comes.

This remedy should be studied along with **Caust.** to which it is very similar.

OXALICUM ACIDUM.

Oxalic acid is both a corrosive and a true poison. If it be taken in the solid form, symptoms of corrosion are the first to appear; this, however may be avoided, by its administration in dilute solution. The taste is a strongly acid taste. In a case of poisoning the first symptoms to appear are sensations of heat in mouth, throat and stomach ultimately turning into an intense burning pain. The pain is accompanied by a sensation of constriction of the throat and a feeling of impending suffocation. Voice becomes fainter and ultimately gets completely extinguished. Persistent vomiting of coffeeground substance is invariably present. Death occurs from exhaustion. The lips, mouth and fauces become ashy-white. There is severe thirst. Persistent hiccough, violent lumbar pains shooting down into lower extremities, and urine surcharged with albumen and pus, and violent spasms of tetanic character are some of the other symptoms of poisoning.

Oxalic acid is obtained by the action of Nitric acid upon sugar and is utilized in commerce in the arts of dyeing, calico-printing and in removing stains of ink and fruits from fabrics.

It has proved itself of immense value in the hands of the homœopath. We use it in lumbago, spinal meningitis, gastrodynia.

myelitis, paralysis, vomiting of pregnancy, loss of voice and in numerous other ailments but always on proper indications. One of the keynote indications of **Oxalic acid** is that it is a leftsided remedy. Like **Lach.** it has a special affinity for the left side. Another strange peculiarity that needs mention, is that out of the whole of the left region, it makes a natural selection of the lower lobe of the left lung. Pain—sharp lancinating pain in left lung is extremely characteristic of **Oxalic acid** and it is so intense that it deprives him of breath for a few seconds. This symptom, wherever present, has repeatedly led to the selection of **Oxalic acid.** It has been prescribed with unwonted success in many cases of angina pectoris when such symptom was present.

Secondly terrible pain in the lumbar region, extending down thigh and over region of both kidneys—a symptom that has been found in almost every case of **Oxalic acid** poisoning is of as great importance as the one first mentioned. An old lady of about 55 who suffered from such a pain and who was absolutely bedridden, slightest movement causing unendurable agony, was relieved instantaneously with a few doses of **Oxalic acid** where **Bryo.** and many other remedies had failed.

The third keynote indication, is aggravation of all symptoms from the mere thought of the disease. As soon as the patient remembers about his pains, they return immediately. This is not only true of pains but of other symptoms as well. When he thinks about his urine it becomes imperative for him to urinate. Thought of stools or diarrhœa brings on an urgent desire to defecate. Such symptoms may not mean much to an Allopath who prescribes on diagnosis, but it is of incalculable value to the homœopath.

In **Oxalic acid** the pains are felt in small spots. In this respect it differs from **Picric acid** a remedy as great as **Oxalic acid** in many varieties of spinal ailments.

PÆONIA.

In ordinary language it is called the Peony. It belongs to the natural order of Ranunculaceæ. The tincture is prepared from the fresh root obtained in the spring as in other seasons the root is supposed to be inert. Although it is a remedy little known and little used, I would not like any homœopath to be altogether ignorant of **Pæonia**. Its indications, though not many are very clear-cut and precise. It is mostly useful in anal abscesses, fissures, fistulæ and boils. The leading indications are intolerable pain during and after stools and the oozing of a kind of moisture from the anus, leaving it constantly damp. Dr. Hering reports of a case of ulceration of the rectum of 18 years' standing that responded most marvellously to the action of **Pæonia**. This patient had been operated on several times, but in vain. His anus and its surroundings were purple and they were covered with thick crusts. On the verge and entrance of the rectum, there were several fissured ulcers with elevated and indurated edges. The pain was atrocious with and after each stool, preventing sleep. He had to walk nearly all night. There was constant oozing. from the fissures.

This remedy compares well with **Graph., Nit. acid, Phos., Ratanhia,** and **Silicea**.

In **Graph.** the pain is violent. The rectum feels, as if it is split with a knife; this makes it quite inconvenient for the patient to take wide steps. There are rhagades at the anus. Every stool is followed by a sensation of constriction.

Nit. acid is also a remedy for fissure of the anus, particularly when there is a feeling as if there were splinters or sticks poking at the anus. The feeling of constriction, as seen in **Graph.** is absent.

Phos. is indicated in bleeding piles. Blood flows profusely with each stool. Violent burning is experienced after stools.

Ratanhia is an excellent remedy for fissure of the anus, and is useful when there is constriction of the anus. Stools are forced with great effort and the anus aches and burns for hours after stools.

Silicea is also as good a remedy for fissure of the anus as **Pæonia**. The patient tries to force the stool but after partial expulsion it slips back again. The hæmorrhoids are intensely painful; the pain goes from the anus to the testicles. There i usually complication of fistula with piles.

Pæonia has a peculiar sensation of splinter in the skin of right great toe when touched.

It is an important remedy for nightmares and dreams of terrifying nature.

PALLADIUM.

It is a metal. In nature it is found in conjunction with platinum and gold.

It must be fully 8 years ago that I was called in to treat a respectable lady who hailed from the district of Dinajpur. She came to Calcutta for the treatment of a huge tumour of the ovary of the right side. She was over a month under the treatment of the teacher of surgery in the Campbell Medical School of Calcutta.

She was very reluctant to go on the surgical table and hence, boric compress, fomentation, douching, injections and many other auxiliary means were tried. Ultimately when all availible means were exhausted and she could not be induced to have the tumour removed by surgical means, she was handed over to the homœopath, with the assurance however, that ultimately after her curiosity had been fully satisfied, she would have to go back to them to be operated on, which was, according to their conviction, the only sensible thing to do. There was hardly any symptom except a sensation of swelling and load on the right side of the pelvis, with an occasional pain of a bearing down character which was, always relieved by pressure. She was, indeed, anæmic and suffered from periodical headaches, which of course, was not suggestive of any particular remedy. I guessed and groped in the dark, and was quite unable to arrive at any satisfactory selection of the remedy. **Mercurius, Bryo.,** and few other remedies were tried on certain stray symptoms, but nothing availed. The tumour was the size of a large orange. The patient was getting restive and impatient in spite of all my assurances, that a tumour of the size of an orange, even while disappearing, would naturally take a reason able course of time to do so. As time progressed and no appreciable improvement was visible I was induced to call in consultation the Late Dr. P. C. Mozumdar of Calcutta. After going through the whole case with me he advised to prescribe a few doses of **Palladium 6.** We were called on again after about a fortnight, when lo and behold, inspite of our utmost scrutiny, the tumour could not be detected anywhere! It was the most marvellous thing I had yet experienced. The tumour was gone—how, when and where no body knew. Science and common sense seemed dumb-founded. The teacher of surgery was sent for and even he had to acknowledge that the tumour was gone. This is how homœopathy works. When the tumour came, it did come without notice and without telling any one, and when it went it disappeared similarly. This seems to be the only rational explanation of this remarkable cure.

Now let us come back to our symptoms again, as it would not do to dismiss this remedy with the mere statement of a case, however instructive. This remedy is very rich in mental symptoms, as all remedies with uterine affections are. The most important characteristic of **Palladium** is a feeling of wounded pride. She is inclined to weep. Everything puts her out of humour; she feels that everything that has been said or done has been done on purpose to exasperate her by wounding her dignity. In this respect she is somewhat similar to **Acon, Cocc., Ignatia., Platin., Pulsat., Nux vom., Staphis.** and **Stram.** We should not find it difficult to differentiate **Pallad.** from these remedies. The sensitiveness of **Acon.,** though great, is not of the type of **Pallad.** In **Platinum,** we have the demonstrative self-exaltation and contempt for others, whereas in **Pallad,** it is self-love and an exasperated notion about the opinion of others. In **Ignat.** and in **Staphis.** there is the disposition to be offended, same as in **Pallad.,** but the other symptoms are guiding.

The headache of **Pallad.** is quite characteristic. It is felt across the top of the head, from ear to ear. The pain is like all pains of **Pallad.** *viz.,* fleeting and transient.

All symptoms are better by touch, hard pressure, and by rubbing. A few peculiar sensations of this remedy are—as if the head had grown taller, as if something terrible would happen, as if something was hanging in the throat and as if the uterus would prolapse.

———————

PAREIRA BRAVA.

Pareira brava ordinarily known as Virgin Vine or Velvet Leaf is a climbing plant and a native of West Indies and South America. It belongs to the natural order of Menispermaceæ. The most important field of action of **Pareira brava** is limited to the urinary organs. It has been proved repeatedly by many eminent men of our profession and they all have found it to be efficacious in diseases of the bladder and urinary organs. The most important symptom is a constant urging for urination but then it is not evacuated easily. Great and violent straining is necessary and even then it is ineffectual. He must get down on all fours to urinate. In his agony, he cries most bitterly and can only emit small quantities of urine by going down on his knees and pressing his head firmly on the floor. In this awkward and uneasy posture, and partially due to the exertion of straining, he breaks out into sweat and then finally urine begins to drop with frequent interruptions, accompanied by tearing burning pain all along the passage. On this symptom it has been used in renal colic, enlargement of prostate, catarrh of the bladder and nephritic colic. A strong pain in glans penis is an important indication. Black bloody foamy urine depositing a brick dust sediment of uric acid, contusive pain in renal region, severe pain in back and bladder with painful retraction of testicles, pain extending down along thigh to big toe and a strong ammoniacal smell of the urine are symptoms too clear and well defined for even a *tyro* in Homœopathy to make a mistake about.

Here is an instructive case of a man of 68 who was pretty well worn out with prostatic affection. Constant urging with entire inability to pass urine was his affliction. His feet and legs were swollen, the only possible way, he could pass urine, was by assuming the peculiar **Pareira brava** attitude mentioned beforehand. **Pareira** gave him rapid relief and removed the swellings and practically put him on his legs to reassume his business.

Chimaphila, Uva ursi, Hydrangea, Sabal ser., Ocim. c., and **Berberis** are remedies bearing great resemblance to **Pareira brava** and it would pay us to study them closely.

PARIS QUADRIFOLIA.

It is also called true love and is a native of Great Britain. It belongs to the natural order of Liliaceæ. It was originally proved by Hahnemann, Stape and others and we have many important symptoms that make it an admirable remedial agent. It has various characteristic symptoms, the most important of which is a sense of expansion felt principally in the head. The head feels as if it is badly distended or as if the skull has become too tight. Such sensations, though uncommon, are also to be seen under **Argentum nitricum, Bell., Bovista, Glon., Nux vom., Nux mos.,** and **Rananculus.** The headache of **Paris** is of spinal origin. It arises from the nape of neck and produces a feeling as if head were immensely large. Pathologically it is due to acute congestion of brain. As is natural in such cases, the headache is aggravated by close thinking. The eyes too, feel as if they are too large for their sockets and that the lids would not cover them. Another peculiar sensation in the eye is a feeling as if the eyes are being tightly drawn backward by means of a string, to the middle of the brain. This symptom has been repeatedly verified and numerous cures have been effected on it.

The next characteristic symptom is loquacity. The patient is garrulous. He jumps from subject to subject in great self-complacency and vivacity. Such talkativeness is also to be seen in **Hyoscyamus, Lachesis** and **Stramonium.**

The third important characteristic is seen in the disorder of the sense of touch. Everything feels rough to touch. This is an important landmark of **Paris.** Numbness and pricking accompany this feeling of roughness.

We notice great sensitiveness in **Paris** to offensive odors. At times this sensitiveness is so exaggerated that the patient experiences foul smell everywhere. Milk, bread, butter and every other item of food are discarded due to the imaginary foul smell of putrid meat everywhere. This can be regarded as another cardinal indication of **Paris.**

Paris has been used in affection of cerebro-spinal nerves, with pain in the nape of neck, increasing at times to great acuteness and associated with numbness, heat and heaviness. The pain, beginning in the nape of neck and shoulder, extends over the whole side and renders even the arm powerless. Moving hand and grasping anything excite pain in the occiput and nape of neck.

Any exertion of memory or intellect causes violent pain in occiput and faintness.

It is antidoted by **Coffea** and is incompatible to **Ferrum phos.**

Case.—Mrs B., aged 45 became insane and was put under Kaviraji treatment. After quite a month when the patient showed no signs of improvement, was put under homœopathic treatment. The symptoms were occasional fits, loquacity; foolish behavior at times, vertigo brought about by thinking about her son, she lost sometime ago; painfulness of whole body especially when touched; coldness of the left side of the body when the right side was hot; dislike for food as everything smelt putrid; eyes looked as if they were bulging out. **Ignatia** was tried in various potencies but proved inefficacious. **Paris** acted quite promptly and the patient was restored to absolute sanity.—Dr. Brojendra Nath Banerjee. *Calcutta Journal of Medicine.*

PASSIFLORA INCARNATA.

This remedy has not been proved sufficiently; for our knowledge of this drug we are mainly indebted to Hale. It is ordinarily called the Passion flower. It belongs to the natural order of passifloraceæ.

It has been highly applauded in ailments like convulsions, trismus, chorea and other spasmodic affections. Dr. L. Phares reports of numerous cures of tetanus with **Passiflora** both in human being and horses. He also reports of having cured a case of chorea in a girl at the age of puberty in whom the menses did not appear. Under the influence of **Passiflora** the menses showed itself and the chorea disappeared.

My experience with **Passiflora** consists in its application in insomnia. It is the most powerful agent we have to induce sleep, but it must be used in big doses. The insomnia in **Passiflora** is not due to any pain or distress but to a sort of nervous erethism. **Passiflora** by reason of its power of inducing sleep helps wonderfully in delirium tremens. Dr. D. C. Buell after having failed with other remedies to relieve symptoms of delirium tremens in an old man resorted to **Passiflora** as a sort of a last measure in teaspoonful doses. This removed his insomnia, craving for liquor and morphia habits.

Covert cured menstrual epilepsy with **Passiflora** tincture in massive doses.

The dose varies from ten drops to one dram of the tincture according to the age of the patient.

It is said that the most important indication of **Passiflora** in any case is a clean tongue; it does not work so well when the tongue is foul.

The above indications of **Passiflora,** though helpful, are not exactly what we as homœopaths, regard sufficiently homœopathic to prescribe on. Finer delineations of symptoms are wanted which with further provings and verifications will in course of time, be arrived at.

PETROLEUM.

Petroleum is the Rock or the Coal Oil. It is a colorless fluid of a peculiar smell, somewhat like that of kerosine oil and is highly inflammable in character. It was originally proved by Samuel Hahnemann. It is a highly potent remedial agent. People, working in **Petroleum** factories, are often seen to suffer from diseases of the skin. malnutrition, anæmia and dyspepsia.

It is one of our leading antipsorics and is very akin to **Graphites** in many of its indications. It is generally indicated in long-lasting wasting diseases with a particular tendency to gastric and intestinal troubles as we shall see pretty soon. Its application in skin diseases is what we intend to take up first, as that is where most of its guiding characteristics are to be found. We notice the same unhealthy condition as in **Hepar sulph., Graphites, Fluoric acid, Silicea, Mercurius, Borax, Psorinum, Calcarea carb., Ammon mur., Sanicula** and **Thuja.** Skin affections of **Petroleum** are characterised by cracks, fissures and rhagades. They are mostly moist because of an amber-colored exudation. This exudation thickens and forms yellow crusts. It chiefly affects the dorsa of hands, the interstices between the toes, and the scalp It has cured the worst variety of eczema caput, the hair gets glued together by the exudation and we have intense itching and uncanny bleeding that prevent the sores from healing. Profuse foul-smelling foot sweat, intense heat and burning on soles of feet and palms of hands, painful itching chilblains and great sensitiveness of the skin are a few of its important indications.

It boasts of a few peculiar and absurd mental symptoms-symptoms often seen in delirium and in insanity. He imagines that another person is lying in bed alongside of him or that there are two babies in the same bed, or that he has got two more legs that would not rest quiet.

Generally speaking, these patients are melancholy, sad and despondent. They feel as if death is very near and they are anxious to settle all affairs in a hurry, thinking that there is hardly any time left to arrange matters.

The headache of **Petroleum** is generally located in the occiput where a sensation of heaviness is felt as from lead. At times this headache becomes so severe as to make him pretty nearly unconscious. It seems as if everything in the brain were alive. The head feels numb like a piece of wood. They also complain of a sensation as of a cold breeze blowing on it.

These patients are subject to vertigo, which comes particularly on stooping and on rising. They feel as if they are intoxicated. Sometimes it is complicated with bilious vomiting.

In the eye, its use is confined to blepharitis marginalis. Loss of eye-lashes, fissure of canthi and scurfy and dry appearance of the skin around the eyes should be considered its leading indications.

Its action on the stomach and bowels should be studied carefully as **Petro.,** as has been mentioned before, is particularly useful in lingering, debilitating ailments affecting those organs. It is particularly useful in gastralgia where its chief indication is amelioration after eating. The pain is felt mostly when the stomach is empty. I have verified this symptom repeatedly; on the strength of this symptom a cure was effected of the most chronic and obstinate gastralgia that defied treatment for years and reduced the patient to mere skin and bone. It is a remedy *par excellence* in dyspepsia but it is a dyspepsia of the atonic type with a tendency to diarrhœa and pain and tenderness in epigastrium. Nausea and qualmishness are very characteristic of this remedy. They are particularly marked in the morning and this makes it difficult to distinguish it from **Nux vomica.** There are the same distaste for food at breakfast and the same accumulation of water in the mouth that prevent them from eating. They are almost as irritable and ugly in temperament as **Nux vom.** Diarrhœa is very often present. The stools are yellow, watery and gushing and contain particles of undigested food. It is caused by indulgence in cabbages and sour-krouts. A peculiar feature of this diarrhœa is that it comes on mostly in the day time. Canine hunger after stool, a feeling of nausea, water-brash in the morning, cold sweat, vertigo and vomiting are accompanying symptoms.

Petroleum is a good medicine for seasickness. All its ailments are aggravated or brought about by riding in carriage or sailing in ships. All its symptoms are worse before thunderstorm **(Rhododendron).**

PETROSELINUM.

In common language it is known as the Parsley. It is cultivated very frequently as pot herbs in many countries, although it is mostly indigenous to the southern parts of Europe. Our medicine is prepared from the whole plant, collected when it is fresh. The juice is extracted and mixed with an equal part, by weight, of alcohol. It belongs to the natural order of Umbelliferæ.

It enjoys amongst us a great reputation as being an effective remedy in the treatment of gonorrhœa, but as we have said again and again this reputation depends solely upon its indications, and the most important indication for this remedy is the sudden urging to urinate which, if not gratified, will at once produce severe pain in the fossa navicularis. This urging is caused by tingling and titillation. Very frequently this grows so intense as to amount to real itching. This itching is so severe that the patient wants to thrust something in the urethra to scratch. This last symptom is quite characteristic. I remember to have cured a very persistent case of gonorrhœa with **Petroselinum** and I was led to its choice by the symptom of intense itching in the urethra. The patient said he felt like tearing it to pieces.

We find this sudden urging also in **Merc., Canth.** and **Cannabis ind.** but they can very easily be distinguished from one another.

In **Mercurius** the inflammatory infiltrations of the prostate and the adjoining parts are present. The chordee is not as violent as in **Canth.** The discharges are purulent, bloody and corrosive, sometimes greenish-yellow. The aggravations too are at night.

There is much burning, but it is during micturition; painful swelling of the lymphatic vessels along the penis and **prepuce is always** present.

Cantharides is needed very much in the acute stage of gonorrhœa. It produces much sexual excitement with unceasing painful erections. There is a violent urging to urination with inability to void more than a few drops, which scalds and burns but mostly before, during and after micturition.

Cannabis ind. is much used in the acute stage of gonorrhœa. Hartman favours the application of the mother tincture. " I continue it three times a day till the pain is entirely gone " he says. The chordee is quite well marked. Burning, scalding and stinging pains before, during and after micturition are very prominent. We find much priapism and nymphomania under this remedy.

The treatment of gonorrhœa is an exceedingly troublesome affair, for the patient soon gets restive and the doctor also is perplexed by the uniformity of the symptoms, but on the whole the symptomatic treatment far excels than other method of treatment which consists in a vigorous cauterization of the urethral canal with Nitrate of silver and Zinc and the administration of large doses of Copaiva and Cubebs, inasmuch as these last-mentioned ways of patching-up of a complex disease simply bring about a series of complications in their train. In treating cases of gonorrhœa we should be very careful about the patient's mode of living. There are certain rules which if observed, will greatly facilitate his cure and alleviate his sufferings. He may take gentle exercise; but should avoid all severe exertions. He should wear from the start a good suspensory bandage to prevent orchitis. He should avoid fatty food, meat, spices, coffea, wine and other intoxicating beverages. Light supper taken in good time will prevent nocturnal erections. The penis should be washed frequently with warm water to prevent balanitis and phimosis. The patient should frequently drink cold water to prevent the urine from getting too concentrated.

Sometimes the physician is sent for in a hurry to attend to a small child jumping up and down with pain and screaming. On inquiry as to the cause of the child's suffering he is informed that the poor thing is unable to pass urine. What to do in such cases? A single dose of **Petroselinum** will relieve all his sufferings and earn for the doctor the gratitude of the whole family.

We think of **Petroselinum** in fevers when it is complicated with chronic urethritis or strictures, but only when the symptoms call for it.

There is a thing called hemeralopia or night blindness. The patient can see very well during the day but at night he cannot see at all. **Petroselinum** is a remedy in such conditions. The other remedies to be thought of in a similar condition are **Bell., China, Hyos., Lycop., Phos., Verat.,** and **Nit. acid.**

PHELLANDRIUM.

This remedy prepared from fine-leaved water-hemlock was proved by Nenning. Although rarely used and very little known, it has a few striking symptoms and that is why I feel, it should have a place in this volume.

The symptom above all others that I would like every homœo-path to remember is that it is a right-sided remedy and that it has got special affinity for the female mammæ, specially the right one. The nipples pain each time the child is put to the breast. The pain shoots inward and backward to the shoulder and to the sacrum. Immediately after nursing she experiences intolerable pain in the right breast along the course of the lactiferous tubes, causing physical and mental distress, so that she loses her strength and is seized with fits of hysterical weeping. This is a very valuable information and will be of great use to us when we come across mothers complaining bitterly of pain each time they nurse their babies. As medical men we must be equal to all emergencies. It will be our duty to relieve suffering whenever possible.

Another indication worth remembering is that it removes abnormal sleepiness in women after child-birth. Usher reports of such a cure with **Phellandrium** in a woman, who would go off to sleep standing over her wash-tub.

It is also very useful in the treatment of bronchitis and phthisis. We notice continuous cough for hours in the morning accompanied by dyspnœa and prostration. Coarse rales are present and they compel the patient to remain in a sitting posture. It relieves the cough even in the last stage of consumption when cavity has formed in the lungs and when œdema of the extremities, copious diarrhœa, difficult respiration and profuse sweat have started as heralds of the inevitable end.

PHOSPHORIC ACID.

Here we have a remedy that deserves mention by reason of its overwhelming importance in diseases characterised by great listlessness, apathy and indifference. This is in my opinion the red-strand of this drug. On this important indication it has been known to have helped cases of chronic diarrhœa, spermatorrhœa, impotence, hysteria, ague and typhoid fever of the worst type. This listlessness also characterises the mental attitude of the patient. Great depression of the sensorium, sadness, grief, incapacity for thought and weakness of memory are prominent points about him.

A second important trait of the remedy is seen in the constitution of the patient. It is generally suited to persons of weak health—persons whose constitutions have been debilitated by loss of vital fluids. Young lives giving full promise of brilliant careers, are often wrecked on the sad shoals of such bad habits, as masturbation and sexual excesses. Their nervous system, originally strong, gives way to the continual drain upon it and we have broken-down, stoop-shouldered, slender, shy almost maidenly coy youths to deal with. These are admirable subjects for **Acid phos.** They tremble in all their limbs at all times. While walking they make mis-steps and stumble easily. Great disinclination for business, utter indifference to affairs of life, constant fainting fits from the slightest cause and total apathy—symptoms betraying absolute neurasthenia—are symptoms to be encountered in **Acid phos.** It thus requires to be studied side by side with **China.** It is very useful in ailments brought about by care, chagrin, grief, sorrow and home-sickness.

As may be naturally expected, we find great perversion of the sexual system. This is where they suffer most. Nightly polutions, sometimes several in one night, devitalise our patient. Impotence is the natural sequence but it is not the total and complete impotence of **Selenium.** The sensibility of the part is still there; erections happen but they are weak and inefficient. To make matters worse they are also troubled with a constant desire to urinate. The urine passed is larger in quantity than usual and is intensely debilitating. At times it is intensely chalky and is cramped full with phosphatic deposits. Due to great thickness of the urine, the flow is interrupted; it stops and flows again. Stringy, jelly-like masses, at times looking like curdled milk or cheesy substance, block the passage. The smell of the urine is none too pleasant. It emits an odor of raw meat. During night he has to get up several times to pass large quantities of urine. This breaks his rest and further accelerates his downward progress. All considered, we do not feel surprised that our patient is so gloomy and takes such despondent view of life.

As is to be expected, these people suffer from a sort of stupefying confusing headache. It is particularly to be thought of in headaches of young girls and students, who grow too fast and who suffer from weak legs. It is mostly occipital. It may also be in the nape of neck and is caused by exhaustion of nerve power or is due to shocks caused by grief, sorrow and chagrin.

Phosphoric acid should particularly be remembered in chest affections of lean, thin, debilitated subjects. The cough which is slight to begin with, is caused by a sensation of tickling low down in the chest, in the region of the ensiform cartilage. A great feeling of weakness is complained of in the chest and it is aggravated by talking and coughing. There is very little expectoration particularly in the evening. The slightest talk brings on dyspnœa. Hoarseness and roughness in throat also accompany this cough. **Phosphoric acid,** if prescribed on these indications, will not only relieve the cough but correct the constitutional weakness of the patient.

We will next discuss the action of **Phosphoric acid** on the bones. Here also the same scrofulous tendency is to be noticed. It is particularly applicable in hip diseases, caries of the vertebra and curvature of the spine. Periosteal and interstitial inflammation of the bones respond readily to the curative influence of **Phosphoric acid.**

Phosphoric acid has strong action over the kidneys as is to be guessed from its tendency to cause polyuria or copious urination. It is an excellent remedy for Bright's diseases and diabetes mellitus. Insatiable thirst and great desire for effervescing liquids, high specific gravity, great muscular weakness, torpor, prostration, sleeplessness and emaciation are important landmarks of this remedy.

In typhoid and typhus the main indication of **Phosphoric acid** consists in a great depression of the vital force. The apathy and indifference, as has been mentioned before, are overwhelming; he takes no notice whatsoever of his surroundings. He desires nothing, asks for nothing; he does not mind even when pinched Question him however much you like no response will be forthcoming. It is so difficult to rouse his slumbering vitality. When however he does answer, we notice want of coherence as of a man slumbering or one much confused. What could be more convincing of his sinking vitality and critical condition than his looks? Sunken eyes, pointed nose, dark blue rings round the eyes, crusty lips, sordes on teeth, fetor oris, glassy and half-closed eyes, indicate the low ebb of his life. He constantly bores his fingers into his nose. His abdomen is distended and bloated. Involuntary defecation containing masses of undigested food, petechia, ecchymosis, decubitus and finally urine loaded with earthy phosphates and albumen, speak of unmistakable signs of disintegration. The nearest remedies here are **Rhus tox, Phosphorus, Arnica, Opium, Baptisia** and **Pyrogen.**

PHOSPHORUS.

Phosphorus, the element is a solid body of the appearance and consistency of white wax. On exposure to air, it gives off white fumes; it is luminous in the dark and is of a disagreeable garlicky odor. It is insoluble in water but dissolves in absolute alcohol at 15°C, ether and fatty oil. It should be kept carefully under water, in a secure and moderately cool place, protected from light or else there is danger of fire.

It is a great local irritant. Even the fumes of **Phosphorus** may inflame exposed mucous membranes, such as the conjunctiva and the mucous membrane of the mouth and the respiratory tract. It has very strong action over the bones and periosteums, particularly the jaw bones where it causes processes of necrosis to take place Taken internally, even in therapeutic doses, it is apt to irritate the stomach, as is shown by loss of appetite, nausea, uneasiness, symptoms of vomiting and diarrhœa. Therapeutically it produces increased activity in the development of bones. Cartilaginous epiphyses ossify with undue speed and completeness; spongy bone tissues increase in thickness and grow compact and hard. On the nervous system also, it sets up morbid derangements of nerve functions and thus, under the principle of Similia Similibus Curantur, rectifies malnutrition and exhaustion of nerve tissues. It is thus a great nerve nutrient.

Under the allopathic system of therapeutics, it is administered on general surmise, for the betterment of the deranged conditions of the nervous and the bony structures. Homœopaths, however, dispense with all surmises and put its application on a more scientific basis, taking into calculation the minutest deviations it causes, when administered to healthy human being and thus measure its capacity for doing good as well as harm in the minutest degree possible. It is no wonder, therefore, in Homœopathy, based as it is on Nature's immutable law of Similars its application is frought with innumerable blessings to the ailing humanity unsullied by any damage or deterioration to the constitution of the patient.

It is generally adaptable to tall, slender persons of sanguine temperament and to young people who grow too rapidly, and are inclined to stoop and show a great tendency to phthisical ailments These are just the kind of people that run into consumption, unless due care is taken and their constitution set right by the timely administration of such constitutional remedies as **Phosphorus, Calcarea carb., Silicea** etc., determined according to the principle of Similia Similibus Curantur. The **Phosphorus** constitution is, at all times, a frail constitution. They are born, as it were, with the stigma of scrofulosis in them. Too rapid a growth is never a normal affair. Nature does not approve of too hasty cell-proliferation in any of its departments. Such abnormality generally means premature decay and extinction. Administered at the proper time and at the proper potency, **Phosphorus** puts a sort of a check on such abnormal working of nature and rectifies the gradually growing anæmia and malnutrition of the patient. **Phosphorus** patients are, as a rule, extremely susceptible to external impressions. Lights, sounds and odors influence their life to a great extent. They are particularly sensitive to electrical changes and thunderstorms. Mentally they are excitable and impressionable and in consequence they easily get into temper. Anxiety, fear and dread are constantly present. The opposite condition of apathy is no less marked. They are indifferent to everything; their home, children and family hold no interest for them.

Phosphorus has a sort of mania that is of particular interest to us Great loquacity and vehemence characterize **Phosphorus** in its delirium. The patient talks on incessantly and uninterruptedly. It may have its origin in sexual erethism or it may be simply the pure flow of idea, due to excessive stimulation of certain cranial centers. Amativeness and shamelessness are as characteristic of **Phosphorus**

as they are of **Hyoscyamus.** She uncovers herself and wishes to go naked as if insane. She lifts up her clothes and kisses hotly all who come near her. She accuses herself of the most obscene action, of which she was never guilty and bursts out simultaneously into hysterical laughing and crying spells. Then again, it is a great remedy for mania of grandeur. Like **Sulphur,** she imagines herself as being a person of regal importance and feels herself surrounded by all sorts of grand objects. She feels incited to take a commanding aspect of things and to treat everybody around her haughtily, as in **Platinum.** It is also used for the bad effects of chronic alcoholism, such as, great mental and physical exhaustion, trembling of limbs, paralysis, idiocy and maniacal attacks of fury and violence.

Now about a few keynote symptoms of **Phosphorus.** The most important one is burning It is felt in spots all along the spine but specially in the region between the scapulae. We notice intense heat and burning in palms of hands, chest, lungs and other organs and tissues of the body.

The second feature worth noticing is a great weak empty all-gone sensation in different parts of the body, such as the head, chest, stomach, abdomen, etc.

The next characteristic point is great weakness and prostration attended with nervous trembling.

Cravings and desires of **Phosphorus** deserve the next place. He wants cold refreshing drinks, such as icecream and lemonade. He feels better after drinking such cooling things but the relief is only fleeting and short-lived as they are vomited out as soon as they get warm inside the stomach.

Phosphorus is a splendid remedy in gastritis, chronic catarrh of the stomach, ulceration of the stomach and even in cancer of stomach when the following symptoms are present:—Pressure in the pit of stomach as from a hard substance; burning cutting pain n stomach relieved by cold drinks; vomiting of acid and bitter mucus, of bile and of blood; regurgitation of ingesta in mouthful; excessive flatulence with frequent palpitation of the heart; earthy color of the face, great weakness and loud borborygmi.

We think of it also in cirrhosis of the liver due to excessive indulgence in strong liquors. Waxy liver, fatty degeneration of the liver with malignant jaundice, also come within its scope. Let us now discuss diarrhœa of **Phosphorus.** Stools pour out of rectum in profusion like water from a hydrant, immediately after eating and drinking. The anus is wide open and there is

a constant oozing of fetid painless watery stool from this open
passage.   The stools may be bloody and purulent or like the
washings of meat and contain undigested food, but the one mostly
seen in **Phosphorus** is a stool that is full of tallow-like pieces that
resemble little particles of sago.   In this respect we should compare this with **Cina** and **Colchicum.**   This diarrhœa is very
debilitating and is worse in the morning.   It is a remedy par
excellence in chronic diarrhœa of nervous and delicate children.

From what has been said let us not think that it is only useful in diarrhœa ; we think of it in its own peculiar type of constipation when the stools are slender, narrow and hard like those
of a dog.   An apt expression for it is ' pipe-stem' stool.

Phosphorus is a great hemorrhagic remedy.   The blood is
very fluid and takes long time to coagulate.   The bleeding is very
profuse and frequent.   When it flows it flows freely and then
ceases for a time.   This hemorrage may come from any part of th.
body.   The hemorrhage of **Phosphorus** is often associated with
Bright's disease.

Now this question of hemorrhage brings to mind the utility
of **Phosphorus** in diseases of the chest, such as bronchitis, pneumonia and tuberculosis; we will take up this discussion just now.
It is an oft-used remedy in bronchitis of tall slender persons.
The fever is high, the pulse is rapid and the patient lies on his
back, breathing fast, the respiration being chiefly abdominal.   He
complains of great tightness across the chest and each act of
coughing is accompanied by tearing pain under the sternum as
if something were torn loose.   Oppression of chest is excessive
Anguish, anxiety and heat in chest are very troublesome
Stitches in various parts of the chest, accompanying each act of
inspiration, make life intolerable.   The cough is constant but i
is aggravated in the evening and this aggravation lasts till mid
night.   It is worse from laughing, reading, talking, drinking
eating, lying on the left side and going from warm to cold air.

When neglect and indiscretion lead these cases on to wha
we call broncho-pneumonia **Phosphorus** may still be our remed
All the above symptoms are more accentuated.   The sense
tightness, the feeling of excoriation in the chest, the dryness
the air passages become more tormenting.   **Phosphorus** affec
principally the right lung specially its lower half, where a du
sound is noticed on percussion.   An important hint, that we w
do well to remember, is that it is rarely indicated in the sta

of hepatization. We think of it mostly when the bronchial symptoms are prominent.

Phosphorus also deserves mention in the treatment of typho-pneumonia. It is our remedy when the lungs become stagnant from extravasation of fluid blood from the veins causing extreme dyspnœa, cold clammy sweat, thready scarcely perceptible pulse, wing-like motion of the alæ nasi and hippocratic distention of face. The sputa is rust-colored and is expectorated with difficulty.

Finally let us take up its indication in tuberculosis of the lungs. Extreme cachectic appearance, hoarseness, aphonia, hemoptysis, and salty purulent expectoration are important symptoms. He feels hungry in the dead of night; must get up and eat something or else he faints right away. He also complains of an empty feeling in the pit of the stomach particularly in the forenoon at about 10 to 11 A.M. The roof of the mouth and tongue is covered with aphthous sores; diarrhœa is common, the odor being like that of lime.

We will now study the action of **Phosphorus** on the bones. It has a special affinity for the lower jaw and we use it extensively in necrosis of that bone. The workers in match factories are commonly seen to suffer from this disease.

It is also useful in caries of the vertebra of scrofulous children. The caries may extend to the cord itself and produce extensive inflammation there.

We use it in rachitis, exostosis of the skull and hipjoint diseases. In this connection we will discuss the indications of a few other similar remedies.

Angustura has exostosis and necrosis of lower jaw. It thus bears great semblance to **Phosphorus** but the tendency in this remedy is for the carious process to pierce the bone and affect the marrow.

Asafœtida is useful in syphilitic affections of the long bones specially those of the legs. The characteristic offensive odor, excessive sensitiveness and a great tendency towards bleeding are present.

Aurum met., the king of such remedies, is thought of in mercuro-syphilitic affections of the mastoid process, nasal bones and the skull.

Manganum aceticum is inferior to none in respect of the great sensitiveness of the bones to touch. The inflammatory affections in this remedy are specially located in the ankles.

Phosphorus is valuable in abscesses of the lymphatic glands specially when they become full of fistulæ and in other phlegmonous inflammations where the hectic ulcers keep on throwing out fetid pus and blood.

Phosphorus is very useful for fatty degeneration of the heart. The symptoms are: palpitation, puffiness of the face particularly under the eyes, and a general aggravation of all symptoms after sleeping. It particularly affects the right side of the heart in preference to the left.

Phosphorus is a valuable remedy in many affections of the eyes, such as amaurosis, momentary blindness, amblyopia, retinitis, glaucoma and hyperemia of the choroid coat. The patient sees all kinds of colours, flashes of light-green halo around candles and black spots and a veil of mist within the field of vision. It also rectifies abnormality in the function of the optic nerve. The patient sees all sorts of abnormal colours, black spots in the air and a sort of a dull veil over things as though he is looking through a mist or fog. Another symptom which it has rectified repeatedly is vision of red color. Every object looked at seems red. Even letters appear red when reading. Like **Silicea, Baryta carb., Conium** and **Calcarea carb.,** it also retards the growth of cataract.

PHYSOSTIGMA.

It is also called the Calabar Bean, a climbing plant indigenous to Africa. It belonges to the natural order of Leguminosæ. The alcoholic tincture is prepared from finely pulverized Bean. It contains an alkaloid called Eserine. It stimulates heart's action and causes increased peristalsis. It also causes contraction of the pupil.

Physostigma is a noted remedy for various affections of the eyes which it is our object to discuss just now. It causes a great contraction of the ciliary muscles and thus induces a kind of short-sightedness. A noted symptom is spasm and twitching of the ciliary ocular muscles. Hence it is very useful in myopia, resulting from ciliary spasm. It is also useful in night blindness and glaucoma. It relieves intra-ocular tension by acting upon muscular tissues of vessels. It is particularly useful when iridectomy has to be postponed for some reason or when tension increases after iridectomy or in some cases of secondary glaucoma. It replaces the prolapsed eyes and is useful even in muscular asthenopia. Dudgeon relates a case of injury to left eyeball by the cork of a soda water bottle causing intense pain, effusion and extremely myopic vision which he rectified with **Physostigma** after other remedies had failed.

Physostigma causes and hence cures muscular weakness and paralysis with tremor. It has been used in myelitis with signal success. Its indications are tremor, staggering gait, and a feeling of weakness passing down from occiput through back to lower extremities. It is also useful in progressive muscular atrophy and general paralysis of the insane.

In the heart we have extreme fluttering, felt sometime in the throat. The palpitation is so severe that beats of the heart become perceptible in the head and the chest. Another important symptom is a great sore feeling at the tip of the tongue.

PHYTOLACCA DECANDRA.

This is also called the Virginian Poke. It is indigenous to North America, Africa, South of Europe and China. It grows in damp places. The fresh root is chopped and pounded to a pulp; from this is made the alcoholic tincture. It belongs to the natural order of Phytolaccaceæ.

It is pre-eminently a glandular remedy. It also powerfully affects the fibrous, the osseous tissues and sheathes and fascias of muscles. Hence it becomes an admirable remedy in rheumatic affections. It helps even when there is a syphilitic taint underlying the rheumatism. There is a general soreness over the whole body and the patient moans and groans every time he moves. It should thus be classed with remedies like **Rhus tox.** and **Bryonia.** But it is more deep-seated in its action than the two remedies named above. It further combines with the pain, intense prostration and great exhaustion. The lassitude that accompanies rheumatism makes him lie down every now and then. The rheumatic pain of **Phytolacca** has a tendency to affect the outer aspect of limbs. It has been used with remarkable success in sciatica and hipjoint disease on this symptom of the pain shooting from sacrum down the outer aspect of thighs to knees and toes. The pain occurs in such quick succession that it renders the leg powerless numb and heavy. It has a special affinity for muscles of the shoulders and arms. The pain like that of **Kalmia** repeatedly shifts its location. It flies from place to place. Lameness, soreness and a bruised feeling are felt all over the body. Each movement elicits groans.

Phytolacca vies with **Lachesis, Lycopodium** and **Mercurius** in the treatment of diphtheria. The tonsils, uvula and in fact the whole fauces become swollen and dark red. Dryness, roughness and burning of throat are intense. It feels like a piece of red hot iron lodged in the throat. The whole place burns like fire. Deglutition becomes painful and difficult. Each attempt at swallowing causes excruciating pain to shoot into the ear. Uvula becomes large and looks translucent. He also experiences great pain at the root of the tongue when swallowing. Hot drinks are aggravating. We notice a great disposition to hawk and clear throat which, however, does not afford him much relief. Regurgitation of food through nostrils proves the passage to be wholly or partially blocked. The irritation extends from posterior fauces into Eustachian tube. The tongue is thickly coated at back and fiery red at tip. It becomes fetid and putrid. The diphtheritic membrane and the exudations are generally ash-colored; sometimes they have a sort of a pearly white appearance. The patient hawks up ropy offensive mucus. The glands of the neck become swollen and tender. A great soreness and a bruised feeling of the entire body associated with intense prostration. high fever and rapid pulse indicate **Phytolacca.**

It is also serviceable in less serious complaints such as, follicular pharyngitis, chronic sore throat and ordinary glossitis and quinsy. The symptoms are a distressing sensation of enlargement of the caliber of the pharynx and the œsophagus, profuse salivation, difficult and painful deglutition, ulceration of the tonsils and great prostration and low-spiritedness. The feeling of burning is quite prominent. Even tongue feels scalded.

Now we come to its action on the glandular tissue—a very important chapter in **Phytolacca.** It is an excellent remedy for mastitis caused by excessive accumulation of milk in nursing mothers. We notice a tendency towards caking from the very start. The hardness is excessive and every time the child nurses the pain goes from the nipple to other parts of the body. **Phytolacca** is specially thought of in cases of threatened suppuration of the breast. The mammæ become hot, painful and swollen. Our friends of the other school, in such instances advocate the use of the breast-pump and the application of a plaster of Belladonna and finally the application of the knife. Time and again, have I seen mutilated breasts, full of fistulous ulcerations in women, who have grown reconciled to a continuous running discharge, as nothing has been found helpful, respond to the action of **Phytolacca.** It is a wonderful remedy in the above condition. It has been found helpful even in caked breasts that have been pronounced cancerous. The nipples look cracked and excoriated. Nodules, hard and painful, felt under the skin, respond to its action and disappear under the action of **Phytolacca.**

A comparison with **Bryonia,** another noted remedy, will not be out of place. It is generally a remedy for an earlier stage when the heat, hardness and pain are not sufficiently pronounced to warrant the application of **Bellad.** The pains of **Bryonia** are sharp and stitching. **Phytolacca** on the other hand is useful either in the cold stage or when suppuration has been threatening or even when suppuration has been complete with deep eating fistulous passages weaving their way in and out through the soft glandular structures of the breast, and discharging a continuous flow of sanius ichorous pus.

The headache of **Phytolacca** is peculiar and should therefore be particularly remembered; it is accompanied with increased sense of hearing.

One more symptom of **Phytolacca** that has been of great help to practitioners is an irresistible inclination to bite the teeth and gums together or bite at anything handy. On this symptom Dr. **Nash** cured a case of persistent diarrhœa during dentition in an **emaciated** little baby.

PICRIC ACID.

Picric acid is a great explosive and like all explosives it combines great energy and potentiality within a small volume. In the material world it is utilized in accomplishing difficult feats, as the blasting of big rocks and other tasks, requiring great use of force and violence. It is no wonder then that such an agent should be employed as medicine to accomplish the much more useful tasks of regulating the deviation of the diseased vital force.

Picric acid exists as bright yellow glistening crystals. It has no odour, but it has a very bitter taste. The crystals are soluble in boiling water and alcohol and in the commercial world it is utilized as a dye to color wool, silk and other animal tissues.

We get **Picric acid** by the action of **Nitric acid** on such organic substances as indigo, silk, etc. But it is generally prepared by gradually adding **Carbolic acid** to strong **Nitric acid,** and then boiling the compound. The yellow crystals found at the bottom of this mixture after cooling are the **Picric acid** crystals. Then one part by weight of this pure **Picric acid** is dissolved in ninety-nine parts by weight of distilled water and we get our first centesimal potency.

The first and the foremost use we think of making of **Picric acid** is in the case of individuals who suffer from great debility, weakness, languor and exhaustion. This prostration is continually on the increase. From a mere fatigue and tired feeling it may amount to real paralysis. At first it manifests itself by headache, vertigo and burning sensation of the spine. The least mental or physical exertion brings on these attacks. As a consequence the patient is disinclined to do work of any kind. He has a rooted disinclination to exertion of any kind. There are other remedies such as **Arsenic, China, Con., Calc., Gels., Iod., Nat. carb., Phos., Phos. ac., Sel.,** and **Sulphur** wherein we find a similar prostration but they are each and every one of them different from each other.

In **Arsenic** the prostration, which is much greater than in **Pic. acid** and of a different sort altogether, is due to organic involvement and our patient is in a real critical condition, whereas in **Pic. acid** it is of a sort of gradual and wholesale decline of vitality which is more of the nature of enervation.

Our **China** patient is very poor in blood and his weakness is due to a great loss of the vital fluid in the shape of seminal emissions, hæmorrhages, diarrhœa and profuse perspiration. It is the remedy for the ill effects arising out of these conditions.

In **Calc. ost.**, the patient exhibits great weakness but this is mostly perceived after an act of coition. Every embrace causes languor, trembling of the extremities, weariness and headache. This exhaustion is felt more in the morning.

Conium combines muscular prostration with nervous exhaustion. The weakness is accompained by trembling. The patient is so weak that he feels exhausted and faints after a short walk. This is to be accounted for by such pernicious habits as masturbation and prolonged attacks of zymotic diseases.

The pot-bellied **Sulphur** and the emaciated **Iod.** complain of exhaustion more during hunger and it disappears when the hunger is satisfied.

Our **Selenium** patient, as a result of indulgence in sexual excesses and venery, suffers from great weakness of the sexual system. Dribbling of prostatic fluid at stool and of semen during sleep is characteristic of **Selenium.** Like the **Natrum carb.** patient he gets particularly exhausted from exposure to the heat of the sun.

Last of all we come to **Phos.** and **Acid phos.** These two remedies go hand in hand in all nervous affections and they resemble **Pic. acid** more closely than any that we have yet mentioned. The weakness and trembling, the burning and the clouding of the sexual atmosphere, speak of the great resemblance in the three remedies.

Phos. acid is the most adynamic of the three remedies. The apathy, the indifference, the listlessness of this drug can hardly be equalled. It is applicable in the chronic effects of many exhausting ailment.

With the weakness **Phosphorus** combines great irritability as shown by its sensitiveness to all external impressions.

The fagged condition of the brain may, if neglected, lead to a more critical state, viz., the softening of the brain. This may induce paralysis according to the region involved. We have watched animals poisoned with this acid. The first symptom to manifest itself is a weakening of the muscular system; this weakness gradually develops into paralysis, especially of the hind legs. Autopsies revealed a general softening of the brain and the spinal cord. Such pathological observations prove beyond doubt that **Picric acid** can be a very powerful agent in the above conditions; but the symptoms are a surer guide to the choice of the remedy indicating it in spinal and cerebral softening. During the first stage the patient complains of intense headache from the least mental exertion. He keeps his legs wide apart when standing and he looks at objects so steadily that it seems he is unable to make them out. His limbs become too weak to support his body and his will-power too seems to be quite suspended. In exaggerated cases we have real mental aberrations. The poor patient looks like a total imbecile, with an entire suspension of reason and memory. He sits still without taking interest in anything.

The one symptom of all symptoms from which he seems to be a constant sufferer, is headache, and it troubles him always. It is generally an occipital headache with the peculiarity of aggravation from the least overwork and excitement. This headache either extends down the back or forwards into the supraorbital foramen and thence into the eyes. It is relieved by lying flat on the back and keeping quiet and becomes worse from motion, especially going up stairs.

We cannot very well afford to lose sight of the sexual condition of the **Pic. acid** patient. The general run-down condition, so characteristic of the remedy, manifests itself in his sexual sphere. Beginning with a morbid excitement he gradually verges towards impotence. In the first stage he suffers from violent, strong and long-lasting erections. They are sometimes so hard that he fears the rupture of his penis. These erections are followed by profuse seminal emissions. With this is combined backache. His back seems to be the weakest part of his body. His lower limbs feel heavy with occasional sensations of formication and needle pricks in his legs.

A few other remedies, noted for priapism are **Canth., Caps., Can. ind., Mygale,** and **Phos.**

Oxal. acid comes very close to **Pic. acid** in its sexual debility. This patient also gets erections but these come on mostly on lying down without any cause. He also complains of pain or rather a sensation of heaviness in his occiput (but the symptoms that help differentiation are that instead of a heaviness in the lower limbs he complains of a dullness and the parts look blue). The pains are in limited areas and they grow worse when he thinks about them. **Picric acid** is highly recommended in diabetes. With the already existing exhaustion the patient combines a high-colored urine of high specific gravity. The urine is full of albumen, sugar, phosphates and uric acid crystals. His feet always cold and chilly, are covered with cold clammy sweat. We must not always run to **Camph.** and **Carbo veg.** on finding a cold limb covered with a cold sweat. The totality of the symptoms should invariably guide us in the selection of remedies.

Dr. Halbert reports of the case of a lady of about 49 years whom he cured with **Pic. acid** 6x. Her system was thoroughly broken down. She suffered from loss of appetite, copious urination, exhaustion, backache and brain-fag. The specific gravity of her urine was 1040, and she had $7\frac{1}{2}$ per cent. sugar.

Dr. Thery of Paris recommends **Pic. acid** very highly for burns of the first and the second degree. A saturated solution (90 grains of **Picric acid** to each 3 ounces of alcohol) diluted with one quart of water is advised. The burnt area is first bathed with this solution and then stripes of sterilised gauze soaked with it are applied to the parts.

Last of all we will discuss skin symptoms of this remedy. Numerous boils appear in the auditory meatus. They are small and painful. **Calc. pic.** too has a similar symptom.

The locations of boils and eruptions are always important considerations in prescribing. Hence it will not be out of place to consider the favourite sites and locations of some of our remedies. **Aconite** and **Ananth.** have boils on tips of nose. **Nat mur's** favourite site is the region over the left eye. **Lyco.** and **Phosphorus** have boils in axilla. **Petroleum** has boils on arms. **Hyoscyamus** and **Ignatia** have boils on thighs. **Silicea's** favourite sites are the calves. **Ratanhia's** choicest locations are soles of feet.

PICROTOXIN.

It is an alkaloid obtained from the seeds of Cocculus Indicus. This is extracted through the help of boiling alcohol, the concentrated solution is cooled, the fat removed, and we have **Picrotoxin**. It may be found either in the crystal or powder form. It is odorless but has a very bitter taste.

The action of **Picrotoxin** closely resembles that of strychnin. It is used generally for poisoning fish. The medicinal employment of **Picrotoxin** consists in its application to relieve night-sweats of phthisis.

J. H. Henry proved it on himself. The symptoms were nausea, intestinal pains, purging, polyuria, cramps and paralysis. I have not used this remedy and cannot therefore say much about it.

PILOCARPUS MICROPHYLLUS.

Pilocarpus is an alkaloid obtained from Jaborandi and is an important diaphoretic. It produces profuse salivation and myosis.

Its property to cause free elimination through skin and other secretive organs is utilised in relieving pressure on the kidney when that organ needs help. A case of **Pilocarpus** cited by Wood is very instructive. It was in a woman three months in pregnancy whose urine had got scanty and who was suffering from extreme nausea and vomiting. The nausea was so intense and the salivation so profuse that she was saturating six to ten handkerchiefs daily with this continuous flow of saliva from her mouth. **Mercury, Ipe., Nitric acid, Kali bi., Hydrastis** and **Actea racemosa** were all tried in succession but nothing brought any relief. In desperation he prescribed a tablet containing ¼ grain of **Pilocarpus,** dissolved in half a glass of water, to be taken a teaspoonful every 2 hours. The improvement was most marvellous and rapid. The very next day, the patient was found sitting cheerful and free from all nausea and salivation.

It is useful in ex-ophthalmic goiter with palpitation, pulsation of arteries, tremor, nervousness, heat and sweating. Its action on the gland makes it an admirable remedy in mumps. It also checks debilitating sweats after diseases.

It is a valuable remedy for eye-strain. We use it in cases where the slightest use tires the eyes. It checks vertigo and nausea when brought about by the use of electric or other artificial lights. It also leads to a contraction of the pupil to pin point. It improves distant sight.

In the ear it is curative of labyrinthine deafness. It is also curative in aural vertigo where it is associated with deafness and tinnitus.

PIPER METHYSTICUM.

It is Polynesian plant used by the natives as a stimulant. Excessive indulgence in its decoction produces a kind of skin disease resembling leprosy. The skin, particularly that of the extremities, assumes the appearance of well-marked ichthyosis, associated with a certain degree of atrophy such as is observed in senile skin. There is an absence of inflammatory symptoms.

One important keynote symptom of this remedy is to be found in the amelioration of its pains, even though for a short time, by diversion of attention as in **Orig.** Another characteristic indication is an irresistible desire to change position which gives little or no relief.

Dr. Skinner cured with this remedy a case of an intense toothache in a young girl who was almost frantic with pain except when she forgot her troubles through some amusement or excitement.

PIX LIQUIDA.

Pix liquida is liquid Pine-tar and it has been found to be of great use in phthisis and chronic bronchitis. Cases of poisoning reveal symptoms of high fever, black vomiting, black stools and dark-coloured urine. Homoeopathic provings, however, bring into prominence a pain referred to the third left costal cartilage, as it joins the rib. This symptom is regarded as a keynote symptom and when associated with expectoration of a purulent matter of offensive odor and foul taste, a great cough and a constant vomiting of blackish fluid with pain in stomach, the indication becomes a certainty.

PLANTAGO MAJOR.

This is a herb growing plentifully in Europe and America. It belongs to the natural order of Plantagiaceæ. It is also called Ribgrass and Way-bread. It is used as food for cage-birds. This is comparatively a new remedy and was first proved by Dr. F. Humphreys of the United States. This fibrous plant grows to a height of one to three feet. The leaves are broad, ovate, smooth and entire. The flowers are white, small, numerous and densely disposed on a cylindrical spike. Tincture is made from the whole plant when coming into flower. Mention is made of this plant in two such old books as **"Herbal of Dodoens"** and **"Theatre of Plants,"** which show that the plant was utilized for medicinal purposes as early as 1558. They used it mostly for bruises, cuts and injuries as also for toothache and earache. In Switzerland they cure toothache by inserting the green threadlike fibres of its leaves into the ears. It is said that where it cures, the fibres turn black needing renewal of the same process, and where it does not they remain green.

The fact that has earned for this remedy an ever-lasting renown, is its efficacy in curing odontalgia and otalgia. The simultaneous existence of toothache and earache and the presence of salivation during an attack of toothache are two very important indications of **Plantago** and they are never known to have failed. The toothache which is of a boring, digging nature, is aggravated by walking in the cold air and by contact. Sometimes the tooth feels elongated. Dr. Reutlinger says that he cured about seven-tenths of the cases of odontalgia that came under his treatment with this remedy and that in about 15 minutes. Drs. Humphreys, Hale and Clarke too, express similar opinions about its efficacy. I also can remember instances from my own practice where **Plantago** rendered very useful service in toothache.

Plantago is also serviceable in neuralgia. It may be in the teeth, ear, nose and face, but most often in the last place. The pain which is of an erratic nature shoots into the temporal, maxillary, and orbital regions. Dr. Clarke recommends the local application of the tincture as also its internal administration. Dr. F. P. Stiles cites a few brilliant cures of neuralgia with this remedy. In each of these cases he applied the tincture locally with the most gratifying results.

We use **Plantago** in nocturnal enuresis of children. In this connection I will quote the remarks of Dr. E. W. Jones.

" It is especially applicable to the nocturnal enuresis of children, particularly when depending on laxity of sphincter vesicæ. In most of these cases the children secrete a large quantity of pale, watery urine, and though great pains are taken to have the bladder thoroughly emptied before retiring, yet the pressure on the weak sphincter will cause its escape before morning. It is of no use when enuresis is due to paralysis of the sphincter."

It will be as well to have a short review of the action of **Bell., Caust., Chloral., Kreo., Lac can., Senega** and **Sepia** in respect to symptoms of enuresis.

Belladonna is invaluable in involuntary micturition where enuresis takes place during deep sleep, generally after midnight and towards morning.

In **Causticum** the enuresis is due to real paralysis or paralytic weakness of the sphincter. The most important feature is that it takes place in the first part of sleep. The trouble is much aggravated in winter.

Chloral is useful where the child persistently wets his bed every night even after great precaution is taken. The enuresis takes place towards the last part of the night.

In **Kreosotum, Lac caninum, Senega** and **Sepia** the child wets the bed while dreaming that he is urinating in a decent manner and in the proper place. It is difficult to rouse him from his deep sleep.

In **Sepia** as in **Causticum** the involuntary urination takes place during first sleep, almost as soon as the child falls asleep.

Plantago is very rich in skin symptoms. The provers had itches and eruptions of various sorts, but the symptom that we deem most important is its tendency to produce erysipelatous inflammations in various parts of the body, especially in the female breast. Hale relates a case of erysipelas of the female breast which he cured with repeated local application of the tincture. He seems to regard **Plantago** far more satisfactory for allaying and arresting the inflammatory process than **Arnica** and **Hamamelis.**

There is also on record another case of a young lady whose hand and a portion of whose face got red, swollen and erysipelaous. She was given **Plantago** internally and then a lotion prepared by adding a teaspoonful of the tincture to a cup of water was applied locally. The relief was prompt and a complete cure resulted within three days.

Plantago is reported to have cured cases of ivy poisoning. The leaves are wilted and applied to the part with immediate relief of the suffering.

Plantago vies with **Calendula** in lacerated and incised wounds and in injuries of various kinds. Its especial indication is the presence of much painful swelling and erysipelatous inflammation around the affected part. Hale cites several cases where **Plantago** wrought wonderful cures. In one case a young man had his finger very badly cut. The injury gradually got worse till at last it was cured by the external application of **Plantago** tincture.

The next case was that of a punctured wound in the palm of a lady from a thrust of the fins of a cod fish. Her whole hand was swollen right up to the shoulder joint and the pain was excessive and agonizing. She applied bruised plantain leaves repeatedly. In about half an hour after the application, she felt so relieved that she fell asleep and slept probably an hour—the first sleep she had had after the accident. In two or three days the finger was well.

PLATINUM.

Platinum is a remedy without which our Materia Medica would be really incomplete. Without it we would find ourselves at sea in the treatment of many arduous ailments especially of the weaker sex, as we shall see presently.

It is a bright metal, white in colour with a slight bluish tinge. It is to be found plentifully in California, South America and Russia. The remedy was proved by Hahnemann.

In the crude state this metal is found mixed up with various other impurities. **Platinum** dissolves in lead and advantage is taken of this circumstance to separate it from other metallic impurities. The alloy of **Platinum** and lead is melted and exposed to a current of hot air in which the lead oxidises and falls off as slags. The precipitated metallic **Platinum** is then triturated.

If the whole feature of this remedy can be expressed in one word, it is sensitiveness. We find this illustrated in both the mental and physical side of the patient. The patient is like some sort of a volatile, highly combustible oil that ignites on the least spark. You dare not approach her. She is proud, haughty and fault-finding. She looms very large in her own imagination while others seem insignificant and small. It is this egotism that makes her so undesirable a companion. Arrogance is marked in every feature of her countenance. She walks straight like a queen, her head erect and her eyes turned away from all contemptible creatures around her. They all seem far too beneath her dignity to be taken notice of. **Platinum,** however, is not the only remedy to claim this symptom. **Lycop., Pall., Sulph** . and **Verat alb.** lay claim to an equally unenviable disposition with of course sufficient peculiarities of their own to facilitate differentiation.

Lycop. for example is vehement, imperious and domineering: but this mood is mostly due to his digestive and hepatic disturbance.

Palladium is very similar to our remedy. The patient is given to as violent a language and as strong a passion as **Platina** and her mental condition like that of the latter remedy, is a sort of a reflex of the ovarian and uterine complaint to which she is a chronic martyr. But the main difference consists in the fact that the **Palladium** patient, delegates great importance to the opinions of others and she feels herself to be constantly slighted. Her irritability is thus the effect of these supposed slights.

The typical **Sulphur** patient is irritable, peevish and quick-tempered. She is of an excitable and obdurate nature, but the redeeming feature of her character is that she becomes easily penitent. Great forgetfulness and benign contentment are some of her characteristic mental symptoms.

Verat alb. has an equally vicious temper. This patient too is a great one for finding out other people's faults and cursing them. There is very often a lascivious bend to her mind; in fact, sometimes we find her vulgar. To crown everything she is an inveterate liar.

The **Platinum** patient is hysterical. Great changeability of mood is as characteristic of **Platinum** as it is of **Aconite, Nux moschata, Ignatia, Crocus** and **Pulsatilla.** This alternating mood generally comes on after intense anger. Another important symptom is a homicidal tendency. Jules Gandy mentions of a case of a woman who could not go to the dining table for fear she would thrust the knife into the bosom of her husband—husband she was passionately fond of. The very sight of the knife brought about the homicidal craving. **Platinum** relieved her symptoms.

Sometimes we find these patients steeped in deep dejection and profound melancholy. Low-spirited and dull, they weep for hours. Very often this takes the apathetic turn. As in **Aurum, Fluoric acid, Phos., Sepia** and **Thuja,** they lose all their interest in the affairs of their life.

A great want of the sense of proportion leads them to the most ridiculous actions. They laugh in the wrong place and laugh most immoderately. At other times they cry at something that throws everybody else around them into a peal of laughter. I remember such an instance in an old man suffering from the after-effects of apoplexy. His sexual passions were highly exaggerated and this is what first drew my attention to **Platinum.** He used to attend minutely to whatever was said or done about him, but what impressed me as being very peculiar was his want of the sense of proportion. **Platinum** removed good many of his unfortunate symptoms.

Another peculiarity which it is worth our while to remember is an irresistible desire to whistle and sing. They whistle and sing in company even though they know that decency condemns it. **Crocus, Carbo animal., Lachesis** and **Stramonium,** also have the symptom.

We also notice in **Platinum** a tendency for violent spasmodic yawning. They are also given to great fear and anxiety. The dread of death constantly haunts them.

The pain of **Platinum** is very peculiar and characteristic. It increases gradually and as gradually decreases. Moreover this pain is accompanied by numbness as in **Aconite, Chamomilla** and **Kalmia.** This pain may be in any organ or part of the body and prescribed on its proper indication **Platinum** will certainly help. On this symptom of pain **Platinum** is reported to have cured many cases of ovaritis. This lead us on to consider the influence of **Platinum** over the sexual system. It is very marked both in the male and in the female sexual sphere. It produces great excitement of the sexual passion both in the males and females. In grown-up people this leads on to excessive venery, whereas in young boys not having the opportunity of their elders, it ushers in the pernicious habit of self-abuse. **Platinum** is rightly recommended by Gallavardin for the impulse to pederasty and sodomy. It also removes the ill-effects of prepubic masturbation. Hence it is used with benefit in epilepsy due to the same cause. In this respect it closely resembles **Bufo.**

It suits young girls with premature development of the sexual organs and instincts. This often leads them on to nymphomania and to similar vicious practices. This is also due to the titillating and tingling sensation in the genitals. Under **Platinum** this instinct of nymphomania becomes more in women in their lying-in state. Another peculiar feature with these **Platinum** cases is the great sensitiveness of the sexual organs. This aggravated sensitiveness makes coition, digital examination, practically impossible. Sometimes we find them fainting during these acts.

Platinum however is not the only remedy with such aggravated sexual cravings. We also find them in **Aster., Apis, Coffea, Grat., Hyos., Kali phos, lili. tig., Murex,** and **Phos.** They have all their distinctive features and we will discuss them below.

In **Aster.** the craving is insatiable and is not removed by coitus.

In **Apis** we have intense sexual desire in widows.

Coffea has excessive sensitiveness about the genitals with voluptuous itching.

In **Gratiola** as in **Platinum** the desire is increased in the lying-in women.

Hyoscyamus has as great an equal sexual craving. The patient is decidedly lascivious and her extreme lasciviousness leads her to impudent exposure of the pudenda. She is also given to smutty talk.

Kali phos. is to be thought of in premature growths of virgin girls. In this remedy the desire becomes intense after each menstrual period.

Lilium tig. is indicated in a similar insatiable desire for sexual gratification in women with ovarian complaints. There is voluptuous itching in the vagina with a feeling of fullness in this part.

No remedy can come near **Murex** as regards the intensity of sexual passions. The desire is insatiable and uncontrollable; it simply drives the patient crazy. The slightest touch renews this craving.

Origanum is indicated in women whom the excessive craving drives to masturbation.

Phosphorous is helpful in nymphomania in widows; in this remedy the excess of desire is due to a condition of forced celibacy. The irresistible desire for coition leads her on to lascivious exposure of the genitals as in **Hyos.**

On these symptoms **Platinum** is reported to have cured ovarian tumors, cystic growths on the womb, uterine fibroids, **sterility,** dysmenorrhœa, leucorrhœa, menorrhagia, puerperal convulsions, hysteria and neurasthenia.

Platinum is helpful in a peculiar type of uterine hæmorrhage. The blood is too profuse and consists of dark, stringy clotted mass as in **Crocus** and **Chamomilla.** They are accompanied by spasms or painful bearing down sensation in the uterine region.

The temperament of the patient, which is generally hysterical in nature, should be particularly helpful in arriving at a decision about the remedy.

Platinum is very helpful in spasm during labor. It is used in eclamptic fits during labour when such is accompanied with extreme sensitiveness of the vagina and external parts.

Platinum is a great remedy for painters' colic. The pain is in the umbilical region and it extends through into back. The patient screams and resorts to every position to get relief. Constipation is a very frequent accompaniment. This constipation however is very peculiar. It is due to intestinal inertia as in **Alumina**. Great straining is necessary and even then the evacuation is very small and unsatisfactory; sometimes the difficulty is so great as to necessitate manual assistance as in **Silicea**. The stools passed after so much exertion are soft and clayey adhering to rectum and anus like soft clay. Such constipation is very frequently met with in emigrants, travellers and in lying-in women.

The postures and attitudes as assumed by the patient are of importance to us, homœopaths, in the selection of the remedy. Hence a short discussion on this aspect of **Platinum** will not be much out of place. She generally lies on her back with her arms over her head, thighs drawn up and knees thrown wide apart. There is also a tendency to kick off the clothes and keep the legs uncovered. This posture is a great pointer and will help us to prescribe this remedy in many serious complaints such as typhoid epilepsy, hysteria, tetanus etc.

Before closing I would draw my reader's attention to another feature of **Platinum.** The physical symptoms and the mental symptoms are antagonistic; that is, when the physical symptoms disappear, mental symptoms appear and vice versa. Dr. Nash reports of a case of insanity that he cured with **Platinum** on the strength of this symptom alone.

We will quote hos own words. "The physical symptom was a pain along the whole length of the spine. This was the symptom alternating with the mental one (fear of death). It was one of the most brilliant cures I ever saw. Improvement began the first day and never flagged and she has remained well now 15 years with never a sign of return."

Case 1.—Miss P., aged nineteen years, features sallow, blue borders around the eyes, is brought to me by her mother, who fears that her daughter suffers from mental disorder. She has a tremorous look, speaks in monosyllables and does not answer any of my questions. Her mother states that menstruation set in regularly when she was seventeen years old appearing every four weeks and continuing for eight days, but accompanied with such excrutiating pains in the uterine region, that the girl acts then more like a crazy woman. The pain begins on the second day, increases on the third, and continues on the fourth. The pains are drawing, pulling labour pains, increasing to convulsions in the form of continual twitchings so that she cannot be kept from screaming; the severity of the pains is so great that the girl begs to be killed, and this idea follows her through the free intervals, taking away her former good humour, so that she looks worn out and melancholy. Prescribed **Platina 2**, a few grains morning and evening; light diet, fresh air and luke-warm sitz-baths were recommended in order to remove the stagnation in the circulation and the nervous irritation resulting from it. It took full four months to eradicate the disease; but then she was also another person; her bright and blooming face, the smiling and pleasing expression of her countenance showed that she enjoyed life once more and that all its functions were in a normal state.—(**Dr. Hirschel. Klinik. Am. Jour. Hom. Mat. Med., vol. iii., p. 127.**)

Case 2.—Lady aged twenty; at twelve, she was attacked with leucorrhœa, which has continued till now; discharge like the white of an egg, uninterrupted day and night, inoffensive, but debilitating; began to menstruate at fourteen; at fifteen, was seized with violent dragging, tearing pain and soreness in the region of the left ovary, the dragging extending through to the small of the back. This pain was especially violent at the time of her menses, and otherwise as permanent as the leucorrhœal discharge. With the pain, the menstrual blood became black; it came in clots, and the flow lasted eight or ten days; violent compressive pain in the temples, and a sense of weight upon the chest, as if it would be crushed by a mass of lead; the soreness in the region of the ovary gradually extended over the whole left side, and was especially violent in the small of the back when it extended across the spine. Excessively painful shootings from the side, along the lower portion of the left mamma, two or three times a day, with nausea and giddiness; unable to rest on the left side on this account. For the last three years, the pain in the region of the left ovary had changed to a dull, heavy, gnawing pain, and the soreness in the side had greatly increased; weak and languid; blue circles around the eyes; aversion to society; extremely melancholy. No improvement under allopathic treatment. **Plat 200**, night and morning aggravated at first, and cured in eight days.—Dr. Hempel.

PLUMBUM METALLICUM.

Medical literature is replete with instances of lead poisoning. This may take place in various ways. Skin, lungs, and mouth may all be the channels of infection. As the compilation of our Materia Medica is greatly helped by a careful and scientific observation of symptoms brought about by the inadvertent use of the poisonous material or of the material in poisonous doses, it behoves us to consider here a case of saturnine intoxication; such procedure will clothe our abstract Materia Medica with the rain-bow hue of reality and vividness. The first sign to appear is the impairment of nutrition or even when the patient experiences no loss of strength, his skin assumes a sallow tint. He experiences a sweetish metallic taste in the mouth. There also appears the gingival line; (also called the lead-line) which is a peculiar bluish hue about margin of gums. Then comes the pain (the lead colic) in and about the navel where the patient experiences a sense of sinking. The colic is mostly accompanied by an obstinate constipation, retraction of abdominal parietes, loss of appetite, thirst, fetid odour of the breath and general emaciation with paralysis of a peculiar kind, affecting mostly the flexors of the fore-arm and causing a dropping of the wrist of manifesting itself in a general paralysis of the limbs. Squinting and amaurosis are occasional symptoms. Albumen is found in the urine in an advanced stage of poisoning. After death, the large and small intestines are found to be much contracted and their coats thickened These changes are especially marked in the colon. Granular degeneration of the kidneys is very common. Now that we have seen how our patient looks and feels and acts after taking a poisonous dose of this metal, we will study the fine shades of symptoms that constitute the chief beauty of the homœopathic therapeutics.

The facial appearance of the patient is particularly striking. It is extremely pale, yellow and ash-colored, almost corpse-like in ugliness. There is a sort of bloatedness that adds to the disfigurement of his appearance. The face is expressive of intense anxiety and suffering. The skin of the face is greasy and shining; this is true of a lot of remedies such as **Sel., Nat. mur., Merc., Bry.** and **Psor.,** but it would not do to base our prescriptions on one symptom alone. There is extreme and rapid emaciation. This emaciation may be either general or partial. There are other remedies having emaciation—such as **Ars., Iod., Abrot., Syph., Tuber.** and **Nat. mur.,** and we must learn to differentiate between them.

In **Ars.** the prostration is more marked than the emaciation and with that prostration we notice the general features of restlessness, burning, amelioration by heat, great fear of death, great thirst and midnight aggravation.

Iod. also has marked emaciation. The patient eats ravenously, but this does not stop the progressive emaciation; arms, hands, the mammary glands, the testicles—none escape the gradual decay. With this there goes excessive mental irritability.

Abrot. is another great remedy for emaciation. It is mostly indicated in marasmus of children with marked emaciation, especially about the legs (**Iod., Sani., Sab.**).

Syphil. has emaciation of the entire body. With this remedy we find great craving for alcohol, falling off of the hair and the general aggravation of all symptoms from sun-set to sun-rise.

In **Tuber.** the emaciation is very rapid and pronounced, but what enables us to distinguish this remedy from other similar remedies is the great tendency of this patient to catch cold, he knows not how or where.

Lastly, we come to **Nat. mur.** The peculiarity here is that the emaciation is most marked about the neck. The little isthmus of the neck connects the two continents of the head and the body. This is accompanied by a strange lachrymal disposition, dryness of mouth and throat, great thirst, obstinate constipation and a tendency towards profuse sweating.

The action of **Plumbum** on the muscles is particularly striking. It causes contraction of the voluntary and involuntary muscles and finally paralysis and atrophy. In the paralytic sphere it has a peculiar affinity for the flexor muscles of the fore-arm causing the "wrist-drop" we so often see in plumbism. **Plumbum** is also a useful remedy in the treatment of local spasms. Dr. Stokes has recorded several cases of cramps of the calves cured by it. It is also a valuable remedy in the spasmodic conditions of the rectum, and the vagina. Teste has put on record cases of retraction of the testicles cured by it.

We will not neglect the mental symptoms of **Plumbum,** since mental symptoms are the ones that play the biggest role in homoeopathic prescribing. The patient is slow of perception; there is intellectual torpor, lassitude and gradually growing apathy.

Plumbum is a good remedy in delirium when it alternates with colic; the patient bites and strikes at those around him like

Bell., but unlike **Bell.** there is tremor of the head and hands and a goodly collection of yellow mucus about the mouth and teeth.

Agaricus has a similar delirium. The patient knows no one, throws things at the nurse, sings, talks but does not answer questions; tries to get out of bed as he sees dead relations, particularly dead sister calling him. He makes grimaces. This reminds us of **Cantharis** in delirium where the patient barks (In **Cuprum** he bellows like a calf) and bleats. There are also confusion of head, anxious restlessness and cold sweats, especially on hands and feet.

We will now discuss the most important symptom of **Plumbum**—the colic. The pain is of a neuralgic and spasmodic character. It is sharp, constant, becoming acute by paroxysms, aggravated by motion, and is worse in the evening and night. It is ameliorated by pressure. The colic is almost always accompanied by obstinate constipation but no flatulence. The unfortunate patient feels that some one is twisting and clawing at his intestines and this pain from the region of the navel radiates upward to the chest and downward to the pubis. There may be vomiting and slight icterus; the abdomen which is as hard as stone is retracted in a concave fashion and he feels as if a string is pulling it towards the spine. The patient in his agony stretches and stretches violently for hours. He assumes the strangest attitudes and positions in bed to find relief which he gets and that only temporarily, from hard pressure. We will in this connection compare it with **Bell., Coloc., Cuprum,** and **Dios.**

In **Bell.** the patient feels as if a spot in the abdomen were drilled with nails. The migrating pain comes on suddenly and disappears just as suddenly. There is a feeling of pain to the slight touch but it is ameliorated by hard pressure. It is aggravated by standing and walking and ameliorated by bending backward.

Colocynth is similar to **Plumbum** in the cutting colic which emanating from a central point in and around the navel radiates all over the abdomen and chest. The patient feels as if his bowels were being squeezed between stones. The pain doubles him up and he finds relief only by pressing his abdomen hard against the bed-post or any other hard object or by lying on his stomach.

Cuprum has violent cramp in abdomen. Like **Plumbum, Zinc., Op.** and **Pod.,** the abdomen is drawn in. It does yeoman's duty in intussusception of the bowels where the intense agony brings about piercing screams from the patient and is attended with stercoraceous vomiting and singultus.

Dioscorea is a notable remedy in abdominal colic. It is just the reverse of **Colocynth**. There is a great deal of flatulence. The pain here is relieved by stretching the body out and from moving about; another peculiar characteristic of this remedy is that the pain in the abdomen suddenly shifts and appears in distant localities, such as the fingers and the toes.

I have used **Plumbum** in constipation with great success. I cannot do better than cite an instance where we had a very gratifying result from its application. Dr. G—of Diamond Harbour, aged 80, contracted a huge lump in the right hypochondrium which was diagnosed as abscess of the liver. He was placed in Allopathic hands and when plasters and blisters failed and the unhappy patient grew decidedly worse, operation was proposed. The distracted patient, scared at such an undesirable contingency, at last decided on homœopathic treatment. Thanks to Hahnemann's wisdom! he came round nicely under the treatment, till we shoaled him on a very severe attack of constipation. There were marked spasms of the rectum. He complained of a sensation as if a string were drawing the anus up into the rectum. Stools consisted of small, hard, black balls like sheep's dung. The passage was entirely blocked by a huge conglomerated mass. He was given Plumb 30, twice, with the result that the constipation permanently disappeared.

We also prescribe this remedy in intestinal obstruction from causes other than mechanical, as in strangulated hernia. Many such instances have been recorded of **Plumbum** saving the patient from the clutches of the surgeon's knife.

Epilepsy is again another trouble which is very trying to our friends of the other school—I mean the physicians who base most of their pretensions on science. Here their science fails them, their knife is not of any use; the most powerful microscopes cannot detect any deviation of the vital force, the real dynamo which governs, protects and prolongs human life. Here homœopathy proves its excellence. It takes into account the very minutest deviation of the " life force " as manifested by symptoms and wins its laurels in the very face of its scientific competitor. We will discuss in this connexion a few of our great remedies, such as **Plumb., Bell., Cic., Cup. acet., Cup. met., Agar., Artemisia** and **Alumina.**

Plumb. does wonderful work in epilepsy from cerebral sclerosis or tumors. The patient feels an almost paralytic heaviness of the legs before the attack and there is often paralysis and prolonged snoring after.

To an Allopathic doctor all cases of epilepsy are the same, but to us, Homœopaths, two cases of epilepsy are as different as are two cases of headache and diarrhœa. We individualise all our patients. We pay very little attention to the diagnostic symptoms, because they are present in every disease having the same denomination. We take note of where the aura begins, how the patient feels before, during and after the attack, what he does, his mental symptoms, the etiology and a lot of other minute details which enable the Homœopath to make the differentiation which is the chief beauty of our system and which marks the distinguished tyro from a Hahnemann, a Hering and a Lippe.

Bell.—It is very useful in fresh cases of epilepsy with pronounced brain symptoms. The aura here is different from that of any other remedy. The patient feels as if a mouse is running over his extremities, or heat is rising from his stomach. The convulsions begin in the upper extremities and extend to mouth, face and eyes. The spasms are excited by the least touch.

Cicuta vir. is useful in epilepsy from concussion of the brain. It is most serviceable in cases where the convulsions are violent. The patient is rigid, opisthotonos or emprosthotonos with fixed staring eyes, bluish face and frothing at the mouth.

In **Cuprum acet.** the aura begins at the knee and then it ascends till it reaches the hypogastric region when unconsciousness supervenes. Like **Lach.** and **Crot. hor.**, the patient continuously protrudes and retracts tongue like a snake during the attack. The patient always grows worse by going into a warm room with high ceiling.

Cuprum met. is a great remedy for epilepsy. The attacks are generally nocturnal; strange to say the fit generally occurs at regular intervals.

In **Agaricus** there is a fit every seven days.

In **Artemisia** the fits are brought about by violent emotions; the convulsions come close together and then follows a long interval of rest.

We think of **Alumina** in cases of epilepsy where the attacks come on mostly while passing stools. This is something that an Allopathic doctor will never take notice of; on the other hand, it will furnish him with a nice ground to laugh at his brethren of the sugar-pill variety; but this symptom will be a nice ground of distinction just the same to us and a good index to cure an obstinate case of epilepsy and then we can laugh last and laugh best at our " Scientific Scoffer."

Case 1.—Mrs. E., forty years old, suffered for a year from severe cardialgia. She complained of pressure in the stomach, as from a heavy weight, increasing to a strangling sensation during the severe colicky paroxysms, and followed by sour and bilious vomiting. External pressure does not incommode her; loss of appetite, but excessive thirst; pains in the back, alleviated sometimes by bending forward, at other time by bending backward; constipation, once a week, a hard, knobby stool; the paroxysms increase in severity and duration, and the patient is already atrophic and anæmic. **Nux.** and **Bis.** did nothing. Taste always sweetish; abdomen compressed, hard, like a board; constriction of the throat; paralytic weakness in the extremities, especially on the right side; hands and feet cold; want of perspiration. Every symptom indicates **Plumbum acet.**, which she took 30, then 6 and 3, producing a perfect cure in a few weeks.—Dr. S. Lilienthal.

Case 2.—Mrs. T., aged thirty years, heretofore in good health, was taken with colic, for which **Aconite** and **Arsenic** were prescribed without affording her relief. Two days later she vomited up dead worms; the colic continued. Prescribed **Cina** and **Nux.**; no relief. On the following day: constant hiccough, with belching of fetid gas; nausea and retching, with immediate vomiting after drinking. Coated tongue, foul taste in the mouth, dryness in the mouth without thirst. Loss of appetite; no fever.; Pressing burning, tearing pains in the lower abdomen; tympanitic condition of the lower abdomen, with a tumor of the size of a fist in the umbilical region, which is sensitive to pressure; the paroxysms of pain seem to start from this tumor. The intestines are full of gas and can be felt singly as the gas moves about; constant rumbling from flatulence. The bowels have not moved for four days, although there has been frequent desire. Forty-eight hours later, vomiting of fecal matter, hiccough with fecal odor, more pain. Prescribed **Plumbum met. 6**, one dose every two hours. Improvement. Stool of hard, small feces, which look as if they were covered with membrane. Return of appetite and recovery.— **(Theuerkauf in Allg. Hom. Zeitg., vol, lvi).**

PODOPHYLLUM.

Podophyllum is a perennial herbaceous plant that grows plentifully on the borders of woods in America. It grows to the height of two or three feet with leaves spread out like an open hand; hence its name **Podophyllum** which means Duck's Feet. It is also called May apple, Mandrake, Indian apple and ground lemon. The medicine is prepared from the fresh root of the plant gathered before the fruit is ripe. It is chopped and pounded to a pulp and then mixed with two parts by its weight of alcohol. The tincture is then separated by decanting and filtering. It was first proved by Dr. Williams of the United States of America. It belongs to the natural order of Berberidaceæ.

Before going into the symptomatology of **Podophyllum** I will mention a few experiments with this drug by Dr. Anstie. He introduced an alcoholic solution of **Podophyllum** into the peritoneal cavity of dogs and a few other lower animals. The duodenum and the rectum were found to be chiefly affected. The lining membrane of the whole of the small intestine was covered with bloody mucus. The liver was found to be congested. When administered to the healthy, it causes griping pain accompanied with vomiting and persistent diarrhœa. In poisonous dosage, it brings on inflammation and ulceration of the intestines, bloody stools, prostration, stupor and death. It stimulates the liver; hence it is extensively used in the digestive disturbances, usually called biliousness. It is thus a great liver and bowel remedy as we will see by the finer shades of symptoms arrived at by Homœopathic proving.

Podophyllum is a great cathartic, hence to the homœopath it is a great remedy for diarrhœa, but it is good for its own kind of diarrhœa. It begins early in the morning, continues through the forenoon and is followed by a natural stool in the evening. The patient thinks he is better but the next morning the same diarrhœa starts again. This diarrhœa is accompanied by a sensation of weakness or sinking in the abdomen or rectum; he feels as if everything would drop down through the pelvis. The stools are painless, very offensive and profuse as if coming from a hydrant. Sometimes they are yellow-coloured with meal-like sediment in it and sometimes greenish-yellow, slimy or bloody. Prolapsus ani before and during stools even from the least exertion, is also a characteristic feature. Very often **Podophyllum** is needed in diarrhœa of children—diarrhœa when the child is being washed. It comes on after eating like dirty water soaking the napkin through. This profuseness of stools is a mystery: every time the patient seems to be drained dry but he fills up again. This ought to convince our brethren of the dominant school about the futility of the idea of "washing, douching and cleaning up the system." Inspite of their grave pretensions to science they seem to forget the most important elementary principle that the human system is not a barrel but a self-acting, autonomous whole, where an all-wise, ever-prudent vital principle fights for self-preservation and deals out its just share to the demands of the minutest parts of our organism.

We will revert to its diarrhœa once more. We must not get confused when we get a case of morning diarrhœa, for like **Podo.** we have morning diarrhœa in **Bry., Nat. sulph., Aloes, Sulph., Rumex** and a few other remedies. Just a little discriminating and a little judgment are necessary to help us out of this tangle. They are all different, each one with its own characteristic symptoms.

We have morning diarrhœa in **Bry.** and **Nat. sulph.** but it comes on after rising in the morning and moving about.

In **Sulph.** and **Rumex** the urging is felt before rising. Pierce makes the differentiation very clear between **Podophyllum** and **Sulphur,** when he says that the "**Podophyllum** patient goes to the closet on the trot, while in **Sulphur** he goes on the run."

In **Aloes** the want of confidence in sphincter ani is a marked feature.

A symptom that I have omitted to mention, is a loud gurgling in the abdomen before stools. During stool the patient experiences great heat and pain in the anus. There is another symptom particularly characteristic of **Podophyllum** and that is a sensation, as if the genital organs would come out during stools. After stools the patient experiences great weakness and exhaustion. The **Podophyllum** diarrhœa is brought about by eating fruits.

Podophyllum is a great fever remedy. It is generally indicated in bilious remittents. The patient wakes up in the morning with a dull throbbing headache, a dry mouth and bad taste. The tongue is heavy with a dirty coating of yellow. Nausea is quite prominent and the patient vomits bilious substance; it is accompanied by a yellow or greenish diarrhœa.

It is also useful in intermittent fevers. The time of the paroxysm is 7 a.m. Backache, gastric and bilious symptoms are marked sometimes for days before the attack. Loquacity is a great feature of this drug which continues all through the chill and partly through the stage of heat. At the zenith of the fever the patient falls asleep and perspires profusely. During chill he complains of pain in the hypochondria, knees, ankles, elbows, and wrists. This symptom may lead to a confusion with **Rhus tox.** and **Eupat.**, but the totality always helps in the decision. The patient forgets everything; no recollection of his loquacity afterwards.

In **Apis,** too, there is the sleeping at the climax of heat and sleeping during the stage of perspiration, but the thirstlessness, the time of the paroxysm which is 3 p.m., and the scantiness of the sweat help differentiation.

In **Calad.** also we have this peculiar symptom of sleep during fever.

The tongue of **Podo.** is foul with the imprint of teeth like **Merc.** and **Rhus.** The breath is offensive but unlike **Puls.** the patient gets disgusted with his own breath.

Sometimes during dentition, we have a hydrocephaloid condition. The child moans, tosses his head from side to side, grinds his teeth and whines. One thinks of **Bell.** in such cases and very often there is an abuse of **Bell.,** being a favourite remedy; but we must not also lose sight of **Podophyllum** in such circumstances.

The headache of **Podophyllum** is, as has been said before, a bilious headache. It begins in the morning with flushed face and alternates with diarrhœa. There is a kind of blurring of vision during headache, objects looking hazy and misty. This headache mostly occupies occipital protuberance and is associated with disgusting nausea and sour vomiting. The pain extends from the occiput down into the neck and shoulder. All the symptoms, as has been said repeatedly, are due to torpidity of the liver and sluggishness of the portal system.

In **Gels.** on the other hand, the pain, which begins in the cervical spine, extends over the head and settles in the forehead and eyeballs causing a bursting sensation.

Podophyllum is called the "vegetable mercury" as it has a lot of symptoms in common with mercury. Like **Mercury** the tongue takes the imprints of the teeth. It is covered with a whitish or yellowish fur; the breath is very offensive and the saliva copious.

The action of **Podophyllum** on the female sexual system should not be overlooked. It is used in ovarian tumors, leucorrhœa, prolapsus uteri and many other kindred troubles. The prolapsus of the uterus is also simultaneous with prolapsus ani. The bearing down sensation is the effect of prolapsus ani and is to be accounted for by indiscriminate lifting or straining. A peculiar symptom is amelioration of pain from lying on stomach. It also relieves morning sickness and excessive vomiting in pregnancy due to a congested condition of the pelvic viscera. Suppression of menses in young females calls for Podophyllum when with the bearing down sensation, felt mostly in hypogastric and sacral regions, there are the concomitant symptoms of chronic prolapsus of the anus, thick transparent leucorrhœa, pain in ovary, nausea, hemorrhoids and relief of pain from lying down.

We will next study the action of Podo. on the liver. It is used in jaundice, chronic hepatitis, hyperæmia of liver and gallstones. It is to be remembered, however, that homœopaths must not prescribe on mere names of diseases. It is perilous to walk on such uncertain grounds. It is safer to base our prescription on symptomatology and the symptoms which indicate Podo. in liver troubles are the following: great fulness, soreness and pain in the region of the liver, amelioration from rubbing the hypochondriac region, stitches in the epigastrium from coughing, sour regurgitation of food, acute burning pain in the region of pyloric orifice, jaundice, bilious nausea, giddiness, dark urine, bitter taste, clayey stools, alternate constipation and diarrhœa, sensation of weight in hypogastric region and piles with prolapsus ani.

We must not, however, be led away with the idea that Podophyllum is our sole and only hepatic remedy. There are others just as important and a short summary of the action of a few amongst them will be useful.

Ptelea trif. has the sensation of great heaviness in the region of the liver, for in reality the liver has grown to an enormous size; when the patient lies on the left side, the liver keeps dragging on its ligaments. The heavy aching pain in the liver becomes relieved by lying on the right side.

Cobaltum has shooting pains in hepatic region and also in spleen, worse taking a deep inspiration; but in Cobaltum the stitches run down the thighs from the liver.

Chelidonium is another great liver remedy. From slight fullness there may be short stitching pains in the region of the liver; this pain may penetrate into the stomach or may go into the back from the posterior part of the liver. But that important symptom of marked pain under the angle of right scapula is always **an index.** The patient awakes in the morning **perspiring,** with **vague** recollection of dreams, with headache from **sleepless-** ness, **with** a tight feeling of constriction in the region **of the** liver preventing free expansion of the chest. His pains are better by eating.

PRUNUS SPINOSA.

Prunus spinosa is prepared from the Black-thorn which is a native of Europe and America. It was first introduced into our Materia Medica by Hale. This remedy, though not so well-known, is of infinite interest to the homœopath. As I have said before, we cannot delegate any remedy to the lumber-room. Every remedy, however unimportant and rare, should be always kept handy if we are to be helpful in every case that comes to us for relief. **Prunus spinosa** has some very characteristic indications on which some fine cures have been made. This remedy is in great demand in the treatment of glaucoma, choroido-retinitis, choroiditis, in ciliary neuralgia and in certain affections of the bladder provided always the indications are present. It is our object to deal thoroughly with the indications that make it so effective a remedy in the treatment of those complaints. The key-note indication of **Prunus spinosa** consists in the direction of its pains. They are outshooting and outpressing; commencing at an internal spot they shoot and radiate outwards. We have sharp pain beginning in the right side of the forehead, shooting like lightning through brain and coming out at occiput. Sometimes the pain presses from within outwards. Sometimes the skull feels as if it would be pressed outwards by a sharp plug. In nose, ears, gums and teeth, in fact everywhere the same type of pain is to be seen. In toothache the tooth feels as if it would be raised out of its socket and thrown off.

Another symptom of **Prunus spinosa,** just as characteristic and remarkable, as the one mentioned above, is the shortness breath to which he very frequently becomes a victim. He sighs constantly as if he were climbing a high or a steep hill. The tight short and difficult breathing, this anxious respiration led Dr. Lippe to prescribe **Prunus spinosa** with remarkable success a case of sprained ankle in a young lady of 16, who jumped from a carriage whilst the horse had bolted. The left ankle and foot were sprained and swollen; but as the swelling and pain abated new symptoms developed; her breath became rapid; she felt great oppression of chest with constant desire to take long breath; it felt as if the air she inhaled did not reach the pit of the stomach, and this necessitated frequent long inspiration and constant yawning.

Another important and peculiar symptom is the strangury caused by pressure of flatus on the bladder. The desire to pass urine is continuous. If this desire is not attended to immediately, violent crampy pains ensue in the bladder. He is therefore, afraid to hold urine long. Sometimes again an opposite condition is to be met with. The urging and imperative call for urination is not always successful; the urine seems to pass forward into the glans penis and then seems to turn back, causing violent spasmodic pain in the urethra. I do not know if any other remedy has this symptom so well marked.

It is an excellent remedy in neuralgia. I have used it with uniform success in cases of ciliary neuralgia on the following symptoms:—

Pain in the eyeball, as if crushed, or pain as if pressed asunder; sharp shooting pain extending through the eye back into the brain; sometimes the pain commences from behind the ear and shoots forward into the eyes.

I have also used this remedy in women during climacteric period, suffering from tachycardia. The beating of the heart is audible and furious. The carotids are distended and their pulsations are visible. The purple lips, the bloated face, the suppressed menstruation and the above-mentioned cardiac symptoms make **Prunus spinosa** a sister remedy to **Lach., Glon., Sang.** and **Amyl nit.**

It is also used in cardiac dropsy. Anasarca, after debilitating chronic diseases, depending on hypertrophy of the heart finds in **Prunus spinosa** an effective remedy. We must not, however, lose sight of the principle of " Similia " that should be our guide in the selection of the remedy.

PSORINUM.

It is a nosode of high remedial agency. It was first brought into life by our great Master Samuel Hahnemann. We have had three different preparations of this nosode since Hahnemann's time. The first was prepared by Hahnemann himself from the sero-purulent matter contained in the scabies. Dr. Gross had a preparation of his own which he calls psora sicca, prepared from the epidermis of efflorescence and pityriasis. The third preparation was by Constantine Hering who utilised the salt derived from a product of psora.

The importance of **Psorinum** is especially marked by its power to meet the inner dyscrasia of some patients who are termed psoric. This I am afraid needs some explanation. This world of ours has been gliding slowly but surely from eternity to eternity. Lives have been bubbling up in their never-ending course and after the short spell allotted to them, full of varied complexities, they are merging back into that pool of eternity called death. We with our limited knowledge have been all along trying to probe into the secret principle that guides this vast concourse of humanity, in their rise and in their fall. The result has been many empiric principles derived from our experiences of centuries handed down by generation to generation with additions and alterations made by each succeeding generation, on to what has been handed to them by their predecessors but in spite of these, almost every now and again, we bump against facts deeper and more inscrutable than others, not reached by any empiric principles laid down for us. About some seven years ago I in company of a friend, went out on a shooting excursion. It was a damp, dreary night. It drizzled, it rained and it thundered all night, and both of us were exposed to the inclemency of the weather. In the morning I found myself miserable, with aches and pains, swollen parotid gland, sore-throat and a temperature of 103°. But my surprise knew no bounds when I found my friend invigorated, refreshed, full of exuberence of life, happier than he has ever been, healthier by far than when the weather was fine, bright shiny and smiling.

A whole family of children went to Darjeeling. After three months they all came back, one of them showing symptoms of goitre, the second with signs of elephantiasis of the leg, a third prostrated with sprue, but the rest of them with the bloom of freshness and roses in their cheeks. Facts like this we encoun everyday and every medical man can recount numerous instances from his own Record-Book of cases, that go contrary to all rules and laws empirical. This divergence of phenomena can only be explained on the basis of some inherent latent poison found in the system of some individuals, sometimes self-acquired other times handed down to them by their predecessors in varying degrees of intensity.

Hahnemann after a life-long search for truth came to the conclusion that the poison found latent in our system, the poison that usually protracts cure and complicates suffering are generally of three varieties, named syphilis, sycosis and psora. This theory seems very plausible and it explains many of the apparent absurdities and complexities that we encounter daily in course of our practice. Although we claim for Hahnemann an exalted position, a claim that is indubitable and world-acknowledged, it would be sheer folly to claim that the great Hahnemann was absolutely infallible. Yet there are amongst us men so bigotted and narrow-minded, so devoid of all principles of logic, as to proclaim that everything laid down by the great master, irrespective of all future discoveries, regardless of all improvements and progress, should be blindly worshipped and Homœopathic science must remain at a stand-still at the place where he left it. I for one, believe in carrying the great standard to fresh fields of glory and science, in unision with all progress and accomplishments. His great law of cure, Similia Similious Curantur, is an eternal, immutable and glorious truth. It has stood all tests so far and it will stand for all ages to come. This is a solid and a glorious foundation on which we must work and try to complete the great edifice started by the great benefactor of humanity. It is for us to investigate, to search, to compare and find out if we can, any better theory to explain, that Hahnemann tried to explain by his Theory of Miasms.

In **Psorinum** we have a remedy that rectifies the latent dyscrasia in psoric diathesis. The glands in these constitutions, are scrofulous and the skin is extraordinarily subject to all kinds of unhealthy rash and eruptions. We notice intolerable itching of the body, specially at night and in bed when it gets warm. The patient scratches until he bleeds. In respect of this mad scratching, it is very similar to **Sulphur**. In fact **Psor.** is a remedy to be thought of in those chronic cases in which **Sulphur seems** indicated but fails to act. The skin is dry, greasy-looking, with yellow blotches. Looking at him, one would feel that he had not a bath for ages. There are eczemas behind ears, on scalps, and in bends of elbows and armpits. These eruptions have a great tendency to bleed and to suppurate; pemphigus, ulcers, moist itches, condylomata, psoriasis syphilitica, copper-coloured pustules, urticaria, boils, tinea capitis and most of the other varieties of skin affections are to be found in abundance all over the body. Eruptions are noticed particularly over the occiput, completely hiding the scalp. The exudation is very profuse, excoriating and offensive. The hair, too, is dry and lustreless and it tangles easily; at times, the discharge from the ugly eruptions on his scalp loosens the hair altogether and makes it most difficult to comb. Altogether we have in **Psorinum** a combination of all our unhealthy remedies, such as **Hep. sulph., Silicea, Borax, Graph., Merc., Mez., Petr.,** and **Sulph.** The greasy appearance of the skin, as if it is bathed in oil should be particularly borne in mind. Although the sebaceous glands are over-worked, the skin is very inactive. It is dry, parchment-like and absolutely devoid of perspiration.

Now that we have discussed the constitution of our patients we will do well to go into the general characteristics of the drug. The first and the foremost point in this remedy is the great filthy odour of the whole body and the carrion-like smell of all the discharges. All excretions are horribly offensive, and the detestable odor follows the patient everywhere. It is an odour, the very remembrance of which will cause nausea and qualmishness. t will not be wise to prescribe this remedy unless this symptom s prominently marked. Its absence is a contra-indication of the lrug.

The second important characteristic, in this remedy, is the great sensitiveness of the patient to cold air. He uses a fur-cap in the hottest weather. As soon as the sky gets cloudy, we see him run indoors and use still warmer materials than what he has on, although what he usually uses is thicker, heavier by far than what is generally used by the common run of people. In fact, he is like a barometer; by looking at him and noting the change in his clothes we may very safely predict, change in the atmospherica condition. In this respect **Psorinum** compares well with **Rhodo Sepia, Silicea** and **Tuberculinum.**

The third prominent feature is to be seen in its modalities There is decided amelioration of all complaints by lying down an by bringing the arms close to the body. I have helped in man cases of bronchitis and asthma on this remarkable symptom of relief from lying down.

I consider this a very striking phenomenon, as usually, in such cases, the patient generally wants to be propped up to the perpendicular posture. Usually this means relief of all dyspnœa and difficult breathing.

The fourth characteristic to which reference has already been made is to be seen in its power to rouse the latent defective vitality in cases very much overwhelmed by inimical diseased forces, wherever a well-selected remedy does not produce the slightest ripple of reaction. It is like the whip that goads the lethargic exhausted vitality, to fresh attempts at self-preservation in its struggles against inimical diseased forces.

Finally we may give unhealthiness of the skin and its susceptibility to all kinds of skin diseases, the fifth place. As I have discussed this part of Psorinum in full, I need not spend any more time over it.

My object next is to peep into the secret chambers of Psorinum's mental state. Here we notice a variegated panorama of ideas, thoughts and sentiments, the most important of which is the great depression of spirit. Despair, melancholia, despondence and downheartedness are the most prominent traits of his character. He makes his own life miserable and those around him very unhappy. Nothing that happens, brings him any ray of light and hope. He takes the sorriest view of everything. His mind is so tainted that he seems to revel in thoughts that are dark, gloomy and sad. In this connection I want to cite a cure of the most marvellous description that Dr. Allen effected while I was yet a student, studying medicine at his feet. It was in the case of a very near and dear relation of mine, who was suffering from a most persistent, distressing colic for years, which various doctors diagnosed, differently and none agreed as to its real nature.

After years of unavailing sorrow and suffering and failure of every other treatment, I, then a medical student in Chicago, brought this to Dr. Allen's notice. He sent one single dose of Psorinum C.M. packed nicely in an envelope to the patient in India. Since that day, and it is about 17 years ago, the patient has been having unfailing health and there has not been a vestige of pain from the time he took that solitary dose of medicine till the present moment. I did not then very well understand the real import of this prescription and took it as a sort of despotism and dictatorship on the part of the great professor. Now after the lapse of so many years, in the light of present experience and knowledge, I find and appreciate the true basis of that inimitable choice. This colic was the after-effect, which none but Dr. Allen appreciated, of a suppression of the most distressing, maddening, tormenting eczema that the gentleman had for years on his scrotum and which he suppressed by the application of many external and soothing ointments. The second reason that probably prompted Dr. Allen to make this choice was the peculiar mental attitude already referred to in this lecture. The patient was in total despair about his recovery and had even a suicidal tendency. I remember how every night, the intense scratching of the scrotum used to drive him almost to despair. The third ground for this prescription was probably the want of reactive power on the part of the patient or else why did he suffer so long and all remedies, even homœopathic ones, prescribed by responsible doctors, some of which were well indicated, failed to bring him the desired relief.

These patients suffer from abnormal appetites. They get up in the middle of the night feeling hungry and look for something to eat to satisfy their hunger. They feel hungry even after a hearty meal. Most of their symptoms vanish while they are eating to start immediately after the meal is over.

Psorinum is very useful in the treatment of tonsillitis and quinsy. Submaxillary glands are swollen, making deglutition painful. The throat is ulcerated and the patient complains of a cutting, tearing pain on swallowing; saliva is profuse and offensive; there is a great accumulation of tough mucus in the throat, necessitating hawking. The patient frequently hawks up small cheesy flakes like tiny globules and these emit an exceedingly, offensive and disgusting odor. Dr. Allen recommends **Psorinum** very highly in the treatment of quinsy. It not only ameliorates all acute symptoms but eradicates the tendency towards quinsy.

As has been already mentioned **Psorinum** has many important symptoms in the respiratory tract. We notice anxious dyspnœa with palpitation and pain in the cardiac region. This dyspnœa gets worse on sitting up, or bringing the arms nearer to the body and is better lying down. The wider apart the patient keeps his arms the better he can breathe. In this connection our attention should be drawn to **Ant. crud.**, **Led.**, and **Spig.** **Psorinum** feels the dyspnœa more in the open air and has to hurry home and lie down in order to breathe. On this important indication, Dr

Hering recommends **Psorinum** even in the state of convalescence,
in many diseases when on going out for a walk the patient
gets very tired and exhausted instead of being invigorated, and
has to **return home** to lie down to be able to breathe easily.

We also notice a dry, hard, tickling cough that returns every
winter. It is **aggravated** in the morning on waking and evening
on lying down. The sputum is solid, green and greenish-yellow.
This cough is sometimes the after-effect of a suppressed itch.
Another very striking feature is that it comes on while drinking.

Psorinum patients are usually very nervous and restless.
They get easily startled; a tired and sleepy feeling is constantly
on them. Very little labour brings on exhaustion. This exhaustion and debility are constantly on the increase. There is also a
tendency to perspiration on the slightest exertion. These patients
are usually well the day before the attack. Before this chapter
on **Psorinum** is closed, a warning is necessary. This remedy
should **not be** prescribed for psora alone or on the supposition of
psoric diathesis. As in the case of other remedies, we must be
always guided by the totality of the symptoms—although special
importance should be given to the striking, prominent and
characteristic indications.

PTELEA TRIFOLIATA.

Ptelea is commonly known as the Hop and the Wafer Ash.
It belongs to the natural order of Rutaceæ.

It is a great liver remedy and as such it should be studied in
close comparison with **Bryonia, Chelidonium, Nux vom., Mag.
mur., Podo.,** and **Mercurius.** It causes great congestion of the
liver, stomach and bowels and is generally indicated in people
with swollen liver who suffer from bitter taste in the mouth and
a dull confused frontal headache as a result of the hepatic disorder. The enlargement causes a sort of an aching distress and
a sensation of heaviness in the region of the liver. This is greatly
aggravated by lying on the left side. The patient exhibits a sort
of repugnance to animal and rich food and complains of a sensation of pressure as of a stone at the pit of stomach. The stools
are generally bilious, thin and offensive; the urine is high-colored,
yellowish-red and scalding. We also find an excess of saliva
in mouth. The pain from forehead to root of nose is characteristic.

Its resemblance to **Bryonia** consists in its amelioration on lying on the right side. The bitter taste and the peculiar thin offensive stools are common in both the remedies. But the characteristic thirst of **Bryonia,** the stitching pain due to inflammation of the peritoneal covering of the liver, the etiological factor of anger and the constant feeling of chilliness of the latter remedy are wanting in **Ptelea.** The stools of **Bryonia** have an odor of old cheese.

Chelidonium is indicated in many affections of the liver beginning from a mere congestion to a positive inflammation. The sharp stitching pain felt at the angle of right shoulder blade, the peculiar tongue taking the imprint of teeth, the craving for milk, the peculiar characteristic bright yellow or clayey stools are absent in **Ptelea.**

PULMO VULPIS.

This is a Sarcode prepared from the fox's lungs. My attention was originally drawn to this remedy by a beautiful cure reported by Dr. Grauvogl in the *Homœopathic News.*

The case in point is that of an elderly lady suffering from asthma of desperate type. She was greatly emaciated. Œdema of the lungs had taken place. Sonorous whistling and coarse rattling were audible from some distance. Heart's action was irregular and death seemed imminent. Great dyspnœa, dropsy of the legs, inability to lie down, slight almost imperceptible relief from a sitting posture and want of expectoration were some of the symptoms. **Pulmo vulpis ix** gr. il, was given and repeated in an hour. Improvement was immediately noticed. After a third dose the patient was able to lie down and she had the most refreshing and invigorating sleep lasting for hours. In eight days' time she was quite well and able to engage in her daily avocations. I have not so far used this remedy but have a mind to do so as soon as occasion arises. I hope others will make good use of this drug and report their successes and their failures to the homœopathic world to lead to a better understanding of the remedy by the profession.

PULSATILLA NIGRICANS.

There are two varieties of **Pulsatilla**, the **Pulsatilla nigricans** and the **Pulsatilla nuttaliana.** It is the former variety we are concerned with just now. It belongs to the natural order of Ranunculaceæ. In common parlance it is known as the Pasque Flower and the Wind Flower. It grows plentifully in the sunny and sandy soils of central and northern Europe. The tincture is prepared from the fresh plant when in flower by adding alcohol to the chopped and pounded pulp. This drug was first proved by our indefatigable master Samuel Hahnemann.

Pulsatilla is one of the polychrests of our Materia Medica. There is scarcely any disease where this remedy is not useful. This proves beyond doubt the wide range of its application, but as has been said of all our remedies, it is only useful when indicated.

You can mark out a **Pulsatilla** patient from a big crowd of people, for none in that large congregation will present such a phlegmonous, mild, yielding disposition as this one. She is so gentle that she can hardly say a cruel word to anybody. People very often take advantage of her sweet disposition. Say what you will to her, she is always the same forbearing, patient creature. A **Pulsatilla** wife never quarrels with her husband. She is very different from those hasty, irritable housewives that return tenfold of what they get. She is a little indecisive in her character. She keeps on brooding for hours as to what course to follow. Promptitude, dogmatism, and vehemence are traits unknown to her. This is one main reason why she is so much loved by everybody that knows her. The only fault in her character is her weeping mood. The least thing throws her off her balance. In fact she cries even when nothing has happened, or at least it is very difficult to account for the reason of her crying at all. Thus for example, when she comes to her doctor for a trivial ailment, which a patient of a more cheerful disposition would overlook, she will almost break her heart crying while telling him about it. We find such patients almost everyday in our practice. This tendency to weep is, I consider, the most important feature of the **Pulsatilla** patient. By this I don't mean that this is the only remedy we have, for lachrymal mood. There are others almost as important; but every one of them is characterised by their distinctive marks of difference.

The **Natrum mur.** patient is equally sad; but in her case the sadness is more noticeable when somebody sympathises with her in her troubles. At ordinary times she can control her tears; but when people console her for the treatment she has suffered or the loss she has sustained or the troubles she has gone through, she loses all control and out gushes the pent up whirlpool of her sadness. This great sadness is accompanied by palpitation and intermittent pulse.

Our **Lycopodium** patient is somewhat similar. It is hard for her to control her tears when she is thanked for some good office she may have performed. When she cries she cries aloud.

The lachrymal mood in **Sepia** is intermingled with great indifference. Things she used to love so much, the baby that was the apple of her eye, the husband to whom she was intensely attached—they all, in a way inexplicable to our ordinary ways of reasoning, lose every charm for her. This mood, in her case, is the reflex of her uterine complications.

Changeableness is another feature of the **Pulsatilla** temperament. Now she is happy, but the very next minute that happiness changes into misery. The mild and complacent temperament very often gives place to wild vehemence, fury and peevishness. It thus bears a resemblance to **Ignat., Nux mosch., Sarsap.** and others.

This changeableness is a general characteristic of this remedy and we find it manifested in all its symptoms. The pains are changeable and erratic. They come and go and keep changing their locations. They are now here but the very next minute they are in a different place. Another peculiarity of the pain is that it is almost always accompanied by chills—the severity of the chills being measured by the intensity of the pain. The association of these two symptoms has always been for us a great index and it has scarcely ever disappointed us. **Bovista, Colocynth** and **Dulcamara** are a few of the others we know of, with a similar association of chill with pain.

In **Bovista** the chill is intense and is accompanied by shuddering and pain. The chill is so great that the unfortunate patient is compelled to seek the warmth of a lighted stove to keep warm. Great weakness of the joints and limbs and a putty condition of the system help differentiation.

Colocynth, though similar to **Pulsatilla** in the former respect is essentially different. The intense, squeezing, cutting, griping nauseating pain, that radiates from the umbilicus to different part of the abdomen and chest, is always a guide.

Dulcamara need not be confounded with **Pulsatilla.** The pain in this remedy is almost always caused by an exposure to cold and rain.

We have strayed a bit from our topic—I mean the delineation of the mental condition of **Pulsatilla.** She is prone to menstrual irregularities and particularly at this time her mental phenomena undergo strange transformations. She becomes gloomy and morose. A sort of dread pervades her whole being—the dread of eternal damnation. The bright light of hope that leads on all human being, gets extinguished as far as she is concerned. At night the world seems to be on fire and the devil dances all round in the light of that unhallowed fire; sometimes he rushes to seize her and she screams and cries, pleading to be rescued.

Occasionally she becomes really insane, subject to the strangest hallucinations. The idea of going to bed is distasteful to her. She imagines that somebody is lying naked, warpped up in the same bed-clothes. Strange as it may seem, such symptoms are not very infrequent. We have other remedies with somewhat similar symptoms.

The **Rhus tox** patient suffers from a similar delusion—that there is somebody in bed with her who, she thinks, is driving her out of it.

Chloralum is another instance where this imaginary person stands at the foot of her bed menacing her all the time.

Euphorbium has a peculiar symptom. The patient sees somebody walking in front of him and as he looks behind, some one seems to him to be following him as well.

These symptoms may occur not in cases of insanity alone, but in delirium as well, and their curative value is very great indeed. Many astounding cures that have been wrought in homoeopathy, have been based on symptoms like these.

For ailments after grief, mortification and sorrow, **Pulsatilla** becomes often indicated, of course the other symptoms corresponding. I remember to have cured a very bad case of diarrhœa in a mild, plethoric and bashful young lady—a diarrhœa that had baffled all treatment for a short period. After many unsuccessful attempts it was brought to my notice that the diarrhœa had its origin in a quarrel that she had with her husband. The maidservant informed me that she had been crying ever since the quarrel. Other remedies to be remembered in such circumstances are **Aurum, Caust., Cocc., Gels., Ign.,** and **Staph.**

The **Pulsatilla** patient very often suffers from bad headache. It is either uterine, or neuralgic in origin. It is located in the frontal or supra-orbital region. The pain is almost stupefying. It is aggravated by mental exertion, by warmth and in the evening. When the pain is neuralgic, it is erratic in nature, wandering from one part of the head to the other. Sometimes the headache is behind one ear as if a nail were driven into the brain. The headache is relieved in the open air (**Phos., Seneg., Sep.,** and **Zinc.**) and by bandaging the head (**Arg. n., Hep. sulp., Sil.**).

There are a few other remedies with sensation as of a nail being driven into the brain and we shall discuss their relation to **Pulsatilla** presently.

In **Coffea** the headache is more of a neuralgic character. It is very severe, almost unbearable, making the patient tearful. Unlike **Pulsatilla** it is worse in the open air. It is brought on by emotional disturbance such as that caused by excessive joy, contradiction, vexation, noise, etc.

Hep. sulph. has a sensation of a nail or a plug in the head, but it is distinguishable by its great sensitiveness to touch, to other impressions of the senses and to draughts of air.

Ignatia is indicated in a similar headache in hysterical and neurasthenic subjects.

Ruta is useful for headaches produced through excessive inebriation. Meat does not agree with these patients as it causes putrid eructations.

Pulsatilla has a great affinity for all the mucous surfaces of our system and it is indicated in the catarrhal affections of the ear, nose. eyes and throat. When it affects the ear, we have a sort of deafness to start with, as if the ears were blocked up; then starts severe pain, darting. tearing and pulsating in nature. In the day time the patient is perfectly at ease; he seems to be suffering from no ailment whatsoever; but at night his troubles start and his pains become almost unbearable. At last a thick, yellow, bloody discharge takes place, giving relief to all his pains. It is also a remedy for otitis externa. The whole ear gets red and swollen.

Coming to the eyes, we find a similar catarrhal condition. The lids become swollen and itchy; the conjunctivæ become full of minute pustules and keep on discharging a bland, thick, yellow or yellowish-green secretion. This patient has a great predilection to styes, especially on the upper lids and **acne** on the face. The lids get glued together.

Very often **Pulsatilla** is our remedy for gonorrhœal ophthalmia. Fistula lachrymalis and ophthalmia neonatorum also find their remedy in **Pulsatilla** as soon as the discharge gets thick and yellow.

Pulsatilla is one of our great remedies for toothache. The pain is very severe The sensation is as if a nerve is stretched to its utmost and then all of a sudden let loose again. This tense, tearing, throbbing, jerking pain shoots into the gum every now and then and makes the eyes water. The pain gets almost unendurable towards evening and early part of the night. The patient dares not pick at her teeth; it brings on the pain and in this respect it is similar to **Sanguinaria**. It will help differentiation to remember that the gum in the latter remedy is spongy, bleeding and in a fungoid condition.

The **Pulsatilla** patient is very reluctant to enter a warm room or a warm bed for fear of the toothache; even rest brings on the pain, so she has to walk about in the open air which brings her decided relief. Other remedies, where locomotion relieves toothache, are **Magn. carb., Phos.** and **Rhus tox.**

Under **Magn. carb.,** the toothache is excrutiating while at rest; the unfortunate patient is compelled to rise from bed and walk about. It frequently starts while driving in carriage.

In **Phosphorus** too the pain comes on during rest, but it can be easily distinguished from the others by reason of one peculiarity, and that is the aggravation of the toothache from the dipping of the hands into water. Peculiar as it may seem, it is a valuable symptom; none of our remedies can lay claim to a similar symptom.

Last of all we come to **Rhus tox.** The toothache in this remedy is caused by working in damp, cold places in winter, and unlike **Pulsatilla,** the pain is relieved by external warmth.

We now come to what we consider the most important part of our remedy—we mean its relation to the diseases and ailments of the female sexual system. The menstruation under this remedy is irregular, delayed and scanty. It flows more in the day time, when walking about, than at night. We homœopaths lay great importance on the time of the flow. It means a great deal to us to know whether it flows in the day time or at night, or in the morning, noon or evening. We place an equal amount of importance on the modalities of the symptoms. In fact these particulars, however insignificant they may seem to our friends of the other school, are the ones that guide us in the selection of our remedy.

In **Causticum** we have the flow during the day only—no discharge taking place at night or when lying down. Another important point which helps differentiation is the intermittent nature of the flow. It flows and after a little while it ceases, then flows again.

Coffea again is another remedy where it flows only in the day-time; but with this distinction, that it is only towards the latter part of the day that the discharge takes place.

In **Hamamelis** the discharge of blood, which is very profuse, takes place as in **Pulsatilla** during the day. At night it ceases altogether. The flow of blood is steady, bright-red or dark-coloured. We find a great deal of dysmenorrhœa under **Hamamelis.** Severe pain is felt, mostly in the lumbar and hypogastric regions, with an accompanying soreness of the abdomen. We will next compare **Pulsatilla** with **Bovista** and **Magnesia carb.,** remedies with symptoms exactly opposite to those of **Pulsatilla.** In both these remedies the flow takes place mostly at night when lying down. It ceases immediately after getting up. Similar though they are in this respect, it is very easy to distinguish between them.

In **Bovista** the menstruation takes place every two weeks and is preceded and accompanied by diarrhœa; there is also a strong bearing down pain.

In **Magnesia carb.** on the other hand, it takes place **at night,** mostly during sleep. The blood is acrid, dark, thick, **viscid** and almost pitch-like. The menstruation is preceded by coryza, obstructed nostrils, and labour-like pains.

The menstrual discharge in **Pulsatilla** is either thick, black, clotted or thin and watery. The general characteristic feature of the remedy, we mean its changeability, also holds good here. Not two discharges are the same. The colour, the consistency, and the other accompaniments vary as well. During menses there is very often fainting. The weeping mood, the chilliness, the trembling of the legs, the nausea and vomiting, the migraine and the difficult breathing are all there to complete the picture.

Pulsatilla is also applicable in suppression of the menses. Very often young, plethoric girls do not menstruate at their wonted time and they don't take their mothers in their confidence; the result is that they become pale and chlorotic and pine away in silence. Such conditions are to be grappled with instantly, otherwise there is danger of the child running into consumption. The suppression may be due to nervous debility, chlorosis, or getting the feet wet. We must get at the cause to be able to remedy the innumerable ailments such as headache, anorexia, dysuria, ophthalmia, nausea, etc., to which the girls become subject at such times

It has been said that the woman is an organism centered around her sexual system. No statement can be truer and it should always be our policy to interrogate, whenever we get a female patient and whatever may be her trouble, about any deviation that there may be in this sphere. It will save many discomfitures to be able to discover the root-cause of women's ailments.

Leucorrhœa is another ailment to which the feminine world is subject and we believe that it is a general complaint with many of them. The leucorrhœal discharge that we find under this remedy is thick and milky-white. This leucorrhœa appears in young girls during puberty or during suppression of menses due to fright or exposure to cold and damp. Sometimes we find leucorrhœa in little children who are mere infants; we have to grapple with such circumstances when they arise and **Senecio aureus** will help us out in such cases.

Pulsatilla is a great remedy in pregnancy. It is a much better instrument in the hands of the Homœopathic physician than forceps and other scientific up-to-date mechanical devices in the possession of the most skilful accoucheur of the other school. Time without number have we rendered unnecessary, by the administration of a single dose of **Pulsatilla** or of any other indicated remedy, the aid of the obstetrician in a case of difficult labour. It needs skill indeed to drag out the fœtus from the pregnant womb, but it needs a much rarer intelligence to make an organism gifted with a self-contained impulse to act in the natural, heaven-gifted, easy way. The indicated remedy selected with much precision and care, stirs up the inert organ and brings into play its wonted action. The irregular, deficient, fitful labour pain grows in intensity and improves in character. To illustrate our point I will cite a case that Dr. Guy B. Stearns of New York City, reported in one Transactions of the International Hahnemannian Association.

" A case in point is that of a woman aged thirty-three who had five children. Every labour lasted from four to five days, and ended with forceps delivery. At the beginning of every labour there seemed to be a spasmodic contraction of the uterus without any progress towards dilatation of the os. Chloroform inhalations and all other measures failed to relax, until finally high forceps had to be used. During every pregnancy her confinement was looked forward to with added dread. Her sixth child was born under homœopathic care, and she commenced labour as she had done in the others. She sat on a chair, her teeth chattering, nervous chills running up and down her back, weeping with constant frantic and ineffectual pains and no sign of progress of the labour. Two doses of **Pulsatilla 12th** were given, fifteen minutes apart. Her chattering and chilliness ceased soon after the second dose. The pains changed their character, becoming effectual, and within two hours the woman was delivered of a normal healthy child. Her recovery was without a symptom, although all of her previous ones had been accompanied by complications."

Medical literature is replete with such instances and they prove beyond doubt the efficacy of homoeopathic remedies in hard and difficult labour.

Pulsatilla promotes expulsion of moles. It is a remedy that has to be used with great caution during pregnancy; injudiciously used it may even induce abortion. It is a remedy that we are called on to use often to prevent abortion. The flow appears every now and then during pregnancy with pains, fainting spells and craving for fresh air. I want to lay especial importance on one general characteristic of **Pulsatilla,** a characteristic that proved itself of immense value to me as well as to others. It is the association of difficult breathing with the diseased condition of parts other than the lungs. Dr. Ballard of Chicago reports of a case of abortion, during the fifth month, that he prevented by the timely administration of **Pulsatilla** on this symptom alone. **Sepia** failed him, but instead of losing courage, he took pains to examine his patient once more and noticed that every pain was accompanied by loss of breath. This was a hint on which to act. To err is human and we will make many mistakes but we can minimise them a great deal by retaining hold of cool judgment in trying and crucial cases.

Pulsatilla corrects wrong position of the foetus in the womb. There is great controversy about this point but nothing is more convincing than facts and we have facts to back us in the statement that it does do so. I will cite a case here in support of this statement from Dr. F. E. Gladwin's report in the Transactions of the International Hahnemannian Association. "The patient was thirty-four years old and this was her first child. She had been in labour about fifteen hours and there was no progress beyond the dilatation of the os; head presented L. O. A.; she was weeping, completely discouraged and begged for instruments. I gave **Pulsatilla,** and waited half an hour but still no progress and still she begged for instruments; so I went home for them. When I returned in about an hour I found the patient, nurse and mother-in-law all smiling. I said 'what's the matter, has the baby been born?' They answered 'no, but he has turned over.' I asked th patient what made her think so and she told me that after I had gone she had two tremendous pains, and it felt as though the baby had turned a somersault. She added, " You can see for yourself that the baby, which has been lying all on the one side is now lying on the other side.' That baby came breech first."

Dyspepsia is almost a general ailment now-a-days; the mode of life and the general circumstances all tend towards it. Rich food, little exercise, sedentary life and the all-engrossing hankering after gold, all point to **Pulsatilla** as the remedy for the ailment they bring on. The digestion is very slow and as a consequence the smell and taste of food remain in mouth very long. There are frequent attacks of vomitting, in which all the foods taken for days are brought out. She complains of pressure in the pit of the stomach as from a stone. This is also associated with a gnawing distress as from an ulceration in the stomach.

We have great deal of flatulence in **Pulsatilla** which rumbles and gurgles in the evening making her quite uncomfortable. Sometimes her abdomen gets so much distended with it that she is forced to unlace. This wind gives rise to a sort of colic which makes her bend double as in **Colocynth.** These conditions are generally brought about by free indulgence in ice-creams, fruits and pastries. All sorts of fat and rich foods disagree with our patient. Her tongue is coated and she is quite thirstless.

Every now and then this dyspepsia assumes acute forms and we have attacks of diarrhœa to deal with. As has been mentioned before, the stools are very changeable in character. Some stools are greenish, some bloody, some again are white. There is no depending on the color. They are different each time. Some are very offensive while others are quite odorless and so on. Very often this diarrhœa changes to constipation. It is accompanied by backache, nauseous bad taste in the mouth and irregular menstruation. The taste in the mouth feels so offensively detestable that the patient rinses his mouth several times a day but to no effect.

Nothing perhaps is fraught with so much danger as suppression of gonorrhœa. It gives rise to complications like orchitis, epididymitis, prostatitis and what not. They all find in **Pulsatilla** a very good remedy. There is great tenesmus and stinging in the neck of the bladder. A pressure is also felt on bladder which gives rise to an ineffectual desire to pass water. Sometimes we meet with hæmaturia. In troubles like these arising from suppression of gonorrhœa we may also think of :—

Argent. nit. in which remedy too as a result of the suppression, the testicles become quite enlarged and indurated. Each urination is accompanied by excessive boring and cutting pain extending clear up to the anus· The discharge, if any, is purulent and excoriating.

Erechthites too has orchitis during gonorrhœa.

Sarsaparilla claims an exactly similar symptom, but the distinctive points are the great swelling of the spermatic cord, much sexual excitement, eruptions on skin and a history of abuse of mercury.

It is hard for the **Pulsatilla** patient to retain the urine. It spurts out on the least movement or strain; she is afraid therefore to go out into company. She soils her clothes even while she is sitting or walking. She is afraid to cough, sneeze or laugh It is a hard job for her to keep clean· Life such as she leads, is wretched indeed. This symptom also reminds us of **Nat. mur. Sep., Caust., Squil**. and **Ferr. met.**

Much has been said and a great deal has been vaunted of the efficacy of quinine in the treatment of malarial fevers. Quinine in great number of cases in which it is prescribed, only check the fever. The reason for which it is such a general favourite with the average run of our physicians, is, that it needs no skill and very little intelligence to prescribe quinine. This tempts even physician of our school to prescribe quinine. To prescribe the right homœopathic remedy requires consummate intelligence, great power of observation, penetrating discrimination and elaborate study, but once the right remedy is prescribed it dispels for ever the ailing incubus of the tortured patient· I know of a homœo pathic physician who, lacking in points that guarantee success got dissatisfied with Homœopathy to cure " chills " and went over to quinine. The result was that all his cases kept on coming back time after time with the recurrence of the disease. Then at last the truth dawned on him; he went back to his own system and gave it the study it deserved and now he is a staunch homœopath.

Pulsatilla is an invaluable agent in the treatment of such fever thus suppressed. Really speaking **Pulsatilla** is good for all types of fevers—simple and compound, quotidian, tertian and quartan. has both morning and evening paroxysms though the evening or at 4 p.m. is predominant. The attack is mostly always preceded by gastric disturbances such as diarrhœa, nausea, vomiting, etc The broad and the large tongue is coated white or yellow and covered over with a tenacious mucus. The statement that I have previously made regarding changeability of symptoms also holds good here. No two paroxysms are alike; the stages of chill, heat and sweat run into each other presenting different aspect on each separate paroxysm. The chill starts at 4 p.m. with vomiting mucus and dyspepsia. The chilliness is flitting in nature; is now here but a while after, the parts feel hot and he feels chilly in a different place. Sometimes it is only one-sided with numbness on the other side.

The next stage is that of heat. It is quite an anxious and an uneasy time with our patient. He feels as if hot water is dashed over him. His hands, his feet and his whole body burn like fire and like our **Sulphur** patient, he is constantly in search of a cold spot. External warmth is intolerable and he complains of the room being too hot and stuffy and wants all the doors and the windows open. The veins are quite distended and his face is red. There is a symptom that may easily mislead us. On entering the sick room we notice that one check of our patient is red and the other pale and we may jump to **Chamomilla** and **Aconite.** They are not the only remedies with such a symptom. **Pulsatilla** has an equal right to it.

Even before the stage of heat is over, sweat appears like beads of pears on the face trickling down in great abundance. Sometimes the sweat is one-sided like the chill. It is worse in the evening and night and during sleep. As soon as the patient wakes up, the sweat stops. This is exactly the reverse of what we find in **Sambucus.** All night long he perspires and his sleep is more like a stupefied slumber. It does not refresh him at all in the morning. All throughout the night in that disturbed, stuporous slumber the **Sambucus** patient talks much.

Now a few words about the thirst of **Pulsatilla.** The general belief of thirstlessness as characteristic of **Pulsatilla** is liable to lead many into errors when it comes to the treatment of fevers. The morning paroxysms are almost always attended with thirst during the entire attack, while the evening paroxysm at 4 p.m. is generally free from thirst.

There is another axiom that we can lay down which is worth our while to remember. If the heat that follows chill, is merely objective it is attended by thirst.

Sometime ago I treated a case of typhoid fever with **Pulsatilla.** The patient, an elderly gentleman of 60, started with chill, headache and backache early one morning. There were great thirst, rest-

lessness, and pain in the chest. Ere long gastric symptoms mani
fested themselves in the form of loose stools and loud empty
eructations. Gradually his consciousness ebbed away and he begar
to spit blood complaining of a very severe pain in the right chest
His pulse was very variable ranging from 90 to 120. In a shorr
while the pain changed its location and character shifting to the
region between the scapulæ and manifesting itself like "stabs'
which elicited painful shrieks from the patient. He had **Acon.
Bellad., Phos.** and a few other remedies but the patient steadily
kept on getting worse.

The delirium became quite marked; he wanted to get out o
bed and run away and saw all kinds of strange fantasies. Th
pain in the meantime had again shifted to the region of th
liver and this time it was like twists.

Taking the case over again .I determined to pay greater im
portance to the vacillation of symptoms. **Pulsatilla** seemed to b
the presiding genius of the case and it was prescribed and th
patient made a steady recovery.

Pulsatilla has a decided prostatic enlargement, so that th
fæces passed are long and flat like ribbons. This is a complair
generally met with in elderly people, with a taint of gonorrhœa
history.

These patients are afraid to lie down; immediately after doin
so they are seized with an irresistible desire to pass water, owin
to the pressure of urine on the neck of the bladder. This desir
they are afraid to satisfy, as micturition is followed by spasmod
pain in the neck of the bladder extending into pelvis and dov
the thighs.

Pulsatilla is an important remedy in rheumatism. The pai
as I have said before, is flitting in character and is attended l
chilliness. It is very similar to **Rhus tox** in its modalities. T
aggravation takes place at night, when at rest in bed and wh
rising after sitting long.

The remedy that is very similar to **Pulsatilla** is **Kali sulph.**
the latter remedy the pain which shifts and changes is alike wor
in warm rooms and in the evening.

Case 1.—Suppression of urinary and lochial secretions; cold perspirati
over the whole body; eyes swollen; hands and wrists cold; could ؛
discern any person; head felt too full, or as if the skull was lifted up; wr
she closed her eyes she saw pictures and all sorts of strange sights; he
all kinds of operatic airs; had to lie constantly on her back; complains
labor-like pains, compelling her to press downward, considered herself dyi

Puls. 200. A large quantity of retained spurious liquor amnii was discharged with relief of all the symptoms.—Dr. Lippe.

Case 2.—T., aged twenty-five, dark complexion, black hair, 12th of December stated that he had felt unwell for some weeks, had no appetite, frequent headaches, and occasional pains in the abdomen. **Nux vom.** 40m. Saw him evening of December 14th. Had been confined to his bed all day; the pains in the abdomen had gradually increased, were constant, with periodical increase of them, and he was then relieved by very profuse vomiting of a green substance (bile), with much transparent mucus, and finally at the close of these attacks of vomiting, a gulping up of a few mouthfuls of bright red blood; abdomen felt sore when touched; no stool for some days; urine scanty; the past twenty-four hours had passed about four ounces of dark red urine; no thirst; mouth dry and clammy; tongue clean; pulse small and hard, eighty; found no relief in any position, but had to draw in his abdomen, as any attempt to stretch himself increased the pains. **Puls.** 50 m. December 15 had a sleepless night; had vomited less often, and no more blood had been gulped up at the cessation of vomiting; pulse was softer; urinary secretions increased; pain in abdomen not severe; the tenderness to touch continued. Day by day he grew better, the pain diminished, the urine became more abundant and cloudy, but he did not sleep, no appetite; no thirst; no movement from the bowels. December 21, took some beef tea, which brought back the pain in the abdomen, **Puls.** 75m relieved him. December 28, not so well **Puls.** cm. and he made a rapid recovery.—Dr A. Lippe.

PYROGEN.

Pyrogen is a nosode, the importance of which it is not possible to over-rate. It is a product of sepsis, as Dr. Allen describes it. It is prepared from beef decomposed in water.

Like **Baptisia** to which it bears great resemblance it is characterised by offensiveness of all the discharges of the body. The stools, the sweat and the other excretions are rendered prominent by this carrion-like smell.

The next feature is a great soreness of the body, in consequence of which, the bed on which they lie down seems hard and uncomfortable. They keep on moving constantly in search of a soft place and a comfortable position. It thus resembles **Arnica, Eupatorium, Rhus tox, Baptisia, Ruta, Medorrhinum** and **Ipecac.**

It is the first remedy to be thought of in a case of septicemia, either puerperal or surgical or from any other cause. It also occupies an important place in every case of blood-poisoning, be it from diphtheria, typhoid, typhus, or any other malignant disease to which human flesh is subject. But as has been emphasized so often we as homœopaths must always look to the totality of symptoms in every case.

Chills that invariably accompany sepsis are another striking feature of **Pyrogen.** They begin mostly in the back between the scapulæ and are very severe, extending deep down to the bones. They seem to bear the patient down and crush life out of him. Sudden rise of temperature, intensely dry burning skin, an abnormally rapid but weary pulse—a pulse that is entirely out of proportion to the temperature of the body, a vacant agonised look, are sure indications of **Pyrogen.**

The appearance of the tongue should not be overlooked. It is large, flabby, lifeless, smooth and shiny as if varnished; it is dry, cracked and fiery red. Articulation is difficult. Taste is sweetish, fetid and puslike. Vomiting is frequent and distressing. The substance brought out is brownish, coffee-ground, offensive and stercoraceous. Stools are painless, offensive and involuntary.

In **Pyrogen** we find complete inertia of the bowels as in **Opium** and **Sanicula.** The rectum becomes glutted with large black hard balls which are extremely offensive and the stools are expelled with great straining often needing manual help.

Dr. J. H. Hunt reports of having cured many cases of varicose ulcerations with **Pyrogen** that refused to heal under other drugs. Bellairs cured with **Pyrogen** a long-standing case of ulcerated leg where **Hepar sulph., Silicea** and other analogous drugs had failed. These facts sufficiently vindicate the truth of Dr. Allen's famous statement—" When the best selected remedy fails to relieve or permanently improve, **Pyrogen** is indicated."

With **Pyrogen,** if administered at the proper time, threatened typhoid can be averted. Numerous cases are on record—cases that were diagnosed as typhoid—which instead of running through a proper course, were definitely cut short with **Pyrogen.** We think of this also in fevers caused by sewer gas poisoning, surgical infections, dissecting wounds, blood-poisoning or absorption of pus. Following cases reported by various medical authorities are very instructive and convincing.

Case 1.—A young German Jewess after a protracted ailment, during which she had been at various medical institutions for treatment, was ultimately placed in the hand of Dr. T. M. Dellingham. Her case was diagnosed as Brights' disease, as most of her symptoms pointed towards it. Her urine was full of albumen and casts. Her feet, legs, and face were swollen and puffy. Throbbing headache, nose bleeding and vomiting, were some of her symptoms. Many remedies were prescribed but the effect was unsatisfactory. On coming to know that the trouble dated from a very large abscess which was badly lanced and cared for, and finding that most of her symptoms started from that date, the doctor gave **Pyrog. cm.** Soon after improvement started, but it took fully five months before she was absolutely cured.

Case 2.—N. B., child 4 years old, resided in a house in which plumbing was being repaired. A few days after was attacked at 2 a.m. with vomiting and purging; stools profuse and watery. Cold extremities, ears and nose; forehead bathed in cold perspiration. Tongue heavily coated, yellowish-gray; edges and tip very red. Great prostration. Great restlessness, mental and physical; pulse 140, small and wiry; temperature 99°. Great thirst for small quantities, but the smallest quantity was instantly rejected. Later in day stool was horribly offensive, of a carrion-like odor; face pale, sunken, bathed in cold perspiration. Tongue dark red and free from the heavy coating of early morning, intense thirst, but water aggravates both vomiting and purging. After **Ver., Ars., Carbo v.** and **Bap.** had been given, with no improvement, the patient evidently sinking, impossible to count the pulse, thinking perhaps sewer-gas poison may have been the factor, and the clean, fiery red tongue called my attention to Dr. Burnett's cures in the Homœopathic World with **Pyrogen.** I gave two doses dry on the tongue with prompt and permanent relief.—Dr. Allen.

Case 3.—An old woman dying with gangrene inoculated one of her nurses; the nurse had chills, high fever and red streaks running up the arm following the course of the lymphatics. **Pyrogen** rapidly removed the whole process.—Dr. Boger.

On the female sexual system its usefulness is very great. We use it in puerperal fever with offensive lochia. It is also thought of in septicæmia following abortion specially when fœtus of secundines are retained and the decomposed inside emitting horrible odour. The following cases reported by Dr. Wakeman illustrate our point.

Case 1.—Mrs. T. B., pale, slender, delicate, but in good health; primipara; was successfully delivered April 10th, 1901. On the 20th found her with a temperature of 102°; lochia scanty, pale, offensive; but she felt well and had no pain. Fever increased in severity gradually for several days, until temperature reached 105° and 106°, with a pulse of 120-130; still she insisted she felt well and would not go to bed. Several remedies, **Bapt., Bell., Ech., Tar.,** were given without effect. Finally a severe shaking chill followed in a few hours by another sent her to bed, and the nurse was recalled. **Pyrogen** was given. Following day temperature was 102°; lochia reappeared in natural colour; the abdominal sensitiveness ceased and in two or three days disappeared entirely. She rapidly recovered.

Case 2.—Mrs. W. S. C., a slender woman; primipara; delivered June 10th, 1896 instrumental. Severe perineal laceration, which was repaired. The morning of the third day had ague; cutting spasmodic pain in uterus, which was swollen and sensitive; lochia dark, profuse, clotted; both iliac region sensitive to pressure, aggravation on left side. **Bell.** gave no relief. **Fever** continued to rise; lochia darker, more offensive, containing threads and clots. The odour and other symptoms indicating approaching sepsis, she received **Pyrogen** with very gratifying results, and a rapid recovery.

Case 3.—Carrie, aged 16 years had been sick two or three months and was under allopathic care. Breath, perspiration, expectoration, menses, urine and fæces horribly offensive, carrion-like; disgust up to nausea about an effluvia that arises from her own body; soreness of the chest and abdomen, menses last but one day and a sanguineous leuchorrhœa, that is of the same odour; pulse 106, with a bad cough, worse coming into a warm room; large, fleshy, pale, greenish or chlorotic face, mother having just died of consumption. **Pyrogen cm.,** one dose, and better in ten hours, and on November 12th cough, odour and soreness nearly all gone; pulse 80, tongue clean. **Sac. Lac.** was continued till she became quite well.

The mental symptoms of **Pyrogen** are many and important. She is inclined to talk all the time during fever, and sometimes talks so fast that it is difficult to follow her. She becomes delirious on closing her eyes; sees men at the foot of the bed.

The following are some of the symptoms that will well repay us to remember and use when the proper time comes:—

Sensation as if she covers the whole bed; knew her head was on the pillow but did not know where the rest of her body was. She feels when lying on one side that she is one person and that when she turns to the other side she is another person; sensation as though she was crowded by arms and legs; as soon as fever came on, she commenced urinating; redness of the face and also of ears as if blood would burst through them; hallucination that she is wealthy.

RADIUM BROMIDE.

The place of **Radium** in the homœopathic therapeutics indicates the progressive nature of the system of treatment. We are keeping up with all the modern inventions of science but we have not deflected from our principle of Similia Similibus Curantur. **Radium** was first discovered in 1898 by Prof. and Madam Curie of Paris. Pure radium is a white metal which oxidizes in water, burns paper, turns black on exposure to air and has the property of adhering to iron. As it is almost impossible to obtain it in the pure form, compounds of radium, especially the compound known as Radium bromide is commonly in use. They give off heat and thus raise the temperature of surrounding bodies. They give off light of which the rays penetrate opaque substances such as lead, gold, silver, aluminium etc. They also give off gas or emanations. These emanations are found in large amount in the rays of the sun and the heat of the sun is believed to be due to enormous deposits of radium in that body. They have also the property of rendering other substances radio-active while brought into contact with them. **Radium** is found in deposits in Bohemia, Cornwall, Portugal, Colerado and California. The richest source of radium is the mineral known as the Pitchblende, an impure oxide of uranium. The purity of radium is determined by the relation of its radio-activity as compared to that of uranium. For homœopathic purposes we triturate **Radium bromide** of the highest radio-activity obtainable. The proving of this drug was done by Drs. J. H. Clarke of London, William H. Dieffenbach and Von der Goltz of New York.

The most important action of **Radium** is seen over the skin and this remarkable agent has been largely used with varying degrees of success in various lesions of the skin such as keloids, nævi, pigmented moles, urethral carbuncle, epithelioma, lupus vulgaris, papilloma, fibroma, sarcoma and carcinoma.

Radium increases the polymorphonuclear neutrophiles. These cells act like so many police men of the blood corpuscles by attacking the invading bacteria and destroying them, hence an increase in their number means a greater resisting power of the vitality. The allopaths use it indiscriminately in every case where surgery portends trouble and operation is deemed inadvisable. The two important points of radio-therapy according to our allopathic brethren consist in the duration of application and the dose. If applied for a short time **Radium** stimulates, if for number of hours it produces paralysis. It has been also observed that small doses stimulate while large doses inhibit cellular activity. In the treatment of malignant growths it is used in overwhelming dose to destroy the nuclei of recalcitrant cells. In some cases a little while after the infection, severe chill with chattering of teeth intervenes, followed by rapid action of the heart and gradual rise of temperature; the higher the fever and the longer the pyrexia the better was the resulting action on malignant tissue. That this is a short-sighted principle and based on a narrow inadequate and fallacious theory of the human system, is amply proved by innumerable cases of failures of radio-therapy in malignant cases.

Here as in other remedies the best principle consists in Similia Similibus Curantur, a principle which rarely fails if strictly adhered to. Drs. Copeland, Crump, Sayre and Stearns have warned against the use of the sixth potency as it is too strong and produces overwhelming aggravations. They recommend the twelfth potency.

The following are a few trustworthy symptoms of **Radium** that will rarely fail if utilized on Hahnemann's principle:—

Severe pain over the entire body making him restless; tossing about relieves the pain; entire body feels as if fire with needle pricks or electric shocks is all over the body; anxiety; fear, apprehension; a feeling as if something is going to happen; fear of being alone in the dark.

Vertigo when rising; when on feet tendency to fall on to the left side and has to support himself. Vertigo better lying down, after a warm bath, on going into open air; worse getting up.

A peculiar metallic taste in mouth with increased salivation. Parched dry sensation in roof of mouth, better from drinking small amount of cold water.

Dysuria during the day; had to wait sometimes before the urine came; brick-dust sediment in urine; faint trace of albumen in urine; granular and hyaline casts in urine; tight constricting sensation about the heart better in open air; sharp pain in the region of the heart, better by walking.

Succession of small boils on forehead and chest; scaly eruption on anterior surface of the right eye; scaly circumscribed eruption on flexure side of the forearm, worse scratching, better dry heat and open air.

Chronic Radio-dermatitis on both hands; eczematous eruptions, cracks and fissures; scaly excrescences that itch and burn most violently.

Shock passes through body during sleep like electric shocks.

Dream of passing urine; dream of comitting suicide in some ridiculous way; awake with fear of being alone and wish for some one to be near; the dreams are vivid and it takes some long time for the patients to realise that visions are not true. During night they awake in the midst of a dream panting as though running with heart pounding like a hammer.

RANA BUFO.

(*See* **Bufo.**)

RANUNCULUS BULBOSUS.

The tincture is prepared from the plant Bittercup. It belongs to the natural order of Ranunculaceæ. The juice of this plant is highly excoriating and irritating to the skin where it gives rise to vesicle, pemphigus, herpes and in extreme cases flat ulcerations. We will discuss its indications in skin diseases later on.

It also has very strong action over the mucous membranes. It produces smarting from eyes as from smoke. There is also a similar smarting in nose and fauces; the eyes run and are painful; mucus runs in torrents from the nose; it thus becomes an important remedy in hay fever. Almost all the symptoms of **Ranunculus** are aggravated towards the evening. The patient complains of a sensation of pressure at the root of nose with tingling and crawling sensation within its cavity. This sensation also extends to posterior nares, causing the patient to hawk and a desire to scratch the affected part. In this respect **Rununculus** should be studied in comparison with **Aconite, Arsenic, Euphrasia, Allium cepa** and **Sambucus.**

Its action on the serous membrane, however, is more important. It causes inflammation, particularly of the pleura or peritoneum, where it sets up acute stabbing pains, accompanied by an effusion of serum into the serous sacs. Thus like **Apis,** and **Bryonia** it becomes an important remedy in pleurisy and pleurodynia. The pains in **Ranunculus** are sharp, stitching and shooting; they come in paroxysms and are also induced by atmospheric changes and sudden exposure to cold. The aggravation, from wet and stormy weather and from touch and motion, is particularly guiding. The patient experiences pressure and tightness across lower part of chest, with fine stitches. This is aggravated on moving, stooping or taking an inspiration. On these indications, it may be prescribed in diaphragmitis, pleurisy, hydrothorax and even in adhesions left after pneumonia and pleuritis. Great soreness is experienced below nipple on taking a deep breath. The sensation is as if something is tearing inside. The pain radiates from the affected area over the whole chest. Even the external surface of the chest becomes sensitive to touch.

We will next consider its application in affections of the muscles. It is particularly indicated in rheumatism of the muscles of the trunk; it is regarded almost a specific in intercostal rheumatism. There is usually great deal of soreness to touch and the whole area feels as if it is bruised and pounded, same as in **Aconite, Arnica** and **Bryonia.**

Ranunculus bulbosus is particularly useful in herpes zoster. Vesicles of dark bluish appearance appear on the skin and soon get inflated with serum. The part looks as if it has suffered from burns. These vesicles are more prone to appear along the course of the supraorbital or intercostal nerves. In this respect it is very similar to **Rhus tox., Arsenicum** and **Mezereum.**

Ranunculus is equally applicable in pemphigus. The blisters are usually large; some of them being as big as four inches in diameter. As the blisters burst they expose raw surfaces underneath, which keep on secreting a foul-smelling, gluey matter. The ulcers of **Ranunculus,** as has been hinted at before, are flat and are attended with great deal of stinging pain.

Ranunculus is one of the most effective remedies we have, for the removal of the bad effects of alcoholic beverages, such as hiccough, epileptiform spasms, delirium tremens etc.

RAPHANUS SATIVUS.

This is the wild radish. It belongs to the natural order oi Cruciferæ. The tincture is prepared from fresh root immediately before flowering and also from the whole plant. This is one of our new remedies.

My experience with **Raphanus** is very limited; it has given me great satisfaction in incarcerated flatus. It is a flatus that does not pass either upward or downward but continues torturing the patient. Some little while ago I was called in to treat an old man who took ill very suddenly. I found him restless, writhing and gasping from excessive accumulation of incarcerated flatus. His abdomen had become greatly swollen, hard and painful to pressure. Vomiting and purging which continued long instead of bringing him relief as expected, made him worse. **Raphanus** cured him.

Great rumblings and gurglings are heard in abdomen particularly at night time. The pains come in paroxysm. It is partially relieved by eating, hence he is obliged to eat all the time during colic. The stools are brown or yellow-brown and are extremely fluid. They are expelled with much force, as in **Gambogia** and **Croton tig.**

Raphanus has marked action on the female sexual system. We use it in hysteria specially when associated with pain in uterus and titillation in genitals forcing her to onanism. The sensation of globus hystericus is also present. A round hot foreign body starting from the fundus of uterus stops at the entrance of the throat and chokes her. As regards nymphomania **Raphanus** ranks equal with **Gratiola** and **Origan.** Great sexual excitement starting in the morning and continuing unceasingly till 11 p.m. is noticed. This brings on a sort of sexual insomnia. The irritation in the sexual organs keeps her awake far into the night. **Raphanus** cures the insomnia by putting a stop to the irritant which is the root cause of the trouble.

Mentally **Raphanus** patient is characterised by a great dislike to her own sex. This is illustrated by her antipathy towards her daughters amongst all her children. She also displays great aversion towards other women. The touch of a woman's hand brings about disgust, fury and capriciousness.

A wider application will lead to better knowledge of the remedy.

RATANHIA.

The **Ratanhia** tincture is prepared from the roots of Krameria triandra, a plant growing in dry argillaceous and sandy soils of Peru. The colour of the tincture is blood-red. It is a great astringent and a styptic and is consequently used in passive hemorrhages. This astringent property of the drug is manifested in the proving by a peculiar contracting sensation as experienced in the stomach, throat, anus, eyes and other parts. This is not an oft-used remedy but its indications are definite and clear-cut. The sphere in which its efficacy has been mostly demonstrated is the fissure of the anus. This is a very distressing complaint. The patient suffers the agonies of death. The anus burns like fire, not only during defecation but also before and after. After each stool he feels as if splinters of glass were sticking in every direction in anus and rectum. Sometimes the straining for stool is so very great that defecation is accompanied by protrusion of hemorrhoids. This burning for hours after each stool is a characteristic symptom, and is only relieved by the application of hot water. One patient whom **Ratanhia** helped had this modality very well marked. He had to sit for hours in a sitz-bath as hot as he could endure to get relief from the intense burning pain. As has been said before, there is quite a bit of constricting sensation in the rectum. The stools are forced with great effort and the anus aches and burns for hours after the stool.

As regards the fissure of the anus we may compare **Ratanhia** to **Æsculus, Nitric acid, Pæonia** and **Thuja.** In all these remedies we find the rectum greatly affected but they have all their distinguishing features.

In **Æsculus** the rectum feels full of small sticks, very much the same as in **Ratanhia** but there is in **Æsculus** the sensation of fullness, dryness and heat in the rectum with severe dull pain in the lumbo-sacral articulation.

Nitric acid too has the sensation of splinters and constriction in the rectum; this remedy should have preference when there is a syphilitic base underlying the constitution.

Pæonia has fissures with much oozing, due to ulceration of the mucous membrane of rectum and anus. The parts are swollen, offensive and moist all the time.

I have forgotten to mention that this tendency for fissures and cracks, is also noticeable in the nipples in nursing women.

Ratanhia is reported to have cured pterygium and twitching of the eyelids. Rummel relates the case of an unlucky girl whose right eyelid used to twitch so very badly as to prevent proper vision. **Ratanhia** cured her permanently.

Ratanhia has a peculiar toothache. The molars feel elongated with sensation as if ice cold air rushes out of them. It is also of great use in toothache during the early months of pregnancy. It is so intolerable as to make our patient get out of bed and walk about. This makes **Ratanhia** very similar to **Magnesia carb.** Dr. Farrington mentions of how a New York doctor unable to cure such a case with **Magnesia carb.** called Dr. Lippe in consultation, who suggested **Ratanhia**, which proved effective. For toothache during pregnancy we can also remember **Chamomilla, Lyssin, Nux mosch., Pulsat., Raphanus, Sepia** and **Staphisagria.**

Ratanhia is said to be a good remedy for pin-worms. Cushing reports great success with it in such cases.

RHEUM.

Rheum is our everyday Rhubarb that grows so plentifully in China from which country it is exported to all parts of the world. The medicine is prepared from the powdered root. It was proved by Samuel Hahnemann.

It is an indispensable remedy, the importance of which it is hardly possible to over-rate. The leading keynote of this remedy is sourness—a sourness that pervades the whole system and characterises all the discharges and exhalations of the body. The stools are sour; the sweat is sour; the taste of the mouth is sour; even the temper is sour. It is a sourness from which there is no escape. Wash the **Rheum** child however much you like, the sour smell will not leave him. From his sweat his pillow and bedsheet smell sour. The milk that he vomits up becomes curdled from the excessive sourness of the stomach. Mentally he is impatient and vehement, ugly and impossible to satisfy. He screams, kicks and makes himself decidedly unpleasant. In appearance too, he is quite sour-looking. There is occasional twitching of the eyelids and the corners of his mouth that gives him the appearance of frowning.

The next characteristic symptom of **Rheum** is the sweat. It is constant and profuse, on scalp, fore-head, face, mouth and nose. In respect of this sweat we may well compare **Rheum** with **Calc. carb., Sanicula, Magn. mur., Silicea** and **Ammon. mur.** It is present whether he is asleep or awake, quiet or in motion. A sopping wet head, associated with night-screaming, is particularly characteristic of our remedy. We must not also forget the symptom of excessive accumulation of offensive mucus in mouth after sleep. There is also a desire for various kinds of food which become repugnant as soon as a little is eaten. In this connection let it be mentioned that the whims and fancies of **Rheum** are quite conspicuous. The restlessness and irritability are as marked as in **Cina** and **Antim. crud.,** but unlike those remedies, the **Rheum** patients find temporary satisfaction after their whims are gratified.

It is a capital remedy for diarrhœa and disordered stomach in children, arising out of eating unripe fruit. The stools are brown slimy, loose, thin, curdled, sour-smelling and fermented; it corrodes the anus. Sometimes it is whitish but turns green on being left on the diaper exposed to the air. During stool there are chilliness and cutting constricting pain in abdomen—a pain that stiffens him and makes him scream most violently. The evacuations are also accompanied by shivering followed by renewed urging There is also cutting colic in the umbilical region. It is so violen that the patient is doubled up with it. Another strange charac teristic about this colic is that it is invariably worse by uncovering either arm or leg.

Rheum has a few urinary symptoms of consequence. Due t great weakness of the bladder, we meet with difficult micturition A great deal of pressure is required to expel the accumulate urine from the inert bladder. It is invaluable in stupor of childre during dentition, associated with distended abdomen, the result c accumulation of urine in the bladder. The pale face covered wit cold sweat, the sopping wet head, twitching of lips, eye-lids ar fingers and above all the peculiar characteristic **Rheum** smell a symptoms that will never lead us astray.

RHODODENDRON.

Rhododendron chrysanthum is an evergreen shrub found growing largely on the mountain tops of Siberia. The tincture is prepared from the dried leaves of this plant. It belongs to the natural order of Ericaceæ. It is also called the Snow-rose.

This remedy deserves a place in our Materia Medica by reason of its extensive application in rheumatic and gouty complaints, and in indurations of testicles due to exposure. The most characteristic indication for **Rhododendron** consists in its aggravation before thunderstorm. It is not so much due to the damp as to the electrical changes in the atmosphere. Toothache, stiffneck, lumbago, neuralgia and many other complaints of **Rhododendron** grow worse by the approach of the thunderstorm. In this respect it resembles **Natrum carb., Phosphorus, Psorinum** and **Silicea.**

Another modality of **Rhododendron** consists in its aggravation during rest and amelioration from motion. Thus it is like **Rhus tox.,** but in **Rhododendron** the pain is felt more in the periosteum and the deeper structures than in **Rhus tox.**

Rhododendron is characterised by great loss of memory. He omits words while writing. We also find sudden vanishing of thoughts. This is manifested by sudden stoppage while in the act of talking; he often desists while in conversation, to enable himself to recall the trend of his thoughts. Although this forgetfulness is nothing compared to the loss of memory as found in **Anacardium** and **Acid phos.,** it becomes quite confusing. Furthermore, it is associated with great deal of vertigo which occurs mostly while lying in bed and is ameliorated by moving about. An intense degree of tinnitus aurium complicates the vertigo.

We will now talk about its application in diseases of the scrotum for which it is such an excellent remedy. Most of its fame arises out of its efficiency in subduing orchitis, both chronic and acute, the result either of suppression of gonorrhœa or of exposure to cold. The testicles become retracted, enlarged and very sensitive to touch. Sharp dragging pains are felt all along the course of the spermatic cord. Even when the acuteness subsides and induration gives way to atrophy, we may still think of **Rhododendron.** The feeling in the gland is as if it were being crushed. It relieves the fever accompanying orchitis and gradually brings in resolution. The pains are worse by touch and sitting up and ameliorated by moving about. It may be so intense at times as to arrest breathing.

The rheumatic swellings of **Rhododendron** are migratory, wandering from joint to joint and from limb to limb. The pains are brought on by damp, cold and wet weather. They mostly affect the small joints. It is particularly important in gouty affection of the great toe-joint. There is usually a fibrous deposit in the affected part. The pains are drawing and tearing in character and are felt in the periosteum. It also affects ligaments of small joints. Like **Causticum, Rhododendron** abounds in arthritic nodes.

Toothache of **Rhododendron** occurs during every change of weather and is accompanied by earache. It is worse at night time and better from application of heat.

RHUS AROMATICA.

Rhus aromatica is a non-poisonous shrub growing from two to six feet high on rocky soils. The medicine is prepared from the bark of the root. It belongs to the natural order of Anacardiaceæ.

My experience with this remedy is very limited but still it deserves a place in our Materia Medica by reason of its great fame as a remedy for diabetes. The urine is pale and albuminous. The quantity of urine passed is very great as in **Acid phos.** and **Acetic acid.** It is frequently characterised by great incontinence due probably to atony of the bladder muscles; hence it is thought of in senile incontinence which it helps to a great extent. We are greatly indebted to Dr. McClanahan who made extensive use of this remedy and cured quite a few cases of diabetes, some of which had gone very far. A case, particularly interesting, is that of a middle-aged lady who contracted diabetes mellitus and became extremely weak due to frequent passing of large quantities of urine, of high specific gravity. Extreme thirst, backache, slight rise of temperature, cough with night sweats and occasional attacks of diarrhœa reduced her to an extreme state of debility. **Rhus arom.** in half teaspoonful doses, every four hours, brought about a speedy and a steady diminution in the quantity of urine passed, till at last the patient was declared thoroughly cured. Numerous other cures of like nature have been reported by other physicians. It, therefore, behoves us to give it a more thorough proving and put it on a more scientific basis.

It has been recommended in painful micturition of children. Like **Lyco.** and **Sarsaparilla,** it has severe pain at the beginning of urination.

Dr. McClanahan also recommends it in hæmorrhages from kidneys, bladder and uterus. Whenever any such discharge is the result of an atonic condition, **Rhus aromatica** should be given due consideration; it is thus a great hemostat. Dr. J. A. McKey relates a case of severe uterine hemorrhage that he stopped with **Rhus aromatica** after all other means had failed. The patient was passing large clots of blood and the condition was getting desperate, till the patient was almost desanguinated. The first dose of **Rhus aromatica** checked the flow which had ceased entirely after the second dose.

RHUS GLABRA.

This plant, also called Smooth Sumach, belonging to the natural order of Anacardiaceæ, is prepared from the astringent bark of the deciduous shrub. This medicine was proved by Dr. A. V. Marshall, on himself with very substantial doses. The most important symptom obtained was a sensation of extreme weakness as found in **China.** This weakness is associated with profuse perspiration. It is **highly** recommended in occipital headache, specially when it is associated with epistaxis. Another symptom worth noting is that these patients are subject to a peculiar dream, as though flying through the air.

RHUS TOXICODENDRON.

This plant is known by various names such as Mercury-vine, Poison-ash, Poison-oak and Poison-vine. It differs from Rhus radican or the poison-ivy in that it is comparatively dwarfish. This shrub grows in fields, woods and along fences in America and Europe. It grows to a height of one to three feet. The plant is very poisonous and should be handled carefully. The fresh leaves are collected after sun-set on a cloudy day from shady places and chopped and pounded and then mixed with alcohol in proportion of 1 to 2 and then filtered and strained. The tincture contains Rhoi-tannic acid and Toxico-dendric acid, two poisonous volatile prin ciples. Night and dampness favour the exhalations of Toxico-dendric acid; hence the above conditions are recommended as being suitable factors in the collection and preparation of the drug.

This remedy rightly deserves an important place in the list of our polychrest remedies. It affects the fibrous tissues very powerfully and is adapted to persons of rheumatic diathesis. We find it useful whenever tendons, ligaments, aponeuroses and connective tissues are inflamed either due to over-exertion or to exposure. It causes erethism, the result of increased circulation in the affected area. Here as in other remedies, the peculiar and characteristic symptoms stand out prominent and our attention is naturally drawn to them.

The first and the foremost feature of **Rhus tox** is the amelioration of all symptoms from continual motion.

The second characteristic feature is the great sensitiveness to open air and to all atmospheric changes; when the sky become cloudy he puts on a warm garment as an act of precaution Exposure to least draft or cold brings on a general aggravation of all the symptoms and getting wet of course is an extrme penalty In this our remedy resembles **Aconite, Bryonia, Dulcamara, Hepa sulph., Colchicum, Psorinum, Rhododendron** and **Tuberculinum** This sensitiveness to cold is so extreme that even when a par of the body is exposed, the troubles are aggravated immensely.

In **Aconite** and **Bryonia** we find aggravation from exposur to cold dry air.

In **Colchicum** and **Dulcamara** the aggravation is noticed fro exposure to cold damp air.

Hepar, Psorinum and **Tuberculinum** are all characterised l extreme sensitiveness to cold either damp or dry

In **Rhododendron** the aggravation is noticed during thunderstorm.

I would give restlessness the third place. This is partially due to the relief that motion brings along with it and partly to the anxiety, apprehension and an uneasy feeling to which he is subject. This is why it finds an important place in the therapeutics of rheumatism, gout and lumbago The limbs feel stiff, numb and painful during rest and on first movement; the stiffness, numbness and pain however become decidedly less after continued motion, but this relief is not usually obtainable on account of great muscular weakness and exhaustion. It must be remembered that **Rhus tox** is not the only remedy, that has aggravation on first movement. **Anacardium, Conium, Capsicum, Ferrum, Lycopodium** and **Pulsatilla** are a few others that have a similar modality.

Rhus tox., has a very strong action on the cellular tissues of the human body. We should think of it in cellular infiltration whenever found secondary to inflammation. In **Rhus tox.** this infiltration very easily gives way to pus formation, whereas in **Apis** the cellular infiltration rarely or never terminates in the same way. Connective tissue inflammation forms as integral a part of **Rhus tox.** as it is of **Aconite** and **Belladonna**—only in **Rhus tox.** the affected parts look dark and red. The swellings may look shiny as in **Bell.** but the differentiating feature is that the inflamed skin of **Rhus tox.** is covered with numerous small painful white vesicles. **Rhus tox.** also has strong action over glands where it sets up inflammation, induration and lastly suppuration. The glands to which it has a special affinity are the axillary and the parotid glands. Another feature of the remedy is a soreness to touch, of the prominent projections of bones.

Rhus tox. has a remarkable action on the skin. The erythema, I like to emphasise again, progresses rapidly on to vesication. Œdema and scab formation are everywhere to be seen. Milk crusts, acne rosacea, impetigo, crusta lactea, eczema, ulcers, corns, abscesses of axillary and parotid glands, herpes zoster, warts, rhagades, chaps and chilblains come under the influence of **Rhus tox.** and are readily helped by it.

Rhus tox., it may be guessed from all that has been said beforehand, is a splendid remedy for phlegmonous erysipelas. The strutures for which it has a special affinity are the scalp, the skin of the face and genital organs. It may affect other parts of the body but generally a partiality is seen for the sites mentioned above. The erysipelatous area is covered with large blebs or smaller vesicles glled with a bloody serum. It generally begins on the left side of the face and spreads on to the right. In **Apis** on the other hand a reverse order is noticed. Great cellulitis always accompanies the inflammatory process. I would like we will compare it with **Lachesis,** another noted remedy for facial erysipeals. In **Lachesis** too, the left side is affected in preference to the right. The color of the affected area, though bright red at first, soon takes on to a darkish bluish hue. The tissues involved in **Lachesis** soon go through degnerative changes. Drowsiness, delirium and a pseudo-excitements with loquacity are prominent symptoms of **Lachesis.** We should take particular care not to confuse **Rhus tox** with **Euphorbium** which too shows preference for the face and the cheeks. In **Euphorbium** too, it is vesicular in nature. Large vesicles, as big as fists, full of a yellowish serum, soon appear on the affected area. Gangrene is,threatened. The pains are intense extending from the gums into the teeth and ear. It is indeed a remedy for a more serious stage of the disease. In **Cantharis** the affection starts on the dorsum of the nose and then spreads to both cheeks. In **Belladonna** the bright red swelling, smooth and shiny, soon shows a tendency towards meningeal complications and spreads rapidly into neighbouring areas and in well-defined streaks.

The mental complex of **Rhus tox** deserves our careful attention. The most prominent trait here is anxiety, but it is an anxiety only arising out of his pains. It is decidedly unlike the anguish of **Arsenicum.** He is restless, apprehensive and tremulous. He feels as if he has come to the limit of his endurance and could not keep up anymore on account of the beating and drawing pains in his limbs. Thoughts of suicide, betraying a great disgust for life, play hide and seek in his mental atmosphere. He weeps with great despondency at the utter helplessness of his condition. We find also a sort of delirium in **Rhus tox.** but it must be mentioned that is a low, mild and muttering delirium. He frequently imagines and in his sleep dreams about feats of bodily exertion. These points will be dealt with more fully in our discussion of typhoid. Suffice to say at present that it lacks all the violence and vehemence of **Aconite, Bell., Cantharis, Hyoscyamus, Stramonium** and **Veratrum viride.** Quite a great deal of weakness characterises **Rhus tox.** All his limbs feel stiff and paralyzed and they tremble. Limbs upon which he lies fall asleep easily.

Causative factor plays an important part in the homœopathic prescribing. **Rhus tox.** fever is frequently the effect of a drenching in rain or bathing in ponds or streams or living in a damp room. Yawning and stretching are the first symptoms to be noticed. The patient feels weary and languid; this soon gives way to a regular aching of the limbs. A dry, teasing, fatiguing cough soon makes its appearance. Such a cough in the prodromal stage is also noticed under **Bryonia, Psorinum, Sabadilla** and **Sambucus.** Then comes the stage of real chill. All symptoms noticed in the prodromal stage are intensified. The stretching becomes more violent, the yawning louder and the pain in the limbs really distressing. The time of the **Rhus tox** chill is about 7 p.m. He shivers with great chilliness and feels as though dashed with ice-water. The least movement as that of eating and drinking aggravates this chill, but still he moves about, for movement eases his pains a bit. The cough that we have noticed in the prodromal stage still lingers on. This chill is soon followed by the real febrile stage. The blood that was so long running like a stream of ice-water through the blood-vessels, feels boiling hot; headache is present, but that teasing cough is no more and in its place we find urticaria breaking out over the entire body with violent itching and great thirst. The patient continues just as restless as ever. He continually changes his place but finds rest nowhere. Then the patient breaks out with profuse odorless perspiration. Let us remember that with the advent of this sweat the urticaria passes off. It will not be out of place in this connection to compare **Rhus tox.** with **Apis, Hepar** and **Ignatia.** Under all these remedies we find urticaria though in different stages.

In **Hepar** urticaria is present before and during the stage of chill.

In **Ignatia** during heat only.

In **Apis** urticaria shows itself as soon as the stage of chill is over.

During the stage of sweat the **Rhus tox** patient sleeps profoundly as in **Podophyllum.**

I have forgotten to mention one peculiar symptom of **Rhus tox** that has helped to score for this remedy many a success—i mean the hydroa on the lip. In this **Rhus tox.** resembles **Natrum mur.**

Rhus tox. is equally serviceable when the fever takes on a typhoid turn. It begins with great weakness and exhaustion, which gradually usher in a sort of a mild delirium. The patient constantly wants to jump out of bed and escape. He is very restless and fidgety; we rarely find him in one posture. He changes his position constantly. He is now on his back but the next minute finds him on his sides. This goes on constantly. We find him also a subject to hallucination. He suspects everybody to be conspiring against his life. He would not take any medicine or food from the attendants for fear they will poison him. To all interrogations his answers are slow, reluctant and petulant. The progressive delirium ends in stupor when we notice a condition somewhat similar to that of **Mur. acid, Phos. acid, Baptisia, Arnica** and **Carbo veg.** Apathy, indifference, involuntary stool, involuntary urination, great thirst, are some of the prominent symptoms noticeable at this stage.

The **Rhus tox.** tongue is characteristic. It is broad and flabby taking the impressions of teeth. It is covered with a brownish tenacious mucus. At other times it is dry, rough and cracked, with red edges and triangular red tip.

The stool is passed unconsciously. It is frequent, fetid and scanty; sometimes it is like blood-stained water, similar to the washings of meat. In dysentery the stools may be jelly-like and odorless. During stool the colic is unbearable and he suffers from nausea, tenesmus and tearing pains down the thighs. His sleep is restless; he dreams of great exertion, as if roaming over fields, climbing hills, swimming in tanks, wading through snow and so on. When this typhoid stage becomes complicated with pneumonic symptoms **Rhus tox.** may still remain our remedy. We hear rales all through the chest but especially in the lower lobe. The cough is at first dry but it soon becomes loose, and has the characteristic blood-streaked sputa.

In scarlatina **Rhus tox.** becomes indicated when it takes on an adynamic type. We are thus able to differentiate it from **Belladonna** where the congestion is more marked, fever higher, and the skin bright red. In **Rhus tox** on the other hand the child slowly grows drowsy and the restlessness becomes very pronounced; the fauces look, dark, red and œdematous. The cervical glands too are swollen more or less. This swelling may even extend to the parotid gland. The glands of the axilla are especially affected in **Rhus tox.**

The other remedies with a similar low stage of vitality are **Ailanthus, Arsenicum** and **Lachesis,** but these remedies generally prognosticate a graver issues and present greater adynamic condition.

Rhus tox. is of value in iritis and in many other affections of the eyes. Strong aversion to light, obscurity of vision, as of a sensation of veil before eyes, redness, swelling and œdematous condition of the eyelids with profuse gushing of hot tears, sac-like swelling of conjunctiva, yellow purulent mucus discharge, pustules and superficial ulceration in cornea, aching and pressive pain in eyes and agglutination of eyes in the morning on waking up are symptoms to indicate it in conjunctivitis, scrofulous ophthalmia, kerato-iritis, orbital cellulitis and mydriasis.

Ptosis of the eyelid and also paralysis of the muscles of the eye-balls due either to exposure to cold or to injury, find in **Rhus tox.** a ready help.

In head we notice a form of vertigo, common in old age which gives our patient a sensation of confusion and dullness. It is aggravated from movement as of rising from a sitting posture and is associated with a feeling of heaviness and dullness in the brain.

Case 1.—W. H. aged seventeen years, had the itch in his childhood. He was carried to me on October 2, 1848, and gave me with the aid of his father the following statement: "I went two and a half years ago, into the forest to help load a tree, and perspired freely while at work. When the tree was loaded I was tried and, to rest, sat down upon the hindmost part of the tree. On the road home, we were overtaken by a snow storm with rain and violent wind. I remained on the tree. On my arrival at home I alighted—being stiff from the tree, and discovered that the right leg, especially in the hip, was lame, and pained me on motion. All possible means were used, but the evil, instead of getting better was aggravated, and I am lame with the leg to this day." Symptoms: a **drawing** pain, with **crepitation** in the hip-joint; pains increased by leaving a chair, after sitting on it long; by sitting down in the cold; by exertion of the leg during walking; in the autumn and by change of weather. The pains are eased by sitting near a warm stove, in the sun, and by continued gentle motion. The leg is lame, that he is obliged to take hold of his pant's leg in the knee, in order to lift it up and move it on, when he wishes to walk, or rather, to limp; while limping, the leg has always been bent in the knee-joint and every time to extend it caused pain, and complete extension was not possible. The limb is stiff in the hip-joint, and every motion is painful and imperfect. Prescribed one dose **Rhus tox 12.** Eight days later, the patient reported again, having **walked** the whole distance to the Doctor's office (five post miles). The patient consisting mainly in a feeling of animation in the leg. On the second day he could raise the leg without being obliged to take the hand for support and the long walk, just taken, was not at all troublesome. He still limped somewhat and received a second dose of **Rhus tox 12,** followed by a complete cure. (This is a remarkable case and is well authenticated.—Ed.).—(Dr. Bolle in the **Allg. Hom. Zeitg., vol. xlvi**).

Case 2.—M., forty-eight years old, robust, tall and strong, who has never been sick before, worked very hard some three weeks ago and was taken with dizziness, aching in the limbs, nausea, etc., culminating in a nervous fever, which was treated allopathically. After three weeks he presented the following symptoms: .Vertigo, when raising himself up or moving, but not when lying quietly; forgetfulness; he demands a drink, receives a glass of water, holds it in his hand and does not know what to do with it. Headache, delirium. Staring, glassy, dull, stupid eyes. Dry tongue, stiff and hard like a board; trembling of the tongue as it is protruded; deafness; dryness of the nostrils. Much thirst for very cold drink. Loss of appetite, nausea with eructations; hardness of the abdomen, constipation; frequent emission of light-coloured urine, depositing a sediment like the dregs of beer; hot fever, with anxiety and dryness of the surface of the body; he cannot perspire; he wants to sleep all the while; he lies in bed, sleeping, snoring and muttering; if he is called loudly, he inquires what is wanted, and sleeps on; his hands are in constant motion, feeling about the bed and picking the cover. He can not stand on his feet; if he is helped out of bed, to arrange its furniture, he faints away from utter exhaustion. Pulse small, hard, eighty beats per minute. Prescribed **Aconite,** with relief after twenty-four hours. **Rhus tox.** followed by a general aggravation of all the symptoms, continuing a day and a night; after three days, the fever, thirst, delirium and deafness improved; on the sixth day he could leave the bed and sit up for hours, and an entire recovery followed soon.—(Gaspary, ann. d. Hom. Klinik., vol. ii., p. 196.)

RICINUS COMMUNIS.

This is our ordinary castor oil plant that grows so luxuriantly in India. The medicine is prepared from the ripe seeds which are coarsely powdered and then covered with five parts by weight of alcohol. For a thorough knowledge of this drug, we are indebted to Drs. Salzer, B. L. Bhaduri, Hale, and McWilliam. The analysis of the seeds shows that they contain an alkaloid recinine to which we may attribute most of the symptoms derived from **Ricinus.**

The most powerful action of this drug is over the gastro-intestinal region. When taken in big doses, it produces symptoms very similar to those of Asiatic cholera such as loose stools, pyrosis, cramp, nausea, vomiting, thirst profound adynamia, albuminuria, etc. It is, therefore, curative in such cases. Dr. Salzer advocates its use in cholera when the stage of diarrhœa is predominant. Its place is thus before **Cuprum** and **Camphor,** two remedies characteristic of the two stages of cramp and collapse.

Ricinus is a great galactagogue. It has the effect of increasing the quantity of milk in nursing women. Its action is more noticeable in women whose breasts are well developed. In others with shrivelled mamma, it acts on the uterus by bringing on the menses or causing an immoderate flow. It thus stands side by side with **Lac defloratum** and **Urtica urens.**

In **Lac defloratum,** the diminution in secretion of milk is due to the atrophy of the mammary gland. The breasts are unusually small.

Urtica urens has always been regarded as the best remedy for non-appearance of milk in women when no apparent cause is noticeable.

Mr. McWilliam mentions a peculiar custom among the women of the Cape de Vere Island who, to increase the flow of milk, use it locally in the form of a decoction. They also foment their breasts with the leaves of **Ricinus** used in the preparation of the decoction. In India also the custom prevails of fomentation of arthritic joints with the broad leaves of this plant.

ROBINIA.

Robinia is prepared from the bark of the 'Locust tree' that grows plentifully in the United States. We can ill-afford to neglect **Robinia** as it is frequently a remedy for one of the most fashionable complaints of the present time, I mean dyspepsia, especially when acidity is the characteristic feature. There is excessive secretion of acid in the stomach as a result of which food soon turns sour. Eructations too are sour and they are accompanied with vomiting of liquid sour ingesta. His digestion is so far disturbed that he has to be extra-careful about his meals. Even the water that he drinks at night is vomited out in the morning in the form of a green, sour, ropy mucus. His body smells sour. The other discharges of his system, such as sweat and stool, also partake of the same characteristic. Flatulence, that ever-present feature of dyspepsia is not wanting. There is constant dull heavy squeezing pain in stomach particularly after meals.

All that has been mentioned does not particularly individualise **Robinia.** There are a host of other remedies like **Æthusa, Calc. carb., Carbo veg., China, Kali sulph., Lycop., Magn. carb., Natrum carb., Rheum** and **Acid sulph,** that can present symptoms greatly similar. What then are the special tracts of **Robinia?** It is the modality consisting of the nocturnal aggravation that characterizes the remedy. In the day time the patient is not troubled so much;

he moves about doing his day's work without much trouble or worry, but as night dawns his troubles start. Acid vomiting, acid eructations, rumbling, gurgling and heartburn, worry him all night and disturb his rest.

Robinia is useful in a peculiar kind of sick headache. The head feels as if it were full of boiling water and that the brain was constantly knocking against the skull particularly when the head was moved. This headache is associated with gastric symptoms mentioned above and is caused by fat, meat, cabbages, turnips, warm bread and pastry.

Robinia is highly recommended in neuralgia of the jaw bone when it spreads to the eyes and forehead. The jaw bone feels as if it is disarticulated. If this neuralgia is associated with the acidity of the digestive tract there is hardly any chance of a mistake.

RUMEX.

This plant is a native of Europe and America; it grows in dry fields and waste lands. It belongs to the natural order of Polygonaceæ. It is commonly called the Curled Dock or the Yellow Dock. It was first proved by Dr. Henry A. Houghton of the United States. The tincture is prepared from the fresh root gathered before flowering. It is chopped and pounded to a pulp and then mixed with two parts by its weight of alcohol, and then after decanting and filtering, we get the tincture. In **Rumex** we have a splendid remedy for cough and I am greatly indebted to it for the relief afforded by it at a crucial moment when many other seemingly indicated remedies failed. It was in a case of persistent cough during pregnancy. The harsh, dry, tickling cough, used to shake the patient's whole being and was regarded almost as a precursor to abortion. A few doses of this remedy removed all her symptoms. I will take this opportunity to emphasise the precious symptom that particularly led to prescribe **Rumex** in this case. It was the extreme sensitiveness of the patient to open air. Almost every time I remember seeing her she was covered up with bed clothes to avoid inhalation of the cold air

This sensitiveness is the grand keynote of the remedy. It holds good even in other spheres. We find even the skin symptoms of **Rumex** aggravated after an exposure to cold air. The urticaria, the itch and the various other cutaneous affections become extremely troublesome during undressing.

We will revert to the cough symptoms of this remedy, as we have not dealt with them thoroughly. The cough is dry, incessant, and fatiguing; it is caused by tickling in the throat-pit extending to the rear of the sternum. This cough is also provoked by pressure on trachea, deep inspiration, inhalation of cold air and talking.

Another useful indication of **Rumex** is "clavicular pain." The patient complains of raw pain under each clavicle while hawking mucus out of the throat. The observations of Dr. C. Dunham on this point are so apt, explicit and convincing that I can hardly do better than quote them.—" **Rumex** diminishes the secretions and at the same time exalts in a very marked manner the sensibility of the mucous membrane of the larynx and trachea, exceeding in the extent of this exaltation any remedy known to us. The cough, therefore, is frequent and continuous to an extent quite out of proportion to the degree of organic affection of the mucous membrane. It is dry, occurs in long paroxysms, or under certain circumstances, and is almost uninterrupted. It is induced or greatly aggravated by any irregularity of respiration, such as an inspiration a little deeper or more rapid than usual; by an inspiration of air a little colder than that previously inhaled; and motion of the larynx and trachea, such as are involved in the act of speech; and by external pressure upon the trachea, in the region of the supra-sternal fossa. The subjective symptoms are rawness and soreness in the trachea, extending a short distance below the supra-sternal fossa, and laterally into the bronchi, chiefly the left, and tickling in the supra-sternal fossa, and behind the sternum, provoking the cough; this tickling is very annoying and very persistent, and is often but momentarily and sometimes only partially relieved by coughing."

Rumex is of great help to us in allaying the cough of phthisis. It relieves the tickling cough that harasses the patient so much. It is also very helpful in asthma of consumptives especially when the aggravation is at about 2 a.m. In this respect it compares well with **Mephitis** and **Sticta**.

Mephitis is indicated in very peculiar constitutions; patients seem to have the power of withstanding extreme cold. While everybody else around is shivering with cold they will not even cover. Bathing in ice-cold water is extremely agreeable.

Sticta is indicated when the asthma is associated with a splitting headache.

Rumex is also a good remedy for morning diarrhœa. The stools are painless, offensive and profuse and the sudden urging drives the patient out of bed early in the morning. It is possible to confuse it with **Aloes, Sulphur, Natrum, sulph, Podophyll.** and a few others. Sometimes this diarrhœa is associated with the tickling cough mentioned above. The following case cited by Dunham illustrates our point. "I have noticed in one case the cessation of a brown watery diarrhœa, after the administration of **Rumex.** A boy of five years had brown watery diarrhœa chiefly in the morning, having five stools from 5 to 9 a.m. attended with moderate griping in the lower part of the adbomen. This continued several days, notwithstanding two prescriptions which I made for it. Observing that the boy had a cough which presented the characteristic feature of **Rumex** I gave that remedy, and both diarrhœa and cough were speedily cured."

Before we close our remarks let us add a few skin symptoms of **Rumex.** Various kinds of skin eruptions are observeable in **Rumex.** We have urticaria, the army-itch, prurigo, psoriasis, eczema, and various other forms of cutaneous rash but the peculiar part of it all is the decided aggravation from exposure to cold air. In this peculiar aggravation **Rumex** is similar to **Natrum sulph.** and **Oleander.**

RUTA GRAVEOLENS.

It is the ordinary Rue, a plant of the order of Rutaceæ. It is a native of south of Europe. The tincture is prepared from the fresh herb gathered shortly before blooming. The plant is chopped and pounded to a pulp, and the juice is extracted by pressure; it is then mixed by brisk agitation with an equal part by its weight of alcohol. Its reputation, as an agent in affections of the eye, was very great even amongst our ancestors. Milton refers to its efficacy in visual troubles when he makes his angels wash Adam's visual nerve with " Euphrasy and rue " to help his sight. It is a powerful local irritant. Taken internally in large doses, it causes violent gastric pain, profound nausea, excessive salivation, swelling of the tongue, prostration and even vomiting of blood.

Like **Arnica, Calendula, Staphisagria** and **Rhus tox.,** it is yet one more of our vulnerary remedies and we think of it particularly in injuries of the periosteum. It is of the same relation to

he periosteum as **Calendula** is to the lacerated wound, **Staphisagria**
o a clear-cut wound, **Rhus tox.** to sprains and **Arnica** to injuries
nd contusions of the soft parts. The symptom that I consider
he red strand of this remedy and that has been verified repeatedly
s the great pain and the soreness as after a fall or a blow which
e experiences all over his body. It causes a bruised feeling all
ver the body from the head to the toe. The whole body is a mass
f soreness and he finds it difficult to lie on any side. The scalp,
he eyes, the thighs, the legs, and the ankles, feel as if they have
een beaten to pulp. He is unable to bend on account of pain
n all his joints and bones. The ankles feel as if they have been
islocated; the Hamstrings feel shortened and weak and knees
ive way going up or downstairs; wrist feels as if they are
prained; even the coccyx bone feels as if it has been injured. In
espect of this soreness **Ruta** bears great semblance to **Arnica,**
Baptisia, China, Eupat. perf., Hepar sulph., Natrum mur. and
Pyrogen.

Prolapse of the rectum immediately on attempting a passage
s the next important symptom. It comes out on the least straining
nd even from the slightest stooping. **Ruta** is a good remedy for
prolapsus after confinement. There are a few other remedies in
which this tendency towards prolapsus ani is equally marked.

Ignatia is one in which we find prolapsus with or without
iles, with sharp stabbing pains shooting into the rectum. It
nnoys him even when the stool is soft. The contradictory feature
f relief during stool and aggravation after is also present. The
rolapsus is more towards evening.

Muriatic acid is a great remedy for prolapsus. The rectum
omes out even while urinating and it is very sensitive to touch.

It would be sheer folly not to discuss in detail the action of
Ruta over the eyes and the ocular muscles. We use it in all com-
laints of that important organ, arising out of excessive use and
training. Amblyopia, asthenopia, choroiditis etc., come under its
nfluence when arising out of overwork or straining of the eyes.

Ruta is rich in urinary symptoms. The patient complains of
constant pressure on the bladder and a consequent desire to pass
rine. This pressure is not relieved after micturition. The desire
o urinate is constant and urgent. He can hardly retain urine; as
on as the desire is felt he has to hurry to the water-closet. If
ver he forcibly retains the water, he finds it difficult to pass it
fterwards and it is attended with severe pain.

Case 1.—Miss M. æt, nineteen; for several months has been unable to use her eyes for reading, sewing, or fine work of any kind, without a great deal of pain; the pain would usually commence inside of twenty or thirty minutes, and would be located not only in but over the eye-ball running backward into the temporal region; she also complained of considerable burning and smarting of the eyes; if she persisted in using her eye after the pain began, a considerable hyperæmia of the conjunctiva would soon be produced, which would be perceptible for some hours, even after she ceased work. These symptoms always came on sooner and were more persistent if the eyes were used by artificial light; at first they would disappear as soon as the work was laid aside; but laterly they would remain some time. Examination revealed Hm. 1-24, although distant vision was perfect without glasses. There was decided objection on the part of the patient to use glasses, notwithstanding they allowed her to use her eyes with perfect ease. As she was anxious for some remedy to be tried, **Ruta** was prescribed though with not much hope of success; inside of a week she reported as being able to use her eyes a longer time without pain, and a persistent use of the remedy for about one month gave her complete relief.—Dr. F. F. Foster.

Case 2.—Mrs. H., thirty-six; suffered for a long time with constant urging to urinate and could hardly retain her water; when that feeling occurred she had to hurry to the water-closet; if she forcibly retained the water, she could not pass any afterward, and suffered very severe pain. Gave twelve powders of **Ruta**, 1, every evening a powder. Cured.—Dr. A. V. Koch.

SABADILLA.

This plant is indigenous to Mexico, Goatimála and Venzuela. The tincture is prepared from the powdered seeds. The drug was first proved by Samuel Hahnemann. The great characteristic of this remedy is periodicity which renders it a leading remedy in the treatment of neuralgia, headache, ague, etc. This periodicity is almost as clocklike and precise as that of **Cedron.** As regards this periodicity we may also compare it with **Aranea, Arsenicum, China, Gelsemium, Lachesis, Nux vomica** and **Sepia.**

In **Arsenicum** the periodicity may be either annual or on the fourteenth day.

In **China** the periodicity is marked on the seventh day.

In **Nux vom** and **Sepia** we notice it on the twenty-eighth day.

Points like these, so seemingly unimportant, help us great at critical periods and are hence worthy of our attention.

The action of **Sabadilla** on the nasal mucous membrane is very remarkable. It brings on fluent coryza and violent spasmo-

sneezing—so violent that once the sneezing commences there is
no knowing as to when it will end. Hence I am justified in calling
it the great sneezing remedy of our Materia Medica. I have
verified this symptom again and again. The sneezing is followed
by profuse lachrymation and a copious watery discharge from the
nose. **Sabadilla** thus compares well with **Ammon. carb., Ammon.
mur., Rhus tox., Mercurius, Hepar sulph., Arum trif., Nux vomica**
and **Allium cepa.** Every one of them affects the nasal mucous
membrane in a similar way and they all have spasmodic fits of
sneezing but in none do we find it affected so powerfully as in
Sabadilla.

It is a good remedy for headaches in students and scientists,
when it is due to too close an application of concentrated attention.
The affections however where **Sabadilla** finds its greatest scope,
are sorethroat, diphtheria, tonsillitis and various other ailments of
the fauces. As a result of the severe cold the tonsils become
swollen and indurated. This readily gives way to suppuration.
Although swallowing is extremely difficult he is compelled to go
through a process of constant swallowing to relieve himself of the
peculiar sensation of a skin or a lump of foreign matter that he
feels dangling in his throat. Warm drinks relieve. As a general
rule throat and fauces are always dry.

As has been mentioned before **Sabadilla** finds an important
place in the therapeutics of ague. The great characteristic points
are the regularity of the paroxysm, commencement of the chill in
the lower extremities gradually moving upwards, and the severity
of the chill. The stages are incomplete; the stage of heat is sometimes absent but the first stage, I mean the stage of chill is
peculiarly prominent. It is so violent that he has to move to the
vicinity of a hot object, a stove, to warm him up. This reminds us
of **Veratrum** where the chill is still greater—so much so that the
proximity of a hot stove or fire does not, in any way counteract his
great chilliness. The stage of chill in **Sabadilla** is characterised
by the absence of thirst. As in **Rhus tox** and **Bryonia** we notice
a dry spasmodic cough with pain in the ribs and tearing in all the
limbs and bones. Tongue feels as if it is scalded and full of
blisters.

In Mexico where this plant grows in profusion it is utilised
for the destruction of lice and vermins. This feature of the drug
also shows itself in the homœopathic proving. We notice violent
itching of the hairy scalp, vertex, anus, rectum, alæ nasi, auditory
meatus and various other parts of the body, as from parasites

This symptom makes it as great a vermifuge as **Cina** and **Teucrium.** Dr. Kent gave it to a pet dog of his on finding great irritation in its anus as manifested by the constant rubbing of the anus against the ground. The dog passed a big lump of worms with subsequent relief of all his symptoms.

Before we close we will mention a few peculiar mental symptoms of the **Sabadilla** patient. He suffers from erroneous impressions as to the state of his body. He imagines himself sick when in fact he is not so. Thus it has been used with success in imaginary ailments of various descriptions. Dr. Hering used this remedy in a female who fancied herself to be pregnant when her abdomen was merely distended with flatus. This symptom has been verified often by many medical practitioners. I had an occasion to use **Sabadilla** in the case of a lady who was labouring under the idea that she had a cancerous growth in her throat which constantly made her hawk. She had been to many doctors but none could help her, until she had **Sabadilla,** which cleared up the delusion.

SABINA.

Sabina is the common savin—a woody shrub growing in Australia, Switzerland, France, Italy and Newfoundland. It belongs to the natural order of coniferæ. This drug was first proved by Samuel Hahnemann. The tincture is prepared from the young fresh tops of branches. It is one of our important hemorrhagic remedies. The characteristic point in **Sabina** is the intermittent and paroxysmal nature of all its symptoms. I consider this the leading feature of **Sabina.** The pains are paroxysmal and labor-like, so is the hemorrhage. The flow is copious, dark, clotted and it comes out in gushes. This hemorrhage of **Sabina** is mostly of uterine origin and it is due to a loss of tone in vessels of the uterus, either from disease or from pressure of fœtus. Thus like **Secale, Ipecac, Crocus** and **Trillium,** it makes a grand remedy for metrorrhagia, menorrhagia and threatened abortion. The distinguishing feature is the nature of the pain that accompanies this hemorrhage. It is a drawing pain, in the small of the back penetrating right through the pelvis to the pubis. It thus differs from **Viburnum,** where the pain commencing from the same region, mean the sacrum, instead of penetrating through, goes round the body to the pubis. The hemorrhage is always worse from the east movement as in **Secale.** These characteristics being present, Sabina will help in any kind of hemorrhage from any cause such as retained placenta, abortion, etc. It not only checks the hemorrhage but also helps greatly in subduing the inflammation of the ovaries or the uterus after abortion or premature labor. As has been said before, it checks any kind of hemorrhage. The blood is either clotted or fluid or bright red, thin and liquid. Sometimes in association with the peculiar pain mentioned above, we have the labor-like pain in the lumbar and the uterine region, shooting down into the thighs. The blood comes out in gushes and is particularly profuse on motion, the os uteri being constantly open. We also use it in menorrhagia during climacteric period in women. There is also profuse leucorrhœa which is milky, starchy, ropy and glairy with the same drawing pain in the broad of the back.

We will next discuss the constitution of the patient. She is subject to arthritic pains and is of very nervous disposition. As in Thuja, Graphites, Natrum carb., Acid phos. and Sepia, we find great intolerance of music in such patients. They simply cannot stand it. It seems to go through their marrow of the bone and makes them fidgety. This nervousness finds further expression in their hysterical mood. They are hypochondriacal, irritable and anxious. They are also given to a peculiar hallucination as if something alive were in their abdomen.

Sabina like **Thuja,** to which it is complementary, is another anti-sycotic remedy. It sets up warts, condylomatous and exuberant granulations in different parts of the body specially in the muco-cutaneous surfaces. In the male it sets up sycotic excrescences on the glans penis.

Sabina resembles **Pulsatilla** in various respects, particularly its modality. We have aggravation from warm air and warm room and amelioration in cool open air.

Sabina is an excellent remedy in rheumatic affections of the heels; the pain suddenly increases and slowly disappears. The pain is also relieved by cold application.

Ammon. mur., Ledum, Pulsatilla and **Graphites** are a few other remedies to be thought of in a similar rheumatic affection of the heels.

SALICYLIC ACID.

Salicylic acid a non-poisonous substance, is found abundantl in the leaves and barks of Willows and in Oil of Winter-green Artificially it is prepared from Carbolic acid and is utilised commercially in the preservation of food stuffs.

It has a very strong action over the bony structures of th human body. Bone tissues, if placed in a light solution of **Salicyl acid,** lose their compactness and become slowly dissolved. destroys dentine tissues as well but is powerless on the enamel teeth. It causes ulceration of the mucous surfaces of the boc and even produces articular rheumatism. The bone to which it particularly destructive is the tibia.

With us it is a great remedy for articular rheumatism, attac ing one or more joints, particularly the elbow or the knee-joir It causes great swelling, redness and high fever; an excessi sensitiveness to touch, motion or jerk is also to be noticed **Salicylic acid.** It suits robust persons of sanguinous temperamer Numerous cases are on record where it rendered yeoman's servi on the following symptoms: intense pain, profuse sour-smelli sweat, heavy sediment in urine, great swelling, sleeplessness a great emaciation with anemia. The pain is quite acute and pierci and is relieved from the application of dry heat.

It is extremely useful in dyspepsia. The symptoms that particularly characteristic are putrid eructations, excessive acc mulation of flatus, acidity of stomach, great belching of gas, anen and despondency. It is even recommended in gastritis and gast ulceration with great deal of pain in the epigastric regi Nausea, gagging, waterbrash and vomiting are frequent. 1 stools are loose, green, acid and putrid-smelling.

It has been recommended in Meniere's disease. Its indicatie are vertigo, noise in the ears, indeterminate giddiness in horizor position, and getting worse on raising the head or sitting up.

Its action on the mouth is considerable. It causes and he cures stomatitis and chancre sores. The mouth feels hot and and the tongue is covered with burning vesicles. The whole mc becomes dotted with white patches of scalding sores and er foul breath.

SAMBUCUS.

The tincture of **Sambucus** is prepared from the fresh leaves
and flowers of the European Elder, a large deciduous shrub found
growing in central and southern Europe. It belongs to the natural
order of Caprifoliaceæ.

In **Sambucus** we have a great remedy, much in demand, for
various types of respiratory complaints, such as influenza, laryngismus, croup, whooping cough and asthma. The grand keynote of
the remedy is to be found in the œdema and dropsical swellings in
various parts of the body. Though the œdema is particularly seen
in leg, in step and feet, it really is the secret of most of its respira-
ory and laryngeal symptoms. It is mainly on account of this that
the breathing is anxious, loud, wheezing and crowing. The suffocative attacks that appear mostly at night time, making the patient
restless, fearful and tremorous, are to be accounted for by the
œdema of the respiratory channel. The child suddenly wakes up
t night time, nearly suffocates, and sits up in bed. He turns blue
and gasps for breath which he finally succeeds in getting. These
are symptoms of asthma and **Sambucus** copes with them successfully, specially when such attacks are mostly nocturnal and are
brought about by lying with the head low.

It is also indicated in spasm of the glottis, a disease of central
origin and of difficult texture. The symptoms are most distressing
and precarious and unless helped quickly, may lead on to fatal
results from suffocation. **Sambucus** like **Chlorine, Calc. phos.,
Iodine** and **Bromium,** is very helpful in such cases. The differentiation between these remedies is not difficult.

Bromium is particularly useful when inspiration seems to be
extremely difficult. In **Sambucus** on the other hand, the difficulty
is seen mostly at the time of the expiration. His gasping becomes
worse, his struggle more acute and he looks more pale and livid
when he exhales.

Iodium is useful when the spasm is due to a sort of a reflex
from the enlargement of the thymus gland.

If such spasms occur during dentition, the child presenting
all the symptoms of scrofulosis, **Calc. phos.** would be a better
remedy.

We have quite a lot of hoarseness in **Sambucus** caused by the
accumulation of tenacious gelatinous mucus in larynx. The
patient presents much dry heat with restlessness. In the inner
chest and the lungs, great deal of oppression is felt, the patient

complaining of great pressure beneath the sternum. The cough
is hollow, dry at night and is mostly suffocative in character. Th
paroxysms are mostly troublesome at mid-night. The mos
important point about all these attacks is the high degree o
dvspnœa. The patient almost suffocates to death. The face, lip;
and the hands turn blue and break up into profuse sweat du
to the high pressure of his suffering. It also relieves, if it doe
not cure, the hectic, choking cough of phthisical patients that o
wakes him up at mid-night with a feeling of sudden suffocation.

Now as regards the general red strand characteristic o
Sambucus, the most important characteristic to take note of,
the great tendency of the attacks to recur. As has been sa
before, the child wakes up at night, suffocated, livid and blu
struggling for his very breath. The attack passes off only to l
repeated again. Similar things happen in laryngismus stridulu
croup and cough. Another characteristic of Sambucus, almo
equally important, is the aggravation from sleep. This too
illustrated in many complaints in which Sambucus is indicated.
thus acquires a place by the side with Lachesis, Spongia, Seleniu
Stramonium, Sulphur and Veratrum.

The next point to be observed is the peculiar nature of tl
sweat of Sambucus. It is profuse and over the entire body b
only during waking hours—as soon as he falls asleep sweat sto
and dry heat returns. In this respect it is similar to Nux vo
Sepia and Sulphur. The remedies that have the opposite sympto
are Antim. crud., Bovista, China, Ferrum, Conium, Pulsat.. a
Thuja.

Sambucus finds its scope in the therapeutics of fever. Its ind
cations are very peculiar, precise and clear-out. In the prodrom
stage, we find deep, dry and a teasing cough, as in Rhus to
Bryonia and Sabadilla, which extends far into the stage of chi
but this dry cough, unlike that of the remedies mentioned, is ass
ciated with nausea and thirst. Sambucus chill starts from han
and feet, which are cold to touch and lasts about half an hou
This limited duration of chill is peculiarly characteristic of San
bucus. Thirst is absent both during the stage of chill and hea
The sweat of Sambucus is very profuse, non-debilitating and
mostly at night. It stands out in drops over the face and t
entire body. During the stage of heat a sensation of burning
felt in the face and body with a peculiar icy-coldness of the fee
but a strange thing is that inspite of such furious heat he co
stantly wants to cover. We may even say that he dreads uncove

ing. There is an admixture of moisture in this heat during his
waking hours—as soon as he falls asleep the heat becomes particularly dry. This symptom, as I have mentioned over and over
again, is very peculiar of **Sambucus** and I can safely say that **Sambucus** is the only remedy in which this symptom is so well marked.

Dr. Dunham has reported a case of fever of quotidian type
that presented such an array of confusing symptoms that he prescribed **Eupatorium, Bryonia, Ipecacuanha, Arsenicum, Caladium**
and **Sabadilla** but in vain till at last 'the hard, dry cough before
the chill,' 'the half-an-hour chill' and 'the profuse non-debilitating
sweat at night' reminded him of **Sambucus** which, when administered, removed the entire train of symptoms.

SANGUINARIA CANADENSIS.

Sanguinaria is a perennial plant that grows profusely in the
United States. The first systematic proving was done by Dr.
Bute. Commonly this plant is known as the Blood-root, a name
very aptly given to it from the vermilion red fluid that exudes
from its root when cut. The tincture is prepared from the fresh
root chopped and pounded and then mixed with two parts by its
weight of alcohol. It belongs to the natural order of
Papaveraceæ.

It is pre-eminently a right-sided remedy. It acts powerfully
on the mucous membrane of the respiratory tract. It causes
great disturbance in the vasomotor circulation of the human
system and this to a great extent accounts for the circumscribed
redness of the cheeks, flushes of heat with burning in palms of
the hands and soles of the feet, distention of veins and many
other symptoms of circulatory type. Many of its mental symptoms too are accountable to the same cause. A great deal of
anxiety is present in **Sanguinaria.** It is more like a feeling of
dread. The great onrush of blood to brain produces a sort of
excitement and this excitement is expressed in the form of
anxiety and anger. The patient also complains of a peculiar sensation as if paralysed. There is a feeling of utter helplessness.
Although fully conscious, she feels she is unable to move. Then
again, we have that peculiar mental state resembling day dreaming.
She lies with her eyes wide-open but still dreaming away, one

chasing another and thoughts constantly revolving round one idea—an idea that causes a sort of nauseous sickness. This circulatory disturbance causes redness of the external ears with a humming and a roaring noise and a great hyperexcitation of the auditory nerve. This circulatory disturbance again, is at the root of the peculiar feeling of confusion and jar; the patient feels a sensation of rapid movement as if in a car or in a vehicle and a peculiar vibratory sensation throughout the body. A great desire to be held, as in **Gelsemium,** is noticed. In **Sanguinaria** the desire to be held, is indulged in simply because it will prevent the sensation of jar and vibration; in **Gelsemium** on the other hand the patient prefers to be held tightly because of the peculiar tremulousness more subjective than objective, to which the patient is a victim.

This circulatory disturbance then is a symptom of utmost importance in **Sanguinaria.** The characteristic that comes next in importance is the offensive nature and the acridity of all the discharges of the body. Oversensitiveness comes in next. She is painfully sensitive to sudden sounds. The sense of smell is equally acute. The least odor produces tendency towards fainting.

The circulatory disturbance on which such stress has been laid, leads to congestion and thus brings **Sanguinaria** into the same category as **Bell., Amyl nitrate, Aconite, Veratrum viride,** and **Opium.** It is this congestion that accounts for the severe headache of **Sanguinaria.** The face looks highly flushed; if we take pains, however, we will notice that the flush of **Sanguinaria,** unlike the flush of **Bell.,** is a carefully circumscribed flush. This circumscribed redness is seen on the cheeks alone. True, the veins of the face are distended and they betray a certain amount of soreness to touch, but we do not find any of that diffused redness that marks each and everyone of the above-mentioned remedies. The headache is periodic in its nature; it returns every seventh day. It is a headache that begins in the morning and continues to get worse during noon and then diminishes with the waning sun. The headache which is bursting in nature begins at occiput and thence spreads upward and forward and settles over the right eye. The sensitiveness, a great characteristic of this patient, is illustrated in his inability to stand, light, odor, jar, and noise. When the headache reaches its acme, the patient begins to vomit food and bile. It is a headache often brought about by the foregoing of an accustomed meal; it also troubles females at the climacteric period. Relief is sought and obtained by lying down on bed and pressing the head against the pillow. Thus, though the similarity is great, it differs from **Belladonna** in that the patient is better lying down and that the headache is associated with a good deal of gastric irritation.

Sanguinaria is indicated in a special variety of neuralgia of the face—a neuralgia that is better by kneeling down and pressing the head firmly against the floor. It generally affects the right eye, being a right-sided remedy. The pain starting from the jaw, extends in all directions and is particularly severe behind the angles of the lower jaw.

Its application in pneumonia is another instance of its power over the circulatory system. Although its efficacy is as great as that of **Aconite** and **Phosphorus**, it is needed in a later stage of the malady. When the lungs are practically impacted with blood and we have what we call the stage of red hepatization, we think of prescribing **Sanguinaria.** It must be clearly understood however that the students of Homœopathy must not be misled into the habit of prescribing on pathology; what is really meant is that at this stage he usually develops many of the symptoms which are characteristically the symptoms of **Sanguinaria,** and that is exactly why **Sanguinaria** should be prescribed and for no other reason. The most prominent symptom in **Sanguinaria** is an unwonted amount of dyspnœa. The patient finds comfort in no position and practically gasps for breath, his lungs inside his chest weighing like lead. The cough is at first dry and is excited by tickling and a crawling sensation in trachea and upper portion of the chest. The sputa look rust-colored. A great accumulation of blood in the lungs also gives a sensation of heat and ebullition. Sharp stitching pains are complained of in the region of the right nipple. **Sanguinaria** disperses the congestion and checks the fever—the patient slowly progressing towards recovery. Another very important symptom is the offensiveness of the sputa. The patient usually prefers lying on his back. The face and the extremities are inclined to be cold. Pressure reveals great dulness. A remedy that is closely associated with **Sanguinaria** and that very aften precedes it in the above complaint is **Veratrum vir.** It is useful when congestion really amounts to regular engorgement of the lung tissue. It is a remedy we think of before hepatization has commenced and there is a lot of arterial excitement. **Veratrum** is still our remedy when the engorgement becomes very profound and threatens paralysis of the lungs. Let me here caution my readers not to prescribe on such pathological basis. My purpose in associating pathology with symptomatology is simply to impress the interdependence of the two. The latter is the safer and the surer guide in prescribing.

Very frequently, in cases like these unless the truly indicated remedy finds application at the proper time, they generally run to what is generally known as phthisis florida. The fever subsides in acuteness but takes on a hectic form. The dyspnœa, though it lessens to a great extent, does not altogether disappear. The cough gradually becomes stringy and every day towards the afternoon, the patient presents a false appearance of health with the circumscribed redness of the cheeks. Emaciation progresses and gradually hæmoptysis sets in. A fast pulse, great offensiveness and putridity of expectoration, felt not only by people nearabout but by the patient himself, and nightsweats make diagnosis easy. Such a catastrophy can be easily avoided but it means careful observation and proper precaution in the initial stage.

We must not forget the application of **Sanguinaria** in polypus. It is reported to have dissolved many such cases in various parts of the body, such as ear, nose, larynx and womb. I can myself testify to many cures of polypus effected with **Sanguinaria** after everything else had failed and surgery was supposed to be the only remedy.

Sanguinaria is useful in rheumatic affections. We think of it in acute muscular rheumatism when the pains are sharp and erratic in nature. It particularly affects the muscles of the neck and back, sometimes extending to the right deltoid muscle, as in **Ferrum** and **Phytolacca**. A symptom very characteristic of **Sanguinaria** and a very important one too at that, is that the pain vanishes from the painful part on being touched and appears in some other part of the body. **Sanguinaria** is rarely useful in rheumatism when it affects the joints. It is also our remedy when as a result of local applications so frequently resorted to by physicians, the patient complains of stitching pain in the cardiac region with irregularity of the heart's action. A last useful hint that I like to drop about **Sanguinaria** in rheumatism is that it helps when the parts that are least covered with flesh are affected.

Next we come to the study of **Sanguinaria** in its action over the female sexual system. It is specially indicated in climacteric disorders such as hot flushes, burning of palms of hands and soles of feet, fetid corrosive leucorrhœa, enlargement of the breasts, vertigo, menorrhagia, metrorrhagia, and a host of similar ailments that generally make their appearance at this critical age. The profuse menstrual discharge which is generally offensive, is sometimes black, at other times bright red. The flow is more profuse at night. The sick-headache already described is generally a frequent accompaniment of all these complaints.

SANGUINARINUM NITRICUM.

It is a brownish red powder—acid, bitter and pungent in taste. Its action is principally confined to the mucous membrane of the respiratory tract where it produces a sort of catarrhal inflammation. It thus causes a sense of obstruction and fullness in those regions, and we have quite a descent accumulation of mucus causing a sense of suffocation, heat and tension. It thus becomes one of our principal remedies in the treatment of influenza, coryza, bronchitis, asthma, Eustachian catarrh, hay fever, laryngitis and even sore throat. The principal symptoms are smarting and burning in throat and chest, lachrymation, pain in eyes, head and scalp, pressure behind center of sternum, a sensation of dryness and burning in throat and bronchi and a constant tickling cough with hoarseness. On these indications it has been known to have effected important cures in the abovementioned complaints. Hale mentions of a very chronic case of laryngitis with postnasal catarrh and bronchitis in an old man who, for eight years, inspite of continuous old school treatment, had been a constant martyr to a series of uncomfortable symptoms and sensations, which at last responded permanently to **Sanguinarinum nitricum** administered in its lower attenuations.

It therefore bears great resemblance to **Aconite, Arum trif., Arsenicum,** and a few more of our catarrhal remedies; the distinction is that it acts better in long drawnout cases where the continuance of trouble had given rise to tissue changes in the affected area and the patient is slowly but certainly veering round towards incurable conditions and states.

SANICULA.

The medicine **Sanicula** is prepared from the water of Sanicula spring of Ottawa, III, U. S. A. This mineral water contains Natrum mur., Calc. m., Calc. carb., Calc. sulph., Alumina, Magnesia mur., and a few other mineral ingredients. Its symptoms are many and it bears great semblance to **Natrum mur., Silicea, Calc. carb., Graphites** and **Borax,** as will be evident from a further study.

If we make a minute observation of this drug certain features will impress themselves on our mind because of their preponderating importance. One of them is emaciation, as a result of which we find skins wrinkled and hanging down in folds. It thus compares with **Abrot., Iodium, Natrum mur., Sarsaparilla, Argentum nit.** and **Syphilinum.** The patients calling for this drug are ill-nourished, weak, scrofulous and of a dirty, greasy appearance. When I say scrofulous, I mean they are of an unhealthy complexion and that they are subject to sores, eczemas, ulcers, eruptions and skin troubles of all kinds. Scaly dandruff over the scalp, eye-brows and other hairy parts testify to a low, debilitated constitution. The face is full of pimples and acne; the hair is dry and lustreless; the digestion is slow and the abdomen is pot-bellied.

Mentally they are forgetful, nervous, irritable and headstrong; fear of some impending evil, as in **Calcarea,** constantly makes them restless and fidgety. They cannot stick to one occupation. They jump from work to work but accomplish little.

The next important feature is the peculiar smell of all the discharges of the body. This smell, so peculiar and so disgusting, follows them everywhere. We can call it a fish-brine smell. The fluid that oozes out from the eczema, the sweat that comes out so profusely over the scalp and feet, the blood that flows during her period are all characterised by this intense, ugly, nauseating smell. Such an offensive smell is also noticed under **Calc. carb., Graphites, Medorrhinum** and **Tellurium,** but they differ in the following points:

The offensive smell in **Tellurium** is particularly noticeable in discharges that take place from the ear.

In **Calc. carb.** and **Medorrhinum** it is the moisture that oozes out from the anus and the rectum that stinks.

In **Graphites** we have the smell from the scabs and the ulcers.

The third point is the changeability of all the symptoms. This gives **Sanicula** a place by the side of **Pulsatilla** and **Lac. caninum**.

The **Sanicula** patient suffers from a peculiar burning sensation in different parts of the body particularly in the soles of feet in consequence of which he constantly keeps them exposed. We find him kicking off bed-clothes even in the coldest winter. It thus belongs to the same category as **Lachesis, Medorrhinum, Sanguinaria, Sulphur, Hepar** and **Calc. carb.** This burning is also felt in the tongue. It is so intense that he frequently protrudes it into open air to cool it. Another important point in **Sanicula** is that the sweat is profuse in the head, hands and feet. The head and neck perspire so freely during sleep as to wet the pillow far around. On the other extremity too it is so constant and free that the legs feel as if they are constantly dipped in water. There is also sweat between toes as in **Silicea**, with consequent ulcerations in those parts. Sometimes a peculiar cold sensation is also felt in the lumbar and the sacral regions, and the parts feel as if a cold cloth were tied around those parts.

The **Sanicula** patient is inclined towards constipation. Inspite of a big accumulation of fæces he hardly has any desire to pass them. The condition is somewhat similar to what we find in **Alumina.** It is due to atony and absence of life in the guts. After great straining he succeeds in partially expelling some of these lumps; but as soon as they approach the rectum they recede back. In this game of hide and seek **Sanicula** resembles **Thuja** and **Silicea.** Sometimes this becomes so annoying that he has to remove them manually. In this respect it is like **Selenium.** The stools are hard, greyish white like burnt lime. As in **Ammon. mur., Magnesia mur.** and **Natrum mur.** we find these greyish balls crumbling when they come near the verge of anus. Although hard and fragile they smell like limburger cheese.

Another strange thing about the **Sanicula** stool, that just escaped my memory, is that the stools are square as if curved with a knife. The symptom is so peculiar and uncommon that it will pay us to remember it.

In diarrhœa the stools are changeable in character and colour. It is sometimes like scrambled eggs, sometimes frothy and grass-green, at other times light-coloured like scum of frog-pond. It excoriates the skin about the anus, perineum and genitals. As in **Aloes,** there is the want of confidence on the sphincter ani. The patient is afraid to pass flatus for fear he will soil his clothes.

Another symptom frequently found in diarrhœa is that the patient frequently crosses his legs to prevent fæces escaping.

On the female sexual system its action is no less striking. There is a great weakness and a bearing down sensation as if the contents of the pelvis would escape and this feeling is aggravated by walking, mis-step and jar. She frequently places her hand against the vulva as if to stop the womb from coming down. She is always better by rest and by lying down. This bearing-down sensation is associated with leucorrhœa of a strong fish-brine odor as has been mentioned before.

SANTONINUM.

A few words about this remedy would, I am sure, not be out of place in this volume. **Santonine** is the active principle obtained from the plant called Levant worm seed or Cina. It is colourless and odorless and of a bitter taste. It is a very powerful remedial agent and one should be very careful in using it. In doses of more than 3 grains, **Santonine** causes poisonous effects; although some people could take 4 or 5 grains with impunity. The symptoms of poisoning are convulsion, unconscious, nervous twitching, foaming and frothing of the mouth and stertorous breathing. We should be careful in its application in cases where we suspect cerebral irritation for those are instances where even a mild dose of **Santonine** would provoke such fearful symptoms.

It is a powerful parasiticide. It is inimical to lumbricious oxyuris and other varieties of intestinal worms. Two or three grains of the first or the second trituration in a spoonful of sweetened milk in empty stomach is sure to kill all intestinal worms. Hale also recommends its application (a few grains of **Santonine** in its lowest trituration in one oz. of warm water) in the form of injection in the rectum when these tiny little thread-worms prove very obnoxious and irritating in the rectum necessitating itching and rubbing of that part.

It has been found very useful in headaches with vomiting and delirium and in cerebral congestion.

It has a specific action over the eyes. It is found to be curative in amaurosis and blindness. This blindness where **Santoninum** is curative, is only a "nervous failure of sight" as

Dr. Hale calls it. It is due to paralysis of the optic nerve. Of the 36 cases where **Santoninum** was used, as many as 26 recovered more or less perfectly. It has also been found to be effective in cases of cataract.

Finally we will discuss its action over the urinary organs. It has been found to be very effective in cases of chronic cystitis. It causes an immediate amelioration of many of the worst symptoms such as sensitiveness and soreness of the bladder, incontinence of urine and dysuria. There is also an immediate increase in the volume of urine that brings great relief to the patient.

In fevers in children who are troubled with worms and where on account of the worms it frequently takes on a remittent turn, a few doses of **Santoninum** will remove irritation and cause the fever to come down and also allow other remedies to act more satisfactorily.

SARRACENIA PURPUREA.

In **Sarracenia** we have a favourite remedy as it is regarded as a sort of panacea for all cases of small-pox. It ought to be a subject of special interest to the Indian homœopaths. Numerous cures with **Sarracenia,** have been cited by doctors from many climes. It behoves us, Indian homœopaths, to give it a special proving and announce to the world its real curative value or expose it as an ephemeral remedy of no great importance. It is a native of Novascotia and Southern parts of Canada. It generally grows in boggy and damp place and is commonly called the Pitcher Plant or the Chief Plant. We are indebted to the Red Indians for our knowledge of this remedy, who used it often and it is said with great success in epidemics of small-pox. Surgeon Major C. G. Logie gave the following as his experience with **Sarracenia** in small-pox.

"Four of the cases in my hospital have seen severe confluent cases; they have, throughout the disease, all been perfectly sensible, have had excellent appetite, been free from pain, and have never felt weak. The effects of this medicine, which I have carefully watched, seemed to arrest the development of the pustules, killing, as it were, the virus from within, thereby changing the character of the disease and doing away with the cause of pitting, and thus avoiding the necessity of gutta-percha and India rubber applications, or opening of the pustules. In my opinion, all anticipation of disfigurement from pitting may now be calmed if this medicine is given from the commencement of the disease.

Dr. Manual Miracas of Spain, who gave it an extensive proving in an epidemic of variola in Barcelona also expressed the following opinion:—

"I had occasion to try the **Sarracenia** homœopathically prepared. This remedy, which I have used in low dilution, has invariably given me the finest results. I have noticed, from my first experiment with the remedy, that it acts with the same efficacy and promptitude in patients differing in age, sex and temperament. In Barcelona, as well as in Sans Sarria, Gracia, Bodalona, etc., many persons owe their safety to this precious remedy, and have escaped the indelible cicatrices which variola so often leaves upon the face." Dr. Taylor, an English physician used this remedy very extensively with equal success. Out of many cases reported by him we shall cite only one—"The first case was a little girl, six years of age. She was seen on the third day of eruption of primary small-pox, and immediately began to take the decoction, four ounces per diem, in divided doses, and in less than twenty-four hours the mother reported her "better ever since she began to take the medicine." The eruptions were very extensive; pustules large, and in some places confluent. The case advanced apparently without interruption until the seventh day, when the pustules began to shrivel, and on the eleventh day the desiccated scales had nearly all fallen off; no pitting; patient convalescent." Every succeeding case was treated in the same manner, and with the same success. Dr. Bilden another homœopathist used **Sarracenia** in 58 cases that came under his treatment; out of which 4 only proved fatal. This remedy has been advocated as a great prophylactic. Hence it should be classed with **Malandrinum** and **Variolinum**. Dr Cigliano has drawn the following conclusion from his numerous experiments as to how **Sarracenia** works in a case of small-pox:—

1. Soon after giving the remedy the temperature increases a little but finally diminishes in direct proportion to the fever usually in a few hours.

2. **Sarracenia** shows its influence at every stage of the disease. In the prodromal stage it breaks up the fever and the disease,

3. In the stage of eruption the temperature oscillates between 37° and 39°C. The whole disease is over by the ninth day, without any suppurative fever.

4. The pulse always diminishes about ten beats a minute. It does not always coincide with the abatement of temperature.

5. The variolous papulæ become vesicular.

6. The vesicles never pass in perfect pustules, but dry up, assuming a semispherical form, and in consequence of it the sup purative stage does not set in, and no depression will be found.

7. The contents of the vesicles are always serous, or at most seropurulent.

8. **Sarracenia** not only develops a curative power, but it is also a preventative against the variolous infection, diminishing greatly the individual disposition of catching the disease.

Now that we have seen so much and heard so much about **Sarracenia,** it is our duty to give it a thorough proving and either confirm or denounce it at its proper valuation. We are placed by Providence in a country where it is possible for us to test its virtue.

SARSAPARILLA.

The remedy **Sarsaparilla** is prepared from the long fibrous roots of several species of the genus smilax indigenous to central America. These plants grow in swampy forests seldom visited by civilised travellers, so they are only imperfectly known to botanists. Since its introduction it has been regarded as a valuable diaphoretic by the Allopaths in chronic rheumatism, syphilis and various skin diseases. The dried root of the Honduras variety is coarsely powdered and mixed with five parts by weight of alcohol and kept for a period of eight days in a well stoppered bottle. The tincture is then poured off and filtered.

Sarsaparilla is our great stand-by in renal and vesicular affections. It will help us to tide over many troubled waters. There is retention and also suppression of urine in **Sarsaparilla.** Great tenderness and distention are felt over the region of the bladder. It is attended by pain and cramps in the bladder with urging and burning. There is severe strangury with discharge of white, acrid, turbid matter. The urine is either too frequent, copious and pale, or scanty, slimy and flaky. At the conclusion of urination, severe, almost unbearable pain is felt. There may be slight distress before and during micturition, but after micturition, it is especially marked. The patient cries through agony. We find a similar symptom under **Berberis, Equisetum, Cantharis, Lithium** and **Thuja.**

In **Canth., Clem.** and **Merc.** the pain is felt more at the commencement of urination.

In **Prunus spinosa** there is an urgent desire to urinate, which, if not attended to immediately, causes sharp crampy pain in bladder. This pain is relieved as soon as the flow of urine is established.

This symptom of excruciating pain at the conclusion of urination is worth its weight in gold. It has been verified hundreds of times. Dr. Case reports of a case of dysuria that he cured with a few doses of this remedy, the symptom to guide him being this peculiarity of the pain. Another symptom that went along with this, was a " shudder that used to go all over her person with the last drop of urine, so that she had to hold on to something tightly at the time."

Another distinctive feature that we must not over-look is that urinary complaints are at abeyance during the menstrual period. The bladder does not trouble during the period of flow; but as soon as the flow ceases, the trouble re-starts and lasts till the next monthly function.

There is one more peculiarity about the urinary symptom of **Sarsaparilla** that we will do well to remember. It is this: When the patient sits, urine dribbles from him; but when he stands up it passes freely.

In **Causticum, Conium** and **Hypericum** it passes best standing. The peculiarities of a few of our remedies and the postures of patients while urinating will reward study.

In **Pareira brava** the patient is in an unenviable fix. Whenever he wants to urinate, he is compelled to take the posture of going down on his knees with his head pressing against the floor.

In **Zincum met.** the patient can urinate only when sitting or leaning back.

There is also, in this remedy, the reverse condition of weakness of the bladder and a consequent difficulty in retaining urine. When sitting the patient must swing her feet constantly or else the urine will escape.

In **Chimaphila** we meet with a different condition. The patient, a sufferer from chronic catarrh of the bladder, is unable to pass urine unless standing with feet wide apart and the body inclined forward.

Some patients suffer from difficulty of urination which no position relieves. They are forced to urge and urge hard till urination starts. **Alum., Caust., Hep., Mag. m., Mur. ac.** and **Opium** are a few remedies where great and constant urging is unavoidable.

In **Mur. acid** he has to urge so hard, to start the flow, that his anus protrudes through the pressure.

Sarsaparilla is one of our best remedies in uric acid irritations, especially in children. Uric acid crystals are noticed very often in urine or on the child's diaper. The child screams before urinating. We notice this also in **Lycop.** and **Bor.** As regards gravel and calculi, we ought to think of remedies like **Benz. ac., Berb., Calc., Canth., Lith., Lycop.** and **Pareira,** for they are all noted for their curative influence in this sphere. There is really no danger of confusion between these remedies.

In **Benz. ac.** the urine is terribly offensive. The smell is like that of horse's urine. It is very high-coloured and it contains an excess of hippuric acid. The specific gravity too is very high.

Berberis vulg. affects principally the left side. The pain is felt mostly in the loins and hips. All the symptoms grow worse from fatigue.

Calc. os. is an important remedy in urinary troubles. The urine of our fat, flabby patient soon turns turbid and deposits a white fatty, flaky sediment on the surface. The trouble is very frequently brought on by the wetting of the feet.

Canth. is an excellent remedy in vesicular troubles. The painful retention of urine, the intolerable tenesmus, the burning pain worse before and after urination are symptoms too prominent to escape the physician's attention.

In **Lithium carb.** the urine turns very turbid through the presence of mucous sediments. It is surcharged with uric acid and pus. When these urinary symptoms are associated with chronic rheumatism and valvular affections of the heart, the indications for the use of this remedy are very positive.

Lycop. has severe pain in the back before urination. There is also a deposit of red, sandy sediments. Greasy particles sometimes float on the surface. The acidity, the heart-burn, the time of aggravation and the flatulence make the selection an easy affair.

The effect of **Sarsaparilla** on the skin is very important. It cures rhagades. Ulcers, the effect of abuse of mercury and of syphilis come within its jurisdiction. Sometimes the ulcers are herpetic. They extend in a circular form.

It will not do to neglect the mental attitude of this patient. Gloominess, despondency and depression are the key-notes of his mental condition. Strange to say that this depression accompanies any pain that may trouble him. It matters not where the pain is located, but if it causes depression, the indications for this remedy will be positive. We know of no other remedy in our Materia Medica that can claim this symptom.

Dr. Taylor reports of a case of backache that he cured with **Sarsaparilla.** It was a case that baffled quite a few other physicians. We have said again and again that it needs keen insight, strong power of observation, and the ability to penetrate into the hidden mysteries of the constitution, to make a sound Homœopath. A simple memorizing of the Materia Medica will not go very far to bring success. We will do well to quote Dr. Taylor's words:

"When in a curable case, we fail, the fault is with us and not with the remedy" and it was so in this case. The patient would frequently declare that he would not mind the pain so much if it did not depress him so. It was this pronounced depression accompanying the pain that so greatly distressed him. Here then was the characteristic feature of the case. He received **Sarsaparilla** 10m. and made a perfect recovery.

Chronic, obstinate constipation sometimes calls for **Sarsaparilla.** An attempt to pass stool is accompanied by an intense desire to urinate. The patient goes to the closet, sits there for a long time, and strains hard till he breaks out into profuse perspiration and faints. Now this fainting during stool is peculiar and hence it is an important symptom. Not many remedies in our Materia Medica have this. **Aloes. Crotalus** and **Sulph.** are the only ones that we know of that can claim similar symptoms.

There is fainting in **Arsen.** and **Digit.,** but then it happens before the stool. We have fainting after the stools in **Aloes, Coccul., Crot. tig., Phos.** and **Tereb.**

We use **Sarsaparilla** often in certain varieties of sexual ills and ailments. The patient's constitution is debilitated by intemperance and undermined by the abuse of mercury. He combines in him all the punishments of his former vices. He is bent double with gonorrheal rheumatism. The syphilitic taint, the long suppressed gonorrheal history make his life none too pleasant and his sexual life too is on the wane. He complains of frequent nocturnal emissions. The least excitement causes emission without sexual feeling. Sometimes they come on even during daytime. These emissions are very prostrating and they depress him very greatly

Sarsaparilla is a great remedy for dyspepsia but only when the patient combines in him the troubles of the urinary sphere with symptoms of indigestion. Like **Lycopodium** he feels full and satiated after partaking of a small meal. Of all food, bread seems to disagree with him the most. We notice this aggravation from bread also in **Bryonia** and **Pulsatilla,** but the totality of the symptoms always helps in the final selection.

Sarsaparilla is useful in marasmus of children. It is characterized by great want of assimilation. The emaciation in **Sarsaparilla** is most marked in the neck.

A few words more about the asthma of **Sarsaparilla** and we will be done with it. It is an asthma from emphysema. He feels a sort of rigor spreading over his body from below upward There are also nausea, vomiting and headache Constant urging with only scanty emission of urine is another distressing feature of this asthma.

Case 1.—A sickly-looking child, a girl aged three, was brought to my office from the country, in the summer of 1872. The child had been in bad health several weeks. The symptoms of the urinary organs were most conspicuous. Two prescriptions had been given by me, without any good result. The mother, an intelligent lady, finally stated that she was confident that every time the child urinated, wind came, with a noise, from the bladder. This symptom, which I never met with in practice before, at once directed my attention to **Sars.** The other urinary symptoms corresponding with considerable accuracy, **Sarsa.** 200, one dose, was administered, and in a few days the case was, in all respects, very much improved. The symptoms mentioned permanently disappeared.—Dr. H. Ring.

SCUTELLARIA LATERIFOLIA.

It is also called the Mad-dig Skull-cap. It belongs to the Natural order of Labiatæ. For our knowledge of **Scutellaria,** we are indebted to Dr. Hale who found it holding a respectable place in the list of remedies used in domestic practice. It has a great calming effect on the nervous system and is hence utilised in brain-fag and nervous exhaustion. Every physician, sometime in his life, comes across cases where though nothing is found to be wrong, everything is seen to be in a state of utmost confusion. It is in instances like these that **Scutellaria** is found to be in its prime efficacy. The following case reported by G. H. Royal is an instance in point. The head of a large school, an unmarried lady of thirty-two, complained of a nervo-bilious headache, located at the base of the brain. Although examination revealed nothing she could not have a night sleep for many a long night and showed symptoms of utter exhaustion, as if she had been altogether used up. Frequent nervous explosions, sick headaches and an utter incapacity were the fore-runner of a complete break-down. Although **Picric acid** and **Phos. acid** gave certain amount of relief, they could not set her completely up on her legs, till at last **Scutellaria** was given in ten drop doses, every half hour. Very shortly sleep returned, headache left and she became her ownself again. In instances of this nature, where organic defect of any kind does not warrant the amount of suffering involved, we should think of **Scutellaria.** Many such instances can be recorded from the practice notes of other physicians.

It has also been recommended in delirium tremens, tetanus, cramps, sleeplessness, night terrors, hysteria and in depression of vital power through long sickness, over-exercise, over-study and long-continued and exhausting labours.

SECALE CORNUTUM.

In damp rainy season rye and grass that grow on damp ill-drained soils become infected with a fungus known as Claviceps purpurea. The rye thus infected loses all its starch and becomes penetrated with the white spongy tissue of the mycelium of the fungus. It is not from the rye but from this fungus that grows at the expense of the rye that our medicine is prepared. It seems to have been known to the medical profession from a very remote period, but Dr. Stearns of Saratoga was the first to bring this drug into importance about the year 1807. Many of the symptoms of this drug has been derived from its poisonous effects. We had terrible epidemics of "Ergotism" devastating different parts of Europe at different times. They were caused by the people using the flour prepared from rye infected with ergot. They died in great numbers and death resulted from gangrene, convulsions and other exhausting hemorrhages and discharges; when it takes on the gangrenous turn, the first symptoms to appear are a heavy aching pain in the limbs, an intense feeling of coldness and a general weariness and languor. Then a dark spot appears on one of the extremities. The toes are the parts that are generally affected. On that dark livid spot, mortification sets in. It may be either dry or moist, but mostly dry. It is of the same nature as the senile gangrene or what is induced by a frost-bite.

In the other variety, we mean the convulsive, rigidity alternates with relaxation. The hands are either clenched or the fingers are kept widely apart.

Secale has a especial affinity for the involuntary muscles. Its specific influence over the unstriped muscular fibres consists in exciting in them a persistent and a long-lasting contraction. These muscular fibres are plentiful in the blood vessels and the uterus and hence the secret of its power there. It is employed by our allopathic brethren " to arrest hemorrhage, to occlude aneurism and varices, to starve fibrous tumors and to diminish congestion of the brain and cord." It is very greatly used in obstetrical practice to hasten the expulsion of the fœtus or the placenta and to stop postpartum hemorrhage, but in our use of the drug we are always guided by that one eternal and immutable law **Similia Similibus Curantur.**

This drug is especially adapted to thin, scrawny women. The face is pale, pinched, ashy, sunken and hippocratic. The eyes are sunken too with blue rings around them. The vision is dim, and the voice is hoarse and creaky. This means a desperate condition and it is really in desperate cases that we are called on to prescribe **Secale.** A mistake in prescribing in such a case means a push to our patient towards his or her grave. In our capacity as physicians and healers we possess unbounded opportunity to minister to people's wants and sufferings, but we must not forget at the same time that in us lies the power of doing an immense amount of harm to our fellow beings. The moment we relax in our effort to master the situation, we fall short of our duty and become guilty of unnecessary suffering to human beings. It behoves us, therefore, to be constantly on the alert and master every secret that our Materia Medica offers.

Secale is one of our great hemorrhagic remedies. This hemorrhage may take place from any outlet, but it is generally from the uterus. The patient is feeble and cachectic, exhausted by a prolonged stay in tropical climates. It takes place from atony of the uterus, especially after miscarriage or protracted labour. The flow is black, fluid, non-coagulable and offensive. It is aggravated by the slightest motion. Our other friends in such critical moments are:—

Aletris far. which too is a remedy for passive flooding due to atony of the uterus. The uterus and ovaries are in a stage of congestion.

China too has atony of the uterus. The patient is debilitated by the loss of vital fluids, such as hemorrhages, excessive lactation, diarrhœa, suppuration, etc. She is a dyspeptic with a great deal of flatulence. Coldness and blueness of the skin, ringing in the ears, vertigo, and vanishing of the senses are some of the important points in this remedy.

Helonias comes in very handy at times. The menorrhagia that we meet with in this remedy, is often caused by ulcers in the cervix. The patient is very gloomy and depressed.

Sarsaparilla is a remedy that we are called on to prescribe often during labour, when the pains are weak or even suppressed and the patient has fainting fits which interrupt the labour still further. Everything seems loose and open but labour does not advance. The labour may be delayed by a series of causes amongst which mal-position is one and even this condition is amenable to our homœopathic drugs. It has been proved time and again. Nothing can be more gratifying than to see the wonderful action of homœopathic medicine in such cases when our friends of the opposite school are preparing for an operation or getting their forceps and instruments ready.

Not very long ago I had occasion to use **Secale** in a case where a lady was suffering from very great after-pains. **Gossypium, Cimicifuga** and **Sabina** w re tried without any appreciable result; **Secale cornutum** at last saved from further embarrassment. Immediately after its administration a big clot was expelled and there was the end of her troubles. It is similarly used in cases of retained placenta where the patient complains of a strong and constant bearing down in the abdomen.

Secale is one of the few remedies that we prescribe for patients who suffer from habitual abortions. It is the worst ill-luck that can befall a pregnant woman. The treatment of abortion resolves itself into a consideration of the symptomatology as also of the etiology. It is also customary to distinguish between predisposing and exciting cause of abortions. Amongst the predisposing causes may be mentioned abnormalities in the development of the embryo, abnormalities of the placenta, infectious diseases, mal-nutrition on the part of the mother and abnormalities in the generative tract, such as displacement of the uterus, retroflexion, prolapsus, etc. Syphilis in the parents is the most potent cause of abortions. Amongst exciting cause may be mentioned injury, over-exertion, and intense mental emotions such as anger, fright, grief, etc. In some women the uterus is in such a state of irritability that the slightest violence, as that caused by an act of coitus, a mis step, tripping over a carpet, or a ride over a rough road, will bring about an abortion. It will be to our advantage to enter minutely into details in a case of this type. It will need all our skill as prescribers to avert the calamity. I remember with regret, how, not very long ago, we disappointed a young lady who got into the habit of losing the imperfected product of her conception precisely at the end of the third month. She had three previous miscarriages and she was so anxious to have a child. I promised to help her. I did my best but as the third month gradually drew towards its close, she complained of slight shows of blood. Gradually the hemorrhage increased and as the month closed she had her usual miscarriage.

It will be a long time before I can forget her disappointment. Such discomfitures are not very rare in the medical profession. May be, she needed a long course of treatment to erase the dyscrasia from her system. Probably I did not enquire into her constitution as I ought to have done.

Now back to our point again, we mean the indications of **Secale** in miscarriage. The miscarriage in this remedy generally takes place about the third month with copious flow of black, bad smelling liquid blood. She gets cramps in her fingers and she holds them asunder. This distresses her more than the hemorrhage. **Viburnum op., Apis, Kali carb., Croc., Sab., Thuja,** and **Opium.** are equally useful in miscarriage and we will go through them minutely to be able to differentiate between them at the critical moment.

In **Viburnum op.** the miscarriage takes place in the first month. The pains are very great, almost labour-like, and of extraordinary severity. This is a symptom that has been verified repeatedly. The spasmodic pains shoot from the uterus into the legs. It is a remedy to be used when miscarriages are early and frequent, so that the ovum is expelled at every menstrual period. It ranks with **Arnica** and **Caulophyllum** in abortions where pain predominates.

Apis comes in for miscarriages at the second month. The stinging and burning pains first start in the ovaries. They get more and more severe till the labour-pains start finally ending in miscarriage. The urine is scanty. The absolute absence of thirst and prolonged and obstinate constipation are two other important indications of **Apis.**

Kali carb. is a remedy where the abortion takes place at the second month. The pains are more of a stitching nature. The patient complains of very severe backache when walking; so that she must sit or lie down. Pain predominates.

In **Croc.** we have miscarriage at the third month. As soon as blood flows from the vulva, it forms into black stringy masses. The patient is of a fickle hysteric temperament. She cries and laughs alternately. This changeability of mood is one of the guiding symptoms of **Croc.**

Sabina is a remedy where symptoms of miscarriage appear at the third month. The pain commences in the small of the back and thence extends to the pubes. It is a remedy where hemorrhage preponderates. The blood is profuse, bright red or dark fluid and clotted.

Thuja is a remedy for those sycotic females where we find a history of habitual miscarriage at the third month. The patient generally has a dirty appearance with brown or brownish-white spots all over her face and body. Large, seedy, pedunculated warts are in great abundance. She sweats much and the sweat is fetid. People sometimes think her to be out of her wits, fo she gets many funny ideas into her head. Very often she is really insane. She suffers from strange hallucinations; she imagines as if an unknown person were standing by her bed-side; as if her soul and body were separated; as if a living animal has invaded and is crying in her abdomen. It is an excellent remedy in puerperal insanity. I remember such a case where the unfortunate patient really believed that she was made of a brittle substance and would not let anybody touch her for fear she would break.

Last of all we come to **Sepia.** Here we have the catastrophy during the last month of pregnancy. The patient is very constipated and complains of a sensation of heaviness in the anus, as if a ball were lodged there. There is an empty all-gone sensation in the stomach with frequent flushes of heat, faintness and transitory attacks of blindness, especially in a warm or closed room. The fætal movements are very feeble and are scarcely perceptible. The constant pressure and bearing down, great despondency and dejection of spirit are some of the characteristic features of this drug.

We have discussed the uterine hemorrhage of **Secale.** It is necessary to state here that there is hemorrhage from every outlet of the body; thus we have hæmatemesis, epistaxis, hematuria and every hemorrhage from the anus, but the one characteristic symptom to guide us in all these troubles is the steady flow of dark, thin blood, which prostrates the patient beyond measure. The pulse becomes thready, and the appearance turns haggard, and woebegone. There are tingling and formication in the limbs. The great desire for fresh air, aversion to be covered, and burning are all important symptoms to be considered.

Secale has very important gastro-enteric symptoms. It produces violent diarrhœa. The stools are watery, offensive, yellowish or greenish, gushing, sometimes involuntary. In the abdomen we have flatulence with great deal of rumbling. The pain in the lower belly is sometimes so great as to force the patient to lie down in bed all huddled up like a bundle. The thirst is unquenchable. He wants cold refreshing drinks, such as lemonade and ice water. It is especially useful in long interminable summer diarrhœa in scrofulous children which resists every remedy. As a consequence the child turns weak and emaciated.

Neglected, these cases turn into cholera with all the symptoms of that dreadful disease. It is more often indicated towards the latter part of the disease I mean the stage of collapse. The vomiting is generally over at this stage or if present, is painless, without effort and followed by great weakness. The whole body is icy cold to the touch but the extremities are particularly so; but inspite of this superficial coldness the patient complains of a great heat and burning inside. Heat makes him feel decidedly worse, consequently he shows a great aversion to being covered. Finding him so cold and clammy, perhaps a fond relation may put a blanket or a sheet over him. He throws it away impatiently.

Herein it differs much from **Arsenic.** This patient, equally cold and clammy, wants to be warmly wrapped up. He is more restless, more anxious and more prostrated. The stomach is in a very irritable condition; the least water he drinks is vomited up. **Arsenic** also lacks the tingling sensation which is almost always present in **Secale.**

Another similar remedy is **Carbo veg.** Very often it is the last remedy. We cannot imagine a condition more critical. The patient scarcely seems to live. His nose, cheeks, and finger-tips are icy cold; his respiration is weak and laboured; his very breath is cold, which shows that the fire of life is pretty nearly extinct. His voice is hoarse or totally lost. At this critical juncture there may come on hemorrhage from every outlet of the body.

Secale is a remedy that is called for in all types of fevers with a tendency to typhoid and typhus. The three stages of chill, heat and sweat are very pronounced. It is ushered in with violent shaking chills. The body feels intensely cold to the touch, particularly the face and the extremities. The thirst is unquenchable. The lips are bluish and the tongue deadly pale.

Camph., Meny., Nux, Phos. and **Verat.** are all noted for great chills and icy coldness of limbs. We will discuss them here in detail. Nothing seems to us to be more difficult than to treat cases of fevers with success. The common belief that homœopathy is incapable to cope with ague, arises from the fact that the homœopathic physicians do not take the care and precaution they should, in prescribing in such cases. We have seen cures that seemed almost miraculous. Cases are on record where hundreds of grains of quinine having failed to check the paroxysm responded to a single dose of the indicated remedy.

In **Camph.** the chill is long-lasting and very severe. The body is cold and blue and the face is pale and death-like. There is no thirst.

Menyanthes is another remedy where the chill preponderates. The lower limbs from the feet to the knees feel icy cold as if the had been emergd in ice-cold water. This icy coldness also extends to the hands and abdomen, but the rest of the body retains its warmth.

Nux vom. is another remedy that deserves to be placed at the head of the list of our cold remedies. The patient, a nervous dyspeptic, burdened with care and worry, spoilt by too little physical and too much mental exercise, gets his chill early in the morning between 6 and 7 a.m. The chill is violent, shaking and long-lasting. He does not seem to get rid of this chilliness at all, for even during the stages of heat and sweat he feels it on the slightest movement and he wants to be covered all the time. So great indeed is the chill that his hands, face and finger-tips turn blue from it.

In **Phosphorus,** the chilliness begins in the evening and it is just as marked as in the previous remedies. He suffers from cold knees which gets very oppressive in bed at night as in **Carb. veg.**

Verat. album. is the last remedy that we will talk now. The patient complains of great internal chilliness, running through the entire body and this is aggravated by drinking water. His very bones seem to shiver from the effect of this chilliness. His skin is cold and clammy. The indications for this remedy are the presence of cold sweat on an ice-cold forehead, great prostration and rapid sinking.

SELENIUM.

Selenium, an element was first discovered in 1818 by Berzelius. It was introduced into our Materia Medica by Hering.

It has marked action on the genito-urinary organs and is quite a favourite remedy with homœopaths for the ills and abuses of the sexual system. The most characteristic feature of this remedy is debility. He seems to be in an eternal state of prostration. Devoid of all energy, ambition and enterprise, he succumbs to a tremendous fit of laziness. We find him lolling about and resting when he should be up and slaving hard. He is incapable of doing anything. A state of utter prostration has seized him from which he even lacks the inclination to extricate himself. Such then is the sad state of the patient. It is not a case of simple bodily exhaustion but a pronounced instance of mental incapacity. In **Arsenicum** the bodily exhaustion is more pronounced than in any other remedy, we know of; but still there is the mental excitability and the turmoil; whereas in **Selenium** we meet with what can be aptly termed a 'nirvana.' The desire is wanting, the ability is lacking and the patient has become inert, lifeless and immobile. When such debility is seen even after a serious sickness, such as typhoid, we must not forget **Selenium.** Such a condition really dawns in all instances where there has been a great loss of the verile element in man due to abnormal loss, arising out of injudicious use of the sexual function. A real impotence is to be seen in all such cases. There is involuntary dribbling of semen or prostatic fluid during sleep. The prostatic juice oozes even while sitting or when straining at stool. What little strength is left is drained swiftly through such happenings. There is no mark of lewd thoughts but due to insufficient and slow erection, the patient is thoroughly incapacitated from fulfiling his sexual obligations. In this respect we would do well to compare it with **Agaricus, Agnus, Aurum met., Caladium, Calc. carb., Conium, Lycopodium** and **Phosphorus.**

In **Agaricus** a great desire for an embrace is present with slight debility and insufficient seminal emission. What is most striking about this remedy is the evil consequence that follows an act of coition. Debility and languor increase greatly after an embrace and we have profuse night sweats following closely at the heel of each action.

Agnus castus is totally different. There is diminished sexual instinct, but each embrace brings with it ease, lightness and a feeling of well-being. The sexual life is at the lowest ebb in this remedy. The penis is exceedingly relaxed. Even voluptuous fancies excite no erection. The testes are cold, swollen, hard and painful. Melancholia, apathy, mental torpor, self-contempt and general debility are characteristic features of **Agnus castus.**

In **Aurum met.,** we notice great deterioration of the testes which hang like two pendent shreads. Penis is constantly relaxed. The melancholia is so pronounced as to assume suicidal tendencies.

Caladium is preferable in advanced cases of sexual weakness. It presents a case of perfect spermatorrhœa which is generally the effect of sexual excesses. Nocturnal dreams are frequent and they occur without any lascivious excitement.

Calc. carb. typifies the bad effects of early masturbation. Every coitus is followed by weakness of mind and body. Ejaculation is tardy and unusual weakness follows indulgence.

Conium, a great remedy for impotence, presents the sad picture of a wreck who suffered simply through sinning against nature. It is a remedy for the bad effects that arise out of suppression of sexual desires.

Lycopodium is a remedy for the cold, nervous patient who pays the penalty of excessive and exhausting seminal loss. This leaves him cold, exhausted and feeble. He falls asleep during an embrace. As a remedy it is greatly needed in cases of old men who, although suffering from strong desires, cannot manage to get up an erection.

Phosphorus too, is a remedy for excesses in venery. He has been drained almost dry so that during an embrace there is hardly any seminal discharge. Like **Conium** it rectifies the evil effects of forced celebacy. We think of it also in excessive voluptuousness in widows.

Selenium is indicated in headache of nervous origin. It is associated with profound melancholy and profuse flow of urine. This headache is brought on by drinking wine, tea or lemonade. It is also caused by debauchery. Headache is located over the left eye and is always aggravated by exposure to sun and from inhalation of strong odors.

Another strange characteristic with these patients, is the falling out of hair from the eyebrows, whiskers, and genitals. The **Selenium** patient shows a marked propensity for ardent spirits. At times this longing almost turns into a maniacal craving. The sleep of **Selenium** is quite characteristic. Like **Sulphur,** he sleeps in catnaps. He awakens several times in the course of the night but falls asleep each time to be roused again by the slightest disturbance.

Selenium has strong action over the liver. It is especially useful in enlargement of the liver, when such enlargement is associated with loss of sleep, white coated tongue, absence of thirst, sharp stitching pain in the region of the liver and the onset of a peculiar rash over the hepatic region.

Its action over the skin is no less marked. It has a kind of itching rash in the folds of the skin and about the joints, particularly the ankle-joints. On the scalp we have a peculiar eczematous eruption which secretes a sort of a serous fluid. Here again **Selenium** resembles **Sulphur.**

The constipation of **Selenium,** like the constipation of **Sulphur,** is due to a sort of atony of the intestinal tract. As in **Silicea,** we notice daily an impaction of the rectum with hard fecal matter which has to be removed manually. Such a condition is due to improper or deficient peristaltic action. Stools of **Selenium** are immense in size and they threaten to tear the anus and hence they are difficult to pass. It takes the patient a long time to evacuate and he becomes exceedingly nervous and agitated from the mere idea of a stool. **Ghaphites, Silicea, Sulphur, Opium** and **Bryonia** are greatly similar to **Selenium** in this respect.

Selenium has a marked action in the larynx. Due to inflammation of the lining membrane, the voice becomes husky and the patient frequently hawks up transparent lumps of phlegm. It is particularly useful in hoarseness after long use of voice. We find these patients constantly clearing their throat due to a frequent accumulation of clear starchy mucus. **Selenium** finds an important place in the more serious condition of tubercular laryngitis. In addition to the symptoms mentioned above, the patient is troubled with frequent expectoration of blood-tinged mucus. The cervical glands become swollen and hard. The accumulation of mucus in the wind pipe causes quite a good bit of dyspnœa.

SENECIO AUREUS.

It is called the Golden Rag-wort. It belongs to the natural order of Compositæ. Here also we are indebted to Dr Hale for whatever knowledge we possess of this remedy.

Its chief action is centered over the urinary and sexual organs both male and female. Quite an important sequence is noticed between the non-appearance of menstruation and a host of other ailments. This seems to be the pivotal point around which everything else in this remedy hangs. As soon as menses appear, everything else seems to clear off. Sore-throat, headache, leucorrhœa bronchitis, hoarseness, cough, and dyspnœa show decided improvement as soon as menstruation commences. Dr. C. M. Fos effected a remarkable cure with **Senecio** 1x in a young girl o about eighteen years of age, who after her period had stopped fo fifteen months showed signs of chlorosis with a dry hacking cougl Even the abdomen had become puffed due to accumulation of serou fluid in the cavity. Tapping had been decided upon but all symp toms rapidly disappeared and the menses reappeared within a shor time after the application of this remedy.

Senecio, as has been said before, has a strong action upon th kidneys and the bladder. It causes congestion and inflammation kidneys, particularly the right one. Pain in the loins, fever a prostration accompany these inflammatory attacks. The urine becomes scanty, high-colored and bloody. Great heat is felt and urging is incessant. These symptoms may be so intense as to suggest the application of **Cantharis, Berberis, Pareira** and **Osimum.** The urine looks red and frequently deposits thick brick-dust sediment. Ascites and œdema of lower extremities when attributable to inflammation of kidneys, find in **Senecio** a ready help. Even headache when associated with irritation of the bladder is relieved by **Senecio.**

An important symptom that has been omitted is the association of menstrual irregularity with vesicle irritation. It is also a good remedy for leucorrhœa particularly when it is preceded by irritation of the bladder. Intense backache accompanies amenorrhœa.

SENEGA.

Senega is commonly called the Seneca Snake-root after the Seneca Indians by whom it was extensively used as a remedy for snake-bite. It belongs to the natural order of Polygalaceæ. The alcoholic tincture is prepared from the powdered root. It is extensively used by allopaths in many of their cough preparations.

In **Senega** we have another catarrhal remedy of high repute. It has a great affinity for the mucous linings of the larynx, trachea and bronchi. It is used in sub-acute or chronic inflammation of the pleura. Hydrothorax, œdema, diseases of the heart, dropsy after albuminuria, hydro-ophthalmia with intraocular compression, and ascites accompanying hepatic diseases have great claim on **Senega,** which invariably checks the progress of the disease and soon relieves the high tension by letting loose the power of free elimination.

Senega acts best in fat, plethoric and phlegmatic persons of lax fibre. As I have mentioned before, its greatest usefulness is seen in catarrhal affections such as influenza, catarrh of the pharynx, irritation in larynx, etc. The leading indications of **Senega** everywhere are, firstly, a great accumulation of clear albuminous mucus difficult to get rid of; secondly, a great soreness of the walls of the chest and finally a pressure on chest, as though the lungs were forced back to the spine. It is particularly useful in harassing cough of old age where there is a great accumulation of phlegm in the chest causing a great deal of rattling and wheezing noise. Thus it greatly resembles **Ammon. carb., Ant. tart., Caust., Ipecac, Kali sulph.,** and **Sepia.** Many interesting cures have been reported on these indications. With a few doses of **Senega** 30 Dr. Clarke relieved a fairly serious condition in an elderly stout lady of phthisical taint, who had pneumonia on both sides. Violent paroxysms of cough with expectoration of ropy blood-tinged mucus, disappeared under its action in an incredibly short time. We also have a report of a cure of a case of pleuro-pneumonia in "Hering's Guiding Symptoms." After **Bryo., Acon.,** and **Bell.** had completely relieved the lancinating pains there still lingered a whole hoast of other unpleasant symptoms, such as oppression of the chest, expectoration of copious phlegm, loose stagnating mucus with rattling in the chest, cold sweat, and great adynamia. **Senega** removed them all after **Ant. tart.** had failed.

It is also used in effusion of the lungs and thickening of the pleura consequent on pleurisy. These sub-acute and chronic stages are critical stages. Negligence often leads to fatal issues. We often hear of patients gradually drifting into phthisis after neglected cases of pneumonia and pleurisy. **Senega** often rectifies the mistakes and inexperience of the initial stage and gradually re-establishes the lost equilibrium and prevents the patient from gradually sinking into an incurable stage.

SENNA.

Senna, a species of Cassia, belongs to the natural order of Leguminosæ. In Bengal it goes by the name 'Sonamukhi., It is a small shrub only growing to the height 30 to 40 inches. Its pod is broad, flat, coriaceous, slightly curved containing about half a dozen seeds. It grows very extensively Central Africa. The leaflets are gathered twice a year by native tribes and carried to Alexandria where they are carefully cleaned and finally exported to the different parts of the world. It also grows extensively in southern India.

It is one of the most satisfactory and generally useful simple cathartics. It empties the bowels thoroughly in ten twelve hours and causes slight griping. **Senna** leaves, chewed daily are a favourite habitual laxative with many people.

With us it is a favourite remedy for infantile colic particularly when the colic arises out of incarceration of flatus. The child is restless and tosses about in agony. Great heat is felt in the palms of hands.

It is also used for oxaluria, phosphaturia and acetonuria. The specific gravity is increased. A great indication of this remedy is exhaustion. The patient breathes hard from the slightest exertion. Examination reveals no organic defect, but the exhaustion goes on uninterruptedly. **Senna** acts almost as a tonic in these cases of simple exhaustion caused purely through an excess of nitrogenous waste. A better proving and a more frequent use will lead to a better understanding of this drug.

SEPIA.

Sepia is a blackish brown liquor found in the contents of the ink-bag of the Cuttle Fish- a fish very common in the Mediterranean Sea. This fluid is utilized by the fish for purpose of self-protection and catching its prey. This is done by darkening the water with this fluid, when it is pursued by its enemy or when it wants to pursue its own prey. This is somewhat on the principle of the smoke-screen theory of the present day navy and the aeroplane warfare. The triturations and tinctures are made from the pure, dried, genuine **Sepia.** It belongs to the natural order of Cephalopoda.

The idea of proving **Sepia** dawned on Hahnemann on having found a complex lot of symptoms in a friend of his, an artist, who was in the habit of wetting his brush containing India-ink with his saliva. This remedy was proved and a whole array of symptoms was arrived at, as a result of the proving. Since then, **Sepia** has proved itself extremely useful and has justly acquired a place in the list of our polychrest remedies. It acts particularly on the portal system and causes great deal of venous congestion. Many of its symptoms are the direct effects of this condition. We find flushes of heat in various parts of the body finally breaking out in pools of perspiration; we have throbbing all over the body and in many of the internal organs due probably to the same cause. The engorged uterus of **Sepia,** the sensation of heaviness in the hepatic region, the burning of the

palms of the hand and soles of feet and the frequent attacks of
headaches are all to be ascribed to the same pathological condition.

Now, we will do well to go through the main characteristic
of our remedy. The symptom that stands out most prominently
is the state of relaxation that is to be found everywhere in this
remedy. The patient is wanting in life, vigour and enthusiasm
This feature is noticed both in the mental and the physical side of
the remedy. The memory is weak and the flow of idea is slow.
On the physical side we notice weakness of the different joints
and the muscles of the body; limbs go to sleep easily; the joints
are all weak and they give way occasionally. The patient faints
very easily after the slightest exertion, as from riding a carriage,
while at prayer in the church, after getting wet, etc. In this **Sepia**
resembles **Gelsemium;** but in **Sepia** it is mostly the result of her
uterine disorder.

The next point, in these patients, is the tendency towards
erethism. The face becomes red and flushed on the least movement or excitement and this is followed by perspiration over the
whole body. This is a frequent symptom in the climacteric period
and so **Sepia** stands side by side with **Amyl. nit., Acid sulph.,
Crotal., Jaborandi, Kali bich., Lachesis, Glonoine, Sanguinaria** and
Sulphur. This erethism is accompanied by a sensation of emptiness in the epigastrium. The patient feels as if her inside is one
big hollow. It can be better described by the term ' goneness.'

Chilliness supplies the next important feature of **Sepia.** It is
characterised by a peculiarity rarely noticed in any other remedy.
A sort of antagonism is noticed in this respect between the lower
and the upper limbs, that is, when the legs become cold, hands
become warm and *vice versa.* She is particularly sensitive to cold
air.

The lower lip is usually swollen giving the patient almost
a vulgar appearence. The face is puffy, pale, yellow, almost
earthy. Over the puffy face there is a marked yellow saddle
across the bridge of the nose. We also notice numerous yellow
spots on face, specially around mouth and lips. She is distinctly
inclined to be flabby and coarse and has, what has been aptly
termed, a fish-woman appearance. She sweats profusely but
especially in and about the genitals, back and axilla. The face
looks woe-begone, blank and listless. The mental condition of
the patient is quite in keeping with her general appearance. The
apathy, the indifference and the sadness are in over-whelming
preponderance to the other traits of her character. She has no

use for any of her dear and near relations. They are no longer the object of her solicitations, as they seem on longer to constitute a part and parcel of her existence. She is irritable, vexed, discontented and out of humour with everybody. Anxiety enters into this intricate mental state to render it still more distressing and intolerable. She is constantly afraid of some impending calamity or of some imaginary trouble. She is discontented, not only with the past and future but with the present as well. This discontentment leads to great depression of mind and makes her very lachrymose. We frequently find her indulging in fits of weeping. Then again, this depression gives in to a spirit of vindictiveness and scolding. She breaks into violent brust of anger and gesticulates furiously. Everything taken together, she is altogether an unenviable, unlovely being. She bears great resemblance to remedies like **Pulsatilla, Nat. mur., Causticum, Lil. tig., Palladium** and **Platina.** They are, all of them, lachrymal in their mood but the points of differentiation are many.

The head symptoms of **Sepia** are very prominent. She suffers from, what we call, hemicrania. This headache is mostly a reflex of her uterine troubles and is neuralgic in character. It begins in the occiput and thence spreads over the whole head to the eyes. It commences in the morning, lasts till noon or evening and is accompanied by nausea, vomiting and contraction of pupils. It is better from rest and in a dark room. The paroxysms are renewed or aggravated by motion, noise and thunderstorm. Malposition of uterus or menstrual disturbance is, as has been said before, the root cause of all these troubles. We also think of it in brainfag caused by prolonged occupation. During headache, a great aversion is noticed to all kinds of food and a feeling of emptiness and goneness is complained of in pit of the stomach. Often this headache of **Sepia** is associated with a great rush of blood to the brain; in consequence apoplexy may be apprehended, particularly in men and women who are addicted to drinking and sexual excesses. These patients, as may be imagined, are subject to arthritic and hemorrhoidal complaints.

We will now consider the action of **Sepia** on the male and the female sexual organs. It causes increased sexual desire but unattended with proper erection. We also notice profuse sweat around the genitals as in **Thuja.** It further resembles **Thuja** in the preponderance of warts and condylomatous growths around the penis. Numerous cures of such growths are ascribed to **Sepia** even after **Thuja** had failed. Speaking about condylomata re-

minds us about its great anti-sycotic properties. It is very efficacious in the treatment of those persistent cases of gonorrhœa
that drag on everlastingly in the face of the most careful treatment. We think of it particularly after the acute symptoms have
subsided. There is hardly any pain and the discharge is only
slight and takes place at night—a few drops of yellowish pus staining the linen slightly. **Sepia** also betrays, as has been mentioned
before, a great weakness. This general weakness gets particularly
augmented after coition.

The female sexual system is particularly amenable to its influence. Like **Pulsatila,** it constitutes one more of our women's
remedies. Its symptoms are many, varied and important. In the
first place. it causes a great sensitiveness of the sexual organs,
which is the root cause of the great dislike towards sexual intercourse, betrayed by these patients. The congestion on which so
much importance has been laid previously leads to induration of
the ovaries with their appendages and of the neck of the uterus.
It is this congestion also that brings into being the great feeling of
downward pressure in the pelvic cavity, compelling the patient
to cross her thighs to prevent protrusion of the already prolapsed
uterus. This is indeed an ineviable state of affairs, which may
be certainly and peremptorily put right by the timely administration
of **Sepia** by the conscientious homœopath who takes pains to go
into the minutest details of symptoms and never grudges patient
application over the long pages of his Materia Medica. This displacement of the womb also causes oppression of breathing and
anxiety and is accompanied by a greenish, yellowish, leucorrheal
discharge of fetid smell and corrosive. nature. Dr. Nash in his
"Testimony of the Clinic" cites a case of one Mrs. Alice W.,
age 56, who was suffering from complete procidentia with all its
accompanying symptoms. A dose of **Sepia cm.** not only removed
all the annoying symptoms but helped to draw the uterus back
into the vaginal cavity. Cures such as these, and they are too
numerous to be mentioned, seem to strike a discordant note in the
credulity of our allopathic brethren who find them smelling of the
improbable and the absurd. But that the wand of homœopathy is
magical and that it renders many such apparent absurdities into
real possibilities, is testified to, by the merest novice in the science
of homœopathy. Our literature is replete with instances of such
kinds. It is up to the disbelievers to put it into practice on the
staunchest principle of Similia and publish to the world their
failures. One such instance, cited by Constantine Hering, is that

of a woman during the twelfth week of her pregnancy. The vaginal portion of the uterus had swollen immensely and it was protruding from between the labias. The os uteri was open admitting point of the index finger. The body of the uterus was quite engorged and heavy practically filling up the pelvic cavity. When efforts at manual replacement proved futile, **Sepia** was administered and the result was comparative ease and partial replacement which enabled the mother to carry her pregnancy into the full term.

Frequently the patient complains of a sensation of weight in the rectum which is not relieved by evacuation. Sometimes stitches or shooting lancinating pains are complained of, in the uterus which go up to umbilicus and the pit of the stomach. **Sepia** has been known to check metrorrhagia during climacteric age or during pregnancy, specially in the fifth and the seventh months and thus prevents abortion. **Sepia** has a very characteristic leucorrhœal discharge. It is bloody, slimy and yellowish. It may be also of a thinner consistency like milk coming profusely after each urination. It is acrid and it gives rise to soreness of pudendum. This leucorrhœal discharge comes mostly at day time and is practically absent at night. It is unceasing and exhausting and it is associated with enlargement of the mammary glands.

We must not also forget **Sepia** in delayed labor with insufficient labor pain. We think of it particularly in cases of clumsy women, full of dark brown spots on face and who suffer from cold feet with flushes of heat in the face. Inspite of the fact of the os being half open, and of the constant bearing down feeling, labor does not progress satisfactorily. The patient shudders with pain and wants to be covered up.

The menses of **Sepia** too, are characteristic and should be carefully borne in mind. It usually comes on very late every month and is preceded by violent aching in abdomen causing faintness, chilliness and shuddering. It is usually scanty, sometimes lasting only a day. During menses, the patient is sad, morose and despondent. Toothache, headache, discharge of plugs from nose, pain in tibia, epistaxis and colicky pains are particularly troublesome during this period.

To have a complete picture of this remedy, we must not neglect the symptoms pertaining to its urinary organs. There is a feeling of fulness in the bladder, as if it is about to overflow, compelling her to urinate frequently. This sensation of fulness and heaviness is particularly characteristic of our remedy. Very often there is really an overflow. As in **Causticum,** the patient finds it difficult to sneeze and cough for each paroxysm is accompanied with a spurting of urine. The **Sepia** patient consequently has a smell of urine on her. It is very fetid with a lot of whitish clayey sediment in it which settles down at the bottom of the vessel when allowed to rest. This sediment adheres to the vessel firmly as if it is burnt on it. Sometimes, though rarely, we may find a reddish sediment as in **Lycopodium.** As regards fetidity of urine **Sepia** is similar to **Indium, Calc. carb., Benzoic acid** and **Nitric acid.** In respect of this spurting of urine **Sepia** may be compared to **Causticum, Pulsatilla, Squilla, Ferrum** and **Natrum mur.**

Sepia is a great friend of the young children. It helps them in nocturnal enuresis, especially when they wet the bed during the first sleep as in **Kreosote.**

We will next consider the action of **Sepia** on the abdominal organs. We find it applicable in a special form of dyspepsia in morbid women suffering from uterine diseases. It is associated with a peculiar sinking, emptiness or goneness at the pit of stomach. The patient complains of a sour or bitter taste in the mouth with a craving for acids and pickles. Great aversion is displaced towards meat, fat, bread and milk.. Emaciation is marked and frequent. Heartburn extending from the stomach to the throat is a constant affair. Waterbrash is also very frequent. She displays a great nausea which is particularly aggravated from the smell of cooking food. The tongue is coated white and the bowels are constipated. The liver generally is enlarged and frequent stitches are complained of in the hypochondrium. The abdomen though distended, has a sensation of emptiness in it. Hemorrhoids are not infrequent. We notice protrusion of varices in the rectum with great heat and burning and a sensation of heaviness in the anus. It is more like a sensation of ball or weight in anus and is not relieved by defecation. The rectum prolapses particularly after smoking. The stools are insufficient and they look like sheep-dung. They also are covered with mucus as in **Graphites.** As in **Silicea** it becomes necessary to render manual assistance. There is also oozing of moisture from the rectum as in **Nat. mur.** and **Antim crud.**

It must not be supposed however that **Sepia** is the only remedy that has this symptom of emptiness and goneness; **Cocculus, Ignatia, Kali carb., Lobelia, Mercury, Petroleum, Phosphorus, Stannum,**

Sulphur and a few others can put in just as valid a claim to this symptom as **Sepia.**

Cocculus is noted for the weakness accompanying the feeling of emptiness. Like **Sepia,** she too, tires very easily. Each exertion seems to aggravate this feeling. We also have aversion to the smell of cooking food. The differentiating feature, however, is to be found in the etiology of this symptom. In **Cocculus** it is generally brought about by loss of sleep and journey by train or steamer.

Ignatia is indicated in nervous hysterical females and the feeling of emptiness is associated with sighing.

Kali carb. shows the same lowered vitality as **Sepia** but under this remedy great relief is obtained after food, which not only removes the emptiness but causes great bloating as well.

In **Lobelia** the emptiness, though felt in the epigastrium, extends up to the heart and is associated with great nausea and profuse perspiration.

Under **Mercury** this symptom of emptiness is not so prominent, though present, and is particularly aggravated from **pressure.**

Petroleum has the emptiness characteristically marked **after** a stool.

Phosphorus, as we all know, is noted for this sensation of emptiness; but under **Phos.** it is particularly associated with nausea.

In **Stannum,** the sensation of goneness and emptiness is felt particularly in the chest behind the sternum—the patient complaining of great weakness while talking.

Sulphur undoubtedly is the king amongst all such remedies. It has torpidity associated with defective reaction. The sensation of emptiness starts, in this remedy, at about 11 A.M. Something must be eaten immediately or he feels he would succumb.

These unfortunate dyspeptics calling for **Sepia,** may suffer from looseness of the bowels. The stools are generally very putrid and are expelled suddenly—the whole quantity coming out at once. This diarrhœa is generally brought on by drinking boiled milk which is always an object of horror to the **Sepia** patient. The stools are jelly-like, whitish, gray and sometimes full of green mucus. We have prolapsus ani during stool and a feeling of smarting and burning after. The characteristic sensation of weight or ball in anus is usually present.

Lastly we will consider the action of **Sepia** over the skin. Like **Silicea, Hep. sulph., Mezereum** and **Borax,** the skin is intensely

unhealthy.   Slightest injury tends to ulceration.   **Sepia** is particularly our remedy for ulceration about joints, specially on the
bends of the knees and elbow-joints and the tips of the fingers.
In this respect too, it is similar to **Mezereum** and **Borax,** the three
together making a great trio for this particular symptom.   We
must also remember that the **Sepia** eruptions generally make their
appearance during pregnancy and nursing.   We notice various
kinds and classes of skin eruptions in **Sepia,** such as herpes carci-
natous, ringworms, nettlerash, acarus itch, pruritus, tetters, warts,
vesicles, pemphigus, pustules, boils and psoriasis.   The usual sites
for these eruptions are the lips and the mouth and the region
near about the genital organs.   The skin is usually covered with
brown red spots.   Pruritus also appears on face, eyelids, hands,
feet, armpit, vulva, anus, ears and scalp.   **Sepia** thus vies with
the best of our remedies applicable in such conditions.   Like **Apis,**
Rhus tox and **Nat. mur.,** **Sepia** excels in nettlerash but it generally
breaks out during a walk in cold air, disappearing as soon as the
patient enters a warm room.   I have used **Sepia** with great satisfaction in ringworms, especially when they are isolated and cover
a small area.   In **Tellurium,** another great ring-worm remedy, we
find a large surface of the body involved and the multiple rings
intersect one another.

These **Sepia** patients are great subjects to gout and to
swelling of the lymphatic glands.   The nails are generally crippled
as in **Graphites** and **Silicea.**   The constitution for which it is particularly suitable is pre-eminently a scrofulous constitution.   Old
pot-bellied women who are irritable, filthy and leucophlegmatic in
nature are proper subjects of **Sepia.**   They usually have dark hair
and are of rigid fibre.

Case 1.—A lady, aged thirty, has been ill nine or ten days; is in a
remittent febrile condition with evening exacerbations, no chill, pulse
ninety-six (at 11 A.M.). Aching weight and soreness in the right hypochondrium, and distress and aching in the right shoulder and scapula; cheeks
flushed; the forehead and conjunctiva yellow; irregular yellow patches on
the forehead; lassitude; the limbs and back ache, obstinate constipation
and occipital headache; anorexia, she loathes fat and milk; thirst; tongue
flabby and indented; great flatulence after food; restless sleep; dry, hot
skin; urine scanty and loaded with urates. Her disease is said to have
been pronounced remittent fever and prescribed for as such.   She has
taken **Podophyllum** and she knows not what else.   I gave **Sepia** 200, in
solution, a dose every four hours. In twelve hours the fever had gone and
did not return; the side was better, the bowels had moved; in a week she
was entirely well.

SEPIA **685**

Case 2.—A girl of twenty-two years, formerly healthy, took a severe cold and ceased to menstruate. She had always menstruated scantily, the periods returning too soon, and the intervals marked by a slight leucorrhœa. Symptoms: Appearance pale, like wax; peculiar expression of apathy in the countenance; she is chilly, without subsequent fever. She has frequent stitching pain in the forehead, increased toward night. Beating and roaring in the head, especially on the right side. Well marked rushing sound in the right carotid, less in the left. Violent palpitation and difficult breathing after the least exertion; the sounds of the heart are normal. For some time she has coughed and expectorated slightly during the night; auscultation reveals nothing abnormal. Loathing of meat and vegetables; meat, especially fat meat, is rejected at once. Stools hardly ever costive. Pricking in the feet, as if they were "going to sleep," caused and aggravated by walking about. She feels particularly bad in the evening; she is then exceedingly weary and sleepy. She was under "regular" care for three months. On December 27th she received three doses of **Sepia** 200 with direction to take one dose each day. On January 2nd she commenced to mensturate, but very scanty. January 24th she is better; she has all the old symptoms, but they are milder. Constant improvement without mensturating, until February 5th. **Sepia** 200, three doses—one dose to be taken each day. February 13th—Menstruates. Constant improvement. March 5th—Her troubles have all disappeared. March 11th—Unwell again. Menstruation continues for three days. Looks fresh and well, but there is still a slight "rushing" in the carotid.—Dr. Ruekert.

Case 3.—Mrs. S., aged twenty-seven, mother of one child. Anteversion of uterus for two years and occasional severe attacks of cystitis, consequent upon pressure. Saw her during one of the attacks. Urine turbid voided five or six times an hour; accompanied by the well-known symptom of "bearing down" and sensation of prolapsus of the pelvic viscera, with desire to "cross the limbs" to prevent protrusion. Had suffered with dysmenorrhœa, also leucorrhœa. **Sepia** 55,000, every two hours. First improvement noticed in less tenesmus. Afterward, urine of better color and passed less frequently. All violent symptoms abated within six hours. Entirely free from pain, and no trace of trouble two weeks after. Two months later, trouble recurred from lifting, again cured by the same medicine.—Dr. W. J. Guernsey.

SILICEA.

Silicea is an oxide of silicon and it occurs in great variety of forms. It is commonly known as silicious earth flint or quartz. It is found in the hair nails, skin, periosteum, nerve sheath and even in the bony tissues. It has a very low rate of thermal conductivity and is used extensively as stuffing for the hollow walls of ice-chests, fire-proof safes, etc. It is also used in the making of dynamite. Though inert in its crude state because of its insolubility, it becomes a very powerful remedial agent when potentized.

Every part and form of human tissue is acted upon by **Silicea.** Connective tissue, bones, mucous membrane, skin and nervous tissues are profoundly influenced by it and hence we find it indicated in a wide variety of ailments, affecting all these different tissues. We will firstly consider its action over the cellular tissue. It produces extensive inflammation of these tissues and this inflammation easily matures into suppuration, but it is a suppuration that is generally indolent and sluggish—by this we mean a suppuration that does not evacuate easily but perpetuates itself into a long drawn-out process which ebbs and flows for months. Various theories have been offered regarding this slow and indolent suppurative process. It is mainly supposed to be due to deficiency of Silicea in the cellular tissues. **Silicea** in the potentized form rectifies this deficiency and helps in the expulsion of foreign or quasi-foreign substance imbedded in the connective tissues. It is for this reason that **Silicea** is widely used in abscesses, carbuncles, boils, sinuses and fistulæ which do not respond to treatment and drag on eternally. In the Biochemic system of treatment this is explained on the basis of **Silicea** augmenting the supply of silicic acid in the connective tissue cells. We, as homœopaths, are more concerned with the indications on which it should be prescribed rather than how it works, when introduced into the human system. Great sensitiveness and over-susceptibility are the two keynote indications on which the prescription of **Silicea** should be based, particularly in suppurative diseases. The part affected is extremely tender to touch and is the seat of a peculiar shooting pain. The pus that **Silicea** either absorbs or lets loose is copious, watery, thin, gelatinous and putrid. Chronicity, as has been mentioned before, is the peculiar hallmark of **Silicea.** The suppurative process in **Silicea** extends to joints, ligaments, tendons and bones and are generally deepseated in character. **Silicea** has also the property of aborting boils and abscesses. It sets up a healthier phenomenon and prevents the dreaded recurrence of the complaints. Any curiosity as to its relation to **Hepar sulphur** and **Mercurius** is justifiable. It usually follows the abovementioned remedies. **Mercury** facilitates maturity; **Hepar sulphur** expels the pus that **Mercury** generates; **Silicea** usually comes in after all the foreign substances are expelled and promotes steady healing.

The aid of **Silicea** is usually called in to disperse cold induarations. Often it happens that after boils and abscesses are partially cured there usually remains a surrounding area of hardness, due probably to the secretion of plastic exudations during the inflammatory process. **Silicea** leads to the absorption of this substance and establishes the normal consistency of tissues. In this connection it should be mentioned that it goes so far as to obliterate even cicatricial tissues. After abcesses are healed, burnt surfaces have gone through process of resolution, we are often confronted with new connective tissue growths in the form of scarred tissues. **Silicea** has the reputation of dissolving these objectionable aftergrowths.

The action of **Silicea** on the bony tissue is the matter of our next consideration. Mal-assimilation, the keynote symptom of **Silicea**, shows its influence on the bony structure of the patient. This particular tissue becomes soft, pliable and spongy. This leads to various types and forms of mal-formations and disfigurements. Curvature and necrosis of the vertebral column, disfigurement of joints, nonclosure of cranial bones, rhachitic disfigurements of the ribs, caries of tibia and fibula, suppuration and caries of hip bones are instances illustrating the action of **Silicea** on the hard tissue.

The mucous membrane too, does not escape from the action of **Silicea**. We have offensive and protracted discharge from various mucous surfaces in **Silicea**. It is serviceable not in the catarrhal, nor in the inflammatory but in the putrefactive stage of various ailments affecting the mucous lining of the different orifices of the human system. We use it in otorrhœa, ozæna, pharyngitis, laryngitis, conjunctivitis, blepharitis and in many other affections of similar nature when they are characterised by chronicity, involvement of neighbouring glands, affection of the sub-mucous connective tissues and periosteum and the presence of a discharge that is thin, ichorous, corrosive and putrid.

The action of **Silicea** on the skin is of paramount importance. It is absolutely unhealthy. It lacks all power of recuperation. A simple scratch festers and turns into an ugly sore; every little injury suppurates; even the nails of the fingers and toes become brittle and crack easily; simple ulcer becomes phagedenic and extends in depth and keeps on secreting its characteristic discharge. The appearance of the skin is wax-like, and earthy. It is covered all over with itching exanthema, pustules, acne solaris and rosacea, eczema, intertrigo, impetigo, herpes, pemphigus and herpetic eruptions. The ulcers of **Silicea** generally appear in membraneous parts. They are, as has been said, phagedenic, flat and bluish white at the base. The edges are high, hard and spongy, bleeding most readily. There is also a sensation of coldness in these ulcers.

The action of **Silicea** on the nervous tissues is no less marked. It causes a tendency to paralysis and paralytic weakness due to defective nutrition of the nerves of the spinal cord and brain. There is a great want of vital warmth even when he takes exercise. A sense of weakness and debility is constantly on him and he wants to lie down most of the time. In tremulousness, nervous debility, drowsiness, lassitude, depression and excessive gaping it so resembles **Gelsemium** that a confusion between the two remedies is very likely. It must be remembered however that most of these symptoms originate from imperfect nourishment and malnutrition in **Silicea**. Furthermore there is always the history of suppression of a natural discharge such as sweat, etc.

Silicea is a great constitutional remedy. It is especially useful for system rendered weak by defective assimilation. The long list of skin troubles, where **Silicea** is curative, clearly shows that it is useful in psoric and scrofulous diathesis. The patient is as a rule emaciated, pale and of light complexion. However much he is fed and cared for, he dwindles down every day. He wears an expression of constant suffering. The head in this patient is disproportionately large but the body is small and emaciated. The face is pale and cachectic and it is covered all over with cracks and rhagades. The large head is almost always covered with profuse sweat although the body remains dry. There is a marked sensibility to touch particularly of the scalp and he objects even to the pressure of a hat; to brush the head is also out of the question owing to the same tenderness. Another strange characteristic, inspite of this great tenderness, is a desire to wrap up the head warmly. This he does to protect himself from catching cold.

Mentally he is weak and feeble. Reading, writing, and thinking bring on fatigue. He experiences great difficulty in fixing his attention on any subject and in consequence he makes many mistakes and becomes quite confused. The other aspect of **Silicea** is irritability. He can be and generally is, as repulsive as **Nux vomica.** With this repulsiveness he also combines obstinacy.

We must not forget that **Silicea** also suffers from certain fixed ideas. However much he tries, he cannot get himself out of certain delusions; for instance he feels as if pins are scattered all over the place and he is in constant dread of stepping on them. He searches for them all the time and even his failure to detect any, does not help him to realise his mistake. In this respect he is similar to **Spigelia.** On this curious symptom Dr. Clarke effected a wonderful cure in a case of post-influenzal insanity. There are a few other ideas that haunt him. He believes as if he were divided into halves; that something alive were in his ears; that his eyes are dragged back into the head by strings; that a hair is on the tip of his tongue; that a pin is lodged in his throat; that his finger tips were made of paper. Symptoms such as these are very helpful and we will do well to take note of them.

Silicea is a splendid remedy for a particular type of headache. It is due to a sort of congestion to the head which gives a feeling of heaviness in the head and a sensation of heat in the face. It must be borne in mind, however, that this congestion is neither as violent nor as acute as that of **Belladonna.** It is caused by excessive study or mental exertion. It is more of the nature of sick headache. It starts from the nape of the neck and ascends to the vertex and finally settles on one side of the forehead, generally the right side. It is generally relieved by the wrapping up of the head and hot compresses as in **Manganum** and **Stront.** The headache is also relieved by the passing of profuse urine as **Gels., Kali bi., Iris,** and **Lachesis.** At the height of the paroxysm there is apt to be nausea and vomiting. This patient is also subject to a peculiar sort of vertigo which too rises from the spine to the head. It may be the effect of suppressed foot-sweat. It is aggravated from motion or looking upward. All these symptoms prove conclusively that the malnutrition hinted at so often in **Silicea,** extends to the nervous structure same as it does to the other tissues of the body.

The visual tract too comes under the dominion of **Silicea.** Amblyopia, keratitis, sclero-choroiditis, irido-choroiditis, parenchymatous iritis and cataract find in **Silicea** a ready help. All these inflammatory processes are, as has been emphasised before, violent in nature. There is usually a tendency to the formation of sloughing ulcers. Photophobia is present in almost everyone of these complaints. Vision becomes dim and letters run together

Black spots or sparks before eyes, haziness of retina. opacity c
the humors, posterior synechiæ and various such complication
respond readily to the timely action of **Silicea**.   The ulcer
wherever they may be situated, have a tendency to perforate
Sloughing with profuse purulent discharge easily gives in to **Silicea**
Hence we use it successfully in pustular keratitis, ophthalmia an
fistula lachrymalis.   In traumatic inflammation too, **Silicea** be
comes useful when foreign particles, lodged in the eye, give ris
to inflammatory symptoms.   It reduces the inflammation by ex
pelling the foreign substance from the imbedded area.

We will now discuss its application in traucoma. Great hy
peræmia, swelling of conjunctiva, copious secretion of tears ar
mucus, violent supraorbital pain and an intense photophobia ar
some of its symptoms.

We use **Silicea** both in constipation and diarrhœa.   In diarrho
the stools are pasty, offensive and painless.   It contains particle
of undigested food and is attended with great exhaustion.
suits tiny, pot-bellied children during dentition who sweat pr
fusely in the head and in whom mal-assimilation is vividly po
trayed by the steady decline of weight inspite of the utmost ca
that is being taken of the child.   It is also extremely serviceable
those persistent cases of diarrhœa that appear after vaccinatio
In this respect it should be compared to **Thuja** to which it
complimentary.

The constipation of **Silicea** is very remarkable.   The stoo
are extremely hard and large and remaining long in the rectum, :
they usually do, they rob the rectum of all its power of expulsio
Though this hard mass of fæces is covered with slime, it takes ;
his strength to force it to the verge of the anus from which pla
it unfortunately slips back again. Ultimately he has to remove
mechanically by inserting his finger into his rectum.   The strai
ing is so violent that even the abdominal walls become sore ar
the patient breaks out into pools of sweat.   Such a constipation, :
is to be expected, brings on hæmorrhoidal complications.   T
whole region beginning from anus to rectum becomes intense
painful.   Tension at the time of passing stool is so great as
give rise to regular constriction of the anus.   The anus al
becomes cracked and fissured due to the passage of such enormo
lumps of fæces.

Silicea as is to be expected, has a very salutary influence
many affections of the womb and its appendages. It reduc
indurations of cervix uteri; it resolves serous cysts in vagina;

disperses periuterine cellulitis; it cures amenorrhœa and leucorrhœa. The indications are: Itching of pudenda, profuse acrid corroding milky flow coming out in gushes from the vaginal canal, cold feet and the discharge of blood between periods. The nipples of the breast are usually disfigured with ulcerations, rhagades and cracks. A very important symptom in **Silicea** is a sharp pain in either the breast or the uterus in mothers while nursing. Several cases of cancer are reported to have been helped on this indication. In this connection it should be mentioned that the funnel-like appearance of the nipples, so often seen in the cancer of the breast, is a great indication for **Silicea**. **Silicea** also moderates the too violent motions of fœtus in the gravid uterus.

Silicea is applicable in all kinds of fevers—intermittent, hectic and typhoid. The causative factor always is the suppression of foot-sweat. Though the various stages are ill-defined, the first stage, I mean the stage of chill, is particularly strong and well-marked. The shaking chill commences at 6 p.m. and obliges the patient to lie down. The slightest movement aggravates the chill and the patient scrupulously keeps his hands and feet in bed nicely covered up. The shivering and the chill are not relieved by the heat of fire. The feet and the legs as far as the knee, are icy cold. Violent heat causing dark redness of the face, is ushered in with strong thirst. The sweat which is always profuse breaks out periodically starting generally from the head and running down the face. It is offensive, sour and debilitating. There is usually loss of taste and appetite with a marked aversion to warm food.

In hectic fever the sweat starts mostly at midnight and wets the pillow far and wide. The profuseness of the sweat is accounted for by the slow suppurative process in the lungs. In typhoid fever, together with the great debility and the profuse sweat we find a strong desire to be magnetised.

Silicea is chronic of **Pulsatilla**, by which it is meant, that it corresponds to the chronic form of such diseases as call for **Pulsatilla** in their acute stage. Many of the symptoms are common. We have the same aversion to fat food, the same oily taste in the mouth and the same lachrymal mood in both the remedies. **Silicea** however is a deeper-acting remedy than **Pulsatilla**. It finishes what **Pulsatilla** leaves half-done. **Pulsatilla** acts similarly on the mucous membrane as **Silicea**, the only difference being that **Pulsatilla** supplies the connecting link between the ultra-acute stage of **Aconite** and the very chronic stage of **Silicea**. In **Aconite** and other catarrhal remedies, the discharge is strictly mucus though extremely thin and watery; in **Pulsatilla** it is thick, yellow and bland but still the mucus character of the discharge is retained; in **Silicea** the character of the discharge degnerates from mucus into purulent matter.

We will close this chapter with a short discussion of the indications of **Silicea** in epilepsy. The convulsions, almost always, start from the solar plexus. The periods at which they usually occur are the full moon and the new moon. The disease is generally ushered in by an overstrain of the mind or emotions. We must however be guided by other constitutional symptoms of the remedy.

Case 1.—A woman, thirty years old, had a tooth extracted on November 1st, she being pregnant. On May 25th of next year she was in the following condition: A cadaverous countenance, pale, thin, fleshless, and dry, bearing the marks of grief and pain; staring, lifeless eyes; the lower jaw was swollen to such an extent that it protruded several inches, as if a large sausage had been tied over it; the teeth of the lower maxillary stood in front of those of the upper jaw; both bones were lying as firmly and immovably upon each other as they are found in fully developed lockjaw. The entire lower jaw, with its covering tissues, was diseased and swollen; fistulous ulcers were advancing towards the bone from the inner and outer surface of the jaw, discharging a large amount of ichor of pestilential odor. A silver probe touched the denuded bone everywhere; it was rough and smooth in places; the probe itself turned black. Four months past she has had the most violent pains, day and night, preventing sleep; she lost her flesh from inability to eat. Prescribed **Silicea 30.** After fifty days the pain had left her; the mouth could be opened far enough to permit the removal of two teeth, to make an opening for the introduction of more solid food. For eighteen months she received one dose of **Silicea** every forty or fifty days. The fistulous openings united after a while; the lower jaw receded from the upper maxillary, while the gums assumed their old position, healed and became firmer and more compact. In September, 1838, the dead jaw-bone was removed; new bone had formed. The final result was a perfect cure.—(*Ibid*).

Case 2.—J. K., aged twenty years; two years ago he received a bruise just above the inner tibial tuberosity; has been under medical care for two years. On January 10, 1876, his condition was as follows: The joint was enlarged to twice its natural size, with constant pain through the joint of a sharp, cutting nature; the patella is immovable and there is almost total immobility of the joint and considerable atrophy of the limbs. Prescribed **Silicea** 30, one grain. Within two hours after taking the first dose the pain increased until it became almost unbearable, when it began to subside. January 24th, **Silicea** 200, one grain. February 17th, some pain, **Silicea** 200, one grain dose. Simple, warm fomentations every evening. March 1st, the pain absent; the patella can now be displaced a very little; the joint is also becoming more flexible. April 10th, has dispensed with the use of the cane, but there remains a slight limp in walking, owing to a shortening of the flexor ligaments. **Calcarea carbonica** 200, one dose.

July 1st.—The case is improving constantly and discharged as needing no more treatment.—(**C. in Cin. Med. Advance July, 1878).**

Case 3.—Mrs. S., during convalescence from spinal meningitis, experienced great trouble from a distressing cough. Marked excitation and aggravation of the cough by the slightest current of cold air from without into and through the room.—Set in motion by the most gentle opening and closing of the doors, as well as by the simple and easy movement of her attendant across the chamber, and whether awake or asleep. **Sil.** 6, every four hours, cured.—Dr. R. Ludlam.

SINAPIS ALBA.

Under this heading we have two preparations—Sinapis Alba and Sinapis Nigra. One is the white mustard and the other is the black mustard.

In India the oil extracted from mustard is a great remedy for all kinds of colds. From birth to death it is a thing of daily use with the Indian. The body is given a daily mustard bath as a precaution against cold. The boy, the adult and the old man have their chest and back rubbed with mustard oil whenever there is the slightest indication of an oncoming cold. In the homœopathic proving, too, this aspect of **Sinapis** has been very well authenticated. It is in the treatment of hay fever, cold and catarrh that it has been found to be mostly useful. The following are some of its important symptoms:—

Dryness of the anterior nares; left nostril stopped up all day; scanty acrid discharge from nose; mucous membrane of nose dry and hot; no discharge; symptoms aggravated in the afternoon and evening; either nostril may be affected alone or alternately with the other. Profuse, thin, watery discharge from anterior nares, excoriating and acrid; wings of nose red and sore; draws considerable mucus into the throat from posterior nares; voice thick, nasal; frequent short, hacking cough, aggravated during day and ameliorated by lying down. Feeling as if the nostrils were stopped up although they discharge profusely; excoriation of nose and lips; itching and smarting of eyelids; post-nasal discharge; continually clearing throat; infrequent hacking cough; dull frontal headache; nasal, voice. Hay fever with suffused eyes; itching and smarting of eyes; nose swollen and discharging continually a thin acrid mucus; oppression of chest, as if movement were impeded; a sensation as if something heavy oppressed her on all sides from her neck to diaphragm; aggravation at night and on lying down; black tongue; ulcers in the mouth, especially on the tongue, with violent burning pain; the whole buccal cavity is so sensitive that even blandest food or drink becomes unbearable;

Sinapis alba cured a woman eight months in pregnancy, who was constantly suffering from burning in the stomach extending up œsophagus to throat and mouth . Her mouth was full of canker sores, and it was with great difficulty that she could either eat or drink.

SINAPIS NIGRA.

Sinapis nigra, the Black mustard, belongs to the natural order of Cruciferæ. This remedy has not been very satisfactorily proved but its efficacy in hay fever with intense coryza, lachrymation and sneezing, can hardly be denied. The discharge is acrid and we have frequent stoppage of nostrils. Great dryness is complained of in the anterior nares. Throat feels hot, inflamed and scalded. The cough which is barking in nature is relieved by lying down. The breath of the mouth is very offensive. Another important symptom is the sweat on the upper lip and forehead.

SLAG.

This medicine is prepared from the pulverised slag of Blast furnace in which iron is melted. It contains **Silicea, Alumina, Calcium, Sulphur, Ferrum** and **Phosphorus,** as its ingredients. This remedy, too, is of recent origin and has not been proved sufficiently, although some of its properties specially its action over the anal mucous membrane and veins justify its inclusion in our Materia Medica.

We are indebted for this remedy to Dr. J. Meredith. The following symptoms are characteristic:—.

Great itching in the anus.

Piles with intense itching.

Soreness of the anus.

Pains in the knee-caps.

Swelling and pain in the patellæ worse on going upstairs.

Flatulent distention in the evening and an oppressed feeling in the heart.

SOL.

Sol is the sun-light. Saccharum lactis is exposed to the concentrated rays of the sun and kept constantly stirred with a glass rod till it is well saturated.

Light is a decided factor in health and is an agent, which combines with fresh air, exercise, and substantial food, prolongs human life and adds to its well being. That sun light has important therapeutic value cannot be denied. The effect of light on living organism is manifested in nature in various ways. It is illustrated by the difference in the tint presented by the same species of plants grown in the shade and in the sun. We also know that people that live in ill-lighted habitation lack the ruddy healthful appearance of those who live in bright sun light and lead an outdoor life. The use of sun baths was in vogue even in ancient time. The skin and soft parts are permeable to the rays of the sun. The bactericidal effect of light has been conclusively proved. The body cells too are stimulated by the rays of the sun, their metabolic activity increased and their power of resistance against inimical bacterial agency augmented. Effort has been made by Wilhelm, Conrad, Rœntgen, Windmark and Finsen to utilize this in the treatment of certain pathological conditions of the skin. Homœopathy, too, is not behind-hand and certain physicians chiefly Thayer, Webster, Swan and Fincke have experimented with the potentized principle of light. The results, though needing further verifications, have not been bereft of good consequences. Webster used it in a case of epithelioma in which the growth was removed by solar cautery with scarcely any scar left.

The symptoms however, have not assumed any definite shape. I recommend further provings, for us to arrive at a clear-cut symptomatology of the drug.

SOLANINUM.

Under this heading we will study the various members of the genus of the Solanaceæ such as **Solanum nigrum, Sol. tuberosum, Sol. aceticum, Sol. arrebenta, Sol. carolinense, Sol. mammosum** and **Sol. oleraceum.**

Solanum nigrum is called the Black night shade. It is a weed that grows mostly in tropical countries and has white flowers and black berries. It is very similar in its action to **Bell** and many of its symptoms are to be found in the other remedy. In delirium we notice the same stammering speech, the efforts to get out of bed and go away, the piercing cries and the convulsions alternating with coma and twitching. The pains too are throbbing and they come and go quickly. The same aggravation from mistep and stooping is to be found here. The face looks highly congested, and betokens great anxiety, fright and terror. The differentiating points, however, are to be found in its action over the skin where it has a tendency to produce blackness. The affected parts become swollen and gradually become darker and darker till they look almost black as if dyed. I had very gratifying results from it in a desperate case of progressive gangrene in the finger tips and knuckles and toes of a young man who had several of his fingers amputated through extension of the gangrenous process. **Lach., Secale** and **Arsen.** failed to bring on any response till **Solanum nigrum** was administered with the effect that the progress of the disease was immediately checked.

Its application in convulsions and spasms is based on a peculiar movement of the hand during the attack. The patient stretches his hands as if to grasp something and then carries them eagerly to his mouth and goes through motions of mastication and swallowing. The varicose veins all over his body look prominent. The patient betrays great sensitiveness to cold air.

Solanum tuberosum ægrotans is the active principle derived from the tubers of diseased potatoes. Potatoes thus affected are sour and of great danger and instances are not rare where they have been instrumental in causing great havoc. Its action seems to be particularly confined to the rectum. It produces and therefore cures prolapsus ani, attended with great pain and ineffectual effort to discharge the contents of the rectum. We also notice a foul odor in the breath as well as the body of the patient. It is reputed to have cured tumours of the rectum that look like decayed potato. Frequent urging to stool, violent burning in anus and rectum, alternate protrusion and retraction of anus during stool and also a sensation of contraction of sphincter ani are important indications of this preparation.

Solanum aceticum.—This preparation of **Solanum** vies with **Ant. tart.** in respiratory paralysis. We have great accumulation of mucus in the larger air passages causing a regular rattling during inspiration. Hence like **Ant. tart.,** it should be particularly thought of in the death rattle of patients, which condition it removes most marvellously by enabling the patient to expel the obstructing phlegm.

Solanum arrebenta grows spontaneously in some of the provinces of Brazil. Like **Bell.,** it produces great redness of the face. Like its sister remedy it is recommended highly in apoplectic attacks where its scope is almost as great as that of **Bell.**

Solanum carolinense is also called the Horse-nettle and it contains a large percentage of solanin. It is reputed to be of great use in convulsions and epileptic seizures, where given in dosage of 30 to 60 drops, several times a day, it checks the virulence of the attacks and gradually brings on a cure. It is of particular value in the grand mal of ediopathic type and in hystero-epilepsy.

Solanum mammosum is prepared from a fruit commonly known as the Apple of Sodom. The chief symptoms are irritability of the mind and an utter inability to think. The mind is not altogether a blank. The comprehension is there but there is a total lack of the power of combining thoughts and expressing them in sentences. Like **Bell.,** we have sleepiness without being able to sleep.

It is also a great remedy for coxalgia and sticking pain in the left hip-joint. This pain gets worse during and after exercise and disappears while standing and sitting down.

Solanum oleraceum is prepared from the flowers of Juquerioba, a herbaceous plant growing in the damp marshes of Brazil. It has been found to be highly efficacious in swelling of the mammary glands attended with profuse secretion of milk. We also have long protracted menses and profuse discharge of white mucus from the vagina. This remedy needs further verification.

SPIGELIA ANTHELMIA.

It is known as the Demerara Pink-root. It is also called the worm-grass because of its anthelmintic properties. There is another variety called Spigelia marylandica, growing in the southern state of North America. Here we are concerned with the former variety. Tincture is prepared from dried herbs.

The name **Spigelia** is, in my mind, very intimately associated with pain. It is a great anodyne for pain of a certain description and we will go into it thoroughly just now. The pain of **Spigelia** is mostly neuralgic. It is burning, tearing, stitching and radiating in character. The pain is distinctly worse by noise, jar, movement and change of weather. The principle seats of pain, though it may affect any part of the body, are head, eyes, face, teeth and heart. Another peculiarity of the pain of **Spigelia** is, as mentioned by Dr. Clarke, outpressing. It begins from some interior portion of the body and shoots outward; sometimes again the direction of the pain is from below upward. We will have ample opportunity to study it further, later on in connection with the various affections for which it is indicated.

The **Spigelia** patients are generally of a rheumatic diathesis. Ascaridæ and Lumbrici, as has been already hinted at, are frequent complications where **Spigelia** is indicated. These patients are, like **Kali carb,** and **Stannum,** very sensitive to touch; the least touch sends shudders throughout the whole frame. They are pale, sickly and bloated in appearance; yellow discolouration around eyes, a marked presence of sweat on face and a general aggravation of all symptoms from sunrise to sunset are special characteristics of **Spigelia.**

The bodily sensitiveness of **Spigelia** is quite in keeping with the mental irritability of the remedy. We notice a kind of restlessness and anxiety and a great disinclination for work and a marked solicitude for the future. But the most striking symptom of all is a fear of pointed things. On this symptom **Spigelia** has been reported to have cured a case of extreme nausea during pregnancy. **Silicea** has somewhat of a similar symptom and should be remembered in this connection.

Spigelia is a very valuable heart remedy. The symptom to indicate it is a pain of a very violent description located in the region of the heart. Sharp stitches sometimes shooting into arm and neck are referred to in the cardiac region. These stitches are synchronous with the pulse. Anxiety of mind and oppression frequently accompany these stitches. On these symptoms al ne it has been prescribed with great success in valvular diseases, endocarditis and pericarditis. Palpitation—violent palpitation frequently complicates the disease. It is so violent that it can be sometimes discerned through the clothing; it shakes the whole chest and even the sound is audible to people near about. The patient complains of a peculiar parrying sensation over the heart. This violent palpitation is frequently a precursor to fainting. The feeling in the heart is as if it were compressed and squeezed.

Even endocarditis with insufficiency of the mitral valve, after acute articular rheumatism and cystolic blowing at the apex have been known to respond to **Spigelia.** Dr. Nash vouches to have not only relieved but cured valvular troubles with this remedy. Dyspnœa and suffocating attacks from the slight movements, have been relieved with **Spigelia.** Aggravation from the slightest movement, as that of raising of an arm or taking deep breath, is a cardinal indication of **Spigelia.**

Spigelia is a first-rate remedy in a certain variety of headache. The headache commences early every morning with the rising of the sun, increases till noon and then gradually declines with the setting of the sun. It starts from the nape of the neck and extending over the head settles over the left eye. The sensation is, as if the head were pressed open along the vertex or as if the brain were forcing itself out through the forehead. It is usually worse from noise, jarring of the body, bright light, opening mouth, speaking aloud, laughing and stooping. The pain is so violent that at times it feels as if the nerves were being torn out by a pain of sharp pincers. The pain located in the forehead and temple extends into the eyes and the malar bones. Profuse lachrymation, photophobia, pulsation of the temporal arteries, coryza, and bilious vomiting accompany this headache.

Our task will be incomplete if we leave out its indications in ciliary neuralgia and prosopalgia. The pain in the eyeball, for which it is indicated oftener than any other remedy, is most intense and intolerable. It feels as if the eyes are too large for their sockets and the pain radiates through eyeball into the back of the head; at times it commences at a certain point and thence radiates into different directions. The eye feels as if it will be pressed out of the socket; every movement hurts. The pain spreads from the eyes into the frontal sinuses and head. There is also great inclination to wink. The above symptoms lead to its application in glaucoma, sclero-choroiditis, rheumatic ophthalmia, gonorrhœal ophthalmia, scrofulous conjunctivitis, keratitis and iritis. Dr. Hering cites of a case of a man suffering from extreme pain over temple and forehead, the effect of an injury caused by a brick striking over the eye sustained years ago. **Spigelia** brought the wished for relief and cure. The symptoms on which it was indicated are better given in his own language. "At irregular intervals extreme pain came over the site of the wound; it was at times so severe that he feared he would lose his reason; the pain came at about 10 a.m. and reached its height at about 3 p.m.; sharp and cutting pain extended over temple and forehead with profuse flow of water from the eyes; he was better in a dark room when quiet and almost entirely relieved at night." A routine prescriber would have run to **Arnica**.

We will next have a short comparison of **Spigelia** with **Ant. crud., Bry., Gels., Kali. bich.,** and **Kalmia.**

In **Antimonium crudum**, the headache starts somewhat similarly. It is a stupefying dull headache, generally the effect of a prolonged bath in flowing water. Aversion to food, nausea, loathing, want of appetite, and vomiting are some of its important symptoms.

Bryonia resembles **Spigelia** in respect of its modality. The headache is always worse on opening the eyes and on movement. It commences in the morning, not on awaking, but after opening eyes and lasting till evening. The headache which is jerking and throbbing in character starts on the forehead and goes backward to occiput.

In **Gelsemium** the headache begins in the nape of the neck, passes over the head and settles over the eyes. It is also a sun headache; the patient finds a sort of blur before his vision before the headache starts and is always better after a copious urination. Dizziness with blurred vision, heaviness of head, nausea, vomiting and cold sweat are prominent features of this remedy.

Kali bichromicum is another remedy in which the headache starts with the sun. Here also blindness precedes the headache but sight returns as the headache increases.

Kalmia lat. too has headache which increases with the ascending sun and decreases as the sun goes down.

Case 1.—M. L., Aged, thirty years, has suffered greatly during the past two years from frequent attacks of neuralgia which, at first of short duration and comparatively slight, have steadily increased in severity and now last as long as three days. The attacks are always preceded by a roaring in the left ear as of a great wind. The severest pain is in the left upper arm. Sometimes preceding, and sometimes accompanying the pain in the arm, is a pain in the left chest, in the cardiac region, which describes a semi-circle corresponding to the border of the right half of the left mamma, and continuing from the upper part of the mamma, in a direct line to the front of the left shoulder; it is continuous with the pain in the arm. The pain about the heart is sometimes attended with a constrictive sensation. The pain in the arm commences above the left elbow, in front, apparently in the bone, and runs in a line up the anterior part of the arm, and in front of the shoulder joint, ascending in a direct line to the mastoid portion of the temporal bone. A streak of pain dips into the left ear. Of late, the pain has gone around the left side of the occiput, and has reached the crown of the head. There is obscuration of vision, especially in the left eye during the paroxysms; the pain increases and diminishes without apparent irregularity. The left upper arm, shoulder and left side of the neck feel as if a great heat were radiating upon them, which are superficially so sensitive that the slightest covering increases the suffering. When the pain is greatest the head is repeatedly jerked to the left side. When she attempts raise her arm, it seems to be drawn down to her side. During the pain there is much sweating, which does not relieve. The hands and feet are always very cold. She is worse at night; the pain prevents sleep. He had severe attacks both in wet and in dry weather, and during all seasons, but the pains have been worse during an approaching thunder-storm—rather easier after the rain has begun to fall. At the menstrual periods the attacks are aggravated apparently from increase of the pain about the heart, but the suffering has not been peculiar to this period. She is worse when sitting up; from application of cold water and from the heat of a fire. There is no amelioration from warm water. She cannot, of course, lie on the painful side. Her menses have been somewhat premature and profuse. Her digestion is not good; she drinks much water at a meal; unless she does this, she has continued hiccough until the food is thrown up. She received **Spigelia,** which broke up the neuralgic pains and improved her general health. She had left some rheumatic pains in the right shoulder and arm.—(Dr. Hamilton Ring in **Ohio Med. and Surg. Reporter, March, 1868).**

Case 2.—A woman, twenty-six years old. She had, after her fourth confinement, spasmodic symptoms, which attacked the chest. After a long time of Allopathic treatment she presented the following symptoms: Constant burning, pressure of painful feeling of "being bruised" in the chest. Shortness of breath and seeming suffocation upon motion, so that she dare not leave the bed. Sensation of constant trembling in the chest and temples, aggravated by every motion of the hand, even knitting, and enforcing absolute idleness. The most violent symptoms are, however, produced when she raises the arms to the head. It causes a feeling as if something was being torn in the chest, with suffocation and anxiety. Touching the chest causes rush of blood to the face with perspiration. Consequently she cannot bear clothes and is only lightly covered with a shirt. There is often a sensation of a spasm which commences in the lower abdomen, extends upward and stops her breath. Again, violent action of the heart, with a sensation as if the heart were compressed; again a feeling of trembling and pain. At other times it seems as if everything in the chest were too short or were loose and tumbling about. She is consequently very cautious when moving down upon the chest, whether she is lying down or sitting up. An attempt to hold it up is followed by anxiety and a feeling as if something in the chest was tearing, with spasmodic inspirations, during which there is spasmodic action of the whole chest; cyanosis of the countenance; stormy action of the heart. Pulse synchronous in all the arteries. When reclining, 80 per minute; sitting up, 92 per minute, and not synchronous with the beat of the heart. The hand detects a feeble, indistinct action of the heart. The ear, especially with the aid of the stethoscope, distinguishes the differences between the systole and diastole by wavy motion rather than by the distinct beat. Prescribed **Spigelia** 30, followed by an aggravation of symptoms; on the following day improvement commenced; she could move the arms without difficulty and even walked a little. On account of some little aggravation the remedy was repeated; followed by a cure. She remained well and soon became pregnant.—**(Bethmann in Allg. Hom. Zeitg., iii., 109).**

Case 3.—Mr. B. was sitting, half-leaning in bed; would not move the least; would hardly speak or take a deep breath, as all this would aggravate the pain; pain fearfully cutting, piercing through the left chest, near the sternum, to the back; heart not beating, but an uninterrupted rush of blood through it; pulse not beating, but appeared to the finger like a thread quickly pulled through the artery; hands icy-cold with cold perspiration; great anguish expressed in the face. He had had rheumatism before. **Verat. alb.,** two doses with benefit. **Spig.** 6, one dose, relief in ten minutes. Next day the beating of the heart and pulse was regular and the pains all gone.—Dr. H. Lehmann.

SPONGIA.

Spongia was introduced into our Materia Medica by Samuel Hahnemann. It is prepared from roasted sponge. The tincture is prepared from the solution of 20 grains of the roasted sponge in 400 drops of alcohol. It contains Iodine and certain other ingredients of minor importance. The great characteristic of **Spongia** is dryness of the mucous membrane of tongue, pharynx. larynx and trachea. We will have ample evidence of this during the course of our discourse on this remedy.

Rawness in the chest characterises the second important keynote of **Spongia**.

Thirdly, we must take note of the excessive sensibility to touch of **Spongia** which, in my opinion, should be given the third place in the list of its characteristic indications.

The following are some of the important indications of **Spongia.**

Mind. Irresistible desire to sing, excessive mirth, followed by sadness.

Paroxysms of anxiety or anguish. Cardiac troubles.

Weeping and inconsolable mood.

Terror and fear: of approaching death; that she will cough; with the heat; with the sweat.

Every excitement increases the cough.

Head. Pressing headache in r. frontal eminence, from within outward, aggravated while sitting, on entering warm room after walking in open air, and from looking at anything sharply; ameliorated when lying in horizontal position,, especially when lying on back.

Throat. Sore throat, aggravated after eating sweet things.

Thyroid gland swollen, even with chin; at night suffocating spells, barking, with stinging in throat and soreness in abdomen.

Throat extremely swollen; suffocating attacks.

Respiration, wheezing, whistling, occasionally sawing; head thrown back, muscles of chest working, abdomen contracted under ribs with very effort to inflate lungs; cold, clammy sweat all over; lies quietly on side, anxious for breath; does not want to be fanned; eyes fixed, pupils dilated; does not notice attendants; loose involuntary discharge from bowels in morning. Diphtheria.

Difficult swallowing. Croup.

Appetite. Thirst. Desires. Aversion. Eating and drinking relieve cough.

Male Sexual Organs. Swollen, painful spermatic cords.

Maltreated orchitis; also after checked gonorrhoea.

Scirrhous testicle.

Female Sexual Organs. Enlargement and induration of ovaries.

Menses too soon, too profuse.

Before menses: colic, backache, soreness in sacrum and craving in stomach, palpitation.

During menses: drawing in all the limbs; awakes with suffocating spells. Violent drawing in upper and lower limbs, during menses.

Voice and Larynx. Trachea and Bronchia. Hoarseness, cough, coryza. Hoarse, voice cracked or faint, choking sensation; whistling inspiration. Feeling of a plug in larynx; larynx sensitive to touch and when turning neck; talking hurts.

Chronic sore-throat, aggravated when reading aloud, talking or singing; aggravated after eating sweet things.

Laryngeal phthisis.

Great dryness of larynx.

Iaryngismus stridulus.

Talking, singing or swallowing hurts larynx.

Inflammation of larynx, trachea and bronchia.

Attacks of mucous rattling in windpipe; at times strangling.

Feeling of stoppage in windpipe;

Starts from sleep suddenly with contraction of larynx.

Region of thyroid gland indurated.

A sound as if a foreign body is audible in larynx or trachea moving to and fro.

Larynx sensitive to touch. Croup. Whooping cough.

Perichondritis laryngea; hollow, barking, dry cough, day and night, constriction in larynx; pain in larynx on touching it, and on turning neck; whistling breathing.

Dry bronchitis, with terrible, hard, dry, racking cough; much dyspnœa and slight expectoration; Aggravated in hot room, ameliorated by eating or drinking.

Cough dry and sibilant, sounding like a saw driven through a pine board. Croup.

Croup aggravated before midnight (aggravated before morning, **Hepar**).

Cough is dry and sibilant, or sounds like a saw driven through a pine board, each cough corresponding to a thrust of the saw; no mucus rattle; cough dry and hoarse, causes pain in throat. Croup.

Asthma: from taking cold, cannot lie down; sibilat ronchi; after menses; breathing always tight, cannot inspire nor expire freely; in consequence of goitre; breathing rattling and panting; after every slight motion loses her breath and becomes faint; blood rushes to her chest and head; hot face, anxious; fears she will die of suffocation; spasmodic, with organic disease of heart; must throw head back; aggravated at full moon.

Cough dry, barking, hollow, croupy; wheezing, asthmatic; caused by burning or tickling in larynx, sensation like a plug or valve, or by feeling of accumulation of mucus and weight in chest.

Heart, Pulse and Circulation. Constricting pain in cardiac region with anxiety; anxious sweat. Angina pectoris. Heart beating a double stroke; pulsating sound in ear.

Attacks of oppression and cardiac pain; aggravated lying with head low.

Rheumatic endocarditis, loud blowing with each heart-beat.

Stinging pressing pains in præcordial region.

Violent palpitation, awakens after 12 P. M.; sensation of suffocation; bellows' mumur; loud cough, which is hard, tight, dry; great alarm, agitation, anxiety, dyspnœa.

Palpitation: violent, with pain, gasping respiration; suddenly awakened after midnight, with suffocation, great alarm, anxiety, valvular insufficiency; before catamenia; with congestion to chest.

Rheumatic endocarditis, valvular insufficiency (usually mitral), systolic murmur.

Angina pertoris; contracting pain in chest, heat, suffocation, faintness, and anxious sweat.

Case 1.—A blooming boy of five years has had a peculiar cough for two evenings. At 9 o'clock of the third evening there were present: red countenance; frequent, full, hard pulse; hurried breathing, short, sawing, labored. Suddenly he jumped up, opened the eyes and nostrils as wide as possible, and, with his face purple, and his mouth wide open, gasped for air. Immediately after, a few short, barking, hoarse coughs and then long, whistling inspiration. During the height of the paroxysms extreme distress, clutching of the throat and throwing back of the head. After it, exhaustion and complaint about pain in the windpipe. Hoarseness. Prescribed **Spongia** incture, six drops in a glass of water, a spoonful every fifteen minutes. mmediate improvement and perfect cure in six days.—(Billig).

Case 2.—Rheumatism had left the lumbar muscles and seized the heart the second similar metastasis with this patient). Was awakened between ' and 2 A.M. by a sense of suffocation, accompanied by violent, loud cough, ;reat alarm, agitation, anxiety and difficult respiration. The action of the neart was violent and rapid, and each beat was accompanied by a loud lowing, as of a bellows. **Spong.**; (Jen). 200. The bellows-sound, which was oud, gradually disappeared, and in a day or two ceased to be heard.—)r. P. P. Wells.

SQUILLA.

Squilla is commonly called the sea onion. It is a bulbous plant bearing a long spike of whitish flowers. It belongs to the natural order of Liliaceæ. It is abundant on the shore of Mediterranean. It is diuretic, expectorant, emetic and cathartic.

My experience with **Squilla** is very limited. I have used it once or twice in a peculiar cough that baffled all treatment and only succumbed to **Squilla.** The **Squilla** cough is very characteristic. There is an abundance of catarrhal symptoms with the cough. Acrid corrosive fluent coryza, sneezing, soreness of the nostril as in **Allium cepa,** spurting of urine while coughing, constant expectoration of mucus and gushing of tears while coughing are characteristic indications of this remedy. The cough is loose in the morning, but it gets dry towards the evening. It is caused by a tickling creeping sensation in the chest. Sometimes this tickling is felt as low down as the region of the spleen. Hence it is recommended very highly in splenic cough. Stitches are felt during cough under the free ribs of the left side. This is supposed to be a very important indication of **Squilla.**

It is also useful in pleuro-pneumonia, specially when we find stitching pains in the left chest. Constant hacking cough, profuse urination, high temperature, rapid pulse and a great abundance of catarrhal symptoms as has been mentioned before are the principal indications. Excessive flow of urine should always draw our attention to **Squilla.** Dr. Boger brought great relief to a patient suffering from angina pectoris on the principal indication of profuse urination accompanying severe heart pains and much loose mucus in the throat and trachea.

STANNUM.

Tin, one of the oldest minerals known, is a component of bronze. An ingot of pure tin is white with a slight tinge of blue, it does not tarnish in the air and is proof against acid liquids. It is imported in big quantities from Cornwall and Italy where it occurs in granite and in the clayish state in association with wolfranite, mica, topaz and other minerals. Bolivia, Peru and Queensland are other sources of our supply of tin.

This remedy was first introduced into our Materia Medica by Samuel Hahnemann. It was used by the ancients in various ailments but up to the time Homœopathy came into the field, the only use made of it by the Allopath was as a vermifuge. The keen intellect of our master is responsible to a very great extent for the wonderful unfolding of the strange properties of this hitherto neglected metal.

We, homœopaths use it for numerous complaints and in each instance, we are guided by the strange, peculiar and the uncommon symptoms. The symptom that stands out most prominent in **Stannum** is, in my opinion, the profound weakness so frequently complained of by these patients. It is a weakness mostly located in the chest. It is more of a nature of nervous exhaustion. The patient has to desist and rest frequently while attending to her usual daily avocations. She stops often while talking as she gets out of breath; she complains of palpitation from the least exertion. This weakness is more of the nature of an empty, all-gone sensation. She feels as if her whole chest is one empty cavity and it is this feeling that takes out all sensations of solidarity from the patient.

This nervous exhaustion is particularly felt when the patient walks down-stairs more than when she ascends; her limbs simply give way under her and she has to drop into the nearest available seat. Mentally too, she is not over-bright.

She manifests great sadness, a strong disinclination to talk and a pronounced aversion to the company of men. She is anxious, weak and irritable. **Stannum** also shows a strong bend towards crime. The lachrymal mood is particularly prominent before menstruation; the distress of mind ceases as soon as the period is established. She does not, however, frequently give way to crying as crying makes her worse. In this connection, it will not be out of place to discuss the attitude favoured by the

Stannum patient. We find her most of the time on her back with one leg stretched and the other drawn up.

The next characteristic of **Stannum** is to be seen in the nature of its pain. It begins slowly, increases gradually to a certain degree of intensity and then as gradually decreases. This pain is generally of neuralgic origin and is ameliorated by pressure as in **Colocynth.** This modality applies to headache, facial and dental neuralgia, abdominal and other pains.

It is a great remedy for intermittent supra-orbital neuralgia after abuse of quinine and in violent neuralgia of face and head where pain steals in a "slow, sure fashion requiring hours to reach its maximum and then begins to decline in exactly the same way." We must also think of **Stannum** in pain of the malar bone and its great sensitiveness to touch as also of its aggravation occurring before and **during menses.**

A third symptom which is of particular interest in **Stannum** is pain, weakness and aching in the deltoid muscle and arm particularly felt when using the voice. This modality is curious and hence important.

In appearance our **Stannum** patient is lean, thin and weakly; dark rings under the eyes are particularly noticeable; pale face, sunken eyes, dulness of intellect, and sickly elongated features are characteristics of **Stannum.**

We will now study its application on the male and female sexual organs. It is essentially a voluptuous remedy. Orgasm in **Stannum** is easily produced. The slightest irritation and the least approach of thoughts bordering on sexual subject bring on emissions. Hence we use **Stannum** frequently in nocturnal emissions, spermatorrhœa and in neurasthenia, especially when such sexual sensitiveness is at a great premium. Emissions take place without the least lascivious dreams; scratching arm produces an intolerable sensation of pleasure in the genital organs which extends to uterus and produces sexual orgasm. It is almost a great a remedy as **Sepia, Platina** and **Belladonna** for prolapsus uteri. It is also used for prolapsus of the vagina. The bearing down sensation in the uterus and vagina is always worse during stool so much so that she is afraid to attempt it.

The menses are too early, too profuse and are preceded by melancholia and pain in the malar bone. Leucorrhœa is profuse; is sometimes yellowish and at other times transparent, like the white of an egg. This constant leucorrhœa helps to aggravate the already existing debility.

Next we will consider the action of **Stannum** in chest, throat and larynx. It is supposed to be a great remedy in affections of the respiratory organs, particularly in tuberculosis of the lungs. There is a marked hectic fever towards the evening with profuse sweat at night. The cough is a deep, hollow and violent shattering cough, generally coming in paroxysms of three cough. It is caused by talking, singing, and laughing; the irritation is felt low down in the trachea. The secretion of sputum is usually abundant; it is like the white of an egg but mostly it is yellowish green with a sweetish and salty taste. Respiration is usually short and difficult due to weakness of the respiratory organs. A sensation of constriction of chest, stitching pain and a certain amount of dyspnœa and hemoptysis are frequent accompaniments of **Stannum.** It is not exactly in a typical case of consumption but generally in neglected cases of catarrh threatening into phthisis, that we are generally called in to prescribe **Stannum.** The one cardinal symptom that must never be overlooked here, as well as elsewhere, is the profound sense of weakness so characteristic of this remedy.

In this respect it will be worth our while to compare it with certain other remedies equally useful in the treatment of phthisis. **Phosphorus** should come in first. Here also is found a great weak, empty, all-gone sensation in the chest as well as in the entire abdomen. But it is generally used in phthisis of people who grow very rapidly, who are of a fine texture and in whom the mind develops more rapidly than the body. Here also we have hoarseness, evening aggravation, copious expectoration and hectic fever but there are usually a more prolonged and frequent hemoptysis, intense and intolerable burning, and profuse diarrhœa. The mouth is full of aphthous sores.

Silicea as a remedy is generally called in more advanced stages of phthisis. It is especially adapted to those who suffer from imperfect nutrition due to deficiency of assimilation. The pale, waxen, cachetic, earthy-looking complexion of **Silicea** with offensiveness of sweat, which is profuse and constant, is a guiding symptom. It has a wonderful control over the process of suppuration and as such it very often checks further progress of the disease.

Pulsatilla is admirably suited to young chlorotic girls with phthisical tendency, where the expectoration is yellow, salty and

offensive and where subclavicular pain, gradual loss of weight,
hectic fever, and a fast and rapid pulse point towards insipient
tuberculosis.

Sepia with its empty and hollow sensation, resembles Stannum to a certain extent but in this remedy the central third of
the right lung (Ars. upper third) is specially affected.

In Kali carb. too, we have a hollow sensation in the entire body.
It is one more of our agents, in our struggle against the great
white-plague. It has been highly spoken of by Hahnemann
for its great efficacy in all cases of phthisis, particularly those
following in the wake of pleurisy and characterized by darting,
stitching chest pains. In marked prostration and weakness, though
it resembles Stannum, it should never be confused with that
remedy; its great anti-psoric properties and constitutional symptoms are too characteristic to lead to any confusion. The globular
sputa, the special 3 A.M. aggravation, great touchiness of soles of
feet, puffiness of eyelids, aphonia, and difficult, wheezing breathing
are symptoms too characteristic to be mistaken.

Lastly we will discuss its application in disorders of digestion.
Nausea and vomiting are characteristically present especially from
odors of cooking food. There is a weak, gone-feeling in stomach
as in Sepia; oppression of stomach in hysterical women with
nausea, pale face and great weakness calls for Stannum. Gastralgia with clawing, kneading pain extending to the umbilicus—colic
relieved by hard pressure—diarrhœa and Monday constipation or
constipation appearing particularly on the day following rest, are
indications calling for Stannum in dyspepsia.

Case 1.—Although a majority of the cases where I have made any
success in the treatment of consumption have been with Sulph., and always
with high potencies, yet I have in my note-book one cured by a trituration
of Stan. 3 hardly less brilliant in its results. The case came to my hands
after being treated by two or three different allopathic physicians. I
learned that she had a scrofulous tumor, dispersed from the neck by Iodine
iust previous to this attack upon the lungs. I found her with a pulse from
50 to 160 per minute, with hectic fever and a racking, exhaustive cough
day and night, causing her to expectorate nearly or quite a quart of tough
glairy mucus mixed with purulent matter every twenty-four hours—the
quantity exceeding anything I ever saw before or since. She was rather
stout-built and of sanguine, bilious temperament and had lost her husband
a few months previous. Auscultation showed a large cavity in the upper
third of right lobe. I first gave her Calc. 30 which improved her so far as
to bring the pulse down to 120 and diminish the expectoration about one-
fourth. In the course of four or five weeks her pulse began to accelerate

and no further improvement was made in cough or expectoration. I then gave her three doses of **Stan. 3** in the course of the next eight days. She was so much improved at my next visit, which was in about ten days, that she called herself well. The pulse had fallen to about 90 and she expectorated very little. She had but two or three doses more to complete the cure.—Dr. G. N. Brigham.

Case 2.—Mrs.........., aged thirty-nine, gravida in the fourth month. Continued anxiety and restlessness; must keep in bed not only on account of bodily weakness, but also on account of her inability to do anything, as she cannot master sufficient courage and is forgetful and absent-minded. Feels like crying all the time, but crying makes her feel worse; great palpitation of the heart and anxiety, especially if she has to give directions in her domestic affairs. Thinking makes her feel wretched, and she cannot get rid of what once gets fixed in her mind. Over-sensitive to smell; vertigo on moving the head; visions in the morning and through the day of all kinds of fancied things; drawing pains in different places; difficult evacuation even of soft stool; urine profuse and pale, and then scanty and brown, sometimes white, like milk; flatus; dry, tiresome cough sometimes. She lies always upon her back with one leg stretched and the other drawn up. **Stan. 200** (lehrmann) changed at once her whole mental and bodily condition. In a few weeks she was able to make a little journey, but the exertions brought on symptoms of abortion, which were promptly removed by **Bell. 3.**—Dr. Kunkel.

STAPHISAGRIA.

In **Staphisagria** we have a remedy that is second to none in its action over the nervous system. This plant is known by various names such as the Lark-spur, Stavesacre and Delphinium staphisagria. It grows plentifully in Southern Europe. The tincture is prepared from macerated ripe seeds which are covered with two-thirds their weight of alcohol. The usual process of stoppered bottle, shaking, straining and filtering has to be gone through.

This is comparatively speaking an old remedy; we find it mentioned in the writings of Dioscorides, but its use, till the time of Samuel Hahnemann was chiefly confined to gout and itch. It is regarded as a great germicide and the Allopaths still use it to destroy lice and itch-mites.

It is necessary to mention that potentization adds to the curative power of a drug. A comparison of the therapeutic value of this remedy as prepared and used by the two schools of Medicine will show the vast superiority of Homœopathy over the other school. The ailments that call for the application of **Staphisagria** are many and various; **Staphisagria** should therefore be rightly placed in the list of polychrest remedies.

Staphisagria is the premier remedy of the 20th century because it is called for the premier vice of the present time, we mean the evil habit of onanism. All the melancholy symptoms that appear in the train of this evil habit find, as we shall very soon see, a great help in **Staphisagria.** These patients look abashed; they cannot look you straight in the face; a guilty conscience is constantly reminding them of their despicable treason against law of nature. Their countenance, which but for their filthy habit might have been full of life and health and happiness, is indicative of total wreckage. The nose is pointed and the eyes are sunken with blue rings around them. Not a ray of hope, not a ray of ambition lighten their brows and their whole expression is one of solid darkness, apathy and indifference. Their memory too has suffered from the great drain on the vital fluid. After short mental work they complain of a sensation of weight between the eyes. In a very short while they so completely forget all that they have studied that they are scarcely able to recall them even after long reflection. We very often come across such sad cases of young men who, through this pernicious habit, get transformed into blank idiotcy and stand sorely in need of remedies like **Staphisagria.** Their sensitiveness is so highly strained that it is a matter of extreme difficulty to live peaceably with them. They cannot brook any slight and when no slight is meant they will construe other peoples' dealings as indicative of such and feel miserable over the supposed slight.

Staphisagria is a very important remedy in ailments from indignation, vexation or reserved displeasure. As has been said before, successful prescribing needs very minute examination and a complete understanding of the case. I will mention an instance in point. Sometime ago I called in to treat a case of persistent diarrhœa in a young boy of 15. Many physicians of both schools had tried and they made a medicine chest of the poor helpless creature but to no avail. I found him very emaciated and irritable. Any little disturbance would throw him into a violent rage and the only way to appease him was to give him some food. I gave him **Sulphur,** as **Sulphur** seemed to cover all the symptoms in the shape of emaciation, and offensive stools. It made little impression. Then a further enquiry revealed that the child had been silently brooding over a supposed slight in being left behind by his father. Ever since he has been morose and irritable. A few doses of **Staphisagria** put a stop to all the unpleasant symptoms. Other remedies of a similar nature are **Colocynth, Ignatia, Anacardium** and **Palladium.**

We must not overlook the great importance of this remedy on the eye and the trouble of vision. It has become classical for styes, nodosities and chalazæ on eyelids. This remedy not only cures them when they actually come but removes the predisposition. Medical literature is full of instances of such marvellous actions of this drug. We have verified this symptom over and over again in our practice.

It is also applicable in marginal blepharitis when the margins of the eye-lids are dry with hard lumps on their borders and the hair follicles are destroyed. It has also been used in iritis when of syphilitic origin with bursting pain in the eye-ball, temple and side of the face; it is worse from evening to morning and upon using the eyes by any artificial light.

Staphisagria is very serviceable in any kind of injury to the cornea. Hering mentions of a case of laceration of the cornea with prolapse of the iris in which **Staphisagria** effected a cure. He also advises its application even in incised wounds of the cornea as in an operation for cataract.

There are on record some cases of arthritic ophthalmia in which **Staphisagria** helped. The pain in such cases, is very severe in the eyes and it extends to the teeth of that side. The eyes burn on the slightest exertion as though they are dry, although constant lachrymation is present.

We will now discuss the relation of this remedy to the bony tissues of our system. We use it in osteitis and in mercurial diseases of the bones; quite a bit of swelling is noticeable in the bones and they become very painful. Sometimes the syphilitic nodes break down and we find ourselves face to face with real caries. The bone in such patients are very fragile and break down easily under the probe.

The teeth also show signs of decay. They turn black or show dark streaks preparatory to a final breakdown; sometimes these decayed teeth ache most fearfully; another peculiarity about this **Staphisagria** toothache is its aggravation during menses, when the pain extends even to the roots of a whole row of sound teeth. The pain is also worse after eating, drinking cold water, drawing cold air into the mouth and also from a simple touch. The gums too are spongy and they present fistulous-looking ulcers.   In this respect we should compare **Staphisagria** with **Mezereum, Kreosotum, Thuja** and **Sepia.**

The decay in **Mezereum** comes suddenly.   The enamel of the teeth gets rough and gradually wears off.   The pain which is drawing, boring and stitching in nature extends to the facial bones and temples and unlike **Staphisagria,** is ameliorated by keeping the mouth open and drawing in open air.

The decay that comes in **Kreosote** is very early; it appears as soon as the teeth make their appearance; **Kreosote** is often a remedy for sycotic children with a whole mouthful of caried teeth.   The odour from mouth is offensive.

In **Thuja** the decay commences at the root close to the gums, the crowns remaining sound.

Sepia is indicated in carious decay of teeth in yellowish complexioned women of dirty habits, bearing the tale-tell face of uterine derangement.

We have given this drug the premier place in an ailment so very prevalent now-a-days—we mean the evil effects of onanism and sexual excesses.   Nocturnal emissions are very frequent and debilitating and they are followed by great chagrin and mortification. Constantine Hering mentions of such a case in his Guiding Symptoms.   We can site several instances from our own practice; but it is not necessary as such experiences are by no means rare.   It is also useful in prostatitis when symptoms of chagrin, mortification and anguish are present.   From the constant debilitating discharges, the testicles atrophy for which condition too this remedy will be useful.

In the female sexual sphere, we find nymphomania with **extreme sensitiveness** to mental and physical impressions.

Staphisagria is a splendid remedy for dyspepsia of the careworn neurastheniacs. In such patients, due to deficiency of muscular tone, the abdomen feels as if it would drop and they feel like holding it up.   In this respect **Staphisagria** is similar to **Abrotanum, Ipecac, Lobelia,** and **Tabacum.**   There is extreme hunger in **Staphisagria.** They want to eat even after a hearty and a substantial meal and the consequence is not very salutary. They suffer from colic and diarrhœa as a result of such indiscretion. The fæcal dicharges are offensive, smelling like rotten eggs.   The diarrhœa or the dysentery is always worse after a meal or after drinking cold water.

Last of all we will discuss the action of this remedy on the skin. We use it both internally and externally for injuries caused by sharp cutting instruments such as knife, glass, etc. We also use it for shocks after a big surgical operation such as lithotomy, ovaritomy, and so on.

Staphisagria gives us great satisfaction in the trial of eczema but we must be very cautious as to the kind of eczema for which we use it. The eruptions may be dry and scabby or moist with yellow crusts discharging a very offensive secretion. The usual site is the head, especially the occiput and the region behind the ears. It is also serviceable in chronic tinea capitis sicca. The whole hairy scalp becomes covered with a dark scaly eruption, where scratching causes bleeding and a discharge of clear, non-glutinous fluid which dries quickly, leaving the whole head covered with the yellow, offensive crusts. We use this remedy even in common itch on these parts but the peculiarity is that when scratching stops in one place it goes to another.

Staphisagria is a great sycotic remedy and we find it very useful in warts, pediculated condylomata, etc. **Staphisagria** also remedies the constitutional effects of mercury.

Case 1.—W. S. J. had been afflicted with a tumor of the lower lid for several years. Had often been advised to have it removed by the knife, but declined. The margin of the upper lid was much thickened by nodules of torsal tumors. Was frequently subject to styes, which always left an enlarged gland after it suppurated. Dark hair, blue eyes. Did a large amount of office work by night, by gaslight. I gave him **Staphisagria 30**, to be taken night and morning for a week, then every morning for a week, when, if any improvement was noticed, medicine was to be discontinued. At the end of two weeks the large tumor was nearly gone, medicine was discontinued, and in a month the borders of the lids were cleared up and tumor gone. This occurred over two years ago. There is no appearance of a new crop of styes and no more tumors.—(Dr. H. C. Allen in **Am. Homœopathist, August. 1878).**

Case 2.—H. V. B., thirty years old, suffers, for several days, each January, from rheumatic gastric troubles, tearing pains in the left side of the face, etc., and was taken, during the winter, with rheumatism, which at last assumed the form of prosopalgia. Symptoms: Tearing pain, starting from a decayed tooth in the left upper jaw, running through all the left upper teeth, causing the most violent pain, increased by touch and slightly relieved by hard pressure. When more than usually severe, the pain extends behind the left ear and runs into the left arm. Sensation of swelling in the cheek, spasm of the œsophagus, drawing colic in the lower bowels. From the severity of the pain weeping-spells, difficult breathing, coldness of the hands and cold perspiration on the face. The paroxysms are often of daily occurrence, without coming on at the same time. **Staphisagria 30** cured the prosopalgia.—(Neumann in **Parkt. Beiträge. i.,** P. 186).

Case 3.—In a very acute case of neuralgia occurring in an old lady, and affecting chiefly the face and forehead on both sides, I found **Staph.** 30 and **12** of great benefit.   The case had for years resisted all treatment, both medical and surgical.   Some branches of the nerve had been divided, with only partial relief.   When I saw the case the patient was unable to put food into her mouth save with her fingers, the least metallic contact with a spoon or fork always brought on a violent attack.   The sensations were as fine cuts with a very sharp knife, beginning at the lips and extending to the eyes and above the orbits.   Mastication was impossible from the pain it induced, and the patient was reduced to living upon soups put in her mouth with her fingers.   The relief afforded by **Staph.** was remarkable, and made her life bearable, though it did not perfectly cure her, which was possibly the combined fault of her age and the continued wrong treatment under which she had suffered.—Dr. W. Bayes.

STICTA PULMONARIA.

This is comparatively speaking a little known and a rarely used remedy but that does not render it any the less important, for those cases that will call for **Sticta** will need **Sticta;** there **Sticta** and none but **Sticta** will help.

Sticta is a form of lichen found growing on the trunks of large trees in the northern mountainous countries of England and in the United States.   It rarely grows in big towns and cities where the atmosphere is surcharged with soot and dust and other forms of impurities as it depends on the atmosphere for nutrition.   Its existence thus is always an indication of salubrity of the locality.

Its preparation is very simple.   The fresh lichen is finely chopped and covered with five parts by its weight of dilute alcohol.   This is allowed to remain in a well-stoppered bottle for eight days after which period the tincture is poured off and filtered.

Sticta is as great a catarrhal remedy as **Aconite, Ammon. carb., Arum trif., Cepa, Euphrasia** and a few others, but this big list need not disconcert us for they are each one of them different in their own way and the symptoms are so distinctly peculiar that there is scarcely any danger of confusion.   Unlike these remedies **Sticta** coryza is strictly dry.   The excessive and painful dryness of the mucous membrane is not due to any want of secretion; for secretions occur but they dry up very rapidly leaving thick crusts behind them.   The whole of the buccal cavity and the throat are so dry, parched and leather-like that our patient finds it hard to sleep. He sits up all night, unfortunate man sneezing and coughing. It is only towards the latter part of the morning when the palate and the throat get a bit moistened that he is able to sleep.

In consequence of this deposit of thick crusts in the nostrils the patient blows his nose violently but to no purpose.

Sticta is almost a specific for hay-fever, if we could have a specific in Homœopathy; what we mean is that the catarrhal symptoms of **Sticta** are so very similar to the symptomatology of hay-fever that we use this remedy with success in that ailment. The peculiarity, as we have already noticed, is the great dryness at night and secretion during day. Dr. Hering says:—

"At night discharges almost cease, air passages become dry, paroxysms of sneezing more frequent, explosions seem to number more at each paroxysm, until sneezing and coughing are almost incessant; very little sleep until morning when hyperæmia gradually subsides, air passages become moist and at sunrise there is again a profuse discharge from eyes and nose which is hot and excoriating, causing rawness and soreness of cheeks, borders of nose and upper lip."

We find quite a bit of coughing in this remedy and the cough is rather dry, incessant and titillating. It has proved very successful in that distressing, teasing cough that follows in the wake of measles and influenza. **Sticta** is also reputed to have a soothing effect in the distressing, hacking cough of consumptives. We know cure is not possible in those cases where the disease has advanced to a critical stage but relief is not denied and it is relief that is sought and Dr. Hale assures us that **Sticta** brings much relief in such cases.

Hale gives **Sticta** a very high place in the therapeutics of rheumatism. Hering also testifies to its great usefulness in that complaint. We use this remedy with success in rheumatism of the right shoulder-joint, wrist-joint, ankle and knee-joints.

The marvellous cures, that this remedy is reported to have made in such cases, at once secure for it a very respectable place in our therapeutics. Wt are told by Hale, of a middle-aged gentleman who used to suffer severely with rheumatism in right shoulder-joint, deltoid and triceps muscles extending at times to his forearm, making him almost helpless towards morning. Improvement commenced immediately after the administration of **Sticta** and he was cured permanently in a wonderfully short while. I have had a similar experience. A lady aged about 45 came to me for a similar complaint. For years she could not lift up her right hand. Various remedies, useful in such cases, were tried but no improvement was noticed till **Sticta** was given when in an incredibly short time she got well. Hering cites a case of bursitis that resulted from a fall on the knee. There was a distinct collection of fluid in the patellar bursa. **Sticta** cured the patient. He mentions another instance of an unlucky patient bed-ridden for six months with intense, darting, lancinating pain in all the joints of the body where **Sticta** proved highly efficacious.

We must not think that this remedy is good only in chronic rheumatic ailments. We use it also in acute inflammatory rheumatism. The symptoms are heat, swelling and circumscribed redness.

It will be an unjustifiable omission to neglect the mental side of this remedy. The patient is very talkative but this talkativeness is different from the garrulity of **Lachesis** and **Stramonium**.

In **Lachesis** it is the great over-flow of ideas that keep him going; in **Stramonium** it is the imbecile garrulity of a deranged mind, whereas under **Sticta** it is due to his inability to keep his tongue quiet. Further he is subject to certain strange ideas. His lower limbs feel so light and airy that they seem to hover in the air. In this respect **Sticta** is similar to **Asarum, Lac can.** and **Valerian**—the only difference is that in these latter remedies it is not part of the body but the whole body that feels light and seems to hover in the air. Peculiar though this symptom may seem it is not a rare one. Such symptoms are very common in hysteria and in hysterical chorea. Before we close our remarks we would like to add that this remedy needs further proving and many of its symptoms stand in need of verification.

STILLINGIA SYLVATICA.

The tincture is prepared from the root of the Queen's Delight, a perennial plant found in Virginia, Florida and a few other neighbouring states.

Stillingia produces symptoms very similar to those seen in secondary syphilis, such as bone pains, nodular growths on forehead and tibia, caries of nasal bones, chronic rheumatism, etc. It has been used with success in many cases where **Mercurius, Aurum** and **Thuja,** failed to do any good. Dr. M. Preston reports of a case of secondary syphilis that he cured with **Stillingia** after other remedies failed. The bone pains were instantaneously relieved. The immense nods on head and leg disappeared and as he says, "From the most deplorably downhearted miserable thin-looking object he changed into a buoyant, joking, rotund-looking fellow."

Stillingia helps even in chronic syphilitic eruptions of torpid, scaly, nature.

It is thus an important remedy not to be over-looked or rightly passed over. As syphilis is such a devastating disease and as it is fundamentally at the root of most of the ailments to which we fall victims it behoves to strengthen our armamentarium by adding **Stillingia** to the powerful list of other antisyphilitic remedies.

STRAMONIUM.

Datura stramonium is one more of our great remedies that has helped us in scoring off many a success. It is known by various names, such as Thorn-apple, Jamestown or Jimson weed etc. It belongs to the natural order of Solanaceæ. It grows plentifully all over the world. In India the two varieties of fastuosa and alba are the ones mostly seen. The poisonous effect of this plant is due to an alkaloid datoorin which resembles hyoscyamine and atropine in its properties. Prof. Landenburg asserts that it is a mixture of both atropine and hyoscyamine. This alkaloid crystalizes in long colorless prisms. It has a bitter and acrid taste.

This remedy is prepared from the ripe seeds. They are powdered and then mixed with five parts by its weight of alcohol

This is filtered after being left in an well stoppered bottle for eight days and we get our tincture from which the attenuations are made. This remedy was first proved by Samuel Hahnemann. Datura, as a remedial agent, was known to the people of India for ages. It is almost as old as Hindu civilisation. One of the characters of Hindu mythology, Bhola Moheswar, proves this beyond question. He is described as a jovial, careless, forgetful, semi-insane personality much addicted to "Datura" and "bhang." The Kabirai who practices the indigenous system of treatment, uses this drug for various purposes, such as mania, sleeplessness and nervous disorders of various kinds.

Instances of Datura-poisoning are very common and they supply us with many of the symptoms, we find recorded in our Materia Medica. We have known quite a few cases of insanity from Datura-poisoning. A boy, almost a grown up lad, got into bad company and acquired the habit of drinkng. His father came to learn about it and stopped all his allowances hoping thus to cure him of his drinking habit. This produced a still worse effect. Goaded by his hankering he began taking a decoction made from Datura seeds, with the result that he became insane. When we come to deal with the mental symptoms of this remedy, we will dilate upon the details of insanity as the result of Datura-poisoning.

Datura is very often resorted to by criminals for the perpetration of their criminal designs. When Thugs used to abound in India, Datura was their favourite poison. Here is an interesting case of a boy aged about five years, who took some Datura seeds with a portion of the plant. In a very short time his face got flushed and he staggered and fell as if intoxicated. His pupils were dilated, his face flushed and he was in a state of raging delirium, biting and beating those around him. He was talking incessantly and incoherently, performing various ludicrous gestures, such as driving away imaginary animals and the like. We can divide a case of **Stramonium-poison** into three stages. The first stage of poisoning is commonly marked by delirium, restlessness, great muscular weakness and giddiness. The patient is unable to stand; he talks incoherently, laughs wildly, tries to run away from imaginary evils, catches at the air and picks at his clothes. Sometimes he appears to be drawing out imaginary threads from the ends of his fingers and he performs various other ludicrous antics. In the second stage we find this delirium merging into complete drowsiness.

stupor, utter insensibility and stertorous breathing. In the third stage the lost consciousness slowly returns or the insensibility turns still more profound ending slowly in death.

On post mortem examination we do not notice much change except congestion of the vessels of the brain and its membrances, congestion of the lungs and a great flaccidity of the heart. Sometimes we notice marks of diffused inflammation about the stomach. The choroid plexus too suffers from a similar congestion.

Stramonium is very rich in mental symptoms; but the one that I deem most important is its desire for light and company. Whenever the patient is alone and in the dark, a sort of inconceivable horror passes through him. This desire for company is more strong at night time and during menses, when solitude becomes especially unbearable. Other remedies with a similar peculiarity are **Ars., Bism., Kali carb.** and **Phos;** but all of them have their points of difference and we will touch on them in passing as we progress.

In **Ars.** and **Phos.** we not only find a desire for company but aggravation of all the troubles during solitude.

Kali carb. desires company and when the patient gets company he treats them most outrageously.

Sepia is another remedy with an exactly opposite symptom. The patient cannot stand company; she must be alone and it is only when alone that she feels relieved.

Ambra grisea must not be over-looked. The patient has a nature somewhat similar to **Sepia;** she hates the presence of strangers, but she hates them most when attending a call of nature.

The symptom of **Stramonium** which we will talk about now as important as the one just mentioned—we mean the beseeching and the praying attitude we so often meet with in young women with suppressed menses. We have seen girls, who are naturally far from a religious bent of mind, turn over-pious on such occasions. They sing pious songs, solemnly utter words of wisdom and even deliver sermons of great virtue. Even their attitude is one of supplication and prayer. They lie on their back with their knees flexed and their hands joined together. This symptom has often led to the administration of this remedy in cases of typhus attended with delirium. These patients in their unconscious delirium jerk up their heads from the pillow and then drop them back again, carrying on such antics for a long time. Very often they see ghosts, strangers and animals. Delusions are not uncommon. They think they are very tall and other objects around them are small and dwarfish. They feel as if they are on an elevation. It is not the impudent pride and self-conceit of **Platinum** that we find here, but a simple sense of physical largeness. We have forgetten to mention that in puer-peral fevers and mania these patients get obsessed with many absurd ideas, such for instance that they are double, that some-body is lying in the same bed with them, or that they are cut into halves. Such absurd fancies are also to be seen under **Bapt., Valer., Petr., Anac** and **Lac. can.**

There is another important symptom that must be mentioned, on which I once cured a very bad case of delirium. This patient had a great desire to hide. When I entered the sick-room, there was no patient to be found. The bed was there and on one of its corners the quilt was all heaped up in a bundle. On enquiry it was found that the patient was concealed in that mass of quilt. Then when the quilt was removed and the patient exposed to view, he looked very frightened and scared. His eyebrows were knitted and he kept looking intently at me till at last he broke out into a scream and grasped at his sister, who was near by, for protection. The patient presented some of the other symptoms mentioned above and the prescription was easy to make and he was cured.

Stramonium is used both in coma and convulsion. The indica-tions are great brightness of the eyes, dilatation of the pupils, twitching of the hands and feet and automatic grasping of the hands towards nose and ear.

Another feature of the **Stramonium** patient is loquacity. She is babbling all the time; there seems to be no end to her talking. There are a few other remedies, such as **Lach., Podo., Hydo., Teucr., Bar. carb., Calad.,** and **Selen.,** where also we note a similar garrulity, but a confusion is impossible to the conscientious homœopath, who takes the trouble to differentiate between them.

The **Lachesis** patient seems to suffer from an overflow of ideas. As soon as she is finished with one subject, she passes on to another, scarcely giving her audience a chance to speak or ask her anything. Like **Stram.** and **Baryta carb.** this talkativeness in the **Lachesis** patient is worse during her menses.

Podophyllum is talkative, but occurs chiefly during the stage of chill.

In **Teucrium** the talkativeness is mostly marked during the stage of heat.

For talkativeness during the stage of perspiration we have **Calad.** and **Selen.**

The next feature to be discussed is painlessness; this is a great point with **Stramonium.** Whatever may be the ailment with this patient, he seems to be free from pains except in hip-joint diseases where the pain is very acute.

The diarrhœa of **Stramonium** is a painless one. The stools are black and very offensive. I cured a case of cholera a long time ago but yet not so long as to elude my memory. The cure was a brilliant one. The unhappy patient was suffering from cholera and it was cholera of the worst type. His stools were very frequent, black, almost jet-black, and offensive. His physician who was an allopathic practitioner pronounced his case hopeless and asked his relatives to be prepared for the inevitable end. Then as a last resource, like the last attempt of the drowning man to catch at a floating straw, the homœopath was called in. To my utter disappointment, as soon as I entered the sickroom, hiccough supervened. He was given a timely dose of **Stramonium** which practically patted him through. The remedies that we naturally hit upon in such a case are **Arsen., Brom., Lept., Merc., Opium.** and **Verat.** They all have black and offensive stools, but in none do we find hiccough so prominent as under **Stramonium. Stramonium** covered the case and **Stramonium** cured it.

Our **Stramonium** patient is a bundle of nerves. He is prone to all sorts of nervous disorders. Convulsion, hysteria, chorea, epilepsy, and catalepsy are all common in **Stramonium.** They are all aggravated by the sight of bright, dazzling objects. The spasmodic motions of **Stramonium** are characterized by gracefulness. The convulsions of **Stramonium** are accompanied by consciousness. Sometimes when drinking or even on attempting to swallow liquid, the patient is thrown into violent fits of convulsions. **Bell., Lyssin** and **Mur. acid** also have a similar characteristic—aggravation from bright light and shining objects. **Stramonium** thus becomes one of our best remedies for hydrophobia. It presents many of the symptoms of that disease.

Stramonium is also indicated in locomotor-ataxia. The patient cannot walk in the dark or with his eyes closed. He reels and falls as if intoxicated on attempting to do so.

Stramonium is good for all kinds of fevers—typhoid, typhus, quotidian, double quotidian, etc., when the indications are there. There is no thirst during chill, but during the stages of heat and sweat, he feels parched and dry. It is a chilly patient that we

have to deal with in **Stramonium.** The chill begins in the back
and extends over the whole body. Hands and feet turn cold, blue
and almost immovable. Gradually his face gets flushed up, eye
half-closed and his pupils dilated. During heat the patient fre
quentl, starts and jerks. Sweat intermingles with heat and ever
during these stages the patient covers up closely like **Nux vom.**

We must say a few words about the difficulty of speech in
the **Stramonium** patient. He utters only single, inarticulate sound:
and that with great difficulty. He has to exert himself a long
time and he makes faces while doing so, which makes his audience
laugh.

Euphrasia has a peculiar kind of stammering; while speaking
he recommences many times, not only repeating the first word
or his sentence but even when finished he begins again with the
same sentence.

Cicuta can articulate the first few words of his sentence with
out difficulty, but while speaking the rest he collapses.

Zinc. met. has what is known as the echo speech. The patien
repeats in a monotonous way the words and sentences he hears
He has very little or almost no control over this. He is not ever
conscious of his sing-song habit.

Spigelia suffers when he begins to speak. All his difficultie
are at the commencement. After he utters the first few word
with difficulty the rest comes on smoothly and well.

Under **Stramonium** the secretion of urine becomes either sup
pressed or scanty; as this condition is often to be met with in
cholera, eclampsia and nephritis, **Stramonium** comes to be o
very great use in the treatment of those troubles.

Other remedies having a similar action on the kidneys ar
Canth., Bell., Hyos., Opium, and **Lactuca virosa.**

In **Stramonium** the urination is accompanied by rigors an
rumbling in the abdomen and with symptoms of cerebra
hyperemia.

Bellad. and **Lact. vir.** are useful when stupor is the leading
symptom.

For acute strangury, with scanty or hot urine mixed wit
blood and albumen and voided drop by drop, we can think of n
better remedy than **Canth.**

Kali bich. and **Merc cor.** are two important remedies for sup
pression of urine. The former is mostly applicable for suppressio
following cholera,

Merc. cor. is useful for suppression of urine, in albuminuria and other cases, where the urine is thickly clouded with filaments, and dark flesh-like pieces of mucus. The intense tenesmus of he bladder, hot burning offensive urine, and the acute pain felt vhile passing urine, are additional points in its favour.

Case 1.—A boy, eleven years old, was greatly frightened some fifteen eeks ato; he experienced, in consequence of this fright, symptoms which eemed to indicate mental disturbance, but terminated, at last, in chorea. ymptoms: He reels, as if dizzy; his walk is staggering; it is impossible for m to walk straight unless he is guided. The head is drawn backward upon e shoulders. Trembling of the arms and legs. Great freedom of motion all the limbs, and yet he is not able to raise himself up. The muscles voluntary motion fail to obey his will force; one can see the useless efforts the patient to moderate the untoward motions of the limbs. He can rdly conduct his hand to the glass; it is still more difficult to raise the ass to the lips, which can be done only after several efforts. He frequently esses his hand upon the small of the back and then bends backward with expression of pain, as if he were suffering from violent distress. The untenance expresses stupidity and a loss of balance as well as great dulliness the special senses. The eye is staring and watery, the pupils enlarged d do not react promptly. Loss of memory; cannot recite verses which knew perfectly, and does not remember occurrences of few days ago. If wants to speak (and he does this only to answer repeated questions) he mmers: shows a visible effort, which is accompanied by a peculiar con-.ction of the facial muscles, especially of the mouth, which is drawn to her side. He complains rarely about pains in the head or in the bowels. e appetite is regular perhaps a little increased; there is violent thirst; bowels are hard. Constipation of several days' standing is followed by rrhœa. Scanty urination. Frequent hawking, as if from a pressure in throat. Occasional nausea but no vomiting. Oppressed and frequent athing. Pulse small and spasmodic. Stiffness and coldness of the hands feet with unusually flushed and full countenance; in fact, there is quite endency to chilliness; uneasy sleep; he lies with his limbs drawn up, ngs the arms about in various directions; snores and makes inarticulate nds. He likes to lie down. In the morning, immediately after rising, cannot distinguish object, although he sees them well enough, he runs inst the table and chairs, as if he were feeling his way in the dark. merly obedient, he is now very stubborn, but withal very shy and timid ore strangers. Prescribed **Stramonium 9**, one drop in the morning. On very next day he spoke of his own accord and dressed himself. the third day he sat down to the table and ate heartily; his movements e passably regular, his gait still irregular, but surer than it had been. conduct and behaviour are nearly natural. Prescribed a second dose of .monium. Within three days all spasmodic action had disappeared. A stray symptoms demanded **China 12**. The cure was permanent. idi in **Archiv., vii., 2, 73**).

Case 2.—Young girl thirteen years of age, of good constitution, sanguine erament, had suffered already from two attacks of facial erysipelas the only disease to which she had been subject. She had experienced for days great nausea and sore throat; great heat and inflammation of the skin; the parts were swollen and those principally on the forehead; want of appetite and great thirst. During the night of the 23d, some vesicles appeared on the skin, and violent delirium set in. **Bell.** every four hours without benefit. **Rhus tox.** every third hour. At my morning visit I was told that the delirium and restlessness had subsided after the first dose. The erysipelas, which was extending to the scalp, ears and neck, was arrested, although a large number of vesicles appeared on the face; medicine continued every four hours. At 8 o'clock in the evening, the state of the case was unchanged, except that the delirium had redoubled in severity towards the evening, and was then at its height. The parents of the patient stated that in two previous attacks the delirium had lasted five days. The character of the delirium was such that the patient endeavoured to throw herself out of bed **Stram. 6** every two hours, to be left off as soon as the patient procured sleep. The delirium ceased entirely after the administration of two doses of **Stram.**; the patient gave rational answer to my questions; she had had a quiet and refreshing sleep. The erysipelas had invaded other regions although retaining the local character mentioned before; seeing this, prescribed **Rhus tox.**; this medicine brought about the desiccation of the vesicles on the seventh day of the attack, the sypmtoms were completely subdued on the eighth, and on the ninth, the patient rose completely cured —Dr. Gifre.

Case 3.—Abdominal typhus, which had not improved, although it had been under skilful homœopathic treatment for over a fortnight; had begun with symptoms of an ordinary gastric fever. The condition of the young man was this: On looking at him he stared at me, then appeared on his forehead and in his emaciated face deep wrinkles; at times he would cry out loud till he became hoarse; mouth and lips were ulcerated to such degree that he declined to drink on account of the severe pain caused by any fluid (or solid) coming in contact with his mouth; the lips were peeling off, and bled when he picked them; abdomen fallen in, tender to contact he vomited occasionally, mucus, with specks and streaks of blood; frequent watery, offensive stools; no sleep; no appetite; urine scanty; pulse very frequent and not regular; great emaciation. **Nux vom., Bryon., Phospho. Mercur., Nitr. acid, Arum. trif.** had been given according to the most prominent symptoms, but the mental symptoms, as expressed in the countenance had remained unaltered, while the pathological condition was worse; the attending physician knew that we had before us "ulcerated Peyer's bodies. **Stram.** covered all the symptoms but that of the sore mouth, but in Hering proving was the symptom: "It feels as if the inner mouth was raw and sore." **Stram. 50m.** cured.—A. Lippe.

STRONTIANA CARBONICA.

This is a small but an invaluable remedy not much known and rarely used. It grows in the form of crystals in massive quantities in lead mines of Strontian, a place in Argyllshire whence it derives its name.

It has a great tendency to produce congestion and it therefore belongs to the same category as **Glonoinum, Amyl nit., Belladona, Verat. vir.,** etc. The arteries dilate to make room for the increased rush of blood and throb with the excitement of the great rush. Such a congestion may be in the heart, the lungs and the head.

The great characteristic of this remedy consists in the aggravation of this congestion from the least movement. There are people whose face becomes livid and flushed every time they move about. These patients are great subjects of apoplexy. Timely administration of **Strontiana carb.** will remove such tendency and save the patient from the impending catastrophy. I have used this remedy scores of times for congestive headaches specially at climaxis. The flushes are frequent and continuous. The symptom that helps greatly to diffierentiate **Strontiana** from **Lachesis** and **Sulphur,** is a great desire on the part of the patient to have the head wrapped up, inspite of the great heat and the warmth. The patient can not bear the least draft of cold. In this respect **Strontiana** is similar to **Silicea** and **Magnesia mur.**

I am ever grateful to **Strontiana,** for the relief it gave me, while still a medical student in Chicago, from an attack of persistent nocturnal diarrhœa to which unfortunately I became a subject. It used to come on every night with a peculiar urging that made me stick to the closet for hours. I would scarcely be off the vessel before I had to return. It used to leave me punctually after 3 a.m. Dr. H. C. Allen prescribed **Strontiana.** I have not suffered from it since.

It is equally great for constipation. The stools are large, hard and are expelled with great effort. Defecation is followed by pain in anus and burning lasting for hours and compelling the patients to lie down.

Strontiana is used in caries of the bones specially of the femur when such affections are associated with diarrhœa.

Lastly let me mention that its efficacy is very great in those cases of chronic sprains particularly of the ankle-joints when other remedies such as **Arnica, Ruta,** and **Rhus tox.** fail. There is almost always a certain amount of œdema associated with this pain due perhaps to interference in the circulation of blood. Dr. C. M. Boger cured with **Strontiana** a case of sciatica on the indication of its being associated with œdema of the ankle of the same side.

STROPHANTHUS.

Strophanthus, an ornamental climbing shrub, a native of Africa, belongs to the natural order of Apocynacæ. It causes great disorders of digestion, intense nausea, vomiting and diarrhœa. This property of **Strophanthus** is utilised in bringing about repugnance to alcohol in dipsomaniacs. An extract of the seeds is used by the natives of Africa in poisoning arrows.

The therapeutical action of **Strophanthus** is directly referable to the heart, and is somewhat similar to the action of **Digitalis.** **Strophanthus** does not contract the arteries as in **Digitalis** and hence none of the gain from cardiac stimulus is counteracted and also there is none of the danger of daming back the blood upon an incompetent heart. It is more prompt, in its action, than **Digitalis.** It strengthens and slows the heart-beat, prolonging the diastolic period and restores more readily the rhythm to an irregular beat. The action of **Strophanthus** however is far less prolonged than that of **Digitalis** and is not cumulative in its action like the latter, hence it is used by our friends of the other school more as an emergency remedy than as a main stay. The principle on which we work, however, is altogether different. With us, the choice of the remedy is based, as everywhere, on the totality of the strange, peculiar, and the characteristic symptoms. Mentally these patients are irritable. We find a certain amount of loquacity in **Strophanthus** though this is not as marked as in **Lachesis.** Nausea without actual vomiting is an important symptom. There is great loathing of food; if however he eats any food, it is actually vomited out. The patient experiences great burning in the œsophagus and stomach.

It is, as has been said before, an important heart remedy. The pluse though weak betrays a weak action of the heart due to great debility of the heart muscles. Quite a lot of dyspnœa is experienced, due probably to the œdema of the lungs. The following case from the diary of Dr. Clarke is not only impressive but instructive. W. G., 16, a delicate-looking boy, was admitted to hospital, having had rheumatic pains about him for three months, and an attack of rheumatic fever two years previously. He had been laid up a month before admission and a week before was taken with cough, shivering and occasional vomiting. When admitted he had a frequent short, dry cough, aggravated by lying down; had to be propped up in bed; had œdema of feet, especially left. Tongue white; unable to retain any food for three days; no pain after food, but much flatulence, eructations giving much relief. Heart greatly dilated, pulsation diffused; double mitral bruit. Dulness at bases of both lungs, moist rales halfway up right lung. Expectoration of bright blood for seven days. **Strophanthus** θ one drop every four hours was given. Improvement in all the symptoms was immediate; sickness, cough, hæmoptysis, and dropsy all disappeared; and the heart sounds had cleared up to a large extent when the boy went home, less than three weeks after admission.

STRYCHNINUM.

Any Materia Medica without a few lines on **Strychninum** will be imperfect as it is such a potent remedial agent. Furthermore, we have such a lot of cases of poisoning with **Strych.** that it behoves us, either homœopath, allopath, kaviraj or hakim, to have a full and thorough understanding of all the symptoms of this remedy. It is an alkaloid obtained from **Nux vom.** and **Ignatia** bean. It is a whitish or grayish-white powder. It is inodorous but excessively bitter with a peculiar metallic taste. The various preparations of **Strych.** are Nitrate of Strych., Acid Phosphate of Strych., Sulphate of Strych. and Valerianate of Strych. The preparation that we will discuss in this chapter is the liquor Strychnine. Strych. was first extracted from the seeds of N.V. in 1819 by Pelletier and Caventen.

Before embarking on a consideration of the therapeutical application of **Strych.** it will be proper to study it in its general physiological and toxical action on the human system. When taken in a very small quantity, enough to produce a physiological effect the first symptoms to appear, are a feeling of restlessness, trembling in the limbs, some slight stiffness in the neck and the jaws, muscular twitchings, a sensation of stricture in throat and chest and a feeling or dread of some impending calamity. When taken in fatal quantity its effects are visible within 10 to 15 minutes of the administration of the drug. Very speedily the head is jerked backward, the limbs get extended, and back arched, so that the body rests on the head and the heels only. In a few minutes the mouth gets drawn and the patient presents all the symptoms of spasmodic tetanus. These symptoms pass off in a few minutes and there is complete relaxation of all the muscles; the spasmodic condition speedily returns however to be relieved again by moments of respite. Hyperesthesia, of all the senses, is an important feature in **Strychnine** poisoning. The slightest noise or touch or a draught of air ushers in this trying and painful condition of tetanic rigidity. Accession and remission of tetanic state ensue so rapidly that within half an hour of the administration of the poison the patient succumbs either through exhaustion or through asphyxiation. Throughout the paroxysm the mind is quite unaffected. The patient's suffering is agonizing.

Now we are in a position to study **Strych.** in its therapeutic aspect to appreciate and to apply this great remedial agent to relieve suffering, according to the principle we follow in regard to our other remedies. The symptoms that stand out as characteristic and guide us as so many beacon lights in the rough and perilous sea of correct prescribing, are the following—(a) great hyperæsthesia of pharynx and œsophagus, (b) a great feeling of stiffness and a marked rigidity of the cervical muscles, (c) spasmodic twitchings and jerkings and a general tremor of almost all the muscles of the body, (d) great relief by lying on the back and continued hard massage and rubbing, (e) aggravation from slight touch and lastly (f) the constant presence of consciousness from the beginning to the end.

There is congestion of the head, so much so, that the face looks bluish black and the veins stand out full and tortuous, the eyes look staring and protruding. The expression on the face is one of extreme terror as if some thing most awful and untoward is going to happen any minute. Hands, lips and tongue get blue and purplish. Ear, nose and eyes burn and itch most violently; deglutition is almost impossible, for each attempt produces spasams of the muscle of the pharynx. In the mouth we have an important symptom such as a great sensation of itching of the roof of the mouth. The taste is bitter. Excessive dyspnœa, a great craving for fresh air, great tension of the muscles on each side of the larynx and tumultuous action of the heart are symptoms too important to be neglected. Another symptom in common with **Nux vom** is a feeling as if head and face were enlarged. This symptom makes this remedy as well as **Nux** applicable after a debauch, when such sensations are very common.

SULPHUR.

This remedy is the king of our anti-psorics. The term anti-psoric needs explanation. We are born with a constitution peculiar to each one of us. This constitution undergoes modifications as we grow older as the result of the varying influences of environments and ailments to which we become subject and by the time we die we turn into quite different individuals from what we first started. So great indeed is the transformation that we would not really know ourselves if we went through an introspection. In many instances these transformations are unfortunately brought about by the long-continued administration of various drastic, harmful medicines to which we subject ourselves through our sojourn of life. As the result of these harmful administrations and to protect the system against entire destruction, nature causes abnormal changes to take place in our organisation. Sometimes, however, chronic miasms lurking in our system work great havoc against which " the best regulated life, and the greatest energy of the vital powers are incapable of coping unless aided by the specific curative remedy." Samuel Hahnemann by diligent application and years of study and research has traced out three such miasms. They are syphilis, sycosis and psora. Now the question is how do we know them? It is very easy. Syphilis discloses itself by chancers; sycosis by cauliflower-like excrescences and psora by a sort of cutaneous eruption characterized by unbearable tickling, voluptuous itching and specific odor. These preliminary remarks bring us to the subject under review. **Sulphur** works wonders in cases where we discover such a psoric base and hence it is called the great anti-psoric.

Sulphur is a non-metallic, yellow, brittle substance. It is found plentifully in Sicily and Italy. In the organic world we meet with **Sulphur** everywhere, this element forming an essential component of the albumenoids, a class of compounds contained in all vegetable and animal structures. Of organic materials rich in **Sulphur** we may mention animal hair and the essential oil of the onion, garlic and mustard.

Sulphur is prepared for homœopathic use in two different ways firstly, the flowers of **Sulphur** washed and cleaned, are mixed with alcohol to form the tincture; secondly, by triturating flowers of **Sulphur** with sugar of milk. This second preparation is by far the best.

If we were called upon to practise medicine with only one remedy, I think I would do well to select **Sulphur.** It is one of the chief remedies of our Materia Medica. Its use is most varied and its cures are wonderful. We will first study the appearance of the **Sulphur** patient and see what he is like. He is spare and stoop-shouldered; he walks and sits stooping; standing is the most uncomfortable position for him; his face is delicate, with long thin eyelashes. In this he is very much like **Phosphorus** which also is indicated in tall slender persons of sanguine temperament. The **Phosphorus** skin too, is fair and the eye-lashes delicate. He too is anemic but he grows rapidly and is inclined to stoop. The similarity is so great that Dr. Nash very aptly says: " If it had equally the psoric element, it would, at sight, seem a counterpart of **Sulphur,** so close, that we could not take them apart."

But really speakeing there is no mistaking a **Sulphur** patient. He has such a stinking odour about him that people know him from a distance. This foul odor is not wholly due to his uncleanliness; wash however, much he may, the odour will not leave him. As is the case with all dirty, filthy people, he has a natural disgust for washing.

In this respect **Sulphur** is very much like **Psorinum.** The latter remedy is as much prone to skin affections as the former. The skin is like parchment, dirty and unhealthy; the sweat emits an unpleasant odour and this unpleasant odour characterises the drug from the beginning to the end. But to distinguish between the two remedies is not difficult. The **Psorinum** patient is very susceptible to cold; he wears a fur coat in the hottest summer; his collar is always up. **Sulphur** on the other hand is a particularly heat-producing remedy; the patient keeps his doors and windows constantly open. While in bed he is always in search of a cold spot whereon to rest his burning hands and feet. There is also burning in vertex, chest, mouth, eyes, vulva, urethra, rectum, and in the internal organs. In fact, this great burning is the most important feature of this remedy. This burning is explained by a sort of local congestion produced by **Sulphur.** There is a rush of blood to the brain and consequently the head feels full and throbbing and the face looks flushed. There is also congestion to the chest with or without hæmoptysis. The patient feels an oppression of breathing and he wants the doors and windows open. The congestion may also be marked in the region of the heart on which case the patient suffers from terrible palpitation; often he feels as if the heart were too large for the thoracic cavity.

The portal congestion in **Sulphur** is most common and hence we come across a lot of hemorrhoidal troubles. This general tendency to congestion is manifested by the redness of the various orifices of the **Sulphur** patient. His lips are vermilion red. The urinary meatus, the vulva and the anus show a similar condition. These are great points to be noted in prescribing. Many a time and often have we been led to prescribe **Sulphur** on solitary symptom of redness of the orifices of the body.

Dr. P. C. Mojumdar of Calcutta mentions a very interesting case in which with a single dose of **Sulphur** 200 he cured a young lady of a great burning sensation which used to come on her frequently. The doctor says: "As I was taking down the history of the case, the lady with a faint cry betook herself to the marble floor and kept on rolling vigorously and said she had great burning over the entire surface of her body. After rolling in this way about a quarter of an hour, she was better and sat up again." There are quite a few other remedies where burning is prominent. Among them are **Acon., Agaricus, Apis. Cantharis, Capsicum** and **Anthraxinum.**

In **Arsenicum** the burning seems almost intolerable, but the strongest part of it is, that this burning is best relieved by heat. **Arsenicum** excels all the rest of them in intensity and is characterised by restlessness, sudden prostration and midnight and midday aggravation.

Phosphorus has a burning sensation all over. sometimes in small isolated spots. The patient is anemic. over-sensitive and phthisical.

The **Aconite** burning is met with in acute inflammatory affections in their first stage. High fever, restlessness, impatience, and thirst are characteristic of the remedy.

In **Apis,** we have redness, swelling and œdema accompanying the burning and stinging pain. Unlike **Agaricus** it is aggravated by heat and relieved by cold.

In **Agaricus** there is burning, itching and redness as if from frost bites and chilblains.

Cantharis burns like fire; it has especial affinity for the urinary tract. There is a constant desire to urinate and every effort to urinate is accompained by intolerable burning.

Everybody is aware of the most important symptom of Cayenne pepper. It is burning—intolerable, intense burning—accompained by smarting.

In **Anthraxinum,** the burning is mostly connected with the ulcers, putrid sores, gangrenes, and malignant pustules.

Having discussed the main trails of **Sulphur,** we will next have a glimpse at his mental condition. His memory is very weak, particularly for names. He remembers with remarkable accuracy the events that occurred a long time ago but not what transpired recently. **Anacardium, Cannabis ind., Glon., Phos.,** and **Acid phos.** betray an equal amount of forgetfulness. **Sulphur** is indifferent and disinclined for work of every description. Nothing appeals to him—work, pleasure, talking, exercise afford him no enjoyment. It is not the indifference of **Phosphorus** and **Sepia** where it is manifested chiefly towards one's own relations and beloved. It is a disgust for everything mundane as he calls it. If there is anything to which he attaches any importance, it is the question of his own salvation and other similar philosophical speculations.

Some cases of insanity call for **Sulphur** where the patient suffers from what is called a sort of fantastic mania. He is very jolly. He has no care, no anxiety, and worry to disturb the peace of his mind. He is an optimist of the first water. Everything seems full of beauty. He dresses himself in the most tattered rags but considers them the most elegant of decorations.

Sulphur acts on the eyes. It is used in retinitis, cataract, keratitis, marginal blepharitis and innumerable other affections.

Sulphur is useful in deafness with humming or hissing in the ears. As regards the hissing noise in the ears, we should compare it with **Causticum, China, Graphites, Acid phos., Petroleum, Kali phos** and **Salicylic acid.**

In **Causticum** we find persistent roaring in the ears while words and steps re-echo in auditory passage.

The roaring in the ears in **China** is a well-known fact due to the extreme debility of the **China** patient. It is a debility brought about by the great loss of the vital fluid. We find this symptom mostly in women after great flooding, in phthisical patients after a severe attack of hemoptysis, and in weak anemic young men suffering from constant loss of the seminal fluid.

Graphites has humming or roaring in the ears accompanying deafness, but the peculiarity about this patient is that he hears best in noise. You tell him something in a quiet and secluded place and it will make no impression on his impaired hearing but in a street-car or in the hum of machinery his power of hearing is at its best.

In otitis too, we have to administer **Sulphur,** but it is mostly in psoric patients with tendency to skin eruptions and after other selected remedies had failed.

Sulphur has decided influence on the nose. There is profuse catarrhal discharge from the nostrils when out of doors, but indoors the patient feels his nostrils blocked-up. It has cured freckles and black spots on the nose and face.

Now we will consider the action of **Sulphur** on the respiratory organs. Beginning with the tongue, we find it coated white with red tip and edges. Sometimes it is full of aphthæ, like what is found in **Borax, Mercurius,** and **Hydrastis.**

Laryngitis, pharyngitis, bronchitis, pneumonia and even phthisis find in **Sulphur** a very powerful remedy. In laryngitis the prominent symptoms are hoarseness and aphonia. This hoarseness is worse in the morning. The more chronic the case, the better is this remedy indicated.

In bronchitis and pneumonia its scope extends from the beginning to the end. In the incipient stage of inflammation a judicious dose of **Sulphur** will relieve the lungs of their hyperemia. It is also used after **Aconite** or **Bryonia** has controlled congestion preventing hepatization and promoting absorption. In those desperate cases where pneumonia assumes a torpid character and threatens to terminate in tuberculosis, where the patient responds but tardily to the indicated remedy, where the complaints keep constantly relapsing, we know of no other remedy that will help more than **Sulphur.** The other symptoms calling for it are:

Oppression in the chest with a sense of heaviness. The patient feels suffocated and wants the doors and windows open, particularly at night. There is a similar sense of weakness in chest when talking as in **Stannum.** That sharp stitching pain through left lung to back, worse when lying on the back and aggravated by the least movement is quite characteristic of **Sulphur.**

All the features of asthma are produced in the pathogenesis of this remedy. Those of us that have inhaled **Sulphur** vapour know very well the great influx of phlegm, the difficulty of breathing, the cough and a series of other unpleasant symptoms produced by it.

Sulphur has the alternation of skin irritation and asthma. There are innumerable cases on record where suppression of eczema brought about violent fits of asthma and the cure of asthma was brought by the restoration of the original asthma.

Dr. Villers mentions of a case of eczema that he cured with a single dose of **Sulphur** C.M. the suppression of which by external ointment brought about a very distressing attack of asthma. The administration of the first dose of **Sulphur** brought about very serious aggravation; the patient had to tear her clothes loose, roll on the floor and scratch till she pretty nearly bled. Shortly after this was established a very excoriating, fetid discharge from the ears and the vulva which terminated in a complete cure of all her ailments.

The **Sulphur** cough is dry and is caused by the rawness of the larynx; it is also excited by a sensation of tickling in the larynx as with a feather. In the evening and night there is no expectoration, but in the morning and day time the patient brings up a sort of darkish bloody sputum. Sometimes it is yellow, greenish, purulent or milkwhite mucus. It tastes sour, nauseating, flat or saltish. The cough is accompanied by pain in chest as if it would burst to pieces. Sometimes there is a peculiar sensation of coldness in the chest as if from a lump of ice.

We must not over-look the action of **Sulphur** on the digestive tract. It produces important symptoms which we can ill-afford to neglect. Our patient is a chronic dyspeptic. He complains of faintness, **great** and a weak gone-feeling at stomach at 11 a.m. This is very characteristic. At other times feels quite fit, but as 11 a.m. approaches, hunger gets hold of him. It is sometimes more than ordinary hunger; he feels a sort of empty sensation in his abdomen accompanied by fainting spells. He must eat something then and there. We remember a case of neurasthenia in an elderly lady. She was bed-ridden for a year. Her physician, an allopathic doctor, finding medicine ineffectual, advised a change of climate at a time when she could hardly move in bed unaided. Amongst a very complex lot of symptoms we noticed that she suffered from this empty, enervated sensation at about 11 a.m. which, she told us, was the worst time for her out of the twenty-four hours. She felt as if she would faint if she did not get something to eat at that hour and that is why she could not wait for the return of her husband from work. This symptom was a great clue to us. The other symptoms she had were an offensive odour permeating the whole body despite frequent washing, unhealthy skin, frequent hot flushes, burning of the hands and feet, redness of the orifices of the body and many other **Sulphur** symptoms. A few doses of **Sulphur** did her a world of good. It had only to be supplemented later on with a few doses of **Zincum** to make the cure a complete one.

Other remedies having closely similar sensations are **Hydrastis, Ignat., Phos., Petrol.,** and **Sepia.**

In **Hydrastis** the empty, all-gone feeling is very characteristic and this symptom frequently leads to its successful application in many cases of gastric affections which otherwise would have turned into gastric ulcerations or even carcinomatous degeneration of the stomach.

Ignatia has the weak, empty enervated feeling observable in hysterical patients; but here eating does not relieve.

Phosphorus has this sensation just as marked as in **Sulphur.** The sensation extends throughout the whole abdomen and is aggravated at night, so much so that the patient must get up and eat something. This remedy is more useful in patients with phthisical tendencies. Very often this sensation comes on during nausea.

Petroleum has similar sensations after stools.

Sepia exhibits identically the same symptom but it is mostly in connection with uterine troubles; there is a strong sensation of bearing down and prolapsus with it. Strangely enough the patient notices it when she thinks of her food and during headache.

Amongst the patient's desires and aversions we notice that he drinks much but eats little. This symptom really helps us to cure many cases of marasmus in children. Oftentimes he is very fond of sweets and he suffers from diseases consequent to eating too many sweets. In this last respect, he is very much like **Argentum nitricum,** but he is not a puny, wrinkled, shrivelled up dot of a child as the **Argentum** baby. It is scrofulous, big-bellied, dirty-looking imp of a child with emaciated limbs.

To return to our dyspeptic again. We must not forget him so soon. He very frequently suffers from incarcerated flatulence. His intestines feel as if strung in knots, worse by bending forward. In this respect **Sulphur** ranks equally with **Carbo veg., Cinchona** and **Lycopodium.**

In **Carb. veg.,** the flatulence collects more in the upper part of the abdomen and in the stomach causing gastralgia. The wind mainly passes upward. It is especially useful in disorders arising from fatty food and pastries, particularly after **Pulsatilla** has failed to relieve.

In **Cinchona officinalis,** the entire abdomen is "packed full" and the wind travels both upwards and downwards. It is very often complicated with spleen and liver affections. The patient is in a weak debilitated condition from loss of vital fluid. Periodicity is well-marked here.

In **Lycopodium,** the flatulence is most marked in the lower bowels and is pressed downwards towards the rectum. Urinary and liver complications are very common with this remedy. The 4 p.m. aggravation should be noted carefully.

Sulphur has a strong desire for alcohol, especially for beer and brandy. The other remedies that we may think of in this connection are **Sulphuric acid, Asarum, Selenium, Syphilinum** and **Medorrhinum.**

The **Sulphur** patient frequently suffers from morning diarrhœa. It drives him out of bed in the early hours of the morning (5 a.m.) with a feeling as if his bowels were too weak to retain their contents. We have a similar morning diarrhœa in **Bryo., Nat sulph., Phos., Podo.,** and **Rumex** and we will differentiate between them.

The morning diarrhœa in **Bryonia** is urgent and it comes on after the patient gets out of bed in the morning.

Natrum sulph. diarrhœa starts when the patient gets up and moves about for a while.

Phosphorus has (chronic) morning diarrhœa in lean slender persons. There is oozing from the constantly open anus and sometimes forcible expulsion—stools pouring as from a hydrant.

Podophyllum too, has diarrhœa in the morning; but the objectionable feature is that it keeps on the whole forenoon. It is accompanied by prolapsus ani, and pain in sacrum. The stools are profuse, watery, whitish and offensive.

Rumex diarrhœa begins in the morning (before rising) and is associated with dry, tickling cough so characteristic of the remedy.

The **Sulphur** stools are brown, watery, fecal, undigested, frothy sour, changeable, fetid, and corrosive. They may be mucus tinged with blood as in dysentery. The odor of the stools like all the excretions of the **Sulphur** patient is quite characteristic. It follows him about as if he has soiled himself. The suddenness and urging in **Sulph.** is characteristic and like **Aloes,** though to a less extent it has that feeling of fullness and weight in the rectum and loss of power of the sphincter ani.

During stools **Sulphur** has prolapsus ani. This reminds us **Ignatia, Podo.** and **Trombid.** We will study it more in detail later on.

Sulphur finds application in dysentery. There is tenesmus after stool and, as in **Colchicum,** the patient falls asleep as soon as the tenesmus ceases. The anus feels excoriated and swollen. Itching urning, pressing, stitching and crawling sensations continue in the rectum for a long time after the stool is over.

The diarrhœa that we have just discussed alternates very frequently with constipation. The stools become hard, dry and black as if burnt. They are mostly met with in hemorrhoidal complaints and in hypochondriac patients.

Sulphur is one of Dr. Guernsey's "big fours" in hemorrhoids. It is good for painless piles. It may be blind or bleeding. The blood is venous.

Sulphur is our great stand-by in scrofulosis. The glands all over the body are swollen. The patient sweats very much on the head, especially during sleep. His fontanelles remain open for a long time from defective osseous growth. He breaks out with boils, itches, and eruptions. He is very subject to caries, rickets, curvature of the spine and hip-joint diseases. It is not because he has a poor appetite that he is so thin and unhealthy. Far from it, he suffers from a voracious appetite. He is eating all the time; but the trouble is he does not assimilate what he eats. Consequently he looks marasmatic. This is very much like our **Iodium** patient who eats all the time but still looks emaciated. We find marasmus in various other remedies, such as **Abrot., Kreos., Sarsa., Nat. mur., Sanic., Tuber.** and so on, but there are points of real difference and so there really need be no danger of confusion.

Now we would like to make a few remarks about the skin symptoms of **Sulphur.** It has a great tendency to expel everything internal out on to the surface. We have seen this while discussing the bearing of **Sulphur** on asthma. The skin is apt to be rough scaly, scabby and coarse. There is very little perspiration; if any, is very offensive or sour. Eruptions appear here and there which itch and burn greatly. Later on they turn into pustules. Rhagades furuncles, ecchymoses, freckles, uritcaria, lichen, corns, crops of boils, herpes, and eczema are plentiful.

We will next consider the application of **Sulphur** in fevers. It is used in cases where the fever assumes a slow type and runs on to the typhoid condition. The torpor with slowness in answering questions, the offensive exhalations of the body and the besotted look of the patient remind us of **Baptisia.** In the latter remedy the case is more desperate—the torpor easily gives place to stupor. The tongue in **Baptisia** is covered with sordes and the blood is actually in a state of decomposition due to sepsis. The conditions calling for **Sulphur** arise more from a miasmatic condition of our

system than from real degeneration as in **Baptisia.** Dr. H. C. Alle
expresses it in the following sentences:

"Intense, persistent, long-continued fever; skin dry, hot an
burning; temperature 103-105, little or no remission day and nigh
patient literally being consumed with fever."

The sinking in the **Sulphur** fevers is due to lack of reactiv
power on the part of the system. The chills are very peculiar
that they constantly creep from the sacrum up the back witho
subsequent heat, worse by warmth of fire.

Chill is mostly internal. It creeps from the sacrum up t
back. Like **Nux vom.** and **Stram.** there is great sensitiveness
open air; the slightest movement brings about shivering. Stran
to say this shivering is not often followed by heat. Duri
shivering there is coldness of the nose, hands, feet, chest, an
back and abdomen. Icy coldness of the genitals is a great in
cation of this remedy. During the stage of heat the patie
complains of frequent flushes in the face, with shivering sensati
over the body. These flushes of heat are only transient; th
end in moisture and faintness.

At night the patient breaks out in profuse perspiration ov
the whole body. The perspiration smells sour and offensive a
it breaks out on the slightest motion or manual labor. This pe
piration makes him very restless and he tosses in bed all nig
rising in the morning unrefreshed and languid. He sleeps
snatches with half-open eyes; sometimes he talks loudly in sle

Now a few words on the sexual system. There is invol
tary discharge of semen with burning in urethra. The semi
secretion is thin, watery and inodorous. The penis is icy c
and sexual power is almost extinct. On attempting coition
orgasm results very quickly. The testicles are relaxed and ha
ing down.

On the female sexual system, the influence of **Sulphur**
quite marked. There is a great congestion to these parts
consequently she complains of a sense of fullness with bear
down in pelvis towards genitals. This pressing down is felt m
acutely when she stands up and as a consequence that post
she is very reluctant to assume. Over and above this, she suff
from leucorrhœa. It is yellow and corroding. The menses
are dark, thick and acrid.

Talking about its menstruation, remember how once it hel
me in a critical case of metrorrhagia. She was about 50 ve
old. The hemorrhage was very profuse, so much so that e

ight one entire piece of "sari" would get thoroughly soaked
a blood. She was long under allopathic treatment and was sup-
osed to suffer from cancer of the womb. Her condition was
ally critical. Emaciation was profound. The reactive power
f the system was at a very low ebb, for no medicine, however
arefully selected, would retain its ground for long. The sense
: burning in the palms of the hands and the soles of the feet
as quite oppressive. She would keep the doors and the win-
ws open otherwise she would feel suffocated. These were some
her symptoms. I prescribed **Erigeron, Hamamelis, Phosphorus,
ina, Sabina, Trill., Ustilago** and a few more of our hemorrha-
c remedies, but all to no effect. The patient was gradually
aking till at last struck on the happy idea of following dear
ahnemann's foot-steps and prescribing on the totality of symp-
ms, instead of going by the routine—a mistake so often com-
tted by novices, a few doses of **Sulphur** were prescribed and
e effect was marvellous. A cyst protruded from the vagina and
rst. That was the end of her trouble and she was cured. Evi-
ntly she was suffering from a cystic growth.

A few words about epilepsy and we will be finished with our
course on **Sulphur.** It is useful in those cases where there is
ne scrofulous taint; such patients are ultra-religious and are
nceited with a sense of their own importance. The aura seems
proceed from the extremities up the back as a creeping sen-
ion or up the leg to the right side of the abdomen. The
ient is apt to fall on the left side.

The treatment of epilepsy is a hard problem and we may
identally mention here that especial attention should be devot-
to the causative factor. If the attacks are caused by the pres-
e of cicatrices upon adjoining nerves, it should be removed
h a knife. Sometimes it is the effect of menstrual derange-
nts, helminthiasis, excessive noctural emissions and so on.
ese matters ought to be attended to before the resultant epi-
sy can be cured.

It may prove useful to mention a few practical hints before
close. We must in the first place be very careful about the se-
ion of **Sulphur.** It is double-edged sword; even when select-
properly we may do almost irreparable harm by an injudi-
s repetition or by the administration of an unsuitable potency.
Farrington says: "I would caution you as to how you
this drug. If carelessly or wrongly given it may precipitate
disease which it was desired to cure. You must not repeat

your doses too frequently and you must never give it unless yo
are certain it is the remedy; for the tendency of **Sulphur** is t
arouse whatever lies dormant in the system."

Brigham's admonition, too, is worth noticing. He says: " I
consumption everything depends upon the potency; the lowe
potencies are pernicious. I once provoked fatal activity of th
secreting vessels in a pulmonary consumption with a thir
potency, so that my patient was absolutely drowned."

Case 1.—I., aged twelve months, had had diarrhœa for nearly a mont
Her flesh was soft and flabby; open fontanelles; tongue coated white
the back. She was thirsty and drank a good deal of milk and water. T
diarrhœa was worse in the morning, beginning about 4 a.m., continui
more or less until the afternoon. It was dark yellow watery; occasiona
greenish white mucus, coming with a gush early in the morning, alm
involuntary during the day when standing. Child cried a little before bow
were moved. There was also a cough, worse on lying down at night, son
times causing her to vomit. Child slept with eyes only half closed. T
patient's appearance suggested **Calc. carb.,** which was prescribed; no bene
resulting, **Sulphur** 6 was given. The diarrhœa ceased, and her health grea
improved in a few days, no other remedy being needed.—Dr. A. E. Hawk

Case 2.—Mrs. W., aged twenty-five. Married, and has two children; t
last was born fifteen months before I saw her, from which time she l
suffered from profuse yellow leucorrhœa, with violent pruritis vulvæ, wo
at night. She has, at the same time, great bearing-down of the won
perfectly incapacitating her from standing or walking, or doing her hou
hold duties, such as ironing or washing. Most violent chronic headaches,
a throbbing and tensive character, and arising from the least worry or fatig
with habitual constipation. Has been under Allopathic treatment two ye
without benefit. The key-note to the cure was as follows: Heat and pr
sure on vertex, throbbing and tensive headaches, more or less constant, a
worse before the menses; worried by trifles, and memory impaired. Flu
ing of face; fainting spells without a cause; sinking, empty exhaus
craving for food; always worse at eleven o'clock in the forenoon; inte
icy coldness of the feet; worse when the head is bad. **Sulphur,** one millio
potency in one dose of five pellets, cured permanently, every sympt
constipation, leucorrhœa, and sensation of prolapsus included, and with
repetition.—Dr. Thos. Skinner.

SULPHURIC ACID

Sulphuric acid is used extensively in the arts and the manufactures, and cases of poisoning by it are very common. There is voilent bu ning and pain extending through the throat and gullet to the stoma h. This is followed by retching and vomiting; the vomited matter contains particles of mucous membrane from the gullet and stomach and in severe cases portions of muscular structures, for it has been known to cause gangrene of the stomach. The mouth is excoriated and its lining membrane and the tongue look as if smeared with white paint. The stomach gets so irritable that whatever is swallowed is immediately vomited up.

It is a remedy that the ancients used as gargles (in dilution) for a series of complaints, such as aphthæ, ulceration of the gums, venereal ulcers, diphtheria, etc. Hahnemann proved it and placed it on a scientific basis. The symptom that **Sulphuric acid** first reminds us is the great acidity which it causes when taken in healthy condition. The eructations are sour and the acidity is so great that it sets the teeth on edge. We all remember the sweet days of our childhood, and the raw mangoes from the wayside trees and the salt, and the setting of the teeth on edge. Our **Sulphuric acid** patient feels exactly this latter sensation without having partaken of that childhood dainty. The other similar remedies are **Calc. carb., Digit., Lycop., Iris** and **Rob.**

Our strumous **Calc. carb.** patient is sour all over. His eructations are sour, his vomiting is sour, his stools are sour and he himself smells sour. He has an aversion for meat and for warm food. He wants his victuals cold. Palpitation of the heart, fulness and bloatedness of the stomach, alternate diarrhœa and constipation, and cold damp feet, are all important symptoms of this remedy.

Digitalis is often needed in cardiac dyspepsia where there is trouble both after and before meals; after eating he feels a sort of sinking sensation in the stomach and spits up mouthfuls of what he has eaten sourer than vinegar. After the stomach is emptied he gets terrible pain and discomfort, so he wants to eat again.

Lycop. is looked upon as one of the great friends of the dyspeptic. There is canine hunger, but satiety after a few mouthfuls, excessive accumulation of flatulence, the amelioration from hot drinks, the debility and the mental attitude of the patient make the possibility of error in prescribing an absurdity.

Iris vers. is a much neglected remedy. **Kali bich.** is often used where **Iris** is indicated and consequently failure is the result. The two remedies are so very similar that a confusion between them is very natural. The sticky, gummy and soapy nature of the discharge is characteristic of both the remedies; but the latter lacks the acidity of the former.

Robinia can aptly be compared to **Sulph. acid.** Perhaps no remedy in our Materia Medica has more marked acidity of the digestive tract than this one. The stomach is intensely acid and the extreme sourness of everything coming from it sets the teeth on edge same as in **Sulph. acid.**

This acidity, which we have just spoken about, is merely a symptom of dyspepsia to which our **Sulphuric acid** patient is a chronic martyr. Another way in which this dyspepsia manifests itself is diarrhœa. The stools are chopped, saffron-yellow, stringy, forthy green and watery. In adults it is caused by eating oysters. In children it may be the effect of dentition.

The dyspepsia that we notice under this remedy is a chronic affair, the result of a long-continued indulgence in intoxicating drinks. The patient's stomach feels cold and relaxed, to relieve which he has recourse to frequent drinks of alcohol. When he partakes of any food, he gets the sensation of a stone in the stomach. Sometimes severe pain, starting from the pit of the stomach and penetrating right through to the region between the shoulder blades, obliges him to desist. He has much sour and bitter eructations, and regurgitation of food. **Ars., Asar., Sel., Op.** and **Nux vom.** are some of the remedies generally thought of in similar conditions, but in none of them do we find such a run down, debilitated and wretched condition as under this remedy.

Another feature of the remedy is the great exhaustion and weakness to which our patient becomes a victim. He seems to be almost overpowered by it. This is one reason why we find this remedy so often indicated in typhoid, typhus, septic and other varieties of pernicious fevers. His face is deathly pale, and his mouth is covered with aphthous sores. We have to ask him the same question often for he is slow in answering. This is partly due to his hardness of hearing and partly to the loss of " elasticity of the parts." The exhaustion of the patient is rendered worse by frequent attacks of epistaxis and hemorrhage from other outlets of the body. The blood is thin and dark and it oozes continuously.

There are two other remedies that vie with **Sulph. acid** in the treatment of typhoid or typhus. One of them is **Acid phos.** It is a remedy called for in all stages of this fearful malady. The precursory stage in **Acid phos.** almost always begins with a gastric disturbance. Great sensitiveness of the abdomen, red miliary eruption in the various parts of the body, weak frequent intermittent pulse, muttering, bland delirium, stupor, and lienteric stools, are all characteristic of **Acid phos.**

But there is another remedy which comes still closer to **Sulphuric acid**, and that is **Muriatic acid.** Under this, the case is more advanced than in the two previously-mentioned remedies. The only remedy in the Materia Medica that can present a graver situation is **Carb. veg.** Dr. H. C. Allen's report to a brother physician who called him in consultation about the prognosis of a case, is worth remembering. He said " My prognosis is **Muriatic acid."** The utterance of that great man has impressed on my mind the gravity of this remedy. The symptoms to indicate it are clear-cut and precise. With moaning and groaning the patient keeps on sliding down the bed and this takes place repeatedly, even after the patient has been placed in a proper position. There is constant muttering when awake with inability to collect one's senses. The mouth and anus are especially affected in this remedy. A sort of paralytic weakness creeps over the tongue so that, even when perfectly conscious, he is unable to articulate as he would desire. The mouth and face are distressingly parched. The pulse intermits at every third beat and he passes large quantities of watery urine almost unconsciously.

We have already spoken of the aphthous sores of this remedy and we will now deal with them in detail. There is no remedy in our Materia Medica where this condition is more marked than in this remedy. The whole buccal cavity is full of these ulcers and they are white or yellow in appearance. It is especially needed in aphthæ of children suffering from exhausting diseases.

Mercurius and **Borax** approach very near to this remedy but they lack the great weakness of **Sulphuric acid.**

Arsenicum comes much closer, but is distinguished by its still greater exhaustion, its restlessness and the peculiarities of its aggravation and amelioration.

We have already spoken of the weakness of **Sulph. acid** but we have omitted to mention its peculiarity. It is a sort of tremulous weakness and this tremulousness is merely subjective. The patient complains of a sensation of trembling without actual trembling. This is like **Gelsemium** and **Ther.**

Sulphuric acid has a very characteristic pain. It increases gradually to a certain degree and then suddenly ceases. We will now discuss the indications of a few other remedies with peculiar pain symptoms.

Stan., Plat. and **Syphil.** are three remedies where the pain begins lightly, increases gradually to the highest degree and then gradually declines.

In **Bell., Kali bich., Nit. acid, Carb. acid** and **Mag. phos.,** shooting pains appear suddenly and disappear just as suddenly.

In **Colocynth** the pains commence suddenly and severely but disappear gradually.

The **Sulph. acid** patient exhibits peculiar mentality. He is obsessed with hurry. Time does not move quick enough to suit him; while eating he just bolts his food; while writing he exhibits a similar impulse of haste and his pen flies over his paper. He can furnish no rational reason for this actuation to hurry. Such impatience should particularly draw our attention to **Sulph. acid.**

Dr. Clarke recommends this remedy in nightmare when occurring before each menstrual period. He says: "With **Sulphuric acid** 30, a dose every night, I gave great relief to a delicate woman" who was suffering from a similar condition.

Sulphuric acid is one of our great remedies for trauma. We use it to remove the bad effects of mechanical injuries, such falls, blows, bruises, etc. Frequently we notice extravasations of blood from the effect of such injuries.

Sulphuric acid is very often needed in the coughs of drunkards and of women in their climacteric years. It is a sort of hacking, dry, constant cough. Very frequently they complain of sudden violent pain in the upper left chest passing through to the scapula on that side. Sometimes a tired and a sore feeling is ascribed to the region between the scapulæ. The cough is a stomach cough ending with belching and always accompanied with foul breath.

We use this remedy for hernia scrotalis when there is a great tendency for the hernia to come down. Dr. Guernsey recommends it for hernia in infants who are profoundly weak.

Some people unfortunately contract the drinking habit, but when at last they realize their pitiful situation and desire to withdraw, they find themselves enmeshed too firmly in the clutch of the drinking mania. Hering recommends them **Sulphuric acid** one part with three parts of alcohol, 10 to 15 drops, thrice daily, for three or four weeks. It subdues their craving for liquor.

SUMBUL.

Sumbul is prepared from Musk-root—an aquatic plant of the order of umbelliferæ. The odour, as its name implies, is similar to that of musk and it is used extensively in adulterating the latter article. It is a native of Central Asia. In its action, too, it is very similar to **Moschus.**

This medicine was originally proved by Dr. Cattell. Being analogous to **Moschus** and other remedies useful in hysteria such as **Castor., Nux mosch., Ambra grisea, Asafœtida** etc., we see quite a few symptoms of hysteria in its pathogenesis. Fits of hysterical laughter and tears, depression of spirits, mirthfulness, fidgetiness, and excitability are some of its mental symptoms. We also notice under its heading a great tendency towards fainting. But the symptom that is considered the key-note symptom of **Sumbul** is the tenacity of the yellow mucous discharges from the nose and throat. From both these orifices, are to be seen a profuse flow of such tenacious mucus. Hence it is curative in the worst form of nasal and pharyangeal catarrh. In respect of this discharge it is similar to **Cubeba., Hydrast.,** and **Pulsat.** Dr. Hale strongly recommends it in the catarrh of children who are nervous, irritable and sleepless.

It has oily pellicle in urine. This floats on the surface although the urine is clear underneath. In this respect it is similar to **Sulph., Pulsat.** and **Petrol.,** under each of which we notice a similar scum on the surface of the urine. I have just got two more symptoms to add—one is climacteric flushings and the other is prurigo specially on head of infants; the spots are round, dry, slightly raised and reddened at edges with brain-like scale in centre.

SYMPHYTUM.

Symphytum is a great vulnerary remedy same as **Arnica** and **Ruta.** Its constituents are mucilage, sugar, asparagine, tannic and gallic acids, and starch. It is also called Comfrey and it belongs to the natural order of Boraginaceæ.

Here is another remedy of very ancient lineage; we find it mentioned in the writings of Dioscorides. It is found all over Europe and in certain parts of America, in fields and near about ditches. It greatly diminishes irritation in sores and ulcerations, lessens suppuration and promotes healing. It therefore facilitates union of fractured bones by favouring production of callus. It is principally used in mechanical injuries caused by blunt instruments.

Medical literature is replete with instances of wonderful cures effected with **Symphytum,** in cases of injuries both to the soft parts as well as to the periosteum and bony tissues. As such it should be compared with **Arnica, Calendula, Cicuta, Conium, Hyper., Led., Rux tox., Ruta, Sulphuric acid** and **Staphis.** It will pay us to look into the domain of each one of these remedies separately. It is because of such remedies as these that we are able to dispense with the knife in many instances where knife seems inevitable; and it is on account of the marvellous effects of these remedies that the belief has gained ground, that in homœopathy knife is superfluous.

Arnica is applicable in bad effects of springs, strains, bruises, concussions, contusions and other mechanical injuries with laceration of the soft parts. Its early application retards suppuration.

Calendula is useful in incised and lacerated wounds. This remedy too, retards suppuration and assists in quickening primary union along incised surfaces. It is specially suitable to cases where there has been loss of soft parts. Bloody and serous infiltrations of cellular tissues meet in **Calendula** a ready help.

Cicuta should be thought of in concussions of the brain or spinal cord. The tissues damaged in this remedy are mostly nerve substance.

Conium is indispensable in indurations of glandular substance due to contusion and bruise.

Hypericum is a splendid remedy for punctured wounds and there is extreme sensitiveness of the affected part. When any part of our body or limb gets smashed and in spinal concussions as is caused by a fall on the coccyx and also in lacerations attended with intolerable pain which shows involvement of the nerve-tissue, we have no remedy to equal **Hypericum.**

Ledum is also a great remedy in fractured wounds and in injuries inflicted with sharp instruments. It gives a cold sensation around the injured parts—a symptom that helps us greatly in differentiating **Ledum** from other similar remedies.

Rhus tox. is invaluable in erysipelas. We also think of it in traumatic lesions attacking the cellular fibres or articular tissues and in bad effects of straining or over-lifting. It has marked actions on ligaments of joints.

Ruta. is useful in sprains, strain or rupture of tendons, wounds of joints, synovitis the result of injuries, injuries to periosteum, and fibrous tissues and in mechanical injuries to tarsal and carpal joints.

Staphis. like **Led.** should be thought of in mechanical injuries from sharp cutting instruments and in clean incised wounds.

Sulph. acid like **Arnica** is useful in contusions and suggillations with a special tendency on the part of blood-vessels to break due to degeneration of the walls of arteries.

Dr. Anshutz has in his "New, Old and Forgotten Remedies" cited a few remarkable cures effected by **Symp.** These cases are very interesting and instructive and I feel it will do, every homœopath, good to go through them. These cases very clearly enunciate the principle that homœopathy, though it does not altogether dispense with surgery, to a very large extent stops the abuse of the knife.

Case 1.—A boy, fourteen years old, broke the bones of the forearm, at the junction of the lower and middle thirds, two years ago. He had twice repeated the fracture by slight falls. The ends of the fragments are now slightly movable on each other, and the arm is weak and admits of little use. Three doses of **Symphytum** effected a perfect cure. The lad became more robust, and has since had better general health than ever before—Translated by P. P. Wells, M. D. from "Connection of Homœopathy with Surgery" by Croserio.

Case 2.—A boy, eight years old, fractured the humerus, near the junction of the condyles and shaft. **Arnica.** 30 immediately arrested the spasmodic jerks of the muscles of the injured arm. This remedy was continued for the first three days, when the traumatic fever had entirely subsided. He then had **Symphyt.** 3, gtt. i., in half a tumbler of water, a teaspoonful every morning and evening. The splints were removed the ninth day, and the bone was found consolidated. The cure was entirely without pain. How much earlier than this the fragments ceased to be movable is not known.

Case 3.—A man who was suffering from a malignant growth in the nose—a malignant tumour of the antrum, which had extended to the nose, saw Dr.

W. H. Thompson, President of the Royal College of Surgeons in Ireland.
An exploratory operation confirmed this diagnosis. We are quoting below in
Dr. Thompson's own language his experience about this case.

" He refused the larger operation. The exploration was made
by Dr. Woods. We found that the tumour did extend from the
antrum, into which I could bore my finger easily. Dr. O'
Sullivan, Professor of Pathology in the Trinity College, declared
the growth to be a round-celled sarcoma. Of that there is no
doubt. The tumour returned in a couple of months, and the
patient then saw Dr. Simon, in London, who advised immediate
removal. He returned home, and after a further delay he asked
to have the operation performed. I did this in May last by the
usual method. I found the tumour occupying the whole of the
antrum. The base of the skull was everywhere infiltrated. The
tumour had passed into the right nose and perforated the septum
so as to extend into the left. It adhered to the septum around
the site of perforation. This was all removed, leaving a hole in
the septum about the size of a florin. He went home within a
fortnight. In a month the growth showed signs of return. It
bulged through the incision and protruded upon the face. Dr.
Woods saw him soon afterwards, as I had declared by letter that
a further operation would be of no avail. The tumour had now
almost closed the right eye. It was blue, tense, firm, and lobula-
ted, but it did not break. Dr. Woods reported the result of his
visit to me, and we agreed as to the prognosis. Early in October
the patient walked into my study after a visit to Dr Woods. He
looked in better health than I had ever seen him The tumour
had completely disappeared from the face, and I could not identify
any trace of it in the mouth. He said he had no pain of any
kind. He could speak well when the opening, remaining after the
removal of the hard palate, was plugged, and he was in town to
have an obturator made. He has since gone home apparently
well."

The patient told Dr. Thompson that he had applied poultices
of Comfrey (or Symphytum) and that was all.

———————

SYPHILINUM.

Other names for this remedy are Lueticum and Luesinum. It is a very powerful nosode. It is of inestimable value to us in our practice. Of all nosodes this seems to be the most far-reaching and oft-needed remedy. It should always be used in higher potencies. Dr. H. C. Allen's immortal advice about this remedy should be carefully brone in mind by every homœopath. "Syphilitics, or patients who have had chancre treated by local means, and as a result have suffered from throat and skin troubles for years, are nearly always benefited by this remedy at the commencement of treatment, unless some other remedy is clearly indicated."

Apart from this we must also take notice of the grand keynote characteristics of **Syphilinum.** The first and the foremost amongst these, is the nocturnal aggravation. All pains, all symptoms and all ailments are worse from darkness to daylight. They begin with twilight and end with daylight. The headache, the neuralgia, the asthma, the cough and every other complaint for which we need this remedy are distinctly and perceptibly worse at this time. So prominent and so certain is this aggravation that the patient simply dreads the approach of the night. This dread is so great, that I have seen patients get into a regular tremor-as, hour by hour, minute by minute, the light of the day lapses into darkness of the night. The feeling of dread is most weird, unreasonable and unconquerable. This unholy and inexplicable dread is almost always present when **Syphilin.** is indicated. We will have enough opportunity to verify this as we proceed. In this respect **Syphil.** is similar to **Merc.** and **Phytol.**

Craving for alcohol in any form is the next important characteristic. Dr. Clarke expresses this idea very cleverly when he says that Bacchus and Venus are close allies. This craving for alcohol is very acute and in this **Syphil.** closely resembles **Asar., Sulp.** and **Sulp. acid.**

Thirdly a constant stream of boils makes up another land-mark of **Syphil.** It breaks out in endless succession, one after the other.

The fourth important point is the fetidity of all the discharges and secretions. The stool, urine, sweat and other secretions normal, as well as abnormal partake of this grand characteristic.

The glandular system is affected throughout and the nutrition of the body is badly impaired; that is why Dr. Burnett advocates **Syphil.** the same he has done with **Medor.** in delicate children with constitutional blight.

The pains of **Syphil.** are very characteristic. They increase and decrease gradually as in **Stann.**

Emaciation is as marked in **Syphil.** as in **Abrot.** and **Iodium**; all bones are affected epecially the bones of the head and tibiæ.

We should carefully compare **Syphil.** with **Aurum., Asaf., Kali iod., Merc., Phyt.** and **Nit. acid** as being similar remedies.

In **Asaf.** we have inflammation and caries with softening of the bones. There is a great tendency towards bleeding and ulcers are intolerably sensitive to touch specially around edges, while the pus discharged is thin, fetid and offensive.

In **Aurum,** the mastoid process and the nasal bones are mostly affected. Swellings of the periosteum and syphilitic exostoses on skulls are characteristically present.

In **Kali iod.** interstitial infiltration of bony as well as soft tissues in mercuro-syphilitic constitution should be our guide.

In **Phyt.** the bones are inflamed and swollen; the joints too are similarly affected. The ulcers have lardaceous bottoms and are punched-like in appearance.

Nit. acid is noted for carious ulcers with irregular edges and exuberant granulations.

In **Syphil.** the bases have a greyish appearance.

Syphilinum is used in certain cases of excruciating headache —headache that causes sleeplessness at night; it makes him restless and keeps him constantly on the move. This tendency to move and walk during severe headache is a key-note indication. Dr. Wildes has given us a very interesting case of a young girl of 16, who suffered from terrible headache. It was so intense that the veins on her temples used to stand out and she had to walk about much of the time; her irritable mood would not stand the slightest opposition, which had the effect of making her almost violent and lose all self-control. She was absent-minded. She had another peculiarity and that was a desire to wash her hands constantly. Her menses were irregular, delayed and scanty and were extremely painful; her sleep was anxious, wakeful and restless **Syphil.** cured her thoroughly.

It also has a kind of a linear headaches, commencing at both angles of the forehead and extending in parallel lines backward. It is a headache that breaks into his continuity of thought and memory. He frequently makes mistakes. Dr. Wildes reported another cure of a similar headache with **Syphil.** 1m.; it was in a book-keeper who had a persistent, piercing headache over his right eye extending deep into his brain. The severity of this headache made him lose all consistency in his thoughts and talks. Under the action of **Syphil.** the whole complaint disappeared within a period of 10 days. His mental faculties regained its full vigour and strength, but within a short period of this cure, his whole eyebrow broke out into a peculiar syphilitic eczema. It practically covered his forehead from temple to temple and went even behind his ear and to the hairy parts. It frequently happens that after contracting syphilitic poison, people would try to get a speedy cure by means of balms, ointments, and washes. The syphilitic rash and ulceration disappear from the surface, and do incalculable damage and harm. This cure reported by Dr. Wildes is an instance in point. The same author cites another instance of a case of ozæna. It was in a bright, brilliant young woman of 26. She had been always delicate from her childhood. A few doses of **Syphil.** cured the ozæna, but brought on a terrible band of inflamed, angry, eczematous rash and syphilitic sores across her forehead, from side to side. This rash also disappeared after proper treatment and the ozæna never returned.

We will now look into the mental trait of the **Syphilinum** patient. Great despondence stands out prominently everywhere. In fact all syphilitic patients suffer more or less from such symptoms. They always fear that their trouble will never get better. Want of concentration of mind, loss of memory, irritability, peevishness and a terrible dread at night—are symptoms to be remembered.

We have good many symptoms of the eyes in **Syphil.** Ptosis paralytica, diplopia, strabismus, chronic recurrent paralysis, keratitis, photophobia, acute ophthalmia neonatorum, conjunctivitis, syphilitic iritis and various other diseases of the eye come under its influence and can be readily cured provided proper indications are not wanting. All these complaints get worse at night and are relieved by cold applications.

The teeth in **Syphil.** undergo various degeneration. They decay at the edge of the gums; the crowns are cup-shaped and serrated. They break off easily and leave lots of stumps behind them. The tongue is coated white and the edges are indented by teeth; the breath is foul; the whole of buccal cavity is studded with numerous ulcerations. I remember having cured a young man of about 20 years of age, who had been suffering for quite a few years with ulcerated mouth. **Antim. crud., Merc. cyn., Merc.**

sol., Sulph., Muriatic acid were all tried.   The sores would go for a little while to reappear again.   This persistence and the apparent failure of other remedies, and the history of heriditary syphilis led me to try **Syphil.** The sores have long disappeared and have not recurred any more.   This proves that the constitutional syphilitic dyscrasia has been up-rooted.   Such instances are not rare in the busy career of a medical practitioner; repeated failures, instead of disheartening us, ought to make us pry more minutely into the secrets of maladies and take measurement of all malignant influences and miasms so that we may be in a position to prescribe the correct constitutional remedy and once for all set at naught the mischievous elements that make disease a permanent tenure with our patients.

With a few more indications of **Syphil.** we will close this chapter.   The leucorrhœa is profuse, so much so that it soaks through the napkins and runs down to the heels.   It is yellow and offensive.   It is mostly aggravated at night time; and it causes violent itching and inflammation of the external organs.

The constipation of **Syphil.** is chronic and is of many years' standing.   This constipation is due to a kind of stricture high up in the rectum.   The rectum feels as if tied up with strictures. The breath of the patient is very fetid.   When constipation is due to constriction or contraction of the rectum and the anus, we should also think of **Chelidonium, Graphites, Lachesis, Lycopodium, Mezereum, Nat. mur., Nitric acid, Nux vomica, Plumbum, Silicea, Theridion** and **Thuja.**

In **Chelid.,** the stools are ash-colored, whitish and lumpy and with constriction is associated intense itching.

In **Graphites,** as we all know, the constriction is mostly due to fissures in the anal cavity.   Each stool means sharp, severe, cutting pain which is followed by constriction and aching for hours together.

Lachesis is a grand remedy.   The constriction here is associated with extreme sensitiveness of the rectum due to innumerable hemorrhoidal knobs protruding therefrom.

Lyco. is second to none in constriction.   It is almost impossible to evacuate stools due to spasmodic constriction of the anus. Even the desire to evacuate is followed by painful contraction.

Mezereum need not be confused with **Syphilinum** or any other remedy as the constriction causes tearing and drawing pain not only at the anus but in the perineum as well and through into the urethra

Nat. mur. is the king amongst remedies for contraction of the rectum and constriction of the anus. There is invariably a feeling of excoriation in the anus after evacuation. The stools are dry and hard and they crumble through the fissured anus which bleeds through the effort.

In **Nitric acid** with the spasmodic contraction which continues many hours after stools, we have intense proctalgia and a constant oozing of fetid moisture from the fissured anus. The pain in the rectum is as if it has been torn or cut with a knife.

In **Nux vomica** the constriction is associated with inactivity of the bowels. We have ineffectual desire for stools and a sensation as if more remains and could not be evacuated.

The other remedies have been dealt with previously and we need not worry any further about them here.

SYZYGIUM JAMBOLANUM.

It is a native of Bengal where it grows most abundantly. The fruit is black in colour, delicious but slightly astringent and is of the size of grape. It is called ' Jumbul ' or ' Jam.' The tincture is prepared from the powdered fruit stones. It is a most useful remedy in diabetes mellitus. It causes a marked diminution of sugar in the urine. Prickly heat in the upper part of the body is an important symptom. Specific gravity of the urine is very high. Great thirst is experienced. The patient emaciates inspite of proper nutritious diet. Weakness and diabetic ulceration in different parts of the body are characteristic indications. Dudgeon cured with **Syzygium** in two drop doses, given thrice daily, a pronounced case of diabetes in an elderly man who was covered all over with prickly heat. The specific gravity was 1036 and the urine was surcharged with sugar. Thirst was great and the flow of urine was profuse, which was being passed every two hours night and day. Under the influence of this remedy the specific gravity steadily declined, sugar disappeared and all the other symptoms subsided.

TABACUM.

Tabacum belongs to the natural order of Solanaceæ. It is a rank hairy plant, 3 to 5 feet high with coarse leaves having a disagreeable odour and taste and turning brown on drying. It was originally a native of America, but is now grown in many parts of the world. The word Tobacco as originally applied by the Spaniards to this weed has persisted all these centuries and is now universally used. It was first introduced into Spain by the followers of Colombus and from Spain it found its way to other European countries. Jean Nicot the French ambassador to Lisbon sent some seeds to Catherine de Medici and thus from Spain it came to France. The name of this gentleman has been perpetuated till eternity; the essential principle of tobacco has been called Necotin after the name of the ambassador. The introduction of tobacco into England is to be attributed to Sir Walter Raleigh.

Its introduction into India is of a slightly later date and is to be attributed to the Portuguese.

The active principle of tobacco as has been said before is Necotin, a volatile oily fluid that is soluble in water. The symptom of tobacco poisoning are nausea, vertigo, vomiting, tremor, salivation, extreme pallor, prostration and clammy sweating. The pulse becomes small and weak. Where death occurs it occurs from respiratory failure.

Tobacco is used by chewing, snuffing, deeping and smoking. The last however is the commonest method of using tobacco. Its dilatory action on the heart is worth studying. The work of the heart is increased to a great extent and in cases of severe smoking we sometimes notice what we call tobacco angina. By far in the greater number of cases the cardiac symptoms of chronic necotin poisoning are functional and there are hardly any pathological changes. Occasionally, however, after long continued use hypertrophy results; fatty degeneration and arteriosclerosis though rare are sometimes evident. The symptoms most commonly met with, are those pointing to " irritable heart." Palpitation, dyspnœa pain, muscular weakness, headache and amnesia are very frequently to be seen.

The effect of tobacco on the eyes is universally recognised. Amblyopia is of frequent recurrence. It also causes sexual weakness. As to the effect of tobacco on the general development it causes a decided loss of weight. The muscles that are mostly affected are the muscles of cheek and back.

As to the argument in favour of tobacco smoking it affords pleasure and mental satisfaction. It is a nervous sedative in times of hardship and anxiety. It also checks the sense of hunger. Doughlas's argument in its favour is very gratifying to the tobacco smokers. "After an usually vexatious day, when I am in that unpleasant condition of mind when it seems as though the slightest word would cause an outburst of passion, nothing else does me so much good as smoking."

We will now study the therapeutic action of **Tabacum.** This remedy like all others has some special characteristics of its own. The main point in **Tabacum** is intense nausea with incessant vomiting. In this respect it vies with **Ipec.** The latter remedy however is wanting in the intense wretchedness of **Tabacum,** neither do we find in **Ipecac,** so prominently, the tremor, the cold clammy sweat, and the pallor of our remedy. Another peculiarity about the nausea and vomiting of **Ipecac** is that the slightest movement causes aggravation of the symptoms; the patient has to remain quiet, inert and inactive to prevent this harassing nausea from getting worse. This intense nausea and vomiting make it an admirable remedy in sea-sickness. These indications also lead to its application in Asiatic cholera.

The second important feature of the remedy is the sinking sensation felt at the pit of the stomach. It is a feeling very hard to describe; it is mostly a sensation of relaxation felt at the stomach with nausea accompanying it; it is a dreadful faint feeling in the stomach. Dr. Hering reports of a case of a lady aged about 70, ailing for upwards of a year. Her complaint was nausea, vomiting and constant pain in the stomach. She often threw up mucus and blood together with the food taken, but what ailed her most was the incessant pain in the stomach and intense and constant feeling of sickness. **Tabacum** relieved her completely.

We must not forget the aggravation and amelioration which form the third differentiating feature of our remedy. There is always a marked amelioration of the symptoms from exposure to draught of open, fresh air and from uncovering. The aggravation from the slightest movement, even that of opening the eyes, is almost as important a symptom as any we know of.

The appearance of the patient is striking. He is extremely emaciated. The death-like pallor of his face is awful. It is also blue, pinched and sunken. The drawn features and deeply sunken eyes, surrounded by blue rings, indicate the agony and the wretchedness of the sufferer.

Tabacum has very pronounced symptom in the region of the heart and it is often used in many serious complaints affecting that organ. It has been recommended in dilatation of the heart and also in angina pectoris. Violent constriction in the throat, tightness across the upper part of the chest with paroxysmal oppression and palpitation, tinnitus aurium, muscæ volitantes and irregular, feeble pulse are some of the symptoms that accompany others already mentioned.

I have never had any occasion to use this remedy in rheumatism but I cannot withhold the temptation of citing a cure effected by Dr. E. T. Blake with **Tabacum.** It was in a middle-aged lady of 40, who had all her joints affected with rheumatism which rendered them rigid. "Whenever she composed herself for sleep, just as she was lapsing into unconsciousness, the knees would attempt to fly up towards the chest with an abrupt jerk, tearing painfully at the acetabular adhesions." Other symptoms were: "Sweating, impaired memory, hypochondriasis, drumming in the ears, facial as well as crural clonus, white tongue, epigastric sinking alternating with nausea and flatulence; heart's action used to increase by day and diminish down to severe fainting during the night. **Tab.** 12 gave three hours' refreshing sleep the first night, more the second, and after the third the leg-jerk departed for good." Remarkable as this cure seems to be it was effected on the following redstrand symptoms:—**Episgastric sinking, intense nausea, and a frequent feeling of faintness at night time.**

It has been recommended in strangulated hernia. I cannot personally vouch for its reliability in such affection as I had no experience with it. It seems plausible considering that, the picture produced by **Tabacum** is greatly similar to the one brought on by the strangulation of guts. Gurgling in bowels, tympanitic abdomen, retracted navel due to constriction in abdominal muscles, coldness, vomiting, deathly nausea, and deathly faintness are all symptoms found in a case of strangulation and they point towards **Tabacum.**

TANACETUM VULGARE.

Tanacetum is a rarely-used drug but we can not dispense with it, for the same reason for which we cannot do without **Nux v.;** in those cases where it is indicated nothing but **Tanacetum** will help. It is indigenous to Europe and Central Asia. It flowers in July and August. The flowers are deep yellow and button-shaped. It belongs to the natural order of Compositæ. Its common name is Tansy, a word which means immorality, from the fact that the plant was mainly utilized for bringing on abortions. Most of our symptoms of **Tanacetum** have been obtained from cases of drugging, done with the intention of procuring abortions.

The fresh plant, when in flower, is chopped and mixed with two part by its weight of alcohol. It is strained and filtered after the usual period of eight days and we have the tincture.

When taken in big doses it produces almost all the symptoms of epilepsy, such as convulsions, frothing of the mouth, clenched fists, and so on. It has been used with success by Dr. Pierson in that disease. He recommends drop doses of the tincture four times daily.

It produces certain strange symptoms of the mind. She assumes all sorts of strange positions and makes funny gesticulations—symptoms generally occurring in hysteria and chorea. She wants to stand on her head; she stretches her limbs and draws them up again. Though her mind seems very clear, she is unable to accomplish anything. There is a sort of "laziness," a malaise and an unconquerable desire to lie down and wait; this sort of mood characterizes the **Tanacetum** temperament.

It retards the development of the fœtus in the uterus. One woman who took the drug to bring on abortion but did not succeed, delivered a child, at full term, of the size of a small kitten.

This remedy needs further proving and our study of its symptomatology will not be complete till a more thorough proving is done and the remedy used a bit oftener.

TARAXACUM.

This remedy deserves mention by reason of its curative value in affections of the liver, such as gall-stone, bilious attacks and jaundice. The tincture is extracted from the Candelion, a perennial herb common in northern countries. It belongs to the natural order of Compositæ.

The best indication of this remedy is seen in its mapped tongue (**Lachesis, Mercurius, Natrum mur., Arsenicum.**). This is caused by little patches of the white coating coming off from different places exposing red tender sensitive surface of the tongue. The taste of the mouth is bitter. As has been said before, the most important action of the remedy is seen in its action on the liver. It becomes enlarged and indurated. Also we notice an irresistible drowsiness after a meal which also speaks of the torpid state of the liver. Often this leads to a sort of a bilious diarrhœa. Another important symptom is chilliness. This reminds us of another important characteristic of **Taraxacum** which is icy coldness of the finger tips.

Taraxacum often finds application in typhoid fever of a low adynamic type—a type represented by **Rhus tox**, with which remedy it is often confounded. We have the same muttering delirium, the same intolerable pain in the lower extremities during rest and as great prostration; but then the differentiating features are to be found in the violent tearing pain in the occiput, great chilliness after eating and drinking, the mapped tongue and the coldness of the finger tips—symptoms that are characteristically indicative of **Taraxacum**.

It is a right-sided remedy.

TARENTULA CUBENSIS.

Tarentula is prepared from the poisonous spider found abundantly in Cuba, Mexico, Spain and South America.

It is useful in various affections like chorea, hysteria, and paralysis. We notice constant movement of arms and legs and twitching of various muscles of the body. This is due to great sensitiveness and irritability of the nervous structure of the system. Constant movement and friction are necessities with these patients; they relieve the hyper-irritation of the terminal points of the nerves. They rub their hands and legs and even their heads against something. They must roll something between their fingers and must put their fingers in their mouth. This extra-irritability of the entire body is the red strand symptom of the remedy, and whenever present, should remind us of **Tarentula.** This also leads to its application in multiple sclerosis, tabes dorsalis, epilepsy, chorea, hystero-mania, paralysis agitance and various other nervous affections which are supposed to be incurable.

I remember a case of chorea in a girl that could hardly stand. She could not keep quiet anywhere or in any position till music soothed her nerves. This feature of amelioration from music is a great characteristic of **Tarentula.**

The next important point is periodicity. Troubles occur at the same time every year.

Hyperesthesia completes the third essential point of importance. Least excitement irritates. This extreme sensitiveness is particularly noticeable on the spine. Slight touch on the spine provokes spasmodic pain in the chest and the cardiac region. Headache, neuralgia and other similar affections are rendered worse by noise, touch and strong light.

It is also useful in abscesses, boils, carbuncles, felons, malignant ulcers and gangrene. There is a great bluish discolouration of the skin as in **Lachesis.** An atrocious burning pain, that reminds us of **Arsenicum** and **Anthraxinum,** is another keynote indication of **Tarentula.**

It causes great hyperemia and hyperesthesia of the female sexual system which lead to extreme sexual excitement. This is the reason why it makes such an important remedy in nymphomania. They are simply forced to resort to this vile habit from the intensity of the excitement. In the male it leads to onanism and imbecility, ending ultimately in insanity.

It is a great remedy for intense unbearable pruritus vluvæ extending into vagina. The itchiness is great indeed at night time; with dryness, heat of the parts, burning and frequent expulsion of gas from the vagina, the patient is almost driven mad every night. The urine generally is thick, hot and full of sediments.

It is a remedy in cystitis; high fever usually complicates the case. The patient experiences great difficulty in passing even a few drops of urine. **Tarentula** relieves the swelling of the bladder, removes the tension and disperses the inflammation from the part.

The following are a few more of its characteristic indications: extreme sensitiveness of the tips of fingers; sore bruised feeling all over the body; aggravation of choreic movement when watched; cough relieved by smoking; stool following immediately on the washing of the head; pain in the ear associated with hiccough.

TELLURIUM.

This element bears a close resemblance to Selenium and is found in combination with minerals like silver, lead and gold. In appearance it resembles silver.

It has been used with great success in ringworms affecting the face, body and the hair roots. The rings are elevated and are marked with minute itching vesicles from which exudes a watery excoriating fluid that smells like fishbrine. The rings intersect each other.

It is also very useful in otorrhœa, and its indication, here as well as elsewhere, is that same fish-brine odor and the discharge setting up angry vesication whichever part it comes in contact with.

It is used with benefit in cases of injury and hence **Tellurium** finds entrance into the category of vulnerary remedies. With **Tellurium** Dr. Kent succeeded in bringing back into consciousness a boy that fell from a great height. Its great indication here is an extreme hyperesthesia of the back; the sensitiveness is so great that the least tactile impression sends vibration of pain to remote parts of the body.

Tellurium patient sweats profusely and the odor of the sweat is offensive and garlick-like.

TEREBINTHINA.

Terebinthina, oil of turpentine, a clear colorless liquid is obtained by the distillation of the exudation from certain varieties of the pine.

It is useful in certain affections of the kidney and the bladder. I would give it a very important place in Bright's disease. In the first stage when blood and albumen are more abundant than casts and epithelium, when the urine though scanty becomes surcharged with albumen, casts and blood discs, when œdema of legs sets in, when the urine becomes dark-colored due to decomposition of blood corpuscles, when due to rupture of the capillaries of the kidney blood pours into the pelvis of the kidney, no remedy can take the place of **Terebinthina.** Violent burning in urethra, great tenesmus of the bladder, dyspnœa, and a peculiar sweetish odor of the urine resembling the smell of violets, are indications of **Terebinthina.**

In addition to the symptoms given above, we find a smooth glossy red tongue devoid of papillæ, excessive tympanites and great drowsiness.

We also use it in fatty degeneration of the kidney, albuminuria and vesicle catarrh. It relieves the general dropsy that follows such kidney complaints. Cures are reported where such dropsical swellings were almost full to bursting, preventing the patient from undertaking the slightest movement. We must not forget the violent burning and cutting pain of **Terebinthina,** experienced while at rest and relieved from walking in the open air. The urine passed is black with coffee-ground sediment in it. Stiffness though universal is particularly pronounced in the loins.

We should not lose sight of **Terebinthina** in uremia and uremic coma. It removes the stupefaction and deep sleep that follow uremic poisoning. Administered in proper time it removes the tendency to syncope and stops the gradual progress of all the symptoms of coma.

Finally let me add that it is one of our great hemorrhagic remedies. It checks hemorrhage from the bowels, kidneys, bladder, lungs, uterus and anus, specially when the ejected blood shows signs of degeneration.

Terebinthina is extremely serviceable in those desperate cases of typhoid fevers where there is a tendency towards hemorrhage. It aborts the danger, removes the tympanites and relieves most of the nervous tension and urinary complications attending the trouble.

It is not possible to portray truly the enormous difficulty to which we, as medical men, are exposed at times. Face to face with a case of convulsion, eclampsia or hemorrhage, the physician feels the same, as the captain of a doomed ship, the play-thing of the mountainous waves, about to be snapped asunder any minute and penetrate to the bottom of the fathomless depth. It reminds me of such a case, that I had lately the misfortune to attend—a case that I lost and which might have been saved had I had the inspiration to prescribe **Terebinthina.** Many such vain compunctions and unavailing remorse might be avoided if we but think of studying our Materia Medica properly.

It has been used with signal success in peritonitis of the worst type following enteritis. Hering cured such a case of peritonitis with **Terebinth.** On the sixth day the patient had become pulseless cold and collapsed. The other symptoms on which the prescription was based, were great agitation of mind, fear of death, difficulty of breathing owing to a tympanitic condition of the abdomen which became enormous in size, not sensitive, but hard and resonant like a drum, and a dry tongue, which looked as if scalded with a hot iron in the center.

TEUCRIUM MARUM VARUM.

It is prepared from the Cat Thyme of the natural order of Labiatæ. The remedy was introduced and proved by Dr. Stapf. It is a remarkable medicine for helminthiasis and for mucous and fibroid growths. It vies with **Cina** and **Santonine** in the treatment of ascarides. We have many of the symptoms of **Cina** present in this remedy, as for example the sensation of crawling in the rectum after stool, itching and creeping in the anus as from ascarides, restlessness at night, excitement of mind, vivid and anxious dreams causing the patient to start, and sleeplessness on account of intense itching in the anus. We also have great emaciation in spite of voracious appetite.

Teucrium has always enjoyed a great reputation, amongst homœopaths, for being a first-rate remedy in the treatment of polypus—nasal, vaginal and recteal. We have a case on record, of a man suffering from nasal polypus, who had it removed yearly for thirty successive years. The roots had extended up to the ethmoid bone and into the antrum of Highmore. After a short course of treatment with **Teucrium** his breathing, which was usually obstructed, became quite free and the sense of smell which had been impaired for 20 years was restored, and for all practical purposes he was cured. Mucous polypus of the nose, as well as, fleshy polypus springing from nostrils or elsewhere when accompanied by a crawling sensation in the nose, stoppage of the nose and a sensation of formication and shooting at the root of the nose finds in **Teucrium** a ready help. The other symptoms are discharge of green scales and clinkers from nose and offensive smell from it. Smooth pedunculated pear-shaped polypus of the vagina, protruding outside, disappears under its influence.

Teucrium has a peculiar cough. It is associated with a mouldy taste in the mouth while hawking up the mucus. This may be considered a key-note symptom of the remedy.

Teucrium is also reputed to have cured hard fibrous growths on the inner side of the eyelids which prevented them from properly closing.

With time and experience, as we have further verifications of **Teucrium,** we will be able to arrive at the proper valuation of this remedy.

THEA.

This is our common Tea. The tea plant as seen under cultivation, is a shrub of two to five feet in height, although it may grow much bigger in the wild stage. It is a native of Asia. It has been in use in China for over thousand years and has become almost a necessity with the Chinese. We use it to a very great extent in India. It is also in use in Europe. Its principal ingredient is an essential oil, from $\frac{1}{2}$ to 1 per cent., and this is the source of its flavour and a good part of its exhilarating effect. It is on account of this essential oil that the tea relieves fatigue, stimulates thought, postpones sleepiness and cheers up the mind. It also contains Thein, from $1\frac{1}{2}$ to 3 per cent. Tannin, present in proportion from 12 to 17 per cent. is the third constituent. This Tannin is the least desirable part of the tea, and it is on account of this constituent that we find tea to be astringent. An infusion of tea when it is made for drinking purposes, should be done quickly, as it gives more fragrance and less bitterness and astringency. The following are some of the principal symptoms of **Thea**:

Nervous, restless, depressed, ill-tempered at about 5 P.M.; all-gone sinking sensation at the epigastrium; suicidal and homicidal mania; impulse to jump out of the window; delirium tremens; desire to cut her baby's throat and throw it downstairs, and talkativeness.

The above symptoms are all verified; hence they are reliable. A few more symptoms may be mentioned, but not being so useful as the foregoing we will abstain from discussing them.

THERIDION CURASSAVICUM.

In **Theridion**, we have another remedy prepared from the spider and hence it belongs to the natural order of Arachnida. It is commonly called the Orange-spider as it thrives mostly in the orange trees. It is found in the West Indies, chiefly in the island of Curacoa. It is usually of the size of a small cherrystone; when young, it is velvety black; the antero-posterior portion of the insect has numerous white pots on them. On the posterior portion of its body are to be seen three orange red spots; on the belly we have a large square yellow mark. It is a highly poisonous insect and should, therefore, be handled very carefully. The symptoms produced by its bite are mostly nervous in nature. It is no wonder, therefore, that **Theridion** should find application in many nervous ailments, such as hysteria, vertigo, nervous cough and irritation of the spinal cord. Before proceeding to deal with these complaints in detail, we will follow our usual practice of looking into the main characteristics of the remedy.

The most prominent trait of **Theridion** is to be seen in its hypersensitiveness to noise and to jar of all descriptions. In this respect, it excels all such remedies in our Materia Medica. Every shrill sound and reverberation penetrate through her entire body, particularly through her teeth and cause giddiness, nausea and sickness. The tearing of a piece of cloth, the sound of footsteps on the pavement, and the shrill whistle of a motor horn seem to jar on her and penetrate into her innermost nature causing a terrible revulsion of feeling. This is amply illustrated in the headache of the remedy which is brought on by the least noise or motion. It is located in the front of the head and it extends from behind the eyes into the occiput. This headache is also associated with weakness, trembling, coldness and anxiety. This sickish feeling is so prominent that it resembles very nearly a case of sea-sickness. It is particularly suitable to such headaches in women at the climacteric period.

The second characteristic of the remedy is to be found in the aggravation from the closing of the eyes. Almost all complaints, in which **Theridion** finds application are characterestised by this peculiar aggravation. Headache, vertigo, fainting, hysteria, morning sickness of pregnancy and toothache exhibit this modality of the drug. Although motion, as has been said before, aggravates to a certain extent, the aggravation is nothing compared to the inconvenience, worry and trouble brought on by the mere closing of the eyelids.

The symptoms leading to its application in hysteria are hilarity, talkativeness, a peculiar feeling as if her head did not belong to her and could be lifted up whenever necessary, luminous vibration in eyes, photophobia and double vision. The spine is in a state of intense irritability; the patient sits sideways in the chair to avoid pressure of the back of the chair against the spine.

It is particularly useful in phthisis florida. The patient complains of violent stitches in the chest beneath left shoulder and a sensation of pressure in œsophagus. Many cases are said to have been averted by the timely administration of **Theridion** in this fatal affliction. Dr. Baruch extolls **Theridion** highly and considers it almost indispensable in that disease. He assures us that it " effects a certain cure if given in the beginning of the disease." Such universal sweeping generalisation sounds unscientific and cannot be supported by the great dictum of Similia. If the patient, labouring under the burden of this dread affection, presents the characteristic indications of **Theridion,** undoubtedly **Theridion** will help and not otherwise. **Theridion** also presents a peculiar characteristic cough. He jerks his head forward and draws his knees up to his abdomen while coughing.

I have had the privilege of verifying one symptom of **Theridion**; with him time passes very slowly. In this respect it is like **Cocculus, Medor., Lac can.** and **Alumina. Argentum nit., Cannabis ind.,** and **Nux moschata** present the reverse symptom. Time with these remedies passes too quickly. From morning to evening they are in a state of constant hurry; they cannot finish their work quick enough.

THLASPI BURSA PASTORIS.

It is an annual plant, growing particularly in Europe. It is also called Shepherd's Purse and it belongs to the natural order of Cruciferæ. The tincture is prepared from the fresh flowering ·plant.

It is one of our great anti-hemorrhagic remedies and as such it deserves special attention and study. It has been, for centuries, a great home remedy in Europe not only for hemorrhage from any outlet of the body, but also for strangury and colic induced by renal calculi. Its effect is instantaneous and marvellous and many a time it renders us yeoman's service, when prescribed on proper Hahnemannian indications. Firstly we will discuss its bearing with respect to hemorrhage. The hemorrhage of **Thlaspi** is mostly to be found in connection with the uterine organs. It may be used both in menorrhagia and metrorrhagia. The peculiar feature of its hæmorrhage is to be seen in the fact that it usually starts very slowly and it gradually grows worse and worse, till the patient is almost ex-sanguinated. On the first day she hardly gets a show; on the second day the slight show turns into a hemorrhage with severe colic, vomiting and expulsion of clots. The flow usually continues long leaving the patient in a state of exhaustion from which she has hardly any time to recover before the next period starts. Very often this hemorrhage is consequent on abortion, and is usually to be seen at the critical age. Such hemorrhage coming particularly at this stage of life, forbodes at times a fatal malady in the shape of cancer of the cervix of uteri. **Thlaspi** often rectifies such conditions and averts the catastrophy. The blood of **Thlaspi** is usually dark and clotted. It is used also in too frequent and copious menstruation in women of relaxed constitutions.

It is an excellent remedy in copious discharge of urinary sand, particularly when the sediment is of brick-dust color. This brings **Thlaspi** very close to **Lycopodium**. Dudgeon cured a lady of muscular pain in various parts of her body that baffled many physicians with **Thlaspi**. He was led to this remedy by the most abundant secretion of coarse sand which formed a thick layer at the bottom of the utensil. **Thlaspi** diminished the sand in a marvellously short time and cured her of a very long-standing complaint to which she had become virtually reconciled as being beyond medical aid.

THUJA OCCIDENTALIS.

It is also called Arbor Vitæ, which means the tree of life. It belongs to the natural order of Coniferæ. This is a north American tree growing abundantly in Canada and the Northern States. It is an ever-green tree with spreading and graceful branches often growing to a height of 40 to 50 feet. It thrives in swampy spots and it assumes a conical form. It is therefore cultivated in gardens as ornamental trees. It contains 1% of a volatile oil, tannic acid and a minute amount of glucoside called thujin.

The Allopaths have very little use for this plant which they consider merely as an astringent, diuretic and expectorant. It is in the hands of Homœopaths alone that most of its intrinsic, life-saving and life-prolonging properties have been unfolded and it has truly become what its name signifies, a real tree of life. The leaves are small and imbricate and are borne on flattened branches which are easily mistaken for the leaves. The leaves give an aromatic odor.

This is truly a monument of Hahnemann's sagacity who was first led to its use by observing a sort of a grayish purulent discharge from the urethra of a theological student who had chewed a few leaves. Thus according to our dictum of Similia, it, makes an important remedial agent in gonorrhœa. We use it when the discharge is thin and greenish and is accompanied with a scalding pain during urination. The urethra is swollen, as a result of which there is always a retention of a few drops of urine which ooze out and soil his cloth some time after the urination is finished. It is oftener indicated in the after-effects of maltreated or suppressed gonorrhœa. Gouty and rheumatic symptoms are to be found abundantly in these patients, as a result of such suppression. Prostatitis, impotence and condylomatous growths are to be seen everywhere. The penis is disfigured by the appearance of these warty excrescences which look like fig-warts. They are present in the inner surface of the prepuce as well as in the point of penis below corona glandis. These warty growths discharge a sort of a viscid fluid, of which the stench is unbearable. They say it smells like old cheese or herring brine. The patient also complains of erosions and rawness between legs and on sides of the scrotum, from which there is always a constant oozing of moisture. This emits a strong sweetish honey-like smell and stains the linen yellow. In women these warts and excrescences, appear about the vulva. They render the parts extremely sensitive. The region, however, where these growths are most frequent is the anus. There. is often such a collection of them at this part that the passage almost gets obliterated rendering the passage of stool almost impossible. These growths generally indicate syphilitic taint. We use it in hæmorrhoids when they are complicated with fissured anus and condylomatous excrescences. As has been mentioned before, the parts are extremely sensitive and on account of pain the patient has to desist while having a stool.

The action of **Thuja** on the human constitution is that of unlimited cell-proliferation and it is on account of this property, that we meet with such a lot of pathological vegetative growths, spongy tumours, and many other varieties of morbid manifestations. It is said to have a strong action over the lymphatic secretions. It also acts very strongly over the nervous system causing disturbance of circulation, which leads to sensations of ebullition and pulsations all over the body, particularly in the præcordial region.

The patient's mental condition is strongly indicative of his deranged nervous state. He is constantly in a hurry. When he talks, he talks in a rush. His movements are hurried and impatient. We also meet with extreme nervousness in this patient. The slightest disturbance puts him off his balance. The merest approach of a stranger sets him on his edges; when spoken to, he answers with tears and sobs. In reading or writing he uses wrong expression and gives one the impression of approaching mental derangement. It is one of our principal remedies for fixed ideas. He is subject to all sorts of insane ideas. **Thuja** is reputed to have set many such patients right. It establishes the lost equilibrium and we find the patient reverting to his normal ways of thoughts and actions. As an instance of his mental aberration we may say that he feels as if a strange person were at his side; as if soul and body were separated; as if his body were made of glass and that he would break readily; as if a living animal were in his abdomen; as if legs were made of woods; as if his lower limbs were elongated. Like **Anacardium** he is subject to a sense of dual personality. He feels that he is under the control of a superior power from which he cannot break away, and that he is bound hand and foot. As a rule this patient is extremely quarrelsome and he gets easily angered about trifles. Loathing of life, depression of spirits, sleeplessness, and dissatisfaction are distinctly marked over his entire feature. He shuns everybody. At times he exhibits a sort of suicidal mania. He attempts to jump out of the window and put an end to his existence. A sort of indifference like what is found in **Sepia** and **Lilium** takes possession of **Thuja.**

Thuja has a peculiar headache in which the patient has a sensation as though a nail were being driven in the vertex or the frontal eminences. Sometimes it is described as that of a pressure by a convex button in one of the aforementioned parts. The headache is always worse from sexual excesses and at night and is distinctly relieved by exercise in open air, looking upward, and turning the head backward. It must be distinctly remembered that there is, in almost every case, where **Thuja** is indicated, a substrata of sycotic or syphilitic history.

We use it in neuralgia as well when the pain is intense and of stabbing character. It seems to begin somewhere in the region of the malar bone and shoots into the head. The pain is worse from sitting—the patient mostly maintaining a horizontal position. The pain of **Thuja** is almost relieved by wrapping up. Another strange thing about this pain of **Thuja** is that it is accompanied by frequent micturition. Whatever may be the location of this pain, particularly when the pain is most intense the patient passes urine very frequently.

From what has been already said, it is naturally to be expected that **Thuja** will make an important remedy in keratitis, syphilitic iritis and ophthalmia. There is, as has been repeatedly mentioned, a syphilitic or a sycotic history. Great photophobia is always present. When cases become chronic and inspite of the utmost care, do not respond to treatment, when the discharge becomes purulent and eyelids agglutinate, when fungus tumours make their appearance in orbit, when styes and tarsal tumours complicate the case, we cannot do any better than prescribe **Thuja** which is a deep-acting and miasmatic remedy.

It should be particularly remembered that **Thuja** is not only a remedy for small-pox but is a prophylactic as well. Applied during suppurative stage it prevents pitting. In the epidemic of 1849 when it was used extensively, it shortened all cases and prevented scars in most cases where it was employed. We also use it to counteract the bad effects of vaccination. Vaccination, though getting into fashion daily, is not devoid of dangers and after-effects. It will be folly indeed to condemn it wholesale, though cases have been known where its application was found to be fraught with dangers. In some people vaccination leaves deep-seated and long-lasting after-effects and that is exactly where **Thuja** comes in, in its capacity of a great counter-agent of vaccination.

Dr. Burnett mentions of an interesting case of an infant almost in the throes of death. The child was in a state of collapse. The only thing to account for this condition was that the wet-nurse whose services were only recently requisitioned, was vaccinated the day before she took charge of the patient and through whose milk the child was imbibing the vaccinal poison. **Thuja 6,** given both to the nurse and the child restored the child to his usual health and dried up the vaccinal vesicles on the nurse's arm.

Thuja has important action on teeth and gums. These are undoubtedly the best and the most reliable index of the human system and it is on these that we find **Thuja** exercising its lasting effect. The teeth decay at roots though the crowns are found to remain in tact. They turn yellow and crumble to pieces. The toothache is always worse in cold or warm room. Like **Belladonna** the pains come suddenly and go as suddenly. The taste of the mouth is sometimes sweet but generally it is like that of rotten eggs. The patient shows great dislike to fresh meat and potatoes. We use **Thuja** to counteract the bad effect of beer, fat, acids, tea, wine and onions.

I have always found **Thuja** a very useful remedy in cases of persistent indigestion and loose bowels. The most important symptoms of the remedy, are distention of the abdomen with flatus and great rumbling, croaking and grumbling noise in the abdomen. The movement of flatus, which gives rise to this peculiar noise, so great as to resemble the quickening of a child in the gravid uterus. The abdomen protrudes here and there from flatus as though something alive were moving inside. In this connection I would speak of a case of morning diarrhœa in one of my assistants which baffled me for a long time. The stools were very urgent. As natural I prescribed **Aloes, Podophyllum** and **Sulphur** but none of them did the least good. My attention was then directed to **Thuja** one day, when, while sitting near me, I could hear sound resembling the pouring of water, from an airtight vessel, in his abdomen. A couple of doses of **Thuja 200** produced the most marvellous effect. The diarrhœa of **Thuja** starts early in the morning after the patient had partaken of a breakfast. The stools are watery, painless and they stream out with much gas. They are generally brown and offensive and the feeling in rectum is that of boiling lead passing through it. Vaccination is frequently at the

oot of this trouble. The anus smarts and burns all day after the
morning diarrhœa. In **Thuja** as in **Laurocerasus** we have drinks
olling into the stomach quite audibly.

Its action on the bladder is somewhat like that of **Nat. mur.**
There is paralysis of the sphincter muscles of the bladder, in consequence of which we have incontinence of urine. The urine spurts
ut while laughing, coughing and sneezing. Another characteristic
vorth remembering is the suddenness of the desire for urination;
when this happens he finds it difficult to retain urine even for a
moment. He runs to the vessel, grasping at his penis and even
hen fails in retaining it. When however he is compelled or when
e makes up his mind, the ability to retain urine is not found
vanting.

The cough of **Thuja** is peculiar inasmuch as it comes on during
he day. It hardly troubles at the night time. It is excited by a
hoking sensation, and is followed by an expectoration of yellow
r green lumps. Sometimes this cough is aggravated after eating.
t is also recommended in asthma of sycotic children.

We will close with a few observations on the skin symptoms
f this remedy. The unhealthiness of **Silicea** and **Hepar sulphur** is
een in an aggravated form in **Thuja.** Moist tubercles, blood boils,
leeding fungus growths, warts, condylomata, pemphigus, impetigo,
hingles, ringworm and other varieties of deadlier cutaneous dis-
rders come within its domain. The skin has a dirty look with
irty brownish discolorations. Another characteristic of **Thuja** is
network of fine capillaries, visible like the veining of a piece of
aarble. The nails too crumble as they are very brittle. They
re absolutely devoid of moisture and of the healthy glow to be
een normally. Like **Silicea** it is a great remedy for ingrowing
e-nails. **Thuja** sweats a great deal but only on uncovered parts,
e covered parts generally remaining dry and hot. We also notice
etid sweat on toes and the genitals.

Case 1.—(Fungus on the lower Jaw.) On December 27 last, Mrs. K.
ought to me her daughter, aged ten, apparently a blooming girl. The
other informed me that her daughter was in the habit of exchanging chewing-
m with the girls of the place, and attributed to this the fact that she now
d something in her left lower jaw, the location being that of the first
olar tooth. The other physicians to whom application had been made
formed her that the tumor or fungus must be cut out with a piece of the
wer jaw bone. Before permitting this disfigurement she decided to try
e. The fungus looked **purplish, bled easily** and had a **stem.** The father
the child I knew to be sycotic, if not more; the mother, on the contrary,

was a woman of fine frame and health, having borne several children. The fungus became more **angry** in **damp weather.** In addition to this, the girl had an eruption like "Zoster around the abdomen." Appetite good, sleeps well, and only fears cutting. Prescribed **Thuja** 6 dec., one dose, morning and night. From this time on the girl improved, and the size of the dose was gradually lessened, till about the middle of February. At this time the mother thought that a little cauterization would accelerate the cure. In order that she might be convinced of her error, I applied **Potassa Caustica.** Like manure to a wheat field, the fungus grew again. From this time to March 20 she never interfered with **Thuja,** which was given about three times a week. Now the fungus or tumor is entirely well; it left a very slight carious exfoliation of the jaw, but it went off after two or three doses of **Silic. 30 trit.** The child is now perfectly well.—Dr. T. Meurer.

Case 2.—September 28, 1876, a gentleman called at my office, whose wife suffered from intense headache. The pains are so severe, that she screams constantly and keeps the whole house awake. She nearly loses her consciousness and is unable to speak. Aggravation of the pains and vomiting when rising up. Rest and horizontol position bring some relief, although the paroxysm is at its height about midnight. Another peculiarity is that the pain prevents the eyes from closing, and thus she had nearly passed two weeks with hardly any sleep, and the few snatches of sleep failed to refresh her. She felt weak and exhausted, especially as she is also troubled with habitual excessive menstruation, appearing too often and lasting too long. Although only twenty-five years of age, she has already passed through five puerperiæ. Thus there is a state of anæmia with its consecutive painful nervous affections. The present attack of headache began with great debility and lassitude, so that she had to go to bed. During the first week the neuralgia was bearable, but steadily increased during the second week. The forehead, the region of the eyes and ears, felt as if stabbed with knives or, as she said, as if knives went tearing round in her brain. She also complained of being chilly. She wanted to be covered up, as her feet and knees felt cold. After short intervals the pain always increased. There was no thirst, but nausea and vomiting when rising up and frequent eructations. Palpitations were frequently complained of. Prescribed **Thuja** 100. Cured —(Dr. Goullon, Jr. Hirschel's Klinik, iii., 1871. Lilienthal's translation).

THYROIDINUM.

This is one more of our rare remedies but as some nice cures are attributed to it, we think it will not be labor thrown away to have a short discussion on it. It is a sarcode. This remedy may be prepared either from the dried triturated thyroid gland of the sheep or calf or from an extract made from it. As homœopaths we use the potentised form instead of the crude drug. To be able to arrive at a proper understanding of its symptomatology we will consider the physiology of the gland. Its function is nutritive. Hyperthyroidism therefore causes acceleration of metabolism and athyroidism on the other hand favours retardation of the same. In the first, we notice a gradual decrease in the weight of the patient, irritability and palpitation. In the latter condition the process of body building comes to a stand still. The tissues stay in their embryonic condition and the result is the arrest of development of bones, soft parts, as also psychic and samatic impairments. The administration of thyroid gland in large doses accelerates proteid and fat metabolism and causes increased elimination of nitrogen, phosphorus chlorine, etc. Clinically polyuria, sweating, tachycardia, tremor, emaciation and glycosuria are observed. The removal of the thyreoid gland on the other hand leads to anæmia, oligæmia, myxœdema, cretinism and obesity.

Thyroidin. has a very strong action over the heart. It produces palpitation and if the dose is excessive it may bring on a fatal weakness of the organ. Syncope and cyanosis are some of the evil consequences of the abuse of this drug. There is close relation between thyroid gland and the reproductive organ as is shown by the enlargement of the gland during pregnancy and menstruation. The hyperplasia of the thyroid gland during pregnancy is a physiological necessity as it provides for the duel metabolism of the mother and the infant. Those cases of pregnancy where such hyperplasia is not seen, end in convulsion, coma and other vital ailments of like nature.

We may regard puffiness, obesity, rapid pulse, it che, nausea, weakness and anæmia, characteristic symptoms of **Thyroidin.** Dr. Clarke speaks of a case of hystero-epilepsy, that he permanently cured with the 3x potency of **Thyroidin.**, given thrice daily. Her eyeballs were prominent, heart-sound feeble and pulse 120. She found it difficult to lie down as such actions distinctly brought on palpitation. Her thyroid gland was very slightly enlarged. **Thyroidin** not only cured the epilepsy but also removed the characteristic prominence of the eyeballs. He also mentions a case of diabetes that responded to the action of the 3x and the 30th potency of **Thyroidin.**

With thyroid feeding H. O. Nicholson is said to have stopped convulsions during pregnancy.

Thyroidin acts as a galactagogue. It is especially indicated when the deficiency of milk is associated with a return of the menses. **Thyroidin** suppresses the latter and increases and enriches the milk.

Thyroidin has been used with benefit in some cases of myxœdema. Some amount of mental aberration, common in these cases, was removed by it. In one case the patient was homicidal. She wanted to strangle everybody by putting her arms very tightly round their necks. The opinion amongst medical men seems to be that **Thyroidin** is useful in melancholia, mania, delusional insanity, insanity of adolescence, climacterium and puerperium precisely when these cases are associated with some derangement of the thyroid gland. Simple parenchymatous form of goitre often yields to thyroid treatment and it is said young people are more often helped with it than old people. The remedy must be continued long to effect a cure. The principle simply is the substitution of the physiological want.

Thyroid feeding has been very frequently resorted to in obesity but this is a process very often fraught with danger. A loss of fat undoubtedly can be brought about rather in anæmic patients than in real plethora but this fat consumption is accompanied by certain amount of proteid assimilation. As obesity is frequently complicated with cardiac disorders, gout, diabetes, kidney lesions, etc., thyroid therapy becomes a positive danger when so applied.

This drug is contra-indicated in tubercular patients for it may most likely bring about further reduction of weight.

It must be admitted however that our experience with this drug has been very limited and that most of the symptoms mentioned in these pages have been derived from Allopathic literature. This remedy needs further proving and more genuine verifications.

TILIA EUROPŒA.

The tincture is prepared from the fresh blossoms of the common lime. It belongs to the natural order of Tiliaceæ.

This is comparatively a new remedy but it can boast of a few characteristic indications, one of which is an intense sore feeling about the abdomen. The whole abdomen feels painful when touched, specially about navel. It is so intense as to give one idea of sub-cutaneous ulceration of that part of the abdomen. This symptom had led to its successful application in peritonitis. The second important indication is the hot sweat, a symptom found under very few remedies. The third and the most important characteristic symptom is the peculiar bearing down sensation felt in the genito-urinary and rectal regions. It is more like a feeling of pressure in that neighbourhood giving rise to the sensation that the uterus is being pressed out of the pelvis. This last-named symptom brings it under the category of **Sepia, Lil. tig.**, **Bell.** and **Platina.**

Another symptom worth recording is a sensation of a veil before the eyes. She feels as if there is a veil of gauze spread before the field of her vision.

TRILLIUM PENDULUM.

Another name for this plant is Birthroot, which sufficiently testifies to its property of being a great hæmostat. This remedy, too, has not been proved sufficiently, but there is hardly any doubt as to its capacity in checking hæmorrhage, be it from nose, kidney, uterus or any other organ. The hæmorrhage may be either active or passive although usually it is bright-red. It has been used with great success in all kinds of hæmorrhage—anti-partum, post-partum and climacteric. It has been used with equal success in hæmorrhage due to fibroid tumours. It, therefore, occupies as great a place amongst hæmorrhagic remedies, as **Acon.**, **Arnica**, **Bell.**, **China**, **Erigeron**, **Hama.**, **Ipec.**, **Millef.**, **Sabina**, **Sang.**, and **Secale**.

The most important characteristic of the **Trillium** hæmorrhage is the association of faintness at the stomach with the bleeding. It has been recommended both in metrorrhagia and menorrhagia. The blood is bright-red in colour and it comes out in gushes at the least movement. The patient is pale, weak, anemic and anxious.

TROMBIDIUM.

Trombidium is prepared from a parasite found upon the common housefly. It is of a bright-red colour. The provings were made under the supervision of Dr. Hering. It is an invaluable remedy with us for the treatment of diarrhœa and dysentery. Its grand key-note is aggravation after eating and drinking. The stools are generally thin, brown and fecal. Crampy pain before, during and after stools are quite characteristic of this remedy. Great tenesmus, prolapsus ani, and burning in the anus, are important landmark of **Tromb.** The stools are generally expelled with great force. They occur generally after dinner or supper; there is hardly any evacuation after breakfast.

An interesting case is on record, in the "Guiding Symptoms," of a man of full habit, slightly disposed to congestion of the liver, who persistently suffered from a peculiar diarrhœa after his dinner at 5 P.M. The dinner was immediately followed by a violent pain in the intestine, which kept on increasing until he had to seek relief in stool; they were sudden and passed with flatus and great tenesmus. The pains did not subside until he had three or four similar passages, when he ceased to suffer till he dined again the next day. Various remedies were tried but they proved ineffectual till **Tromb.** relieved him permanently. Of course, a similar aggravation is to be seen in **Aloes, Apis, Argent. nit., Arsen., China, Colocyn., Crot. tig., Ferrum met., Gamb., Lycop., Kali phos.** and **Nat. sulp.,** but a proper differentiation between them all is not a difficult matter.

In **Aloes** the want of confidence in the sphincter ani, the early morning diarrhœa driving one out of bed, the aggravation in hot-damp weather, the feeling of fullness and weight in the pelvis, the jelly-like mucus looking like frog-spawn, the rumbling in the abdomen, the desire for juicy things, and the simultaneous escape of stool and urine should easily enable us to pick it out of a whole host of other apparently similar remedies.

Apis mel. is indicated mostly in painless diarrhœa. The stools are involuntary, same as in **Aloes.,** oozing out constantly from the half-open anus. Gradual increasing prostration, smarting and rawness of the anus, sensitiveness of the abdominal wall, history of suppressed exanthemata, and thirstlessness are symptoms that would help us out of many a dilema.

In **Argent. nit.,** although the aggravation is the same as in **Tromb.,** we have the additional feature of stools coming after excitement. It is more or less a nervous diarrhœa and is usually caused by excessive indulgence in sugar and sweets. The nocturnal aggravation, the greenish slimy bloody stool, the deep sighing and breathing are reliable indications of **Argent. nit.**

Arsen. has the aggravation after meals in a marked degree but this remedy is generally indicated in cases where we have grave reasons to be anxious and worried—the case being one of serious nature, as is manifested by a rapid dissolution, sudden loss of strength, anguish, putridity of the evacuation and the peculiar blackish stools, which really mean internal hæmorrhage and rapid disintegration. We also use **Arsen.** in diarrhœa due to septic conditions, same as **Carb. veg., Crotal. hor., Lach., Pyrogen** and **Sulph.**

China is particularly useful in diarrhœa after meals. It is painless and mostly nocturnal. We think of it particularly in diarrhœa caused by eating fruits. Trembling, debility, fermentation in the bowels and the presence of undigested particles of food in the white papescent stool are factors favouring the administration of **China.**

Colocynth can be easily differentiated by the presence of intense colic, amelioration from pressure and the aggravation from emotional excitement.

Crot. tig. is usually indicated in acute cases; the stools are copious, yellow, watery and they come out forcibly. Although we have the aggravation from eating and drinking, same as in **Tromb.,** we must not forget the amelioration of this remedy from warm water. The most guiding of all symptoms is the aggravation from movements. The slightest movement of the body renews fresh desire for stools.

In **Ferrum met.,** the patient can hardly wait till the meal is finished. It is almost simultaneous with eating and drinking. The stools are undigested and mostly nocturnal. It is generally indicated in chronic cases where the evacuations are mostly painless and where the diarrhœa is sort of a precursor to some other impending disease, such as phthisis etc.

Gambog. is particularly indicated in diarrhœa of old people; the urging is excessive and the stools are expelled all at once with considerable force followed by a feeling of general relief.

Lycop. has chilliness in the rectum before stools. Constant sensation of satiety, fermentation in the abdomen, and an aversion to warm boiled food, meat, coffee and smoking are characteristic indications of **Lycopodium.**

Kali phos. is usually indicated in white putrid diarrhœa with adynamic conditions. The breath is extremely offensive.

Nat. sulph. is usually indicated in chronic diarrhœa when it starts some little time after the patient has risen from bed in the morning and after he has moved about a little. **Nat. sulph.** is thus very different from **Sulph.** where the urging drives the patient out of bed long before it is time for him to leave his bed.

TUBERCULINUM.

Another name of this remedy is **Bacillinum.** The medicine is prepared from a pure cultivation of Tubercle Bacilli found in tubercular abscesses. It is therefore a nosode. We are much indebted to Drs. Burnett and Swan for many of its symptoms are their verifications. This remedy is prescribed both on indicated symptoms and on constitutional basis. It is difficult to state which is the correct procedure. Numerous cures are claimed for **Tuberculinum** on both these theories. I feel sure it will be better to combine the two. It is generally adapted to persons of light complexion, and blue eyes. They are tall, slim, stoop-shouldered and flat-chested. Mentally precocious, they are very weak physically, and disposed to catch everything that is in the air. Its three main characteristics are:

Firstly—Changeability of symptoms; no symptom lasts for any appreciable time. Symptoms go through rapid kaleidoscopic transformations. We do not know why it is so; perhaps the miasmatic diathesis may explain this phenomena—but as we are concerned with facts only we will do well to go on with the symptomatology of **Tuberculinum.**

Secondly—A great sensitiveness to cold. In spite of every precaution taken, they keep on getting a fresh cold without knowing how or where.

Thirdly—A pronounced and rapid emaciation; they keep on constantly loosing flesh although the best of nourishments are being taken.

Mentally, though naturally of a sweet disposition, they turn taciturn, sulky, snappish, fretful and irritable. They are given to constant whining and complaining. Glands are indurated everywhere. Crops of boils, intensely painful, keep on appearing successively in different parts of the body, specially on the nose. The pus discharged is generally greenish and fetid. The skin is very unhealthy; eczema mostly tubercular, covers the entire body; itching is most intense and unbearable at night when undressing; eruptions behind the ears, in the hair, in the folds of the skins and axilla and in the groins, render him an unsightly object. Huge quantities of white band-like scales are shed. It is very similar to **Sulph.** and it is difficult to distinguish between these two remedies as far as the skin symptoms are concerned. A persistent summer diarrhœa, excessive night sweats, rapid emaciation, a hideous hacking cough, an easily detachable nonviscid expectoration, flush of cheeks, shortness of breath, moist rales in lungs, an increased vocal resonance, pronounced endocardial bruit, strawberry tongue, anemia and a constant harassing fever, are symptoms that clearly point to one ailment and that is tuberculosis. A few doses of **Tuber.** aptly prescribed at the initial stage, have been known to have averted the dreaded catastrophy.

This remedy is indicated for a very severe type of headache. The intensity of the pain is so great that the patient becomes almost unconscious with it. He becomes like a maniac. He screams, tears at his hair, and hits his head with his fist and tries to dash it against the wall or the floor. Dr. Swan reports of having cured with it a headache of 45 years' standing. This headache used to begin at the right frontal protuberance and extended gradually to the right occipital region. It is also used for school girls' headache—a headache that is always worse after study and even slight mental exertion.

I have used **Tuberculinum** in morning diarrhœa where the attacks are sudden and imperative, after failure of **Sulph.** The stools are dark, brown, watery and offensive. They are discharged with great force.

Dr. Burnett has averted several cases of threatened and incipient phthisis with **Tuberculinum** and I am sure with the judicious application of **Tuberculinum** other homœopaths will be able to do the same.

Not only tuberculosis but various other complaints have been helped by **Tuber.** The following cases are very instructive as well as interesting and will enable us to form a proper conception of the deep-acting nature of this remedy.

Case 1.—A case of cancer of the breast, so diagnosed by best allopathic authority in Boston; no history of grief or traumatism. The most peculiar symptoms about it were the tubercular nodules in the gland which looked like a superficial string extending to the axilla. Previously had suffered from severe headaches: since the growths appeared, headaches ceased. The nipple was retracted. On account of the tubercular character of the growth, the history of former headaches, which were similar to those of **Tuberculinum**, I gave the patient one dose of the remedy. In 48 hours, burning, lancinating pain began in the growths; had previously suffered from burning pain which was palliated by sedatives. The burning, lancinating pain continued two or three days, then gradually disappeared. The retraction of nipple was less marked, the tubercles softened, the pains disappeared and general health promptly improved.—Dr. Allen.

Case 2.—In September, 1905, I was called to see a little Irish girl, named Mary Gilbert, ten years of age, who was suffering with what I thought was an attack of pneumonia. The temperature was 104°, and there was a dry cough with severe pain in the chest. I treated her with the usual remedies, viz., **Belladonna, Bryonia,** etc., with only an apparent amelioration of symptoms. But the child lost flesh and seemed to develop an empyema. About the third week there was a profuse discharge of foul smelling pus-like matter, greenish in colour, from the mouth.

Dr. Pugh, who had attended the mother a year previously, in pneumonia, of which she died, was called in consultation; he made a careful examination and left the following note.

"I think you are completely right. She has I think some empyema on right side (not much), but she has pulmonary tuberculosis of both lungs. I doubt that the hospital would do any good."

I had thought of sending her to the hospital as she had the poorest of care at home; but the doctor said it was of no use, nothing could save her. I quite agreed with him, but bethought myself of **Tuberculinum.** Here was a chance to try it, surely it could do her no harm. She was given a number of doses of the 200, and later higher potencies till I reached the cm., and with continual improvement. The cough diminished, the hectic spots left her cheeks after a number of weeks, but before the real spring came she was a plump and rosy child. All this, too, in a cold, bad winter and with the most insanitary surroundings.—Dr. Allen.

Case 3.—Howard L., 28 years of age, a resident of Attleboro, Mass., was indisposed in the fall of 1898, troubled with hoarseness and gastric ailments. A neighbouring physician was called who had attended the young man's family for many years. This physician commenced in September, 1898, to inject Tuberculin (Koch's), and up to December had injected his toxin twice a week for several weeks, and then once in two weeks the remainder of the time.

And what was the result? At the time of the commencement of this treatment Mr. L. could work and eat comfortably; soon his stomach rebelled against food and the bowels became constipated, his hoarseness increased and distressing, suffocative spells set in every forenoon, lasting an hour or so; he would then be able to breathe well the rest of the day.

In January, 1899, I was summoned hastily in the night and found him labouring for breath, the noise of his breathing audible from the street. His

first words were; "My God, help me; relieve me, Doctor, or I shall die."
Expectoration was scanty, dark green and lumpy. Examination of the throat
revealed a larynx full of tubercular nodes. I saw that his end was near, and
told his parents with whom he lived that they would rather call their family
physician. But as they insisted on my keeping the case, I prepared some
medicine which relieved him, but the next morning he was again worse, and
from that time onward was in agony from his efforts to get breath. To
relieve him, intubation (through the mouth) was resorted to, but he could
not keep the tube in. He died that afternoon, his great agony being ameliorated only by resort to chloroform applied locally. This man had been wild
in his youth, had had gonorrhœa several times, and was of tubercular diathesis.
I asked him if he had told his former physician these things and he said he
had. This case is typical as far as the use of **Tuberculinum** by injection is
concerned, of a score I could mention who have died under the hypodermic
use of **Tuberculinum** in this vicinity the past two years.—Dr. Allen.

Case 4.—A boy aged 13 had diphtheria with fearful headache extending
from neck to vertex, with swelling in back of neck and occiput, due, it was
supposed, to an affection of the middle ear. Seven weeks passed without
improvement. Paracenthesis of the tympanum resulted in the evacuation of
pus for a day or two. At this stage Dr. Nobel was called in, who found
the patient's face bloated and his strawberry tongue coated white at the
root; mastoids were not sensitive to even strong pressure. Swelling of occiput and neck down to fifth dorsal vertebra was prominent. If the boy wanted
to move his head he had to seize it with both hands and turn it slowly, with
painful distortion of facial muscles, until it reached the position desired.
Even the slightest pressure on first, second, or third cervical vertebra was
painful; the skin on them was reddened and the periosteum was swollen;
the glands in the neck were enlarged. Tuberculosis of atlas and second and
third vertebræ, consequent on diphtheria, was the diagnoses. **Tuberculinum**
m., was given, five grains, during the day. Two days after the dose the boy
could move his head more freely, the swelling of the neck diminished, appetite
returned, and in a short time he was able to get up and run about. Five
weeks after the dose, the swelling had altogether gone, and the boy's condition was altogether changed.

URANIUM NITRICUM.

Uranium nitricum is a salt prepared from the Pitch Blande. It is also found in combination with lead and silver in the mines of Bohemia, Saxony, Bavaria, and France. Although it is a remedy of small repute, we cannot possibly leave it out of our Materia Medica. Its chief action is marked over the kidneys. We are indebted for our knowledge of this remedy to doctors Hale and Blake. Their attention was drawn to it by certain experiments of Leconte, a French Psychologist of note, who poisoned some dogs with it. The urine of these poisoned animals showed traces of sugar. This led to further experiments and verifications and they have served to establish its utility and efficacy in controlling both diabetes mellitus and insipidus. The kind of diabetes in which it is specially successful in hepatogenic. The symptoms generally are great languor, debility, cold feeling, vertigo, profuse urination, complete loss of sexual power, dryness of the mouth, tenacious salivation, coated tongue and great thirst. Many cases of diabetes have been relieved and cured by **Uranium nitricum.** Dr. Clarke testifies to its usefulness and cites an instance of a case of diabetes insipidus in a young girl, where **Uranium nitricum** in the 30th potency gave greater relief than any other remedy he had used. He considers excessive thirst, polyuria and dry tongue the guiding keynotes of this remedy.

Uranium is also useful in gastric and duodenal ulcerations. The symptoms calling for it are, boring pain in the pyloric region, sinking at epigastrium, eructations, gnawing sinking feeling at the cardiac end of the stomach a short while after dinner and recurring hematemesis. These are grave symptoms but they are invariably relieved by **Uranium nitricum.** In **Uranium nitricum** threfore we have a splendid weapon to contend against the deadliest of maladies to which the human race is subject. It should be more extensively used by homœopaths all over the world and their successes and failures made known so that we can definitely launch out against a malady regarded as incurable and fatal.

Uranium nit. is extremely poisonous, acrid and should, therefore, be used with great deal of care and caution. Indiscriminate use of the low potency is likely to lead to serious consequences.

Case 1.—A corpulent man of temperate habits, gradually verging on old age, noticed progressive debility and emaciation. Gradually the sense of weariness in the lower extremities slowly resulted into œdema of the legs his tongue was coated with a thick white fur. A sensation of dryness of the mouth and fauces caused an intense thirst. This was followed by a secretion of an enormous quantity of urine of which the specific gravity was found to be 1044. The urine was found to be surcharged with sugar to the extent of 85 grains per litre. He was extremely dispirited and morose. His appearance became extremely haggard with the cheek bones showing prominently and dark rings appearing under the eyes. The case gradually progressed from bad to worse till it resulted in extreme anemia. There was hardly any trace of blood in his lips, tongue, ears and eyes. After **China, Acid phos.,** and **Laurocerasus** had failed, he was given **Uranium nitricum** in the 30th potency three times a day. In a short time the progress of the disease was arrested. The secretion of urine became normal. Sugar, albumen and casts disappeared, and the patient went back to his usual avocations of life and as far as I know he is alive up to the present moment.—Dr. N. M. Choudhuri.

UREA.

Urea, the chief nitrogenous constituent of urine, is the product of tissue metamorphosis. When the kidney fails to eliminate these waste products, uremic intoxication, delirium, coma and convulsions become the inevitable consequence. Naturally therefore, the homœopathic provings have brought out a series of important symptoms and it is our intention to discuss in this chapter a few characteristic symptoms of **Urea.**

Most of the symptoms of **Urea** have a special bearing on the kidney and the bladder. There is a strong urging to urination; this urging begins at the root of the penis. The urine is thin and is of low specific gravity. These symptoms lead to its application in albuminuria and diabetes. **Urea** also removes renal dropsy and general anasarca, and this is done by the increase in the quantity of urine secretion.

URINUM.

The dilution and the potentization of human urine give us our remedy of **Urinum.** From time immemorial in various countries and climes crude urine has been used for therapeutic purposes with various degrees of success. All sorts of claims have been propounded in its favour. It cannot be denied that like various other objects it has real remedial properties. Proving—regular systematic proving—is necessary to render its symptoms more definite, clear and scientific.

URTICA URENS.

Urtica urens is a remedy of a very ancient lineage. We find this remedy mentioned in the writings of Dioscorides, who extolled it very highly as a great cleansing agent. In our time Dr. Burnett has taken it up and given it a very extensive proving.

Urtica urens is prepared from the " stinging nettle." The fresh plant is utilized in making the tincture.

Dr. Burnett used **Urtica urens** in acute gout associated with fever. He, however, used it in five-drop-doses of the mother tincture in a glass of warm water, every two or three hours Under its influence, urine became free and plentiful and the patient made a steady progress until complete recovery ensued.

It is an excellent remedy for nettle rash. Great irritation of the skin was noticed in all the provers. It causes intense itching and burning of the skin with a sensation as if the part is scorched Red and raised blotches appear in different parts of the body and they are characterised by a constant desire to scratch. These blotches generally precede an attack of rheumatism. They are also periodical. They affect the patient every year at the same season. A great peculiarity about **Urtica urens** is that both the eruption and the itching disappear as soon as the patient lies down and reappears immediately on rising from the recumbent posture. The association of rheumatic pain and continued fever with nettle rash, already hinted at, is an important key-note symptom and has led to many wonderful cures. This remedy seems to have a special affinity for the deltoid muscles; we have used i successfully in rheumatism of the arm when the deltoid muscle is affected. The case of Dr. W. H. Procter is an instance in point He was seized with sudden pain in his right deltoid muscle and high fever. After hypodermic injection of morphia and atropia had failed, and the poor doctor had been in bed for over three weeks, not knowing how or where to get relief, he placed himself under the treatment of a Homœopath. The intense burning of the skin after sleeping, great dread of sleep which almost invariably entailed greater suffering, led to the prescription of **Urtica urens.** After three doses of it had been given, he fell into a restful sleep to awake free from all irritation.

Urtica urens is one of our best remedies for causing free flow of milk, when that has been impeded. It has been used re peatedly in insufficiency or entire want of milk secretion (agalactica) with almost astounding results.

Dr. Clarke, in his Dictionary, reports a case of a woman with a lump in her left breast of many years' duration, who after childbirth, was altogether lacking in milk secretion. She had severe pain in the whole of her right lower limbs, breasts, chest, sacrum and in the muscles of her neck. **Urtica urens** was given and after three doses the breasts were full of milk together with a general relief of all the pains in all her limbs.

It is used in pruritus valvæ with great stinging and itching and œdema of the parts. Dr. Nothingham's report of a cure, in a lady who had the most agonising eczema on the vulva is quite interesting. The itching and burning were indescribable. The labia had thickened considerably. There were innumerable fissures and a lot of dry scaly eruptions. **Urtica urens** removed all the local symptoms together with the indescribable sexual excitement induced by constant rubbing.

It is also used in burns of the first degree, when the integument and the subjacent tissues are not destroyed and when the injury is confined to the top-skin. This can be used both locally and internally.

It has also been highly extolled in stings of insects specially of the bee. In this **Urtica urens** resembles **Apis.** Some of the symptoms mentioned above have not been verified thoroughly. A more extensive use will lead to a better understanding and verifications of many of its symptoms.

USTILAGO MAIDIS.

This is a fungus that grows on the Indian corn; hence it is very similar to our remedy **Secale cornutum.** Many symptoms are common to both these remedies. The affinity between these two remedies, is more marked in their action on the female sexual system. It is also known by the names of Maize-smut and Corn-smut.

This fungus sometimes grows as large as an orange, often larger. It is covered over by a surface of dark, gray or brown epidermis. On ripening this epidermis bursts. We make triturations as well as tinctures from this fungus. In making the tinctures we add five parts by weight of alcohol to the powdered fungus. For the proving of this drug we are indebted to Dr. Burt of the United States.

As we have said a while ago, the most valuable symptoms of this fungus are to be found in its action on the female generative organs. It is a noted abortifacient. Dr. Burt administered two drachms of **Ustilago** to two pregnant bitch dogs and in both it caused abortion. Mention is also made of cows aborting fed on Indian corn infected with this parasite.

We use **Ustilago** for passive hemorrhage from retention of secundines after miscarriage. The blood that keeps oozing for days and weeks, is darkish and coagulated. The uterus itself is enlarged and the cervix tumified; the patient complains of a constant bearing-down pain. There is profuse discharge of blood from the enlarged uterus and the flow is accompanied by backache and sharp pain across the lower abdomen from hip to hip. This flow of blood is sometimes intermittent. It stops and then on slightest excitement reappears. Other similar remedies are, **Ambra gris. Bov.,** and **Calc. ost.,** and a brief differentiation will be to our advantage.

In **Ambra grisea,** we have the same intermittent flow. It is also similar to **Ustilago** that the hemorrhage that shows itself frequently between periods, is caused by the least bit of exertion. A short ride, a little cycling, a long walk, lifting of a light weight and going down-stairs or up-stairs a little oftener bring on a discharge of blood. This remedy is marked by a great varicose condition of the veins. During menses the left leg looks almost blue from distended varices. Itching of the pudenda, swelling of the labia, dyspnœa, palpitation and anguish are further indications of **Ambra grisea.**

In **Bovista,** another great remedy for menstrual irregularity, the blood shows itself between periods as with the former remedies, but the distinctive point is that the flow takes place mostly during night and towards morning when she is lying down. During day when she is on her feet and moving about, the flow is hardly present. In this remedy the menstrual discharge is always ushered in with diarrhœa. A puffy condition of the whole system is particularly characteristic of **Bovista.**

In **Calc. ost.** our fat and flabby patient, the period shows itself several times during the same month but in **Calc. ost.** it is due more to mental excitement than to over-exertion. A slight mental excitement as that caused by a little anger, grief, worry, anxiety, is sufficient to cause a show of the period.

Ustilago causes neuralgia of the testicles. The patient complains of a constant, aching distress in the testicles, more specially in the right. **Hamamelis** has a similar symptom. The pain is very severe, and it shifts suddenly to the bowels; the pain is accompanied by nausea and cold sweat on the scrotum. It is particularly useful in orchitis after gonorrhœa when the disease becomes chronic and the acuteness of the pain gives way to a feeling of soreness in the testicles. In this connexion we should not lose sight of **Oxalic acid** a remedy where the neuralgic pain in the spermatic cord becomes almost unbearable. The patient avoids all movement inasmuch as the pain becomes aggravated by the slightest motion.

The **Ustilago** patient suffers from frequent attacks of tonsillitis. The tonsils seem to be his weakest parts. They are congested and enlarged. The left tonsil is especially affected. It looks large and dusky and the pain on swallowing is intense. It is of a lancinating character and it extends from the tonsil to the ear. The throat is dry and there is the feeling of a lump behind the larynx which makes her swallow constantly.

There is one other feature of **Ustilago** that has so far escaped our notice and that is alopecia. We find a complete loss of hair under this remedy. Dr. Hurndall relates of a case of alopecia in a bitch dog that he cured with **Ustilago** 3x in five-drop-doses given three times a day. The symptoms which led to this prescription were her tendency to abort and the hemorrhage to which she was a frequent subject. His surprise knew no bounds when the above symptoms subsided and a perfect coating of hair sprang up in three months' time. We give below the indications of a few other remedies noted for loss of hair.

Aurum met. is applicable mostly to syphilitic patients.

Carb. veg. is useful when the trouble starts after severe disease, abuse of mercury and during parturition. The falling of the hair is most marked on the occiput.

Lycopodium is a great remedy for alopecia after abdominal diseases and after parturition. The scalp is full of eruptions and thick crusts, which itch and burn particularly after exercise which generates heat and warmth.

URVA URSI.

Uva ursi is prepared from the fresh leaves of the plant known as Beer-berry. Its application is very limited and its margin of utility very meagre; but still we cannot afford to leave it altogether out of our Materia Medica, for it has its own scope of action and within that scope, it is all important and all powerful. One single experience of mine, an experience that I am going to narrate just now, will prove the truth of the above statement. An old man, to be more precise, a man about to verge into old age, who looked sallow, emaciated, wane and œdematous came to me for relief. He was ailing, as he said for years and had every sort of treatment, but nothing brought him any relief. His trouble was located in his bladder. He had very frequent urination, and this left him hardly any time for rest. Even at night time he had to get up 3 or 4 times every hour to pass urine and each time it took him 10 to 15 minutes to finish, although the quantity of urine passed was very meagre. Urination was preceded by continued spasms of the bladder. Great straining, burning in the glans, depression of mood, and dribbling of urine were some of the other symptoms. The urine passed was muddy and foul-smelling, and there was always a great abundance of grey slimy sediment and a big quantity of membraneous flaky deposit. **Chimaphila, Cannabis indica, Canth.** and a few other remedies were tried, but none seemed to bring him any lasting relief. I was feeling quite disheartened, till at last my attention was directed to one symptom which had escaped my attention all along. After careful study of the symptom I was prompted to use **Uva ursi.** It was administered and the result more than surpassed my fondest expectation. Fully 75 per cent. of all his symptoms disappeared within 24 hours. The urination became free and less frequent. He kept on passing huge quantity of foul-smelling sediment but without much pain or hardship. Appetite returned, the wane sallow complexion disappeared till after few months he looked his ownself again. The symptom on which **Uva ursi** was prescribed, was the comparative ease with which urine was passed in a lying-down posture. I had seen him several times in all sorts of postures and attitudes, but it never struck me till the last that everytime he wanted to pass urine he had to lie down. Observation is a great thing in homœopathy. Its importance cannot be overrated. The physician, that watches everything and takes proper valuation of every symptom presented, is the one that will score in the long run.

VALERIANA.

This perennial herb, a native of Europe and Asia, is a familiar object in our gardens. Its important constituents are volatile oil, Valerianic acid and resin. It has a great intoxicating action on cats, who, as is natural everywhere, seem to have an irresistible craving for it. Animal nature is the same everywhere. The dominant spirit of refractoriness that prevailed and ultimately spoiled " The Garden of Eden," rules everywhere. Things that should not be done have more allurements and this seems to be the only explanation that we can produce, for this irresistible craving for **Valeriana** on the part of the cats.

Valeriana is generally indicated in patients that suffer from emotional unbalance, hysterical and nervous disturbance, headaches and other pains due to same nervous cause. " It calms the nervousness, abates the excitements of circulation, removes wakefulness, promotes sleep and induces a sensation of quiet and comfort."

It has a peculiar fetid odour due probably to the presence of Valerianic acid. In the days of Hahnemann it was largely used by the ladies of Germany, in the form of a decoction. Its use has since then been abandoned due to the fact of its being the cause of extreme nervousness in the ladies of that age. When we look at the long list of symptoms mostly of nervous origin caused by **Valeriana,** we do not wonder that it brought on emotional disturbances and hysterical symptoms in those that used to indulge in it.

Valeriana produces an exalted state of the sensorium. All the organs and senses are in a state of nervous excitement and over-sensitiveness. The vision becomes extremely acute. He seems to see even in darkness. His hearing too is in a state of hyperæsthesia. Slightest exertion causes violent headaches; slightest pain ushers in fainting.

Mentally those patients are very intellectual. Their brains are cramped with ideas and they pass from subject to subject with the greatest ease. They are hysterical, over-excitable and changeable. Hallucinations and delusions are plentiful. They frequently see figures of animals, men, etc. Erroneous ideas are very common. If the patient happens to be a woman she labours under the peculiar idea that she is some one else and removes to the edge of the bed to make room for herself. She imagines animals to be lying near her which she fears may hurt. The other peculiar sensations are—as if flying in the air; as if eyes would be pierced from within outward; as if smoke were in her eyes; as if a thread were hanging down throat; as if something forcing a passage through the pit of the stomach; as if suffocating on falling asleep; as if something warm were rising from stomach.

Restlessness of **Valeriana** is a very prominent feature. She cannot keep still for long. She is in a state of nervous irritation, moving from place to place, changing from one subject to another and never finding contentment in any of her occupations.

Valeriana has a strong affinity for the tendo-achillis. Numerous instances are on record where after the failure of many other remedies, **Valeriana** helped to remove the pain in the heels. The most important point to remember about its indication in such pain, is the peculiar aggravation and the amelioration. The pain is worse standing and letting the foot rest on the floor. A certain amount of relief is obtained by resting the foot on a chair or in lying down. The pain comes and goes quickly as in **Bellad.**   In this connection, I am citing a case reported by Bœninghausen in the preface to his Pocket Book. It is not only interesting but instructive.   It shows the way of a master homœopath in the handling of a case.   The observation, the scrutiny, the fine differentiation and the splendid grasp of the case ought to be like a beacon light to every homœopath, to show them the proper way as to how a difficult case should be pilotted.

Case.—E. N., æt 50, of blooming, almost florid complexion, usually cheerful, but during his most violent paroxysms inclined to outbreaks of anger with decided nervous excitement; had suffered for four months with a peculiar violent kind of pain in the right leg after the previous dispersion, allopathically, of a so-called rheumatic pain in the right orbit by external remedies; this last pain attacked the muscle of the posterior part of the leg, especially from calf to heel, but did not involve the knee or ankle-joint. This pain was described as being extremely acute, cramping, jerking, tearing, frequently interrupted by stitches and extending from within outward; but in the morning hours, when the pain was generally more endurable, it was a dull, burrowing with a bruised feeling. The pain became aggravated towards evening and during rest especially after previous motion, while sitting and standing, particularly if he did it during a walk in the open air. While walking the pain often jumped from the right calf to the left upper arm, if he put his hand into his coat pocket or his breast and kept the arm quiet; it was ameliorated while using the arm, and then the pain suddenly jumped back again into the right calf. The greatest relief was experienced while walking up and down the room and rubbing the affected part. The concomitant symptoms were sleeplessness before midnight, frequently recurring attacks during the evening, sudden flushes of heat with thirst without previous chill, a disgusting, fatty taste in the mouth with nausea in the throat, and an almost constant pressing pain in the lower part of the chest and pit of the stomach as if something were there forcing itself outward. **Valeriana** radically cured.

Lastly, with the mention of two very characteristic indications, I will bring this article to a close. One is the vomiting in infant of curdled milk in large lumps, as soon as they have nursed, after anger of mother. The second is a symptom on which Dr. Hering lays great importance and stress and it reads " Red parts become white."

VARIOLINUM.

Variolinum is prepared from the pus obtained from small-pox. Its provings are very fragmentary, but clinical experience attests to its efficacy and usefulness. It has been extolled very highly in small-pox, both as a prophylactic and as a remedial agent. This much is certain, that it does not produce the bad effect of vaccination nor does it anywhere or to any extent produce the usual sequelæ of vaccination. The cardinal symptoms of **Variolinum** are—

Morbid fear of taking small-pox.

Intolerable pain in the occiput.

When asleep tongue protruded, black coating; when raised it is with difficulty drawn back; looks like a mass of putrid flesh.

Intense backache, worse in the lumbar region.

Pharynx and fauces exhibit deep purplish crimson, with gangrenous appearance.

Breath horrible and offensive.

Jaw falling when asleep, with trembling when aroused.

The following experience of Dr. Clarke clearly proves the prophylactic nature of the remedy—" **Var.** 6 (three pilules) was given to the mother and children of a family, one of whose members was taken with small-pox and removed to an insolation hospital, with his mother to nurse him. The patient (who did not receive **Var.**) was dangerously ill for a month. Neither the mother who nursed him nor any of the other children took small-pox. Vaccine was sent by the Government and all the family were vaccinated, but it did not take with any of those who had taken **Var.,** although the vaccination was repeated.

Dr. H. C. Allen advocates the application of **Var.** in those types of small-pox that are comparatively free from pain and where the patients do not show symptoms of sepsis, in short in mild types of small-pox.

VANADIUM.

Vanadium is a rare metallic element of which the atomic weight is 51. It is derived from Vanadis, a goddess of Scandenavian mythology. It is obtained from the iron ores of Sweeden. It is analogous to Chromium. It is a light gray powder which, under the microscope, appears crystalline and exhibits a silvery lustre. The most remarkable of its chemical properties is the readiness with which it combines with nitrogen gas.

Vanadium is supposed to be a great oxidant that stimulates organic combustion and restores health, appetite, strength and weight. Dr. Burnett reports of having cured a case of fatty degeneration of the liver and atheroma of the arteries through the agency of **Vanadium** in an old man of seventy. It is true it stimulates liver and is applicable in all sorts of degeneration of tissues but a real homœopathic proving will illucidate more of its properties of which we are ignorant at the present moment.

VERATRUM ALBUM.

Veratrum album, in common parlance known as the White Hellebore or European Hellebore, belongs to the natural order of Liliaceæ. It grows throughout the year, in the mountainous parts of central Europe and Siberia. It was first proved by Hahnemann. The tincture is prepared from the roots of this plant, which are first dried and powdered, and then mixed with alcohol. The whole is allowed to remain in a well-stoppered bottle for a few days and then the tincture is poured off and filtered.

Human nature is typically conservative. It clings to the old and dreads all innovations. When years of failure, disappointment and disaffection led Samuel Hahnemann, the thinker, to investigate into the law governing human health and sickness and made him come out with the principle of ' Similia,' he was, like Christ, ostracised by the then philistines of medicine. Truth always survives but it took the world a long time to understand and to appreciate the new system of treatment brought into existence by our master. The narrative of its success is long and painful. Belief came gradually with slow but the sure unfolding of the truth of homœopathy. The first battle of this great war of homœopathy against the other systems of treatment was fought and won by **Veratrum.** Due to its marvellous effect over the digestive tract it easily won over the credulity of the public in the potential efficacy of homœopathy in combating all sorts of bowel complaints. In India particularly, which has become the second home of this new system of treatment, people started believing in homœopathy because they came to realise that homœopathy was best adapted to combat against cholera and is superior by far to the other systems of medicine that were in vogue.

It is of cholera then that we shall speak first. It is a dreaded disease, and in India is synonymus with death. **Veratrum album** meets it on equal ground. It is mostly in the advance stage of the disease that **Veratrum album** is needed. The patient's appearance is pre-eminently distorted and disfigured by the ravages of the disease. He is cold, blue, and collapsed. The nose becomes pointed and of a leaden hue; dark rings make their appearance around the eyes. The eyes are sunken, the lips and nose become blue and extremities cold as ice. We notice beads of perspiration over the cold clammy limbs particularly on the forehead. Circulation seems to have stopped altogether. Heat is totally absent in all his limbs; even the tongue feels cold and the breath is chilly like the cold Alpine breeze. The voice is feeble and hoarse and pulse is altogether imperceptible. Though so cold and lifeless, the patient is instinct with the restlessness of the final struggle. He tosses constantly and exhibits great anguish in all his features. His eyes are turned upward showing only the whites. If at times the pupils become visible, they look lustreless, fixed and full of woes. Such then is the condition of our patient. He looks more like one that has half-crossed the border. This is not all. Great nausea and still greater vomiting drain the patient of the little vitality, that is still left in him. He vomits large quantities of watery, blackish, yellowish bilious substance; sometimes little particles of ingesta may be found mixed with it. Thirst is excessive but it only serves to aggravate the nausea and the vomiting. Stools are watery and inodorous. The most important symptom of all is the huge quantity of the evacuations. They are too frequent and profuse and they simply drain him thoroughly. It seems almost a wonder how and where these evacuations come from. Another symptom worth recording is the simultaneous purging and vomiting in the **Veratrum album** patient. These stools are better described as rice-water stools. To make his agony insupportable we find violent cramps in calves, thighs and masseter muscles. Then again we must not forget the terrible colic that usually accompanies these evacuations. It is felt mostly near the umbilicus and is so severe as to give him the sensation that his bowels would be torn open. This colic is the most important feature of cholera in **Veratrum.** It is rarely indicated in cases that are painless.

Some physicians regard **Veratrum** as a great prophylactic against cholera and advocate its use in the very early stage. We prescribe on symptoms and as soon as we find the symptoms of diarrhœa and vomiting with the cold sweat on the head we will have ample justification for its use.

Bæhr recommends **Aconite** as a great specific for cholera. He says:

"We have prescribed from fifteen to twenty drops of the tincture of *Aconite* in six to eight ounces of distilled water, a teaspoonful of the same to be taken every ten, twenty, or thirty minutes according to the intensity of the symptoms. Under its influence, the patient begins to revive, the circulation of the blood returns to the normal condition, the pulse rises, the internal heat ceases, the thirst is allayed, and the vomiting and diarrhœa arrested."

We will next compare **Veratrum** with **Camphor, Arsenic, Carbo veg., Cuprum ars.,** and **Hydrocyanic acid**—remedies greatly similar to **Veratrum.**

Camphor comes very close to **Veratrum alb.** Hahnemann recommends its use in the first stage as a prophylactic. The pale face, the ashy color, the sunken eyes, the cold clammy skin and the wild unconscious look are equally characteristic of this remedy, but the great point that helps distinction is the suddenness of the onest. The prostration is overwhelming and the collapse is sudden. There is a very virulent type of cholera known as cholera sicca or the dry cholera to which· this remedy is particularly adaptable, because of the suddenness of the attack and the great and rapid sinking of strength of the patient.

Arsenicum alb. is another that presents an exactly similar picture, only it adds a further amount of restlessness to the patient, and greater burning and discomfort. We rarely find a rice-water stool in this remedy. The stool is generally dark, scanty and offensive.

Carbo veg. is administered in the asphyxiated stage where both vomiting and diarrhœa have stopped and yet the patient is sinking. The abdomen is puffed up with flatulence and the patient presents a more complete picture of collapse. The icy hands of Death have a very firm grip over him and every minute his life-force seems to be ebbing away. His breathing is fast and laboured, his pulse is nearly absent and his voice gone. When he speaks at all he speaks in that suppressed, husky tone which sounds like the voice of the grave. The lungs are half collapsed and he calls for a lot of external aid. He wants but this must be done from a distance, as it interferes with his difficult breathing.

The type of cholera where **Carbo veg.** is most useful is cholera hemorrhagica, where the red corpuscles pass out with the serum and tinge the stool red.

Cuprum ars. is a remedy we can scarcely do without in a case of cholera, for almost invariably there comes a stage where the patient is troubled with dyspnœa. In that state it is the one remedy that will be needed.

The next remedy we will consider is **Hydrocyanic acid.** It is one of our last agents in the treatment of cholera. It is very similar to **Carbo veg.,** but it differs from it by the violence and rapidity of the onset. "It is indicated if the attack at once assumes the highest degree of intensity so that but a few hours intervene between the commencement of the attack and the moment when death seems to be lurking on the threshold. **Carbo veg.** may be sufficient if the failing of the strength is less rapid."

The next swing of the pendulum brings us to the constipation of **Veratrum album.** It is inferior to no remedy in the treatment of this disease. The constipation under this remedy is very pronounced.

It is a sort of chronic constipation. Like **Opium** and a few other remedies, the rectum seems to be inert and hence the difficulty in expelling the stools, the first portion of which is large and the latter part consists of thin strings. He has to urge and strain so hard each time that he breaks out with cold sweat on the forhead and he feels quite weak and exhausted.

Alumina is a remedy that presents a similar torpor of the rectum; this is so bad that even a soft stool requires a great deal of straining and exertion.

The importance of **Veratrum** on the mental sphere can hardly be overlooked. We find various shades of mental aberration in this remedy—all sorts of moods from the most lively gaiety to the profoundest melancholy. The form of insanity for which this remedy is especially useful is "mania de grandeur." He believes himself to be a man of very great importance and enormous wealth and he squanders his money. To start with, they are considered perfectly sane as they present no other deviation from the normal.

Veratrum suits women in a certain form of puerperal insanity. They become extremely affectionate and exhibit great love for everybody. They kiss everybody they come in contact with. From the affectionate nature they may merge into an amorous and lascivious state. They talk about indecent things, make impudent gestures and gesticulations. This may pass on to real vehemence and fitful rage. They will curse and complain, and tear and cut. Phenomena like these are very often caused by the suppression of the catamenia.

In short the patient combines in her person the wildest vagaries of the religious enthusiast, the amorous frenzies of the nymphomaniac and the execrative passions of the infuriated demon, each of these manifestations struggling for ascendency and cause her to writhe and struggle with her mental and physical agonies; after short anguish the patient passes from this frenzy into one of deepest melancholy, abject despair of salvation, imbecile taciturnity and complete prostration of mind and body.

We will next consider the indications of **Veratrum album** in febrile affections. It is particularly efficacious in all varieties of pernicious fevers accompanied by general exhaustion, rapid sinking of strength and profuse diarrhœa. On these indications it is useful in quotidian, tertian and quartan fevers. The time of the paroxysm is generally 6 a.m. The stage of chill is very promiment; it starts with great severity, with icy coldness of the entire body. Inspite of great chilliness the patient craves for cold, and refreshing drinks. As soon as heat succeeds the stage of chill, his face gets congested and his brain becomes confused but gradually, even before the heat thoroughly subsides, cold, clammy sweat bursts forth over his forehead; then as the heat declines, his face that was red and congested a while ago, turns pale and woe-begone and haggard.

Elaterium comes very close to **Veratrum album.** Here, as in the last remedy, the fever starts with cholera-like symptoms. He is very chilly and he gapes and stretches all throughout this stage. With the beginning of the stage of heat, start nausea, vomiting, cutting colic and copious frothy stools. His thirst is very great. This patient is very subject to urticaria which appears with the suppression of the chill and it itches intolerably.

As regards the 6 a.m. paroxysm we may compare **Verat.** with **Arn., Bov., Fer., Hep.** and **Nux v.**

We have epistaxis under this remedy. It comes on during sleep at night, but only from the right nostril. The other remedies in which we find epistaxis during sleep are **Merc., Nit. ac., Bry.** and **Nux vom.**

In **Mercurius** the blood discharged from the nose is black and it hangs down the nose like black icicles just exactly as we find in **Croc.** and **Kali bich.** Of course the glandular swelling, the sore mouth, the profuse saliva, and the indented tongue are all very characteristic of **Merc.**

Under **Nitric acid** we find very exhausting hemorrhage of the venous blood. The gums are swollen, dark-red and bleed easily; the patient complains of a splinter-like pain in the nose.

Under **Bryonia** the hemorrhage is mainly vicarious. It comes on in place of the menses. It takes place mostly in the morning after rising from bed, and sometimes during sleep.

Nux vom. is an oft-used remedy for epistaxis. It is always worse in the morning and sometimes during sleep. It is preceded or accompanied by frontal headache. The **Nux vom.** temperament is always guiding.

Veratrum has a very pronounced action over the female sexual system. It produces great irritation in the parts and turns them into nymphomaniacs. Whenever we find extreme irritation in the sexual organs that causes intense excitement and many unholy desires, whatever the cause may be, our attention should be drawn to **Veraturm album.** It soothes and thereby removes all abnormal cravings from the mind of the patient. The menses in **Veratrum** occur too early and they are too profuse. Like **Bryonia,** we notice vicarious blood-spitting during menses. At this time the mental condition of the patient goes through certain transformations and we notice an extra amount of partiality towards religion and religious matters. It also successfully copes with convulsions, and eclamptic fits during parturition.

The indications are pallor, collapse, anemia, violent cerebral congestion, shrieking and tearing of the clothes.

Veratrum album is useful in the spasmodic variety of cough. It is caused by a sensation of titillation in the throat. This symptom also leads to its application in whooping cough particularly in its convulsive stage. It helps even in those cases where it does not cure. The symptom is tickling in bronchi that excites paroxysms of deep, hollow, ringing cough. At night there is no expectoration but in the day-time the patient coughs up a sort of yellow, tough, tenacious mucus of bitter, saltish, sour or putrid taste. Sometimes the paroxysms are so violent that the unlucky patient has got to stand up in bed and cry from the severity of his cough. Great exhaustion is a keynote symptom. Children take a long time to recover strength after one of these attacks. Cold perspiration, emission of urine when coughing and vomiting of tough stringy mucus are characteristic indications of **Varatrum album** in whooping cough. Rattling of mucus, either in the passage or in the bronchial tubes, as in **Antim. tart.,** is a notable symptom. The cough is definitely relieved by lying down.

For incarcerated hernia, and for intussusception of bowels we may need **Veratrum album.** The indications are hiccough, cold sweat, nausea, anguish, rapid sinking of strength and fainting. When we fear gangrene of the hernial tumor, remedies like **Arsen.** and **Lach.** come in.

In **Arsen.** restlessness and anguish are more marked than in the latter. Exceeding sensitiveness of the parts and a dark mottled appearance of the skin over the hernial tumor indicate **Lach.**

In **Plumbum** colic and fecal vomiting are marked features of the intussusception. The abdominal wall feels drawn, as if by a string, to the spine.

Serious cases of gastrodynia sometimes call for **Veratrum album.** The pain starts in the epigastrium. It is at first dull but it grows almost agonizing, subsiding slowly again. It is a pain that radiates from the epigastrium both upward and sideways reaching the back between the lowest points of the scapula. It is accompanied by shaking and cold sensation.

It vies with **Colocynth** for abdominal colics and neuralgic pains. They result from abuse of quinine and indulgence in fruits and vegetables. The abdomen gets swollen up with incarcerated flatus which passes neither way and feels very sensitive. The pain is of a burning, twisting, cutting nature with nausea and vomiting and the patient frequently breaks out in cold sweats.

Hahnemann in his Lesser Writing mentions a case of a compositor who used to suffer from terrible colic after partaking of carrots, cabbages, sourcrout, and after every species of fruits, pears in particular. He used to feel a certain movement about the navel followed by pinching as if by pincers. There occurred also a sensation of constriction above and below, so that the flatus could not pass any way. Along with this he had nausea, vomiting, cold sweat, stupefaction and profound exhaustion. "He lay many hours stupefied, unconscious, with a swollen face and protruded eyes without sleep. After wind passed up and down it went away. **Veratrum alb.** four powders each containing four grains of powdered roots, caused a dreadful aggravation followed by a perfect cure."

This is indeed a model cure; for it presents a perfect picture of our remedy. The skill of the master homœopath consists in recognizing this picture.

Case 1.—F., aged twenty-two, a well-proportioned, robust-looking man of florid complexion, complained of "pains in the chest when taking his breath," accompanied by much shortness of breath, from which he had been suffering at times for the past four years. His countenance indicated much real distress; of late the pain and dyspnœa had very sensibly increased. He had for days together been unable to attend to his usual work. He attributed the onset of his disorder to strain in lifting and carrying heavy weights. He had never been the subject of acute rheumatism, nor confined to his bed with other serious disease, was a careful man in his diet and general habits, never smoked or committed excess in drinking. On three occasions he had indulged in a swim, but was always the worse for it. There had never been cough or expectoration. On examining the chest, there were signs of some thickening and hypertrophy of the heart. There was a loud murmur following the second sound, which was distinctly audible over the greater portion o the chest, and even moderately in the arteries of the neck. No evidence o material obstruction to the course of the blood through the arteries an veins. I am satisfied that the distress was not caused by simply a function disturbance. There was valvular disease present and I judged it to be aorti not mitral. Pulse intermittent, scarcely accelerated. **Tincture of Aconite** firs centesimal three times a day, did not relieve. The murmur was as loud an as distinct as before. **Veratrum alb.** in the same dose and strengt After a week's trial, said he was feeling better, and could get his breat more easily. The murmur was much longer, when the patient reported him self as being much better; he was now able to do light work without distres **Ars. alb. 3,** finished the cure.—Dr. W. Prowse.

Case 2.—Child, aged eighteen months, awakens at 11 a.m., with a viole cough and continuous vomiting of mucus; forehead and face covered wi cold perspiration; face looks and feels like white marble; hands and fe cold; great prostration. **Verat. alb. 34m** relieved very soon, and cured in s hours. The child had eaten a large quantity of ice cream the day previous. Dr. Ad. Lippe.

VERATRUM VIRIDE.

Veratrum viride is the American species of Veratrum a is found growing in swamps, wet meadows and along mounta creeks all the way from Canada to Carolinas. It belongs to t natural order of Melanthaceæ. The plant is a large conspicuo swamp herb, having a simple upright leafy stem. The hairs Veratrum are slightly irritating to the skin and hence it is cal the itch-weed. It is very similar in appearance to **Veratr album,** a sister plant growing in the continent of Europe. poisonous properties were known to the aboriginal Indians, w used to taste their strength in the selection of a leader with "He whose stomach made the most vigorous resistance soonest recovers from its effects, was considered the stoutest the party and entitled to command the rest."

Its action has been studied with care by several Ameri physicians amongst whom we note doctors Osgood, W. C. N wood, Henry, Pope, Jackson, Hale and Burt. Besides conta ing resin and starch, it also has certain alkaloids—Jervin Veratroidine, both strong poisons. It is an intense card sedative, acting both directly upon the muscle of the heart its ganglia and indirectly through the general vaso motor syst It reduces the force of the heart beats and the ulterior press to a great extent. Its utility, therefore, is very great in cases of violent congestion. Quick hard bounding pulse, febrile excitement, and high temperature, are conditions that justify its use. Hence it is generally applicable in the early stages of acute febrile diseases in robust or plethoric patients. It is often used with great success in the beginning of pneumonia, pleurisy, rheumatism etc. It is never used in typhoid, septic and other adynamic febrile conditions.

Cases of poisoning with **Veratrum viride** are numerous. To come face to face with such a case is to have a very distinct impression of the drug. Hence I feel it will not be important time uselessly thrown away to discuss a case of poisoning with **Verat. virid.** The case that I feel will be most appropriate is that of the accidental poisoning of Dr. Burt's little baby and we give below the actual summary of the case in Dr. Burt's own language.

Case 1.—My little girl, aged twenty-one months, got hold of my pocket-case, and I found her sitting down eating medicine. She had a vial of **Veratrum viride** in her hand, with the cork out, and its contents emptied. It contained one-eighth of a drachm of the tincture. She could not have had the case more than five minutes before I discovered her, but in about two minutes she commenced vomiting. I immediately gave half a cup of coffee, and then went for some camphor; returned in about five minutes. Her jaws were then rigid and nothing could be put in her mouth; pupils of the eyes widely dilated; face blue; hands and feet cold; no pulse could be found at the wrist. Bathed her bowels and back with camphor for a few moments, when she went into a spasm, with violent shrieks; breathing suspended for several seconds; lasted about two minutes; remained easier for a few moments, and then went into another spasm similar to the first. I then placed her in a tub of warm water, which soon relaxed the whole muscular system; vomiting kept up, with severe retching every few minutes, for three hours, when it gradually subsided. The matter vomited was a white, ropy mucus. The interval between vomiting for three hours, was not at any time longer than five minutes, and most of the time did not exceed one minute. She remained pulseless all the time, with blue, hippocratic face; hands and feet shrivelled up, as if they had been in water for a long time. When she was not vomiting, she lay in a stupor; pupils of the eyes widely dilated. After three hours the pulse could be counted; it was thirty-six; very feeble. In three and a quarter hours after taking the **Veratrum** she went to sleep, and slept quietly and soundly for three hours, and then awoke well, except being a little weak.

The leading symptoms in this case were: constant vomiting of a white, ropy fluid; dilatation of the pupils; blue, comatose state of the brain; great congestion of blood to the lungs; blue, pinched up, hippocratic face, with cold nose, hands and feet; spasm; trismus; no pulse for three hours; pulse 36, very weak and soft.

I would call special attention to the spasms, and the effect it had on the brain and lungs. When I proved **Veratrum viride,** one of the leading symptoms was, constant aching pain in the back of the neck and shoulders, so that it was almost impossible to hold the head up. I believe **Veratrum viride** has a special affinity for the cervical portion of the spinal cord and base of the brain, but especially the spinal cord. The spasms my little girl had were in her thorax and back (Opisthotonos). The amount of medicine taken must have been small, probably only a few drops; the whole amount of medicine in the vial would have poisoned her fatally in a short time.

In this connection it is worth our while to mention that toxicological symptoms, though immensely important are not everything to a homœopath. Other shades and symptoms that evolve from the provings of finer attenuations and that are products of later verifications are equally important inasmuch as they supply the differentiating touches that help us to individualise and characterise our remedies. It is not the outline alone that specializes the products of a master artist; shades, touches and delineations that are by themselves of no importance and that carry no special artistic value in themselves when dissociated from the outline sketched by the master hand, assume signal importance and etherealize and elevate the jumbled mass of line, shades and colours into a super-product that the whole world looks up on as the work of supernatural genius. Hence the necessity of the other symptoms that we will discuss now.

Veratrum viride is a remedy par excellence for congestion. The sensation of fulness, the dusky engorged appearance, buzzing in the ears, the feeling of oppression and constriction in chest and other organs of the body—point towards intense congestion. For this reason it has been used in cerebral congestion; the feeling in the head is as if it would burst open. This congestion may be the effect of extreme plethora, vascular irritation, alcoholism, teething or suppression of some natural discharge. The throbbing of the arteries, stupefaction, increased sensitiveness to sounds, buzzing noise in the ears, excitability, delirium, blood-shot eyes, and thick speech are natural consequences of a great onrush of blood and congestion. This congestion may affect any part or organ of the body. On these indications **Veratrum vir.** becomes of use in congestive headache, apoplexy, acute inflammatory meningitis, eruptive fevers, pneumonia, pleurisy, acute pelvic cellulitis, dysmenorrhœa, puerperal fever, mania, and in various others ailments of congestive origin. We will discuss the special indications of **Veratrum viride,** in these complaints later on. Here we are concerned with just the outline of the drug. One curious feature of the congestion of **Verat. vir.** is the concomitance of nausea and vomiting with the congestion. The patient complains of feeling sick and he often vomits during the attack. This key-note symptom enables us to differentiate **Veratrum vir.** from other remedies noted for great hyperæmia, such as **Bell., Ferr. met., Gels., Glon., Helleb., Lach., Melli., Phos.** and **Sang.**

Suddenness is another feature that characterises **Veratrum vir.** The patient is at her very best but all of a sudden there comes on an attack of fainting. Headache, prostration, nausea, and vomiting are all prominent by the suddenness of their onset. The peculiar appearance of the tongue gives us the third key-note of the remedy. It may be white or yellow, dry or moist but there is the characteristic red streak down the middle of the tongue. Numerous cures have been effected on this symptom alone. On various occasions during my own practice, when I could not come to the similimum, when puzzled, worried, distracted I did not know what to do or what medicine to prescribe, this peculiar red band running longitudinally through the length of the tongue drew my attention to **Verat. vir.** and saved me from further embarrassment. The peculiar sensation of the tongue, as if scalded is a symptom of equal importance and should be carefully remembered.

The mental symptoms of **Verat. vir.** are very characteristic. Stupefaction, confusion, loss of memory, and depression of spirit are prominently marked. It has been highly advocated in puer-eral mania, on the symptoms of silence and suspicion. The patient is mortally afraid of being poisoned. She refuses to see her physician as he seems to terrify her. This antipathy and aversion towards the medical man to whom she was accustomed is almost a guiding symptom. The following case reported by Dr. Atlee is interesting:

"The labour had been preternatural, child delivered and, by podalic version. She did well until ten days after con-finement, when she became silent, suspicious, and distrustful of those about her, without any obvious cause. In the hope that the change was temporary, opium and perfect rest, with careful watching, was enjoined. Two days after, symptoms of puerperal mania were still more developed; it was impossible for the doctor come near her, his presence seemed to terrify her, and her husband told him that since the last visit she expressed strong apprehensions that the doctor had poisoned her and meditated her destruction. She had slept or none, and it was difficult to keep her confined to her bed and room. In the hope that some benefit might result by controlling the general circulation and diminishing the nervous excitement, five drops of the tincture of **Veratrum viride** were given every three hours, as long as it did not produce nausea, vomiting, or prostration. On the following morning, on entering the room, he found his patient lying quietly and calmly on the bed, with a total absence of the sinister expression of the day before. She answered him slowly, but in a whisper, put out her tongue, and left him feel her pulse without resistance. Upon enquiry he found that soon after the administration of the third dose of **Veratrum** on the previous evening, she had become calm, had rested quietly, and had remained so. The pulse was fifty-six per minute. She was cheerful and obedient, conversed rationally and freely, and without allusion to her previously unhappy condition. She recovered in a few days."

It has been prescribed with equal success in insanity. Loquacity, exaltation of ideas, and exalted opinion of her own ideas and powers are characteristic indications. She understands everything. She knows everything that is going about. No one is clever enough to steal any thing from her. No explanation is necessary to help her comprehension. Such attitude of the mind resembling somewhat the mental state of **Platinum** though wanting in the aggressiveness of the latter remedy, is particularly characteristic of **Veratrum vir.**

Now we shall discuss the relation of this remedy to the female sexual system. As has been mentioned previously, it causes congestion of the pelvic organs. It is used in metritis, ovaritis cellulitis and in inflammations of other appendages provided we have high fever accompanying such inflammation. It is an important remedy for dysmenorrhœa and menstrual colic in plethoric women prone to cerebral congestion. Bloodshot face, pulsation in the head, neck and face and high fever accompanying menstrual colic, lead us to prescribe **Veratrum vir.**

It is successfully employed in congestive dysmenorrhœa **Apis, Bell., Bry., China** and **Sulph.** are not our only remedies fo such conditions. The following case from Dr. Hale's own experience illustrates its usefulness:

"A young, stout and very plethoric servant girl had intense congestive headache at each menstrual period (th menstrual flow was very scanty and painful). The attacks wer almost apoplectic, rendering her delirious or insensible, with dar purple redness of the face, throbbing of the carotids, epistaxi nd partial paralysis of motion, and sometimes cramps. No ysterical complication was present. After taking five drops of eratrum viride, ix, three times a day during the inter-menstrual eriod, and every hour during the attack, she was much benefited, ne menstruation being more abundant, and the headache slight. he second period was much more natural, with very little eadache."

Now we come to a controversial point in **Verat vir.** We have een asked by some authors to use it exclusively in every cases f high fevers. We have been advised by others never to use it a pain of incurring fatal results. It is, indeed, a mistake to use with the object of bringing down the pulse or control the heart's ction or to reduce the fever as is sometimes done by many who escribe remedies on the pathological standpoint. Here as well everywhere the golden principle to be followed is the totality the symptoms. No harm can ever come when this dictum is llowed. If the symptoms of **Veratrum vir.** are there, its iministration brings on the most marvellous results. Rapidity its action when thus employed, is certainly the root cause of hy some medical men go off at a tangent with the idea that it is most a panacea for all kinds of febrile affections. When the ver is accompanied by drowsiness, throbbing of the temporal teries, a full frequent hard pulse, vomiting of mucus and bile d show a tendency to spasms, **Veratrum vir.** ought to be a great medy.

If pulmonary congestion is apprehended during the eruptive age of measles as manifested by dyspnœa, cough and pain in the est, **Veratrum vir.** makes a splendid remedy. So in scarlet ver, variola, and other exanthematous ailments, our attention ould be particularly directed to **Veratrum vir.** by the intensity the arterial excitement. Hardness and fulness of the pulse, rest- ssness, dyspnœa sensation of constriction in the chest, and great d high temperature are sure indications for this remedy. If on e other hand the febrile symptoms assume a low or asthenic pe, remedies such as **Rhus tox., Arnica, Baptisia, Pyrogen, Mur.** id and **Acid phos.** should be thought of.

We should discuss **Veratrum vir.** in its relation to the eatment of pneumonia. There was a time when it was regarded crime not to prescribe **Veratrum vir.** in the initial stage in eumonia. From theoretical stand-point, the argument, that by ason of its power to control the action of the heart it prevents rther engorgement of blood into the already congested lungs, and gives the lungs chance to free themselves of all inflammation, sounds quite logical and plausible. Certainly, in many cases of pneumonia it does effect a speedy cure. I mean in those cases where **Veratrum vir.** becomes indicated by reason of the totality of the symptoms. But it will be nothing short of a real catastrophy to prescribe it in each and every case of pneumonia and where other remedies are indicated on the principle of **Similia Similibus Curantur.** The following remarks of Dr. E. B. Nash on this subject carries great conviction.—" I was a young physician and thought I had found a prize in this remedy. But one day I left a patient, relieved by this remedy of an acute and violent attack of pneumonia, to go to a town five miles distant, and when I returned found my patient dead. Then I watched others treated with this remedy, and found every little while a patient with pneumonia dropping out suddenly when they were reported better."

Now as to the symptoms that call for **Veratrum vir.** in pneumonia —chilliness, great heat and oppression of the chest with sensation of a heavy load on it, rapid laborious breathing, full, hard, bounding pulse that cannot be obliterated by pressure of the finger, high fever, flushed face, vomiting, expectoration of pus and florid blood and nausea. These are sound indications and we may safely depend on them. Prescribed on these symptoms, **Verat. vir.** reduces the inflammation and favours quick expectoration and the result is a rapid, easy and a marvellous cure—a cure that will enthral and astound—the like of which is seen only in that one system of treatment based on the principle of " Similia Similibus Curantur."

No remedy is prompter and more reliable, in checking convulsion whether hysterical, epileptiform or puerperal, than **Verat. virid.** When given in a big dose to the healthy individual it causes contortions of the muscular system, particularly of the muscles of the face, neck, finger and toes. The head is drawn to one side, the mouth gets drawn at one corner and the facial muscles get affected with violent convulsive twitchings. These convulsions may be both tonic or clonic.

At other times the action of **Verat vir.** stimulates a series of galvanic shocks. From these it is easy to deduce that **Verat. vir.** should make a first-rate remedy in convulsions and choreic disturbances. I have used this remedy in numerous instances with gratifying results. The following cases reported by Dr. Hale in his " Therapeutics of New Remedies " are very instructive. They prove beyond doubt the infinite superiority of the homœopathic system of treatment in grappling with violent cases of convulsions where blood-letting and other heroic forms of treatment had signally failed.

Case 1.—A case of hysterical or epileptiform, convulsion. The patient was a stout, healthy man, of sober habits. I found him sitting on the side of the bed, seemingly well and perfectly intelligent, unaware, however, that he had had convulsions. All that I could ascertain of his previous history was, that he had been similarly affected in childhood. While conversing with him he was suddenly, and without apparent premonition, seized with a frightful convulsion, occasioning frothing at the mouth, and the most violent jactitations of all the voluntary muscles. I immediately opened a vein and bled him profusely, but without the desired result, for, after the lapse of a certain period, with as perfect a return of consciousness as before, there occurred another convulsion of equal intensity. In this emergency the excessive muscular relaxation capable of being produced by **Veratrum viride** occurred to my mind, and I reflected that such an effect could only be produced by an influence primarily exerted upon the cerebro-spinal system of voluntary nerves. I administered **Veratrum** in full and repeated doses, desiring, and confidently expecting to produce the same train of distressing symptoms that so alarmed me some years previously; there were nausea, vomiting, purging (rarely observed), muscular relaxation, and coldness of the surface. In this I was disappointed; for, though the convulsions were arrested, there occurred no other symptom than a relaxed skin, with profuse perspiration. Since then I have administered the **Veratrum** in numerous cases of eclampsia of children, with such satisfactory results as to establish, beyond all doubt, the power of this agent to arrest convulsions .—Dr. Baker, ,'Southern Medical and Surgical Journal."

Case 2.—A case of chorea in a young lady—When first visited, her symptoms were distressing to the last degree, the entire muscular system being in continuous and tumultuous motion. The case passed on from bad to worse, notwithstanding the most assiduous attention and energetic treatment. Tonics, anti-spasmodics and anodynes were exhausted without avail; the spine and nucha were cupped and blistered, without benefit; chloroform was administered internally and by inhalation; opium and its preparations seemed to make her worse; so, after all the family had given up all expectation of recovery, upon the suggestion of a medical friend, who had twice used the **Veratrum viride,** in two cases of chorea, with the most satisfactory results, he at once commenced its administration, and as she was gradually brought under its influence the turmoil began to cease; the face, which had been changed by its muscles into the most ludicrous and horrible distortion, became placid and intelligent; the head ceased its everlasting jerking, the extremities lay still, the body left off writhing, and the patient quietly passed into a peaceful and profound slumber. This sleep was deep and long, as it was the first, with few and slight exceptions, that she had had in nearly two weeks, and the quiet that the muscles now received was all that had occurred, save during those few and short slumbers. At a subsequent visit, I found the family cheerful and hopeful, and the patient quiet and sleeping, the pulse but little depressed. There had occurred no vomiting. I roused her, and, to my great satisfaction, when awake, there was no jactitation of the extremities, and but very little twitching of the muscles of the face. The **Veratrum** was continued; and for the first few days, if withheld, the commotion began to return. Under the quiet induced, the sleep was so continuous at the outset, that the family called the preparation "the laudanum mixture." After a time the convulsions ceased altogether, and the patient was restored to health under a course of tonics.—Dr. Barker.

Case 3.—A case of chorea in a child aged twelve.—It had been confined to bed for three weeks, and was reported to have been under treatment for about six weeks; first for worms, with **Spigelia**, wormseed, etc.; and subsequently for chorea, with **Cimicifuga, Racemosa, Iron, Quinine,** and the usual routine treatment, until the child was apparently dying. It is not in the power of language to convey a proper conception of the truly pitiable state in which I found this child. It had slept not at all, nor had taken any nourishment for days. It was evidently dying from exhaustion and inanition. The muscular commotion was violent, universal and unaffected by sleep; the lips embossed with foam, worked up by a continued champing of the teeth. Three drops of the tincture of **Veratrum viride** were administered every three hours, the vehicle being gum water. In twenty-four hours I had the gratification to see the symptoms greatly improved; the muscles were much quieter, and the child could swallow without difficulty. The trouble in this respect had constituted the greatest embarrassment in the treatment. At the end of the fourth day, all convulsive action had ceased.—Dr. Terry.

Case 4.—A case of continual nodding of the head. A woman, aged 36, childless, and subject to menorrhagia, immediately after an attack of which she had a continual nodding of the head and violent convulsive action in one arm, together with jactitation of one leg. In this case, six drops of the tincture of **Veratrum viride** were given every three hours. The fourth dose occasioned slight nausea, and after the fifth dose the convulsive action ceased, when the **Veratrum** was withheld. In eight or ten hours the symptoms returned. Upon resuming the medicine, they again disappeared; the doses were then reduced. The case recovered.—Dr. Terry.

Case 5.—A case of cerebro-spinal meningitis.—I was called one night to see a child about four years old, and found her suffering from an attack of pneumonia. The febrile affection which was excessive, accompanied with some delirium; I succeeded in reducing with the usual remedies, and with good results, as in the morning I found her quite comfortable, with the exception of a severe cough; the skin was moist, the pulse about natural, and all the symptoms denoting a decided check to the disease, which was so alarming the night previous. This condition continued until evening, when the febrile symptoms came on again, with considerable pain in the stomach and bowels. Bowels tympanitic and very sensitive to touch. Ordered an injection, but got no relief from a very copious one; then gave olive oil and **Podophyllum,** and in a few hours got a good evacuation, and the removal of the tympanites; bowels still sensitive. In the morning, bowels still sensitive; pulse quick and weary; pupils dilated, and the muscles of the back of neck contracted, drawing the head back on the shoulders. Considerable delirium; cough dry and spasmodic; gave **Aconite, Bryonia** and **Hyoscyamus.**

In the evening the symptoms were increased; the tetanus still continued extending to the trunk. At about 12 o'clock she had a convulsion or a clonic spasm, drawing the head almost to the heels. These spasms continued as often as once in five, ten, or fifteen minutes, with relaxation of the muscles of the back for five days, when, after using all remedies recommended by the authors, and finding the patient almost gone, I asked for counsel, and Dr. Fowle was called. He advised emesis and injections, but with no effect, with the exception of some nausea. On the sixth day of convulsions we used Chloroform, but got no effect.

Dr. Wood came in, and the decision of all was that she must die. During this time, the pupils continued to dilate, bearing the strongest light without changing. It was a complete case of opisthotonos, like that produced on the dog by **Gelsemium**. Not having any **Gelsemium**, I did not give it. During the spasm the heels almost touched the head, forming a hoop of the body.

From the third to the fifth day, the body was covered most of the time with a cold, clammy sweat. On the fifth day there was a marked febrile action; it came on about noon, and went off in the evening. On the sixth, seventh and eighth days it was the same, when I concluded to put her on **Veratrum viride**. Accordingly, about two o'clock in the afternoon, commenced with one-half drop doses every hour; continued this course until twelve o'clock, when there was some nausea. On a close examination, found that the muscles were somewhat relaxed; continued **Veratrum viride** until morning, when there being no fever, I stopped it. I found then, however, that the muscles of the trunk were completely relaxed and the spasms ceased. In the afternoon there had occurred no return of fever, but the muscles of the neck still continued contracting; pupils were natural, but very sensitive to light. I again gave **Veratrum viride**, as before, and to my joy the next day found her able to lie on either side or back. Improvement went on from this time. I gave her **Nux vomica** and other medicines, and in two weeks discharged her.—Dr. C. A. Williams, of Joliet, Illinois.

Case. 6.—A case of violent convulsion—A boy, aged four and a half years, had for several days a croupy cough, and at night considerable fever. The cough yielded to **Phosphorus**, but the feverish state increased until it became nearly or quite a continuous one; tongue coated white; urine scanty and bowels irregular, and pulse 160 to 170. About six days after the attack, he had in the evening a very violent convulsion, which lasted about fifteen minutes, and considerable insensibility for an hour afterwards; after this had passed off mostly the fever began to increase very rapidly, and in four hours the pulse ran into a flutter, and the respiration had increased to 76 per minute. I determined to try **Veratrum viride**, which I prepared at the rate of six drops fluid extract to one-half tumbler of water, repeated every hour, one teaspoonful; in three hours he was asleep, and in the morning quite comfortable and wanted to eat. Continued the medicine from one to three hours during the two following days, and has had no fever since the night in which he had the convulsions, which was decidedly epileptiform. He has made a good convalescence, and is now quite well.—Dr. M. A. Tinker, of Schenectady, N.Y.

VERBASCUM THAPSUS.

Verbascum thapsus is also called the Great Mullein. The plant belongs to the Figwort family and the natural order of Scrophulariaceæ. It is an exceedingly coarse stout herb growing in North America and Europe. The tall stems and leaves are woolly and the flowers yellow at a cylindrical spike. The alcoholic tincture is prepared from fresh plant chopped and pounded to a fine pulp. Mullein oil, so widely used by homœopaths in deafness and earache, is extracted from the pounded yellow blossoms or by saturating the blossoms in oil which gradually absorbs the essence of the blossoms.

It has been spoken of highly in spasmodic, rough, deep-sounding night cough. The attacks are frequent and the deep hoarse cough sounds like a trumpet. It is caused by tickling in larynx and chest. It occurs mostly in children during sleep.

It has also been recommended in piles, specially when they are accompanied by an intense itching in the rectum. Dr. Clarke considers **Verbascum** the best known remedy for itching hæmorrhoids and pruritus ani. The complaint, where it is supposed to do much good, is, neuralgia of the face. The agony is so intense that the patient howls, as if mad. It is mostly a left-sided neuralgia, seated in the supra-orbital nerve. The sensation is as if one were violently pressing upon left malar bone as far as ear. Dr. E. E. Case reports a case of neuralgia in a middle-aged widow that he cured with **Verbascum.** The tearing, stitching pain was mostly located about left ear and it pressed downward and inward. Everything proved futile, till **Verbascum** 1 m. was prescribed This brought lasting relief.

VERONAL.

Veronal is a white crystalline powder of faintly bitterish taste. It is soluble in 145 parts of cold water and 12 parts of boiling water. It is a great hypnotic. In the allopathic therapeutics it is regarded as one of the most important members of their great sleep-producing. It resembles Trional to which it is infinitely superior. It is used as a sedative in 0·5 gm. doses in cases of maniacal excitements. They often resort to this after bromides, chlorals, trionals and warm baths have failed. It should not be given in doses exceeding 1 gm., although in chronic cases of alcoholism, delirium tremens and dementia more has been found necessary. One gramme of **Veronal** is supposed to be equal to ¼ of a grain of morphia as a pure hypnotic.

It is thus a great sedative to the nervous system. It produces a sleep resembling the natural. The patients are easily roused but they soon fall asleep again. It is generally administered in hot milk or in capsule.

We as homœopaths however, should not make this the basis of our prescription. Like other drugs, this should be subjected to a thorough and reliable homœopathic proving and symptoms should be elucidated which alone should be our guide in the administration of this remedy.

VESICARIA

The tincture is prepared from the whole plant collected fresh; it is Vesicaria communis. It belongs to the natural order of Cruciferæ. It has been an old home remedy in various parts of Germany for various forms of urinary troubles attendant on gonorrhœa, gravel, cystitis, nephralgia, prostatitis etc. Its main indication is a great burning and smarting along the course of the urethra with a frequent desire to pass urine. Strangury is also particularly marked. It should, therefore, be studied in close comparison with **Thlaspi, Berberis, Sarsaparilla, Chimaphila** and **Cantharis.**

The following cases reported by George R. Shafer are instructive and should give us food for further thought.

(1) T. S., 67, suffering from nephralgia, for which he had received **Morphia** injection in former attacks.   Received **Vesicaria** θ, in 15-drop doses every fifteen minutes. This gave marked relief in two hours, and a complete cure in six hours. (2) S. B. 57, was suffering from cystitis due to exposure to cold; high fever sweating and burning pain while voiding urine, were prominent symptoms.   The urine passed was in drops only.   **Vesicaria** θ in 10-drop doses, cured in two days. (3) A Lady, aged 39, was in severe pain in the back; there was a goodly collection of brick dust sediment in the urine; her hands and feet were so swollen she could neither close her hands nor walk. **Vesicaria** θ, cured (4) A man, aged 65, was suffering from irritable bladder; he had to rise twenty to thirty times in the night.   **Vesicaria** θ, in 20-drop doses, relieved quickly and cured in six weeks. (5) C. M. aged 89, was suffering from chronic cystitis, and was passing large quantities of muco-pus. The bladder was at first washed out with Boric acid solution, then **Vesicaria** θ, was administered in 20-drop doses every two hours. Improvement followed, and in two hours the Boric acid washing was stopped and **Vesicaria** given every four hours. This finally cured.

It also helps in suppression of urine.   Dr. Davison used it in a lady patient in whom uremic spasms had set in as a consequence of total suppression of urine, **Vesicaria** θ, prescribed in fifteen drop doses established the secretion of urine and finally saved the patient's life.   I have not had any occasion to verify these symptoms, but I put it to the profession as demanding of greater attention and study which will gradually elucidate finer and better homœopathic indications to further consolidate the just demand of this remedy.

VESPA.

Under this name we have three varieties—**Vespa vulgaris** (the wasp), **Crabro** (the hornet) and **Vespa maculata** (the Yellow-jacket). The tincture is prepared from the live insect. It belongs to the natural order of hymenoptera.

We have a few skin and female symptoms well marked in this remedy. There are the prurigo-like pinkish spots over the body which itch intensely; we also have erythematous blush, boils, wheals, and macules; they burn intensely and the burning is relieved by bathing them with vinegar.

As regards its action on the female sexual system, we find that menstruation is preceded by a period of depression and constipation. It has got a special affinity for the left ovary which is markedly affected. Urination is frequent and is accompanied with burning. This remedy also has erosion around the external os.

Another symptom worth remembering is the erysipelatous inflammation of lids accompanied with chemosis of the conjunctiva. In this respect it is very similar to **Apis.**

VIBURNUM OPULUS.

It is a shrub belonging to the honey suckle family and is usually called the High Cranberry Bush. It was first proved by Dr. H. C. Allen. Its berrys are red and sour and are utilized in making jelly. The tincture is prepared from the bark of the roots, shrub and its limbs.

It is a great remedy for women's complaints, specially in spasmodic dysmenorrhœa for which complaint it is specifically indicated. A great sickish feeling, severe pain in the back going around to the loins and across to the pubic bones, a bearing down sensation with a feeling as if the body from the waist downwards would collapse, severe aching in rectum, a great depression of spirit, amelioration of all symptoms from lying down and aggravation from movements are the keynote symptoms of **Viburnum.** The menstrual flow is thin, light-coloured and scanty. Before the onset of the menstrual flow the patient complains of a severe bearing down sensation and a drawing pain in the anterior muscles of the thighs. Both the sacral and pubic regions have a heavy aching feeling.

It is equally useful in severe false pain preceding normal labour; its utility in the after-pains is just as great. Administered before the rapture of the membrane, it prevents threatened miscarriage. Dr. Hering reports of a case of a woman, 5 months in the family way, who while out driving, received a severe strain. Three days later, severe bearing down pain began in the abdomen and the back, and a colicky crampy pain started, which penetrating through the abdomen went into the prominences of the hip bone and thence downward into the vagina. She also complained of nausea and dizziness when rising from cough. Urging to urinate was great. **Viburnum** removed all the disturbing symptoms and averted the threatening miscarriage.

Viburnum also disperses pelvic congestion. The following cure effected by Dr. Susan J. Fenton is worthy of our attention— Miss F., 25, housekeeper, medium height, rather slender, blonde, sanguine, was strong till late in 1891, when she had severe pelvic congestion and was fifteen months under treatment and most of the time in bed. In June, 1892, double oophorectomy was performed with great relief; but attacks of pelvic congestion with severe pain still persisted, at first every two to four weeks, later less frequently, causing impairment of general health and strength. The symptoms were: excruciating pains through lower abdomen, with bearing down sensation and a feeling as if the body from the waist to the lower part of pelvis would collapse; an indescribable sick feeling all over with severe aching in rectum; great depression of spirits; and a general sense of amelioration when lying down. **Vib.** θ.—was taken in three-drop doses thrice daily. After taking it for three days she lost all her symptoms and felt "perfectly well for the first time in over four years."

VINCA MINOR.

It is also called the Lessor Periwinkle. This remedy is noted or skin affections of various kinds but the most important field f its action is located on the scalp. It has been used with great uccess in crusta lactea, favus, plica polonica, eczema, and alopecia. Humid eruptions with intense itching and burning, are numeous on the head. There is an oozing of moisture that mats the air together. Sometimes the whole head gets full of vermin. he dirtiness and the filthiness of **Vinca minor** vie with those of **Mezereum** and **Graph.** I believe it is in the power of every medical man to adduce proofs in support of this. The skin of the whole body is highly sensitive and tends to break out into redness and soreness from the slightest rubbing.

There is a curious symptom, in connection with the nose, that ought to be mentioned here. The slightest excitement or mental emotion throws a quantity of blood into the nose and it looks almost purple. It also has a sort of moist eruption on the septum of the nose which keeps on throwing out a viscid matter that forms into crusts and practically blocks the nose and makes exceedingly rough, ugly and tender. Another symptom that should be recorded is the excessive flow of blood during menstruation. It is so excessive as almost to amount to hæmorrhage. It flows like a stream and causes great debility. Such hæmorrhage due either to fibroid growths or climaxis, finds in **Vinca minor** a remedy and a helpful agent.

VIOLA ODORATA.

Viola odorata, our Sweet Scented Violet, has a specific action in the ear. Numerous cures are on record of obstinate cases of otorrhœa and deafness that after resisting every sort of treatment, had at last to give in to **Viola odorata.** The following case reported by Dr. Cooper speaks of its marvellous efficiency in curing chronic running of the ear. A baby, 17 months old, affected with otorrhœa of both ears from birth, received one dose of **Viola odorata** mother tincture. This brought out a great quantity of offensive discharge from one of the ears and the child steadily improved till all its drowsiness and restlessness vanished as if under magic."

The most characteristic symptom to remember about **Viola odorata** is a sensation of tension felt by the patient everywhere. He complains of tension in forehead, occiput and scalp. This feeling of tension originally begins in the scalp; from there it extends to the upper half of the face, forehead and temples as far as the ears, alternating with a similar sensation in the occiput and the cervical muscles. The patient constantly knits his brows and if asked as to the cause, he will tell you plainly that this inclination to knit is due to an uneasy sensation of tightness on the forehead. The skin feels stretched and tight. A peculiar burning sensation in the forehead is equally characteristic. Great weakness is felt in the muscles of the nape of the neck; the head feels too heavy to be carried straight. It frequently sinks forward.

Viola odorata is very useful in many affections of the eyes particularly in choroiditis. Sensitiveness to light, painful forcible drawing together of lids as from irresistible sleep, illusions of vision, visions of fiery serpentine circles, intense headache, and tension beneath the eyes are symptoms that indicate **Viola** in many affections of the eyes. A case of choroiditis cured by Dr. Cooper is illustrative of its great usefulness in that complaint. This patient was for 20 years a victim of fearful headache, that used to assail her every now and then without any premonitory warning. The pain was intense around temples and eyes. The case was diagnosed to be a case of chronic choroiditis by a prominent oculist. **Viola odorata,** mother tincture, was given at intervals with the effect that she was cured radically. She became healthy, strong and cheerful and her sight became quite normal.

Viola odorata is an important rheumatic remedy. It affects principally the right side, specially the right deltoid muscle, and the right carpal and metacarpal joints. It is also indicated in rheumatism of the wrist. Dr. Constantine Hering cured a case of rheumatism of the joints of right hand in a robust young man of 31. The right wrist was swollen and the hands and fingers of the same side, were affected with intense pain. The affected parts were very hot and the agony rendered the slightest motion impossible. **Viola odorata** brought on a radical cure.

We will discuss one more symptom of **Viola odorata** before closing. It is a symptom I will always remember with pleasure. A short while ago I was asked to relieve a young girl, a primipara suffering from an unusual discomfort of breathing. The discomfort was not at all in proportion to the development of the gravid uterus. She was barely in her

4th month of pregnancy; the distension of the abdomen due to the enlarged uterus, did not warrant the dyspnœa, anxiety, restlessness and the uneasy feeling to which she became a victim. Various remedies such as **Arsen., Acon.** etc. were tried and nothing brought any lasting relief till **Viola odorata** was prescribed which dispersed all the trying symptoms.

VIOLA TRICOLOR.

In **Viola tricolor** we have another remedy prepared from a flower. It is our Pansy, also called Jacea and Heartsease. It belongs to the natural order of violaceæ.

Pansy was proved by Samuel Hahnemann and his provers.

It is one more of our great remedies for eczema and impetigo but its chief characteristic consists in the concomitants of urinary symptoms with skin affections. Urinary disturbances, such as either too copious urination or sudden arrest of urinary secretion, company most of its skin symptoms. The eruption, though generally confined to face, may extend to the scalp. Yellowish brown crusts with much itching and exuding a sort of thick yellow fluid which agglutinates hair, are common features of Pansy. We may, therefore, compare it with **Antimonium crudum., Calc. sulp., Cham., Cicuta, Dulc., Graph., Lyco., Merc., Mez., Nitric acid, Oleander** and **Petroleum.**

Another feature of Pansy which should not escape our attention, is its action over the male sexual organs. It causes involuntary seminal discharge with lewd dreams. The dreams in **Viola** are very vivid and the loss of seminal fluid causes a certain amount of exhaustion and weariness of mind. The urine passed is cloudy and it has a strong smell resembling that of cat's urine as in **Aspar.** and **Caj.** The smell of urine is at times, of great help to the homœopath. Many a time it directs his erring up to the indicated remedy.

Remedies noted for great offensiveness of odor in urine are **Asafœtida, Benz. acid., Bufo, Daph., Dulc., Fluo. acid, Nitric acid,** and **Sepia.**

It has also been recommended in syphilis. Prominent yellowish greenish ulcer in throat, extending from the Vilum Palati to tonsils, chancred ulcers on the posterior surface of the fauces and soft palate, venereal ulcers with swellings of the prepuce.

syphilitic pustules on the labia, and ulcers about breasts, are common occurrences in **Viola tricolor.** It is therefore, just as deep-acting a remedy as some of our preparations of Mercury and Potassium. Evidently we need not, on the slightest suspicion of syphilitic taint, run to a list of stereotyped remedies noted for efficacy in the treatment of venereal affections.

VIPERA TORVA.

This is a comparatively little known remedy, but the benefit we derive from it from time to time, in some very trying cases, which were if not for **Vipera** might have ended fatally, warrants us in discussing the symptomatology of this drug. The fresh poison of the German viper is triturated with sugar of milk. There are various other preparations such as the **Vipera berus,** the common viper of England, the **Vipera redi,** the Indian viper etc., but our discussions in these pages will be simply confined to the **Vipera torva.**

It is reputed to be a great remedy for varicose veins and acute phlebitis and its chief indication is a bursting sensation in the affected limbs when allowed to hang down. We consider this very characteristic of **Vipera.** On this symptom alone I saved an arm from being amputated. The trouble, which originated in a trifling whitlow, threatened mortification of the whole of the forearm. The patient had to keep his arm constantly in a sling. The red swollen hand felt as if it would burst each time it was allowed to hang down. **Vipera** not only removed the symptoms but cured the hand in an incredibly short time.

Allen mentions a case of enlarged and painful liver with jaundice, fever, green and bloody stools. The pain that used to radiate into the shoulder and from there down to the hip, was excruciating. **Vipera** removed the pain and reduced the liver to its normal size. With **Vipera** I also helped, in a case of an ugly sore on the tip of the finger of a diabetic, with a similar history of aggravation from the downward position.

VISCUM ALBUM.

Viscum album is the common mistletœ. It was superstitious-ly respected by the Druids of old who regarded it, as possessed of all kinds of mysterious virtues. This parasitic plant grows upon the oak, elm, apple and other fruit trees. It is sustained by the juices drawn from these plants through the medium of its simple roots piercing the barks. Equal parts of the fresh berries and leaves are chopped and then mixed with two parts by its weight of alcohol. After eight days the tincture is separated by decanting, straining and filtering.

It is one of our little known and rarely used remedies, but nevertheless we cannot afford to neglect it, for in its own field it renders yeoman's service. Like **Aconite, Bryonia** and **Rhus tox.,** it is one of our foremost anti-arthritic remedies. The tearing pain is very characteristic of this remedy. Dr. Huber is of opinion that **Viscum** invariably relieves wherever such pain may exist. It is also effective in neuralgia of a gouty nature. "Dr. Ivatts reports of a case of rheumatism, in an old man with pains in the wrist, ankle, knuckle-joints and back. The distress was very great and the aggaravation was very similar to that of **Rhus tox.,** but **Rhus tox.** failed to help. **Viscum** on 5 drop-doses administered twice daily cured him in a short time.

The next important action of the remedy is on the female generative organs, especially the womb. It is very useful in slow labor. Dr. E. M. Holland reports of quite a few cases in the "Medical Summary" of 1898, where with teaspoonful doses of a mixture of 30 drops of **Viscum** in water he hastened many difficult cases of slow, painful and protracted labour. It is also a remedy of the climacteric years when chronic or periodical hemorrhages are met with.

One of the provers, Mr. Proell by name, developed symptoms of epilepsy from **Viscum.** The aura was peculiar. It felt like a glow of fire rising from the feet to the head. He also felt a sensation of a large spider crawling over the hands. Dr. Clarke in his "Dictionary" mentions a case of a breeder who had a fine stock which became epileptic at the age of four or five. He cured them with a tincture of the fresh leaves bruised in a mortar.

XANTHOXYLUM.

Xanthoxylum is also called the " Prickly Ash " and the "Toothache-tree." It will indeed be a shame to leave out such a remedy from our Materia Medica. It is of great use in many of the complaints of women. We may call it, like **Sepia,** a great women's remedy. It is generally suited to women of spare habits, nervous temperament and delicate organization. It acts upon nervous system especially upon the sensory nerves and causes a sort of a smarting sensation in the mucous membrane, as from pepper.

It is an excellent remedy in dysmenorrhœa of **nervous** women. The pain is almost agonizing along the course of the genito-crural nerve. It almost drives the patient to distraction. It shoots down as low as the knee and no position really relieves. There is a symptom which I have found of great use in **Xanthoxylum** and that is a desire to take deep breath during pain. Another important symptom is a sensation of weakness in the lower limbs; the patient wants to sit or lie most of the time. The menstrual flow is too early and it is always accompanied with pain down thighs. Ovarian pain, with scanty and retarded menses, extending down genito-crural nerves and associated with great backache also calls for **Xanthoxylum.** Leucorrhœa coming on when it is time for menses to appear is another important indication of the remedy. The menstrual blood is almost black, coming in strings and clots and intermitting every other day and generally lasting two weeks.

Xanthoxylum has been used with signal success in chlorosis particularly in these cases where severe œdematous swelling had appeared in the face and the legs and all symptoms pointed to a fatal end. The indications of course, here as well as everywhere consist of sharp, severe, neuralgic pains that radiate downwards from the sciatic crests into the knees.

Professor O. B. Gause recommends it very warmly in after pains; in this respect it occupies almost and the same place of honour as **Arn., Caulo., Chamo., Coffea, Morph. acet., Secale** and **Viburnum.**

Arnica used after the close of labor entirely averts the after-pain.

Caulophyllum is indicated in the spasmodic pain of labor felt in the lower abdomen; it extends into the groins.

The **Chamomilla** pain is distressing to the utmost; it makes the patient ill-natured and irritable. There is also a great desire for fresh air in the **Chamomilla** patient.

Morphia acet. is one of Dr. Marsden's favourite remedies in labor; he used it often with invariable success.

Secale is indicated in after-pains in thin, scrawny, elderly women who have bore many children.

Viv. op. is indicated in nervous, hysterical women and the pain is crampy in nature.

Case 1.—An emaciated feeble, worn-out, woman of 56, was suffering from a fibroid tumour of the size of an orange. The mensturation had stopped some 15 years ago and while it lasted it has always been profuse, painful and was followed and preceded by leucorrhœa. A fetid yellowish discharge from vagina was continuous. The patient was nervous, depressed and sleepy most of the time. The patient had been advised by his Allopathic physician to undergo an operation. The patient was put on **Xanthoxylum 3x** morning and night. In the first week there was an appreciable improvement in the pain and the vaginal discharge. The medicine was continued 4 weeks, at the end of which time the tumor was found much softer and smaller. In six months it had altogether disappeared.—P. C. Mozumder.

YOHIMBINUM.

Its utility is great in that frequent and noxious of ailments—impotence. It is a crystalline alkaloid obtained from the bark of Yohimbeha, a tree of the Cameroons. It throws a great rush of blood into the sexual organs, face, ears and nose and produces great excitement of those parts and of the central nervous system. It also produces a great hyperæmia in the milk glands and stimulates their function. Its indication, homœopathically, consists of lasting erections which is merely a precursor of the opposite condition of sexual neuræsthenia. The desire is absent; the organ becomes limp and the testicles show signs of hypertrophy. Sleepiness and tremor accompany the above conditions. It resembles **Picric acid, Phos., Phos. acid.** and **Cantharis**.

YUCCA FILAMENTOSA.

Yucca filamentosa is known as the Bear Grass. It belongs to the natural order of Melanthaceæ. In this we have one more of our hepatic remedies. It was originally proved by Rowell; since then it has been extensively used by various other doctors and every one of them has confirmed its utility in biliousness. Its symptoms are very much like the symptoms of **Chelidonium**—the patient complaining of sharp cramping pain in the liver, which penetrates straight through to back. There are also bad taste in the mouth and an excess of bile in the stools, which becomes loose and diarrhœic. The tongue which is coated yellow takes the imprint of teeth same as **Chelidonium.** To be exact and this is where **Yucca** differs from **Chelidonium,** the tongue is rather of a bluish-white color than yellow. The Patient passes much flatus by rectum while having stools and complains of a dull, frontal or temporal headache most of the time.

Yucca is also administered in gonorrhœa and urethritis. The patient complains of a sensation of burning while urinating and of a raw sensation at all times. The meatus looks œdematous, red and swollen. The specific gravity of the urine is very high.

ZINCUM METALLICUM.

Zincum met., is a polychrest of a very high order. It is an element belonging to the Magnesium group. It was first introduced into our Materia Medica by Franz, but the real proving was done by Hahnemann himself. It is an immortal monument of our master, a monument that has been built on the solid foundation of innumerable lives, which it has saved in the past—a monument eternal and enduring, as with age it will solidify further having lessened the toll on human lives which time demands of mankind.

In poisonous doses it acts deleteriously on the nervous system, which it enfeebles, exhausts and deteriorates. This action may be more aptly described as enervation. It causes a sensation of formication as of ants walking over the body. A sensation of tremulousness gradually comes on developing later on into a regular tremor. Vertigo, fainting and even convulsions may supervene till death ensues. Muscular sensibility is greatly lessened though the reflex irritability is highly exaggerated.

In the homœopathic therapeutics its main application is centered on its enervating and depressing influence. The patient is in a state of complete enfeeblement. This is reflected in his want of the power of reaction. Nothing stimulates. His brain is too feeble to understand and to remember. If she happens to be a woman, she does not even get her period due to the same cause. There is also the inability to expectorate and urinate. This proves the low state of our patient. Although it is nothing like prostration of **Arsenicum,** where the devitalised state is extreme, it still shows a process of disbandment, which if allowed to proceed unhampered, will ultimately lead the patient on to the **Arsenicum** condition. The patient in **Zincum** is exposed to the malignant influence of some devitalising disease; this inimical influence penetrates into his system and attacks his vitality but due to extreme depression and the want of power of reaction on the part of the vitality, the disease is not thrown out on the surface; it spends its force on the internal organs where it gnaws, corrodes and eats into the most vital part of the system. Thus in **Zincum** we have to fight with a hidden foe and that is why, unless we take cognizance of this fact, we are placed at a great disadvantage. This explains why so many of us fail. The task of a real physician is serious indeed. He must steer clear of all hidden minds and pitfalls and avoid dangers unforeseen and unthought of. This reminds me of a case, I treated while yet a novice, of a little baby, grandchild of a sea-captain. The baby started with a heavy cold and fever. I was called in and according to symptoms prescribed **Aconite.** Progress was appreciable but before convalescence ensued, one day all of a sudden the temperature went up very high. Symptoms indicated **Bell.** which the child received but the fever would not come down. This state of affair continued for 7 or 8 days till the parents decided to put the child in the hands of an allopath and so I lost all track of the case till after a fortnight I was sent for again. The condition of the child, as I saw for the second time, was pitiable indeed. The fever was ranging between 105 and 106. There were distinct symptoms of meningitis, the child being in continuous spasms, tonic and clonic, lasting practically twenty-four hours. The eye had become lustreless and there were distinct ulcerations of the cornea due to extreme enfeeblement and inanition.

I wasted no time but immediately called in consultation the late Dr. P. C. Mozumdar, the great oracle of Homœopathy in India. There was nothing of hurry or haste on him. I remember distinctly how sedately and quitely he sat and went into the minutest details of the case from beginning to end. Nothing escaped his attention. Spellbound, I saw the working out of the case. How he made out that the disease was due to suppression of an eruption of measles, due to the nurse having given the child a tepid bath, which has inexplicably thrown the fever up in the initial stage of the disease, escaped my understanding, but the correctness of the diagnosis became evident when after the administration of three doses of **Zincum metallicum,** the child broke out into general rash all over his body. The vitality of the child had so far gone that inspite of the appearance of this suppressed rash, the poor baby ultimately succumbed to his ailment.

Zincum met. produces a sort of paralysis of the brain as a result of which there are complete unconsciousness, jerking of the whole body, twitching of single limbs, grating of teeth, encephalic cry, automatic motion of different parts of the body and fidgetiness of the lower extremities. These symptoms indicate it in meningitis and hydrocephalus. We have known of instances where the trembling has been so violent as to be required to be held tightly. The encephalic cry mentioned above is caused by a sort of pressing tearing pains in the base of the brain, whence they shoot into the eyes and different parts of the head. These complaints are, more or less, the result of non-development of an eruption.

It is also prescribed in dentition of children who are puny, weak and badly developed. The teeth fail to appear inspite of the hardening of the gums—the child showing great weakness and prostration. The pulse usually is slow and the child soporous and drowsy. It lies with the back of the head pressed deep into the pillow and eyes half-closed and squinting. Great greediness is exhibited by these children while drinking. It rolls the head from side to side as in **Bell., Podo., Teucrium** and **Helleborus.**

Zincum is useful in headaches. A great symptom is pressure on root of nose. This headache is either brought on by indulgence in wine or is aggravated by it. It also increases after dinner. **Zincum** cannot tolerate liquor of any description; this is considered an important indication of the remedy.

Whatever may be the complaint it always brings on aggravation. The most important point to remember in **Zincum** is that it causes and hence cures anemia of the brain and brain-fag. This headache which can be better described as cerebral exhaustion is also accompanied by depression of spirit.

From what has been said above, it may be guessed that the **Zincum** patient is extremely forgetful. He forgets even those things that have been done in the course of the day. The cerebral exhaustion referred to above, makes mental operations extremely difficult. He finds it difficult to grasp ideas and co-ordinate thoughts. Evening is usually the time of aggravation. It is useful even in delirium·tremens—the patient exhibiting great fear of persecution for crimes, which he has never done. He stares as if frightened. We find him, like **Bell.**, attempting to get out of bed and run away. Constant trembling of hands, fidgetiness of feet and coldness of the extremities are guiding symptoms of this remedy. One very important symptom, a symptom that has been verified often, is a tendency to repeat questions before answering them.

We will next discuss the action of **Zincum** on the digestive tract. In the first place we find ravenous hunger at about 11 a.m. This is more like a sensation of weakness or goneness in the stomach. This symptom, as has been said often, is also to be found under **Phos., Nat. carb., Nat. phos., Sulphur** and **Hydrastis.** The patient exhibits great greediness and hastiness in swallowing. There is great aversion to meat, fish and sweet things, particularly to veal. The taste in the mouth is bitter and there is intolerance of water. Heartburn is also present and this is aggravated from wine. We also notice great tympanites with a consequent distention of abdomen. It causes griping pain about the navel and is so severe that it takes away breath. It is accompanied by nausea and running of water from mouth. The feeling in the abdomen is of a heavy pressure backwards as though the abdomen were drawn backwards towards the spine. Sometimes the patient would describe it as an internal induration. It is aggravated by external pressure and drawing in abdomen.

Zincum is an invaluable remedy in a serious type of diarrhœa accompanying typhoid, typhus, meningitis, hydrocephalus and other varieties of adynamic diseases. The stool is foamy, profuse, soft, papescent thin. At times it is almost pitch-like; it is expelled involuntarily. The diarrhœa is mostly accompanied with

stupor generally reminding one of **Opium.** In fact **Zincum** come;
in after **Opium** has failed to set up any reaction. Cerebra
symptoms are very prominent in these cases but **Zincum** is bes
indicated when with cerebral complications we notice great de
ficiency of nerve power and the absence of high temperature.

In cholera **Zincum** finds application in the later stages whe
symptoms of hydrocephalus gradually supervene. The patien
shows signs of great fright, rolls head from side to side, start
jumps and cries while in sleep, bores the nostrils with his finge
and constantly pulls at his cracked and fissured lips. His eye
are staring, pupils contracted and his face looks pinched an
worn out.

It is as great a remedy for constipation as it is of diarrhœa
The stools are generally large in size and are evacuated with grea
effort of abdominal muscles. They crumble to pieces due to grea
dryness. After stool the patient complains of a pressure and
clawing sensation in the anus. This unusual dryness of stool is a
much characteristic of **Zincum** as it is of **Bryonia, Graphites** an
Plumbum. Like **Sulphur** there is great burning in anus afte
stool. Due to the dryness there is often discharge of blood fror
the anus. **Zincum** is almost a specific for constipation in new
born babies.

Last of all we shall discuss the application of **Zincum** in th
male and the female sexual organs. On the male sexual side i
produces great relaxation and depression of the parts. There i
usually a history of abuse with the inevitable consequence tha
follows all excesses. The sexual organ becomes lax, flaccid an
dorment. It is easily excited and emission follows rapidly afte
an embrace. **Zincum** also rectines copious discharge of pros
tatic juice without any apparent cause. The appearance of th
patient is pale and sunken like that of **Acid phos.** and **Coniun**
Blue rings around the eyes belie exhaustion, waste and lowere
vitality.

On the female sexual system it has the two opposite extreme
of irresistible craving and absolute want of desire. There is to b
seen a complete loss of sexual desire as befits a patient in a stat
of **extreme** enervation. Then again we have nymphomania, th
result of intense sexual erethism. The menses usually appear to
early and are too profuse. She passes lumps of coagulated bloo
mostly when walking. The flow is most profuse at night time
As in **Ferrum met.,** we notice alternation of paleness and rednes
of the face. There is always a flow of profuse leucorrhœa whic

auses itching of vulva and a consequent burning in pudenda. The itching is so excessive as to lead to masturbation. There is enerally to be seen a great varicose condition of the external enitals. During menstruation the mammæ become swollen and ore to touch. The hair falls out from the genitals both in the male and the female.

Zincum. has important action over the circulation of blood. t produces great stagnation of blood in the veins of the legs particularly during pregnancy. It also sets right the intense heartburn in pregnant women after taking sweet things. There s usually difficulty in passing urine which is apt to pass more eadily, when the patient is in the standing posture.

The cough of Zincum is spasmodic and is accompanied by severe pain in the chest. The patient during a violent fit of coughing, puts his hand to his genitals. It is aggravated by taking wine and during menstruation. The cough is excited by a tickling sensation in larynx and trachea as far down as the middle of the chest. The sputum is yellow, purulent, tenacious, bloodtinged, sweetish, putrid and metallic.

One more observation and we will be finished with Zincum. Like Lachesis there is general amelioration of all symptoms from the establishment of any discharge or flow from the system.

Case 1.—I——,a boy seven years old, went through an attack of scarlatina, so mild in its symptoms that medical aid was not sought. During convalescence, however, the child was exposed to a severe snow-storm. The face and abdomen œdematous, urine scanty, Arsen, 200, every three hours in water. In the evening of the same day convulsions set in: Head hot, eyes wild, staring; biting, striking those around; Bell. 200, in water, every two hours. No relief in twenty-four hours. A more careful study of the case discovered the following: Convulsions followed by stupor; **occiput hotter than the fore-**; screams before the spasms; trembling of the muscles; **constant motion of the feet** between attacks; urine scanty, bloody. Zinc. 200, in water, every three hours. In twelve hours consciousness returned, and the spasms ceased. **A rash appeared** over the body in irregular patches; speech remained thick. A return of the convulsions the next day was checked by a repetition of Zinc. 200. Recovery complete; urine abundant and of natural colour.—Dr. E. A. Farrington.

Case 2.—Dr. C. Hering relates the following case: Liver hard, enlarged, sore to the touch, could be felt much more to the left, and above the navel as a small, hard lump; several hard lumps in the abdomen; the abdomen enlarged and soft; softest around the navel, sore pains all over the belly. most around the navel; hectic fever, unquenchable thirst, when swallowing he feels a small, hard lump in the throat; sometimes like a worm creeping up from the pit of the stomach into the throat, which makes him cough; frequent gagging and vomiting of : little blood phlegm or thin blood; sometimes pus, of a salty taste, particularly with coughing; the cough worse at night, with a shooting in the scrobiculum; a weak, but very deep cough; has to cough until it raises; stool either in little lumps or frothy; rumbling in the bowels; cannot lie on the left side; during the night a dull moaning; feels so weak that he talks with difficulty; his feet commence to swell, and the swelling rises gradually upward. **Zincum 30** restored him almost completely. (**Am Jour. Hom. Mat. Med., iii., 29.**)

ZINGIBER OFFICINALE.

Zingiber is our common ginger. It is a native of Asia and is used very extensively in cooking as a condiment. The dried root is powdered and then covered with five times by its weight of alcohol. It is poured off, strained and filtered.

This drug was first proved by Franz. The genito-urinary and the respiratory tracts were strongly affected in the provers. When taken in big quantities for a long time, it interrupts the function of the kidneys, hence Farrington recommends its use in infants and in people suffering from Bright's disease. **Zingiber** is reputed to be a good remedy in diarrhœa when caused by drinking impure water, melons and bread.

It is also indicated in humid asthma. The patient feels great difficulty of respiration. He sits up all night but the peculiarity lies in the absence of all anxiety. Even on face of threatened suffocation he seems to be quite cool and collected.

This is all I can safely say about this remedy. It needs further proving and verification.

ZIZIA.

The tincture is prepared from the meadow Parsnip, a plant growing plentifully along moist shady banks of streams.

My knowledge of this remedy is simply confined to cases of chorea in women suffering from uterine congestion and who are subject to migraine. These patients suffer from profuse menstrual flow followed by long and acrid leucorrhœa. This chorea is peculiar inasmuch as the convulsive movements continue even after the patient falls asleep. It should therefore be studied with remedies like **Mygale, Agaricus, Actæa racemosa, Tarentula, Ignatia** and **Stramonium.**

In the first-mentioned remedy the choreic movements are very violent. The head is often jerked to one side, the face muscles twitch, the speeches are indistinct and are thrown out with difficulty rather jerkily. She is unable to raise her hand to her head as each attempt at touching the head is followed by the hand being thrown backward violently.

In **Tarentula** the convulsive movements are mostly on the right-hand-side. Great reslessness, trembling of the body, excessive hyperæsthesia, relief from music, and paralysis with complete loss of movements, are important indications.

Actæa racemosa, like **Zizia,** is useful in chorea in women suffering from uterine displacements and rheumatic troubles.

Stramonium like **Mygale** is useful in chorea characterised by violent movements. These patients rotate arms overhead, jump upon tables and chairs, throw head alternately backward and forward and laugh and cry alternately. The tongue moves involuntarily, rendering speech difficult, oftentimes impossible. Fright is often an important causative factor. Sardonic grin, alternate weeping and laughing, great sexual excitement, strange and absurd fancies, great fear of darkness, at the same time objection to any bright glittering light, loquacity, and frothing at the mouth are symptoms too important to be overlooked in **Stramonium.**

REPERTORY

AGGRAVATION.

DURING THE DAY: Ferr., Nat. m., Nit. ac., Puls., Rhus t., Sang., *Sepia*, Sul.

MORNING: Acon., Agar., Aloe, Ambr., *Am. m.*, Anac., Ant. cr., Ant. t., Arg., Arg. n., Arn., Ars., *Ars. iod.*, *Aur.*, Bap., Bor., Bov., Bry., *Calc. c.*, Calc. phos., *Carbo v.*, Chel., Chrom. ac., *Cina*, Coca, Con., Corn. c., *Croc.*, Dig., Dios., Dros., Dulc., Eup. per., Euphr., Ferr., Gam., Gel., Guai., Hep., Hydras., Ign., *K. bi.*, K. carb., K. iod., K. *nit.*, Kalm., Kreo., *Lach.*, Merc., Merc. i. f., Nat. c., *Nat. m.*, Nat. s., Nit. ac., *Nux v.*, Onos., Petro., *Phos.*, Phos. ac., Phyt., *Podo.*, Pso., Puls., Ran. b., Rheum, *Rhodo.*, *Rhus. t.*, Rumex, Sabi, Sal. ac., Sang., Sele., Senec., Seneg., *Sep.*, Sil., *Spig.*, Spo., Squ., Stan., Staph., Stram., Sul., Tar., *Valer.*, Verat. al., Verat. v., Verb.

FORENOON: Arg., Bry., *Cannab. s.*, Car. v., *Guai.*, Hep., Laur., Mang., Mar., *Nat. c.*, *Nat. m.*, Nux m., *Podo.*, Ran. bul., Rhus. t., *Saba.*, Sep., Sil., Spig., *Stan.*, Staph., Sul., ac., Valer, Vio. t.

AT NOON: Arg., Nux m., Valer.

AFTERNOON: Agar., Aloe, *Alum.*, Ambr., Am. carb., Am. m., Ant. c., Apis., Arg., Arg. nit., Ars., Asaf., Asar., *Bell.*, Bism., Bry., Calc. phos., Canth., Chel., Cic., Cimic., Coloc., Dig., Dulc., Ign., *K. nit.*, Laur., Led., Lyc., Mar., Meny., Merc., Mos., Mur. ac., Nit. ac., Nux v., Phos., Phos. ac., *Puls.*, Ran. b., *Rhus t.*, Rumex, Sang., Sars., Sele., Seneg. Sep., *Sil.*, Sin., Staph., Still, Sul., *Thuja*, Valer., Vio. t. Zinc.

EVENING: Acon., All. c., *Ambr.*, Am. carb., *Ant. cr.*, Ant. t., Arg., Arg. nit., *Arn.*, Ars., Asaf., Asar., Bap., *Bell.*, Bor., Bry., Calad., Calc. c., *Caps.*, Carb. an., *Caust.*, Cham., Cimic., Cocc., *Colch.*, Coloc., Con., Croc., Cyc., Dulc., *Euphr.*, Ferr., Gam., Guai., *Hell.*, Hep., *Hyos.*, Ign., Iod., Ipe., Jat., K. bi., K. carb., *K. nit.*, Kalm., *Lach.*, Laur., Led., *Lyc.*, *Mag. c.*, *Mang.*, *Meny.*, Merc., Merc. i. r., *Mez.*, Nat. c., Nat. m., *Nit. ac.*, Nux m., Par., Petrol., *Phos.*, Phos. ac., *Plat.*, *Plumbum.* Puls., Ran. b., Ran. s., Rhodo., Rhus t., *Rumex*, Ruta. Sabi., Samb., Sang., Sars., Seneg. Sep., *Sil.*, Sin., Stan., Stra., Sul., Sul. ac., Tab., Tar., Thuj., *Valer.*, Zinc.

NIGHT: *Acon.*, Amb., Am. m., Amm. c., Ant. cr., Ant. t., Aral., *Arn.*, *Ars.*, Ars. iod., Asaf., Aur., Bar. c., Bell., Bov., Bry., Calc. c., Calc. ph., Camph., Cannab. ind., Cannab. sat., Canth., Caps., Carb. an., Caust., *Cham.*, *Chel.*, *Chin.*, Cina, Cod., Coff., *Colch.*, Coloc., Con., Croc., Crotal., Cup., Dig., Dros., *Dulc.*, Euphr., Equis., Ferr., Fl. ac., Gam., *Graph.*, Hell., *Hep.*, *Hyos.*, *Iod.*, Ipe., K. br., K. carb., K. iod., K. nit., *Lach.*, Led., Lil. tig., Lyc., *Mag. c.*, *Mag. m.*, *Mang.*, Merc., Merc. cor., Mer.i.f., Mez., Nat. m., Nat. s., *Nit. ac.*, Nux v., Oleand., Op., Ox. ac., Petrol., Phyto., Pic. ac., *Phos.*, *Puls.*, Rheum, Rhus t., *Rumex*, Saba., Samb , Sars., Sec. c., Sele., *Sep.*, *Sil.*, Spig., Spo., Stan., Staph., *Stro.*, *Sul.*, Sul. ac., *Tell.*, Vio. t., Zinc.

FOREPART OF NIGHT: Ant. t., *Arg. n.*, *Ars.*, Bell., Bry., *Carb. v.*, Caust., Cham., *Coff.*, Cup., Graph., *Led.*, *Lyc.*, Mang., Merc., Mez., Mur. ac., Nit. ac., *Phos.*, Phos. ac., Pod., Puls., *Ran. s.*, Rhus t., *Rumex*, Ruta, *Saba.*, Sep., Spig., Spo., Stan., Staph., Valer.

AFTER MIDNIGHT: *Ars.*, Bry., Calc. c., Cannab. s., Chel., Cup., Dros., *Ferr.*, Gel., Ign., *K. carb.*, *K. nit.*, Mag. c., Mang., Merc., Mez., *Nux v.*, Phos., Phos. ac., Pod., Puls., Ran. s., *Rhus t.*, Samb., *Sil.*, Squ., Sul., Thuj.

PERIODICALLY: Alum., Anac., Ant. cr., *Arg.*, Arn.,

PERIODICALLY.
Ars., Asar., Bar. c., Cact., Calc. c., Canth., Caps., Carb. v., *Ced.*, Chin., Ign., *Ipe.*, K. nit., Lyc., *Nat. m.*, *Nit. ac.*, Nux v., Phos., Plum., Puls., Rhodo., Rhus t., Sab., *Sep.*, *Sil.*, Spig., Stan., Staph., Sul., Verat. al.

ALONE, When: Ars., Dros., Sul., Verat. al.

ANGER FROM: *Aco.*, Aur., Bell., Bry., Caust., Cham., Coff., Coloc., *Hyo.*, Ign., Lyc., Nat. m., *Nux v.*, Op., Phos., Phos. ac., Plat., *Puls.*, Staph., Stram., Verat. al.

ANIMAL FLUIDS, from loss of: Calc., Chin., Puls., Sep., Staph.
Carbuncle (a large circumscri

ANTHRAX, poison from: *Ars.*, Lach.

ANXIETY: Aco., *Ars.*, Bell., Cham., *Ign.*, Nux v., Op., Phos. acid., Plat.

ARSENIC, poisoning from: Ipe., *Merc.*, Verat.

ASCENDING: Am. carb., *Ars.*, Bar. carb., Bor., Bry., *Calc. c.*, Calc. ph., Cup., Glon., K. iod., K. nit., Kalm., Merc., Nat. mur., Nux. v., Ox. ac., Phos., Ruta, Seneg., Sep., Spig., *Spon.*, Stan., Sul., Tab., Zinc.

An eminence: Ars., Aur., Bry., Spong., Stan., Zinc.

A height: Calc., Conv., Oleand., Spig., Sul.

Steps: Acon., Alum., Ang., Calc., Carb. veg., Nux, Plat., Plum., Rat., Rhus t., Stan., Sulph., Thuja.

ASPHYXIA: Carbo veg., Chin., Coff., Nitr. ac., Op., Phos.

AUTUMN, in: Chin., Colch., *Rhus t.*, Verat. al.

AWAKING, on: *Ambr.*, Am. carb., Am. mur., Arn., Ars., Calc., Carb. an., Carb. veg., *Caust.*, Chin., Cocc., Dig., Graph., *Hep.*, Ignat., Ip., Kali. b., Kali carb., Lach., Lyc., Merc., Nat. mur., *Nit. ac.*, Nux., *Phos.*, *Puls.*, Rhus t., Samb., *Sep.*, Sil., Staph., *Sulph.*

BATHING: Ant. cr., Ars. iod., Nit. ac., Phos., *Rhus*, Sep.

Cold: Ant. cr., Bell., Caps., Nit. ac., *Rhus*, Sep.

Sea: Ars., Mag. m., *Rhus*, Sep.,

BED, in: Acon., Ambr., Ars., Calc., Caust., Daph., Graph., Hep., Ign., Kali carb., *Led.*, Lyc., Mag. car., *Merc.*, Nux, *Phos.*, Puls., Rhod., Rhus t., Sep., Sil., Staph., Spon., Sulph., Thuja, Verat. al.

BEER, from: Ars., Asaf., Bell., Coloc., Euph., Ferr., Kali b., Lyc., Mez., Nux, Puls., Rhus t., Sep., Stan., Sulph., Thuja, Verat. al.

BENDING: Am. mur., Bell., Bry., Chin., Cic., Crot. tig., Hep., Mur. ac., Nat. m., Phos., Ran. b., Rhus t., Sele., Spon., Stan., Sul.

Affected part: Amm. m., Ant. cr., Arn., Bell., Bry., Calc., Chel., Chin., Cic., Coff., *Ign.*, K. carb., Lyc., Mag. c., Nat. m., Nux., Phos., Puls., Rhus t., Ruta., Sang., Sele., Sep., Sil., Spig., Spon.

BENDING, affected part.

Backward: Anac., Bar. c., Calc. c., Con., Ign., K. carb., Nit. ac., Plat., Puls., *Sep.*, Sul.

Backward and Forward: Chel., Coff.

Inward: Ign., Stan.

Outward: Caps.

To right: Spig.

Sideways: Bell., Calc. c,, K. carb., Nat. m.

Head backward: Cic., Puls., sep. Forward: Rhus t. Sideways: Spo.

BITING TEETH TO-GETHER: *Am. carb.*, Guai., Hep., Ip., Mez., Puls., Rhus t., Sep., Verb.

BREAKFAST, after: Amm. m., Bry., Calc. c., Caust., *Cham.*, Con., Dig., Graph., K. carb., K. nit., Nat. c., Nat. m., *Nux, Phos.*, Sep., Sul., *Zinc.*

BREATHING: Acon., Amm.m., Anac., Bell., Bry., Calc. c., Cannab. s., Caps., Cina, Cocc., *Colch.*, Hep., K. carb., K. nit., Led., Mag. c., *Merc.*, Mur. ac., Nat. m., Nit. ac., Phel., Puls., *Ran. b.*, Rhus t., Saba., Sele., *Sep.*, *Sil.*, Spig., *Stan.*, Sul.

Deep: *Acon.*, Agn., Arn., Asc. t., *Bor.*, Brom., *Bry.*, Dig., Graph., Hell., K. carb., K. nit., Lyc., Meny., Merc., Oleand., Phos., *Rhus t.*, Rumex., Saba., *Sabi.*, Sang., Sil., *Spig.*, Squ., Sul.

When not: Ign., Merc.

Holding breath: K. nit., Spig.

BRUISES: Arn., Con., Ruta, Sul. ac.

BRUSHING TEETH: Coc. c., Staph.

BURNS: Ars., Carb. veg., *Caust.*, Kre., Stram.

CARESSES by: Bell., Calc., Chin., Ign., Plat.

CATARRH owing: Amm. m., *Ars.*, Calc., Carb. v., *Cham.*, Graph., Lach., *Lyc.*, *Merc.*, Nux, Puls., Sabad., Sep., Spig.

Suppressed from: *Bry.*, *Calc.*, Chin., Dulc., Nit. ac., *Nux*, Puls., Sep., Sil.

CHANGING POSITION: *Caps.*, Carb. veg., Chel., Con., *Euphor.*, Ferr., Lach., Lyc., Phos., *Puls.*, Samb.

CHANGE OF Temperature: Ars., Carb. veg., *Puls.*, *Ran. b.*, Sabi., Verb.

Weather: Bry., Mang., *Nux m.*, Phos., *Rhodo.*, Rhus t., Sil.

CHARCOAL from: Arn., Bov.

CHEWING, when: Alum., *Am. carb.*, Am. m., Arg. n., Bor., Bry., Chin., Euphr., Guai., Hep., Hyos., Ign., *Meny.*, Merc., Nat. m., Nit. ac., Oleand., Petro., Phos., Phos. ac., Puls., *Rhus.*, Sabi., Sep., Staph., Thuja, Verb., Zinc.

After: Sabi., Staph.

CINCHONA, abuse of: Ant. t., *Arn.*, Ars., Bell., Calc. c., *Carb. veg.*, Cina, Dig., Ferr., Hell., *Ip.*, Lach., Nat. m., Phos. ac., Puls., Sep., Sul., Verat. al.

CLEAR WEATHER: Bryonia.

CLIMACTERIC, during: *Lachesis.*

CLOSING EYES: Bell., Bry., Chin., Clem., Dub., Hell., *Lach.*, Led., Mag. m., Puls., Sep., Sil., Ther., Thuja.

Mouth: Mezereum.

CLOUDY WEATHER: Cham., Chin., Mang., Nux m., *Rhus t.*, Sep.

CLUTCHING ANYTHING: Amm. carb., Bry., Calc. c., Carb. v., *Caust.* Cham., Lyc., Puls., Sil.

COFFEE from: Canth., Caust., Cham., Ign., Nux v.

COITION, during: Canth., Graph., K. carb., Sele.

After: *Agar.*, *Bov.*, *Calad.*, *Calc. c.*, Chin., *K. carb.*, Nat. c., Petro., Phos., Sele., *Sep.*, Sil.

COLD in general: Acon., Agar., Amm. carb., *Ars.*, Aur., Bar. carb., Bell., Bor., Bry., Camph., *Caust.*, Cic., Cocc., Con., *Dul.*, Hell., *Hep.*, Hyos., Ign., *K. carb.*, Mag. c., Mang., Menth., *Mos.*, Nux m., *Nux v.*, Petro., Puls., Ran. b., Rhodo., Rhus. t., *Saba.*, Sil., Stro.

COLD air: Acon., Agar., *All. c.*, *Amm. carb.*, Ars., *Aur.*, Bar. c., Bell., Bry., Calc., *Camph.*, Caps., Carb. veg., *Caust.*, Cocc., Colch., Con., Dulc., *Hell.*, *Hep.*, Hyos., Ign., Ip., K. bi., K. carb., Mang., Merc., *Mos.*, *Nux. m.*, *Nux v.*, Osm., Petro., Phos., Plan., Puls., *Rhodo.*, *Rhus.*, *Rumex*, *Saba.*, Sep., *Stro.*, Sul., Verat.

Dry: Acon., *Asar.*, Bry., Caust., *Hep.*, *Ip.*, *Nux v.*, Saba., Spo.

COLD, air.

Wet: *Amm. c.*, *Calc. carb.*, *Colch.*, *Dulc.*, Lach., Lyc., Mang., Merc., *Nux m.*, *Rhus t.*, Ruta, Stro., Sul., Verat. al.

COLD, becoming: Arn., *Ars.*, *Aur.*, Bry., Camph., Caust., Cocc., Dulc., Graph., Hep., Hyos., *K. carb.*, Lyc., *Mos.*, Nux *v.*, Phos., *Rhus.*, *Saba.*, Sep., Stro.

A part of the body: Bell., Hell., *Hep.*, Rhus. t., Sep., *Sil.*

After: Acon., Ant. t., *Bell.*, Bry., Calc. c., Calc. ph., Carb. veg., *Cham.*, Chin., Coff., Coloc., Con., Cyc., *Dulc.*, Graph., Hep., *Hyos.*, Ip., K. carb., Lyc., Mang., Merc., Nat. mur., Nit. ac., *Nux v.*, Phos., *Puls.*, Rhus t., Sep., *Sil.*, *Spig.*, Sul., Verat. alb.

In head: *Bell.*, *Sep.*

In feet: Puls., *Sil.*

COUGHING, after: Cina., Hyos., *Phos.*, Sep.

Before: Cina.

CUTTING HAIR: *Bell.*, Sep.

DANCING, when: Borax.

After: Spongia.

DARK, in the: Amm.m., Calc., Carbo an., Phos., *Stram.*, Valer.

DENTITION, during: Ars., Bell., Borax., *Calc.*, Calc. ph., *Cham.*, Cina., Coff., *Ign.*, Mag. c., Mag. m., *Nux*, Pod., Rheum, Sil., Stan., Sulph.

DESCENDING: Bell., *Bor.*, Bry., Con., Ferr., Rhodo., Ruta, Verat. al.

DISORDERED STOMACH: Acon., *Ant. cr.*, Ars., Bry., Carb. veg., Coff., *Ipe.*, Nat. ca., *Nux vom.*, *Puls.*, Staph.

DISTORTION OF FACIAL Muscles: Bry., Spig.

DRAFT OF AIR: Bell., *Calc. c.*, Caps., Chin., Hep., K. carb., Sele., *Sil.*, Sul.

DRAWING IN THE AIR: Ant. cr., Bell., Merc., Nux, Puls., Sabi., Sele., Sep., Sil., Spig., Staph.

DRINKERS, for hard: Agar., Ant. cr., Ars., Bell., Calc. c., Chel., Chin., Coff., Ign., *Lach.*, Led., Lyc., Nat. c., Nat. m., Nux. mos., *Nux v.*, Op., *Ran. b.*, Rhodo., Rhus. t., Ruta., Sil. Spig., Stram., Verat. al., Zinc.

DRINKING when: Bell., Bry., Canth., Cina, Hyos., Iod., Lach., Phos., Stram.

After: Acon., Ant. t., Apoc. can., Arg. n., Arn., *Ars.*, Bry., Caps., *Chin.*, Cic., Cocc., Coloc., Con., Croc., Crot., Cup., *Eup. perf.*, Ferr., Hep., Mar., Nat. m., Nit. ac., *Nux v.*, Pod., *Puls.*, Rhus t., *Sil.*, Sul., *Verat. al.*

DRIVING, in a wagon: Arg., Bor., *Cocc.*, Hep., Ign., Nux m., Petro., Rumex, Sele., *Sep.*, Sil., Sulph.

After: Nit. ac., *Sil.*

DRY WEATHER: Aco., *Asar.*, Caust., *Hep.*, *Ipe.*, Nux *v.*, Saba., Spo.

EATING, before: Ambra., Bov., Calc. c., Cannab. s., Chel., Chin., Croc., Ferr., Graph., *Iod.*, Lach., *Laur.*, *Nat. c.*, *Phos.*, Plum., Puls., Rhus t., Saba., Stro., Sul., Tar.

When: *Amm. carb.*, Bar. c., Bry., Calc. c., *Carbo an.*, Carb. ac., *Carbo veg.*, Caust., Cham., Cic., Cocc., Con., Graph., Hep., *K. carb.*, Lyc., Mag. m., Nat. c., Nat. m., *Nit. ac.*, Oleand., Phos., Puls., Rumex., Sep., Sul.

Fast: Ipe., Nux v.

After: Aloe, Amm. mur., Anac., Apis, Arg. n., *Ars.*, Bell., *Bis.*, *Bry.*, *Calc. c.*, Carb. an., Carb. veg., *Caust.*, Cham., Chel., *Coloc.*, Con., Crot. tig., Cyc., Dulc., Ferr., Gran., Graph., *K. bi.*, *K. carb.*, Lach., *Lyc.*, Mez., Nat. c., *Nat. m.*, Nit. ac., *Nux v.*, Ox. ac., Petro., Phos., Phos. ac., Pod., Puls., Ran. bul., Rheum, Rhus t., Rumex, Seneg., *Sep.*, *Sil.*, Sul., Tar., Verat. al., Zinc.

After eating to satiety: Calc. c., Lyc., *Puls.*, Sul.

ELEVATION, when on: Sulphur.
EMISSIONS: Alum., Iod., *K. carb.*, *Nux vom.*, Sep., Staph.

ERUCTATIONS, from: Agar., Cannab. sat., *Cham.*, Cocc., Lach., Phos., Rhus t., Sep., Verb., Zinc.

ERUPTIONS, suppressed: Ars., Bell., Caust., Cham., Hep., Ipe., Lyc., Nat. c., Bry., Nux m., *Phos. ac.*, Puls., Rhus t., Sep., Staph., Sul.

EXCITEMENT, emotional: Acon., Arg. nit., Atrop.,

EXCITEMENT, emotional.

Aur., Bell., Bry., Caust., Cham., Coff., *Coloc.*, Hep., *Hyos.*, *Ign.*, Lyc., Nat. m., Nux., Op., Phos., *Phos. ac.*, Plat., Pod., Puls., *Staph.*, Verat. al.

Contradiction: Aur., Bry.

Fright: *Acon.*, Arg., Bell., Caust., Coff., Cup., Hyos., *Ign.*, Nux v., *Op.*, Plat., *Puls.*

Grief and sorrow: Coloc., Hyos., *Ign.*, Phos. ac., Puls., *Staph.*, Verat.

Jealousy: *Hyos.*, Ign.

Joy: Coff., Puls.

EXCITEMENT, Love unhappy: Coff., *Hyos.*, *Ign.*, Phos. ac., Staph.

Mortification: Cham., *Coloc.*, *Ign.*, *Ipe.*, *Nat. mur.*, Phos. ac., Seneg., *Staph.*

Reproaches: Ign., *Op.*, *Syph.*

Madness of others: Colch., Staph.

Scorn: Aur., *Bry.*, Cham., Coloc., *Nux v.*

Vexation: Acon., Ant. t., Ars., Bell., Bry., Calc., Cham., *Coff.*, Coloc., *Ign.*, Lyc., Nux v., Op., Phos., *Plat.*, Puls., *Staph.*

With indignation: Coloc, Nux v., *Staph.*

EXERTION mental: Anac., *Calc. c.*, Cocc., Colch., *Ign.*, Lyc., Nat. mur., *Nux v.*, Oleand., Phos. ac., Pso., Saba., *Sep.*, Sil.

Physical: *Arn.*, *Ars.*, *Bry.*, Cannab. s., Cocc., Kalmia, Lyc., Merc., *Nat. mur.*, Nux

EXERTION, Physical.

v., Ox. ac., Phos., Pic. ac., Rheum, *Rhus*, Ruta, Sabi., Sang., Sep., Sil., Sulphur, Zinc.

Of vision: Asaf., Aur., *Calc. c.*, Carb. v., Caust., Cic., Cina, Croc., Graph., *K. carb.*, *Lyc.*, *Nat. c.*, *Nat. mur.*, Phos., Rhodo., Rhus, *Ruta*, Sars., Seneg., Sep., *Sil.*, Spig.

FOOD AND DRINK, alcoholic stimulants in general: Agar., Ant cr., Arg. nit., Ars., Bell., Calc. c., Chel., Chin., Coff., Con., *Lach.*, Led., Lyc., Nat. c., Nat. mur., *Nux v.*, *Op.*, Puls., *Ran. b.*, Rhodo., *Rhus*, Ruta, *Sele.*, Sil., Spig., Stram., Verat., Zinc.

Brandy: Ars Hep., *Nux v.*, *Op.*, Ran. b., Rhus t., Stram., Zinc.

Breakfast: *Puls.*

Butter: Ars., *Carb. veg.*, Cyc., Hep., Puls., Sep., Tar.

Cabbage: *Bry.*, Chin., *Lyc.*, *Petro.*, Puls.

FOOD, eggs: Colchicum.

Odour of: Colchicum.

Fat: Ars., Asaf., *Carbo veg.*, Colch., *Cyc.*, Dros., *Ferr.*, Hell., Mag. mur., Nit. ac., *Puls.*, Sep., Spo., Sul., Thuja.

Fish: Plumbum.

Fruit: *Ars.*, Bor., *Bry.*, Calc. ph., Carbo veg., *Chin.*, Coloc., Mag. mur., Nat. c., *Puls.*, Sele., Sep., Verat. alb.

Garlick odour of: Saba.

Honey: Nat. carb.

Lemonade: Sele.

FOOD.

Meat: Colch., Ferr., Kali bi., Puls.

Milk: Ars., Bry., *Calc. c.*, Carb. veg., Cham., Chel., Chin., Con., Cup., K. carb., Lyc., Nat. c., Nat. mur., *Nit.*, ac., Nux v., Phos., *Sep.*, Sul.

And drink, odor or, and of the cooking: Cocc., *Colch.*

Oil: Bry., Puls.

Onions: Thuja.

Pears: Verat. alb.

Pepper: Cina, Sil.

Smoked: Calc., Sil.

Tobacco: Ant. cr., Bry., Cham., Cocc., Cyc., Euphr., Gel., Hell., *Ign.*, Ipe., Lach., Menth., Meny., Nat. mur., *Nux v.*, Par., Phos., *Puls.*, Ruta, Sele., *Spig.*, *Spo.*, Staph., Tar.

Chewing: Ars.

Vegetables (green): Bry., Hell., Nat. c.

Vinegar: *Ant. cr.*, Ars., Bell., Ferr., Sep., Sul.

Warm: Ambr., Anac., Bar., Bell., *Bry.*, Carb. v., Cham., Cup., Euphor., Kali carb., *Lach.*, Mez., Nit. ac., Phos., Phos. ac., *Puls.*, Rhus tox.

Water, cold: Alum., Ant. cr., Ars., Bell., Canth., Croc., *Ferr.*, Ign., Lyc., Nux v., Rhodo., *Rhus t.*, Spig., Sul.

Wine: Ant. cr., Arn., Ars., Bor., Calc. c., Coff., Lach., *Lyc.*, Nat. c., Nat. mur., Nux m., *Nux v.*, *Op.*, Ran. bul., Rhodo., Saba., Sele., *Sil.*, Zinc.

GONORRHŒA, suppressed:
Agn. c., Aur., Benz. ac.,
Brom., Clem., Daph., Merc.,
Mez., Nit. ac., Puls., Sars.,
Verat., Zinc.

GRASPING, anything tight:
Rhus t.

HANG DOWN, letting limbs:
Alum., Am. carb., Calc.
carb., Sabi., Vip.

HOUSE, in the: Acon., Agn.,
All. c., Aloe., Alum., Amyl.,
Anac., Ant. c., Arg., Ars.,
Asaf., Asar., Atrop., Bry.,
Cact., Cannab. in., Chel.,
Chlorum, Cimic., Coff., Con.,
Croc., Dios., Gam., Hell.,
Hydro. ac., K. bi., Mag.
carb., Mag. mur., Mill.,
Mez., Osm., Phos., Phyt.,
Puls., Ran. s., Rhus t., Saba.,
Sabi., Seneg., Spo., Tab.,
Vib. op., Zinc.

HUNGER: Iod., K. carb., Sil.,
Spig.

INJURIES (includes blows, falls
and bruises): Arn., Con.,
Dul., Hep., Iod., Lach.,
Phos., Puls., Rhus t., Ruta,
Staph., Sul., Sul. ac.

Cuts: Arn., Staph., Sul. ac.

Stabs: Carb. veg., Nit. ac.

Of soft parts: Arn., Con., Puls.,
Sul. ac.

INSPIRATION: Acon., Agar.,
Anac., Arg., Arn., Asar.,
Bor., Bry., Calc.,
Caps., Cham., Chel., Dros.,
Guai., Ipe., K. carb., K. nit.,
Kreo., Lyc., Menth., Meny.,
Merc., Osm., Ran. b., Rhus,
Saba., Sabi., Sele., Seneg.,
Sil., Spig., Spo., Squi., Stan.,
Valer., Zinc.

INTOXICATION, after: Am.
m., Bry., Carb. veg., Cocc.,
Coff., Laur. Nux v., Puls.,
Spo., Stram.

Laughter: Bell., Bor., Carb.
veg., Chin., Mang., Phos.,
Plumb., Stan., Sul.

LIFTING: Arn., Bor., Bry.,
Calc. c., Graph., Lyc., Nat.
c., Phos. ac., Rhus t., Sil.

LIGHT, in general: Acon., Ant.
cr., Bar. c., Bell., Calc. carb.,
Chin., Col., Con., Croc.,
Dros., Euphr., Graph., Hep.,
Merc., Nat. c., Phos., Phos.
ac., Puls., Sep., Sil., Stram.,
Sul.

LIGHT, candle or lamp: Bar. c.,
Bell., Calc., Con., Croc.,
Dros., Graph., Hep., Ign.,
Lyc., Merc., Phos., Phos. ac.,
Ruta, Sep., Sil., Stram.

Day: Ant. cr., Calc., Con.,
Dros., Euphr., Graph., Hep.,
Nux v., Phos., Sep., Sil.

Of fire: Ant. cr., Euphorb.,
Merc., Zinc.

Sun: Ant. cr., Bar. c., Calc. c.,
Chin., Con., Euph., Graph.,
Ign., Nat. c., Nux, Phos. ac.,
Puls., Sul.

LOOKING AROUND: Cic.,
Con.

At distant objects: Ruta.

Downwards: Calc. c., Oleand.,
Spig., Sul.

Straight forward: Oleander.

Over a large surface: Sepia.

At a bright light: Bry., Calc.,
Mag. mur., Merc., Phos.

Long at anything: Aur., Nat.
mur., Ruta, Spig.

LOOKED.

At running water: *Bell.*, *Ferr.*, Hyos.

At shining objects: *Bell.*, Hyos., Stram.

Sideways: Bell., Spig.

At something turning round: Lyc.

Upwards: *Calc.*, Chel., Cup., Phos., Puls, Saba., Sele.

LOSS OF FLUIDS: Ars., Calad., *Calc. c.*, Carbo veg., *Chin.*, Con., Iod., K. carb., Merc., *Nux v.*, Phos., *Phos. ac.*, *Puls.*, Sep., Sil., Squ., *Staph.*, Sul.

LYING: Acon., Ambr., Amm. m., Apis, Arg., *Ars.*, Asaf., Aur., Bapti., Bry., *Caps.*, *Cham.*, Con., Cyc., Dros., Dulc., Euphorb., Euphr., Ferr., Glon., Hell., *Hyos.*, K. nit., Lyc., Mag. m., *Meny.*, Mos., Mur. ac., Nat. c., *Nat. s.*, Nux v., *Phos.*, Phos. ac., *Plat.*, Pb., *Puls.*, Rab. b., *Rhodo.*, Rhus t., *Rumex*, Ruta, Saba., *Samb.*, Sang., Sep., Stram., Sul., Tar., Valer., Verb., Zinc.

Down after: *Ambr.*, Am. carb., Arg., *Ars.*, Asaf., *Aur.*, Caps., Cham., Clem., Cyc., *Dulc.*, Euphorb., Euphr., Ferr., Hyos., K. Carb., Mag. c., Mag. m., Meny., *Plat.* Pb., *Puls.*, Rhus., Saba., *Samb.*, Sep., Sil., *Stron.*, Sul., Sul. ac., Tar.

In bed: *Ambr.*, Am. carb., Ant. t., Arg., *Ars.*, Aur., Bor., Bry., Clem., Coloc., Dros., Euphorb., Ferr., *Iod.*, K. carb., Kalm., Lach., Led., Lil. t., Lith., Lyc., Mag.

LYING, in bed.

carb., Mang., *Merc.*, Merc., i.f., Mez., Nat. mur., Nux v., *Phos.*, Phos. ac., Plat., Pb., Puls., Rhodo., Rhus t., *Rumex*, Sang., Sars., Sele., Sep., Sil., Spig., Stro., *Sul.*, Tell., Verat. a., Zinc.

On back: Amm. m., Ars., Caust., Cham., Coloc. Cup., Iod., K. nit., *Nux v.*, Phos., Rhus, Sep., Sil., Sul.

With head low: Ant. t., Arg., Ars., Chin., Colch., Hep., K. nit., *Puls.*, Spig.

On side: *Acon.*, *Anac.*, Bry., Calc. c., Carb. an., Cina., Con., Ferr., Ign., Ipe., K. carb., Kreo., *Lyc.*, Merc., Merc. cor., Par., Puls., Rhus, Seneg., Stan., Sul.

Left: Acon., Am. carb., Bar. c., Cact., Colch., Nat. c., Nat. mur., Nat. sul., Par., *Phos.*, *Puls.*, Sep., Sul., Thuja.

Right: Amm. m., Benz. ac., Bov., Mag. m., *Merc.*, Nux v., Phos., Rumex, Spo.

Painful: Acon., Am. carb., Ars., Bap., *Bar. carb.*, Bry., Calad., Chin., Dros., Graph., *Hep.*, Iod., Lyc., Mag. c., Mag. m., Merc., Mos., Nit. ac., *Nux mos.*, Nux vom., Par., Phos., Phos. ac., Rheum, Rhus, Rumex, *Ruta*, Saba., Spon.

Painless: Ambr., Arg., *Bry.*, Calc. c., Cham., Coloc., Ign., K. carb., *Puls.*, Rhus t., Sep., Stan., Vio. t.

MEASLES, after: Bell., Hyos., Puls., Rhus.

MERCURY, abuse of: Ant. cr.,
Arg., Asaf., *Aur.*, Bell.,
Calc. c., *Carb. v.*, Chin.,
Clem., Colch., Cup., Euph-
orb., Guai., *Hep.*, Iod.,
Lach., Led., Mez., *Nit. ac.*,
Puls., Sars., Sil,. *Staph.*,
Sul.

Fumes of: Chin., Stram.

MOON, new: Caust., Cup., Sep.
Full: Graph.. Sep. Sul.
Waning: Ant. cr.

MOTION: Acon., Agn., Apis,
Arg., Arn., Ars. iod., Asaf.,
Asar., Aur., *Bell.*, *Bism.*,
Bry., Calad., Camph., Can-
nab. s., Caps., Carb. an.,
Chel., Cimic., Cocc., Coff.,
Colch., Croc., Dig., Eup.
per., Ferr., Glon., Graph.,
Hell., Hep., K. carb., K. nit.,
Kalm., *Led.*, Lil. t., Mill.,
Merc., Nat. m., Nat. s., Nit.
ac., *Nux v.*, Onos., Ox. ac.,
Phos., *Puls.*, *Ran. b.*,
Rheum., *Sabi.*, Sang., Sars.,
Sele., Sep., *Sil.*, *Spig.*, Squ.,
Stan., Staph., Stro., *Sul.*,
Ther., Verat. alb.

After: *Agar.*, Anac., *Ars.*, Can-
nab. s., Carb. v., Croc., Hyos.,
K. carb., *Puls.*, *Rhus t.*,
Ruta, *Spo.*, *Stan.*, Stram.,
Valer., Zinc.

Of affected part: Acon., Æsc.,
Ant. t., *Arn.*, Bell., *Bry.*,
Cannab. s., Caps., *Cham.*,
Chin., Cocc., Coloc., Gels.,
Glon., Kalm., *Led.*, Merc.,
Mez., Nux v., Puls., Ran. b.,
Rheum., Rhus t., Sabi.,
Sang., Sars., *Spig.*, Stan.,
Sul.

MOTION of head: Arn., Bell.,
Bry., Calc. c., Caps., Cup.,
Hell., *Lach.*, Lyc., Mez.,

MOTION, of head.
Mos., Nat. c., Rhus, Sep.,
Spig.

Of eyes: Bell., Bry., Caps.,
Cham., Cup., Hep., *Nux v.*,
Op., Spig., Sul., Valer.

Of eye-lids: Coloc.

Of arms: Acon., Anac., Dig.,
Led., Ran. b., Rhus, Sul.

MUSIC: Acon., Cham., Coff.,
Dig., *Nat. c*, *Nux v.*, Phos.
ac., Sep., Vio. o.

NARCOTICS: Bell., Cham.,
Coff., Dig., Graph., Hyos.,
Ipe., *Lach.*, Lyc., *Nux v.*,
Op., Puls., Sep., Valer.

NARRATING SYMPTOMS,
while: Calc. c., Mar.

NOVIES: Acon., Arn., Bell.,
Calc. c., Cham., *Coff.*, Colch.,
Con., Ign., Lyc., Nat. c.,
Nux v., Phos. ac., Sep., Spig.,
Ther.

NURSING CHILDREN: Bell.,
Bor., Bry., Calc. c., Cham.,
Chin., Dulc., Phos. ac.,
Puls., *Sep.*, Staph.

ODORS, strong: Acon., *Aur.*,
Bell., Cham., Chin., *Coff.*,
Colch., Graph., *Ign.*, *Lyc.*,
Nux v., *Phos.*, Sul.

Of wood: Graphites.

ONANISM: Arg., *Calc.*, Carb.
v., *Chin.*. Con.. Iod., Lyc.,
Merc., Nat. m., Phos., *Phos.
ac.*, Puls.. Sele., *Sep.*, Spig.,
Staph., Sulphur.

OPEN AIR: Acon., Agar., Ant.
t., Ars., Bry., Camph., Carb.
an., Carb. v., Cham., Chel.,
Chin., Clem., Cocc., Coff.,
Con., Ferr., Guai., Hell.

OPEN AIR.

Hep., Kre., Lach., Mar., Merc., Mur. ac., Nat. m., *Nux m., Nux v.*, Petro., Phos., Poly., Rhus, *Rumex,* Sele., Seneg., Sep., *Sil.,* Spig., Stram., Sul., Valer.

PIANO, playing the: Nat. c., Sep.

PREGNANCY: Asar., *Bell.,* Bry., Calc., Caps., Caust., *Cham.,* Cocc., Croc., Hyos., Ipe., Nux m., Plat., *Puls.,* Rhus, *Sabi.,* Sec. c., *Sep.,* Sul.

PRESSURE, of clothes: Bry., Calc. c., Caps., Carb. v., Caust., Hep., *Lach.,* Lil. t., *Lyc., Nux v.*, Sars., Sep., Stan.

PUNCTURES: Carb. v., *Nit. ac.,* Hep., Sil.

READING: Agn., Asaf., Bell., *Calc. c.,* Carb. ac., Chin., Cina, Cocc., Con., Dulc., Graph., Hep., K. carb., Lyc., *Nat. mur.,* Nux v., Oleand., Op., Puls., Rhodo., *Ruta,* Seneg., Sep., Sil., Sul. ac., Verb.

Aloud: *Carb. v.*, Mang., Menth., Par., *Phos.,* Verb.

REST: Acon. Aloe., Amm. m., *Ars.,* Atrop., *Aur.,* Bry., *Caps.,* Cocc., Coloch., *Con.,* Cyc., *Dios.,* Dros., *Dulc.,* *Euphor., Ferr.,* Fl. ac., *Gam., Lyc.,* Mag. m., Meny., Merc. cor., Merc. i. f., Mos., Phos. ac., Plat., *Puls., Rhodo., Rhus, Saba.,* Samb., Sep., *Sul., Tar., Valer.,* Verb., Vib. op., Vio. t., Zinc.

ROCKING: Borax, Carb. v.

ROOM, full of people: Hell.; Lyc., Mag. c., Phos., Puls., Sep., Sul.

RUBBING: *Anac.,* Bism., Calad., Caps., Caust., Coff., Con., Led., Mez., Puls., *Sep.,* Sil., Stro., Sul.

Gently (stroking): Mar.

SALTS, (salty food): Carbo veg., Dros.

SEXUAL EXCESSES: Agar., Bov., Calc. c., Carb. v., Chin., Con., Iod., K. carb., Merc., Nat. c., *Nux v.,* Phos., *Phos. ac.,* Puls., Sep., Sil., Spig., Staph.

Desire suppressed: *Con.*

SEXUAL, excitement: Bufo., Lil. t.

SOCIETY: Bar. c., Lyc.

Strangers, among: Sep, Stram.

Storm, approach of a: *Rhodo.*

Thunder during: Nat. c., Rhodo., Sil.

SUN, in the: Agar., *Ant. cr.,* Bar. c., Bry., Camph., Euphr., Lach., *Nat. c., Puls.,* Sele., Valer.

SWALLOWING: Acon., Æsc., Ant. t., *Apis*, Ars., Atrop., Bar. c., *Bell., Brom., Bry.,* Canth., Cocc., Croc., Dol., Gel., *Hep.,* Hydras., Iod., Lach., *Merc.,* Merc. c., Merc. d., Merc. i. f., Mur. ac., *Nit. ac.,* Nux v., Perol., Phos., Phyt., Pb., Puls., Rhus, Sang., Sep., Sil., Stan., Staph., *Stram.,* Sul., Thuja, Wye.

SWALLOWING.

Empty: Bar. c., Bry., *Cocc.*, Hep., *Lach.*, Merc., Puls., Rhus.

Of food: Bar. c., *Bry.*, Hep., Nit. ac., Nux v., Petrol., Phos., Rhus, Sep., *Sul.*

Liquids: *Bell.*, Canth., Iod., *Lach.*, Merc., Merc. c., *Phos.*, Stram.

SWEAT, suppressed: *Bell.*, Bry., *Calc. c.*, Cham., *Chin.*, Lyc., Merc., Nux v., Phos., Rhus., Sep., *Sul.*

TALKING: Acon. Ambr., *Anac.*, Arg., Arn., Arum t., Bell., Bry., *Calc. c.*, Cannab. s., Carb. v., Cham., *Chin.*, Cimic., *Cocc.*, Dros., Dulc., Ferr., Graph., Iod., K. bi., Mag. m., *Mang.*, Menth., *Nat. c., Nat. m., Phos. ac., Rhus.*, Sars., *Sele.*, Sep., Sil., Spig., *Stan.*, *Sul.*, Verat. alb.

THINKING, of his disease: Bar. c., Nux v., Ran. b., Saba.

Of something else: Camph., Hell.

UNCOVERING: Acon. Ars., Atrop., Aur., Bry., Cic., Clem., Cocc., Colch., Con., Dulc., *Hep.*, Nux m., Nux v., Rhodo., *Rhus*, Rumex, Samb., Sil., Squ., Stro.

WARMTH: Agar., All. c., Ant. t., Apis, Bism., Bry., Dros., *Iod.*, Led., Nat. m., *Puls.*, Sec. c., Seneg., Sul.

Of bed: Alum., Apis, Carb. v., *Cham.*, Cocc., Coc. c., *Dros.*, Graph., Iod., *Led.*, Lyc., *Merc.*, Nux m., Phos. ac., *Puls.*, Sabi., Sec. c., Spo., Sul., Thuja, Verat. alb.

Of room: Agn., Alum., Anac., Ant. cr., Asar., Brom., Bry., Croc., *Iod.*, Lil. t., Nat. c., Pic. ac., *Puls.*, Sabi., Senag., Spo.

WEEPING: Arn., Bell., Croc., Cup., Mar., Verat. alb.

WET APPLICATION: *Amm. carb.*, Ant. cr., Bell., *Calc. c.*, Canth., Carb. v., Cham., *Clem.*, K. nit., Lyc., Merc., *Rhus*, Sep., Spig., Stro., Sul.

Getting: Bell., Bry., Calc. c., Colch., Dulc., Hep., Ipe., Lyc., Nux m., Puls., *Rhus*, Sars., Sep.

Head: Bell., Puls.

With sweat: Acon., Dulc., *Rhus*, Sep.

AMELIORATION.

ALONE, when: *See* Aggravation from society.

ASCENDING: Con., Ferr., Rhodo.

ATTENTION, paying: Camph., Hell.

BATHING: Amm. m., Apis, *Asar.*, Bor., Caust., Chel., Euphr., Pic. ac., Pso., *Puls.*, Spig.

BENDING BACKWARD: Bell., Cham., Cocc., Lach., Rhus, *Seneg.*, Thuja.

Inward: Bell., Sabina.

Sideways: Puls., Sep.

Head backward: Cham., Hep.

BITING: Staph.

BLINKING EYES: Euphr.

BORING in with finger (Ear or Nose): Chel., Nat. c., Phos., Spig., Thuja.

COLD, in the: (*See* aggravation from warmth).

Being: Bry., Cham., Dros., *Iod.*, Led., *Lyc.*, Merc., *Puls.*, Sabi., Sec. c., Verat. alb.

DARKNESS: Acon., Ant. cr., Bar. c., Bell., *Calc. c.*, Chin., Con., Croc., Dros., *Euphr.*, *Graph.*, Hep., Ign., Lyc., Merc., Nat. c., Nux v., *Phos.*, Phos. ac., Puls., Sep., Sil., Stram., Sul.

DRIVING in a wagon: Graph., *Nit. ac.*

EATING, on: Alum., Ambr., *Anac.*, Caps., Chel., Croc., *Ign.*, *Lach.*, Mer., Sep., Spig., Zinc.

After: Anac., Bov., Bry.

To satiety: Iod.

ERUCTATIONS: Ant. t., Arg. n., Aur., Bar. c., Bty., Canth., *Carb. v.*, Chel., Cocc., Dig., Dios., *Graph.*, Ign., K. *carb.*, Lyc., Nat. c., Nit. ac., Nux v., *Sang.*, *Sep.*, Sil.

EXERTING BODY: Ign., *Rhus*, Sep.

FASTING (before breakfast): Bry., Caust., *Cham.*, Chin., Con., Dig., K. carb., *Nat. m.*, Nux m., Phos. ac., Sil., Zinc.

FOOD AND DRINK:

Bread: Caust., Nat. c.

Coffee: Ars., *Cham.*

Fruit: Lach.

Meat: Verat alb.

Milk: Arsenic.

Salt: Mag. c.

Tobacco: Hep., Sepia.

Water, cold: Ant. t., Asar., Bry., *Caust.*, Clem., Cup., Phos., Puls., *Sep.*

Warm: Lyc., Nux v., Rhus.

Wine: Acon., Canth., Carb. ac., Con. Op.

INSPIRATION: Chin., *Colch.*, Cup., Dig., *Ign.*, Lach., Oleand., Puls., Seneg., *Spig.*, Stan.

LEANING, against anything: Carb. v., *Ferr.*, Sep.

Against anything hard: Rhus, Sep.

LIGHT: Carb. an., Carb. v., Plat., *Stro.*

Bright: Amm. m., Calc. c., Carb. an., Plat., *Stro.*, Valer.

LOOKING DOWNWARD: Saba.

Intently: Nat. c.

Sideways: Oleander.

Straight ahead-Bell.

LOOSENING Clothes: Bry., *Calc. carb.*, Cannab. i., Caps., Carb. v., Caust., Hep., *Lach.*, *Lyc.*, *Nux v.*, Sars., Sep., Stan.

LYING: Amm. m., Arn., Asar., Bell., Bry., Calc., Calc. phos., Canth., Carb. an., Colch., *Ferr.*, Glon., Led., Nat. m., *Nux v.*, Spig., Spo., Squ., Verat. alb.

After: *Ars.*, Bell., Bry., *Calc.*, Canth., Carv. v., Cina, Croc., Graph., Hep., Lach., Merc., Nat. m., Nit. ac., *Nux v.*, Oleand., Puls., Sep., Spig., *Squ.*, Staph., Stram., Sul.

LYING, in bed: Bry., Canth., Caust., Cic., Cocc., Coc., c., Con., Hep., Lach., Lyc., *Nux v.*, Rhus., Sil., *Squ.*, Stan., Staph., Stram.

In bed hard: Rhus.

LYING.

On back: Anac., *Bry.*, Calc., Carb. an. K. carb., Lyc., *Merc. c.*, Phos., *Puls.*, *Rhus*, Sang., Stan.,

On side: *Cocc.*, *Nux v.*, Phos., Sep.

On side (left): (See aggravation lying on right side).

On side (right): (See aggravation lying on left side).

On side (painful): *Bry.*, Calc. Cham., Coloc., Puls.

MOISTENING, affected parts Amm. m., *Asar.*, Bor., Caust., Chel., Euphr., *Puls.*, Spig.

MOTION: (*See* aggravation rest).

READING: Nat. carb.

REST: (*See* aggravation motion).

RUBBING: Alum., Amm. m., Arn., Ars., Asaf., *Calc. c.*, *Canth.*, *Carb. ac.*, Cyc., Dros., Guai., Ign., Merc., Mur. ac., Nat. c., Nux v., *Phos.*, Ruta, Sul., Thuja, Zinc.

SEXUAL SUPPRESSION: Calad.

SOCIETY: (*See* aggravation, alone, when).

STOOL, after: Amm. m., Ars., Asaf., Bor., *Bry.*, Colch., Coloc., Con., Lept., Oxyt., Puls., Rheum, *Rhus*, *Spig.*, Sul.

SUNLIGHT: Plat., Stro.

SWALLOWING: Ambr., Arg., Arn., Caps., *Ign.*, Lach., Led., Nit. ac., Nux v., Spon.

SWEAT, during: Bov., Calad., Cup.

After: Acon., Bry., Calad., Canth., *Cham.*, Graph., Hep., Olean., *Rhus,*

Cold: Nux v.

TWILIGHT, in the: Bry., Phos.

WARMTH, in general: (*See* aggravation cold in general).

WARMTH, of bed: *Ars., Bry.,* Caust., Coloc., Hep., K. carb., *Lyc., Nux v.,* Rumex. Saba.

WEEPING: Lycopodium.

MIND AND DISPOSITION.

ABSENT-MINDED: Acon., Alum., Amm. c., Anac., *Apis*, Arn., Aur., Bar. c., Bell., Bor., Calad., Cann. i., *Caust.*, *Cham.*, Cic., Cocc., Colch., Cupr., Graph., Hell., Hyos., Ign., Kali br., Kali carb., Kali phos., Kreos., Lac. c., *Lach.*, Lyc, Mag. c., Merc., *Mez.*, *Nat. m.*, *Nux m.*, *Plat.*, Plb., Puls., Rhus, Sep., Sil., Sulph., Verat.

When reading: Nux m.

ABSORBED: Arn., Caps., Cocc., *Mez.*, Nat. m., *Nux m.*, Onos., Op., Puls., *Sulph.*

ABUSIVE: Anac., Bell., Hydroph., Hyos., Lyss., Nux v., Petro., Seneg., Sep. Verat.

Scolds until the lips get blue and eyes stare and she falls down fainting: Moschus.

AFFECTIONATE: Croc., Ign., Nat. m., Puls.

ANGER: *Acon.*, *Anac.*, Apis, *Ars.*, Ars i., *Aur.*, Bell., Bry., Calc., Calc. phos., Caps., Carb. an., Carb. s., Carb. v., Caust., *Cham.*, Cocc., Coff., Coloc., Con., Croc., Dulc. Graph., *Hep.*, Hyos., *Ign.*, *Kali.* c., Kali p., Kali s., Led., Lyc., Mez., Mosch., Mur. ac., *Nat. m.*, Nat. s., Nit. acid., *Nux v.*, Pall., Petro., Phos., Phos.

ANGER.

ac., Psor., Rhus t., *Sep.*, Stann., *Staph.*, Stront. *Sulph.*, Tarent., Thuja, Zinc.

AILMENTS, after anger: Acon., Ant. t., Apis, Ars., Aur., Aur. mur., Bell., Bry., Calc. phos., *Cham.*, Cocc., Coff., Coloc., Gels., *Ign.*, *Ipecac.*, Kali. ph., Lyc., Nat. m., *Nux v.*, *Op.*, Phos., Phos. ac., *Plat.*, Puls., *Staph.*

CONTRADICTION, from: Anac., *Aur.*, Bry., Ferr., Ign., *Lyc.*, Nicc., Nux v., Sep., Sil., Thuja.

Suppressed from: Ign., *Staph.*

ANGUISH: Acon., Anac., Apis., Arg. n., Arn., *Ars.*, Aur., Bism., *Bell.*, Calc., Cann. i., Carb. v., *Caust.*, Coff., Cupr., *Dig.*, Graph., *Hep.*, Kali. ar., Mag. c., Phos., *Plat.*, Psor.

ANSWER, aversion to: Agar., Arn., Coloc., *Glon.*, Hyos., Kali p., Manc., Nat. m., Phos. ac., Phos., Puls., Sec., Stann., Sulph., Sul. ac.

Refuses to: Agar., Arn., Camph., Chin., Cimic., Hell., Hyos., *Phos.*, *Sulph.*, Sul. ac., Verat.

Stupor returns quickly after: Arn., *Hyos.*

ANXIETY: Abrot., Acon. f., Acet. ac., Æth., All. c., Alum., Ambr., Amm. c., Anac., Ant. c., Ant. t., Arg. m., *Arg. n.*, Arn., Ars., *Ars. i.*, Asar., *Aur.*, Bar. c., Bar. m., Bell., Bism., Bor., *Bry.*, *Cact., Calc., Calc. ph.*, Calc. s., *Camph., Cann. i.*, Canth., Carb. an., Carb. o., *Carb. s., Carb. v.*, Caust., Cham., Chel., Chin., Chin. a., Cimex, Cocc., Coff., Coloc., Cupr., *Dig.*, Dros., Euph., Ferr., Ferr. ar., Ferr. i., Flu. ac., Gra., Hell., Hep., Ign., Iod., Jatr., *Kali. ar.*, *Kali. carb.*, Kali i., Kali nit., *Kali ph., Kali s.*, Lach., Laur., Led., Lil. t., *Lyc.*, Mag. c., Mag. m., Mag. s., Merc., Merc. c., *Mez.*, Mur. ac., *Nat. a., Nat. c.*, Nat. m., Nit. ac., Nux, Op., Petr., Ph. ac., *Phos.*, Plat., Plb., *Psor.*, Puls., Pyrog., *Rhus, Ruta, Sabad, Sabina*, Samb., Sec., Seneg., Sep., Sil., Spig., Spong., Stan., Stram., *Sulph.*, Tab., Thuja, *Verat.*, Zinc.

Air, in open: Acon., Anac., Ant., c., Arg. m., Bar. c., Bell., Cact., Cina, Hep., Ign., Plat., Spig., Tab.

Conscience, of (as if guilty of a crime): *Alum.*, Amm. c., *Ars., Aur.*, Carb. v., Caust., Chel., Cocc., Con., *Dig.*, Ferr., Graph., Ign., Med., Merc., Nat. m., Nux v., *Psor.*, Sil., Sulph., Thuja, Verat., Zinc.

Menses, before: Cocc., Graph., Ign., Nat. m., Nit. ac., Nux v., Stan., Sulph.

During: Bell., Nat. m., Plat.

ANXIETY.

Salvation, about: Ars., Aur., Calc., Camph., **Graph.**, *Lach., Lil. t.*, Lyc., **Med.**, Mez., Psor., Puls., Sulph., Thuja, *Verat.*

Stool, before: Ars., Bor., **Merc.**

During: Verat.

After: Calc., Caust., Nit. ac.

Storm, during a thunder: Nat. c., Nit. ac., *Phos.*

Suicidal: Aur., Dros., Merc., Puls., Rhus.

Urination, before: **Alum., Dig.**, Phos. ac., Sep.

During: Acon., **Cham.**

After: Dig.

AVARICE: *Ars., Lyc., Puls.,* **Sep.**

AVERSION, approached, to being: Iod.

Everything to: Puls.

Friends, to: Ledum.

During pregnancy: Conium.

Husband: Glon., Sep.

Members of family to: Calc., Crot. tig., Flu. ac., Nat. c., *Sep.*

Persons, to certain: Calc., *Nat. carb.*

BAD NEWS, ailments from: Apis, *Calc.*, **Gels.**, Ign., Med., Nat. m., Pall., Sulphur.

Barking: Bell., Canth.

BITING: *Bell.*, Calc., Camph., Canth., Carb. s., Hyos., Lach., Lyss., Phyt., *Stram.*, Verat.

Blood, cannot look at, or a knife: *Alum.*

CAPRICIOUSNESS: Ars., Bell., *Bry.*, *Cham.*, *Cina*, *Coff.*, Dulc., *Ipecac*, *Kali c.*, Puls., Rheum, *Staph.*, Sulph.

CAREFULNESS: Iod., Nux v.

CARRIED, desires to be: Ars., *Cham.*, Cina, Lyc., Kali c., Rhus t., Verat.

CHEERFUL (gay, happy): Acon., Arg. m., Aur., Bell., Cann. i., Carb. an., Cinnab., *Coff.*, *Croc.*, Fl. ac., *Hyos.*, Ign., *Lach.*, Lyc., *Nat. c.*, Nit. ac., Nux m., Nux v., Op., Phos., Plat., Sars., Sulph., Sul. ac., Tarax., Verat., Zinc.

CHILL, during: Cann. s., Puls.
Coition after: Nat. m.
Constipated, when: Calc., Psor.
Menses, before: Acon., Fl. ac., Hyos.
During: Fl. ac.
Stools, after: Bor., *Nat. s.*

CHILDISH BEHAVIOUR: Apis, Arg. n., *Bar. c.*, Bar. m., Carb. s., *Cic.*, Croc., Ign., Nux m., Stram.

CLAIRVOYANCE: Lyss., Nux m., Phos.

CLINGING, child awakens terrified, knows no one, screams, clings to those near: Stramonium.

COMPANY, aversion: Aloe, Ambr., Anac., Aur., Aur. s., *Bar. c.*, Bell., Bry., Cact., Calc. p., *Carb. an.*, Cham., Chin., Cic., Coloc., Con., Cupr., Dig., Ferr., Gels., Hell., Hep., Hipp., Hyos., *Ign.*, Iod., Lac. d., Lach., Led., Lyc., Nat. c., *Nat. m.*,

COMPANY.
Nux v., Oxyt., Plat., Puls., Rhus t., Selen., Sep., Stann., Sulph.

COMPANY. aversion to:
Dread being alone, yet: Clem., Con.
Menses during: Plat., Sep.
Pregnant, when: Lach.
People intolerable to her during stool: Ambra. gr.
During urination: *Nat. m.*
Desire for: Apis, *Arg. n.*, Ars., Bism., Calc., Camph., Clem., Con., Elaps., Gels., *Hyos.*, Ign., Kali ar., *Kali c.*, Kali p., Lil. t., *Lyc.*, Mez., Pall., *Phos.*, Stram.

CONFIDENCE, want of self: *Anac.*, Aur., Bar. c., Bry., Chin., Kali c., Lac. c., Lyc., Puls., Sil.

CONFUSION OF MIND: Acon., Æsc., Æth., Agar., Alum., Anac., Ant. t., Apoc., Arg. n., Arn., Ars., Asar., Aur., Bapt., Bar. c., Bar. m., *Bell.*, Bism., Bor., Bov., Bry., Bufo., *Calc.*, Calc. p., *Cann. i.*, Cann. s., Canth., Carb. an., Carb. s., *Carb. v.*, Chel., *Cocc.*, Coff., Coloc., Con., Croc., Dros., Dulc., Fago., Ferr., Gels., Glon., Graph., Hell., Hyos., Hyper, Kali c., Kreos., Lac. c., Lach., Laur., Lyc., Mag. c., *Merc.*, Mez., Mosch., Nat. c., *Nat. m.*, Nux m., *Nux v.*, Onos., Op., *Petr.*, Ph. ac., Phos., Plb., Psor., Puls., *Rhus t.*, Sabad., Sec., Seneg., *Sep.*, *Sil.*, Spig., Stap., Stram., Sulph., Tab., **Thuja**, Verat., Zinc

CONFUSION.

Heat, during the: Bapt., Hyos.

Injury to head, after: *Nat. s.*

Loses his way in well-known streets: *Glon.*, Nux m., Petr.

Menses before: Cimic., Sep.

during: Am. c., Cimic., Cocc., Lyc., Phos.

after: Graph., Nat. m.

Sprituous liquors from: Alum., Con., *Nux v.*

CONFUSION, sun, in the: Nat c.

Warm room, in: Iod., *Lyc.*, Puls., Sulph.

C O N S C I E N T I O U S-NESS ABOUT TRIFLES:
Ars., Bar. c., *Ign.*, Lyc., Mur. ac., Nat. c., Nux v.

CONSOLATION, agg.: Ars., Bell., Calc. p., Ign., Lil. t., *Nat. m.*, Nit. ac., Plat., *Sep.*, Sil.

CONTEMPTUOUS: Ars., Chin., *Cic.*, Ip., Lyc., Nux v., Plat.

Self: Agn., Cop.

Contradiction, disposition to: Aur., Canth., Caust., Lyc.

Is intolerant of: *Aur.*, Bry., Cocc., Ferr., Helon., *Ign.*, *Lyc.*, *Sep.*, Sil.

COWARDICE: Acon., Bar. c., Bry., Chin., *Gels.*, *Lyc.*, Puls., Sil., Verat.

CURSING: *Anac.*, Hyos., Lac. c., Lil. t., Nit. ac., Verat.

All night, and complains of stupid feeling: Verat.

Convulsions, during: Ars.

DEATH, desires: *Aur.*, Kreos., Lach., Merc., Nat. m., Rhus t., Sil., Sulph.

Presentiment of: *Acon.*, Agn., *Apis*, Arg. n., Bell., Cench., Chel., Graph., Hep., Lach., Lyc., Med., Nit. ac., Nux v., Phos., Plat.

Predicts the time: Acon., Arg. n.

DECEIPTFUL: Arg. n., Bufo, Chlor., Coca, Dros.

DELIRIUM: Acon., Act. sp., Æth., *Agar.*, *Ars.*, *Arum. t.*, Aur., Bapt., *Bell.*, *Bry.*, Calc., Camph., Cann. i., Canth., Carb. s., Cham., *Chel.*, Cic., China, Colch., Con., Crot. tig., Cupr., Dig., Dulc., Gels., *Hyos.*, Ip., *Lach.*, Meli., Merc., Merc. c., *Nit. ac.*, Nux m., Nux v., *Op.*, Petr., Phos., Plb., Puls., *Rhus t.*, Sec., *Stram.*, Sulph., Tereb., *Verat.*, *Verat. v.*

DELIRIUM, Apathetic: Phos. ac., Verat.

Arms throws about: Bell.

Attacks people with knife: Hyos.
Bellows like a calf: Cupr.

Changing subject rapidly: *Lach.*
Cheerful: Bell.

Chill, owing: Arn., Bell., *Nat m.*, Sep., Verat.

Closing the eyes, on: Lach.

Erotic: Canth., Lach., Phos., Stram.

Fantastic: Bell., Stram., Sulph.
Fierce: Stram.

Alternating with language, sighing, whistling, crying etc.: Stram.

Laughing: Bell., Hyos., Ign., Stram.

DELIRIUM.

Loquacious: Bell., *Cimic.*, Cupr., Hyos., *Lach.*, *Lachn.*, Op., Phos., Plat., Rhus t., *Stram.*, Verat.

Maniacal: Æth., *Bell.*, Camph., Canth., Coff., Cupr., Hell., *Hyos.*, Op., Sec., *Stram.*, Verat.

Mouth, moves lips as if talking: Bell.

Picking at nose or lips with: Arum. t.

Quiet: *Bry.*, Carb. v., Chel., *Hyos.*

Raging, raving: Acon., Act. sp., Æth., *Agar.*, Ant. t., *Bell.*, Camph., *Canth.*, Carb. s., Cimic., Cupr., Hell., *Hyos.*, Lyc., Merc., *Nit. ac.*, Op., Plb., Pub., Sec., Sol. n., Stram., Tab., *Verat.*

Religious: Verat.

Repeats the same sentence: Camph.

Water, jumping into: Bell., Sec.

Wedding, prepares for: Hyos.

DELUSIONS, IMAGINATIONS, HALLUCINATIONS, Illusions: Acon., Æth., Ambr., Ars., *Arg. n.*, Aur., Aur. m., Bapt., *Bell.*, Calc., Camph., *Cann. i.*, Cann. s., Cocc., Coff., Glon., Hell., *Hyos.*, Ign., Kali bromatum, *Lach.*, Lyc., Merc., Nit. ac., Op., *Petr.*, Phos. ac., Phos., Plat., Psor., Puls., Rhus, *Sabad.*, Sec. Sil., Staph., *Stram.*, *Sulph.*, Valer., Zinc.

Affection of friends, has lost: Aur.

Alone, she is in the world: Plat., Puls.

DELUSIONS.

Animals of: Æth., Ars., Bell., Calc., Cimic., Colch., Crot. h., Hyos., Med., Op., Plb., Stram., Valer., Thuja.

Black, on walls and furniture sees: Bell.

Rats, mice, insect etc.: Æth., Cimic., Med.

Arrested, is about to be: Zinc.

Assaulted, is going to be: Tarent.

Beautiful: Cann. i., Lach., Sulph.

Rags, seem even: Sulphur.

Birds, sees: Bell., Kali c., Lac. c.

Black objects and people: Stram.

Body, greatness of, as to: Cann. i., Plat.

Lighter than air: Lach., *Op.*, Thuja.

Scattered about bed, tossed about to get pieces together: Bapt., Phos.

Cancer, has a: Verat.

Castles and palaces, sees: Plb.

Child, thinks he is again a: Cic.

Chin, too long is: Glon.

Corner, sees something coming out of: Phos.

Corners of houses seem to project so that he fears he will run against them while walking in the streets: Arg. n.

DELUSIONS, dead persons, sees: Anac., Ars., Bell., Hep., Hyos., Kali br., Kali. c., Lach., Mag. c.

All her friends are dead and she must go to a convent: Lac. d.

Dead brother and child: Con., Plb.

husband: Plb.

sister: Agar.

DELUSIONS.

That he himself was dead: Lach.
her child was dead: Kali br.
his mother is dead: Lach.

Deserted, forsaken: *Arg. n.,*
Cycl., Kali br., Plat., Stram.

Despised, that he is: *Arg. n.*

Devils, sees: Anac., Bell., Plat.,
Puls.

Disease, that he has every:
Aur. m.
is incurable: Arg. n., Sabad.

Divided into two parts: Bapt.
or cut into two: Plat.

Divine, thinks he is: Cann. i.,
Stram.

Dreaming when awake imagines
himself: Bell.

Emperor, thought himself an:
Cann. i.

Encaged in wires: Cimic.

Enemy, everyone is an: Merc.

Enlarged: Cann. i., Op., Plat.
Eyes are: Bell., Op.
objects are: Cann. .
scrotum is swollen: Sabad.
Tall very, is: Op., Pall.,
Stram.

Faces, sees: Bell., Calc., Sulph.
On closing eyes: Arg. n.,
Bell., Bry., *Calc.*

Fire houses, on: Bell., Hep.,
Stram.

DELUSIONS, Fire, room is on:
Stram.

World is on: Hep.

Floating in air: Lach., Nux m.

Fortune, that he was going to
loose his: Psor., Staph.

Glass, that she is made of:
Thuja.

Goitre, imagines he has a: Indig.

DELUSIONS.

Grave, that he is in his: Stram.

Great person, is: Cann. i., Plat.

Halves, left half does not belong
to her: Sil.

Happy, that he will never be,
in his own house: Ars.

Head, belongs to another: Ther.
Can lift it off: Ther.
Seems too large: Acon.
Two, thinks she has: Nux m.

Heaven, is in: Cann. i., Op.

Home, thinks it at, when not:
Cann. i., Hyos.
Thinks is away from: Bry.,
Coff., Op., Rhus.

Husband, thinks he is not her:
Anac.

Identity, errors of personal:
Alum., Ant. c., Bapt., Cann.
s., Gels., Lac. c., Lach.,
Petr., Phos., Plb., Pyrus.,
Stram., Thuja, Val.

Insane, that she will become:
Acon., Chel., Cimic., Manc.
That people think her: Calc c.

Labor, pretends to be in, or
thinks she has pains: Verat.

Marble statue, felt as if he
were: Cann. i.

Mind and body separated:
Anac., Thuja.

Money, as if counting: Alum.,
Bell., Cycl., Mag. c., Zinc.

Murder, thinks she is about to,
her husband and child:
Kali br.

Murder, that he has to. some
one: Ars.

Murdered, that he would be:
Op.

Murderer, that everyone around
him is a: Plb.

DELUSIONS.

Music, fancies he hears: Cann. i., Lach., Stram.

sweetest and sublimest melody: Lach.

Naked, thinks is: Stram.

Narow, everything seems too: Plat.

People converses, with absent: Stram.

Poisoned, thought he had been: Hyos.

that he was about to be: Rhus t.

medicine being: Lach.

Pregnant, thought herself: Sabad., Verat.

Prince, he is a: Verat.

Pursued, police by: Hyos., Kali br.

Queen, thinks she is: Cann. i.

Room, garden is a: Calc.

Shoot, tries to, with a cane: Merc.

Sick, imagines himself: Ars., Calc., Iod., Kali c., Lyc., Sabad., Sepia.

Snakes in and around her: Hyos., Lac. c.

Sold, as if would be: Hyos.

Soldiers, sees: Bel.

Soul, fancied body was too small for: Anac., Cann. i., Thuja.

Spectres, ghosts, spirits, sees: Ars., Bell., Camph., Hyos., Nat. c., Op., Stram., Sulph.

on closing eyes: Bry., Calc., Lach., Sulph., Thuja.

Thieves, sees Nat. m.

after a dream, and will not believe the contrary until search is made: Nat. m.

DELUSIONS.

dreams of robbers, is frightened on waking, and thinks dream is true: Verat.

Thieves, houses in: Lach., Nat. m.

Three persons, that he is: Nux m.

Time, exaggeration of: Cann. i., Cann. s., Nux m., Onos.

Tongue made of wood: Apis.

Violence, about: Kali br.

Visions: Bell., Calc. s. Cann. i., Carb. s., Hep., Hyos., Lach., Nat. m., Op., Puls., Sil., Stram., Sulph.

beautiful: Cann. i., Op.

closing the eyes, on: Arg., Bell., Calc. c., Bry., Chin., Ign., Lach., Puls., Sulph.

grandeur, of magnificent: Carb. s., Coff.

monsters: Bell., Stram.

Walk, cannot walk, must run or hop: Apis, Hell.

someone walks beside him: Calc. c.

someone walks behind him: Crot.

Walls, is surrounded by high: Cann. i.

Wife is faithless: Hyos., Staph., Stram.

DESPAIR: Acon., Ambr., Ars., Ars. i., Arg. n., Aur., Calc., Cann. i., Caust., Coff., Cocc., Con., Crot. t., Graph., Hell., Ign., Lach., Lil. t., Lyco., Merc., Mez., Nat. a., Nat. c., Nat. m., Nit. ac., Psor., Puls., Rhus t., Stram., Sulph., Verat.

Recovery: Acon., Ars., Bry., Calc., Hell., Sep.

convalescence, during: Psor.

DESTRUCTIVENESS: Bell., Camph., Cupr., Hyos., Stram., Terent., Verat.

DICTATORIAL: Camph.

DISCONTENDED, Displeased, Dissatisfied., etc.: Amm. m. Anac., Ars., Aur., Bism., Bor., Bry., Cham., Chel., Chin., Cina, Colch., Cupr., Hep., Kali c., Lyc., Merc., Nat. m., Nit. ac., Nux v., Op., Pall., Plat., Puls., Rhus t., Sep., Sil., Stram., Staph., Sulph., Thuja.

DULLNESS, SLUGISHNESS, Difficulty of Thinking and Comprehending: Acon., Agar., Alum., Ambr., Anac., Apis, Arg. m., Arg. n., Bapt., Bar. c., Bar. m., Bell., Bov., Bry., Calc., Calc. p., Calc. s., Cann. s., Carb. v., Caust., Cham., Chel., Chin. s., Cic. v., Clem., Cocc., Colch., Con., Crot. h., Dig., Gels., Glon., Graph., Hell., Hep., Hydr. ac., Hyos., Kali b., Kali c., Kali s., Lach., Laur., Lyc., Mag. m., Merc., Merc. c., Mez., Nat. a., Nat. c., Nat. m., Nat. p., Nat. s., Nit. ac., Nux m., Nux v., Op., Petr., Phos., Ph. ac., Pic. ac., Plb., Psor., Puls., Rhod., Rhus t., Sars., Sec., Sel., Seneg., Sep., Sil., Spig., Spong., Stann., Staph., Stram., Sulph., Tab., Thuja, Tub., Verat., Zinc.

Think long, unable to: Gels., Phos., Pic. ac.

Understands questions only after repetition: Caust., Phos., Sulph., Zinc.

EAT, refuses to: Croc., Hyos., Kali chl., Phos. ac., Phyt., Verat., Vio. o.

ECSTACY: Acon., Agar., Ant. c., Cocc., Coff., Lach., Op., Phos.

Amorous: Op., Pic. ac.

EGOTISM: Calc., Lach., Pall., Plat., Sil., Sulph.

Ailments from egotism: Calc., Lyc., Pall., Sulph.

EMBRACES COMPANIONS: Agar., Plat.

ESCAPE, attempts to: Æsc., Agar., Ars., Bell., Bry., Cocc., Crot. h., Cupr., Dig., Glon., Hyos., Nux v., Op., Stram., Verat.

ESTRANGED, family, from her: Nat. carb., Nat. m., Nit. ac., Sep.
Flies from her own children: Lyc.
Society from: Anac.
Wife, from his: Ars. Nat. s., Plat., Staph.

EXCITEMENT: Acon., Anac., Apis, Arg. n., Arn., Ars., Ars. h., Ars. i., Asaf., Asar., Aur., Aur. m., Bell., Bry., Calc., Calc. p., Camph., Cann. i., Carb. s., Caust., Cham., Chel., Chin., Cic. Cob., Coff., Daph., Dig., Ferr., Ferr. p., Gels., Glon., Graph., Hyos., Ign., Iod., Kali ar., Kali br., Kali p., Kali s., Lach., Lith., Lyc., Mag. m., Merc., Mosch., Naja, Nat. c., Nat. m., Nit. ac., Nux v., Op., Petr., Phos., Ph. ac., Plat., Podo., Psor., Puls., Sep., Sil., Spong., Stram., Stan., Sul. ac.,

EXCITEMENT.

Sulph., Tarent., Teucr., Thea, Thuja, Valer., Verat., Viol. o.

Emotional: Arg. n., Arn., Aur., Calc., *Caps.*, Caust., Cist., Cob., Cocc., *Coff.*, Con., Gels., Glon., Kali br., **Kali p.**, Lyss., Nat. m., Nux v., Pall., Phos., *Ph. ac.*, Psor., *Puls.*, *Staph.*, Verat., Zinc.

Menses, before: Kreos., Nux v. during: Mag. m., Tarent. after: Ferr.

Perspiration, during: Acon., Bell., *Cham.*, Cocc., *Coff.*, Con., Lyc., Sep., Teucr.

EXHILARATION: Agar., Bell., Cann. i., Car. s., Cinnab., Coca, *Coff.*, Fl. ac., Form., Graph., *Lach.*, *Op.*, Ox. ac., Pip. m., Stram.

EXTRAVAGANCE: Bell., Caust., Con.

FANCIES, absorbed in: Arn., Cupr., Sil., Stram.

Exaltation of: Abies, Acon., Agar., Ambr., Am. c., Anac., Arg. n., Ars., Asaf., *Bell.*, Bry., *Cann. i.*, Canth., Carb. s., Cham., Chin., Coff., Graph., *Hyos.*, Lach., Lyc., Merc., Nux m., Op., Petr., Phos., Plb., Sil., *Stram.*, Sulph., Zinc.

Lascivious: Ambr., Chin., Graph., Lyc., Op.

Sleep, preventing: Arg. n., Phos.

FEAR: *Acon.*, Alum., *Árg. n.*, Ars., *Aur.*, Bar. c., *Bell.*, *Bor.*, Bry., Cact., Calc., Caps., *Carb. s.*, Carb. v., Caust., Coca, Con., Cupr.. Dig., Form., Gels., *Graph.*,

FEAR.

Hep., Hyos., *Kali ar.*, Kali br., Kali c., Lyc., Lyss., Mag. m., Merc., Mosch., Nat. a., Nat. c., Nat. m., Nat. p., Nux v., Onos., Op., Petr., *Phos.*, Phyt., *Plat.*, *Psor.*, Puls., Rhus t., Spong., Stann., *Stram.*, Stront., Sul. ac., Sulph., Tab.

Heart, disease of: Aur., Lil. t. will cease to beat unless constantly on the move: Gels.

High places: Arg. n.

Husband, that he would **never** return, that something **would** happen to him: Platinum.

Imaginary things: *Bell.*, Phos.

Insanity, of: Alum., Calc., Cann. i., Chel., Cimic., Dig., Graph., Kali b., Lac. c., Lit. t., *Manc.*, Merc., Nat. m., Nux v., Phos., *Puls.*, Sep., Stram.

menses before: Acon.

during: Nat. m.

Mirrors in room of: Canth., Lyss., Stram.

Misfortune of: Anac., Calc., *Chin. s.*, Clem., Graph., Psor., Puls.

Noise, from rushing water: *Lyss.*, Stram.

Physicians, will not see him: he seems to terrify her: Iod., Thuja, Verat. v.

Pins, pointed things: Spig.

Poisons, of being: Bell., Hyos., Kali br., Lach., Rhus t.

Poverty: *Bry.*, Calc. i., Psor., Sep.

Pregnancy, during: Cimic.

Robbers, of: Arg. n., *Ars.*, Con., Ign., Lach., Merc., Nat. m., Phos.

FEAR.

Thunder storm, of: Bry., Gels., Nat. c., Nat. m., Nit. ac., *Phos.*, Rhodo., Sep.

Walking across busy street: Acon.

in the dark: Carb. s.

Women, of: Puls.

FIRE, wants to set things on: Hep.

FORGETFUL: Acon., Agn., Ambr., Anac., Arg. n., Arn., Aur., *Bar. c.*, Bell., Calc., Calc. p., Canth., Carb. an., *Carb. s.*, Carb. v., Caust., Chel., Cic., *Cocc.*, *Cloch.*, Con., Croc., Dig., Ferr. p., Fl. ac., Gels., Glon., Graph., Gua., Kali br., Kali p., Lac. c., Lach., *Lyc.*, *Merc.*, Mil., Nat. m., Nat. p., *Petr.*, *Phos.* Phos. ac., *Plat.*, Rhus t., Sulph., Thuja, Tub., Zinc.

Name, his own: Med.

Purchases, of, goes off and leaves them: Lac. c.

Sexual excesses, after: Nat. p., Phos. ac.

Words of, while speaking: Arg. n., *Arn.*, Bar. ac., *Cann. i.*, Kali br., Lach., Lyc., Med., Nat. m., Nux v., Onos., *Ph. ac.*

GESTURES, makes: Bell., Cocc., Hyos.

Hands, of the, grasping or reaching at something: Bell., Bor., Cham., Hyos., Lyc., Ph. ac., Psor., Sol. n., *Stram.*, Zinc.

Picks at bed clothes: Arn., Bell., Cina, Colch., Hell., *Hyos.*, Iod., Kali br., Lyc., Mur. ac., Nat. m., Op., Phos., Ph. ac., Psor., Rhus t., *Stram.*, Zinc.

GESTURES.

Plays with his fingers: Hyos.

Ridiculous or foolish: Bell., *Hyos.*, Lach., Mosch., Sep., Stram.

GRIEF: *Aur.*, *Caust.*, Coloc., Graph., *Ign.*, Lach., Lyc., *Nat. m.*, Nux v., Ph. ac., Puls., Staph.

Ailments from: Apis., *Aur.*, Calc. c., *Caust.*, *Cocc.*, Coloc., Gels., Graph., Hyos., *Ign.*, Lach., *Nat. m.*, Nux v., *Ph. ac.*, Puls., *Staph.*

Cannot cry: Gels., *Nat. m.*

Silent: *Ign.*, *Nat. m.*, Puls.

HATRED: Aur., Calc., Lac. c., Lach., Led., Nat. m.

HAUGHTY: Caust., Ip., Lach., Lyc., Pall., *Plat.*, Staph., Stram., *Sulph.*, *Verat.*

HIDE, desire to: *Bell.*, *Hell.*, Puls., Stram.

HOME-SICKNESS: Aur., Caps., *Carb. an.*, Caust., Clem., *Ign.*, Kali p., Merc., Nat. m., *Ph. ac.*, Sil., Staph.

Ailments from: Caps., Clem.

Red cheeks, with: Caps.

HURRY: Acon., Arg. n., Ars., Ars. i., Bar. c., Bell., Bry., Camph., Carb. s., Hep., Ign., Iod., Kali c., Lach., *Lil. t.*, *Med.*, Merc., Nat. m., Nux v., Ph. ac., Puls., *Sul. ac.*, *Sulph.*, Thuja.

Eating, while: *Caust.*, *Hep.*, *Lach.*, *Sul. ac.*

Mental work, in: Kali c., Sul. ac., Thuja.

Movements, in: Bell., Hyos., Stram., Sulph., Syl. ac., Thuja.

HURRY.

Cannot do things fast enough: *Sul. ac.*

Desires to do several things at once: *Lil. t.*

Walking, while: *Arg. n.*, Sulph., *Sul. ac.*, Thuja.

HYDROPHOBIA: Bell, Canth., Cur., *Hyos.*, Lach., Lyss., Stram.

iDEAS ABUNDANT, clearness of mind: Ars., Bell., Bry., *Chin.*, Chin. s., *Coff.*, *Lach.*, Lyc., Nux v., *Op.*, Phos., Puls., Sulph.

IDIOCY: Æth., Bar. c., Bar. m., Carb. s., Hell., Phos.

IMBECILITY: Alcc., Ambr., Anac., Arg. n., Ars., Aur., Bar. c., Bar. m., *Bell.*, Calc., Cann. s., Caps., *Carb. s.*, Caust., Chel., Cocc., Con., Dios., Flu. ac., Hell., *Hyos.*, Ign., Kali br., Kali p., *Lach.*, Laur., *Lyc.*, Med., Merc., Mer. c., Nat. c., Nat. m., Nux m., Nux v., Op., Oxyl., Par., Petr., *Ph. ac.*, Phos., Pic. ac., Plat., Plb., Puls., Rhus t., Sabad., Sabina, Sep., *Sil.*, Spig., *Stram.*, Sulph., Ther., *Verat.*

IMPATIENCE: Acon., Apis, Ars., Ars. h., Ars. i., Bry., Calc., *Cham.*, Coloc., Dulc., Hep., Hyos., *Ign.*, Iod., Ip., Kali br., Kali c., Lach., Lyc., Med., Nat. m., *Nux v.*, Plat., Posr., Puls., Rhus t., Sil., Sul. ac., *Sulph.*

IMPETUOUS: Anac., Bry., Carb. v., Cham., *Hep.*, Kali c., Nat. m., *Nit. ac.*, *Nux v.*, Staph., Sulph., Zinc.

INCONSOLABLE: Acon., Ars., Cham., Chin., Nat. m., Nux v., Petr., Puls., Spong., Verat.

INDIFFERENCE, Apathetic: Acon., Agar., Anac., *Apis*, Arg. n., Arn., Ars., Bar. c., Bell., Bov., Calc., Cal. ph., Carb. an., Carb. s., *Carb. v.*, Cham., Chel., *Chin.*, Cimic., Cocc., Con., Crot. h., Cycl., Gels., Graph., Hell., Hyos., Ign., Lach., *Lil. t.*, Lyc., Meli., Merc., *Mez.*, *Nat. m.*, *Nit. ac.*, Nux m., Onos., Op., *Phos.*, *Phos. ac.*, Phyt., Pic. ac., *Plat.*, Psor., *Puls.*, Sec., *Sep.*, *Sil.*, *Staph.*, Sulph., Thuja, Verat., Viol. t.

Business affairs to: Sep., Stram.

Chill, during: Op., *Phos.*, *Phos. ac.*

Desire, has no, no action of the will: Hell.

Everything, to: Acon., *Carb. v.*, Cina, Phos., Sep.

Exposure of her person: Hyos., Phos., Phyt., Sec.

Fever, during: Arn., Con., *Op.*, *Ph. ac.*, Puls., Sep.

Loved ones, to: Acon., Fl. ac., Phos., Sep.

Music, which he loves, to: Carb. v.

Onanism, after: *Staph.*

Opposite sex, to: Thuja.

Perspiration, during: Ars., Calc., Lach.

Personal appearance: Sulphur.

Pleasure, to: Ars., Cham., Chin. s., Nat. m., Puls., Sulph.

Relations, to: Fl. ac., Phos., Sep.

her children: *Phos.*, *Sep.*

INDIGNATION: Ars., Coloc., Staph.

Bad effects following: Coloc., Staph.

INJURE, fears to be left alone, lest he should, himself: Merc., Nat. s.

Satiety, must use self-control to prevent shooting himself: Nat. s.

INSANITY, MADNESS: Agar., Alum., Amm. c., Anac., Apis, Arg. n., Arn., *Ars.,* Aúr., Bar. m., *Bell.,* Calc., Camph., Canth., Cic., Cimic., Cocc., Con., Croc., Crot. c., Cupr., Cycl., Dulc., Clon., Hell., Hep., *Hyos.,* Ign., Kali br., Kali chl., Lach., Lil. t., Lyc., Manc., *Merc.,* Nat. m., Nux m., Nux v., Op., Ox. ac., Phos., Plat., Psor., Puls., Rhus t., *Stram., Sulph.,* Tarent., *Verat.*

Busy: *Apis.*

Erotic: Apis, *Nat. m.,* Hyos., Phos., *Plat.,* Puls., Sulph., *Verat.*

Puerperal: Aur., Bell., Camph., Cimic., Cupr., Hyos., Lyc., Plat., Puls., Stram., Verat.

Suppressed eruption, after: Caust., Sulph., Zinc.

Touched, will not be: Thuja.

IRRITABILITY: Acet. ac., *Acon.,* Æsc., Æth., Agar., Ail., Aloe, *Alum.,* Amm. m., Anac., *Ant. c.,* Ant. t., Apis, Arg. m., Arg. n., Arn., Ars., Ars. i., Art. v., Asaf., Asar., Bar. c., *Bell.,* Bism., Bor., *Bov.,* Bry., Calc., Calc. p., *Calc. s.,* Canth., Caps., Carb. ac., Carb. s., Carb. v., Carl.,

IRRITABILITY.

Caul., *Caust., Cham.,* Chin., Chin. a., Clem., Cocc., Coff., Colch., Coloc., Con., Crot. h., Dig., Dulc., Ferr., Gamb., Gels., Gran., Graph., Helon., *Hep.,* Hydr., Indig., Iod., Ipe., Kali br., *Kali c., Kali i.,* Kali p., *Kali s.,* Lach., Led., *Lil. t.,* Lyc., Mang., Med., Merc., Merc. c., Merc. i. r., Mez., Mur. ac., Murex., *Nat. c., Nat. m., Nat. s., Nit. ac.,* Nux v., Op., Pall., Petr., *Phos., Ph. ac.,* Phyt., *Plat.,* Psor., Puls., Ran. *b., Rhus t.,* Ruta, Sabad., Samb., Sars., *Sep.,* Sil., Spig., Stann., Staph., Stram., Sul. ac., Sulph., Tarent., *Thuja,* Verat., *Verat. v.,* Viol. t., Zinc.

After coition: *Calc.,* Chin., Kali c., Nat. c., Petr., Phos., Selen., *Sep., Sil.*

Consolation aggravates: Bell., Cact., Calc. p., *Ign., Nat. m.,* Nit. acid, Plat., *Sep., Sil.*

Menses, before: Caust., Cham., Lyc., Nat. m., Nux v., Sep. during: Cham., Nux v., Sulph.

Noises, from: Ferr.

Sends the doctor home, says he is not sick: Apis, *Arn., Cham.* the nurse home: Fl. ac.

the nurse out of the room: Cham.

Stool, before: Bor., Calc.

JEALOUSY: Apis, Calc. s., Cench., *Hyos., Lach.,* Nux v., Puls.

KICKS: Bell., Lyc., Stram. Child is cross, kicks and scolds on walking: Lyc.

KILL, desire to: Ars., Ars. i.,
Hep., *Hyos.*, Iod., Nux. v.,
Phos., Stram.

Kill the person that contradicts
her: Merc.

Sight of a knife: Plat.

of knife or gun: Alum.

Something urges her to, her husband, of whom she is very
fond: Merc., Nux v.

KISSES EVERYONE: Croc.,
Verat.

Menses, before: Verat., Zinc.

KLEPTOMANIA: Art. v., Cur.,
Nux v.

LAMENTING, BEMOANING,
Wailing, etc.: Acet. ac.,
Acon., *Aur.*, Bell., Bism.,
Bry., Calc., Canth., Cham.,
Chin., Cic., Cina, Coff.,
Coloc., Cor. r., Lach., *Lyc.*,
Mosch., Nux v., Op., Puls.,
Sulph., Verat., Verat. v.

LASCIVIOUSNESS: Ambr.,
Apis, Calad., Calc., Camph.,
Canth., Carb. v., Chin., Con.,
Dig., Fl. ac., Graph., *Hyos.*,
Lach., *Lil. t.*, *Orig.*, Phos.,
Pic. ac., *Plat.*, Selen., Sep.,
Sil., *Staph.*, Stram., Tarent.

LAUGHING: Aur., Bell., Bor.,
Calc., *Cann. i.*, Croc., Ferr.,
Hyos., *Ign.*, Lach., Lyc.,
Nat. m., Nux m., Phos.,
Plat., Sep., *Stram.*, Tarent.

Immoderately: Cann. i., Nat. m.,
Nux m.

Loudly: Bell., Hyos., Stram.

Serious matters, over: Anac.,
Nat. m., Plat.

LOOKED AT, cannot bear to
be: Ant. c., Ant. t., *Ars.*,
Cham., Chin., Cina, Iod.

LOQUACITY: Arg. m., Bell.,
Camph., Cann. i., Carl.,
Cimic., Cocc., Croc., Cupr.,
Gels., *Hyos.*, Kali i., *Lach.*,
Lachn., Mur. ac., Nat. c.,
Op., Phos., Plb., Podo.,
Pyrog., Stram., Verat.

Changing quickly from one subject to another: Cimic., *Lach.*

Chilly, during: Podo.

Heat, during: Lach., Podo.,
Teucr.

Menses, during: Bar. c., Lach.,
Stram.

Perspiration, during: Calad.,
Selen.

LOVE, ailments from disappoint-
ed: Aur., Calc. p., Cimic.,
Coff., Hell., *Hoys.*, *Ign.*,
Lach., *Nat. m.*, *Ph. ac.*,
Staph.

Love-sick: Ant. c., Til.

MARRIAGE, the idea of un-
endurable: Lach.

MEMORY ACTIVE: Agar.,
Aloe, Aur., *Bell.*, *Coff.*,
Gels., *Hyos.*, *Lach.*, Nux m.,
Op., Phos., Sul. ac.

Weakness of: Acon., Agn.,
Alum., Ambr., *Anac.*, Apis,
Arg. n., Arn., Ars., Aur.,
Bar. c., Bell., Bov., Bry.,
Bufo, *Bufo. s.*, Calc., Calc.
p., *Carb. s.*, Carb. v., *Caust.*,
Chin., Chin. a., Chlor., Clem.,
Colch., Con., Crot. h., Cupr.,
Cycl., Dig., Fl. ac., Gels.,
Glon., Graph., Gua., Hell.,
Hep., *Hyos.*, Kali br., *Kali
p.*, *Lach.*, Laur., *Lyc.*, Med.,
Merc., Merc. c., Mez., Nat.
a., Nat. c., Nat. m., Nat. p.,
Nit. ac., *Nux m.*, Nux v.,
Op., Petr., *Ph. ac.*, Phos.,
Pic. ac., *Plb.*, Rhus t., Selen.,

MEMORY, weakness of.

Sep., Sil., Spig., Stan., Staph., Stram., Sulph., Syph., Thuja, *Verat.*, Viola. o., Zinc.

MOANING, GROANING ETC.: Acon., Apis, Ars., Bar. c., *Bell.*, Bry., Calad., Camph., *Cann. i.*, Carb. ac., Cham., Cina, Cic., Cocc., Colch., Cupr., Hyos., Ign., Ip., Kali br., *Kali c.*, Mur. ac., Nux v., Phos., Sec., Stram., Zinc.

MOOD, agreeable: Abrot., Ant. t., Croc., Ign., Lach., Meny., Plat., Sul., ac., Zinc.

Alternating: Acon., *Alum.*, Bar. c., *Bell.*, *Bov.*, Carb., an., Chin., Croc., Dros., *Ferr.*, Ferr. p., Graph., *Ign.*, *Iod.*, Kali c., Mur. ac., Nux v., Phos., Puls., Sec., Stram., Zinc.

Changeable, variable etc.: Acon., Alum., Apis, Ars., Aur., Bar. c., Bor., Calc., Chin., Cocc., Croc., Cupr., Ferr., *Ign.*, Kali c., Lyc., Mag. c., Merc., *Nux m.*, Petr., Phos., Plat., Psor., *Puls.*, Sars., Sep., Stann., Stram., Sul. ac., Valer., Zinc.

MOROSE: Agar., *Anac.*, Arn., Art. v., *Aur.*, Bism., Bry., Calc., Carb. s., Colch., Coloc., Con., Crot., Cycl., Dig., Ip., Kali p., Led., Lyc., Merc., Mez., Mur. ac., *Nux v.*, Phos., Ph. ac., Plat., Plb., *Puls.*, *Sil.*, Sulph., Zinc.

MORTIFICATION, ailments after: Arg. n., Aur., Aur. m., Bry., Cham., Coloc., *Ign.*, *Lyc.*, Lyss., Nat. m., Op., *Pall.*, *Ph. ac.*, Puls., Seneg., Staph., Sulph.

MUTTERING: Apis, Arn., Bell., Cocc., Crot. h., Hep., *Hyos.*, Lach., Lyc., Merc., Op., Phos., Rhus t., Sec., Stram., *Verat.*

NAKED, wants to be: Bell., *Hyos.*, Phos., Sec., Stram.

NYMPHOMANIA: Ant. c., Apis, Brom., Bell., Calc. p., Cann. i., Cann. s., Canth., Chin., Coff., Dig., Fl. ac., Grat., *Hyos.*, Lach., Lil. t., Lyc., Merc., Murex, Nux v., Orig., Phos., *Plat.*, Puls., Raph., Sabad., *Stram.*, Tarent., Verat.

Menses before: Phos., Verat. during: Hyos., Plat., Sec., Verat.

suppressed: Murex, Plat.

Metrorrhagia, during: Mosch., Murex, Plat., Sec.

QUARRELSOME: Acon., Arn., Ars., Aur., Bell., Bov., Brom., Bry., Camph., Caust., Cham., Con., Croc., Cupr., Dulc., Hyos., *Ign.*, Kali c., Lach., Lyc., Merc., Mosch., Nat. m., *Nux v.*, *Petr.*, Phos. ac., Psor., Ran. b., Sep., Staph., Stram., *Sulph.*, Thuja, Verat.

QUIET DISPOSITION: Alum., Bell., Cic., Gels., Hyos., Ign., Lach., *Phos. ac.*, Plb.

During heat: Bry., Gels.

RAGE: Acon., Æth., *Agar.*, Arn., Ars., Bell., Camph., Canth., Carb. s., Colch., Cupr., Hell., *Hyos.*, Lach., *Lyc.*, Merc., Nat. m., Op., Phos., Puls., Sec., Sol. n., Stram., Sulph., Tab., *Verat.*

Violent: *Bell.*, *Hyos.*, Stram.

RECOGNISE, does not, his relatives: Anac., *Bell.*, Glon., *Hyos.*, Lach., Stram., Verat.

RELIGIOUS AFFECTIONS: Arg. n., Ars., Aur., Bell., Calc., Carb. v., Cham., Chel., Graph., *Hyos.*, Ign., Kali p., Lach., Lil. t., Lyc., Med., Meli., Mez., Plat., Psor., Puls., Sep., Stram., *Sulph.*, *Verat.*, Zinc.

REMORSE: Ars., Aur., Bell., Cocc., *Coff.*, Cupr., Dig., Hyos., Ign., Med., Puls., Sil., Verat., Zinc.

RESTLESSNESS: *Acon.*, Agar., Anac., Ant. t., Apis., *Arg. m.*, *Arg. n.*, *Ars. h.*, *Ars. i.*, *Ars. m.*, Art. v., Asaf., Aur. m., *Bapt.*, *Bell.*, Bov., Calc., *Cal. p.*, Calc. s., *Camph.*, Cann. s., Carb. s., Carb. v., Caust., Cham., Chin., Cimic., Cina, Cic. v., Cocc., Colch., *Coloc.*, Cop., Cupr., Dig., Dulc., *Ferr.*, Ferr. ar., Ferr i., Graph., Hyos., Ign., Iod., Ip., Kali. b., Kali. c., Kali n. Kali p., Kali s., Lac. c., Lach., Led., Lil. t., *Lyc.*, Mang., Med., Nux v., Op., Ph. ac., Plat., Plb., Psor., *Puls.*, *Rhus t.*, Rhus v., Rumex, Ruta, Samb., Staph., Stram., Sul. ac., *Sulphur*, Tab., Tarent., Tell., Thuja, Valer., Zinc.

Alone, when: Phos.

Copulation, after: *Calc.*

Convulsions, before: *Arg. n.*

Menses, before: Kreo., Nux v., *Sulph.*

at the time of: Acon., Ars., Calc., Cham., Coff., Cycl., Nux v., Puls., Rhus t., Sep. Stram.

RESTLESSNESS, menses.

after: Mag. c.

Music, from: Nat. c., Tarent.

RUDENESS: Hyos., *Lyc.*, Nux v., Stram., *Verat.*

SADNESS: Abies n., *Acon.*, Æsc., Agn., Alum., Ambr., Anac., Ant. c., Arg. m., Arg. n., Arn., *Ars.*, *Ars. i.*, Asaf., Aur., Aur. mur., Bar. c., Bell., Brom., Bry., Bufo, Cact., *Calc.*, *Calc. ars.*, *Calc. s.*, Carb. s., **Carb. v.**, Camph., Cann. s., Canth., Caps., Carb. an., Caust., Cham., Chel., *Chin.*, Chin. a., Chin. s., Cic., Cimic., Cina, Clem., Cocc., Cupr., Coff., Coloc., Con., Cor. r., Croc., Crot. h., Cycl., Dig., Dros., Dulc., *Ferr.*, Ferr. ar., *Ferr. i.*, Ferr. f., Gels., Graph., Grat., *Hell.*, Helon., Hep., Hipp., Hydr., Hyos., *Ign.*, Indig., Iod., Ip., Kali br., Kali c., Kali i., *Kali p.*, Lac. c., Lac. d., *Lach.*, Laur., Lil. t., *Lyc.*, Manc., Mang., *Merc.*, Merc. i. r., *Mez.*, Nat. a., Nat. c., Nat. m., Nat. p., Nat. s., *Nit. ac.*, Nux v., Ol. an., Petr., Phos., Ph. ac., Phyt., Plat., Plb., *Psor.*, Puls., *Rhus t.*, Rhus v., Ruta, Sabina, Sep., Sil., Spig., Spong., Stann., Staph., Still., Stram., Sul. ac., *Sulph.*, Tab., *Thuja*, *Verat.*, Verat. v., Zinc.

Labor, during: Cimic, Ign., Nat. m., Puls.

Menses, before: Calc., *Caust.*, Con., Lyc., Nat. m., Nit. ac., Murex, *Puls.*, Sep., *Stann.*, Verat.

SADNESS, manses.

> at the time of: Caust., Nat.
> m., Petr., Puls., Sep.
> following: Ferr.
> Suppression: Ars., Aur., Calc.,
> Cimic., Con., Croc., Cycl.,
> Nat. m., Nux m., Nux v.,
> Ph. ac., Phos., Puls., Sep.,
> Sil., Staph., Sulphur.

Pregnant females, of: Lach.

SENTIMENTALITY: *Ant. c.*,
Calc. p., Cocc., Coff., Cupr.,
Ign., Phos., Psor., Sulph.

SEXUAL EXCESS, mental
symptoms as a result of: Bov.,
Calc., Carb., v. Chin., Con.,
Iod., Kali c., *Lyc.*, Merc.,
Nat. c., *Nux v.*, *Phos.*, *Ph.
ac.*, Puls., Sep., Staph.

SHAMELESS: *Hyos.*, *Phos.*,
Secale, Verat.

SIGHING: Æsc., Bry., Cham.,
Cimic., Cocc., *Ign.*, Ip.,
Rhus t., Sec., Stram.

> Heat, during paroxysms of:
> Arn., Cham., Coff., Ign.

Menses, before: Ign., Lyc.

SOMNAMBULISM: *Acon.*,
Anac., Art. v., Bry., *Nat.
m.*, *Op.*, Phos., Sil., Spong.,
Stram., Sulphur.

SPEECH, disconnected: Merc.
c., Op., Stram.

Flattering: Arg. n.

Hasty: Bell., Camph., *Hep.*,
Hyos., Ign. Lach., Merc.,
Mosch.

Incoherent: Agar., Anac., Arg.
n., Bapt., Bell., *Bry.*,
Camph., *Cann. i.*, Crot. h.,
Gels., *Hyos.*, Lach., Morph.,
Nux m., Ph. ac., *Phos.*,
Rhus i., Stram., Sulph.

SPEECH.

Prattling: Anac., *Bry.*, *Hyos.*,
Stram.

Slow: Arg. n., Kali br., *Lach.*,
Ph. ac., Phos., Plb., Sec.,
Sep., Thuja.

Unintelligible: *Bell.*, *Hyos.*,
Merc., Ph. ac., Sec.,
Stram.

SPITTING AT OTHERS:
Bell., Calc., Cupr., Stram.,
Verat.

STRIKING: Arg. m., Bell.,
Cupr., Glon., *Hyos.*, *Ign.*,
Kali c., Lyc., Plb., Stram.,
Tarent., Verat.

STUPEFACTION: Ant. t., Ap.,
Arn., Ars., *Bapt.*, *Bell.*,
Bov., *Bry.*, Calc., Camph.,
Cic., *Cocc.*, Coc. c., Con.,
Crot. h., Cupr., Dulc., Gels.,
Hell., *Hyos.*, Lyc., Nat. p.,
Nux m., *Nux v.*, Op., Petr.,
Ph. ac., Phos., Puls.,
Rheum, *Rhus i.*, Sec.,
Stann., *Stram.*, Sulph., Thu-
ja, Verat., Visc., Zinc.

SUICIDE, disposition to commit:
Anac., Ars., *Aur.*, *Aur. mur.*
Calc., Caps., Chin., Cimic.,
Hep., Hyos., Kali br.,
Lac. d., Lach., *Nat. s.*,
Nux v., Psor., Puls., Sep.,
Spig., Stram., Zinc.

Marked dread of an open
window or a knife with:
Merc.

Menses, at the time of: Merc.,
Sil.

Perspiring when: Ars., Aur.,
Calc., Merc., Spong.

Wants to drown herself: Bell.,
Puls., Rhus t., Sil.

Wants to hang herself: Ars.
poison herself: Lil. t.

SUICIDE, wants to.

shoot herself: Ant. c.

throw himself from a height: Arg. n., Aur., Nux v.

throw himself from a window: Æth., *Aur.,* Carb. s., Glon.

use knife to commit suicide: Ars., Calc., Merc.

SUICIDAL THOUGHTS: Ant. c., *Aur.,* Hep., Ign. Merc., *Nat. s., Psor.,* Puls., Rhus.

SUSPICION: *Acon., Anac., Arn., Ars., Aur.,* Bapt., *Bar.* c., Bar. m., Bell., Bor., Bry., Cact., Calc. p., *Cann. i., Caust.,* Cench., Cic., Cimic., Crot. h., *Dig.,* Dros., Hell., Hyos., Kali br., *Kali p., Lach.,* Lyc., Merc., Nat. a., Nat. c., Nit. ac., Op., Phos., Plb., Puls., *Rhus t., Sec.,* Sep., Stann., *Stram.,* Sul. ac., Sulph., Verat. v.

TALKING, people, who are dead, with: *Calc. sil.,* Hyos.

Nothing, but fine, rats and murder, of: Calc.

Of only one subject: Arg. n.

War: Agar., Bell., Hyos.

To himself: Ant. t., Hyos., Kali bi.

Swallows his words, when: Staph.

TEARING THINGS: *Bell.,* Camph., Kali p., Stram., Verat.

Will tear his genitals: Sec.

Will tear her hair: Bell., Lil. t.

Will tear himself: Stram.

Will tear her pillow with teeth: Stram.

TIME, passing too slowly with him: Alum., Arg., *Cann. i.,* Cann. s., Cench., *Glon.,* Med., Merc., Nux m., Nux v.

Passing too quickly with him: Cocc., Ther.

TOUCHED, don't like to be: Acon., Agar., *Ant. c.,* Ant. t., Arn., Bell., Bry., *Cham.,* Chin., Cina, Kali c., Kali i., Lach., Med., Sil., Thuja.

TRAVELLING, a desire for: *Calc. p.,* Hipp., Iod., Tub.

UNCONSCIOUS: Acon., Ail., Alum., Anac., Apis, Arg. n., Arn., Ars., Arum t., Aster., Bapt., Bar. c., Bar. m., *Bell.,* Bry., Cact., Calad., Camph., Cann. i., Canth., Carb. o., Carb. s., Carb. v., Caust., Cham., Cic., Cina, *Cocc.,* Coff., Colch., Cupr., Cycl., Dig., Gels., Glon., *Hel.,* Hep., *Hydr. ac.,* Hyos., *Ign.,* Kali br., Kali c., Lac. d., *Lach.,* Laur., Led., Lyc., Merc. c., Mosch., Mur. ac., Nat. m., *Nux m.,* Nux v., Op., Petr., Ph. ac., Phos., Plat., Plb., *Puls.,* Rhus t., Sec., Sil., Sol. n., Stram., Sulph., Tereb., Verat., Zinc.

WANDERING ABOUT Naked: Hyos.

Wrapped up in fur during summer: Hyos.

Insane, senseless: Nux v.

WEARINESS OF LIFE: Ars., *Aur.,* Bell., Chin., Kali p., Nat. m., Nit. ac., Nux v., *Phos.,* Rhus t., Sil.

WEEP, inclination to, a tearful mood: Acon., Alum., Ant. c., Ant. t., Apis, Arg. n., Bell., Bry., Cact., Calc., Calc. s., Carb. s., Carb. v., Caust., Cham., Chel., Chin. s., Cic., Cimic., Cina, Cocc., Coff., Con., Cupr., Crot. h., Graph., Hell., Hep., Ign., Iod., Kali bi., Kali br., Kali c., Kali p., Lil. t., Lyc., Mag. m., Mang., Meli., Merc. i. r., Nat. m., Nat. p., Nat. s., Nit. ac., Nux m., Nux v., Pall., Petr., Ph. ac., Phos., Plat., Puls., Rhus t., Sep., Spong., Staph., Sul. ac., Sulph., Verat., Viol. o.

WEEPING AND LAUGHTER

alternate: Acon., Aur., Calc., Coff., Hyos., Ign.. Lyc., Merc., Nux m., Phos., Plat., Puls., Stram.

Anger, follows: Nux v.

Cause, without any: Apis, Cina, Graph., Lyc., Nat. m., Puls., Sulph., Zinc.

Chill, during the stage of: Aur.. Bell., Calc., Carb. v.. Cham., Lyc., Petr., Puls., Viol. o.

Consolation increases her trouble: Calc. p., Nat. m., Plat.. Sep., Sil.

Contradicted. when: Ign.. Nux v.. Stram., Tarent.

Cough. associated with: Bell., Bry., Hep.

Involuntary: Alum., Aur.. Bell., Caust., Ign., Nat. m., Plat., Puls., Rhus t., Sep.

WEEPING and laughing.

Joy, on account of: Coff., Plat.

Looked at, if: Nat. m.

Menses, previous to: Cact., Lyc., Phos., Puls., Zinc.

at the time of: Ars., Cocc., Coff., Ign., Petr., Phyt. Plat., Puls., Stram.

Mortification, following: Coloc., Puls.

Music, from hearing: Graph., Kreos., Nat. c., Thuja.

Narrating her ailments, when: Kali c., Med., Puls.

Perspiring, while: Bell., Calc., Camph., Cham., Cupr., Lyc., Op., Petr., Puls., Spong., Stram.

Pregnancy, during: Mag. c.

Spoken to, if: Med., Nat. m., Plat., Staph.

Thanked, after he was: Lyc.

Touched, if: Ant. c., Ant. t., Cina.

Urination, before: Bor., Lyc.. Sars.

during: Erig., Sars.

Vexed. from being: Zinc.

Violently: Hydr. ac.. Stram.

WILL NOT COMPLAIN, she thinks she is quite well, when really she is very sick: Apis. Arn.

WOMEN, he does not like: Dios.. Lach., Puls.

YIELDING, pliable mood: Lyc.. Puls., Sil.

HEAD

ACHING, undefined pain, headache in general: Alum., Amm. c., Ant., c., *Apis*, Arg. m., Arg. n., Arn. *Ars.*, Aur., Bapt., *Bell.*, Bor., *Bry.*, Calc., Caust., Cham., *Chin.*, Chin. s., Cimic., Cinnab., *Cocc.*, Coloc., Dig., Dios., Dros., Dulc., Ferr., Ferr. p., *Gels.*, *Glon.*, Graph., Hell., Hep., Hyos., Ign., Iod., *Iris*, Kali bi., Kali c., Kali n., Kreos., Lac. d., *Lach.*, Led., Lyc., Mag. m., Manc., Meli., *Merc.*, Mez., Nat. c., *Nat. m.*, Nat. s., *Nit. ac.*, Nux m., Nux v., Petr., *Phos.*, Ph. ac., Podo., Psor., Puls., Rhus t. Sep., Sil., Sol. n., Spig., Staph., *Sulph.*, Thuja, Zinc.

Comes and goes with the sun: Kalm., Nat. m., Spig.

Increases and decreases with the sun: Kalm., Nat. m., Phos., Spig.

Alcoholics: *Agar.*, Ant. c., Ars., Bell., Calc., Chel., Chin., Coff., *Gels.*, Ign., *Lach.*, Led., Lyc., Nat. m., Nux m., *Nux v.*, Op., Phos., Puls., *Ran. b.*, Rhod., Rhus t., Ruta, Selen, Sil., Spig., Stram., Sulph., Verat., Zinc.

Sprituous liquors ameliorate her headache: Ign., Kreos.

Alternates with cough: Lach.

with diarrhœa: Podo.

with hemorrhoids: Abrot., Aloe.

Anger, followng: Bry., Cham., Lyc., Nat. m., Nux v., Petr., Phos., Plat., Staph.

Animal fluid, following loss of: Calc., Carb. v., Chin., Nat. m., Nux v., Phos. ac., Puls., Sep., Sil., Staph., Sulph.

Profuse uterine hemorrhage, following: Glon.

Arthiritis: Ars., Asar., Aur., Bell., *Bry.*, Caps., Caust., Cic., *Coloc.*, *Dulc.*, Eug., Gua., Nat. m., Nit. ac., Nux v., Phos., Puls., *Rhus t.*, Sang., *Sep.*, Verat.

Ascending steps, while: *Bell.*, *Bry.*, *Calc.*, Carb. v., Cupr., Glon., Kalm., Lach., Lyc., Mosch., Nux v., Phos., Rhus t., Sep., *Spong.*, Sulph., Tab.

Bath, following a: Ant. c., Bell., Calc., Nit. ac., Rhus t., improves after a: Lac. ac.

cold: *Ant. c.*, Bell. Caps., Nit. ac., Rhus t.

Blinding: Bell., Caust., Gels., *Iris*, Nat. m., Phos., Psor., Sil., Stram.

Blindness after severe headache, headache growing worse, but sight gradually returning: Kali bi.

before breakfast: Calc., Cimic., Ind., Rumex.

Catarrhal: All. c., Alum., Ars., Aur., Bry., Calc., Carb. v., Chlor., *Dulc.*, Euphr., Ferr.,

ACHING, catasihal.

> Gels., *Graph.*, *Hep.*, Iod.,
> Kali bi., *Kali c.*, *Kali i.*,
> Lach., Lyc., *Merc.*, Nux v.,
> Stict., Sulph.

> Chronic: Ars., Caust., Sil.,
> Sulph.

> people, of old: Iod.

> Climaxis, during the: Carb. v.,
> *Lach.*, Sang., Sep.

> Coffee, from: Bell., Bry., Cham.,
> Cocc., Guar., Ign., Nux v.

> Coition, after: Bov., Calc.,
> *Kali c.*, Nat. c., Petr., Phos.,
> *Sep.*, *Sil.*

> Constipated, when: Aloe, *Bry.*,
> Lac. d., Nat. m., Nux v.

> Continued, constant: Cimic.

> it is fixed, lasting for weeks,
> months and years with rare
> or no intermission: Tereb.

> Coryza, when suffering from:
> *Acon.*, Æsc., Agar., All. c.,
> Arg. n., Aur., *Bell.*, *Bry.*,
> Calc., Chin., Ferr., Gels.,
> Iod., Kali bi., Kali c., Kali
> i., Lach., *Lyc.*, *Merc.*, Merc.
> i. r., Nux v., Phos., Puls.,
> Sang., Sep., Sil., Spig.,
> Sulph., Thuja.

> from suppressed coryza:
> Acon., Calc., Nux v., Sil.

> Cutting of hair, following: Bell.,
> Sep.

> Dancing: Arg. n.

> Debauch, after a: Nux v.

> Descending while: *Bell.*, Ferr.,
> Rhus t.

> Dinner before: Indig., Nux v.

> Eating, before: Sil.

> at the time of: Graph., Ph. ac.

> after: *Alum.*, Bry., Calc.,
> Calc. p., Carb. v., Cham.,
> Cocc., Coff., Graph.,

ACHING, eating, after.

> Hyos., Lith., Lyc., *Nat.*
> *c.*, *Nat. m.*, Nux v., Petr.,
> Phos., Ph. ac., Rhus t.,
> Sil., *Sulph.*, Zinc.

> Eruption, after suppressed:
> Ant. c.

> Exertion of body, from: Cact.,
> *Calc.*, Calc. p., Nat. m.,
> Valer.

> Fall, after a: Arn., Hyper.,
> Rhus t.

> Fasting, on account of: Cist.,
> Kali c., Lyc., Phos., Sil.

> Fatty food, from: Carb. v.,
> Puls.

> Feet getting cold, from: Sil.

> Foot-steps, from: Coff., Nux v.,
> Sil.

> Fright, following a: *Acon.*, Arg.
> n., Coff., Cupr., *Ign.*, Nux
> v., Op., Plat., *Puls.*

> Gastric: Anac., *Ant. c.*, Arn.,
> *Bry.*, Calc., Calc. p., Caust.,
> Carb. v., Coff., Eup. per.,
> *Ipe.*, *Iris*, Lyc., *Nux. v.*,
> Phos., *Puls.*, Sep., Sil.,
> Sulph., Tab.

> Girls, young or school in: Calc.,
> Calc. p., Nat. m., *Ph. ac.*,
> Puls.

> Hammering: Amm. c., Ars.,
> Chin., Chin. s., Cocc., *Ferr.*,
> Hep., Lach., *Nat. m.*, Psor.,
> *Sil.*, *Sulph.*

> Injuries, mechanical following:
> Arn., Bell., Cic., Hep.,
> Hyper., Nat. m., Nat. s.,
> Phos., Rhus t., Staph.

> Ironing, due to: *Bry.*

> Jar, from any: Bell., Bry., Calc.,
> Carb. v., Chin., *Glon.*, Hep.,
> Kali c., Led., Lyc., Nat. m.,
> *Nit. ac.*, Nux v., Phos., Rhus
> t., Sep., Sil., Spig., Sulph.
> Ther.

ACHING.

Light in general, cannot look at
it: Ant. c., Ars., *Bell.*, Bor.,
Bry., *Calc.*, Chin., Cocc.,
Ign., Lyc., Nat. c., Nat. m.,
Ph. ac., Phos., Sang., Sep.,
Sil., Stram., Sulph.

which are artificial, from:
Glon., Sang., *Sep.*, Sil.,
Stram.

Madden him, pain will: Acon.,
Ars., *Bell.*, Calc., Chin.,
Ipe., Nat. m., Nit. ac.,
Stram.

Meat, from taking: Puls.

Menses, previous to: Acon.,
Amm. c., Asar., Bell., Bor.,
Bov., Brom., Bry., Calc.,
Carb. v., Cimic., Cinnab.,
Gels., *Kreos.*, Lach., Lyc.,
Nat. c., Nat. m., Nux m.,
Plat., Puls., Sulph., Verat.,
Xanth.

headache is relieved during:
Lach.

at the time of: Arg. n., *Bell.*,
Bov., Bry., Calc., Carb.
v., Caust., Cocc., Gels.,
Glon., *Graph.*, Hyos.,
Ign., Kali c., *Kreos.*, Lac.
d., Laur., *Lyc.*, Mag. c.,
Murex, Nat. c., *Nat. m.*,
Nit. ac., Nux m., Nux v.,
Phos., Plat., Puls., Sang.,
Sep., Sulph., Verat.

following: Bry., Chin., Ferr.,
Nat. m., Puls., Sep.

Mental application from: Anac.,
Arg. n., Aur., Bry., *Calc.*,
Calc. p., Chin., Cocc., Colch.,
Con., Dig., Gels., *Glon.*,
Ign., Lach., Lyc., Mag. c.,
Nat. c., *Nat. m.*, Nat. s.,
Nit. ac., Nux m., *Nux v.*,
Par., Petr., Phos., *Ph. ac.*,

ACHING, mental application from.

Pic. ac., Psor., *Puls.*, Sabad.,
Sep., *Sil.*, Spig., Staph., Sulph.

Music, from hearing: *Coff.*,
Phos., Ph. ac.

Nervous type: Agar., Arg. n.,
Ars., Asar., *Asaf.*, Cact.,
Calc., Cham., *Chin.*, *Coff.*,
Gels., Ign., Ipe., *Nat. m.*,
Nux v., Petr., *Phos.*, Ph. ac.,
Plat., *Puls.*, Sep., Stram.,
Ther., Valer., Verat., Zinc.

Old people, belonging: Ambr.,
Amm. c., Iod.

Periodical: Æth., *Alum.*, Apis,
Ars., Cact., Calc., Carb. v.,
Cedr., *Chin.*, Chin. s., Ferr.,
Ign., Kreos., Lach., Lyc.,
Nat. m., Nit. ac., Nux v.,
Phos., Puls., Rhus t., *Sang.*,
Sep., *Sil.*, *Spig.*, Sulph.

every seven days: Lac. d.,
Phos., Sang., Sulph.

fourteen days: Ars., Sulph.

Pulsates: Acon., Amm. c., Apis,
Ars., Asar., *Bell.*, Bor., Calc.,
Calc. p., *Carb. v.*, Cham.,
Chel., Chin., Chin. s., *Ferr.*,
Gels., *Glon.*, Hep., *Lyc.*,
Ign., Kali c., Lach., Morp.,
Nat. m., Nux m., Op., *Psor.*,
Puls., Rhus t., Ruta, Sang.,
Sul., Sil.

Rheumatic: Bry., Cimic., *Dulc.*,
Kalm., Lach., *Merc.*, Nit.
ac., Phyt., Ran. b., Sang.,
Sil.

Scarlatina, following: Bry.,
Merc.

Sexual excesses, following: *Agar.*,
Bov., *Calc.*, Chin., Nat. c.,
Nux v., *Sep.*, *Sil.*, Staph.,
Sulph., Thuja.

Sleep, from loss of: Carb. v.,
Laur., Nux v.

ACHING.

Smoking tobacco, on account of: Ant. c., Gels., Ign., Puls.

Wandering, shifting pain: Puls., Sang., Spig.

Warm room will aggravate her headache: All. c., Alum., Apis, Arn., Bell., Bov., Carb. v.. Caust., Croc., Iod., Led., Lyc., Mosch., Nat. m., Phos., Plat., Puls., Seneg., Spong., Sulph.

relieve her headache: Amm. c., Ant. c., Calc., Nux m., Rhus t., Sep., Sulph.

Weather, in cloudy: Calc., Cham., Chin., Dulc., Mang., Nux m., Rhus t., Sep.

in cold: Agar., Amm. c., Ars., Aur., Bell., Bry., Calc., Camph., Caps.. Caust., Colch., Dulc., Hell., Hep., Kali i., Merc., Mosch., Nux m., Nux v., Phos., Rhus t., Sabad., Spig., Stront.. Sulph.

in damp cold: Amm. c., Bry., Calc., Carb. v., Dulc., Lach., Lyc., Mang., Merc., Nux m., Nux v., Rhod., Rhus t., Sil., Spig., Sulph., Verat.

in dry cold: Asar., Caust., Hep., Nux v., Spong.

in winter, known as winter headaches: Aur. m., Bism., Sil., Sul.

BORES HIS HEAD INTO THE PILLOW: Apis, Bell., Bry., Hell., Stram.

COLD, sensitive to: Bell., Chin., Graph., Hep., Kali c., Merc., Mez., Nat. m., Nux v., Phos., Psor., Rhus t., Sep., Sil., Stront

CONCUSSION: Arn., Cic., Hell., Hyos.

CONGESTION, fullness, hyperæmia etc.: Acon., Ambr., Anac., Ant. c., Apis, Arg. n., Arn., Ars., Aur., Bell., Bor., Bry., Cact., Calc., Camph., Cann. s., Canth., Carb. an., Carb. v., Cham., Chin., Cimic., Cinnab., Coff., Con., Cupr., Cycl., Dulc., Ferr., Ferr. p., Gels., Glon., Graph., Grat., Hell., Hyos., Iod., Kali bi., Kali br., Kali c., Kali i., Lach., Laur., Lyc., Mag. c., Mag. s., Meli., Merc., Mill., Nat. c., Nat. m., Nat. s., Nit. ac., Nux v., Op., Phos., Ph. ac., Psor., Puls., Ran. b., Rhus t., Sang., Sep., Sil., Spong., Stram., Sulph., Sul. ac., Tab., Verat., Zinc.

Bed, in: Sulph.

Warm room, in a: Apis, Carb. v., Cocc., Puls., Sulph.,

ERUPTION: Agar, Ars., Bar. c., Calc., Calc. s., Carb. an., Carb. v., Clem., Graph., Hep., Kali br., Lyc., Mag. c., Merc., Mez., Nat. m., Nit. ac., Petr., Phos., Psor., Rhus t., Sep., Staph., Sul. ac., Sulph.

Margin of hair: Nat. m.

Occiput: Clem., Lyc., Petr., Sil., Staph., Sulph.

Boils: Arn., Ars., Calc., Hep., Kali c., Kali i., Mer, Psor., Sul.

Burning: Ars., Graph., Sars., Sulph.

Carbuncles: Anthr., Ars., Hep., Lach., Sil., Sulph.

Coppercolored: Carb. an.

Cracks and fissures: Petr.

Dry: Calc., Mez., Psor.

ERUPTION.

Moist: Bar. c., Cham., Cic., Graph., Hep., Hydr., Merc., Mez., Nat. m., Petr., Psor., Rhus t., Sars., Sep., Sil., Staph., Sulph., Thuja, Viol. t.

ERYSIPELAS: Apis, Ars., Chel., Chin., Eupr., *Graph.*, Lach., Ph. ac., Phyt., Ruta.

EXOSTOSES: *Arg. m.*, Aur., Calc., Calc. f., Kali i., Mez., *Phos.*

FALLING BACKWARD OF HEAD: Agar., Colch., Dig., Ign., Led., Op., Spig.

FULLNESS: Acon., Amm. m., *Apis, Arg. n.*, Bell., Bor., Bry., Calc., Calc. p., Carb. v., Carls., Cinnab., Cycl., Dig., Ferr., Fl. ac., Gels., *Glon.*, Ham., Hyos., Lac. d., Merc., Nicc., Nit. ac., Nux m., Pæon., Petr., Phos., Psor., Ran. b., Ran. s., Rhus t., Sang., Spong., *Sulph.*, Sul. ac., Tereb., Xanth.

HAIR:

Baldness: Anac., Apis, *Bar. c.*, Fl. ac., Graph., Phos., Sep., Sil.

Patches, in: Graph., Phos.

Dark: *Acon.*, Ars., Arn., Bell., Carb. v., Caust., Dulc., Guai., Kali c., Mos., Nat. m., *Nit. ac., Nux v., Phos., Phos. ac., Plat.*, Puls., Sep., Staph., Sul.

Light: Agar., Ang., Bor., Bry., *Calc. c.*, Caps., Cham., Clem., *Cocc.*, Con., Dig., Graph., *Hyos.*, Iod., Kali bi., Lach., Lyc., Merc., Mez., Petr., Rhus t., Saba., *Selen.*, Seneg., *Sil.*, Spig., Spo., Sul., Sul. ac., Thuja.

HAIR.

Falling out: Amb., Ars., Bell., Calc., Carb. v., Ferr., *Graph.*, Hep., *Kali c.*, Merc., *Nat. m.*, Petr., *Phos.*, Rhus t., Sars., Sep., Staph., *Sul.*

Bunches, in: Phos.,

Forehead, from: Ars., Merc., Nat. m., Phos.

Occiput, from: Carb. v., Petr.

Sides of, from: Graph.

Temples, from: Kali c., *Nat. m.*

Vertex, from: *Bar. c.*, Graph., Sep.

Pregnancy during: *Lach.*

Gray: Lyc.

Tangled: Bor., Mez.

HAT, does not like: Iod., Led., Lyc.

HEAT: Acon., All. c., Alum., Ambr., Ant. t., *Apis, Arn., Ars.*, Aur., Bell., Bor., Bry., *Calc.*, Calc. p., Carb. v., Chel., Cocc., Coloc., Con., Crot., Cur., Cycl., Dros., Ferr., Gamb., Gels., Glon., *Graph.*, Hell., Ign., Ipe., Kali chl., Lach., Lac. d., Laur., Mag. c., Mag. m., Mang., Mez., Mosch., Nat. c., Nit. ac., Nux m., *Nux v.*, Op., Phos., Phyt., Plb., Podo., Sep., Sil., Stann., Stram., Stront., Sulph., Verat., Xanth.

Bed, in: Nux v.

HEAVINESS: Acon., Agar., Alum., Amm. m., *Apis*, Arg. n., Arn., Ars., Bell., Bry., Cact., Calc., Camph., Cann. i., Canth., Carb. ac., Carb. an., Carb. v., Card. m., Cham., Chel., *Chin.*, Chin. s., Clem., Colch., Con., Corn., Crot. t., Cupr., Dig., Dros.,

HEAVINESS.

Dulc., Elaps, Gamb., *Gels.*,
Glon., Hell., Hyos., Ign.,
Ipe., Kali bi., Kali i., Kali
n., *Lach.*, Laur., Lyc., Mag.
m., Mag. s., Mang., Men.,
Merc., Mur. ac., Nat. c., *Nat.
m.*, Nicc., Nit. ac., *Nux v.*,
Op., Petr., Phel., Phos.. Ph.
ac., *Pic. ac.*, Plb., Puls.,
Rheum, Rhus t., Sabin., Sars.,
Sec., Seneg., Sep., Sil.,
Spong., Stann., Stron., Staph.,
Sulph., Sul. ac., Tab., Tarax.,
Thuja, Viola t., Zinc.

INJURIES OF THE HEAD:
Arn., Hyper., Nat. m.,
Nat. s.

SCALP:
Adhesion, feeling of: Arn.,
Berb.

Beaten feeling on scalp: Hell.,
Ip., Petr., Ruta.

Blood vessels, distention of:
Bell., Sang., Thuja.

Boils: Hell., Led., Merc., Nux..
Petr., Puls., Ruta, Sep., Sil.

painful: Hell., Hep., Kali c.,
Merc., Mez., Nux., Puls.

painful to touch: Ars., Hep.,
Kali c., Ruta.

of a burning, bitting type,
sensitive to touch and cold:
Ars.

suppurating type: Calc.,
Kali c.

Coldness on scalp: Agar., Calc.,
Iris., Sabad., Sep., Sulph.,
Verat.

sense of coldness: Acon.,
Agar., Ambr., Arn., Bell.,
Calc., Canab., Chelid.,
Lach., Laur., Mosch.,
Phos., Verat.

sense of coldness on forehead:
Cinnab., Merc.

SCALP.

sense of coldness on one side:
Ruta.

circumscribed area, in: Sulph.

from nape extending: Chelid.

from vertex, down to sacrum:
Laur.

Contraction of: Nat. m., Plat.,
Ran. s., Rhus.

in the skin of forehead: Gels.

feeling of: Carb. v., Chin.,
Plat., Sulph.

Creeping sensation: Arg. n.,
Bar. c., Cinnab., Staph.

Cutting pain: Sars.

Daily pain, experienced in the
scalp: Nat. c.

Drawing pain: Canth., Chenop.,
Chin., Graph., Lach., Mag.
n., Meny., Nit. ac., Petr.,
Phos. ac., Puls., *Rhod.*,
Rhus, Ruta, Sars., Sep.,
Staph., Thuja.

Drawing pain, extending to face:
Mag. m.

extending to glands of throat:
Graph.

extending to teeth: Graph.,
Mag. m., Petr.

extending to temples and forehead: Petr.

Furrows on forehead: Cham.,
Hell., Lyc., Rheum, Rhus,
Sep., Stram.

Furruncles: Bar. c., Bell., Calc.,
Kali c., Led., Mag. m., Mur.
ac., Nit. ac., Rhus.

Immobility: Arn., Berb.

Lice: *Psor.*, Sabad.

Lumps, tubercles: Calc., Daph.,
Hell., Ign., Petr., Puls.,
Rhus, Ruta, Sep., Sil.

painful: Hell., Nux., Puls.,
Ruta.

suppurating: Calc., Kali c.

SCALP.

Painful: Ars., Bar. c., Bell.,
Carb. a., Carb. v., Caps.,
Chin., Kreos., Ferr., Lith.,
Nat. s., Nit. ac., Nux, Petr.,
Rhus, Sars., Selen., Sil..
Staph., Tar., Thuja.

from pressure of hat: Agar.,
Carb. a., Carb. v., Crot.,
Nit. a., Sil.

from scratching: Bar. c., Caps.
in small spots: Aloe.

from touch: Agar., Ambr.,
Arg., Ars., Bar. c., Bov.,
Bufo, Chin., Cinnab.,
Cupr., Ferr., Merc., Mez.,
Nat. m., Nat. p., Nit. ac.,
Nux m., Nux v., Par.,
Petr., Rhus, Selen., Sil.,
Sulph., Thuja, Zinc.

Scabs, Scurfs: Ars., Bar. m.,
Bov., Bry., Calc., Carb. a.,
Chelid., Graph., Hep., Nat.
m., Oleand., Petr., Rhus,
Ruta, Sil., Sulph.

Sore spots: Bov.

SENSATION:

Constriction, menses during:
Gels., Helon., Iod., Lyc.,
Merc., Plat., Sulph.

Constriction while passing stool:
Coloc.

Elongated: Hyper.

Empty, hollow sensation: Arg.
m., Ars., Carb., Cocc., Cor.
r., Cupr., Graph., Manc.,
Phos., Puls., Seneg., Sulph.

Enlarged: Arg. n., Arn. Bell.,
Berb., Bov., Cimic., Cor. r.,
Dulc., Gels., Glon., Hyper.,
Lac. d., Mang., Nat. m.,
Nux m., Nux v., Par., Plat.,
Ran. b., Sil.

Formication: Acon., Agar.,
Arg. m., Arg. n., Calc. p.,

SENSATION, formication, of.

Cycl., Ferr., Pic. ac., Rhus
t., Sulph.

Fullness: Acon., Amm. m., Apis,
Arg. n., Bell., Bor., Bry.,
Calc., Calc. p., Carb. v.,
Cinnab., Con., Cycl., Dig.,
Ferr., Fl. ac., Gels., Glon.,
Ham., Hyos., Lac. d., Merc.,
Nicc., Nit. ac., Nux m.,
Petr., Phos., Psor., Ran. b.,
Ran. s., Rhus t., Sang.,
Spong., Sulph., Sul. ac.,
Tereb., Xanth.

Itching: Agar., Alum., Amm.
c., Amm. m., Bar. c., Bor.,
Calc., Carb., ac., Carb. an.,
Caust., Clem., Crot. h., Ferr.,
Fl. ac. Form., Graph., Laur.,
Lyc., Merc., Merc. i. f.,
Mez., Nat. m., Olnd., Petr.,
Phos., Sars., Sep., Sil.,
Staph., Sulph., Sul. ac., Tell.

Numbness: Bry., Graph., Nit.
ac., Plat.

Swollen: Apis, Arg. n., Bell.,
Glon., Nux v., Ran. b.

Tingling: Coloc., Cupr., Rhus t.

Sweat, perspiration: Agar.,
Anac., Ant. t., Apis. Bell.,
Calc., Calc. p., Carb. v.,
Caust., Cham., Chin., Graph.,
Gua., Kali c., Hep., Lyc.,
Mag. m., Merc., Mez., Mur.
ac., Nit. ac., Petr., Phos.,
Puls., Rheum, Sil., Stram.

forehead: Ars., Brom., Cact.,
Calc., Cann. i., Carb v.
Chin., Guaj., Hep., Ip.,
Kali bi., Kali c., Laur.,
Led., Merc. c., Nat. c.,
Nit. ac., Op., Phos., Sars.,
Stann., Tab., Verat.,
Zinc.

occiput: Calc., Ph. ac.,
Sanic., Sep., Sil., Sulph.

SENSORIUM.

CLOUDY: Bell., Bry., Calad., Cocc., Crot., Lact., Laur., Mag. m., Merc., *Nux, Op.,* *Phell.*, Rheum, Samb., Valer.

Dull: Calc., Caust., Kali c., Phos., Sil.

with an attack of cough: Rumex.

with an attack of diarrhœa: Gels.

DIZZINESS, CONFUSION, INDISPOSITION: Acon., Æth., Asar., Bry., Calc., Nux m., Nux v., Plat., Rhod., Sep., Tar.

Gloomy: Arg., Calad., Clem., Dig., Meny., Merc., Mez., Nat. m., *Nux,* Op., Phos. ac., Puls., Rheum, Samb., Thuja, Valer.

Long-continued: Calc.

Seminal emission, as after: Caust., Mez., Ph. ac.

Unrefreshed sleep as if: Ruta.

Watching all night, after: Ambr. Bry., Chin., *Nux,* Puls.

FATIGUE of the head, by mental labor: Aur., Calc., Nat. c. Nux, Puls., Sil.

VERTIGO: Acon., Æsc., *Agar.,* *Ail.,* Aloe, Ambr., Amm. c., Ant. c., *Apis, Arg. m.,* Arg. n., Arn., Ars., Ars. h., Aster., Aur., Aur. m., *Bapt.,* Bar. c., Berb., *Bell.*, Bry., Cact., *Calc.,* Calc. p., *Calc. s.,*

VERTIGO.

Camph., Cann. i., Cann. s. Canth., Carb. an., Carb. s., Carb. v., Caust. Cedr., Cham., Chel., Chin., *Chin. s.,* Cic., Cimic., Cocc., Coff., Coloc., *Con.,* Cupr., *Cycl.,* *Dig., Dulc.,* Elaps., Ferr., Ferr. ar., Ferr. p., *Gels.,* Glon., Graph., Guara., Hep., Hydr., Hyos., Iod., Kali bi., Kali br., Kali c., Kali i., Kali n., Kali s., Kalm., Lach., Led., *Lyc.*, Manc., Merc., Mer. c., Mez., Mosch., Mur. ac., Mygale, Nat. a., Nat. c., *Nat. m.,* Nat. p., Nat. s., Nit. ac., Nux m., *Nux v.,* Onos., Op., *Petr.,* Ph. ac., Phos., Phyt., Plat., Podo., Psor., *Puls.,* Ran. b., Rhod., *Rhus t.,* Rhus v., *Sang.,* Sec., Seneg., Sep., *Sil.,* Spig., Spong., Stann., Stram., Stront., *Sulph.,* Tab., Tereb., Ther., Thuja, Urt. u., *Valer.,* Verat. v., Zinc.

Air open, in: Agar, Caust., Glon., Kreos., Mur. ac., Podo., Ran. b., Sep.

relieved: Amm. m., Camph., Caust., Grat., Kali s., Mag. m., Nat. s., Phell., Puls., Sanic., Sul. ac., Sulph., Tab.

Ascending: Bor., Dirc., Sulph. an eminence: *Calc.,* Kali bi. stairs: *Calc.*, Kali b.

VERTIGO.

Bath, following a: Phys., Samb.

Bed, on going to: Nat. m., Sabad., Stram.

Breakfast, at: Con.

   after: Bufo, Gels., Lyc., Phos., Selen., Tarent.

   relieved after: Alum.

Closing eyes, on: Alum., Ant. t., Apis, Arg. n., *Arn.*, Ars., Chel., Hep., *Lach.*, Ph. ac., Sep., Sil., Stram., *Ther.*, Thuja.

   relieved: Pip. m.

   with nausea: Lach., Ther.

Coition, after: Ph. ac., Sep.

Colic, alternates: Verat.

Coughing, while: Coff., Kali bi., Mosch.

Crossing a bridge: Bar. c., Brom.

   running water, flowing water: Arg., Arg. m.

Crowd, in a: Nux v.

Descending, while: Bor., Ferr.

Epilepsy, before: Caust., *Hyos.*, Lach., Plb., Sulph.

Erection, during: Tarent.

Floating, with a feeling as if: Calc. ar., Hyper., Lac. c., Lach., Manc., Mez., Nux. m., Op., Sep., Valer.

High places: Arg. n., *Calc.*, Sulph., Zinc.

VERTIGO: Hungry, when he feels: Kali c.

Lifting a weight on: *Puls.*

Looking with eyes turned: *Spig.*

   at high buiildings: Arg. n.

      moving things: Agar., Con., Cur., Jab., Sulph.

VERTIGO, looking.

right or left, either ways: Con., Spig.

Steadily: Caust., Cur., Kali c., Lach., *Nat. m.*, Phos., Sil., *Spig.*

   upwards: Calc., Caust., Cupr., Graph., Lach., Nux v., Petr., *Phos.*, *Puls.*, Sang., Sil., Tab., Thuja.

Lying down, on: Bell.

   while: Apis, Carb. v., Caust., Cham., *Con.*, Lach., Nit. ac., Puls., Rhus t., Samb., Thuja.

   back: Alum., Merc., Puls., Sil

Menses, previous to: Calc. p., Con., Lach., Puls., Verat., Zinc.

   when the flow is on: Acon., Calc., Caust., Con., Croc., Cycl., Ferr. p., Gels., Iod., Kali bi., Lach., Ph. ac., Phos., *Puls.*, Sec., Sulph.

   suppressed: Acon., *Cycl.*, *Puls.*

Mental application: Agar., Arg. n., Bor., *Nat. c.*, *Nat. m.*, *Nux v.*, Ph. ac., Puls.

Motion, from: Agar., Am. c., Aur., Bell., *Bry.*, Calc. p., Carb. v., Chin., Coff,. Con., Glon., Graph., Hep., Kalm., Mag. c., Med., Phos., Puls., Sil.

Nauses, coming on with: *Acon.*, Alum., Alumn., Amm. c., Ant., c., Bapt., Bar. c., Bell., Bry., Calc., Calc. p., Calc. s., Camph., Carb. an., Carb. v., Caust., Cham., Chel., *Chin.* s., Cinnab., Cocc., Con., Cycl., *Ferr.*, Ferr. ar., Glon.,

VERTIGO, nausea coming on with.

Graph., Ham., Hell., Hep., Ind., Kali bi., Kalm., Lac. c., Lach., Lob., Lyss., Lyc., Merc., Mosch., Nat. m., Nat. s., Nit. ac., Nux m., Nux v., *Petr.*, Phos., Puls., Rhus t., Sang., Sep., Sil., Spig., Staph., Sulph., Tab., Tereb., Ther., Verat., Verat. v., Zinc.

Noise, from: Ther.

Pregnant woman, in a: Gels., *Nat. m.*

Rising. on: Ambr., *Bell.*, *Bry.*, Caust., Con., Dulc., Gamb., Lyc., Mag. m., Nat. m., Nit. ac., *Phos.*, *Puls.*, *Rhus t.*, Spig.

better: Caust., Rhus t.

after: *Lyc.*, Nit. ac., *Phos.*, *Tell.*

Shave, after a: Carb. an.

Sleep, during: Sang., Sil.

after: Calc., Carb. v., Chin., Dulc., Graph., Kali c., *Lach.*, Lact., Med., *Nux v.*, Sep., Spong., Ther.

Sprituous liquors. alcoholic drinks: *Coloc.*, *Nat. m.*, *Nux v.*

VERTIGO.

Stool, before: Alum., *Lach.*

during: Caust., Cocc.

after: Caust., Nat. m.

better from: Cupr.

Stoops, while he: Alum., Arg. n., Aur., Bar. c., *Bell.*, Bry., Cact., Calc., Camph., Carb. v., Caust., Cham., Glon., Graph., Guare., Ham., Hell., Ign., Iod., Kali bi., Kali c., Kalm., Lach., Lyc., Merc., Merc., c., Nit. ac., *Nux v.*, Petr., Phos., *Puls.*, Sil., Staph,. *Sulph.*

Urinating, while: Acon.

profusely, better: Gels.

Walking on: Carb. v., Chin., Dulc., Graph., Kali bi., *Lach.*, Nat. m.,

Warm room, in a: Croc., Grat., Lyc., *Nat. s.*, Ptel., Puls., Sanic.

Washes his feet, when he: Merc. in warm water: Samb.

Water, while crossing running: Arg. n., Bell., Ferr., Hyos., Sulph.

Wine: Alum., Con., Nat. c., Nux v., Zinc.

FACE.

AFECTIONS, troublesome, of the face:

Abscess: Bell., Hep., Kali. i., Merc., Phos., Sil.

on the lip: Anthr.

upper: Bell.

parotid glands: Ars., Lach., Phos., Rhus t., Sil.

submaxillary glands: Calc., Lach., Phos., Sil.

Acne rosacea: Kali bi., Rhus. t.

Boils: Alum., Arn., Bell., Bry., Chin., Laur., Led.

Cancers: Ars., Aur., Carb. ac., Con., Kali ar., Phos.

lips, on the: Ars., Aur. n., Carb. an., Cic., Cist., Con., Kreos., Lach., Lyc., Sep., Sil.

lupus: Arg. n., Ars., Carb. c., Hydrc., Kali bi., Psor., Sep., Sil.

epithelioma: Ars., Kali s., Lach., Phos., Sep., Sil.

Caries of bones: Aur., Phos.

lower jaw: Aur., Aur. m. Aur. m. n., Con., Fl.. ac., Kali i., Merc., Nit. ac.. Phos., Phyt., Sil.

Cracked lips: Agar.. Ail., Amm. c., Amm. m., Arn., Ars.. Arum. t., Bapt., Bov.. Bry.. Calc., Calc. s., Caps., Carb. an., Carb. v., Cham., Croc., Graph., Hell., Ign., Kreos.. Lach., Merc.. Merc. c., Mez.. Nat. m.. Plat.. Rhus t..

AFFECTIONS, cracked lips.

Sil., Stram., Sulph., Verat., Zinc.

lower lip: Nat. c., Nit. ac., Phos., Sep.

upper lip: Kali c., Nat. m.

Corners of mouth: Arum. t., Cond., Graph., Hell., Hydr., Merc., Mez., Nat. m., Nit. ac., Sep., Sil., Zinc.

Erysipelas: Anthr., Apis, Aur., Bell., Bor., Camph., Canth., Carb. an., Carb. v., Caust., Cham., Chel., Chin., Cupr., Echi., Euph., Graph., Hep., Jug. c.. Lach., Led.. Mez., Nit. ac., Puls., Rhus t., Rhus r., Sulph., Sul. ac.

types, erratic, wandering: Puls.

gangrenous: Ars., Lach.

oedematous: Apis. Rhus t.

phlegmonous: Acon., Apis. Arn., Bell., Crot. h., Hep., Hippoz., Graph., Lach., Rhus t., Sil., Sulph.

Freckles: Amm. c.. Ant. c.. Calc., Dulc.. Graph.. Kali c., Lyc., Nat. c.. Nit. ac.. Nux m.. Phos.. Puls.. Sep.. Sul.

Necrosis of the lower jaw: Hep.. Phos.. Sil.

CHANGE OF COLOUR: Acc., Alum., Aur., Bell.. Caps.. Carb. a.. Cham.. Chin.. Cina. Croc.. Ferr.. Graph.

CHANGE, of colour.

Hyo., *Ign.*, Led., Mag. c.,
Oleand., *Phos.*, Phos. ac.,
Plat., *Sul. ac.*, Zinc.

Discoloration, ashy: Ars., Bad.,
Chlor., Cic., Ferr., Phos.,
Plb.

blacky: Chin., Cor. r., Lach.,
Tarent.

bluish: Agar., Ail., Apis,
Arg. n., *Ars.*, *Asaf.*, Aur.,
Bapt., Bel., Bry., Cact.,
Camph. Cann. i., Canth.,
Carb. an., Carb. s., Cham.,
Croc., *Graph.*, Hel., Ign.,
Lach., Merc., Merc. c.,
Mez., Nat. m., *Op.*, Phyt.,
Puls., Samb., Spong.,
Staph., Stram., Sulph.,
Tab., Tarent., *Verat.*,
Verat. v., Vip.

chill, during: Cact., *Nux v.*,
Stram., Tub.

cholera, in: Camph., *Cupr.*,
Verat.

coughing, while: Apis, Coc.
c., Cor. r., *Dros.*, *Ip.*,
Mag. p., Verat.

laughing, while: *Cann. i.*

menses, previous to: Puls.

pregnant woman, in a: *Phos.*

lips get blue: Acet., ac.,
Acon., Ant. t., Apoc.,
Arg., *n.*, Ars., Aur., Bar.
c., Cact., *Camph.*, Cedr.,
Chin., Chin. s., Colch.,
Crot. h., *Cupr.*, Dig.,
Dros., Hep., *Hydr.*, ac.,
Iod., Ip., Kali i., *Lach.*,
Lyc., Nat. m., *Nux v.*,
Phos., Prun.

cyanosis: Ars., Aur., Cact.,
Cupr., Nat m.

dark: Ail., Apis, Bap.,
Carb. v., Gels., *Nit. ac.*,
Op., Sulph.

CHANGE, of colour.

dirty: Apis, *Arg. n.*, Caps.,
Chel., Cupr., *Lyc.*, Mag.
c., Merc., *Psor.*, Sanic.,
Sulph.

greenish: Ars., *Carb. v.*,
Chel., Ferr., Iod., Med.,
Puls.

red: Acon., Agar., Ail.,
Amyl. n., Anac., Ant. c.,
Ant. t., *Apis*, Arg. n.,
Aur. m., Bad., *Bapt.*,
Arn., Ars., Asaf., Aster.,
Bar. c., *Bell.*, Bov., *Bry.*,
Camph., Canth., *Caps.*,
Carl., *Caust.*, Cedr.,
Cham., *Chel.*, *Chin.*, Chin.
s., *Cic.*, *Cina*, Coc. c.,
Cocc., Coff., Coloc., Croc.,
Crot. h., Crot. t., Cupr.,
Eup. per., *Ferr.*, Ferr. i.,
Dig., Dros., Dulc., Elaps.,
Gels *Clon.*, Grat., Guai.,
Hell., Hep., Hyos., Hy-
per., Ign., Jab., Kali i.,
Lach., Lyc., Meli., Merc.,
Merc. c., *Mez.*, Mur ac.,
Naja, Nat. c., Nat. m.,
Nux v., *Op.*, Petr., Phos.,
Plan., Plat., Plb., Puls.,
Pyrog., Ran. b., Rhus t.,
Sabad., Samb., *Sang.*, Se-
nec., Sep., Sil., Spig.,
Spong., Stann., Stram.,
Stront., Sulph., Sul. ac.,
Tab., Tarax., Thuja,
Verat., *Verat v.*

redness and circumscribed:
Ant. t., Ars., *Chin.*,
Colch., Dulc., *Ferr.*, Kali
ci

red, dark: Bapt., Bar. c.
Bell., Bry., Camph., Chel.,
Coloc., Gels., Hyos., *Op.*,
Sang., Sec., Tarent.,
Verat.

CHANGE, of colour.

yellow: Ambr., *Arg. m.*, *Ars.*,
Bapt., Bell., Bry., *Calc.*,
Calc. p., Canth., Carb. v.,
Card. m., Caust., Cham.,
Chel., Chin., Chin. s.,
Chion., Con., Corn. c.,
Croc., Crot., h., Dig.,
Elaps, *Ferr.*, Ferr. ars.,
Ferr. p., Gels., Graph.,
Hell., Hep., Iod., Ip., Kali
c., *Lach.*, Lyc., Mag. c.,
Mag. m., Med., *Merc.*,
Myric., Nat. m., Nat. s.,
Nit. ac., *Nux v.*, Op.,
Petr., Phos., Phyt., *Plb.*,
Puls., Sars., Sec., *Sep.*,
Sil., *Sulph.*

CHEWING MOTION OF
THE JAW: Acon., Bell.,
Bry., Calc., Hell., Merc.,
Phos., Stram.

CRACKING IN JAW, while
chewing: Amm. c., Lac. c.,
Lach., Meny., Mez., *Nit. ac.*,
Rhus.

COUNTENANCE, besotted:
Bapt., Bry., Bufo, Cocc.,
Crot. h., Gels., Lach., Nux
v., Stram.

Idiotic: *Agar.*, Calc., Lach.,
Laur., Lyc.

Old, aged look: Abrot., *Arg.
m.*, Ars., Ars. h., Aur. m.,
Bar. c., *Calc.*, Fl. ac., Gua.,
Iod., Kreos., *Nat. m.*, Op.,
Sars., Sep., Sulph.

Stupid: Arg. n., Arn., Ars.,
Cann. i., Gels., Ferr., Hell.,
Hydr., Hyos., Nux m., Stram.

FALLING OF WHISKERS,
from the side of face: Calc.,
Graph., Kali c., Nat. m.,
Ph. ac.

HIPPOCRATIC: Æth, Amm. c.,
Carb. v., Chin., Colch., Cupr.,
Ant. c., *Ant. t.*, *Ars.*, Camph.,

HIPPOCRATIC.

Lach., Phos., Ph. ac., Plb.,
Sec., *Tab.*, *Verat.*

INFLAMMATION:

Bones of face: *Aur.*, Calc., Fl.
ac., Mez., Nit. ac., Ph. ac.,
Ruta, Sil., Staph., Sul.

Parotid gland: Amm. c., Ars.,
Arum. t., Aur., *Bar. c.*, *Bell.*,
Calc., Carb. an., Carb. v.,
Cham., Cist., Coc., Con.,
Crot. h., Ferr. p., Hep., Kali
bi., Kali c., Lach., *Merc.*,
Nat. m., Phos., *Puls.*, Rhus,
Sil.

Periosteum: Aur., Calc., Fl. ac.,
Merc., Mez., *Nit. ac.*, *Phos.*,
Ph. ac., Ruta, Staph.

Submaxillary gland: Bell., Dulc.,
Lach., *Merc.*, Phyt., Psor.,
Puls., *Rhus t.*, Sil., Sulph.,
Sul. ac.

PARALYSIS: Agar., Bar. c.,
Cadm., *Caust.*, Cocc., Cupr.,
Cur., Dulc., Graph., Kali
chl., Nux v.

One-sided: Bar. c., Caust.,
Cocc., Graph., Kali chl.

Wet, after he got: Caust.

SADDLE, across the nose: Carb.
an., *Sep.*

SARDONICUS, risus: *Bell.*,
Caust., Colch., Hyos., Sec.,
Stram.

SENSATIONS:

Cobwebs: Bar. c., Brom.,
Graph., Mag. c., Ran. s.

Hairs: Graph.

Large, face getting: Acon.

Long, as if elongated: Stram.

SHINY, face: Apis, Aur., Lyc.,
Nat. m., Plb., Psor.

SORDES ON THE LIPS:
Ars., Colch., Hyos., Phos.,
Stram.

EYES AND SIGHT.

AILMENTS, common:

Bleeding from the eyes: Arn., Calc., Carb. v., Cham., Crot. h., Kali chl., *Lach.*, *Nux v.*, Phos., Sulph.

Retinal hæmorrhage: Bell., Crot. h., Lach., Phos.

Cataract: Amm. c., Apis, Bar. c., *Calc.*, Calc. f., Calc. p., Cann. s., Carb. an., Caust., Chel., Colch., Con., Euph., Jab., Kali c., Lyc., *Mag. c.*, Nit. ac., Phos., Puls., Sec., Sep., *Sil.*, *Sulph.*, Zinc.

capsule, of the: Amm.m.

cortical: Sulphur.

lenticular: *Mag. c.*

old age, in the : Carb. an., Sec.

Chemosis: Acon., *Apis*, Arg. n., Con., Euph., Guare., Hep., Ip., Kali bi., *Kali i.*, Lach., Nat. m., *Rhus t.*, Vesp.

Condyloma: Calc., Merc., Nit. ac., Thuja.

iris: *Cinnab*, Merc.

Fistula of the cornea: Sil.

lachrymation: Apis, Arg. n., Aur. m., Brom., *Calc.*, Fl. ac., Hep., Lach., Lyc., Nat. m., Nit. ac., *Petr.*, Phyt., *Puls.*, Sil., Stan., Sulphur.

Granular lids: Alum., Apis, Arg. n., *Ars.*, Aur., Bor., Caust., Graph., Kali bi., *Lyc.*, Merc. c., Merc. i. f., Merc. i. r., Nat. a., Nat. m., Nat.

AILMENTS, granular lids.

s., Nux v., Puls., Sang., Sep., Sil., Sulph., Thuja, Zinc.

Lachrymation: Acon., Agar., Ail., *All. c.*, Alum., Apis, Arg. n., Ars., Asar., Aur., Bell., Brom., *Calc.*, Caps., Carb. ac., Carb. v., Caust., Chel., Colch., Con., Croc., Crot. c., Crot. h., Elaps., Eup. per., Euph., *Euphr.*, Ferr., Fl. ac., Graph., Ham., Hep., Ign., Iod., Kali bi., Kali c., Kali i., Lach., Led., Lyc., Nat. c., Nat. m., Nat. s., Nit. ac., Nux v., *Op.*, Par., *Phos.*, Psor., *Puls.*, Rhod., Rhus t., Ruta, Sabad., Sang., Seneg., Sep., Sil., Tarax., Thuja, Verat., Zinc.

coryza, during: *All. c.*, Anac., Arg. n., *Carb. v.*, Chin., Euphr., Chin., Kali c., *Nux v.*, Phos., Phyt., Puls., Sabad., Sang., *Tell.*, Verb.

cough, with: Agar., Eup. per., *Euphr.*, Graph., *Nat. m.*, Phyt., *Puls.*, Sabad., *Squil.*

Opacity of the cornea: Apis, *Arg. n.*, Aur., Aur. m., Bar. i., *Cadm.*, Calc., Cann. s., Caust., Chel., Chin., Cinnab., Cocc., Colch., Con., Crot. t., Euphr., Hep., Kali bi., Kali s., Lach., Lyc., Mag. c., Merc. i. f., Merc., Nit. ac., Seneg., Sil., *Sulph.*, Tarent., Zinc.

AILMENTS.

Pannus, vascularization of the cornea: Apis, *Arg. n.*, Aur., Bar. c., Calc., Caust., Euphr., Graph., Hip., Merc. i. f., Nit. ac., Sulphur.

Photophobia: *Acon.*, Agn., Ail., All. c., Alum., Ant. t., Apis, Arg. n., Arn., *Ars.*, Arum. t., Asar., Aur., Aur. m., *Bar. c.*, Bell., Bry., Calc., Calc. p., Caust., Cham., Chel., *Chin.*, Chin. a., Chin. s., Cic., Clem., Coff., *Con.*, Croc., Crot. h., Crot. t., Dig., Euphr., Eup. per., Gels., Glon., *Graph.*, Hell., Hep., Hyos., Ign., Kali ar., Kali bi., Kali c., Kali n., Kali p., Lac d., Lach., Lact. ac., Led., Lili. t., Lith., *Lyc.*, Mag. p., Merc., Merc. c., Nat. c., *Nat. m.*, Nat. s., *Nux v.*, *Op.*, Phos., Phyt., Psor., Puls., *Rhus t.*, Sanic., Sep., Sil., Spig., Stram., *Sulph.*, Tab., Verat., Zinc.

Pterygium: Ambr., Arg. n., Ars., Calc., Euphr., Form., Lach., Nux m., Psor., Rat., Sulph., Zinc.

Spots, specks, etc., on the cornea: Apis, Ars., Aur., Cadm., *Calc.*, Calc. f., Calc. p., Caust., Chel., Colch., *Con.*, Euphr., Form., Hep., Kali c., Merc., Nux m., Nit. ac., Puls., Ruta, Seneg., Sil., Sulph., Symph.

Strabismus: Alum., *Apis*, Bell., Calc., Canth., Chel., Chin. s., Cic., Cina, Con., *Cycl.*, Gels., Hell., Hyos., Kali br., Kali i., Lyc., Mag. p., Merc., Merc. c., Nat. m., Nux v., Stram., Tab., Zinc.

AILMENTS, strabismus.

convergent: Cic., *Cycl.*

divergent: Agar., Con., Jab., *Nat. m.*

Styes: Apis, Aur., Chel., *Con.*, Graph., Lyc., Merc., Ph. ac., Psor., Puls., Rhus t., Sep., Sil., *Staph.*, Sulph., Thuja.

Ulceration, conjunctiva: *Alum.* Caust., Crot. t., Hydr.

corneal ulcers: Agar., *Apis*, Arg. n., Ars., Asaf., Aur., Bar. c., *Calc.*, Calc. f., Calc. p., Calc. s., Chin., Clem., Con., Crot. t., *Euphr.*, Form., Graph., Hep., Ipe., Kali bi., Kali c., Lach., Merc., Merc. c., Merc. i. f., Nat. c., Nat. m., Nit. ac., Psor., Puls., Rhus t., Sang., Sanic., Sil., Sulph., Thuja.

ATROPHY OF OPTIC NERVE: Nux v., *Phos.*

CLOSURE:

Involuntary: Caust., *Chin. s.*, Con., Gels., Grat., Merc., Nat. c., Rhus t., Sep., *Sulph.*

Spasmodic: Alum., *Ars.*, Bell., Calc., *Coloc.*, Con., *Merc.*, Merc. c., *Nat. m.*, Psor., Rhus t.

CLOSED, cannot open them: Calc., Cocc., Grat., Lachn., *Rhus t.*

CRUSTY MARGINS OF LIDS: Arg. n., Aur., Graph., Sanic., Sulph.

ECCHYMOSIS: Acon., *Arn.*, Bell., Cact., Con., Crot. h., Cupr. ac., Glon., Ham., Kal chl., Lach., *Led.*, Lyc., Nux v., Phos., Sul. ac.

FALLING OF LIDS: Alum., Bell., Caust., Gels., Lyc., Op., Viol. t.

INFLAMMATION: *Acon.*, Act. sp., Agar., *All.* c., Alum., Ambr., Ant. c., Ant. t., *Apis*, Arg. n., *Arn.*, *Ars.*, Asaf., Aur., Bad., Bar. c., Canth., Bar. m., *Bell.*, Bor., Bry., *Calc.*, Calc. p., *Calc. s.*, Caust., Cham., Chin., Cinnab., Clem., Colch., Coloc., Con., Dulc., Eup. per., Euph., *Euphr.*, Form., Gels., Glon., Graph., Grind., Hep., Ign., Iod., Ipe., Iris, Kali c., Kali chl., Kali i., Kalm., Lach., Led., Lith., Lyc., Mag. c., Merc., Merc. c. Mez., *Nat. m.*, Nat. s., Nit. ac., Nux v., Petr., Phos., Phyt., *Psor.*, *Puls.*, *Rhus t.*, Sang., Sep., Sil., Spig., Staph., Stram., *Sulph.*, Sul. ac., Ter., Thuja, Zinc.

Burns, from: Canth.

Catarrhal, due to cold: *Acon.*, *All. c.*, Apis., Arg. m., *Ars.*, Aur., Bell., Bry., *Calc.*, Calc. p., Cham., Chlor., Dig., *Dulc.*, *Euphr.*, Graph., Hep., Hydr., Iris., Kali br., *Merc.*, Merc. c., Mez., Nux v., Petr., *Psor.*, Puls., Sang., Sep., Sulph., Thuja.

Erysipelatous: Acon., *Apis*, Bell., Graph., Hep., Led., Merc., Merc.c., *Rhus t.*

Foreign bodies, from: Acon., Arn., Calc., Puls., *Sil.*

Gonorrœa: Ant. t., Merc., *Nit. ac.*, *Puls.*, Spig., Sulph., Thuja.

Menses, when the flow is on: Ars., Zinc.

INFLAMMATION.

Scrofulous: Ant. c., Apis, *Ars.*, Arg. m., *Aur.*, Arum. m. n., Bad., Bar. c., Bar. m., Bell., Cadm., *Calc.*, *Calc. s.*, Calc. p., *Caust.*, Cham., Cinnab., Cist., Con., Dulc., Euphr., Fl. ac., *Graph.*, *Hep.*, Hyos., Iod., Kali bi., Kali i., Lith., Mag. c., Merc., Merc. c., Nat. m., Nat. p., Nat. s., *Nit. ac.*, Nux v., *Petr.*, *Puls.*, *Psor.*, *Phyt.*, Rhus t., Sars., Sep., Sil., Spig., *Sul.*, Sul. ac., Tell., Viol. t., Zinc.

Syphilitic: Ars., *Asaf.*, Aur., Cinnab., Clem., Graph., Hep., *Kali i.*, *Merc.*, Merc. c., Merc. i. f., *Nit. ac.*, *Phyt.*, Staph., Syph.

PARALYSIS:

Lids: Alum., Ars., Cadm., Cocc., Con., Graph., Guare., Merc. i. f., Plb., *Sep.*, *Spig.*, Verat.

upper: Alum., Ars., Cadm., Caust., Cocc., Con., Dulc., Euphr., Gels., Graph., Led., Mag. p., Med., Merc., Morph., Nit. ac., Nux m., Phos., Plb., *Rhus t.*, Sec., *Sep.*, Spig., Syph., Verat., Zinc.

Muscles of eye-balls:

external recti: Caust.

internal recti: *Agar.*, *Con.*, Jab., *Nat. m.*, Ruta, Seneg.

superior oblique: Arn., Seneg., Syph.

cilliary: Acon., Arg. n., Con., Dub., *Ruta*, Seneg.

Optic nerve: Arg n., Ars., Aur. m., Aur. m. n., *Bell.*, Bov., Calc., Caust., Chel., Chin.,

PARALYSIS, optic nerve.

Con., Elaps, Ferr., *Gels.*,
Hyos., Kali s., Lyc., Meny.,
Merc., *Nat. m.*, Nux v., Op.,
Phos., Ph. ac., Plb., Psor.,
Puls., Rhus t., Ruta, Sec.,
Sep., *Sil.*, Stram., Sulph.,
Thuja, Zinc.

PUPILS:

Contracted: Acon., Anac., Apis,
Arn., Ars., Aur., Bell., Calc.,
Camph., Chel., Chin. s.,
Daph., Grin., Hell., Hyos.,
Merc., Merc.c., Mez., Mur.
ac., Nat. m., *Op.*, Phys.,
Plb., Puls., Rhus, Sep.,
Stann., Thuja, Verat., Zinc.

Dilated: Acon., Æth., Agar.,
Agn., Ail., Anac., Apis, *Arg.
n.*, Arn., *Bell.*, *Calc.*, Camph.,
Carb. an., Cedr., *Chin.*,
Chin. s., Cic., Cina, Cocc.,
Coff., Colch., Coloc., Con.,
Cor. r., Croc., Cycl., Dig.,
Gels., Glon., Gua., Hell.,
Hyos., Hyper., Iod., Kali
br., Kali i., Laur., Led.,
Mang., Merc., Mosch., Nat.
c., Nat. p., Nit. ac.,
Nux v., Op.; Phos., Ph. ac.,
Puls., Sang., *Sec.*, Spig.,
Stram., Verat.

Insensible to light: Arn., Bar.
c., *Bell.*, Camph., Chel.,
Cic., Colch., Cupr., Dig.,
Hell., *Hyos.*, Kali br., Kali
i., Merc., Merc. c., *Op.*,
Plat., Stram.

SENSATIONS:

Hair of, in eye: Puls.

Heaviness: Æsc., *Aloe.*, *Arn.*,
Carb. v., Com., Sulph.

lids: Calc., *Caust.*, Cocc.,
Con., Ferr., Form., Gels.,
Graph., Hell., Hydr., Kali

SENSATION, heaviness of.

bi., Lac. c., Lac. d., Lyc.,
Merc., Nat. c., Nat. m.,
Nat. s., Nux m., Nux v.,
Phos., *Rhus t.*, Sep.,
Spong., Sulph., Verat.,
Zinc.

SIGHT:

Blurred: Aur., Con., *Gels.*,
Glon., Lil. t., *Nat. m.*, Nux
v., Phys., Plat., Psor.,
Rhus t.

Colors before the eyes: Bell.,
Bry., Calc., Camph., Cic.,
Cina, Con., Cycl., Dig., Iod.,
Kali bi., Mag. p., Nat. m.

black: Arn., Clem., Lac.,
Merc., *Nat. m.*, Phos.

black, flickerings: *Lach.*

black, floating: Chel., *Phos.*

blue: Aur., Bell., Bry., Cina,
Crot. c., Lach., Lyc.,
Stram.

dark: Anac., Bell., Calc.,
Chin., Cocc., Con., Euphr.,
Merc., Nit. ac., Phos.,
Sep., Sil., Stram., *Sulph.*

green: Ars., Cina, Cycl., Dig.,
Lac. c., *Phos.*, Ruta,
Stront.

red: Bell., Cact., Con., Dig.,
Hep., Hyos., Kali bi.,
Nux m., Phos., Stront.,
Sulph.

violet: *Cina.*

white: Dig., Kali c., Ph. ac.

yellow: Bell., Canth., Cina,
Crot. h., Cycl., Dig., Kali
bi., Kali c., Sepia.

Diplopia: Agar., Alumn., Arg.
n., *Aur.*, Bell., Caust., Chel.,
Cic., Con., Cycl., Daph.,
Dig., Gels., Graph., Hyos.,
Iod., Kali cy., Lyc., Lyss.,

SIGHT, diplopia.

> Merc., Morph., *Nat. m.,*
> Nicc., *Nit. ac.,* Nux v., Plb.,
> Puls., Seneg., Spong., Stram.,
> Sulph., Thuja, Verat.

> pregnant woman, in a: Gels.

Hemiopia: Ars., Aur., Calc.,
> Cocc., Glon., Lith., Lyc.,
> Nat. m., Sep., Stram.

Hyper metropia: Æsc., *Arg. n.,*
> Bell., Calc., Carb. an., Chin.,
> Coloc., Con., Dros., Hyos.,
> Lyc., Lil. t., Nat. m.,
> Nux v., Petr., *Sep.,* Sil.

Large, objects appear: *Hyos.,*
> Laur., Nat. m., Nicc., *Nux*
> *m.,* Onos.

> small objects appear large and
> he will raise his foot high
> while stepping over those
> small objects: *Onos.*

Letters running together: Art.
> v., Camph., *Cann. i.,* Chel.,
> Chin., Con., Dros., Ferr.,
> Graph., Lyc., *Nat. m., Ruta,*
> Seneg., *Sil.,* Staph., *Stram.*

Loss of sight, periodic: Ant. t.,
> Chel., Dig., Euphr., Nat. m.,
> Phos., Puls., Sep., Sil., Sulph.

Myopia: Agar., Amm. c.,
> Anac., Arg. n., Carb. v.,
> Chin., Con., Euphr., Gels.,
> Graph., Hyos., Jab., Lach.,
> Lyc., Mang., Meph., Nat. c.,
> Nat. m., Nit. ac., Petr.,
> *Phos.,* Ph. ac., *Phys.,*Pic. ac.,
> Puls., Ruta, Stram., Sulph.,
> Sul ac., Thuja, Valer.

SIGHT, myopia.

> Nearer, objects appear: Bov.

> Net, before eyes: Carb. an.,
> Chin. s.

> Small, objects appear: All. c.,
> Aur., Glon., Hyos., Kali
> chl., Lyc., Merc., Merc. c.,
> Plat., Plb.

SWOLLEN: Acon., Anac., *Apis,*
> Ars., Bry., Cedr., Cham.,
> Chlor., *Gua.,* Hep., Ign.,
> Ipe., Kali c., Mag. c., Nat.
> a., Nit. ac., Nux v., *Rhus*
> *t.,* Sep., Stram.

Lower lids: Dig., *Kali ar.,* Phos.

Under the lids: *Apis, Ars.,* Hep.,
> *Kali c.*

Upper lids: Apis, Con., Cycl.,
> Ign., *Kali c.,* Med., Nat. c.,
> Petr., Squilla, Syph.

Œdematous lids: *Apis,* Arg. n.,
> Arn., *Ars.,* Crot. t., Cycl.,
> Graph., Kali ar., Kali bi.,
> *Kali c.,* Kali i., Merc. c.,
> Nat. a., Phos., Phyt., Psor.,
> *Rhus t.,* Tell.

WINKING: Apis., Bell., Caust.,
> Croc., *Euphr.,* Fl. ac., Ign.,
> Mez., Nux v., Spig.

YELLOWISH: Ars., Aur. m.,
> Bell., Canth., Card. m.,
> Cham., *Chin.,* Chion., *Crot.*
> *h.,* Dig., Dios., Eup. per.,
> Gels., Hep., Iod., Ipe., Kali
> br., Lach., Mag. m., Nat. s.,
> *Nux v.,* Phos., Plb., Podo,
> Sang., *Sep.,* Verat.

EARS AND HEARING.

AILMENTS, common:

Abscess behind: *Aur.*, Bar. m., Caps., Nit. ac., *Sil.*

in meatus: *Calc.* s., *Hep.*, Mag. c., Puls., *Sil.*

Catarrh:

Eustachian tube: *Ars.*, *Calc.*, Caust., Hydr., Iod., Kali chl., *Kali* s., Mang., Merc., Nat. m., Nit. ac., Petr., Phos., *Puls.*, Sang., Sil.

Eruptions: *Bar.* c., Calc., Cic., Cist., Fl. ac., Graph., Kali bi., Lyc., Petr., Phos., *Psor.*, Sep., Sulph.

blisters: Kreos.

boils: Sulph.

eczema: Kali s.

excretions: *Kali bi.*, Merc., Petr., Sulph.

moist: Calc., *Graph.*, Kali bi., Lyc., Merc., Psor.

purulent: Kreos., *Psor.*, Sulph.

scurfy: Iod., Lach., Lyc., *Psor.*

those extending to the face: Graph., Sep.

those are about the ears: Cic., Cist., Hyper., Mez., Sulph.

those are behind the ears: *Bar.* c., Calc., *Caust.*, Cic., *Graph.*, Hep., Kali s., *Lyc.*, Merc., Mez., *Petr.*, Psor., Puls., Sep., *Sil.*, *Staph.*, *Sulph.*, Viol. t.

Fungus growth: Merc.

Lupus on the lobes: Nit. ac.

AILMENTS.

Otalgia: Acon., All. c., Anac., Arg., Ant. c., Apis, Arg. n., Ars., Aur., Bar. c., Bar. m., Bell Bor., Calc., Cal. p., Calc. s., Cann. i., Caps., Carb. v., Caust., *Cham.*, Chel., Cimic., Cur., Dulc., Fl. ac., Form., Gels., Graph., *Hep.*, Kali bi., Kali c., Kali p., Kali s., Kalm., Lach., Lyc., Mag. p., Mang., Merc. i. f., Merc. i. r., Nit. ac., Nux v., Petr., Phel., *Phos.*, *Ph. ac.*, Plan., Plb., *Puls.*, Rhus t., Sep., Sil., Spig., Spong., Sul., Thuja, Verb., Zinc.

cold, due to: Dulc., Gels., Kalm., Merc., Puls.

faceache, with: *Bell.*

Menses, when the flow is on Kali c.

motion, on: Sil.

noise, from: Bell., *Con.*, Cop., Phos., Sang., Sil., *Sulph.*

swallow, on an attempt to: *Apis*, Calc., Con., Elaps, Lach., Merc., Nit. ac., *Nux v.*, Par., Petr., Phyt., Sulph.

toothache, with: Glon., Plat., *Rhod.*

worse from warmth of bed: *Merc.*, Nux v.

worse from warmth of bed and if wrapped up, it seems relieved: Cham., Dulc., *Hep.*, **Mag.** p., Sep.

AILMENTS.

Otorrhœa: All. c., Alum.,
Alumn., Ant. c., Apis, Ars.,
Ars. i., Asaf., Aur., Bar. m.,
Bell., Bor., Bry., Calc., Calc.
s., Carb. an., Caust., Carb. v.,
Cham., Cist., Con., Crot. h.,
Elaps., Fl. ac., Graph., Hep.,
Hydr., Kali ar., Kali bi., Kali
c., Kali s., Lach., Lyc., Merc.,
Merc. c., Nat. m., Nat. s.,
Nit. ac., Petr., Phos., Psor.,
Puls., Rhus t., Sang., Sel.,
Sep., Sil., Sulph., Tell.

blood: Arn., Bell., Chin.,
Cic., Crot. ·h., Elaps,
Ham., Op., Petr., Phos.,
Rhus t.

bloody: Calc., Calc. s., Chin.,
Crot. h., Graph., Hep.,
Lach., Merc., Nit. ac.,
Petr., Psor., Puls., Sil.,
Sul., Tell.

excoriating: Ars. i., Calc. p.,
Carb. v., Fl. ac., Hep.,
Lyc., Merc., Nat. m.,
Rhus t., Sulph., Syph.,
Tell.

fetid: Ars., Ars. i., Aur.,
Bov., Calc., Carb. ac.,
Carb. v., Cist., Elaps,
Hep., Kali ar., Kali bi.,
Merc., Merc. c., Nit. ac.,
Psor., Sulph., Tell.

gluey: Graphites.

green: Elaps, Hep., Kali i.,
Merc.

ichorous: Ars., Carb. an.,
Carb. v., Lyc., Nit. ac.,
Psor., Sil., Tell.

measles, following an attack
of: Carb. v., Crot. h., Lyc.,
Nit. ac., Puls., Sulph.

offensive: Ars., Aur., Bar.
m., Bov., Calc., Carb. v.,
Caust., Chin., Cist., Fl.

AILMENTS, otorrhœa, offensive.

ac., Graph., Hep., Hydr.,
Kali ar., Kali bi., Kali p.,
Kali s., Lyc., Merc., Merc.
c., Nit. ac., Psor., Sil.,
Sulph., Thuja.

cadaverous odor: Ars.

fish-brine like: Graph., Tell.

putrid meat-like: Kali p.,
Thuja.

rotten cheese like: Bar. m.,
Hep.

purulent: All. c., Alum.,
Alumn., Amm. c., Asaf.,
Aur., Bar. m., Bor., Bov.,
Calc., Calc. s., Caps., Carb.
v., Caust., Chin., Cist.,
Con., Graph., Hep., Hydr.,
Kali bi., Kali c., Kali p.,
Kali s., Lach., Lyc., Merc.,
Merc. c., Nat. m., Nit.
ac., Petr., Psor., Puls.,
Sep., Sil., Sulph., Zinc.

purulent, after abuse of mercury: Asar., Aur., Hep.,
Nit. ac., Sil., Sulph.

scarlet fever, following: Apis,
Asar., Aur., Bar. m.,
Carb. v., Crot. h., Graph.,
Hep., Kali bi., Lyc.,
Merc., Nit. ac., Psor.,
Puls., Sulph., Verb.

suppression, after: Aur.,
Calc., Carb. v., Cast.,
Graph., Hep., Merc.,
Puls.

thick: Calc., Calc. s., Carb.
v., Hydr., Kali bi., Kali
ch., Lyc., Puls., Sil.

thin: Graph., Kali s., Psor.,
Sep., Sil., Sulph.

watery: Carb. v., Cist., Elaps,
Graph., Kali s., Merc.,
Sil., Syph., Tell.

yellowish: Ars., Calc., Calc.
s., Crot. h., Hydr., Kali

AILMENTS, otorrhœa, yellowish.

　　　ar., Kali bi., Kali c., *Kali
　　　s.*, Lyc., Merc., Nat. s.,
　　　Puls., Sil.

INFLAMMATION: Apis, Bell.,
Bry., Cact., Calc., Fl. ac.,
Kreos., *Merc.*, Merc. c., Pic.
ac., *Puls.*, Rhus t.

Erysipelatous: Apis, Carb. v.,
Crot. h., Kali bi., Merc.,
Petr., Puls., Rhus t., Rhus
v., Sep., Sulph.

Eustachian tube: Calc., Iod.,
Kali s., Mang., Merc., Nat.
m., *Puls.*, Sang., Sil., Sulph.

Margin of the ear: Sil.

MOISTURE BEHIND THE
EARS: *Graph.*, Petr.

NOISES IN THE EAR: Æsc.,
Agn., Ambr., Arg. n., Arn.,
Ars., Asar., Aur., Bar. c.,
Bar. m., Bell., Bor., Bry.,
Cact., Calc., Calc. s., *Cann.
i.*, Carb. v., Carls., *Caust.*,
Chel., Chin., *Chin. s.*, Cic.,
Coc. c., Con., Cupr., Dig.,
Eup. per., Glon., *Graph.*,
Ign., Iod., Kali c., *Kali i.*,
Kali p., Kali s., Kreos., Lac.
c., Lach., *Lyc.*, Merc., Nat.
m., Nat. p., Nat. s., Nit. ac.,
Nux, Op., Par., Petr., Phos.,
Ph. ac., Plat., Plb., *Psor.*,
Puls., Rhod., Sal. ac., Sang.,
Sec., Sep., Sil., Spig., *Staph.*,
Tab., *Tub.*

Buzzing sound in the ear: Amm.
c., Arg. m., *Arg. n.*, Arn.,
Ars., Aur., Aur. m., Bar. c.,
Berb., Cact., Calc., Camph.,
Cann. i., Carb. v., Caust.,
Chin., Chin. s., Coff., Con.,
Dulc., Elaps., Eup. per.,
Ferr. p., Ham., Hyos., Iod.,
Kali c., Kreos., Lac c.,

NOISE, buzzing sound.

Lach., Laur., Lyc., Mag. c.,
Mur. ac., Nat. m., Nux m.,
Nux v., Op., Petr., Pic. ac.,
Phos., *Plat.*, Psor., Sep.,
Spig., Sulph., Taren.

Chirping noises: Caust., Lyc.,
Nux v., Puls., Rhus t., Sil.,
Tub.

Cracking: Bar. c., Calc., Com.,
Form., Graph., *Kali c.*,
Lach., Nat. m., *Nit. ac.*,
Petr., Psor., Puls.

Fluttering sounds in the ear:
Bar. c., Bell., Calc., Graph.,
Kali s., Mag. m., Merc., Ph.
ac., *Plat.*, Puls., *Spig.*,
Sulph.

Hissing: Calc., Cann. i., Graph.,
Lach., Nux v., Pic. ac.

Humming: Acon., Alum., Amm.
c., Arg. n., Arn., Ars., Aur.,
Bell., Canth., Carl., Caust.,
Chin., Chin s., Con., Croc.,
Cycl., Dros., Fer., Graph.,
Lyc., Mur. ac., Nat. m.,
Nit. ac., Nux v., Op., Petr.,
Phos., Psor., Puls., *Sep.*,
Spig., Stry., Sulph.

Reverberating: Bar. c., Caust.,
Cic., Graph., Lach., *Lyc.*,
Nit. ac., Nux v., *Phos.*, Ph.
ac., Puls., Rhod., Sars., Sep.

Ringing: Æsc., Agar., All. c.,
Arg. n., Ars., Aur., Bar. c.,
Bell., Bor., *Cact.*, Calc.,
Calc. s., Camph., *Cann. i.*,
Canth., Carb. o., Carb. v.,
Carl., Caust., Cham., Chel.,
Chin., Chin. s., Cic. v., Clem.,
Cocc., Con., Cycl., Dig.,
Dulc., Euph., Ferr., Fl. ac.,
Form., Gran., Graph., Ham.,
Hell., Hydr., Ign., Ipe., *Kali
c.* Kali i., *Kali s.*, Led.,
Lyc., Mag. c., Meny., Merc.,
Mez., Nat. m., Nat. s.,

NOISE, ringing.

Nux m., Nux v., Osm.,
Par., Petr., Phos., Ph. ac.,
Plat., *Psor.*, Puls., Rhod.,
Sang., Sep., Sil., Spig.,
Stann., *Sulph.*

Roaring: Acon., Agn., Ambr.,
Anac., Ars., Asar., Aur.,
Aur. m., *Bar. c.*, Bar. m.,
Bel., Bor., Bry., Calc., Calc.
s., Camph., Canth., Carb. v.,
Carl., Caust., Cham., Chel.,
Chin., *Chin. a.*, *Chin. s.*,
Cinnab., Cocc., Colch.,
Coloc., Con., Cycl., Dros.,
Elaps, Ferr. i., Gels.,
Graph., Hell., Hep., Iod.,
Kali c., Kali s., Lach., Laur.,
Led., *Lyc.*, Mag. c., Mag.
m., Merc., Merc. c., Nat. m.,
Nat. p., Nat. s., Nit. ac.,
Nux v., Op., Petr., Ph. ac.,
Phos., Plat., *Puls.*, Rhod.,
Sal. ac., Staph., Sul. ac.,
Sulph., Ther., Verat. v.

NOISE.

Synchronous with pulse: *Puls.*

Singing: Ars., Camph., Carb.
s., Caust., *Chin.*, Chin. a.,
Con., Graph., Hyos., *Kali c.*,
Kali p., Lach., Lyc., Nat.
c., Nux v., Psor., Sang.,
Stram.

Wistling: Ambr., Nux v.

Wheezing: Arg. n., Caust.,
Hep., Lach., *Lyc.*, Mag c.,
Mang., Mur. ac., *Petr.*,
Plat., Sulph.

SUPPURATION:

Middle ear: Calc., *Calc. s.*,
Caps., Carb. v., Caust., *Hep.*,
Kali bi., Kali p., *Merc.*,
Puls., Sul. Spong.

SWEAT: Puls.

Behind ears: Cimicifuga.

WIND:

Sensitive to: Cham., Lach., Mez.

NOSE AND SMELL.

AILMENTS, Common:

Catarrh: Acon., Agar., Alum., Amm. m., Ant. c., Ant. s., Apis, Arg. n., *Ars.* Ars. i., Asaf., Arum. t., *Aur.*, *Aur. m.*, Bar. c., Bar. m., Bell., Bor., Bov., *Brom.*, *Calc.*, Calc. p., Calc. s., Carb. ac., Carb. an., Cast., Cist., Con., Eup. per., *Euphr.*, Ferr., Ferr. ar., Fl. ac., Form., *Graph.*, *Hep.*, Hippoz., Hydr., Iod., Kali ar., *Kali bi.*, Kali c., Kali chl., Kali i., Kali p., Lach., Lyc., Mag. m., Mang., Med., *Merc.*, Merc. c., Merc. i. f., Merc. i. r., Mez., Nat. a., Nat. c., *Nat. m.*, Nat. s., Nicc., Nit. ac., Nux v., Nux m., Osm., *Petr.*, Phos., *Psor.*, *Puls.*, Rhus *t.*, Rumex, Sabad., Samb., Sang., Sars., *Sel.*, *Scp.*, Sil., Spig., Squil., Stict., *Sulph.*, Teucr., Ther., Thuja, Tub.

Polypus: *Calc.*, Kali s., Lach., Lyc., Merc., Phos., Teur., Thuja.

HEARING:

Acute: *Acon.*, Anac., Asar., Aur., *Bell.*, Bor., Cann. i., Chin., Cic., Cocc., *Coff.*, Colch., *Con.*, Graph., Hep., Iod., Kali c., Kali p., Kali s., *Lach.*, Lyc., *Nat. c.*, Nat. m., Nat. p., Nux m., *Nux v.*, *Op.*, Phos., Ph. ac., Plan., Puls., Sep., Sil., Spig., Stry., Sulph., *Tab.*, Ther.

music, to: *Acon.*, Cact.,

HEARING, acute.

Cham., Coff., Lyc., Nat. c., Nux v., Sep., Tab.

noises, to: *Acon.*, Ars., *Aur.*, *Bell.*, Calc., Chin., Cic., Cocc., Coff., *Con.*, Ferr., Gels., Ign., Iod., Ipe., Kali c., Lach., Lyc., Mur. ac., Nat. c., Nat. p., Nat. s., *Nit. ac.*, Nux, Op., Ph. ac., Sang., Sep., Sil., Spig., Sulph., *Ther.*, Zinc.

Defective, impaired: All. c., Ambr., Amm. c., Amm. m., Anac., Ang., Apis, Arn., Ars., Asar., Aur., Bapt., Bar. c., *Bell.*, Bov., Bry., *Calc.*, Calc. p., Carb. an., Caust., Chel., *Chin.*, Cic., Cocc., Con., Crot. t., *Cupr.*, Cycl., Dros., Elaps, Ferr., Fl. ac., Form., Gels., Glon., *Graph.*, Hep., Hydr., *Hyos.*, Iod., Ipe., Kali bi., Kali br., Kali c., Lach., Lact., Laur., Led., *Lyc.,* Mag. c., Mag. m., Mang., Merc., Mur. ac., Nat. c., *Nat. m.*, Nat. s., *Nit. ac.*, Nux v., Petr., *Phos.*, *Ph. ac.*, Plb., Psor., *Puls.*, Rhus t., Ruta, Sabad., Sabin., Sul. ac., Sec., Sep., *Sil.*, Spig., Spong., Staph., Stram., *Sulph.*, Sul. ac., Tell., Verat., *Verb.*

measles, following: Carb. v., Merc., *Puls.*, Sil., Sulph.

menses, previous to: Kreos.

when the flow is on: Calc., Kreos.

HEARING, defective.

noise, hearing improves in: *Graph.*

paralysis of the auditory nerve, due to: Bar. c., Bell., Caust., Glon., Hyos., Op., Ph. ac., Puls., Sil.

riding in carriages, will improve his hearing: Graph., *Nit. ac.,* Puls.

scarlet fever, following an attack of: *Carb v.,* Crot. h., Graph., Hep., Lach., *Lyc.,* Nit. ac., Puls., Sil., *Sulph.*

sexual excesses, after: Petr.

suppressed intermittents, due to: Calc., Chin. s.

typhoid fever, after an attack of: Apis, Arg. n., Ars., Nit. ac., Ph. ac.

Distant, sound seems: All. c., Cann. i., Cham., Coca., Euph., Lac. c., Nux m., Petr., Sol. n.

ITCHING: Agar., Amm. c., Anac., Ars., *Aur.,* Bar. c., Bov., Calad., Calc., Calc. s., Caps., Caust., Cist., Cycl., Elaps., Fl. ac., *Hep.,* Ign., Kali ar., Kali bi., *Kali c.,* Kali p., Kali s., Laur., Lyc., *Mang.,* Merc., Mez., *Nux v., Petr.,* Phos., Psor., Sars., *Sep., Sil.,* Spig., *Sulph.,* Tell.

Behinnd ears: Agar., *Graph.,* Mez., *Nux v., Petr.,* Phos., Sars., *Sep., Sil.,* Spig., *Sulph.* Tell.

External ear: *Agar.,* Alum., Arg. m., Calc. s., Carb. v.,

ITCHING, external ear.

Coloc., Con., Graph., Kali c., Petr., *Puls., Rhus t., Sulph., Tell.*

Eustachian tube: Calc., *Nux v.,* Petr., Sil.

Coryza: Acon., Æsc., Agar., *All. c., Ambr.,* Amm. c., Amm. m. Anac., Apoc., Arg. m. Arg. n., Ars., Ars. i., Arum. t., Asar., Aspar., Aur., Aur. m., Bell., Benz. ac., Berb., Bor., Brom., Bry., Cact., Calc., Carb. ac., *Carb v.,* Caust., Ceon., Cham., *Chel.,* Chin., Chlor., Cic., Cina, Cinnb., Colch., Cor. r., Cycl., *Eup. per., Euphr.,* Ferr., Ferr. ar., Ferr. p., Gels., Graph., *Hep.,* Hydr., Iod., Jab., Kali ar., Kali bi., Kali c., Kali chl., *Kali i.,* Kali s., Lac. c., Lach., Lyc., Mag. c., Mag. m., *Merc.,* Merc. c., Merc. i. r., Mez., Nat. c., Nat. m., *Nux v.,* Osm., Petr., Senec., Phos., Ph. ac., Phyt., *Puls., Rhus t.,* Rumex, Sabad., Sang., Sep., *Sil.,* Spong., Squilla, *Staph.,* Stict., *Sulph.,* Teucr.

dry, with a discharge: Acon., Amm. c., Amm. m., Anac., Ant. c., Ars., Bell., Bry., Cact., *Calc.,* Camph., Caps., Carb., an., Carb. o., *Caust., Chin.,* Chin. a., Graph., Ign., Ipe., Kali c., Lyc., Mag c., Mang., Nat. m., Nit. ac., Nux v., *Phos.,* Plat., Puls., *Samb.* Sep., Sil., Spig., Spong., *Stict.,*

fluent: Acon., Æsc., Agar., *All. c., Amm. c.,* Amm. m., Ant. t., Arg. m., Ars., Arum. t., Aspar., Bar. c., Bor., Bov., Brom., Bry.,

ITCHING, coryza, fluent.

> Calc., Camph., Caps.,
> Carb. an., Carb. v.,
> Caust., Chin., Chin. a.,
> Graph., Ign., Ip., Kali c.,
> Lyc., Mag. c., Mang. Nat.
> m., Nit. ac. Nux v., Par.,
> Phos., Plat., Puls., Samb.,
> Sep., Sil., Spig., Spong.,
> Sticta, Sulph., Sul. ac.,
> Thuja.

Cracks in nostrils: Ant. c., Aur.,
Aur. m., Graph., Petr.

Epistaxis: Acon., Agar., All.
c., Ambr., Amm. c., Ant. c.,
Arg. m., Arn., Bapt., Bar.
c., Bell., Berb., Bov.,
Brom., Bry., Cact.,
Calc., Cann. s., Caps.,
Carb. an., Carb. v., Caust.,
Cham., Chin., Chin. s., Cina,
Cinnab., Con., Cop., Croc.,
Crot. h., Cupr., Dig., Dros.,
Dulc., Elaps, Erig., Ferr.,
Ferr. ar., Ferr. p., Glon.,
Graph., Ham., Hekla, Hep.,
Hydr., Hyos., Iod., Ipe.,
Kali bi., Kali c., Kali
i., Kali n., Kreos.,
Lac. ac., Lach., Led.,
Lyc., Mag. c., Med., Meli.,
Merc., Merc. c., Mez., Mill.,
Mosch., Nat. c., Nat. m.,
Nat. p., Nit. ac., Nux m.,
Nux v., Petr., Phos., Ph. ac.,
Puls., Rat., Rhod., Rhus t.,
Rumex, Sabina, Sang., Sars.,
Sec., Sep., Sil., Spong.,
Stann., Sulph., Sul. ac., Ter.,
Thuja, Trill., Ust., Verat.

Bed in: Caps., Carb. v.

Blood, bright: Acon., Bell.,
Car. ac., Chin., Dulc., Elaps,
Erig., Ferr. p., Hyos., Ipe.,
Lach., Mill., Phos., Ph. ac.,
Rhus t., Sabin.

BLOOD.

coagulated, clotted: Arg. n.,
Bell., Cham., Chin., Croc.,
Ferr., Ferr. m., Ipe., Merc.,
Nat. m., Nit. ac., Phos.,
Plat., Puls., Rhus t., Sec.,
Sulph., Tarent.

dark black: Arn., Bell., Carb.
v., Cham., Cina, Croc.,
Crot. h., Elaps, Ham.,
Kali n., Kreos., Lach.,
Merc., Nit. ac., Nux m.,
Nux v., Ph. ac., Puls.,
Sep., Stram.

stringy: Croc., Cupr., Merc.

viscid: Croc., Sec.

Climaxis, during: Lach., Sulph.,
Sul. ac.

Cough, whooping, with: Arn.,
Bry., Cor. r., Crot. h., Dros.,
Ipe., Merc., Mur. ac.,
Nux v.

Diphtheria: Carb. v., Chin.,
Crot. h., Hydr., Ign., Kali
chl., Lach., Merc. cya., Nit.
ac.

Epistaxis:

typhoid fever, in: Arn., Bapt.,
Bry., Chin. s., Crot. h.,
Lach., Ph. ac., Rhus t.,
Ter.

headache, during: Acon.,
Agar., Bry., Cinnab.

menses, previous to: Bar. c.,
Lach., Nat. s., Puls.,
Sulph.

when the flow is on: Nat. s.,
Sep., Sulph.

menses, in place of: Bry.,
Lach.

menses, Suppression: Bry.,
Cact., Con., Croc., Gels.,
Lach., Phos., Puls., Rhus
t., Sabin., Sep.

EPISTAXIS.

sleeping, while: Bry., *Merc.*, Nit. ac., Nux v., Verat.

stooping, while: Ferr., Nat. m., Nux v., Rhus t.

vicarious: Bry., *Ham.*, Lach., *Phos.*, Puls.

washing his face, when: *Arn.*, Kali c.

Gangrene: Ars.

Necrosis: Phos.

Nodosities: *Ars.*, *Aur.*

Ozœna: Alum., Amm. c., Arg. n., Ars., *Asaf.*, *Aur.*, *Aur. m.*, Aur. m. n., *Calc.*, Calc. fl., Calc. p., Carb. ac., Carb. an., Con., Elaps, Graph., *Hep.*, Hippoz., Hydr., *Kali bi.*, *Kali i.*, Kali ph., Kali s., Lach., *Merc.*, Merc. c., Merc. i. f., Myric., Nat. c., Nat. m., Nat. s., Nit. ac., Petr., Ph. ac., Phyt., *Puls.*, Sang., Sep., *Sil.*, Stict., Sulph., Syph., Teucr., Ther.

Polypus: All. c., Apis, *Calc.*, Calc. p., Con., Graph., Kali bi., Kali n., Merc. i. r., Phos., Psor., *Sang.*, Sep., Sil., Sulph., *Teuc.*, Thuja.

Snuffles: Asc. t., Aur., *Lyc.*, Nux v., Sang.

Ulcers: Anthr., Fl. ac., Kali bi., Kali c.

inside: Alum., Arn., Ars., *Aur. m.*, *Aur. m. n.*, Calc., Cham., Fl. ac., Graph., Hippoz., Iod., *Kali bi.*, Kali i., Mag. m., Merc., Merc. c., *Nit. ac.*, Nat. c., Petr., Phos., *Sep.*, Sil., Squil., Sulph., *Thuja.*

septum of nose, round ulcers: Aur., Fl. ac., Hippoz.,

ULCERS, septum of nose.

Kali bi., Kali i., Nat. c., Sil., *Thuja.*

tip of nose: Bor., Bry., Caust.

wings: *Puls.*, Sanic.

wing, right: Ars.

wing, left: Dulc., Fl. ac., Kali bi., Kali c.

wing, borders: Kali bi.

Veins, varicose: Carb. v., Crot. h.

DISCHARGE:

Excoriating: *All. c.*, *Ail.*, Alum., Amm. c., *Amm. m.*, Ars., Ars. h., *Ars. i.*, *Arum. t.*, Aur. m., Brom., Calc., Calc. s., Carb. v., Caust., Cham., Con., Ferr., Gels., *Graph.*, Hep., Hippoz., Hydr., *Iod.*, Kali bi., Kali c., Kali i., *Kreos.*, Lac. c., Lach., Lyc., Mag. m., *Merc.*, Merc. c., Mer. i. f., Mur. ac., *Nit. ac.*, *Nux v.*, Phos., Phyt., Ran. b., Rhus t., Sang., Sil., Sin. n., Squilla, Sulph., Zinc.

Glue-like: Merc. c., Psor., Sulph.

Gray: *Ambr.*, *Lyc.*

Greenish: Alum., Ars. i., Berb., Bor., Bry., Calc. f., Carb. v., Kali bi., Kali c., Kali i., Merc., Nat. c., Nit. ac., Phos., *Puls.*, Rhus t., Sil., Stict., Teucr., Ther., Thuja.

Greenish black: *Kali i.*

Greenish brown: Hydr. ac.,

Ichorous: *Ail.*, Lyc., Nit. ac., Rhus t.

Offensive: Asaf., Aur., Aur. m., Bar. c., *Calc.*, Calc. f.,

DISCHARGE, offensive.

Calc. s., Carb. ac., Elaps,
Graph., *Hep.*, Hippoz., *Kali
bi.*, Kali c., Kali p., Kali s.,
Lach., Lyc., Mag. m., *Merc.*,
Nat. c., Nit. ac., Phos.,
Psor., *Puls.*, Sep., Sil., *Sulph.*,
Ther.

Purulent: Alum., Arg. n., Ars.
iod., Asaf., *Aur.*, Aur. m.,
Berb., *Calc.*, Calc. s., Cocc.,
Coloc., *Con.*, Ferr., Ferr. ar.,
Ferr. p., Graph., *Hep.*, Hip-
poz., Hydr., Iod., *Kali bi.*,
Kali c., Kali i., Kali p., *Kali
s.*, *Lyc.*, Mag. m., *Merc.*,
Nat. c., Nat. m., Nat. p.,
Nat. s., Nit. ac., Petr.,
Phos., Ph. ac., Psor., Puls.,
Rhus t., Sang., Sep., Sil.,
Sulph., Stic., Thuja.

Thick: Alum., Amm. m., *Ars.*,
Arum. t., Aur., Bad., Bar.
c., Calc., Calc. fl., Calc. s.,
Carb. v., Coc. c., Hep., Hip-
poz., *Hydr.*, Kali ar., *Kali
bi.*, Kali c., Kali i., *Kali p.*,
Kali s., *Lac. c.*, Mur. ac.,
Nat. c., Nat. m., Nat. p.,
Nat. s., Phos., *Puls.*, Rhus
t., Ran. b., Sabad., Sang.,
Sep., Sil., Spong., Stann.,
Staph., Sulph., Sul. ac., Ther.,
Thuja.

Viscid: *Bov.*, Cann. s., Canth.,
Caust., Cham., Colch.,
Graph., Hippo., *Hydr.*, *Kali
bi.*, Kali i., *Kali s,.* Mez.,
Nat. a., Par., Phos., Plb.,
Psor., Ran. b., Sabad.,
Samb., Sep., Sil., Spon.,
Stann., Sulph.

Yellow: Alum., Arg. n., *Ars.*,
Ars. i., Ars. m., *Arum. t.*,
Aur., Aur. m., Bad., Bar.
c., Berb., *Calc.*, *Calc. s.*, Cic.,

DISCHARGE, yellow.

Cist., Graph., *Hep.*, *Hydr.*,
Iod., *Kali bi.*, Kali c., *Kali
i.*, Kali s., *Kali p.*, Lach.,
Lyc., Mag. m., Mez., Nat.
a., Nat. c., Nat. m., Nat. p.,
Nat. s., *Nit. ac.*, Phos., *Puls.*,
Sep., Sil., Stram., Sulph.,
Ther., Thuja.

Yellowish green: Alum., Aur.
m., Calc. f., Calc. s., Hep.,
Hydr., *Kali bi.*, Kali c.,
Mang., Merc., Nat. c., Nat.
s., Phos., *Puls.*, Sep., Sil.,
Thuja, Ther.

FROST-BITTEN NOSE: Agar.

ITCHING: Agar., Arg. n., *Arum.
t.*, Aur., Bov., Calc., Calc. p.,
Calc. s., Carb. v., *Caust.*,
Cham., Chel., Cina, Kali c.,
Kali n., Mag. m,. Merc.,
Mez., Nit. ac., Nux v., Ph.
ac., Sil., Spig., *Sulph.*, Teucr.

Tip: *Caust.*, Chel., Con., Petr.,
Sep., Sil.

Wings: *Caust.*, Nat. s.

OILY: Hydr.

PICKING NOSE: *Arum t.*,
Cina.

SHINY: *Phos.*

SMELLING:

Acute: *Acon.*, Agar., Anac.,
Ars., *Aur.*, Bar. c., *Bell.*,
Calc., Cham., *Cin.*, Cocc.,
Coff., Colch., Con., *Graph.*,
Hep., Hyper., *Ign.*, Kalm.,
Lyc., Lyss., Nux m., *Nux v.*,
Op., *Phos.*, Plat., Plb., Sep.,
Sulph.

headache, during an attack:
Phos.

sensitiveness of smelling to the
odour of broth: *Colch,*

SMELLING, acute.

sensitiveness of smelling to the odour of cooking food: *Colch.*, Dig., Eup. per., Sep.

sensitiveness of smelling to the odour of eggs: *Colch.*

sensitiveness of smelling to the odour of fish: *Colch.*

sensitiveness of smelling to the odour of flower: *Graph.*, *Nux v.*, *Phos.*

sensitiveness of smelling to the odour of food: *Ars.*, Cocc., Colch., Ip., *Sep.*

sensitiveness to strong odours: Acon., *Aur.*, *Bell.*, Cham., Chin., Cocc., *Coff.*, Colch., Con., *Graph.*, Hep., *Ign.*, Lyc., Lyss., *Nux v.*, *Phos.*, Sep., Sulph.

SNEEZING: Acon., Æsc., Agar., All. c., Amm. m., Anac., Ant. t., Arg. m., Arg. n., *Ars.*, Ars. i., Bar. c., Bell., Brom., *Bry.*, Calc., Calc. p., Camph., Caps., Carb. an., *Carb. v.*, Caust., Chin., Cic., *Cina*, Cist., Con., Cycl., Dros., Dulc., Euphr., *Eup. per.*, Ferr. ar., Ferr. p., Gamb., Graph., Indig., Iod., Ip., Kali ar., Kali bi., Kali

SNEEZING.

i., Kalm., *Kreos.*, Lac. c., Lach., Lyc., *Merc.*, Nat. c., Nat. m., Nat. p., Nat. s., Nit. a., Nux m., Nux v., Osm., Petr., Phos., Ph. ac., Plan., *Puls.*, Rhus r., *Rhus t.*, Rumex, *Sabad.*, Sal. ac., Sang., Senec., Seneg., Sep., Sil., Spong., Squil., Staph., *Sulph.*, Tarax.,Teucr.

Paroxysms, in: Agar., Gels., Ip., Kali i., Nat. m., Rhus t., Sabad., Stram., Sulph.

Sleeping, when: Nit. ac., Puls. wakes him from: *Amm. m.*

Violent: Ars., Bar. c., Bry., Cina, Gamb., Ind., Ip., Kali c., Kali i., Nat. c., Squilla, Thuja.

SOOTY NOSTRILS: Ant. t., Chlor., Hell., Hyos., Lyc., Zinc.

SWALLOW, liquids come out through the nose, when he makes an attempt to: *Arum t.*, Bar. c., Carb. ac., Kali ar., *Lach.*, *Lac. c.*, *Lyc.*, Merc., Merc. c., Merc. cy., Nat. m., Phyt., Plb., Sul. ac.

WINGS OF NOSE, on constant motion: Amm. c.

Fan-like: Ant. t., Brom., Chel., Iod., *Lyc.*, Phos., Spong.

MOUTH.

AILMENTS, common:

Aphthæ: *Ars.*, Arum t., *Bapt.*, Berb., Bor., Calc., Carb. ac., Carb. an., Carb. v., Dig., Hell., Hep., Iod., Jug. c., Kali ar., Kali bi., Kali br., Kali c., *Kali chl.*, Kreos., Lach., Lyc., Mag. c., *Merc.*, *Merc. c.*, *Mur. ac.*, Myric., Nat. m., Nit. ac., *Nux v.*, Plb., Staph., *Sulph.*, *Sul. ac.*

bleed easily, that: *Bor.*, Lac. c.

children, in: *Bor.*, Kali chl., *Merc.*, Mur. ac., Nux v., *Sulph.*

gangrenous: Ars.

hue, of a bluish: *Ars.*

palate: Calc., Hep., Nux m., Phos.

Cancer, affecting the palate: Hydr.

Cancrum oris: Alum., Ars., Asar., Ast., Bapt., Calc., Canth., Carb. v., Chlor., Crot. h., Carb. v., Dulc., Ferr., Kali bi., Kali chl., *Kali i.*, Lach., Merc., Merc. c., Nat. m., Nux, Podo., Sep., Sil., Sulph., Sul. ac.

Condylomata on palate: Arg. n., Gangrene: Crot. h., *Lach.*

Membrane, false (in the buccal cavity): *Arum t.*, Merc. cy., Mur. ac., *Nit. ac.*

palate affected: Lac. c., Lach., Merc., Mur. ac. Nit. ac.

MEMBRANE.

Paralysis, palate: Gels., Lach., Plb., Sil.

Ulcers: Agn., Alum., Anac., *Ars.*, Bapt., Bor., Canth., Caps., Cic., Dulc., Fl. ac., Graph., *Iod.*, Kali bi., Kali chl., *Kali i.*, Lach., Merc., Merc. c., Merc. cy., *Mur. ac.*, Nat. c., Nat. m., Nit. ac., Merc. cy., *Mur. ac.*, Nat. c., Nat. m., Nit. ac., Nux m., Phos., Phyt., Psor., Staph., Sul. ac.

base, black: Mur. ac.

base, lardaceous: Hep., *Merc.*, *Nit., ac.*

base, milky: *Kali i.*

palate: Apis, *Aur.*, Aur. m., Cinnab., Kali bi., Lach., Lyc., *Merc.*, Nat. m., Nit. ac., Phos., Ph. ac., Phyt., Sang.

palate, sloughing: Kali bi., Lach., Merc. c., Nit. ac., Phos., Syph.

palate, syphilitic: *Aur.*, *Aur. m.*, Hep., Kali i., Syph.

type, gangrenous: Ars., Bapt., Bor., *Lach.*, Sul. ac.

type malignant: *Ars.*, Lach., Phos.

type mercurial: Iod., Nit. ac.

type painful: Ars., Fl. ac., Merc., *Nit. ac.*

type phagedenic: Caps., Merc., *Nit. ac.*, Sul. ac.

MOUTH, ulcers.

> type syphilitic: Aur., Aur.
> m., Fl. ac., Hep., Kali bi.,
> Kali i., Lach., Merc. i. r.,
> Phyt., Syph.

COLD BREATH: Camph:
Carb. v., Cedr., Chin., Cop.,
Phos., Verat.

DISCOLORATION:

Blueness: Merc., Plb .

Paleness: Chin. s., Nat. m.

Redness: Apis, Bor., Canth.,
Cupr. ac., Cycl., Hydr.,
Hyos., Kali bi., Kali chl.,
Merc., Nat. c., Nit. ac.

Yellow paleness: Nit. ac.

DRYNESS: Acon., Alum., Amm.
c., Ant. c., Ant. t., Apis,
Arg. m., Arn., Ars., Ars. h.,
Ars. m., Arum. t., Atro.,
Bar. c., Bell., Bor., Bry.,
Calc., Camph., Cann. i.,
Cann. s., Canth., Caps.,
Carb. v., Caust., Cham.,
Chel., Chin., Cinnab., Cocc.,
Coloc., Cupr., Dulc., Ferr.,
Ferr. ar., Gamb., Gels.,
Graph., Hyos., Hyper., Ign.,
Kali ar., Kali bi., Kali c.,
Kali chl., Kali i., Kali n.,
Kali p., Lach., Laur., Lil. t.,
Lyc., Mag. c., Mag m.,
Myric., Naja, Nat. c., Nat.
Myric., Naja., Nat. c., Nat.
m., Nux v., Op., Petr., Phos.,
Phyt., Psor., Puls., Rhod.,
Rhus, Sars., Seneg., Sep.,
Sil., Stram., Stront., Sulph.,
Verat., Verat. v.

FINGERS IN THE MOUTH,
sometimes little children will
put: Calc., Cham., Ip.

ODOR, offensive: Agar., All c.,
Ambr., Anac., Arn., Ars.,

ODOR, offensive.

> Aur., Bapt., Bar. c., Bell.,
> Bry., Calc., Caps., Carb. ac.,
> Carb. v., Carl., Caust.,
> Cham., Chel., Chin., Cimic.,
> Clem., Croc., Dulc., Fl. ac.,
> Gels., Graph., Hep., Hyos.,
> Iod., Kali bi., Kali c., Kali
> i., Kali p., Kreos., Lac. c.,
> Lac. d., Lach., Lyc., Manc.,
> Merc., Merc. c., Mer. i. f.,
> Mur. ac., Nat. m., Nat. s.,
> Nit. ac., Nux m., Nux v.,
> Petr., Ph. ac., Phyt., Plb.,
> Puls., Sep., Sulph., Sul. ac.,
> Tub.

Putrid: Anac., Apis, Arg. m.,
Arg. n., Arn., Ars., Arum. t.,
Aur., Aur. m. n., Bapt.,
Caps., Carb. ac., Carb. v.,
Cham., Chlo., Crot. h., Dulc.,
Graph., Hell., Ign., Kali bi.,
Kali chl., Kali p., Kreos.,
Lach., Lyc., Mang., Merc.,
Merc. c., Mur. a., Nat. m.,
Nit. ac., Nux v., Ph. ac.,
Phyt., Puls., Rhus t., Spig.,
Tub.

SALIVA, bitter: Ars., Chel.

Bloody: Bell., Bufo, Carb. v.,
Crot. h., Dros., Hyos., Kali
i., Mag. c., Merc., Merc. c.,
Nat. m., Nit. ac., Nux v.,
Phos., Rhus t., Sec., Sulph.

Cotton, feels like: Berb., Nux
m., Puls.

Fetid: Dig., Iod., Manc.,
Merc., Merc. i. f., Nit. ac.,
Petr.

Saltish: Ant. c., Carb. an.,
Cycl., Euph., Hyos., Kali i.,
Lyc., Merc., Merc. c., Nat.
m., Phos., Sep., Sulph.

Sour: Calc., Calc. p. Ign., Kali
chl., Sulph.

SALIVA, sour.

Viscid: Ars., Berb., Chel., Cupr., Kali bi., Lach., Merc., Merc. c., Phyt., Puls., Stram.

SALIVATION: Alum., Amm.
c., Anac., Arum. t., Asar., Aur. m., Bar. c., Bar. m., Bell. Bor., Brom., Calc., Calc. p., Camph., Canth., Caps., Carb. v., Caust., Cham., Chel., Chin., Cic., Cinnb., Clem., Coc. c., Colch., Cupr., Dros., Dulc., Fl. ac., Gamb., Glon., Graph., Hell., Hep., Ign., Iod., Ipe., Iris, Kali c., Kali chl., Kali i., Kreos., Lac. c., Lach., Lyc., Manc., Mer., Merc. c., Merc. i. r., Mur. ac., Nat. c., Nat. m., Nat. s., Nit. ac., Nux m., Nux v., Ol. an., Petr., Phos., Phyt., Plb., Podo., Puls., Seneg., Sep., Sil., Stram., Sulph., Sul. ac., Verat., Zinc.

SENSATIONS:

Burning in mouth: Ars., Arum. t., Asar., Asaf., Calc., Cham., Coloc., Cupr., Gels., Gymno., Hipp., Hyper., Iris, Jatr., Kali chl., Mag.

SENSATIONS, burning in mouth.

m., Merc. sulph., Merc., Mez., Nat. s., Nux, Plat., Scilla, Seneg., Sulph., Verat.

on palate: Camph., Carb. v., Cinnab., Dulc., Hipp. m., Ign., Mag. c., Merc. c., Nat. s., Ran. b., Scill., Seneg.

Burning from mouth to stomach: Brom., Camph., Merc. c.

Dry: Nux m.

Hairy, in mouth: Ther.

Hair, on palate: Kali bi.

SPEECH:

Stammering: Acon., Bell., Bov., Bufo, Cann. i., Caust., Cupr., Euphr., Glon., Kali br., Lach., Mag. c., Mag. p., Merc., Nat. c., Nux v., Phos., Plat., Sec., Selen., Spig., Stram., Sulph.

cannot speak a syllable, though he will be making effort: Cimic.

coition, after: Cedr.

has to exert himself long, before he will utter a word: Stram.

TONGUE.

ILMENTS, Common:

Aphthæ: *Bor.*, Jug., Lach., Merc., Merc. cy., Mur. ac., Nat. m., Phos., Sulph., Sul. ac.

tip of tongue: Bry., Ham., Lach.

Atrophy of tongue: Mur. ac.

Cancer: Alumn., Apis, Ars., Aur. m., Carb. an., Con., Hydr., Lach., Mur. ac., Nit. ac., Phos., Phyt., Sil.

Condylomata: Aur., Aur. m. n., Lyc., Mang., Staph.

Gangrene: Ars., Lach., Sec.

Nodosities: *Carb. an.*, Sil.

Paralysis: Acon., Arn., Apis, Bar. c., Bell., Cadm., *Caust.*, Cocc., Con., Cupr., Dulc., Hell., Hydr., Hyos., Lach., *Lyc.*, Mur. ac., Nux m., *Op.*, *Plb.*, Rheum, Rhus t., Stram.

Ulcers: Apis, Ars., Aur., *Bapt.*, Bar. c., Caps., Calc., Chin., Dig., Fl. ac., Kali bi., Kali chl., *Kali i.*, Kreos., Lach., Lyc., Merc., Merc. i.r., Mur. ac., Nat. m., Nit. a., Plb., Phyt., *Psor.*, Sin. n., Staph., Sulph.

type phagedenic: Agar., Caps., Fl. ac.

type, syphilitic: Kali bi., Kali i., *Merc.*, *Nit. ac.*, Phyt.

underneath the tongue: Fl. ac., Graph., *Lyc.*, Plb., *Sanic.*

COLD: *Camph.*, Carb. v., Cedr., Chin., Cop., Phos., *Verat.*

CRACKED, Fissured: *Ail.*, Apis, Ars., *Arum t.*, Bapt., Bell., Benz. ac., Bor., Bry., Calc., Camph., Carb. v., Cham., Chin., Crot. h., *Fl. ac.*, *Hyos.*, Kali bi., Lach., Lyc., Mag. m., Merc., Mur. ac., Nat. a., *Nit. ac.*, Phos., Plb., Podo., Pyrog., *Rhus t.*, *Spig.*, Sulph., Verat., Zinc.

DISCOLORATION:

Black: Arg. n., Ars., Carb. ac., *Carb. v.*, *Chin.*, Chin. a., Chlor., Kali c., Lach., Lyc., *Merc.*, Merc. c., Merc. cy., Nux v., *Op.*, *Phos.*, Sec., Verat.

Blue: Agar., *Ant. t.*, Ars., Carb. v., *Dig.*, Iris, Mur. ac., plat., Podo.

Brown: *Ail.*, Anthr., Apis, Arn., Ars., Bapt., Bell., *Bry.*, Cadm., Carb. ac., Carb. v., Chel., Chin., *Chin. a.*, Colch., Crot. h., Cupr., Dig., Hep., *Hyos.*, Kali bi., *Kali p.*, Lac. c., *Lach.*, Lyc., Merc., Merc. i. f., Nux v., Op., *Phos.*, Plb., Pyrog., *Rhus t.*, Sec., Sep., Sil., Spong., Sulph.

Dirty: Camph., *Chin.*, Kali chl., *Nat. s.*

Green: *Nat. s.*, Nit. ac., Plb., Rhod.

gray: *Nat. s.*

yellow: Calc., Caust.

DISCOLORATION.

Red: Acon., *Apis*, *Ars.*, Aur.
m., Bapt., *Bell.*, Bism., Calc.,
Calc. s., Camph., Canth.,
Carb. v., Cham., Colch.,
Crot. h., Cupr. ac., Ferr. p.,
Gels., Hydr., Hyos., Kali
bi., Kali c., Lach., Lyc.,
Mag. m., *Merc.*, Merc. c.,
Nat. s., *Nit. ac.*, *Nux v.*,
Phos., Plb., Pyrog., *Rhus t.*,
Sulph., Verat.

fiery: Apis, Bell., Canth.

glistening: *Kali bi.*, Lach.,
Phos.

striped down center: Arg. n.,
Bell., *Caust.*, Cham., Kali
bi., Phos., Ph. ac., Seneg.,
Verat. v.

edges: Ars., Bapt., Canth.,
Chel., Crot. h., Fl. ac.,
Gels., Iris, Kali bi., Lach.,
Lyc., Merc., Merc. i. f.,
Nit. ac., Phos., Plb.,
Rhus t.

tip: Apis, *Ars.*, *Arg. n.*, Fl.
ac., Lach., Lyc., Nit. ac.,
Phyt., *Rhus t.*, *Rhus v.*

White: Acon., Æsc., Ant. c.,
Ant. t., Apis, Arg. n., *Ars.*,
Ars. m., Bapt., *Bell.*, Bism.,
Bry., *Calc.*, Carb. ac., Carb.
v., Cham., Chel., Chin.,
Cimex, Cocc., Colch., Coloc.,
Dig., Eup. per., Ferr., Fl.
ac., Gels., Glon., Graph.,
Hyos., Hyper., Kali ar., *Kali
bi.*, Kali chl., Kali i., Kali
n., Kali p., Kalm., Kreos.,
Lach., Lyc., *Merc.*, Merc.
c., Merc. i. f. Mez., Mur.
ac., Nat. c., Nat. m., Nat.
s., *Nit. ac.*, Nux m., Nux v.,
Op., Petr., Phos., Ph. ac.,
Podo., Psor., *Puls.*, Rhus,
Rumex, Sabad., Seneg.,
Sil., *Spig.*, Stann.,
Sulph., *Tarax.*

DISCOLORATION, white.

milky: *Ant. c.*, Bell., Glon.

pale, with red insular patches:
Nat. m.

silvery: *Ars.*

silvery, red stripe down center:
Verat. v.

Yellow: Æsc., *Ant. c.*, Apis,
Arn., Aur. m., Bapt., Bol.,
Camph., Carb. v., *Chel.*,
Cham., Chin., Cocc., Colch.,
Coloc., Crot. h., Eup. per.,
Gels., Hell., Hep., Hyper.,
Ip., Kali bi., Kali s., Lach.,
Lept., Mag. m., *Merc.*, Merc.
c., Merc. l. f., Merc. i.r.,
Mez., Nat. a., Nat. p., Nit.
ac., *Nux m.*, Nux v., Phos.
Phyt., Plb., Podo., Psor.,
Puls., *Rhus t.*, Sep., *Spig.*
Stann., Sulph., Verat.,
Verat. v.

base: Merc., *Merc. i. f.*, Nat.
p., Nux v., Sanic., Sin. n

dirty: Ars., Kali chl., Lach.
Mag. c., *Merc.*, *Merc. c.*
Merc. i. f., Myric., Op.
Sep.

white: Arg. n., Ars., Cocc.
Cupr., Gels., Hydr., Kali
bi., Rhus t.

DRYNESS: *Acon.*, Ail., *Agar.*
Ant. t., *Apis*, Arg. n., Arn.
Ars., Ars. h., Arum t., Bapt.
Bar. m., *Bell.*, *Bry.*, Calc.
Calc. p., *Camph.*, Carb. an
Carb. v., *Caust.*, *Cham.*
Chel., *Chin.*, Cic., Cist.
Cocc., Crot. h., *Cupr.*, Dulc.
Fl., ac., *Hell.*, Hydr., *Hyos.*
Iod., Ip., Kali a., Kali bi.
Kali i., Kalm., Kreos., Lac
ac., *Lach.*, Mag. m., *Merc.*
Merc. c., Merc. i. r., *Mur.
ac.*, Nat. c., Nat. m., Nit.
ac., Nux v., *Nux m.*, Phos

DRYNESS.

Ph. ac., Phyt., Pic. ac., Plb.,
Podo., *Psor.*, *Puls.*, *Rhus t.*,
Sec., Sep., Spong., Stront.,
Sulph., Sul. ac., Verat.,
Verat. v.

FLABBY: *Camph.*, Cub., Hydr.,
Lyss., Lycop., Mag. m.,
Merc., Ph. ac., Sep.

INDENTED: Ars., Ars. m.,
Carb. v., *Chel.*, Hydr., Iod.,
Merc., Podo., *Rhus t.*, Sep.,
Syph.

MAPPED: Ars., Kali bi., Lach.,
Nat. m., Ran. ac., Rhus t.,
Tarax., Ter.

PROTRUSION: Apis, *Crot. h.*,
Hell., Lach., Lyc., **Merc. c.**,
Phyt.

Difficulty, with: Hyos., *Lach.*,
Lyc.

catches on the teeth while protruding: Apis, Hyos.,
Lach.

Impossible: Apis, Lyc., **Merc.
c.**, Nux v., Plb.

PROTRUSION.

Oscillating: Hell., Lyc.

Rapidly, going in and out like
a snake's: *Cupr.*, Lach.

SENSATIONS:

Burning on tongue: Acon., Apis,
Asar., Bar. c., Bell., Bov.,
Calc., Carb. v., Caust., Cocc.
c., Colch., Hipp. m., Hyos.,
Ind., Iod., Jac. c., Kali chl.,
Mag. m., Merc., Nat. s., Ol.
an., Ox. ac., Phos., Ph. ac.,
Plat., Plb., Ran. sc., Rat.,
Rhod., Seneg., Sulph., Verat.

on tip of tongue, with ptyalism: Chin.

Hair on tongue: Kali bi., Nat.
m., *Sil.*

TREMBLING: Agar., Apis,
Aur., Bell., *Camph.*, Canth.,
Crot. h., Gels., Hell., Hyos.,
Ign., *Lach.*, Lyc., *Merc.*,
Op., Ph. ac., Plb., Tarax.

VARICOSE VEINS: Fl. ac.,
Ham., Puls., Thuja.

TEETH

AILMENTS, common:

Aching of the teeth, excited by cold air: Alum., Agar., Bell., Calc., Cham., Caust., Hep., Mag. c., Mag. p., Merc., Nux m., Nux v., Phos., Puls., Rhus t., Sars., Sep., Sil., Spig., Staph., *Sulph.*, Sul. ac., Ther.

cold air ameliorates: Clem., Nat. s., Nux v., *Puls.*

nervous patients, in: Acon., Ars., Bell., *Cham., Coff.,* Gels., Mag. p., Puls.

nursing mothers, while the infant nurses: Chin.

pregnant women, in: Acon., Bell., Calc., Cham., Hyos., Lyss., Mag. c., Merc., Nux m., Puls., Rat., *Sep.,* Staph., Tab.

sleep, while he goes to: Merc.

sound teeth in: Acon., Cham., Coff., Mag. c.

suddenly begins and goes: Bell.

tobacco-smoking, excited by: Bry., Caust., Cham., Ign., Merc., Nux v., *Spig.*

warm drinks, excited by: All. c., Bry., Carb. v., *Cham., Coff.,* Dros., Ferr. p.,

TEETH, aching.

Lach., Merc., Nat. s., Nit ac., *Puls.,* Sep.

warm drinks ameliorate: Ars. Lyc., Mag. p., Nux v. Rhus t.

warmth, external, excited by Bry., *Coff.,* Cor. r., Ferr. Ferr. p., Phos., *Puls.*

warmth, external, ameliorat es: Ars. h., Calc., Cast. Chin., Com., Kali ar., Kal c., Lyc., *Mag. p.,* Merc. Mur. ac., Nat. c., Nu m., *Nux v.,* Puls., Psor. *Rhod., Rhus t.,* Sil., Sul ac.

wrapping the head up wil relieve her toothache: *Nu. v., Sil.*

warmth of bed will increase her toothache: *Cham.* Mag. c., *Merc.,* Ph. ac. *Puls.*

warmth of bed will relieve he toothache: Lyc., Nux v. Sil.

warm room, aggravated in a All. c., Cham., Hep., Iris Kali s., Mag. c., *Puls.*

washer women, in: Phos.

drawing: Ambra., Amm. c. Anac., Bell., Bov., Bry.

TEETH, aching.

Calc., *Carb. v.*, Caust., *Cham.*, Chel., Clem., Coc. c., Cocc., Coloc., Con., Glon., *Graph.*, Kali c., Lach., Mag. c., Merc., Merc. c., Nat. m., Nux v., Plat., Puls., Ran. s., Rhod., Sep., Staph., Sulph.

cold, excited by: *Nux v.*, *Sep.*

menses, when the flow is on: *Amm. c.*, Sep.

warm fluids, excited by: *Sep.*

warm room, in a: *Puls.*

pain that extends to ear: Amm. c., *Kreos.*, Nat. m.

stooping, while: Ferr., Nat. m.

neuralgic: Bell., Carb. s., Cham., Chel., *Coff.*, Coloc., Iris, Kali p., *Mag. p.*, Nux m., Plan., Phyt., Sil.

stitching pain—extending to ear: Nat. m., *Sep.*, Sulph., *Thuja.*

tearing pain: *Acon.*

feels as if nerves were stretched: *Puls.*

Caries, decayed, hollow teeth: Ambr., Amm. c., *Ant. c.*, Bar. c., *Bell.*, *Bov.*, Calc., Calc. p., Calc. s., Carb. v., Cham., Chin., *Fl. ac.*, Glon., Hecla, Hep., Hyos., Kali bi., Kali c., Kali i., Kreos., Lach., Lyc., Mag. c., *Merc.*, *Mez.*, Nat. c., Nit. ac., Nux v., Phos., Ph. ac., *Plb.*, Puls., Rhod., Rhus t., *Sep.*, Sil., *Staph.*, Sulph., Tarax.

decay of teeth suddenly: *Mez.*
decay of teeth as soon as they appear: Kreos.

TEETH, caries.

decay of teeth premature in children: Calc., **Calc. f.**, Calc. p., Fl. ac., *Kreos.*, Staph.

decay of teeth rapid: Calc., Calc. p., Carb. v., *Fl. ac.*, Sep.

Dentition, difficult: *Calc.*, *Calc. p.*, *Cham.*, Ign., Kreos., **Phyt.**, Podo., Rheum, *Sil.*

Looseness of teeth: Amm. c., Carb. v., Merc., Nit. ac., Nux v., Sec. c.

Nerves, injured: Hyper.

Sordes: *Ail.*, Apis, *Ars.*, *Bapt.*, Bry., Cact., Camph., Carb. ac., Carb. v., *Chin.*, Dig., Gels., *Hyos.*, Iris, Kali p., Merc., Merc. c., Mur. ac., *Phos.*, *Ph. ac.*, Pod., Pyrog., *Rhus t.*, Stram., Sul. ac.

CLINCH TOGETHER, constant tendency to: Hyos., Lyc., *Phyt.*, Podo.

DISCOLORATION:

Black: Arg. n., *Chin.*, Chlor., Con., *Merc.*, Nit. ac., Squil., Staph., Thuja.

Yellow: All. c., Iod., Lyc., Merc., Sil., Thuja.

GRINDING: Acon., *Apis*, Arn., Ars., Art. v., *Bell.*, Bry., Calc., Canth., Carb. ac., Caust., Cham., Cic., Cina, Crot. h., Cupr. Grat., Hell., *Hyos.*, Laur., Lyc., Merc., Plb., Pod., Sep., Stram., Sulph., Verat., Zinc.

Chill, during: Calc.

GRINDING.

Convulsive: Bell., Caust., Coff., Zinc.

Epileptic: Bufo., *Hyos.*

SENSATIONS:

Edge, feeling as if on: Amm. c., Aur., Dulc., Iod., *Lach.*, *Mez.*, *Nat. m.*, Sep., Sulph., Sul. ac., Tarax., Zinc.

Elongated, sensation as if: Alum., Amm. c., *Ant. t.*, Ars., Aur., Bor., Bry., Calc., Camph., Carb. c., *Caust.*, Cham., Colch., Glon., Hep.,

SENSATIONS, elongated.

Kali i., *Lach.*, Lyc., *Mag. c.*, Merc., Merc. c., Merc. i. f., *Mez.*, Nat. m., Nit. ac., Nux v., Phyt., Plan., Rhus t., Sep., Sil., Staph., Sulph., Zinc.

TENDER, sensitive: Acon., Bell., Calc., *Nat. m.*

Cold water to: Arg. n., Ars., Bry., Calc., Lach., Nux v., Sil., Stap., Ther.

Touch, to: *Lach.*, Lyc., *Nat. m.* Warmth, to: *Lach.*, *Nat. m.*

FAUCES, PHARYNX AND OESOPHAGUS.

AILMENTS, common:

Abscesses on tonsils, small, painful, frequent: Plb.

Anæsthesia: Acon., All c., Gels., Kali br.

Aphthæ: Æth., Bell., Bry., Canth., *Ign.*, Kali chl.

Cancerous: Carb. an.

Choking: Acon., Æsc., Alum., Apis, Arg. n., Ars., Bapt., Bar c., *Bell.*, Brom., *Cact.*, Calc., Calc. s., Canth., Carb. v., *Caust.*, Cham., Cimex. Cocc., Coc. c., Con., Crot. h., Crot. t., Cupr., Ferr., Fl. ac., Gels., Glon., Graph., Hell., Hep., *Hyos.*, Ign., Iod., Ip., Kali c., Kali s., *Lach.*, *Laur.*, *Lyc.*, Mag. p., Manc., Mez., Mosch., *Naja.*, Nat. m., *Nux v.*, Phyt., Plat., Plb., Puls., Rhod., Sep., *Spong.*, Stram., *Sulph.*, Tab., Thuja, Verat., Zinc.

oesophagus: Æsc., Alum., Alumn., Arg. n., Ars., Bell., Cact., Calc., Carb. ac., Cic., Cimex, Colch., Cupr. ac., *Ign.*, Kali c., *Merc. c.*, *Nat. m.*, Phos., Sabad.

Diphtheria, formation of membrane, exudation etc.: Acet. ac., Amm. c., *Apis*, *Ars.*, Arum. t., Bapt., *Brom.*, Caps., Carb. ac., Crot. h., Echi.,

DIPHTHERIA.

Elaps. Iod., *Kali bi.*, *Kali chl.*, Kreos., *Lac. c.*, *Lach.*, Lachn., *Lyc.*, Merc., Merc. c., Merc. cy., Mur. ac., Nat. m., Nit. ac., *Phyt.*, *Rhus t.*, Sang., Sec., Sulph., Sul. ac., Thuja.

fauces: Caps., Merc. cy.

pharynx, posterior wall: Am. caust., Canth., Merc. i. f., Mur. ac., *Sulph.*

tonsils: Apis, Kali bi., Kali i., Lac. c., *Lach.*, *Lyc.*, *Nit. ac.*, *Phyt.*

uvula: Apis, Kali bi., Nit. ac., *Phyt.*

Gangrene: *Ail.*, Amm. c., Anth., Ars., *Arum. t.*, Carb. v., Chin., *Crot. h.*, Kali p., Kreos., Lach., Merc. c., Mur. ac., Nit. ac., Phyt., Sec., Sil., Sulph.

Paralytic: Apis, *Ars.*, Caust., Cocc., Gels., *Lac. c.*, Lach., Lyc., Nat. m., Nux m., Op., Phyt., Plb., Rhus t., Sil., *Stram.*

oesophagus: Alum., Alumn., *Ars.*, Bapt., Caust., Gels., Hydr. ac., Kali c., Nux m., Op., Plb., Stram., Verat.

pharynx: Apis, *Ars.*, Caust., Cocc., Rhus t., Sil., Stram

GUMS.

AILMENTS, common:

Aphthæ: *Nat. m.*, Sul. ac., Hep.

Bleeding: Agar., Alum., Amm. c., Ant. c., Arg. n., Ars., *Bar. c.*, Bell., Bov., *Calc.*, *Carb. v.*, Caust., Chel., *Crot. h.*, Graph., Ham., Hep., Iod., Kali p., *Lach.*, Mag. m., *Merc.*, Merc. c., Myric., Nat. m., *Nit. ac.*, *Nux m.*, Nux v., Phos., Ph. ac., Psor., Sang., Sec., *Sep.*, Sil., Staph., Sulph., Sul. ac., Ter., Zinc.

extraction of tooth, **profuse** following: *Arn.*, Kreos., Ham., *Lach.*, *Phos.*

Boils: Staph.

Cracks in: Plat.

Fistula of: Aur., Aur. m., Bar. c., Calc., *Caust.*, *Fl. ac.*, Kali chl., Lyc., Nat. m., *Sil.*, Staph., Sulph.

Gangrenous: Lach., *Merc. c.*, Sec.

Mercurial affections: Carb. v., Hep., Merc., Nit. ac.

Putrid: Nat. m.

Scorbutic: Alum., Amm. c., Anac., Ant. c., *Ars.*, Aur. m. n., Bov., Brom., Calc., Camph., Carb. an., *Carb. v.*, Dulc., Hep., Iod., Kali c., *Kali chl.*, Kali i., Kali n., Kali p., *Kreos.*, Lyc., *Merc.*, *Mur. ac.*, Nat. m., Nit. ac., Nux m., Nux v., Phos., Ph. ac., Psor., Staph., Sulph., Ter., Zinc.

Separated, detached from teeth: Amm. c., Ant. c., Aur. m. n., Bapt., Calc., Camph., *Carb. v.*, Cist., Dulc., Graph., Iod., Kali c., Kali i., Kali p.,

GUMS, separated.

Kreos., *Merc.*, Merc. c., Nat. s., Phos., Ph. ac., Staph., Sulph.

Swelling: Alum., Apis, *Ars.*, Bar. c., *Bor.*, Calc., Calc. s., Camph., Caps., Carb. an., Carb. v., *Caust.*, *Chin.*, Chin. a., Cist., Crot. h., Dol., Gels., Glon., *Graph.*, Ham., Hep., Iod., Kali bi., Kali c., Kali i., *Lach.*, Lyc., Mag. c., Mag. m., Merc., Merc. c., Merc. cy., Merc. i. r., Mur. ac., Nat. m., *Nit. ac.*, Petr., Phos., Ph. ac., *Plb.*, Puls., *Sep.*, Sil., Staph., Stront., *Sulph.*, Sul. ac.

Ulcers: Calc., Carb. v., Cupr., Hep., Iod., Kali bi., Kali i., *Kreos.*, Lach., Lyc., Merc., Merc. c., *Nat. m.*, Nux v., Phos., Ph. ac., *Psor.*, Sep., Sil., Sul. ac., Staph.

COLOR:

Black: Merc.

Bluish: Lac., Plb.

Bluish-red: *Kreos.*

Blue line on margins: *Plb.*

Brown: Colch., Plb., Phos.

Dirty: Alum.

Pale: Chel., Cycl., Ferr., *Merc. c.*, *Plb.*, Staph.

Red: Apis, Aur., Bell., Carb. an., Cham., Dol., Dulc., Iod., Lach., *Kreos.*, *Merc.*, Merc. c., Nat. s., Nit. a.

White: Crot. h., *Merc.*, Ferr., Kali bi., Nit. ac., Ph. ac., Staph.

Yellow: Carb. v., Merc.

INDURATED: Carb. v.

PHARYNX, paralytic.

as a sequel of diphtheria: Apis, *Ars.*, Caust., Cocc., Gels., Lac. c., *Lach.*, *Naja*, Nat. m., Plb.

Suppuration of tonsils: Alumn., Anac., Apis, Bar. c., *Bar. m.*, Bell., Calc. s., Canth., Cham., Gua., Hep., Kali bi., **Lac.** c., Lach., Lyc., Manc., *Merc.*, Merc. i. f., *Merc.* i. r., Plb., Sabad., Sang., Sep., *Sil.*, Sulph.

Syphilitic affections: Alumn., *Apis, Ars., Arum. t., Aur. m.*, Bapt., Calc., Calc. s., **Caps.**, Cinab., Elaps., Fl. ac., *Hep.*, Iod., Kali bi., Kali chl., Kali i., Lac. c., Lach., Lyc., Manc., *Merc.*, *Merc. c.*, Merc. cy., Merc. i. f., Merc. i. r., Mur. ac., Nit. ac., Phyt., Psor., Sang., *Sil.*, Sulph.

COLOR—(Fauces and pharynx):

Black: Merc. sul.

Copper-colored: Kali bi., *Merc.*

Dark: Æsc., Bapt., *Phyt.*

Pale: Bar. c.

Purple: *Ail.*, Bapt., Kali bi., *Lach.*, Merc., Nat. a., Nux v., Puls.

Red: *Acon.*, Æsc., Ail., Apis, *Arg. n., Bell.*, Calc. p., Calc. s., Caps., *Carb. ac.*, Cist., Fl. ac., Gels., Hyos., Kali bi., Kali chl., Lach., *Lyc.*, Merc., Merc. c., Merc. i. f., Mur. ac., Nat. a., Nit. ac., Nux v., Petr., *Phyt., Stram.*, Sulph.

DRYNESS: Acon., Æsc..

Agar., All. c., Alum., Amm. c., Anac., Apis, Arg. n., Ars., Asaf., Atro., Bar. c., *Bell.*,

PHARYNX, dryness.

Berb., Bov., *Bry.*, Bufo, *Calad., Calc.*, Cann. i., *Canth.*, Carb. v., *Caust.*, Chel., Sic., Cimex, Cinnab., *Cist., Cocc.*, Coc. c., Colch., Coloc., Con., Cor. r., Crot. h., Dros., Gels., Hep., Hyos., Ign., Iod., Ip., Iris, Kali ar., *Kali bi.*, Kali c., Kali chl., Kali i., Kali s., Kalm., Lach., Lachn., *Lac. c., Lyc., Mag. c.*, Mag. m., Manc., *Merc.*, Merc. c., *Mez.*, Mur. ac., Naja, Nat. a., Nat. c. *Nat. m.*, Nat. p., Nit. ac., *Nux m.*, Nux v., Op., *Phos.*, Phyt., Plat., Podo., Psor., *Puls., Rhus t., Sabad.*, Sabin., Sang., Sars., Sene., Seneg., Sep., *Sil.*, Stann., *Stict.*, Stram., Sulph., Thuja, Verat., *Verat. v.*, Zinc.

ELONGATED UVULA:

Alumn., Apis, *Bar. m.*, Caps., Coff., Croc., *Crot. t.*, Hep., *Hyos.*, Iod., Kali c., *Kali i.*, Lac. c., *Lach.*, Manc., Merc., Nat. m., *Phos.*, Sulph.

ENLARGED TONSILS:

Alumn., *Bar. c., Bar. m.*, Calc. i., Calc. p., Cedr., Chen. ac., Ferr., Hep., Kali bi., Kali c., Lacn., *Lyc.*, Merc., Nat. m., Nit. ac., Phyt., Sep., Sil., Staph., Sulph., Syph.

HAWKING DISPOSITION:

Ail., Alum., Arg. m., *Arg. n.*, Ail., Alum., Arg. m., *Arg. n.*, Arum. t., Bar. c., Bell., Bry., Carb. an., Carb. v., Caust., Cimex, Cist., Coc. c., *Cor. r., Crot. t.*, Dulc., Fl. ac., Gels., Graph., Gua., Hep., *Kali bi.*, Kali c., *Lach.*, Lil. t., *Lyc.*, Mag. m.,

HAWKING, disposition.

Merc. i. f., Mez., Nat. a.,
Nat. c., Nat. m., Nat. s.,
Nit. ac., Nux v. Phos.,
Phyt., Psor., Rumex, Sabad.,
Sel., Seneg Sil., Stann..
Stram., Sulph., Thuja, Zinc.

INDURATED TONSILS:
Agar., Bar. c., Bar. m., Ign.,
Nit. ac., Plb., Stap.

SENSATIONS:

Hair: Kali bi., Sil., Sulph.

Plug or lump: All. c., Alum.,
Ambr., Ant. c., Arg. n.,
Asaf., Bar. c., Calc., Caust.,
Cina, Coc. c., Con., Crot. h.,
Ferr., Gels., Graph., Hep.,
Ign., Kali bi., Kali c., Lac.
c., Lach., Led., Lob., Merc.
i. f., Nat. m., Nux v., Nux
m., Phyt., Plb., Psor., Saba.,
Sep., Sil., Sulph., Thuja.

Plug or lump as if rising: Ars.,
Asaf., Chel., Con., Gels.,
Ign., Kalm., Lac. d., Lob.,
Lyc., Mag. m., Mosch., Nat.
m., Nux m., Nux v., Plat.,
Plb., Puls., Sep., Stram.,
Sulph., Valer.

Narrow: Alum., Bell., Calc.,
Caust., Mez., Nux v.

SWALLOWING, difficulty in
Acon., Æsc., Alum., Alumn.,

SWALLOWING, difficulty in:

Amm. c., Apis, Arg. m.,
Arg. n., Ars., Aur., Bapt.,
Bar. c., Bell., Brom., Cact.,
Calc., Canth., Caps., Carb.
v., Caust., Chel., Chin., Cocc,
Colch., Con., Crot. h., Cupr.,
Dulc., Elaps, Gels., Hell.,
Hep., Hyos., Ign., Iod., Ip.,
Kali c., Kali n., Kalm.,
Lac. c., Lach., Lyc., Merc.,
Merc. c., Nit. ac., Op.,
Phyt., Plb., Rhus t., Sabad.,
Sep., Sil., Stram., Sul. ac
Tab., Wyeth.

Drink, has got to, in order to
swallow: Bell., Cact., Nat.
c.

Fluids, he can swallow only,
solid food gags: Plb.

Liquids: Canth., Cupr., Hyos.,
Ign., Iod., Lach., Lyc.,
Merc., Lyss., Stram., Upa.

Solids: Alum., Alumn., Apis,
Arg. n., Bapt., Bar. c.,
Bell., Carb. v., Cham., Crot.
h., Kali c., Nat. m., Nux v.,
Plb., Rhus t.

Impossible: Alum., Alumn.,
Ant. t., Arum t., Bell.,
Camph., Carb. v. Cic.,
Cina, Gels., Hyos., Lac. c.,
Lach., Nux v., Nit. ac., Op.,
Phos., Plb., Sabad., Stram.,
Sulph., Tab., Verat.

STOMACH.

AILMENTS, Common:

Aching: Abrot., Acet. ac.,
Acon., Æsc., Æth., Ant. c.,
Ant. t., Apis, Arg. m., *Arg.
n.*, Ars., Asar., Asaf., Bar.
c., Bar. m., *Bell.*, *Bism.*,
Brom., *Bry.*, Cact., Calc.,
Camph., Canth., Caps., Carb.
ac., Carb. an., *Carb. v.*,
Card. m., *Caust.*, Cham.,
Chel., *Chin.*, Chin. s., Cina,
Cocc., *Colch.*, *Coloc.*, Con.,
Corn., Crot. h., *Cupr.*, Cupr.
ac., Cupr. ar., Dig., Dios.,
Ferr., Ferr. ar., Gels., *Graph.*,
Grat., Hydr., Hyos., Ign.,
Iod., Ip., Iris, Kali ar., Kali
bi., Kali c., Kali n., Kali s.
Kalm., Kreos., Lach., Laur.,
Lob., *Lyc.*, Mag. c., Mag.
m., Mag. p., Manc., Merc.,
Nat. c., Nat. m., Nat. s.,
Nit. ac., Nux m., *Nux v.*,
Op., Petr., Phos., Phyt.,
Plb., Ptel., *Puls.*, Sang.,
Sec., Sep., *Sil.*, Spig., Staph.,
Stram., *Sulph.*, Sul. ac.,
Tab., Ter., *Verat.*, Verat.
v., Zinc.

Aura epileptic Calc., Cic.,
Indig., *Nux v.* Sil.

Empty feeling, weakness, faintness, goneness, hungry feeling: Æsc., Agar., All. c.,
Ambr., *Ant. c.*, Aran., Arg.
n., Ars., Asaf., Bapt., Bar.
c., Brom., Bufo, Calc., Calc.
p., Camph., Caps., Carb. an.,
Carl., Caust., Chin., Cic.,
Cina, Cocc., Coloc., Croc.,

STOMACH, empty feeling.

Crot. h., Crot. t., *Dig.*,
Elaps, Fl. ac., Gamb., Gels.,
Glon, Graph., Hipp., *Hydr.*,
Hydr. ac., Ign., Kali ar.,
Kali c., Kali chl., Kali fer.,
Kali p., Lac. c., Lach., Laur.,
Lob., Lyc., Mag. c., *Merc.*,
Mur. ac., Nat. c., Nat. m.,
Nat. p., Nat. s., Nux v.,
Olnd., Op., Petr., *Phos.*,
Podo., *Puls.*, Rhus t., Sang.,
Sep., Stann., *Sulph.* Sul. i.,
Tab., Teucr., Tub., *Verat.*,
Zinc.

after eating: *Sep.*

at 11 a.m.: Asaf., Nat. c.,
Phos., *Sulph.*, Zinc.

Cancer: Acet. ac., *Ars.*, Ars.
i., *Bism.*, Caps., Carb. ac.,
Carb. an., Carb. v., *Con.*,
Crot. h., *Cond.*, Hydr.,
Kreos., Lach., Lyc., Merc.
c., *Mez.*, *Phos.*, Sep., Sil.,
Staph.

Empty feeling:

during headache: Phos.,
Sang., Sep.

not relieved by eating: Ant.
c., Arg. m., Ars., Carb.
an., Carb. v., *Cina*, Hydr.,
Ign., *Lach.*, *Lyc.*, Merc.,
Mur. ac., Nux m., *Phos.*,
Sep., Staph., Teucr.,
Verat.

Indigestion: Alum., Ars., *Bar.
c.*, *Bar. m.*, Bism., *Calc.*,
Calc. s., Carb. an., *Carb. v.*,
Chel., Chin., Coff., Ferr. p.

THROAT EXTERNAL.

AILMENTS, Common:

Goitre: Ail., Ambr., Apis, Aur., Brom., *Calc.*, Calc. f., Calc. i, Carb. an., Carb. s., Caust., Cist., Fl. ac., Hep., *Iod.*, Kali i., Lycop., Lyc., Merc. i. r., Nat. c., Nat. m., Phos., Sil., *Spong.*

exophthalmic: Aur., Cact., Ferr., Ferr. i., Lycops., Nat. m., Phos., Spong.

AILMENTS, throat.

Torticollis: Caust., Cupr., Hyos., Lachn., *Lyc.*, Nux v., *Phos.*, Rhus t.

Tumors:

sides, on the: Brom.

cystic: Brom.

fatty: Bar. c.

STOMACH, indigestion.

Graph., *Hep.*, Homar.,
Hydr., *Ip.*, Lach., *Lyc.*,
Mag. m., Merc., *Nat.* c.,
Nat. m., Nux m., *Nux v.*,
Olnd., Petr., Ph. ac., Ptel.,
Puls., Sep., *Sulph.*

coffee: Cham., *Nux v.*

ice-cream: Ars., Carb. v.,
Puls.

milk: Æth., Ant. c., *Chin.*,
Calc., Iris, Mag. c., Mag.
m., Nux v.

pork: *Cycl.*, Ip., *Puls.*

THIRST, extreme.

potatoes: *Alum.*

vexation: *Cham.*, *Ip.*

Inflation: Ars., Calc., Caps.,
Con., Dulc., Hell., Ip., Lyc.,
Nux v., Nux m., Op., Rat.,
Sabin.

Narrow, pylorus feels too: Lyc.

Obstruction of Pylorus, sensation of: Lach., Nux v., Phos.

Ulcers: Arg. n., Ars., Calc. ar.,
Kali bi., Mez., Nit. ac., Nux
v., *Phos.*

APPETITE.

CAPRICIOUS: *Bry.*, *Chin.*, Cina, Hep., Ign., Ip., Mag. m., Phos., Puls., Sang., Ther.

INCREASED: Abies, c., Acon., Agar., All. c., Alum., Alumn., *Arg. m.*, Ars., Aur., Bar. c., Bar. m., Bell., Berb., *Calc.*, Calc. p., *Cann. i.*, Carb. an., Caust., *Chin.*, Chin s., *Cina,* Cinnab., Cocc., Elaps, Ferr., Ferr. ar., Fl. ac., Gels., Graph., Guare, Ign., *Iod.*, Kali s., Lac. c., Lach., *Lyc.*, Mag. m., Merc., Merc. c., Mur. ac., Nat. c., *Nat. m.*, Nat. p., Nat. s., Nux m., Nux v., *Olnd.*, Op., *Phos.*, Ph. ac. Pic ac., Psor., Puls., Rat., *Sabad.*, Sep., Sil., Stann., Staph., *Sulph.*, Teucr., *Verat.*

At 11 a.m.: Iod., Nat. m., *Sulph.*, Zinc.

During fever: Chin., Cina, *Phos.*

During headache: Kali c., *Phos.*, Psor., Sep.

Vanishes, when he attempts to eat: Sil.

Vanishes at the sight of food: Phos., *Sulph.*

INSATIABLE: Arg. m., *Iod.*, *Lyc.*, Sec., Spong., Zinc.

RAVENOUS HUNGER (Canine, excessive appetite) Agar., All. c., Alum., Amm.

RAVENOUS, c., Anac., Arg. m., *Ars.*, Aur., Berb., Bry., *Calc.*, *Calc. s.*, *Cann. i.*, Carb. an., Caust., *Chin.*, Chin. a., Cina, Cocc., Coc. c., Coff., Colch., Coloc., Con., Elaps, Eup. per., Ferr., Ferr. ar., Fl. ac., Graph., Gua., Ign., *Iod.*, Kali n., Lach., *Lyc.*, Merc., Merc. c., Mez., Mur. ac., Nat. c., *Nat. m.*, Nat. p., Nat. s., Nux m., *Nux v.*, *Olnd.*, Op., Petr., *Phos.*, Ph. ac., *Plat.*, Podo., *Psor.*, *Puls.*, Rat., Rhus t., Sabad., Sec., Sep., Sil., *Spong.*, *Stann.*, Staph., *Sulph.*, Thuja, *Verat.*, Zinc.

emaciation, accompanying: Abrot., *Calc.*, *Iod.*, *Nat. m.*, *Petr.*, Phos., Sulph., Tub.

marasmus, accompanying: Abrot., Bar. c., *Calc.*, Calc. p., Caust., Chin., Cina, *Iod.*, Lyc., Mag. c., *Nat. m.*, Nux v., Sil., Sulph.

Returning of appetite after eating a mouthful, in persons suffering from anorexia: Calc., Chin., Sabad.

Satiated, easily: Amm. c., Carb. s., Caust., *Chin.*, Cic., Clem., Colch., Cycl., Dig., Ferr., Gels., Ign., *Lyc.*, Nux m., Nux v., Op., Phos., Plat., Podo., Rhod., Sec., Sil. Sulph., Thuja.

TASTE.

ACRID: Aur., Berb., Hydr. ac., Laur., *Lob.*, Rhus.

ACUTE: Bell., Camph., *Chin.*, *Coff.*, Lyc.

ALKALINE: Kalm.

BAD: All. c., Ang., Ars., Bapt., Bry., *Calc.*, Calc. p., Calc. s., Cann. s., Coc. c., Crot. t., Gels., Graph., Hydr., Kali ar., Kali bi., Kali c., *Merc.*, Merc. i. r., *Nat. s.*, Nux v., Phyt., *Puls.*, Sars., *Sulph.*, Sul. ac.

BITTER: *Acon.*, Alum., Amm. c., Amm. m., Ang., Ant. c., Apis, Arg. n., Arn., Ars., Aur., Bar. c., Bell., Bor., Bov., *Bry.*, Calc., Canth., Carb. an., Carb. v., Card. m., Caust., Cham., *Chel.*, *Chin.*, Chin. a., Cocc., Coc. c., Colch., *Coloc.*, Con., Corn., Crot. h., Dig., Dulc., Elaps, Euph., Eup. per., Graph., Grat., Hell., Hep., Ign., Jab., Kali ar., Kali c., Lach., Lept., Lyc., Mag. c., Mag. m., Mag. p., Mag. s., Manc., Merc., Merc. c., Mez., Merc. i. r., Mur. ac., Myric., Nat. c., *Nat. m.*, *Nat. s.*, Nit. ac., Nux m., *Nux v.*, Par., Petr., Phos., Plb., Podo., Prun., Psor., Ptel., *Puls.*, Raph., Rheum, Stram., *Sulph.*, Tarax, Verat.

Water, everything except: *Acon.*, *Stann.*

BLOODY: Amm. c., Ars., Bell., Ferr., Ip., Lil. t., Nat. c.

BURNING: All. c., Daph., Kali chl., Osm.

EARTHY: Ferr., Ip., Nux m.,

EGGS, like rotten: *Arn.*, Ferr., *Merc.*, *Mur.* ac., Sil.

GREASY (fatty): Asaf., Caust., Cham., Kali i., Lyc., Mur. ac., Psor., Puls., Sil.

INSIPID: Alum., *Anac.*, Aur., Bapt., Bry., Caps., Chin., Cocc., Colch., Ferr., Gua., Ip., Kali c., Merc., Nat. c., Nat. m., Petr., Psor., *Puls.*, Rheum, Sanic., Stann., Staph., Sulph., Thuja.

METALLIC (Coppery): Æsc., Agn., Amm. c., Arg. n., Ars., Calc., Canth., Cinnab., *Cocc.*, Coc. c., Coloc., Cupr., Cupr. ar., Cupr. s., Lach., Lyc., *Merc.*, Merc. c., *Nat. c.*, Nux, Phyt., Plb., *Rhus t.* Seneg., Sep., Sulph., Zinc.

NAUSEATING: All. c., Carb. an., Ip., Myric., *Puls.*, Sulph.

PUTRID: Acon., *Anac.*, Arn., Ars., Aur., Bry., *Calc.*, *Caps.*, Carb. v., Caust., Cham., Cinnab., Cocc., Dros., Ferr., Ferr. ar., Hep., Hyos., Ign., Iod., Kali bi., Kali c., Lac. c., Merc., Mur. ac., Nat. m., *Nux v.*, Petr., Phos., *Psor.*, Podo., *Puls.*,

PUTRID.

Pyrog., Rhus. t., Sep., Sulph., Sul. ac., Verat.

SALTISH: Ars., Calc., Carb. v., Carls., Cycl., Graph., Hyos., Kali chl., *Merc.*, *Merc. c.*, *Nat. m.*, Nux m., Nux v., Phos., Ph. ac., Puls., Rheum, Sep., Sulph., Tarax, Zinc.

SHINY: Arn., Cham., Chel., Chin., Merc., Merc. c., Nat. s., Nux m., Nux v., Petr., Phos., *Puls.*, Rheum, Sep., *Valer.*

SOUR: Alum., Alumn., Ant. c., *Arg. n.*, Ars., Bar. c., *Calc.*, Calc. s., Caps., Carb. ac., Caust., Cham., Chin., Chin. a., Chel., Cocc., Croc., Crot. h., Graph., Hep., Ign., Kali chl., Kalm., Lach., *Lyc.*, *Mag. c.*, Mag. m., Mang.,

SOUR.

Merc., Mur. ac., *Nat. c.*, Nat. m., *Nux v.*, Ox. ac., Petr., Phos., Ph. ac., Puls., Sars., Sep., Sil., Stann., Sulph., Tarax.

SWEETISH: Acon., All. c., Alum., Alumn., Ars., Bell., Bry., Chin., Coc. c., Coff., Cupr., Dulc., Kali c., Kali i., Lyc., Merc., Mur. ac., Phos., Plat., Plb., Podo., *Puls.*, Pyrog., Sabad., Sars., Squil., Spong., Stann., *Sulph.*, Thuja, Zinc.

TASTELESSNESS: Anac., Ant. t., Apis, Aur., *Bell.*, Bor., Bry., Calc., Canth., Crot. h., Cycl., Hep., Hyos., Kali bi., Mag. m., Merc., Nat. m., Nux m., Nux v., Par., *Phos.*, Psor., *Puls.*, Sep., *Sil.*, Sulph., Sul. ac., Ther., Verat.

THIRST

THIRST: *Acet. ac.*, *Acon.*, Agar., All. c., Amm. m., Anac., Ant. c., Apoc., Arg. n., Arn., *Ars.*, Bapt., Bar. c., Bar. m., Bell., Berb., Bor., Bol., *Bry.*, *Calc.*, Calc. ar., Calc. s., Camph., Canth., *Caps.*, Carb. ac., Carb. v., *Cham.*, *Chel.*, *Chin.*, Chin. a., Chin. s., Cic., Cimic., Cina, Cocc., Coc. c., Colch., Coloc., Con., Croc., Cupr., Cupr. ac., *Dig.*, Dros., Dulc., *Eup. per.*, Ferr. p., Fl. ac., *Hell.*, Hep., Hyos., Iod., Kali bi., Kali c., Kali i., Kali p., Kali s., Kalm., Lach., Led., Laur., Mag. c., Merc., Merc. c., Merc. i. f., Mez., *Nat. c.*, *Nat. m.*, Nat. p., Nit. ac., Nux v., *Op.*, *Phos.*, Plb., Podo., Ran. b., Raph., Rat., *Rhus t.*, Sec., Sil., Stram., Sulph., Ther., Thuja, *Verat.*, Verat. v., Zinc.

Constant: Acet. ac., Acon., Apis, *Ars.*, Bar. c., Bell., Bry., Calc., Camph., Carb. s., Crot. h., Dulc., *Eup. per.*, Ferr., Kali p., Lach., Merc., Nat. m., Op., *Phos.*, Rhus t., Sulph., Verat.

Extreme: *Acet. ac.*, *Acon.*, Æsc., All. c., Amm. m., Ant. c., Ant. t., Apis, *Arg. n.*, Arn., *Ars.*, Ars. h., Bell., Bor., Bry., Cadm., *Calc.*, *Calc. s.*, Camph., Carb. ac., Carb. v., Caust., Cedr., *Cham.*, Chel., *Chin.*, Colch.,

THIRST, extreme.
Coloc., Cop., Croc., Crot. t., Cupr., Cupr. ar., Cycl., *Dig.*, Dulc., Elaps, *Eup. per.*, Ferr., Graph., *Hell.*, Hep., Iod., Ip., Kali c., Kali i., Kali p., Kalm., Kreos., Lac. ac., Laur., Led., Lyc., Lycop., Lyss., Mag. c., Mag. m., Med., *Merc.*, *Merc. c.*, Nat. c., *Nat. m.*, Nat. p., Nat. s., Nit. ac., Nux v., Olnd., Petr., *Phos.*, Ph. ac., Podo., *Pyrog.*, Raph., Rhus. t., Rob., Sang., Sep., Sil., Sul. ac., Ter., *Verat.*, Zinc.

MODALITIES:

Chill, during the stage of: Acon., *Apis*, *Arn.*, Bry., Calc., Caps., Carb. v., Chin. s., Cina, *Eup. per.*, Eup. pur., Ferr., *Ign.*, Kali c., Lach., Led., *Nat. m.*, *Nux v.*, Op., Pyrog., Rhus t., Sec., *Sep.*, Sil., Sulph., *Tub.*, Verat.

following: *Ars.*, *Chin.*, Cimex, *Dros.*, Nat. m., *Puls.*, Sabad., Sep.

previous to: *Ars.*, Caps., *Chin.*, *Eup. per.*, Eup. pur., Hep., Nux v., *Puls.*

Heat: Acon., All. c., Anac., Arn., *Ars.*, *Bell.*, *Bry.*, Calc., Canth., Caps., Cedr., Cham., Chin., Chin. s., Cina, Cocc., Coff., Coloc., Con., Croc., Elat., *Eup. per.*, Geis., Hep., Hyos., Ip., Kali ar., Kali c.,

MODALITIES, heat during.

> *Nat. m., Nux v.,* Phos., Podo., Psor., Puls., Pyrog., Ran. s., Rhus t., Sec., Sil., Stram., Sulph., Thuja, Tub. following: China.

Large quantities, for: Acon., *Ars., Bry.,* Chin., Cocc., Eup. per., Ferr. p., Lac. d., Lycop., Merc., Merc. c., *Nat. m., Phos.,* Stram., *Sulph., Verat.*

Perspiration, during: Acon., *Ars.,* Bry., *Chin.,* Chin. a., Chin. s., Coff., Iod., Ip., *Nat. m.,* Op., Ph. ac., Rhus t., Sep., *Stram.,* Thuja., *Verat.*

Phthisis, in: Nit. ac.

Spasm, during: Cic.

With arrest of breathing, during drinking: Anac.

MODALITIES.

Without desire to drink: Ang., Mez.

THIRSTLESS: Æsc., Amm. m., Ant. c., *Ant. t., Apis,* Arg. n., Ars., Asaf., Bell., Bov., Camph., Chin., Con., Cycl., Ferr., *Gels., Hell.,* Hydr. ac., Ip., Kali c., Lyc., Mang., *Meny., Nux m.,* Olnd., Op., *Ph. ac., Puls., Sabad.,* Samb., Sep., Staph.

Heat, during the stage: Æth., Alum., Ant. c., Ant. t., *Apis,* Calc., Caps., Carb. v., Caust., Cimex, *Cina, Dros.,* Ferr., *Gels.,* Ign., Ip., Kali c., Led., Mur. ac., Nit. ac., Nux m., Ph. ac., Puls., *Sabad.,* Samb., *Sep.,* Spig., Sulph.

ERUCTATIONS.

ERUCTATIONS: Acon., Agar., Æsc., All. c., Ambr., Ant. c., Ant. t., Arg. n., Arn., Ars., Asaf., Asar., Bar. c., Bell., Bism., Bry., Calc., Camph., Canth., Carb. ac., Carb. an., Carb. v., Caust., Cham., Chel., Chin., Cinnab., Croc., Cupr., Cycl., Dros., Croc., Cupr., Cycl., Drios., Dul., Eup. per., Ferr., Fl. ac., Gels., Graph., Gua., Helon., Hep., Hydr., Ign., Iod., Ip., Jug., Kali c., Kali p., Kali s., Kalm., Lac. ac., Lac. d., Lach., Laur., Lyc., Mag. c., Mag. m., Merc., Mez., Mur. ac., Nat. c., Nat. m., Nat. p., Nat. s., Nit. ac., Nux v., Ox. ac., Petr., Phos., Ph. ac., Plb., Psor., Puls., Ran. b., Ran. s., Rhus t., Ruta, Sabad., Sars., Sep., Sil., Squil., Stann., Staph., Sul. ac., Sulph., Tarax., Thuja, Valer., Verat., Verb., Zinc.

Acrid: Ambr., Apis, Calc., Calc. s., Cann. s., Carb. ac., Caust., Dig., Fl. ac., Graph., Lac. ac., Lach., Lyc., Merc., Nit. ac., Nuph., Nux v., Phyt., Rhus t., Sang., Sep., Sul. ac.

Bitter: Aloe., Alum., Ambr., Amm. c., Amm. m., Apis, Arn., Berb., Bry., Calc., Calc. s., Cann. s., Carb. v., Carl., Chel., Chin., Chin. a., Chion., Cocc., Ferr. m., Grat.,

ERUCTATION, bitter.

Ign., Lyc., Merc., Merc. i. r., Nat. s., Nux v., Ph. ac., Pic. a., Podo., Puls., Sars., Sep., Stann.. Sul. ac.

Food (regurgitation): Æsc., Arg. n., Arum. t., Bell., Bry., Calc., Calc. p., Calc. s., Cham., Carb. v., Caust., Chin., Con., Cop., Dig., Ferr., Ferr. p., Hep., Kali bi., Lach., Lyc., Merc., Mez., Nat. m., Nux v., Phos., Ph. ac., Podo., Puls., Rhus t., Sulph.

Foul: Ant. t., Arn., Asaf., Berb., Bism., Car. v., Cocc., Dig., Ferr., Fl. ac., Graph., Hep., Kali bi., Plb., Psor., Puls., Sep., Sulph., Sul. ac.

Greasy: Cycl., Mag. c., Puls.

Loud: Arg. n., Asaf., Bism., Carb. v., Chin., Coca, Coloc., Merc. i. r., Phos., Plat., Puls., Sil.

Sour: Acet. ac., All. c., Alum., Ambr., Arg. n., Ars., Bar. c., Bry., Cadm., Calc., Calc. p., Calc. s., Canth., Carb. ac., Carb. an., Carb. s., Carb. v., Caust., Cham., Chel., Chin., Chin. a., Chion., Cimex, Cocc., Con., Cycl., Dig., Dios., Ferr., Ferr. ar., Ferr. m., Ferr. p., Gels., Graph., Hep., Hydr., Ign., Iod., Kali c., Kali s., Lac. d., Lach., Lith., Lob., Lyc., Mag. c., Nat. c., Nat. m.,

ERUCTATION, sour.

Nat. p., *Nat. s.*, Nit. a., *Nux v.*, Op., Petr., *Phos.*, Ph. ac., Podo., Psor., Puls., Rob., Sep., Sil., *Sulph.*, *Sul. ac.*, Zinc.

WATERBRASH:

Alumn., Amm. c., Amm. m., Ant. t., Apis, *Ars.*, *Bar. c.*, Bism., Bry., Calc., Calc. p., Calc. s., Caps., Carb. an., *Carb. v.*, Caust., Chin., Cic., Cina.

WATERBRASH.

Cocc., Daph., Dros., Graph., Hep., Ign., Ip., Kali c., Led., *Lyc.*, Mag. m., Merc., Mez., Nat. c., Nat. m., Nat. s., Nit. ac., *Nux v.*, Par., *Petr.*, Phos., *Puls.*, Ran. b., Rhod., Rhus t., *Sabad.*, Sang., Sars., Sep., *Sil.*, *Staph.*, *Sulph.*, Sul. ac., *Verat.*

Pregnancy, during: Lac. ac. Nat. m., Nux m., Tab.

HEART-BURN.

HEART-BURN: Æsc., Alum., *Ambr.*, *Amm. c.*, Anac., Apis, Ars., Berb., Bry., *Calc.*, Calc. s., Canth., Caps., Carb. an., *Carb. v.*, Caust., Chel., Chin., Chin. s., Cic., Con., *Croc.*, *Ferr. p.*, Fl. ac., Graph., Hep., Iod., Iris, Kali c., Lach., Iod., Lyc., *Mag. c.*, Merc., Nat. c., Nat. m., Nat. s., *Nux v.*, Phos., Podo., *Puls.*, Rob., Sabad., Sabin., Sep., Sil., Sin. n., Sulph., Sul. ac., Syph., Valer., Verat. v., Zinc.

Acids, after: Nux v.

Bed, after going to: Con.

HEART-BURN.

Dinner, after: Acon., Calc. p., Crot. t., Ham., Kali bi., Lyc., Merc. i. r., Sol. n., Sulph.

Drinking, after: Alum.

Drunkards, when complained of by: Nux v., Sul. ac.

Eating, after: Æsc., Amm. c., Calc., Calc. p., Chin., Graph., Iod., Nat. m., Nit. ac., Nux v.

Pregnant women, in: Caps., Merc.

Wine, when he has drunk: Bry., Coc. c., Zinc.

NAUSEA.

REMEDIES: Acon., Æsc., Aeth., Agar., All. s., Alum., Amm. m., Anac., *Ant. c., Ant. t.*, Aran., Arg. m., *Arg. n., Ars.* Asar., Bapt., Bar. c., *Bell.*, Berb., Bism., Bol., Bov., Bry., Cadm., Calc., Calc. p., Calc. s., Camph., Canth., Caps., Carb. ac., Carb. an., Carb. v., Card. m., Caust., *Cham.*, Chel., Chin., Chin. s., Chion., Chr. ac., Cimic., Cist., *Cocc.*, Cod., Colch., Coloc., Con., Crot. h., Cub., Cupr. a., Cupr. s., Cycl., *Dig.*, Dios., Dros., *Dulc.*, Echi., Elat., Euph., Eup. per., Ferr., Ferr. ar., Ferr. p., Fl. ac., Form., Gamb., Gels., Gran., Graph., *Hell., Hep.*, Hydr., Ign., Iod., *Ip., Iris, Iris. f.*, Kali ar., Kali bi., Kali c., Kali s., Lac. c., Lach., Laur., *Lob., Lyc.*, Mag. m., Mag. p., Merc., Merc. i. f., Mez., Mosch., Mur. ac., Nat. c., Nat. m., Nat. p., Nit. ac., *Nux v.*, Ox. ac., *Petr.*, Phos., Ph. ac., Plat., Plb., Podo., Prun., Psor., *Puls.*, Ran. b., Ran. s., Raph., Rheum, Rhod., *Rhus t.*, Rhus v., Sabad., Samb., Sang., Sars., Sec., Seneg., *Sep., Sil.*, Squil., Stann., *Sulph.*, Sul. ac., *Tab.*, Tarax., Ter., Ther., Thuja, *Valer., Verat.*, Verat. v., *Zinc.*

MODALITIES:

Breakfast, previous to: Berb., Bov., Calc., Lyc., Nit. ac., Sep., Tub.

Constant: Ant. c., Ant. t., Dig., Ip., Lac. c., Lyc., *Nux v.*, Sil.

Cough, during: Calc., Coc. c., Ign., *Ip.*, Kali bi., Kali c., Merc., Nux v., Ph. ac., *Puls.*, Sep., Verat.

Deathly: Ars., Cadm., Camph., Crot. h., Dig., *Ip.*, *Tab.*

Drunkards, when complained of by: Ars., Asar., *Kali bi.*, Sul. ac.

Fainting: Arg. n., *Cocc.*, Glon., *Lach.*, Nux v.

Food, when he looked at his: Colch., Kali bi., Kali c., Lyc.

  smell of food: Ars., Cocc., *Colch.*, Dig., Ip., Sep., Thuja.

  thought of: Ars., Chin., *Cocc., Colch.*, Sars., Sep., Thuja.

Ice-cream: Ars., Ip., *Puls.*

Intermittent: Ant. c., *Ant. t.*, Cina, Dros., Sep., *Tab.*

Motion on: Arn., Bry., *Cocc.*, Eup. per., Ip., *Kali c.*, Kali bi., Lac. ac., Op., Tab., Verat., Zinc.

Pregnancy, during: Ant. c., Ant. t., Ars., *Asar.*, Bry., Carb. an., Colch., Con.,

NAUSEA, during pregnancy.

Hell., Ip., Iris, Jatr., Kali c., *Kreos.*, Lac. c., Lach., *Lac. ac.*, Lob., Lyc., Mag. c., Mag. m., Nat. m., Nux m., *Nux v.*, Ox. ac., Petr., Phos., Psor., Puls., *Sep.*, Sil., Sul. ac., *Tub.*

Reads, when he: Arg. m.

Riding in a carriage, while: Calc., *Cocc.*, Con., Glon.,

NAUSEA, riding in a carriage.

Kali bi., *Nux v., Petr.*, Sep., Staph., *Tab.*

Sun, from heat of: Carb. v.

Sweets: *Graph.*, Ip

Warm drinks: Bism., Lach., Phos., *Puls.*

room in a: *Lyc.*, Mez., *Nat. c.*, Phos., Puls., Tab.

water, if he puts his hands in: *Phos.*

VOMITING.

REMEDIES: *Acon.*, *Æsc.*, *Æth.*, Agar., Amm. m., Anthr., *Ant. c.*, *Ant. t.*, *Apis*, Apoc., *Apom.*, *Arg. n.*, Arn., Ars., Asar., Bar. c., Bell., Bism., Bor. Both., *Bry.*, Cact., *Cadm.*, Calc., Calc. s., Camph., Canth., *Cham.*, Chel., *Chin.*, Chin. s., Cimic., Cina, Cocc., Coc. c., *Colch.*, Con., Cub., *Cupr.*, Cupr. ar., Cupr. s., Dig., Dor., Dros., Dulc., Eup. per., Euph., *Ferr.*, Ferr. ar., *Gamb.*, Gran., Graph., Grat., Hell., Hep., Hyos., Ign., Iod., Ip., *Iris*, Kali bi., Kali i., *Kreos.*, Lach., Laur., *Lob.*, Lyc., Merc., Mez. Nat. m., Nit. ac., Nux m., *Nux v.*, Ox. ac., Petr., *Phos.*, *Plb.*, Psor., *Puls.*, Samb., Sang., Sec., Sep., *Sil.*, *Sulph.*, *Tab.*, Ter., Ther., Tub., Valer., *Verat.*, *Verat. v.*, Zinc.

MODALITIES:

Chill, during the period of: Caps., Cina, Dros., *Eup. per.*, Ign., Ip., Nat. m., Puls., Verat.

following: Aran., Bry., Carb. v., *Eup. per.*, Ip., Lyc., *Nat. m.*,

previous to: Ars., Cina, Eup. per., Ferr.

Coughing, on: *Alum.*, Anac., *Ant. t.*, Arg. n., Arn., Ars., Ars. i., *Bry.*, Carb. v.,

VOMITING, coughing on.

Cham., Cimex, Coc. c., Cupr., Daph., Dig., *Dros.*, Ferr., Form., *Hep.*, Hyos., *Ip.*, Kali ar., *Kali c.*, Kali p., Lach., Meph., Nat. m., Nit. ac., Nux, Ph. ac., Puls., Sabad., Sep., Sil. Sulph.

Drinking, after: Acon., Ant. t., *Ant. c.*, Arn., *Ars.*, Bism., Bor., Bry., Cadm., Cin. a., Cina, Cupr. ac., Dulc., Eup. per., Ip., Kreos., Lyc., Nux, Op., *Phos.*, Sec., Sil., Sul. ac., *Tab.*, *Verat.*, Verat. v.

Drinking, cold water: Bry., Cupr., Dulc., Eup. per., Kali c., Lyc., Sil., Sul. ac., Verat., *Verat. v.*

Drinking, immediately after: Ars., Bism., Bry., Cadm., Eup. per., Nux v., Zinc.

Drinking, smallest quantity: Ars., Bism., Bry., Cadm., Phos.

as soon as water gets warm in stomach: Phos., Pyrog.

Drunkards, when complained of by: Alumn., *Ars.*, Cadm., Caps., Carb. ac., Crot. h., *Kali bi.*, Kali br., Lach., Nux v., Sang., Sul. ac.

Forcible: Con., Nux v., Petr., Sanic., *Verat.*

Headache, during: Æth., Apis, Ars., Bell., Bry., Cact., Calc., Caps., Coff., Crot. h., Form., Gels., Graph., Grat., Ip.,

VOMITING, headache, during.

Iris, Lac. d., Lach., *Meli.*, Nat. m., Nat. s., Nux m., Nux v., Phos., *Puls.*, Plb., *Sang.*, Sep., Sil., Stann., Stram., Ther.

Heat, during the stage of: Ant. c., *Ant. t.*, Ars., Bry., Cham., Cina, Cocc., *Eup. per.*, Ip., Lyc., *Nat. m.*, Stram.

following: Eup. per.

Incessant: Arg. n., Ars., Cadm., Iod., Ip., Merc. c., Nit. ac., Phos., Plb.

Menses, when the flow is on: Amm. c., Amm. m., *Apoc.*, Calc., Carb. v., Cupr., Graph., Kali c., Lach., Lyc., Phos., Puls., Sulph., Verat.

following: Bor., Canth., Gels., Kreos., Nux v., Puls.

previous to: Calc., Kreos., Nux v., Puls.

Milk: Æth., *Ant. c.*, Ars., Calc., Iod., Iris, Ph. ac., Podo., Sep., *Sil.*, Sanic Valer.

Motion: Ant. t., Ars., Bry., *Cadm.*, Colch., Cupr., Ferr., Lac. d., Lach., Lob., Nux v., Petr., *Tab.*, Verat.

Perspiration, during: *Ars.*, Eup. per.

Pregnant woman, in a: Ant. c., Apis, Ars., *Asar.*, Bry., Calc., Cadm. Canth., Caps., Carb. ac., *Chel.*, Cic., Colch., Con., Ferr., Ferr. p., Ip., Iris, *Jatr.*, Kali br., *Kreos.*, Lac. ac., Lil. t., Lyc., Mag. m., Nat. m., Nat. s., *Nux m.*, *Nux v.*, Op., Ox. ac., Petr., Phos., Ph. ac., Podo., Psor., Puls., Sep., Sil., Sulph., Sul. ac., *Tab.*, Verat., Verat. v.

VOMITING, pregnant woman in a.

Riding in a carriage, while: Ars., *Carb. ac.*, *Cocc.*, Cloch., Ferr., Hyos., *Petr.*, Sil., *Tab.*

Vertigo, during: Ars., Canth., Chel., Glon., Graph., Hell., Lach., Merc., Nat. s., Nux v., Petr., Puls., Sang., *Verat.*, Verat. v.

Violent: *Ars.*, Cic., Cina. Colch., Crot. t., Cupr., Ferr., Iod., Jatr., *Phos.*, Plb., *Tab.*, Verat., Verat. v.

TYPES:

Bilious: Acon., Ant. c., Apis, Arg. n., *Ars.*, Bell., Bism., *Bry.*, Cadm., Calc., Cham., *Chel.*, Chin., Chin. a., Chion., Cic., Coff., *Colch.*, Coloc., Crot. h., Cupr., Dig., *Eup. per.*, Ferr. p., Grat., Ign., Iod., *Ip.*, Iris, Kali ar., Kali bi., Lach., Lept., Lyc., *Merc.*, Merc. c., *Merc. cy.*, Morph., Nat. c., Nat. m., *Nat. s.*, Nux v., Op., Petr., *Phos.*, Plb., Podo., *Puls.*, **Pyrg.**, Sabin., *Sang.*, Sec., *Sep.*, Sulph., Ter., *Verat.*, **Verat. v.**

chil, before: Eup. per.

chill, during: Ant. c., **Ars.**, Cham., Cina, Dros., *Eup. per.*, Nux v., Puls.

coughing, when: *Chin.*, Puls.

fever, during the: Ars., Cham., Chin., Cina, *Eup. per.*, Nat. m., Nux v., Puls.

headache, attended with: Bry., Calc., *Chel.*, *Ip.*, *Iris*, Lob., Nat. s., Plb., Puls., *Sang.*

sweat, during: Ars., *Cham.*, Chin., Nux v.

SWEAT, during.

Bitter: Acon., Ars., *Bry.*, Carb. s., Cham., Cocc., Coloc., Crot. h., Eup. per., Grat., Kali bi., Merc., Nat. c., Nat. m., Nat. s., *Nux v.*, Petr., *Phos.*, Plb., Puls., *Sang.*, Sars., Sep., Stann., Sulph., Verat.

Black: Arg. n., *Ars.*, *Cadm.*, Calc., Chin., Chin. a., Con., Crot. h., Hyos., Ip., Lach., Lyc., Nat. s., *Nux v.*, Petr., *Phos.*, Plb., Sec., Sulph., *Verat.*

Blood: Acon., Amm. c., *Arn.*, Ars., Bry., *Cact.*, Calc., Canth., *Carb. v.*, Caust., *Chin.*, Chin. a., Cic., *Crot. h.*, Cupr., Cycl., Erig., *Ferr.*, Ferr. ar., Ferr. p., *Ham.*, Hyos., *Ip.*, Lach., Merc. c., Mill., Nat. a., Nit. ac., Nux v., Petr. *Phos.*, Phyt., Plb., Podo., Puls., *Sabin.*, Sang., Sec., Sep., Sil., Stann., Sulph., Verat., Verat. v., Zinc.

Food: Amm. c., Ant. t., Arn., *Ars.*, Bell., *Bry.*, Cact., Cadm., Calc., Carb. v., Cham., Chel., Chin., Cina, Cocc., Colch., Crot. h., Cupr., Cycl., Dros., Eup. per., *Ferr.*, *Ferr. ar.*, Ferr. p., Hydr., Graph., Hyos., *Ign.*, Ip., Iris, Kali bi., Kali c., Kali p., Kreos., Lach., Laur., *Lyc.*, Nat. m., Nux v., Op., Phos., Ph. ac., Plb., *Puls.*, *Sang.*, Sec., Sep., Sil., Stann., Sulph., *Verat.*, Verat. v

immediately after eating: Apis, Ars., Bry., Ferr., Ferr. p., Graph., Kali bi.

intervals of days after food has filled the stomach: *Bismuth.*

VOMITING, food.

indigested food two or three hours after eating: *Kreos.*

indigested: Ferr., Ip., Kali bi., *Kreos.*, Lyc., Merc. c., Nux v., Podo., Puls., *Verat.*

Glairy: Arg. n., Ars., Iris, Jatr., Kali bi., Sil., Verat. v.

Green: Acon., Æth., Arg. n., *Ars.*, Cann. s., Canth., Card. m., Cocc., Coloc., Crot. h., Dig., Dulc., Hell., Hep., Ip., Lach., Lyc., Merc., Merc. c., Nat. s., Nux v., Op., Petr., Phos., Plb., Puls., Sabin., Stram., Teucr., *Verat.*

Milk: Æth., Ant. c., Calc., Iod., Iris, Podo.

curdled: Æth., Ant. c., *Calc.*, Nat. m., *Sil.*, Sulph., *Valer.*

Milky: *Sep.*

Offensive smelling: Ant. t., *Ars.*, Bry., Canth., Cupr., Ip., *Nux v.*, Op., Phos., *Sep.*, Stann., Sulph.

Sour: Ant. t., Ars., Bell., Bor., *Calc.*, Camph., Carb. v., Card. m., *Caust.*, Cham., Chel., *Chin.*, Chin. a., Cimic., Daph., Ferr., Ferr. ar., Ferr. p., Graph., Grat., Hep., Ip., *Iris*, Kali bi., Kali c., Lac. ac., *Lyc.*, *Mag. c.*, Manc., Mez., Nat. m., Nat. p., Nat. s., *Nux v.*, Op., *Phos.*, Ph. ac., *Psor.*, Puls., Rob., Sang., *Sulph.*, Sul. ac., *Tab.*, *Verat.*

Stringy: Arg. n., Chel., *Cor. r.*, Dros., Kali bi., Kreos., Merc. c., Nat. m., Nit. ac., Sil.

Sweetish: *Kreos.*, Plb., Iris.

HICCOUGH.

REMEDIES: Agar., Alum., Amm. m., Arn., Ars., Bar. c., Bell., Bry., Calc., Cham., Chin., Chin. s., Cic., Cocc., Coff., Cycl., Dios., Dros., Euph., Gels., Hyos., Ign., Iod., Kreos., Lach., Laur., Lyc., Mag. m., Mag. p., Merc., Mosch., Nat. c., Nat. m., Nicc., Nux m., Nux v., Op., Par., Psor., Puls., Ran. b., Ruta, Sars., Sec., Sep., Spong., Stann., Stram., Sul. ac., Teucr., Verat., Verat. v., Verb.

MODALITIES:

Alchoholic drinks, after: Ran. b.

Convulsions, with: Cic., Hyos., Ran. b.

Evening: Kali i., Lob., Nicc.

Night: Hyos.

Violent: Amm. m., Cic., Cycl., Lyc., Mag. p., Merc. c., Nat. m., Nicc., Nux v., Stram.

INTESTINE.

AILMENTS, common:

Abdominal pains: Æsc., Æth., All. c., Aloe., Alum., Amm. m., Apis, *Ars.*, Asaf., Asar., Bell., Bol., Brom., Bry., Calc., Calc. p., Calc. s., *Canth.*, Caps., Carb. v., *Cham.*, Chel., Chin., Cina, Cimic., *Cocc.*, Coff., *Colch.*, *Coloc.*, Cop., *Cupr.*, Cupr. ac., Dios., *Dulc.*, Euph., Ferr., Gran., *Graph.*, Hydr., *Ip.*, Iris, *Kali ar.*, *Kali c.*, Kali n., Laur., Led., Mag. m., Meph., Merc. c., Mez., Nat. c., Nat. m., Nat. s., Nux m., Nux v., *Op.*, Ox. ac., Petr., *Phos.*, Psor., *Puls.*, Ran. b., Raph., Rheum, Rhus t., Rumex, *Sec.*, Seneg., Senn., *Sep.*, Sil., Stann., Staph., Sulph., Ter., Thuja, *Verat.*

bend double he must: Bry., Caps., Caust., Cham., *Coloc.*, Iris, *Puls.*, Rhus t.

bending double, relieves pain: Bell., Bov., Caust., Chin., *Coloc.*, Colch., Cop., Iris, *Kali c.*, Lach., Mag. p., Puls., Stann.

coming and going quickly: *Bell.*

eating, after: All. c., Alum., Ars., Carb. v., Cham., Chin., Cocc., Coc. c., Colch., Coloc., Ferr., Gran., *Graph.*, Kali c., Kali p., Lyc., Mag. c.,

AILMENTS, eating, after.

Nat. c., Nat. m., Nux m., Nux v., Phos., Ph. ac., Psor., Puls., Rhod., Rhus, Sars., Stann., *Staph.*, Stront., Sulph., Sul. ac., Thuja, *Verat.*, Zinc.

feels ameliorated after eating: Bov., Nat. c., Psor.

fruits, after taking: Calc. p., Chin., *Coloc.*, Merc. c., Puls., *Verat.*

lying, while: Bell., Phos., Puls.

lying on abdomen ameliorated: *Bell.*, Bry., Coloc., Phos., Stann.

lying on back: Ars.

lying on back ameliorated: Kalm.

menses, previous to: Alum., Amm. c., Bell., Calc. p., Caust., Cham., Cocc., Coloc., Croc., Cupr., Ign., *Kali c.*, Kali p., Lach., Lyc., Mag. c., Mag. p., Nux v., Phos., Plat., *Puls.*, Sep., Sil., Spong.

menses, when the flow is on: Amm. c., Bar. c., Bell., Bor., Brom., *Calc.*, *Calc. p.*, Caust., Cham., Chin., Cimic., Cocc., Coff., Coloc., Con., Cupr., Cycl., *Graph.*, Ign., Kali c., Kali n., Lac. c., Lach., Mag. c., Mil., Nat. m., Nat. s., Nicc., Nit. ac., Nux m., *Nux v.*,

AILMENTS, during menses.

Phos., Plat., *Puls.*, *Sabin.*,
Sars., Sec., *Sep.*, Sil.,
Stram., *Sulph.*, *Vib.*

Paroxysmal: Alum., Bell.,
Cham., Cocc., *Coloc.*, *Cupr.*,
Cupr. ac., Cycl., Dios., Ign.,
Mag. p., Nux v., Plb., Stann.

pressure aggravates her pain:
Bell., *Coff.*, Lac. c., Lach.,
Mez., Nit. ac., Nux v.,
Ran. b., Sulph., Zinc.

pressure ameliorates her pain:
Bell., *Coloc.*, Mag. p.,
Nat. s., Plb., Podo., Stan.

radiating: Ip., Mag. p., Plb.

radiating to all parts of the
body: *Plb.*

radiating across anus: Coloc.,
Crot. t., Ip., Nat. m., Nux
v., Sulph.

warm drinks ameliorate her
pain: Chel., Mag. p.,
Spong.

warmth ameliorates her pain:
Æth., *Ars.*, Bar. c., Carb.
v., Cham., Coloc., *Mag.
p.*, *Nux m.*, *Nux v.*, Podo.,
Puls., *Rhus t.*, Sabin., Sep.,
Sil.

Ascites, dropsy: Agn., *Apis*,
Apoc., Arg. n., *Ars.*, Aur.,
Aur. m., Bry., Calc., Card.
m., Chel., Chin., Chin. a.,
Colch., Dig., Dulc., Fl. ac.,
Graph., Hell., Kali c., Kali
chl., Led., *Lyc.*, Merc.,
Phos., Prun., Sulph., *Ter.*

Flatulence: Agar., *Amm. m.*,
Ant. c., Apis, *Arg. n.*, *Ars.*,
Aur., *Calc.*, Caps., Carb. ac.,
Carb. an., *Carb. v.*, Cham.,
Chel., Chin., Chin. a., Chin.
s., Coca, Cocc., *Colch.*,
Coloc., Con., Cop., Crot. h.,
Dios., Elaps, Fl. ac., Form.,

FLATULENCE.

Gels., Graph., Gua., Hydr.,
Iod., Kali c., Kali n., Lac.
ac., Lac. d., Lach., Lyc.,
Mag. c., Mag. p., Merc.,
Mur. ac., Nat. c., Nat. m.,
Nat. s., Nit. ac., *Nux m.*,
Nux v., *Olnd.*, Op., Phos.,
Ph. ac., *Pic. ac.*, *Plat.*, Podo.,
Psor., Puls., Sep., *Sil.*, *Sulph.*,
Syph., Thuja, *Verat.*, Zinc.

Intussusception: Acon., Arn.,
Ars., Bell., Bry., Coloc.,
Cupr., Lach., Lob., Lyc.,
Merc., Nux v., *Op.*, *Plb.*,
Rhus t., *Verat.*

DISTENTION: Abrot., Acon.,
Agar., All. c., Aloe., Alum.,
Anac., Ant. c., Ant. t., Apis,
Apoc., *Arg. n.*, Arn., Ars.,
Asaf., Bapt., Bar. c., Bar.
m., Berb., Bov., Brom., Bry.,
Calc., Canth., Caps., Carb.
ac., Carb. an., *Carb. v.*,
Caust., Cham., Chel., Chin.,
Chin. a., Chin. s., Cic., Cina,
Cist., *Cocc.*, Colch., Colocy.,
Con., Croc., Crot. h., Crot.
t., Cupr., Cycl., Dig., Eup.
per., Gamb., Graph., Hell.,
Hep., Hyos., Iod., Jatr., Kali
ar., Kali bi., *Kali c.*, Kali i.,
Kali n., Kali p., Kali s.,
Kreos., Lac. c., Lach., Lil.
t., Lyc., Mag. c., Mag. m.,
Meny., Merc., Merc. c.,
Mez., Mur. ac., Murex, Nat.
c., Nat. m., Nat. p., Nat.
s., Nit. ac., Nux v., Op.,
Petr., *Phos.*, *Ph. ac.*, Plat.,
Psor., Puls., Raph., Rhod.,
Rhus t., Sec., Sep., Sil.,
Stann., Staph., Stront., *Sulph.*,
Ter., Thuja, Til., Valer.,
Verat., Zinc.

Menses, previous: Lyc., Puls.,
Zinc.

FLATULENCE.

Menses, when the flow is on:
Chin., *Cocc.*, Graph., Kali c.,
Nat. c., Nicc., Sulph.

Milk, after: Con.

Tympanitic: Ant. t., Arg. n.,
Arn., *Ars.*, Brom., Bry.,
Calc., Canth., *Carb. v.*,
Cham., *Chin.*, Chin. a.,
Cocc., *Colch.*, Coloc., Cupr.,
Eup. per., Graph., *Hyos.*,
Kali bi., Kali p., Kreos.,
Lach., *Lyc.*, Merc., Morph.,
Mur. ac., Op., *Phos.*, Ph.
ac., Podo., Sec., Stram.,
Samb., *Ter.*, Thuja.

GURGLING: Agar., *Aloe.*, Ars.,
Crot. t., Lyc., Nat. m., Nux
v., *Olnd.*, Phos., Ph. ac.,
Podo., Psor., *Puls.*, Sil.,
Sulph.

Stool, before: *Aloe.*, *Olnd.*,
Podo.

RETRACTION: Alum., Ars.,
Bar. c., Carb. ac., Cocc.,
Cupr., Dros., Hydr., Iod.,
Nat. m., *Plb.*, Tab., Verat.,
Zinc.

Umbilicus: Alum., Chel., *Plb.*

RUMBLING: Acon., *Agar.*, Ail.,
Aloe., Alum., *Anac.*, Ant. t.,
Arg. m., Arg. n., Arn., Ars.,
Bell., Bism., Bry., Calc.,
Canth., Carb. ac., Carb. an.,
Carb. v., Cast. v., *Caust.*,
Cham., Chel., *Chin.*, Chin. a.,

RUMBLIING.

Cic., Cocc., Colch., Coloc.,
Crot. t., Cycl., Dios., Dulc.,
Gamb., Gels., Glon., Graph.,
Hell., *Hep.*, *Hydr.*, Ign.,
Jatr., Kali bi., *Lyc.*, Mag. c.,
Mag. m., Manc., Merc.,
Mez., Olnd., Op., Petr.,
Phos., Nat. m., Nat. p., Nat.
s., Nit. ac., Nux m., *Nux v.*,
Ph. ac., Phyt., Plb., Psor.,
Puls., Ran. s., Rumex,
Sabad., Sars., Sep., *Sil.*,
Spig., Squil., Staph., *Sulph.*,
Thuja, Verat., Zinc.

Flatus, passing of ameliorates:
Carb. v., Lyc., Nat. s.

Menses, previous to: Zinc.

Stool, during: Iris.

following: Crot. t., *Jatr.*, Lyc.

previous to: Asc. t., Jatr.,
Mag. c., Mur. ac., Nat.
m., Phos.

SENSATION:

Alive, sensation of something:
Croc., Cycl., *Thuja.*

Weakness: Aloe., Calc. p., *Ign.*,
Nat. m., Petr., *Phos.*, Podo.,
Psor., Sep., Staph., *Sul. ac.*,
Verat.

SENSITIVE TO CLOTHING:
Apis, *Arg. n.*, Bov., *Calc.*,
Carb. v., Caust., Crot., h.,
Lyc., Nat. s., *Nux v.*, Sars.,
Sep., Spong., Stann.

RECTUM AND ANUS.

AILMENTS, Common:

Abscess: Calc., Calc. s., Hep., Merc., Sil.

Aphthous condition of anus: Bapt., Bor., Kali chl., Merc., Merc. c., Mur. ac., Nit. ac., Sulph., *Sul. ac.*

Cholera: Ars., *Camph.*, Carb. v., *Cupr.*, Grat., Laur., Podo., Sec., Tab., *Verat.*

Condylomata: Arg. n., Aur. n., Caust., *Cinnab.*, Euphr., Lyc., Nat. s., Nit. ac., Staph., Thuja.

Constipation: *Aesc.*, Aeth., Agar., Arn., Aloe., *Alum.*, *Alumn.*, Ambr., Amm. c., Amm. m., Anac., Anag., *Apis*, Arg. m., Arg. n., Ars., Ars. i., Aur., Bar. c., Bar. m., Berb., *Bry.*, Cact., Caust., Chel., Chin., Chim., *Clem.*, Coca, *Cocc.*, *Coff.*, *Coll.*, Con., Cop., Crot. h., Daph., Dig., Dios., Dulc., Elaps, Ferr., Ferr. ar., Ferr. i., Fl. ac., Form., Gamb., Graph., Hydr., Hydr. ac., Ign., Iod., Iris, Jab., Kali ar., Kali bi., Kali c., Kali chl., Kali. i., Kali s., Kreos., *Lach.*, *Lac. d.*, Laur., Lept., Lil. t., Lyc., Mag. c., *Mag. m.*, Manc., Meny., Merc., Merc. i., Mez., Mosch., Mur. ac., Nat. a., Nat. c., Nat. m., *Nit. ac.*, *Nux v.*, Nux m., Op., Ox. ac., *Phos.*, Phyt., Plb., Plat., Podo.,

CONSTIPATION.

Psor., Ptel., Puls., Seneg., Sep., Pyrog., Raph., Sabad., Sanic., Sars., Sec., Sel., *Sil.*, Spong., Stann. Staph., Stram., *Sulph.*, *Sul. ac.*, Tab., Tarent., Ther., *Thuja*, Tub., Verb., Verat., Vib., Zinc.

difficult stool: Lac. d., Mag. m., Mur. ac., Nat. m., Op., Sanic., *Sil.*, Thuja.

can pass stool while urinating, only: Aloe., Alum.

drugs, after abuse of: Bry., *Coloc.*, Hydr., *Nux v.*, Op.

dryness of rectum, due to: Alum.

incomplete, insufficient stool, (unsatisfactory): Aloe, Alum., Alumn., Anac., Arn., Bar. c., Benz. ac., Bry., *Card. m.*, Cham., Gamb., Ign., Iod., *Kali c.*, Kali s., Lyc., Mag. m., *Nat. c.*, *Nat. m.*, *Nit. ac.*, Nux m., *Nux v.*, *Op.*, Plb., Pyrog., Sars., Sep., Sil., Staph., Sulph., Thuja, Zinc.

leans far back to pass a stool: Med.

old people, of: Ant. c., Bar. c., Bry., Calc. p., Con., Lach., Op., Phos., Phyt.

pregnant women, of: Agar., Alum. Ant. t., Apis, Bry., Con., Dol., Hydr., Lyc.,

CONSTIPATION, pregnant women, of.

Nat. s., Nux v., Op., Plb., Plat., Podo., Sep., Sulph.

sedentary habits, from: Bry., Lyc., Nux v., Op., Plat., Podo., Sulph.

standing in the easiest posture to pass a stool: Caust.

stool remains long in the rectum to produce awful anxiety: Tarent.

straining without any effect: Æsc., All. c., Ambr., Arn., Anac., Ars., Bar. c., Bell., Bry., Calc., Calc. s., Cann. s., Caps., Carb. an., Carb. v., Caust., Chim., Cocc., Coloc., Con., Ferr., Graph., Ign., Iod., Kali bi., Kali c., Kali s., Kalm., Lach., Lil. t., Lyc., Mag. c., Merc., Nat. c., Nat. m., Nat. p., Nit. ac., Nux v., Op., Phos., Plat., Puls., Rat., Ruta., Sanic., Selen., Sep., Sil., Stann., Sulph., Thuja, Verat., Zinc.

while travelling: Nux v., Plat.

will not pass stool before other, unable to pass stool before other: Ambr.

DIARRHŒA:
Acet. ac., Acon., Æsc., Agar., Aloe., Alum., Ant. c., Ant. t., Apis, Aran., Arg. n,, Arn., Ars., Asar., Bapt., Bar. c., Bell., Benz. ac., Bor., Bov., Brom., Bry., Calc., Calc. ar., Calc. p., Canth., Caps., Carb. s., Carb. v., Casc., Caust., Cham., Chin., Cina, Cist., Coff., Colch., Coloc., Con., Crot. h.,

DIARRHŒA.

Crot. t., Cupr., Dig., Dulc., Echin., Ferr., Ferr. i., Ferr. ar., Ferr. p., Ferr. s., Fl. ac., Gamb., Graph., Grat., Hell., Hep., Hydr., Ign., Iod., Ip., Iris, Jatr., Kali ar., Kali bi., Kali c., Kali s., Lach. Lac. c., Lac. d., Lept., Lil. t., Lyc., Mag. c., Mag. m., Merc., Merc. c., Nat. a., Nat. c., Nat. m., Nat. p., Nat. s., Nit. ac., Nuph., Nux m., Nux v., Olnd., Petr., Phos., Ph. ac., Podo., Psor., Puls., Rheum. Sang., Sanic., Sec., Sep., Sil., Stann., Sulph., Sul. ac., Thuja, Verat., Zinc., Zing.

acids, after: Aloe., Ant. c., Brom., Ph. ac., Sulph.

alcoholic liquors: Nux v.

anger, following: Aloe., Calc. p., Cham., Coloc., Nux v., Staph.

anticipation, on account of: Arg. n., Gels.

bad news, from: Gels.

bath, following a: Podo.

beer, after he drank: Aloe, Chin., Gamb., Kali bi., Lyc., Mur. ac., Sulph.

breakfast, after: Arg. n., Nat. s., Rhod., Thuja.

chargrin, after: Staph.

children, in: Acon., Æth., Agar., Arg. n., Ars., Benz. ac., Bov., Calc., Calc. p., Calc. s., Cham., Cina, Crot. t., Dulc., Ip., Iris, Merc., Mez., Phos., Podo., Psor., Puls., Rheum, Sil., Staph., Stram., Sulph., Valer.

damp grounds, standing on: Dulc., Rhus t,

DIARRHŒA.

debauch, after a: *Nux v.*

dentition period: Acon., Æth., Apis, Arg. n., *Ars.*, Bell., Bor., Calc., Calc. p., Cham., Cina, Coff., Coloc., *Dulc.*, *Ferr.*, Gels., Hep., Ip., Kreos., Mag. c., Merc., Podo., Psor., *Rheum*, Sep., *Sil.*, Sulph.

drinks, after: *Ars.*, Caps., Carb. v., Dulc., Ferr., Hep., Lyc., Nat. s., Nux m., Ph. ac., Puls., Rhus t., Sil., Staph., Sul. ac.

drinking water: Aloe, Apis, Arg. n., *Ars.*, Asaf., Cina, Crot. t., Elap., *Ferr.*, *Ferr. ar.*, Grat., *Nux v.*, Podo., Trom.

drinking water, just after: Arg. n., Crot. t., Podo.,

drunkards (old), in: Apis, Ars., *Lach.*, Phos.

emaciated people, in: Calc., Calc. p., *Sil.*, Sul. ac.

suppression of eruptions: Hep., Lyc., Psor., *Sulph.*, Urt. u.

typhoid: Agar., Apis, Ars., Bapt., Bry., Calc., *Hyos.*, Lach., Mur. ac., Nit. ac., Op., *Phos.*, Ph. ac., Rhus t., Stram., Sul. ac.

Food:

milk, after taking: Calc., Kali ar., Kali c., Lyc., Nat. a., *Nat. c.*, Nicc., Nux m., Sep., Sil., Sulph.

oyster, after taking: All. c., Brom., Lyc., Podo., Sul. ac.

pastry, after taking: Ip., Kali ch., Lyc., Nat. s., Ph. ac., *Puls.*

pears, after taking: Verat.

DIARRHŒA, after taking pears.

pork, after taking: Puls.

Potato, after taking: Alum.

sweet, after taking: Calc. ar.

sugar, after taking: Arg n., Merc., Sulph.

vear, after taking: Kali n.

vegetables, after taking: Lyc., Nat. m., Nat. s.

cabbage, after taking: Bry., Petr., Podo.

cider, after taking: Ant. c., Calc. p., Podo.

coffee, after taking: Cist., Cycl., Thuja.

ice-cream, after taking: *Ars.*, Carb. v., Puls.

fright, after: Arg. n. *Gels.*, Kali p., Op.

fruits, after taking: Aloe, *Ars.*, Bor., *Bry.*, Calc. p., Carb. v., *Chin.*, Chin. a., Cist., *Coloc.*, Crot. t., Ferr., Ip., Iris, Lyc., Mur. ac., *Nat. s.*, Olnd., Ph. ac., Podo., *Puls.*, Rhod., *Verat.*

fruit, unripe: Ip., Sul. ac.

melon, after taking: Zing.

grief, from: Coloc., Gels., Ign., Ph. ac.

hydrocephalus, during: Apis, Calc., Hell., Zinc.

indignation, from: Coloc., Ip., Staph.

jaundice, while suffering from: Chion., Dig., Merc., Nat. s., Nux v., Sulph.

joy, from sudden: Coff., Op.

measles, after: Car. v., Puls..

menses, following: Lach.

menses, when the flow is on: Amm. m., Bov., Caust.,

DIARRHŒA, during menses.

Kreos., Nat. p., Phos., Sars., Tab., Verat., Vib.

menses, previous: Amm. c., Bov., Cinnab., Lach., Sil., Verat.

motion aggravates her diarrhœa: Bell., Bry., Colch., Crot. t., Ferr., Ferr. ar., Nat. m., Nux v., Podo., Verat.

noise, from: Nit. ac., Nux v.

nursing, after: Crot. t., Nux v.

nursing women, in: Chin.

over-heated, after being: Ant. c., Puls.

painless: Aloe., Apis, Ars., Bapt., Bism., Bor., Calc., Camph., Cham., Chel., Chin., Cocc., Coff., Crot. t., Dul., Ferr., Ferr. ar., Ferr. p., Gels., Grat., Hep., Hyos., Kali ar., Kali c., Lyc., Nat. m., Nat. p., Nat. s., Nuph., Olnd., Phos., Ph. ac., Podo., Psor., Pyrog., Rhus t., Sil., Squil., Sulph., Verat.

periodical, on alternate days., Alum., Chin.

periodical, at the same hour: Apis, Sabad., Sel., Thuja.

pregnant women, in: Ant. c., Chel., Chin., Lyc., Nux m., Phos., Puls., Sep., Sulph.

septic condition, with: Ars., Carb. v., Crot. h., Lach., Pyrog., Sulph.

small-pox during: Ars., Chin.

standing aggravates her diarrhœa: Aloe., Cocc., Sulph.

urinating aggravates Aloe., Alum.

DIARRHŒA.

vaccination: Thuja.

vexation, from: Calc. p., Coloc., Petr., Staph.

weakness, without: Ph. ac.

weaning, after: Chin.

wet, after getting: Acon., Calc., Rhus t.

Dysentery: Acon., Æth., Aloe, Apis, Arg. n., Arn., Ars., Bapt., Bell., Bry., Canth., Caps., Carb. s., Carb. v., Cham., Chin., Cinnab., Colch., Coloc., Dirc., Dulc., Hep., Ign., Iod., Ip., Iris, Kali bi., Kali chl., Lach., Lil. t., Mag. c., Merc., Merc. c., Nit. ac., Nux m., Nux v., Op., Ox. ac., Petr., Phos., Phyt., Psor., Puls., Rhus t., Sulph., Sul. ac., Ter., Trom., Zing.

Eruption about anus: Agar., Calc., Caust., Graph., Hep., Nat. m., Nat. s., Nit. ac., Petr., Staph., Sulph.

Fissure: Agn., All. c., Carb. v., Caust., Cham., Cund., Fl. ac., Graph., Hydr., Ign., Lach., Merc., Nat. m., Nit. ac., Nux v., Pœon., Petr., Phos., Phyt., Plb., Rat., Sep., Sil., Sulph., Thuja.

Fistula: Aloe., Alum., Aur. m., Berb., Calc., Calc. p., Carb. v., Caust., Fl. ac., Graph., Hep., Hydr., Kali c., Kreos., Lach., Lyc., Merc., Nit. ac., Petr., Phos., Sep., Sil., Staph., Sulph., Syph., Thuja.

Hæmorrhoids: Æsc., Agar., Aloe., Amm. c., Ant. c., Apis, Ars., Ars. i., Bar. c., Bell., Brom., Cact., Calc., Calc. p., Calc. s., Caps., Carb. an., Carb. v., Card. m.,

HÆMORRHOIDS.

Caust., Chel., Cimex,
Coca, Coff., Dios., Ferr.,
Ferr. ar., Fl. ac., Graph.,
Hep., Ign., Iod., Kali ar.,
Kali bi., Kali c., Lyc., Merc.,
Merc. i. r., Mur. ac., Nat.
m., Nat. s., Nit. ac., Nux v.,
Petr., Phos., Phyt., Podo.,
Psor., Puls., Rat., Rhus t.,
Ruta, Sep., Sil., Staph.,
Sulph., Sul. ac., Thuja, Zing.

alternates with palpitation:
Coll.

blind: Æsc., Calc. p., Nux
v., Puls., Rhus t., Sulph.

bluish in color: Æsc., Carb.
v., Lach., Mur. ac., Sulph.

chronic: Æsc., Aloe., Carb.
s., Lyc., Merc. i. r., Nit.
ac., Nux v., Phos., Podo.,
Sulph.

congested: Acon., Aloe., Bell.,
Caust., Cham., Hep., Kali
c., Merc., Mur. ac., Nux
v., Paeon., Puls., Rhus t.,
Sulph.

menses, during: Aloe,
Carb. s., Carb. v., Coll.,
Graph., Ign., Lach., Puls.,
Sulph.

milk aggravates her hæmorrhoidal troubles: Sep.

parturition aggravates the same:
Ign., Kali c., Mur. ac.,
Podo., Puls.

pregnant women, in: Æsc.,
Amm. m., Caps., Coll.,
Lyc., Nat. m., Nux v.

riding ameliorates her piles:
Kali c.

standing aggravates her
hæmorrhoidal troubles:
Æsc., Amm. c., Caust.,
Sulph.

HÆMORRHOIDS.

stool, prevented by: Æsc.,
Caust., Pæon., Thuja.

stool protrude during: Amm.
c., Calc., Calc. p., Kali
bi., Nit. ac., Sil.

strangulates: Æsc., Aloe,
Bell., Ign., Lach., Nux v.,
Pæon., Sil., Sulph.

suppurating: Carb. v., Hep.,
Ign., Merc., Sil.

touch aggravates her hæmor-
rhoidal troubles: Bell.,
Carb. s., Caust., Hep.,
Mur. ac., Sulph., Thuja.

urination, protrude during an
act of: Bar. c., Bar. m.,
Mur. ac.

walking aggravates her hæmor-
rhoidal troubles: Æsc.,
Brom., Carb. an., Caust.,
Mur. ac., Sulph.

walking, better by: Ign.

Paralysis: Alum., Bar. m., Bell.,
Calc., Gels., Graph., Hyos.,
Laur., Mur. ac., Phos., Sec.,
Tab.

Polypi: Calc. p., Nit. ac.,
Phos.

Prolapsus: Æsc., Apis, Ars.,
Asar., Bell., Calc., Calc. s.,
Carb. s., Colch., Coll., Dig.,
Dulc., Ferr., Gamb., Gels.,
Graph., Hep., Ign., Iris, Kali
bi., Lach., Lyc., Mag. m.,
Mang., Merc., Merc. c.,
Mur. ac., Nat. m., Nat. s.,
Nit. ac., Nux v., Phos.,
Podo., Ruta, Sep., Sil..

diarrhœa, during an attack
of: Calc., Dulc., Merc.,
Podo.

parturition, after: Podo.,
Ruta.

urinating, while: Mur. ac.,
Valer.

HÆMORRHOIDS

Worms:

ascarides: *Bar. c.*, Calc., Ferr., Ign., Mag. s., *Nat. m.*, Nat. p., Rat., *Sabad.*, Sep., Sin. n., Spig., Spong., Sulph., Teucr., Valer.

lumbricoides: Chel., *Cina*, Ferr. s., Sabad., Sil., *Spig.*, *Sulph.*

CONTRACTION, CLOSURE, CONSTRICTION ETC:

Æsc., Bell., Cact., Camph., Cann. s., *Caust.*, Chel., Cocc., Colch., Fl. ac., Form., Hyos., *Ign.*, Kali bi., *Lach.*, *Lyc.*, Nat. m., *Nit. ac.*, *Nux v.*, Op., Phos., *Plb.*, Sep., Tab.

Painful: Caust., Cocc., *Lach.*, Lyc., Mang., Mez., *Nux v.*, *Plb.*, Sil.

Spasmodic: Hipp., Lach., Lyc., *Nit. ac.*, *Nux v.*, *Op.*, *Plb.*

stool, following: *Ign.*, *Lach.*, Mez., *Nit. ac.*, Phos., Sep., Sulph.

stool, during: Alum., Ars., Chel., Kreos., *Nat. m.*, Nux v., *Plb.*, *Sil.*, Thuja.

stool, previous to: Nat. m., Nux v.

stool, preventing: Berb., Chel., Lach., *Lyc.*, Nat. m., Nit. ac., Nux v.

EXCORIATION FROM THE STOOL: *Aloe.*, *Apis*, Ars., Bapt., Kreos., Merc., *Nit. ac,*. Nux v., Sulph.

FULNESS: Æsc., Aloe, *Ham.*, Lach., *Nit. ac.*, *Sulph.*

HÆMORRHAGE FROM

Anus: *Acon.*, *Æsc.*, *Aloe.*, Alumn., Amm. c., Ant. c., Apis, *Ars.*, *Bar. c.*, Bell., Bism., Bor., *Cact.*, Calc. c., Calc. p., Canth., Caps., Carb. s., Carb.v., Casc., Cham., Chin., Cocc., *Coll.*, Ferr., Graph., *Ham.*, Hep., Ip., Kali ar., Kali bi., Kali c., Kali chl., *Lach.*, *Lyc.*, Merc., Merc. c., Mill., Mur. ac., *Nat. m.*, Nat.s., *Nit. ac.*, Nux m., *Nux v.*, *Phos.*, Phyt., Podo., Puls., Sep., *Sulph.*

PULSATION: Ham., *Lach.*, Nat. m., Sulph.

REDNESS OF ANUS: Petr., *Sulph.*, Zing.

RETRACTED: Bapt., Bry., Kali bi., Plb., Tell.

SENSITIVE: Aloe., Bell., Caust., Graph., Hep., Lach., Lyc., *Mag. m.*, *Mur. ac.*, *Nit. ac.*, Podo., Sep.

SPASMS: Caust., Colch., Tab.

STRICTURE: Aloe., Bor., **Calc. s.**, Camph., Lach., Lyc., **Nat. m.**

SWEAT, perspiration about anus and perinæum: Alum., **Hep.**

STOOL.

BALL-LIKE: *Alum.*, *Mag.m.*, Med., *Merc.*, Mez., *Nat. m.*, *Nit. ac.*, Nux v., *Op.*, *Plb.*, Sulph.

BLACK: Alum., Arg. n., *Ars.*, Berb., Brom., Bry., Calc., Caps., Card.m., Chin. a., Chion., Cina, Crot. h., Hep., Kali s., Lach., *Lept.*, *Merc.*, Merc. c., Nat. m., Nit. ac., Nux v., Op., Phos., Plat., *Plb.*, Podo., Pyrog., Rumex, Stram., *Verat.*

BLOODY: Acon., Aloe., *Alum.*, Alumn., Amm. m., Apis, Arg. n., Arn, *Ars.*, Bapt., Bar. m., Bell., Bry., Calc., *Canth.*, *Caps*, Carb. ac., Caust., Cham., Chin., *Colch.*, Coll., Coloc., Con., Crot. h., Graph., Hydr., Ip., Kali ar., Kali bi., Kali c., Kali chl., Kali p., Kreos., Lac. d., Lach., Lyc., Mag. m., *Merc.*, Mur. ac., Nat. a., Nat. c., Nit. ac., Nux m., *Nux v.*, *Phos.*, Phyt., Plb., Podo., Puls., Rhus t., Sars., Sep., Sel., Sulph., Sul. ac., Thuja, Verat.

BLUISH: Bapt., Colch., Phos.

CEASELESS DISCHARGE: Apis, Phos., Trom.

CHANGEABILITY: Dulc., Podo., *Puls.*, Sulph.

CHOPPED: Acon., Cham.

CLAY-COLORED: Berb., Card. m., Chel., Gels., Hep., Iod., Kali b., Merc., Nat. s., Nit. ac., Ph. ac., Podo.

CLAYEY: *Calc.*, Podo., Sil.

COFFEE-GROUND: Crot. **h.**, Dig.

COLD: Lyc.

COPIOUS: Aloe., Ant. t., Apis, Apoc., *Ars.*, Asaf., *Bapt.*, Benz. ac., Calc., *Camph.*, *Carb. v.*, *Chin.*, *Coff.*, *Crot. t.*, Dulc., Elat., Ferr. **ar.**, Grat., Iod., Ip., Jatr., **Kali** chl., Kali p., Kreos., Lach., Lept., Lyc., Merc., **Mez.**, *Nat. s.*, Nux m., Olnd., **Ox.** ac., Phos., *Ph. ac.*, *Podo.*, Psor., Ran. b., Rumex, *Sec.*, Sep., Sil., Sul. ac., Thuja, *Verat.*, Verat. v., Vib.

CRUMBLING: Amm. m., **Mag.** c., *Mag. m.*, Merc., *Nat. m.*, Op., Plat., Podo., Sulph., Tel., Zinc.

CURDLED: Calc., Nit. ac., Rheum., Stann., *Valer.*

DARK: Æsc., *Alum.*, Arn., **Ars.**, Bapt., Berb., Bry., **Chion.** Graph., Nat. a., Nat. s., **Nux** v., Plb., Rhus t., Sec.,

DOG, like that of a: Cimex, *Phos.*

DRY: Amm. c., Ant. c., Arg. m., Arg. n., *Bry.*, Calc., Cimex, Con., Cupr., Ham., Hep., Kali bi., Kali s., Lac. d., *Lyc.*, *Nat. m.*, Nit. ac., *Nux v.*, *Op.*, *Phos.*, Plat., *Plb.*, Podo., Prun., Sanic., *Sil.*, Stann., Sulph., *Zinc.*

FATTY, greasy: Caust., Iod., Phos.

FLAKY: Arg. n., Chel., Dulc., Ip., Nit. ac., Phos., *Verat.*

FLAT: Merc., Puls.

FORCIBLE: Apis, Apoc., Arg. n., *Crot. t.,* Cupr., Dulc., Ferr., Gamb., Grat., Jatr., Kali bi., Mag. m., *Nat. c., Nat. m.,* Nat. s., Ox. ac., Phos., *Podo.,* Ran. b., Raph., *Sec.* Sep., Sulph., Thuja, Verat.

FROTHY: Arn., Benz. ac., Bor., Calc., Caps., Coloc., Graph., Grat., Iod., Kali ar., *Kali bi.,* Lach., *Mag. c.,* Merc., Nat. m., Op., Plan., *Podo.,* Raph., Rheum, Rhus t., Sil., Squil., *Sulph.*

GRAY: Ars., Aur., Calc., Carb. v., Chel., Dig., Hydr., Kali c., Lach., *Merc.,* Nat. m., Op., *Phos., Ph. ac.,*

GREEN: Acon., Æth., Agar., Amm. m., Apis, *Arg. n.,* Asaf., Bell., Bor., Calc., Calc. p., Canth., Caps., Cham., **Chin.,** Chion., *Coloc.,* Con., *Crot. t.,* Cupr., Dulc., Elat., *Gamb.,* Grat., Hep., Hydr., *Ip.,* Iris, Kali br., Laur., Lept., Lyc., *Mag. c.,* Mag. m., *Merc., Merc. c.,* Mur. ac., *Nat. m.,* Nat. p., *Nat. s.,* Nit. ac., Nux v., Phos., Ph. ac., *Plb., Podo.,* Psor., *Puls.,* Rhus t., Sanic., *Sec.,* Sep., Stann., *Sulph.,* Sul. ac., Ter., *Verat.*

Like olives: Apis, Sec.

HARD: Agar., Agn., *Alum., Alumn., Amm. c., Amm. m., Ant. t.,* Apis, Arg. n., Ars., Aur., Bar. c., Bar. m., Bell.,

HARD.

Bov., Bry., Calc., Calc. p., Carb. v., Card. m., Caust., Carb. v., Carb. m., Caust., Chel., Cimex, Cina, Cocc., Con., Coloc., Con., Ferr., Ferr. i., Gamb., *Graph.,* Grat., Gua., Ham., Hep., Ign., *Lac. d., Lach.,* Kali c., Kali n., Kali s., Kalm., Laur., Lyc., Mag. c., *Mag. m.,* Merc., Mez., *Nat. m.,* Nat. s., *Nit. ac., Nux v.,* Op., Petr., *Phos.,* Ph. ac., Plat., Sanic., *Sel.,* Seneg., Sep., *Sil.,* Stann., Stront., Sulph., Tarent., *Verat., Verb., Zinc.*

Burnt, as if: *Bry.,* Plat., *Sulph.*

First portion, then fluid: *Bov., Calc., Lyc.,* Sul. ac.

Menses, during: Amm. c., Apis, Nat. m.

Tough and greasy: Caust.

HOT: *Cham.,* Aloe., Calc. p., Merc., *Merc. c.,* Staph., Sulph.

KNOTTY, in nodules, lumps: Æsc., *Alum.,* Alumn., Ant. c., Aur., Bar. c., Calc., Calc. s., *Carb. s.,* Caust., *Chel.,* Coll., Con., Cycl., Glon., *Graph.,* Hydr., Iod., Kali bi., Kali c., Kali s., Lach., Lept., Lil. t., *Lyc., Mag. m.,* Merc., Nat. s., Nux v., Ph. ac., Plat., *Plb.,* Sil., Stann., *Sulph.,* Thuja.

Green: Chin., Stann.

Mucus, covered with: Alum., Graph., Mag. m., Plb., Spig.

LARGE: Æsc., Alum., Alumn., Agn., Ant. c., Apis, Arg. n., Asaf., Aur., *Bry.,* Calc., Cob., Coloc., Dulc., *Elat.,* Graph., Ign., Kali bi., *Kali c.,*

LARGE.

Kali s., Kalm., Lac. d., Lept., Mag. m., Mez., Nat. m., Nux m.. Petr., Phos., Podo.. Raph., Rhus t., Rhus v., Sel., Sep., Sil., Sulph., Thuja, Verat., Vib., Zinc.

LIENTERIA: Æth., Ant. c.. Apoc., Arg. n., Arn., Ars., Bry., Calc., Calc. p., Carb. s., Chin., Chin. a., Cina, Coloc., Con., Elaps, Ferr., Ferr. ar., Ferr. p. Gamb., Graph., Hep., Iris, Lept., Lyc., Mag. c., Mag. m., Merc., Nit. a., Nux m., Olnd., Petr., Phos., Ph. ac., Plat., Podo., Raph., Rhod., Rhus t., Sang., Sec., Sil., Sulph.

LONG, narrow: Alum., Bor., Caust., Graph.. Mur. ac., Phos.

LUMPS (chalky): Calc., Podo.

MEMBRANEOUS: Arg. n., Brom., Canth., Carb. ac., Colch., Coloc., Ferr., Nit. ac.,

MUCUS, slimy: Æth., Amm. m., Apis, Arg. n., Arn., Ars., Asar., Bapt., Bell., Berb., Bor., Brom., Bry., Calc. p., Canth., Caps., Carb. ac., Caust., Cham., Chel., Colch., Coloc., Corn., Crot. t., Dulc., Gamb., Graph., Hell., Hep., Hyos., Iod., Ip., Kali bi., Kali c., Kali chl., Kali s., Merc., Merc. c., Mur a., Nat. s., Nit. ac., Nux v., Phos., Ph. ac., Phyt., Plb., Podo., Psor., Puls., Rhus t., Sec., Sil., Squil., Stann., Sulph., Sul. ac., Verat.

Bloody Acon., Æth., Aloe., Ars., Bar. m., Bry., Canth., Caps., Carb. ac., Cinnb., Coloc., Dulc., Iod., Kali chl.,

MUCUS, bloody.

Lach., Mag. m.. Merc., Merc. c., Nat. c., Nux v., Podo., Psor., Puls., Sulph.

Chopped eggs and spinach: Cham.

Colorless: Hell.

Covered with mucus: Alum., Mag. m., Plb., Spig.

Green: Acon., Æth., Ant. t., Apis, Arg. n., Ars., Bell., Bor., Bry., Calc. p., Canth., Cast., Cham., Cinnb.

Jelly-like: Aloe., Apis, Asar., Bar. m., Cadm., Chel., Colch., Coloc., Hell., Jatr., Kali bi., Plat., Rhus t.

Tenacious: Asar., Canth., Caps., Crot. t., Hell., Kali bi.

Transparent: Bor., Colch., Hell., Nat. m., Rhus t.

White: Ars., Bor., Cham., Dulc., Graph., Hell Iod., Kali chl., Nat. m., Sulph.

resemble little pieces of popped corn: Cina.

Yellow: Apis, Asar., Bor., Cham., Colch., Cub., Dulc., Kali s., Rhus t., Sul. ac.

ODOR:

Cadaveric: Ars., Bism., Carb. v., Chin., Kali p., Lach., Ptel., Rhus t., Sil.

Eggs, like that of rotten: Ars., Calc., Carb. ac., Cham., Psor., Staph.

Putrid: Apis, Ars., Asaf., Bapt., Benz. ac., Bor., Bry., Carb. v., Chin., Coloc., Kali p., Lach., Mag. c., Merc. c., Nat. s., Olnd., Podo., Pyrog., Sil., Posr., Stram.

ODOR.

Sour: Arn., *Calc.*, Camph., Coloc., Colost., Dulc., *Hep.*, Jalap., Mag. c., *Merc.*, Nat. c., Nat. p., Nit.ac., Phos., *Rheum*, Sulph.

SCRAPINGS OF INTES-TINES, resembles: Bry., *Canth.*, Carb. ac., Colch., Coloc., Ferr., Merc.

SHEEPDUNG, like: *Alum.*, *Alumn.*, Bar. c., Berb., Carb. an., Caust., *Chel.*, Coll., Graph., Kali c., Kali s., Lach., *Mag. m.*, *Merc.*, *Nat. m.*, Nat. s., *Nit. ac.*, Nux v., Op., *Plb.*, Sep., Spig., *Sulph.*, Sul. ac., Verat., Verb.

SPLUTTERING: *Aloe.*, *Nat. s.*

STRINGY: Asar., Carb. v., *Grat.*, *Sul. ac.*

TARRY: Chion., Lept.

WHITE: Ant. c., Apis, Ars. i., Aur. m. n., Bell., *Benz. ac.*, Bor., Calc., *Canth.*, Cast., Caust., Cham., Chel., Cina, Colc., Cop., Crot. h., Dig., Dulc., Form., Graph., **Hep.**, Hell., Iod., Kali chl., *Nux m.*, Nnx v., Phos., *Ph. ac.*, *Puls.*, Rheum, Rhus t., Sanic., Sep., Spong.

Chalk, like: *Calc.*, Chel., **Dig.**, *Podo.*, Sanic., Sil.

Milk, white like: Æsc., **Calc.**, Card. m., *Chel.*, Chin., *Dig.*, Hep., Kali bi., **Mag. c.**, *Merc.*, *Podo.*, Sanic.

LARYNX AND TRACHEA.

AILMENTS, common:

Catarrh: **All.** s., **Amm.** c., **Amm. m.,** *Ant. t.,* **Ars.,** Bad., Bar. c. Brom., Calc., Calc. p., *Carb. s., Carb. v.,* Cham., Chin., Coc. c., Coff., Colch., Dulc., Ferr. p., Hep., Hippoz., Kali ar., Kali bi., *Kali* c., Kali s., Lyc., *Mang.,* *Merc., Nat. m., Nux v.,* Phos., Ph. ac., Rhod., Rumex, *Sang.,* Sil., *Stann.,* *Sulph.*

Condylomata: Arg. n., Merc. c., Nit. ac.

Croup: *Acon.,* Ant.t., Ars., Ars. i., Bell., *Brom.,* Calc., Calc. s., Canth., Carb. ac., Carb. v., Cham., Chlor., Hep., Iod., Kali bi., Kali chl., Lach., Lob., Nat. m., Phos., Samb., Sang., *Spong.,* Stil.

exposure to dry cold air, following: *Acon., Hep.*

CROUP.

membraneous: Apis, Arum. t., *Brom.,* Carb. ac., Hep., Iod., *Kali bi.,* Kali chl., Lac. c., Lach., Merc. cy., Merc. i. f., Nit. ac., *Phos.,* Sang.

Paralysis: **Alum.,** *Caust.,* Cina, **Gels.,** *Lach.,* Plb., Stram.

Phthisis (laryngeal): Agar., Arg. m., Calc., Carb. an., Carb. s., Carb v., Caust., Dros., Hep., Iod., Kali bi., Kali i., Lach., *Mang.,* Merc. i. r., Nit. ac., Phos., Sel., Seneg., Sil., *Spong., Stann.*

trachea: Ars., Calc., Carb. an., Carb. v., Dros., Stan.

SENSATION:

Of some foreign substance in larynx: Arg. n., *Bell.,* Calc. f., Dros., Hep., Lach., Phos., Sang., Sil., Thuja.

VOICE.

APHONIA: Acon., Alum., Alumn., *Amm. caust.*, Ant. c., Ant. t., *Arg. m.*, Arg. n., Arum t., Bapt., Bar. c., Bell., *Brom.*, Carb. ac., Carb. s., *Carb. v.*, *Caust.*, Chlor., Cina, Cupr., Dros., Ferr., Gels., Hep., Hyos., Ign., Kali a., Kali bi., Kali c., Kali i., Kali p., Lach., Merc., Merc. c., Naja, Nat. m., Nit. ac., Nux m., Nux v., *Phos.*, Phyt., Puls., Rhus t., Rumex, Sang. Sel., Seneg., Spong., Stann., *Stram.*, Sulph., Verat.

HOARSE: *Acon.*, Æsc., All. c., Alum., Ambr., Amm. c., Amm. m., Ant. c., Ant. t., Apis, *Arg. m.*, Ars., Arum t., Bar. c., *Bell.*, Brom., Bry., Cact., *Calc.*, Calc. p., Calc. s., Camph., Canth., Caps., Carl., Carb. an., Carb. s., *Carb. v.*, Caust., Cham., Chin., Chlor., Coc. c., Coff., Colch., Coll., Con., Crot. h., Crot. t., Cupr., Dig., *Dros.*, Dulc., Euphr., Ferr., Ferr. p., Ferr. i., Gels., Graph., Hep., *Iod.*, *Kali bi.*, Kali c., Kali chl., Med., Kali i., Kali p., *Lach.*, Laur., *Merc.*, Merc. c., Merc. i. r., Mez., Mur. ac., Nat. c., Phos., Nat. m.,

HOARSE: Nit. ac., Nux m., Nux v., Op., Osm., Par., Petr., Ph. ac., Phyt., Plb., Psor., Puls., Rhod., Rhus t., Rhus v., Rumex, Samb., Sang., Sel., Seneg., Sep., Sil., *Spong.*, Stann., Still., Sulph., Sul. ac., *Tell.*, Thuja, Verat., Zinc.

Evening, in the: Carb. an., Carb. s., *Carb. v.*, Graph., Kali bi., Mang., *Phos.*, Rumex, Sulph.

Morning, in the: Acon., Apis, Bor., *Calc.*, Carb. an., *Caust.*, Coff., Dig., Euphr., Iod., Mang., Nat. m., *Phos.*, Sil., Sulph.

Overused, voice when: Arg m., Arn., *Arum t.*, *Caps.*, Caust., Kali p., Mang., Nat. m., Phos., *Rhus t.*, Selen., Still.

Singing, while: *Agar.*, Arg. m., Arg. n., *Arum t.*, Bry., Mang., Nat m., Selen.

Talking: Alum., *Arg. m.*, *Arum t.*, Calc., *Caps.*, Carb. v., Coc. c., Ferr., Kali bi., Mang., Nat. m., Nit. ac., Phos., Ph. ac., Rhus t.

CHEST

LUNGS AND ITS COMMON AILMENTS:

(1) Abscess *Calc.*, Crot. h., *Hep.*, Kali c., Lach., Led., Lyc., Mang., Merc., *Phos.*, Plb., Psor., *Sil.*, Sulph., *Tub.*

(2) Gangrene: *Ars.*, Carb. an., Carb. v., Chin., *Kreos.*, Lach., Phos., Plb.

Hæmorrhage: Acal., Acet. ac., *Acon.*, Alum., Ant. t., Apoc., *Arn.*, *Ars.*, Bell., Bry., *Cact.*, Calc., Calc. p., Card. m., *Chel.*, Chin., Coc. c., Colch., Cop., Croc., Dig., Ferr., Ferr.ar., Ferr. i., *Ham.*, Hyos., *Ip.*, Kali c., Kali chl., Kali i., Kreos., Lach., Led., Mill., Nat. a., Nit. ac., Nux m., Nux v., Phos., *Ph. ac.*, Puls., Rhus t., Sabin., Sang., *Sec.*, Senec., *Stann.*, Stram., Sul. ac., Ter., Urt. u.

(3) Hepatization: Brom., Cact., Camph., Chel., Kali c., Kali Chl., Kali i., Lach Lob., Lyc., Nux v., *Phos.*, Sang., Sulph., Ter., Tub.

right: Kali c., *Kali i.*, Phos. upper right half: Chel.

left: Lach., *Lyc.*, Myrt., Sulph.

Phthisis pulmonalis: Acet. ac., *Agar.*, Ars., Ars. i., Bar. m., Bufo, *Calc.*, *Calc. p.*, Calc. s., Carb. an., Carb. s., Carb

PHTHISIS PULMONALIS.

v., Dros., Dulc., Elaps, Ferr. p., *Hep.*, Iod., *Kali c.*, Kali n., Kali p., *Kali s.*, Kreos., Lac. d., Lach., *Lyc.*, Med., Merc., Myrt., Nat. m., Nit. ac., *Phos.*, Ph. ac., Plb., *Psor.*, *Puls.*, Sang., Senec., Seneg., Sep., *Sil.*, *Spong.*, *Stann.*, Sulph., *Ther.*, **Tub.**, Zin.

Paralysis: Amm. m., *Ant. t.*, Arg. n., Ars., *Bar. c.*, Calc., *Carb. v.*, Chin., Cupr., Gels.. Iod., *Lach.*, Laur., *Lyc.*, Mosch., Phos., Stann.

EMPHYSEMA: Amm. c., *Ant. t.*, Ars., Bell., Brom., Carb. v., Chlor., Dig., *Hep.*, Ip., *Lach.*, *Lob.*, Merc., Nat. m., Phel., Phos.

EMPYEMA: Ars., Ars. i., Calc., *Calc. s.*, Carb. s., Carb. v., Chin., Chin. a., Hep., Kali c., *Kali s.*, Lach., *Merc.*, Nat. a., Phos., Sep., *Sil.*, *Sulph.*

Respiration, asthmatic: *Acon.*, Agar., Ambr., Amm. c., Ant. t., Apis, *Arg*, Ars., Ars. i., Asaf., Aur., Bar. c., Bell., Blat., Bov., Brom., Bry., Cact., Calad., Calc., Cann. s., Caps., Carb. v., Chin., Chin. a., Cic., Coff., Colch., Con., Crot. h., *Cupr.*, Dig., Dros., Dulc., Euph., Ferr., Ferr. ar., Gels., Hippoz., Ign., Iod., *Ip.*, *Kali*

EMPYEMA, respiration, asthmatic.

ar., *Kali c.*, Kali chl., *Kali n.*, Kali p., Kali s., Lach., Laur., Led., *Lob.*, Lyc., Med,. Meph., Mosch., Nat. m., Nat. s., Nit. ac., Nux v., Op., Phos., Phyt., Psor., *Puls.*, Ruta, *Samb.*, Sang., Seneg., Sep., *Sil.*, Spong, Stann., Still., *Stram.*, *Sulph.*, Sul. ac., Thuja, Verat.

children, in: Acon., *Cham.*, *Ip.*, Mosch., *Nat.* s., *Puls.*, Samb.

coition; during: Æth., Ambr.

coition, following an act of: Asaf., Cedr., Kali bi.

eructations ameliorate: Nux v., Carb. v.

eruption, after suppressed: Apis, Ars., Carb. v., Dulc., Ferr., Ip., *Puls.*, Sulph.

hay asthma: Amb., Art., Ars., Ars. i., Bad., Carb. v., Dulc. Euphr., *Iod.*, Kali i., Naja, Nat. s., Nux v., Sabad., Sil., Sin. n., Stict.

hysterical: Mosch., Nux m., Nux v., *Puls.*

menses, during: Kali c.

menses, previous to: Sulph.

old people, in: Ambr., *Ars.* Bar. c., Carb. v., Con.

gasping: Acon., Amm. c., Ant. t., *Apis*, Apoc., Ars., Brom., Chlor., Cic., Coff., Colch., Coloc., Dig., Dros., Hell., Hydr. ac., Hyper., Ip., Laur., *Lyc.*, Med., Mosch., Naja, Phos., Spong., Stram., Tab,

EMPYEMA, respiration gasping.

rattling: Acon., All. c., Amm. m., *Ant. t.*, Apis, *Apoc.*, *Ars.*, Ars. i., Art. v., Bar. c., Bar. m., Bell., Brom., Cact., Calc., Calc. p., Calc. s., Cann. s., Carb. an., Carb h., Carb. v., Caust., Cham., Chel., *Chin.*, Chin. a., Cina, Coc. c., *Cupr.*, Dig., *Dulc.*, Ferr., Graph., Hep., *Hippoz.*, Hyos., Iod., *Ip.*, Kali c., Kali chl., *Kali s.*, Lach., *Lyc.*, Manc., Mur. ac., Nat. m., Nat. s., Nit. ac., Nux m., Nux v., Op., *Phos.*, Ph. ac., *Puls.*, Pyrog., Ran b., Sang., *Seneg.*, Sep., Sil., Spong., Stann, Stram., Sulph., Tub., Verat., Zinc.

rough: Ant. t., *Bry.*, Hep., Kali bi.

crowing: *Bry.*, Chlor., Chin., Cupr., Gels., *Samb.*, *Spong.*

sawing: Ant. t., *Brom.*, Con., *Iod.*, Kaol., Sang., *Spong.*

sighing: Acon., Arg. m., Ars., Aspar., Bov., *Bry.*, *Calad.*, Calc., *Calc. p.*, Camph., *Carb. v.*, Caust., Cham., *Dig.*, Ferr. Gels., Glon., Hell., *Ign.*, *Ip.*, Lyc., Merc. c., *Op.*, Phos., Phyt., Puls., *Sec.*, Spong., *Stram.*

snoring: Brom., Camph., Carl., Cham., Chin., Cupr., Hep., Ign., Lach., Nux v., *Op.*, Rhus t., Stram., Sulph.

stertorous: *Amm. c.*, Ant. t., Apis, Arn., Ars., Camph., Carb. ac., Chin., Gels.,

EMPYEMA, respiration, stertorous.

Glon., Lach., Laur., Lyc., Nit. ac., Nux v., Nux m., Op., Puls., Spong., Stram.

whistling: Ambr., Ant. t., Ars., Carb. v., Cham., Chin., Hep., Kali c., Lyc., Manc., Samb., Sil., Spong., Sulph.

MAMMÆ, common affections of:

Abscess: Bell., Bry., Camph., Cist., Crot. h., Hep., Lach., Merc., Phos., Phyt., Sil., Sulph.

Atrophy: Chin., Con., Iod., Kali i., Kreos., Nat. m., Nit. ac., Nux m., Sec.

Cancer: Apis, Arg. n., Ars., i., Aster., Aur. a., Bad., Bell., Brom., Bufo, Carb. an., Chim., Clem., Con., Cund., Graph., Hep., Hydr., Lach., Lyc., Merc., Merc. i. f., Nit. ac., Phos., Phyt., Psor., Sang., Sep., Sil., Sulph.

Hardness: Bell., Bry., Cham., Clem., Con., Sil., Sulph.

right: Con.

left: Sil.

Induration: Aster., Bell., Bry., Calc., Carb. an., Carb. s., Cham., Cist., Clem., Con., Crot. h., Crot. t., Cupr., Graph., Iod., Kreos., Lac. c., Lyc., Merc., Phyt., Sep., Sil., Sulph., Thuja.

Milk, absence of: Agn., Asaf., Bell., Bry., Calc., Caust., Coff., Form., Ign., Lac. c., Lac. d., Mill., Urt. u., Zinc.

blood, with: Cham., Lyc., Merc., Sep., Sulph.

MILK.

bloody: Cham., Phyt.

cheesy: Bor., Cham., Phyt.

disappearing: Agn., Arn., Asaf., Calc., Camph., Caust., Chel., Chion., Dulc., Lac. c., Phel., Plan., Plb., Puls., Rhus t., Sef., Urt. u., Ust., Verat. v., Zinc.

increased flow of: Acon., Bell., Bor., Bry., Calc., Puls., Rhus t.

non-pregnant women, in: Asaf., Cycl., Merc., Puls., Urt. u,

suppressed: Agn., Bry., Carb. v., Caust., Cham., Hyos., Iod. Lach., Merc., Puls., Rhus t., Sec., Sil., Sulph., Urt. u.

Pain: Bell., Bor., Bry., Bufo, Calc., Carb. an., Cham., Con., Dulc., Lac. c., Merc., Phel., Phos., Ph. ac., Phyt., Rhus t., Sil., Sulph.

menses, when the flow is on: Con., Merc., Phel., Phos., Phyt.

menses, previous to: Calc., Con., Lac. c.

nurses, while child: Crot. t., Puls., Sil.

pregnancy, during: Sep.

that extends to back: Phel.

radiating over whole body: Phyt.

while nursing: Crot. t., Merc. c., Nux v., Phyt.

Retracted nipples: Nux m., Sars., Sil.

Tumours: Carb. an., Con., Cund., Lach., Phos., Phyt., Sil.

HEART:

Oppression: Acon., Agar.,
Ambr., Amyl. n., Apis, Ars.,
Ars. i., Aur., Aur. m..
Brom., Cact., Calc. ar.,
Carb. v., Caust., Chin., Dig.,
Gels., Glon., Iod., Ip., Kali
c., Lach., Laur., Lil t.,
Lycops., Merc., Naja, Nat.
a., Nat. s., Nux m., Nux
v., Puls., Spig., Tab.

ascending stairs, while: Aur.,
Aur. m.

exertion, on least: Brom.,
Laur., Nat. a.

lying relieves: Laur., Psor.

lying with head low: Spong

lying on left side: Colch.,
Lach., Naja, Spig.

sitting: Nat. s.

Orgasm of blood: Amyl. n.,
Carb. v., Ferr., Glon., Lach.,
Lil. t., Merc., Mill., Nit.
ac., Phos., Sep., Sulph.,
Thuja.

Palpitation: Acon., Agar.,
Alum,. Ambr., Amm. c.,
Amm. m., Amyl. n., Ant. t.,
Apis, Arg. m., Arg. n., Arn.,
Ars., Ars. i., Asaf., Aur.,
Aur. m., Bad., Bar. c., Bar.
m,. Bell., Bism., Brom., Bry.,
Cact., Cadm., Calc., Calc.
ar., Calc. p., Camph., Cann. i.,
Cann. s., Carb. an., Carb. s.,
Carb. v., Caust., Cedr.,
Cham., Chel., Chin., Chin. a.,
Cocc., Coff., Colch., Coll.,
Con., Crot. h., Cupr., Cycl.,
Dig., Dios., Elaps, Eup. per.,
Ferr., Ferr. ar., Ferr. i., Ferr.
p., Gels., Glon., Graph.,
Gua., Hep., Hydr., Hyos.,
Ign., Iod., Kali ar., Kali bi.,
Kali c., Kali chl., Kali fer.,

HEART, palpitation.

Kali i., Kali n., Kali p., Kali
s., Kalm., Lac. d., Lach.,
Laur., Lil. t., Iob., Lyc.,
Lycops., Mag. m., Manc.,
Mang., Med., Meli., Merc.,
Merc. c., Merl., Mill.,
Mosch., Naja, Nat. a., Nat.
c., Nat. m., Nat. p., Nit. ac.,
Nux m., Nux v., Ox. ac.,
Olnd., Ph. ac., Plat., Plb.,
Podo., Prun., Psor., Puls.,
Rhus t., Sars., Sec., Sep., Sil.,
Spig., Spong., Stram., Sulph.,
Sul. ac., Tab., Ther., Thuja,
Verat., Verat. v., Viol. t.

climacteric period: Crot. h.,
Lach., Tab.

coition, during: Lyc., Phos.,
Ph. ac.

coition, following: Dig., Sep.

eating after: Abies. c., Acon.,
Bov., Calc., Camph.,
Carb. an., Carb. v., Ign.,
Lyc., Nat. c., Nat. m.,
Nit. ac., Nux v., Puls.,
Sep.,

fever, during: Acon., Ars.,
Calc., Cocc., Nit. ac.,
Puls., Sars., Sep.

lying, while: Benz. ac., Cact.,
Ferr., Lach., Nux v., Ox.
ac., Puls., Sulph.

motion, from: Amm. c.,
Apoc., Arg. n., Arn., Aur.,
Calc., Cann. s., Carb. s.,
Carb. v., Cimic., Cocc.,
Con., Dig., Ferr., Graph.,
Hyos., Lach., Naja, Nat.
m., Phos., Prun., Psor.,
Sil., Spig., Staph., Stram.

pregnant women, in: Arg. m.,
Con., Lil. t., Nat. m., Sep.

sleep, on going to: Calc.,
Carb. v., Nat. m., Sulph.

HEART, palpitation.

stool, during: Ant. t., Sulph.
stool, after: *Ars. Con.*

tumultuous: Agar., Amm. c.,
Amyl. n., Ang., Apis, Arg.
n., Ars., Aur., Aur. m.,
Calc. ar., Carb. s., Carb.
v. Chin., Chin. a., Coca,
Colch., Cycl., *Dig.*, Ferr.
m., *Glon.*, *Iod.*, *Kali. c.*,
Kali i., Kali n., Kali. p.,
Kalm., Lach., Lycops.,
Naja, *Nat. m.*, Nux. m.,
Olnd., Phos., Plb., *Puls.*,
Sep., Spig., Spong., Staph.,
Sulph., Tarent., Verat.

vexation, from: Aur. m., Ign.,
Nat. m., Ph. ac.

HEART, palpitation.

visible: Ars., Aur., Carb. s.,
Carb. v., Kalm., Lach.,
Spig., Staph., Sulph.,
Verat.

walking: Apoc., Aur. m.,
Cact., Kali i., Naja, Sep.,
Staph.

walking ameliorates his palpitation: Arg. n., Mag. m.,
Nux m.

walking rapidly: Aur. m.,
Nat. m., Phos., Ph. ac.,
Puls., *Sep.*

walking rapidly ameliorates:
Aur. m., Nat. m., Phos.,
Ph. ac., *Sep.*, Puls.

BLADDER.

ACHING: Berb., *Caps.*, Equis., Eupat. pur., Flour. ac., Hell., Nux v., Sep.

Biting pain: Prun. sp.
Aggravation, lying from: Nux v.
Aggravation, at night: Bell.
Urination, after: Cal. ph.
Coition, after: Cepa.
Urinating, before and after: Fl. ac.

AIR, escapes from: Sars.

BURNING: Acon., Apis, Ars., *Berb.*, Camph., *Canth.*, *Caps.*, Cham., Eupat. pur., Sep., *Tereb.*
Neck of bladder: Berb., Canth., Cham., Cop., Elat., Nux v., Puls., Staph.

   with cystitis: Acon., Ars., *Canth.*

CALCULI: Aspar., Benz. ac., Berb., Calc. c., Cann., *Canth.*, Cinch., Chim., Cocc., Colch., Hydr., Ipom., Lach., Lith. c., *Lyc.*, Nat. s., Nux v., Par. br., Phos., Puls., Sars., Sep., Sil.

   After operation for stone: Arn., Calend., Staph.

CATARRH: Ant. c., Apis, *Benz. ac.*, Calc. c., Canth., Carb. an., Carb. v., Caust., Chim., Coloc., Con., Cop., *Dulc.*, Equis., Gels., Ham., Hydr., Kali mur., Lach., *Lyc.*, Nux v., Par. br., Petr., Puls., Sil., Sina. n., Sina. alb., Sulph., Tereb.

CATARRH.
Chronic: Ant. c., Calc. c., Carb. v., Eucal., *Kali mur.*, *Lyc.*, Par. br., Phos., Sars., Senega, Sulph., Tereb., *Uva. u.*

CONSTRICTION: Berb., Nux v., Ph. ac., Puls., Sars.
Sensation of: Berb., Cact. gr., Canth., Caps., Cocc., Puls., Sars.
   kidney towards bladder, from: Lyc.
   painful: *Sars.*
   region painful: Puls.
Spasmodic: *Caps.*

CRAMPS: Berb., Nux v., Op.
Preceded by colic: Zinc.
Sphincter, of: Op.
Stitch-like: Carb. s.

CRAMP-LIKE PAINS: Berb., Lyc., Sars.

CUTTING PAINS: Berb., Canth., Caps., Cub., Kali c., Lach., Lyc., Nux v., Puls., *Tereb.*
Neck of bladder: *Canth.*

DISTENTION: *Apis*, Ars. Canth., Equis., Eupat. pur. Sep., *Stram.*, Zinc.

DISAGREEABLE FEELING *Apis*.

EMPTY FEELING: Dig. Stram.
   Unable to empty: Helon., Hep. Staph.

FERMENTATION: Sars.

HÆMORRHOIDS: Acon., Canth., Ham., Nux v., Puls., Sulph.

Bleeding: *Calc. c.*, Ham.

HÆMORRHAGE: Ant. t., *Apis*, Arn., Ars., Aur. met., Berb., *Cact.*, *Cal. c.*, Camph., Cann. s., *Canth.*, Caps., Caust., *Chim.*, Colch., Con., Cop., Crot. Cub., Cup. m., Ferr., Ferr. mur., Fer. p., Ham., Ipec., Kreos., Lyc., *Merc. cor.*, Mez., Mill., Nat. m. Nit. ac., Nux v., Op., Par. br., *Phos.*, Phos. ac., Plumb., Pul.., Sars., Scilla, Sec. c., Sep., Sulph., Sul. ac., Ter., Thlas.

Abdomen, with cutting pain in: Ipec.

Albuminuria: Merc. cor.

Blood, black and ropy: Tereb.

Blood, thick: Sec. cor.

Bright red: Ham., Nitric acid.

Blood clots: Alum., Chim., Ipe., Lyc., *Mill.*, Ph. ac., Plat.,

Burning heat in lower bowels as if hot water were poured there: Ipec.

Calculi from: Lyc., Erig.

Chilliness: Caps., Mill.

Exertion, from every: Petr.

Kidney with pain in: Mill., Nux v., Phos., Puls., Senecio, Tereb.

Nausea, with: Ipe., Senec.

Spasmodic pain, with: Nux v., Puls.

Tenesmus, with: Merc. s.

Urethra, with burning in: Acon., Ars., *Canth.*, Caps.

HEAVY FEELING: Canth., Lyc., Nat. m.

INJURIES: Arn., Staph.

INFLAMMATION (Cystitis): *Acon.*, *Ant. t.*, *Apis*, Arg. n. Arn., Ars., Bar. m., *Bell.*, Berb., Calad., Calc. c., Cann. i., Cann. s., Canth., Caps., Caust., Chim., Con., Cop., Cub., *Dig.*, Dulc., Equis., Eupat. pur., Gels., Hell., Hydr., Kali phos., *Lach.*, *Lyc.*, Merc. c., Merc. s. Nit. ac., Nux v., Par. br., Petr., *Puls.*, Sars., Sep., Sulph., *Tereb.*

Chronic: Ars., Con., Cub., Dulc., Lyc., Pareira, Sar., Sep.

Causes convulsions: Hell.

Causes nausea and vomiting: Canth., Ars.

IRRITABLE: Actea, r., Apis, Bell., Benz. ac., *Canth.*, Chim., Colch., Cop., Cub., *Erig.*, Lept., Nux, Pod., Plant., Puls., *Sep.*, Staph., Sulph., Zinc., Vespa.

NEURALGIA: Clem., Elat., Mag. ph., Sars.

PAIN: Berb., Calc. ph., *Canth.*, Carb. v., Caust., Chel, Equis., Lith. carb., Lyc., Phyt., Puls., Tarent. Zinc.

Dull, in: Chim., Cub., *Equis.*, Lyc., Nux v., Puls.

Spasmodic: Berb., Canth., Caps., Caul., Cop., Puls.

PARALYSIS: *Ars.*, Bell., Cact. gr., Camph., Cann. s., Canth., Carb. an., *Caust.*, Cic. v., Cupr., *Dulc.*, *Gels.*, Hell., Hyos., Kali ph., *Nux v.*, Op., Plum., Puls., Rhus t., *Sec. c.*, Sil., Stram., Sulph., Thuja, Zinc.

From over exertion: Ars., *Caust.*, Hell., Nux v,

PRESSURE, painful: Ant. t.,
  Apis, Borax, Cepa, Chim.,
  Coloc., Con, Dig., Dulc.,
  Lyc., Prun. sp., Puls., *Sep.*,
  Sulph.

  Neck: Canth., Caps., Carb. v.,
  Nux v., Puls.

SENSATIONS:—

  Bursting: Caps., Sanic., Zinc.
  during cough: Caps.

  Constriction: Berb., Nux v., Ph.
  ac., Puls., *Sars.*

  Disagreeable: *Apis.*

  Drawing: Berb.

  Dragging: Chelid.

  Fullness: Arn., Ars., Calad.,
  Chim., *Dig.*, *Equis.*, Lact. ac.,
  Nux v. Op., *Puls.*, *Sep.*, Zinc.
  desire without, to urinate:
  Calad.

  desire constant, to urinate:
  Dig., Ruta.

  urination, after: Eupat. pur.

  Pressure: Ant. t., Apis, Borax,
  Caps., Cepa, Chim., Coloc.,
  Com., Dig., Dulc., Lyc.,
  Prun. sp., Puls., *Sep.*, Sulph.

  Scalding: *Apis*, Canth.

  Soreness: Bell., Calad., *Canth.*,
  Cepa, Equis., Eupat. pur.,

SENSATION, soreness.

  Lit. c., Merc., *Puls.*, Sep
  Tereb.

  Stinging: Apis, Calad., Canth.,
  Nat. m., **Pallad.**, Puls.,
  Sulph.

  Stitches: Berb., Caps., Chelid.,
  Con., Kali c., Lyc., Nux v.,
  Puls., Sulph.

  neck: Canth., Caps., Guai.,
  Lyc., Puls.

  Weakness: Alum., Cepa.

TENESMUS: Acon., Alum.,
  Apis, *Arn.*, Bell., Calc.,
  Canth., Camph., *Caps.*,
  Caust., Chim., Clem., Coc. c.,
  Colch., Cop., Gel., Hyos.,
  Lith. c., Lyc., Merc., *Merc.
  cor.*, Nux m., *Nux v.*, Op.,
  Prun. s., *Puls.*, Rhus t., *Sars.*,
  Sil., *Tereb.*

  Dysentery, in: *Caps.*, Merc. c.

  Rectum and bladder, simultaneously: Caps.

WEAKNESS: *Alum.*, *Ars.*,
  Canth., *Caust.*, Cepa, Equis.,
  Gels., Hell., *Hep.*, Hyos.,
  Mag. mur., Mur. ac., *Op.*,
  Ph., ac., Rhus t.

KIDNEYS.

AILMENTS, common:

Abscess: Ars., Berb., Bry. Canth., Hep., *Merc.*, Sil., Tere.

Addison's disease: Arg. nit., Ars., Bell., Ferr., Ferr. iod., *Iod.*, Kali c., *Nat. m.*, Nit. ac., *Phos.*, Sep. *Sil.*, Spig., Sulph.

pressing sensation, with: Calc. c., Iod., Nit. ac., Nux v.

Bright's disease (Albuminuria, including): Apis, *Ars.*, Aur. mur., Aur. m. n., Berb., Brach. r., *Calc. ar.*, Calc. c., Cann. s., Canth., Cheliod.. Chin.., Colch., Cop., Crot. h., Cupr. m., Dig., Dulc., Ferr. ph., Gels., *Glon.*, Hell., Helon., Hep., Iod., Kali bi., Kali c., Kali i., Kali p., Kalm., *Lac. d.*, Lach., *Lyc.*. Merc. cor., Merc. cy., Mer. i. r., *Nat. m.*, Nit. ac., Nux v., *Ph. ac.*, Phyt., Sec. c., Sulph., *Tereb.*, Uran. n.

alcohol, from abuse of: Ars., Berb., Carb. v., Crot. h., Lach., Merc. c., Nat. c., Nux v.

amaurosis, with: Apis, Ars., Gels., Hep., *Merc. c.*

back, pain in: Kali nit., Kalm.

convulsions, with uræmic: *Cupr. met., Kali br.*

degeneration, with atheromatous, fatty, granular: Arg.

BRIGHTS DISEASE, degeneration with.

nit., *Ars.*, Calc. c., Dig., Glon., Kali i., Ph. a., Phyt., *Plumb.*, Tereb.

contracted kidney with: *Plumb.*

dropsy, with: Apis, Ars., Calc. ar., Cop., Cupr., Dig., Hell., Kalm., Daph., *Lac. def.*, Tereb.

drugs, after taking strong: Camph., Nux v., Phos.

eyes, swollen: Apis, Arn., Kali c., Lycop. v.

eyes, sacculated lids with: Kali c.

exposure to cold, after: Calc., Colch., *Dulc.*, Kali c., Merc. c., Nux v., Rhus t., Sep.

heart, with complications of: Ars., Ars. iod., Aur met., Colch., Crot., Cupr. met., Dig., Glon., Kali bi., Kali mur, Kalm., Lach., *Lycop. v.*, Ph. ac.

hydrothorax, with: Ars., Bry. Colch.

mercuro-syphilitic, cases in: Aur. met., Kali iod., Nit. ac.

pulmonary complications: Apis, Canth., Chelid., Colch., Crot. h., Kali iod., Kali p., Phos., Tereb.

weakness, with great: Ars., Phos.

COLIC.

Colic, renal: Apis, Arg. nit., Arn., Ars., *Bell.*, Benz. ac., Berb., Canth., *Carb. an.*, Colch., Coloc., Ind., Kali c., *Lyc.*, Nit. ac., Nux m., Nux v., *Ocim.*, Op., *Par. br.*, Plumb., *Sars.* Verat. alb.

bloody urine, with: Arg. nit., Canth., Cocc. c., Colch., Nux.

calculi, with passage of: Aspar., Canth., diosc., Ipom., Lyc., Nux v., Ocim., *Sars.*

nausea, with retching and vomiting: Canth., Ipom., Lyc., Nux v., Ocim., Op., Verat. alb.

contracted, cirrhosis of: Aur. mur., *Ars.*, Clem., Dig., Glon., Nit. ac., Phos., *Plumb.*

Hæmorrhage, renal: Arn., *Canth.*, Ferr. mur., Ham., Ipec., Lyc., Nat. m., Nux v., Par. br., Phos., Senecio, Tereb.

caused by gravel: *Canth.*, *Lyc.*, Ocim., Par. br.

Inflammation: Acon., *Apis*, Arg. n., *Arn.*, Ars., Aur. met., Bell., Ben. ac., Berb., Bry., Cann. i., *Cann. s.*, *Canth.*, Caps., Cepa, Chelid., Colch., Hell., Helon., Hep., Kali c., Kali i., Kali mur., *Lyc.*, Merc. c., Merc. s., Nux v., Par. br., Phos., Phyt., Puls., Rhus t., Sars., Senecio, Sulph., Tereb., Zinc.

backache, with: Benz. ac., Berb., Colch., Par. br.

chest pain, with: Benz. ac.

damp places, caused by living in: Tereb.

INFLAMMATION.

headache with: Chelid.

Nephralgia: Arg. nit., *Sars.*, Tereb., Zinc.

PAIN: Apis, Arg. n., Arn., *Berb.*, Bry., Cainc., Calc., Cann. s., *Canth.*, Caps., Chelid., Chenop., Cinnab., Clem., *Colch.*, Dios., Ferr., Helon., Hep., Kali bi., Kali mur., Lyc., *Nat. m.*, Nux v., Phos. ac., Phyt., Plumb., Puls., Sars., Selen., Sep., Tereb.

Bruised: Berb., Mancin., Par. br.

Constant pain, a sort of: *Berb.*, Calc. c., Canth., Eupat. pur., Hydr., *Lyc.*, Tereb.

right kidney: Crotal., Helon., Kali bi., Sabad.

left kidney: Acon., Agar., Cinch., Cocc. c., Cund., Elat., Pallad.

Dull, heavy: Apis, Benz. ac., Berb., Cann. i., Canth., Equis., Eu. pur. Ferr., Nat. s., Phos., Tereb.

Extends to abdomen: Berb., Canth., Ipec., Nux v.

Extends to back: Berb., Cepa, Colch., Ipom., Kali bi., Kali c., Kalm., Lyc., Mancin., Nux v., Par. br., Ph. ac., Tereb.

Extends to bladder: Arg. n., Bell., Berb., Canth., Cepa, Ipom., Lyc., *Sars.*

Extends to calves: Berb.

Extends to chest: Benz. ac., Cocc. c., Ferr.

Extends to glans penis: Cann. i., Canth.

Extends to genitals: Nux v.

PAIN.

Extends to groin: Cepa, Par. br.

Extends to hypogastrium: Colch.

Extends to hips: Arn., Beib., Nux m., Nux v., Tereb., Polygon.

Extends to ilium: Caust., Dios.

Extends from left to right side and down the right thigh: Nux v.

Extends to loins: Arg. n., Berb., Calc. c., Canth., Colch., Coloc., Nux v.

Extends to lumbar region: Berb., Par. br., Tereb.

Extends to prostate glands: Graph.

Extends to rectum, from, to bladder: Thuja.

Extends to spermatic cord: Syph.

Extends to thighs: Berb., Ipec., Kali bi., Lac. def., Nux v.

PAIN.

Extends to testicles: Nux v.

Extends to ureters: Arg. nit., Ars., Berb., Canth., Chelid., Ipom., Lyc., Par. br., Sars., Tereb.

Extends to urethra: Berb., Canth.

While urinating: Puls.

SORENESS, SENSITIVE-NESS, TENDERNESS: Arg. nit., Asaf., Berb., Cann. s., Canth., Chelid., Cocc. c., *Graph.*, Helon., Hep., Hydras., Nux v., Par. br., Tereb.

To pressure or touch: Apis, Arg. nit., Berb., Canth., Merc., *Nux v., Puls.*

VOMITING WITH KIDNEY TROUBLES: Ipom.

PROSTATE.

ENLARGEMENT OF, Hypertrophy of: Aloe., Amm. mur., Apis, Aur. mur., *Baryta.* c., Benz. ac., Calc. c., Chim., *Con.*, Dig., Ferr. mur., Hyos., Iod. Lyc., Merc. s., Nat. s., Nat. c., Nit. ac., *Puls.*, Sil., Spong., Staph., Sulph., Thuja.

Chronic: Calc., *Con.*, Bar. c., Nat. c., Spong., Sulph., Thuja.

Senile: Aloe., Benz. ac., *Bar.* c., Con., Dig., Iod., Staph.

Urine, dribbling of, with: Aloe., Dig., Par. br., Puls., Staph.,

Retention of urine: Chim., Par. br., Tril. rep.

PROSTATORRHOEA: Anac., Apis, Calc. c., Chim., Elaps, Eryng., Hep., Nit. ac., Phos., Ph. ac., Puls., Sel., Sil., Spig., *Staph.*, Sulph.

PROSTATITIS, acute inflammation: *Apis*, Caust., Chim., Cop., Cub., Dig., Hep., Kali bi., Lyc., Merc. dul., Merc. sol., Petrol., Puls., Selen., Sil., Thuja.

Agony on urinating with: Apis, Par. br.

Anus, oozing from, with: Caust., Nit. ac.

Anus, pain in, with: Nit. ac., Lyc., Staph.

Ball, sitting on a, sensation of: Chim., Sep.

Pain, in bladder, with: Apis, Cact, g., Calc. ph., Caust., Cepa, Pul.

PROSTATITIS.

Emissions, seminal with: Merc. s., Selen.

Heat in prostate gland, with: Puls.

Induration of, with: Con., Cop., Iod., Selen., Sil.

Pain in, with: Bell., Caps., Calc. ph., Cepa, Cub., Cop., Par. br., Staph.

Pain, burning, with: Cop., Merc. Iod., Ph. ac.

Urethritis: Par. br., Puls.

Urine, involuntary escape of (drop by drop): Cop., Dig.

Urinary stream, small: Chima., Graph., Spong., Staph., Sulph., Zinc.

Urination delayed, with (Slow in starting): Apis, Cact., Cann. i., Hep.

Urination, difficult, with: Apis, Chim., Cop., Hep., Par. br.

Urinating efforts, ineffectual: Apis, Dig., Par. br., *Puls.*, Staph.

Urging to urinate, with: Cact., Dig., Par. br., Puls., Staph.

Urging to urinate, constant, with: Apis, Cact., Par. br., Puls.

Urging to urinate, even after he has passed water: Apis, Cact., Caust, Dig., Hep., Merc. s., Nat. c., Puls., Staph.

PROSTATIC FLUID.

EMISSION OF: Agnus, Apis, Chim., *Con.*, Daph., Hep., Lyc., Mag. c., Nat. m., *Ph. ac.*, Selen., Thuja.

Emotion, from: Con., Puls.

Erections, after: Ph. ac.

Erections, without: Nat. m., Phos., *Sil.*

Excesses, sexual, after: *Staph.*

Lascivious thoughts: Nat. m.,

Milky: Iod., Nat. m.

Onanists: Gels., Staph.

Penis relaxed, from: Aur. met., Bell., Lyc., Nat. m.

Stool, before: Cycl.

Stool, during: Calc., Caust., Con., Hep., Ign., Kali bi., Nat. c., Nit. ac., Nux v., Phos., Ph. ac., Selen., Sep., Sil., Staph., Sulph.

EMISSION.

Stool, at the end of: **Calc.**, Caust., Daph., *Hep.*, Iod., Kali c., Nat. c., Nit. ac., Selen., *Sulph.*

difficult: Con., Hep., *Nit. ac.*, Sep.

first portion hard, latter portion soft: Bovista.

soft: Ars.

straining for, while: Agnus, Carb. v., Gels., Hep., **Nat. c.**, **Phos.**, Ph. ac., Sil.

Urination, before: Psor.

Urination, during: *Hep.*, Nat. c., Sep.

Urination following an act of: Calc. c., Daph., Hep., Kali c., *Sulph.*

Walks, while he: Selen.

URETHRA.

CLOSED ALMOST, by swelling: Rhus t.

CONTRACTION, spasmodic: Bell., Canth., Clem., Cop., Gels., Nit. ac., Nux v., Plumb., Prun. s., Sec. c.

CONSTRICTION: Arn., Berb., Clem., Lyc., Verat. a.

INFLAMMATION: Arg. n., Ars., Aur. m., Cann. s., Canth., Hep., Nux v., Par. br., Petr., Tereb.

Chronic: Kali iod., Petr.

Painful: Arg. n., Cann. s., Cub., Merc. c., Petros., Thuja.

INSENSIBLE TO FLOW OF URINE: Caust.

MUCUS CLOGS THE URETHRA: Cann. s., Merc. s., Sep., Uva. ur.

OBSTRUCTION OF, by gonorrhoeal mucus: Cub.

PAIN: Arg. nit., Berb., Cann. s., Canth., Caps., Caust., Clem., Nux v., Rhod., Tereb.

Burning: Ant. c., Ant. t., Apis, Arg. nit., Ars., Berb., Bry, Calc. c., Camph., Cann. s., Canth., Caps., Carl., Caust., Cepa, Clem., Colch., Con., Hep., Kali c., Kali iod., Lith. c., Merc. cor., Merc. sol., Nit. ac., Nux v., Petr., Prun. s., Puls., Rhus v., Sars., Sep., Sil., Sulph., Staph., Tereb., Thuja, Uran. n.

PAIN, burning.

and biting: Cann. s., Merc. s., Prun. s.

with discharge of blood: Graph., Kali c., Nux v., Sulph., Uva ur.

coition: Agar., Canth., Clem.

coition, after: Caust., Sep., Sulph.

emission, seminal: Clem., Sep., Sulph.

erection (before, with or after): Canth., Nit. ac.

gonorrhoea, in: Arg. nit., Merc. cor.

itching, and: Cop., Thuja.

scalding, and: Apis, Benz. ac., Cann. sat.

stitching and, with urging to urinate: Canth., Caps., Phos., Sulph.

stool, during: Coloc.

urinate, with frequent desire to: Cann. ind., Canth., Phos.

urinate, with urging to: Canth., Sulph.

Biting: Caps., Clem., Equis., Graph., Merc., Petros.

urinate, with frequent desire to: Cann. i., Calc. p., Pru. s., Sulph.

Cutting: Berb., Calc. c., Calc. Ph., Canth., Caps., Chelid., Con., Dig., Equis., Ipec., Lach., Merc. s., Nit. ac., Nux v., Sep., Sulph., Thuja.

PAIN, cutting.

    emission, after seminal: Nat. m.

    stitches: Calc. c., Sep., Lyc. stool: Staph, Sulph.

    Lacerating: Cann. s., Colch., Ign., Kali c., Mez., Nat. c., Ruta, Sars, Sep., Sulph.

    Lancinating: Thuja.

    Smarting: Apis, Ars., Berb., Cann. s., Canth., Caps., Chim., Cop., Lil. t., Nat. m., Phos., Sep., Tereb., Teuc., Thuja.

    Splinter, as from a: Arg. nit., Nit. ac.,

    Sticking: Berb., Cann. s., Caps., Lach.

    Stinging: Cann. s., Caps., Lach., Merc., Merc. c., Puls., Sulph.

    Stitching: Apis, Berb., Calad., Cann. i., Cann. s., Canth., Caps., Chin., Clem., Hep., Lach., Merc. s., Merc. c., Nat. m., Sars., Sep., Sulph. coition, after: Nat. m. erections, during: Nit. ac.

SENSATIONS:

    Biting: Cann. s., Canth., Clem., Graph., Merc. c., Merc. s.,

    Contraction of: Canth., Carb. v., Chin., Clem, Cop., Dig., Graph, Indig., Petr., Puls.

    Crawling: Canth., Lyc., Ph. ac.

SENSATION.

    Cylinder, tube thrust along: Stram.

    Drawing: Berb., Cann. s., Cic., Kali bi., Merc., Mez., Petros., Puls., Sabad., Thuja.

    Drop running along, of a: Dig., Sep., Thuja.

    Drops remaining behind: Arg. n., Gels., Kali bi.

    Itching: Amb., Chim., Kali mur. Led., Lyc., Mez., Nit. ac., Pet., Petros., Sep., Sulph., Thuja.

    erections, during: Selen.

    gleet, with: Petr.

    pus, preceding a discharge of: Con.

    urination, during: Amb., Lyc., Mez., Nux v.

    Pressure: Lach., Ph. ac., Thuja.

    Prickling: Arg. nit., Cann. i., Caps., Chin., Nit. ac., Ph. ac.

    Scraping: Ign.

    Tickling: Petros., Sulph., Thuja.

    Tingling: Cann s., Cupr. ars., Clem., Petros., Thuja.

STRICTURE: Apis, Arg. nit., Berb., Calc. c., Canth., Cann. s., Clem., Kali iod., Petr.

    Spasmodic: Gels., Nux v.

URINE

CHARACTER:

Acid: Amyl. n., *Arn.*, *Benz. ac.*, Bell., Calc. c., Card. m., Caust., Chelid., Colch., Cop., Cupr. m., Graph., Lyc., Merc. c., Merc. s., Phyt., Plumb., Sulph.

Acrid: Benz. ac., Calc. c., Caust., Dig., Graph., *Hep.*, *Mer. s.*, Nat. m., Phos., Plant., Rhus. t., Sars., Seneg., Staph., *Sulph.*

Albuminous: *Apis*, Arg. n., Ars., Atro., Aur. met., Barch. r., *Calc. ar.*, Calc. c., Canth., Carb. ac., Cepa, Colch., Dulc., Eupat., Ferr., Ferr. sul., *Glon.*, *Hell.*, Helon., Hep., Iod., Kali mur., Kalm., *Lac. def.*, Lach., Lyc., Merc., *Merc. c.*, Nat. c., Nit. ac., Nux v., Pet., Phos., Ph. ac., Phyt., *Plumb.*, Rhus t., Sec c., *Tereb.*

blood, containing: Apis, Merc. cor., Sec. cor., *Tereb...*

casts, with: Canth., Merc. c., Tereb.

convulsions, with: Plumb.

diphtheria in: Hep., Lach., Merc. cor.

dropsy: Apis, Ars., Eupat. pur., Lach.

eclampsia: Glon.

gouty subjects: Berb., Colch.

iritis, with: Sil.

ALBUMINOUS.

pregnancy during: *Apis.*, Ars., Ars. i., Aur. mur., Canth., Chin., Gels., Helon., Kali c., Kalm., Lyc., *Merc. cor.*, Nat. mur., Tereb.

retinitis, with: Apis, Ars., Merc. cor.

Alkaline: *Bapt.*, *Benz. ac.*, Canth., Carb. ac., Fl. ac., Kali bi.

Bloody: Alumen, Ant. t., *Apis*, *Arg. n.*, Ars., Ars. hy., Aur met., Bell., Cact. gr., *Calc. c.*, Camph., Cann. s., *Canth.*, Caps., Carb. v., Caust., *Chim.*, Cocc., Con., Cop., Crot., Cub., Cupr. m., Ferr., Ferr. mur., Ferr. ph., *Ham.*, Hep., Ip., Kreos., Lyc., Merc., *Merc. c.*, Mez., Mill., Nat. m., Nux., Oci., Op., Par. br., *Phos.*, Ph. ac., Plumb. ac., *Puls.*, Rhus t., Sars., Scilla, Sep., Sulph., Sul. ac., Terab., Thalas., Thuja, Uva. ur.

Foaming, frothy: Apis, *Cepa*, Chelid., Cop., Cub., Laur., Lyc., Par. br., Spong., Thuja.

Milky: *Apis*, Aur. met., Aur. mur., Calc. c., Cina, Dulc., *Hep.*, Lyc., Merc., Nat. m., Nit. ac., *Ph. ac.*, Sulph.

brick-dust sediment with: Phos.

MILKY.

blood, and: *Chim.*, Cop., Dulc., Hell., Puls.

Mucus, ropy: *Chim.*, Kali bi., Lyc.

thick: *Chim.*, Cop., *Par. br.*

Muddy: Kali c., Nat. m., **Rhus t.**

Phosphates, in the: *Benz. ac.*, Canth., Ferr. mur., Kali br., Mag. p., Phos., Raph.

Slimy, viscid: Ant. c., Arg. nit., Cann. i., Chim., Coloc., Cupr. m., Dulc., Hell., Nux v., *Par. br.*, Sars., Uva ur.

Specific gravity, too high: *Arn.*, Ascl., Eupat. pur., Helon., Nat. s., Phyt., Puls., Senecio, Uran. n.

too low: Eup. pur., Puls.

Stains clothing: Cupr. m., Elat., Merc. s., Sep.

Stiffens clothing: Ham., *Helon.*

Sugar in the: Amyl. n., Arg. m., Ars., Chin., Cod., Curare, *Helon.*, Kali bro., Kali mur., Lact. ac., Lyc. v., Mosch., Nat. s., Phos., Ph. ac., Tarent., Tereb., Thuja.

Thick: *Arn.*, Ars., Artem. v., Canth. Chim., Coloc., Con., Cop, Daph., Dig., Hep., Iod., Lac. def., Lyc., *Merc. cor.*, Mosch., Nux v., Par. br., Phos., Psor., *Sabad.*, *Sep.*, Stram., Sulph., Tereb., Verat.a.

getting so after standing: Berb., Bry., Cina, Coloc. Hep., Merc. s., Nux v.

butter milk, like: Aur met.

curdy: Ph.ac.

THICK.

glue like: Coloc.

jelly-like: Coloc., Crotal.

milky and: Lyc.

oil, like: Cocc. c., Dulc., Lil. tig., Stram.

Turbid when first passed: Abr., Coloc., Dulc., Hepar., Sep.

soon becomes: Ant.t., *Ars.*, Berb., ~~Bry.~~, Cham., Chel., Chin. sul., *Graph.*, Kreos., Lyc., Nat. m., Rhus t., Sars, Seneg.

standing, after: Amb., Amm. c., Apis, Berb., *Bry.*, Calc., Caust., Cham., Cina, Coloc., Con., Cupr. m., Dig., Graph., Hep., Kali nit., Laur., Lyc., Mancin., Meph., Merc., Merc. s., Mez., Nit ac., Paris q., Petr., *Ph. ac.*, Plat., Rhus t., Sars., Sep., Sulph., Sul. ac.

cloudy, smoky: Amb., Amm. benz., Anac., Ant. c., Apis, Arg. n., Ars., Aur. met., Bell., Benz. ac., *Berb.*, *Bry.*, Cact. gr., Calc. c., Cann. s., Canth., Caust., *Cham.*, Chel., Chim,. Cina, Coca, Colch., *Con.*, Crot. t., Cupr. m., Cycl, Graph., Grat., Hep., Kali c., Kreos., Lith. c., Lyc., Merc. c., *Merc. s.*, Mosch., Nat. m., Nit. ac., Nux v., Op., Phos., Ph. ac., Plumb., Psor., Puls., Rhus t., *Sabad.*, Sep., Sil., *Sulph.*, Sul. ac., *Tereb.*

COLOR:

Black or blackish: Ars. hy., Canth., Carb. ac., Chion. vir.,

COLOR, black or blackish.

Colch., Dig., Kali c., *Lach.*, Par. br., Sec. c., *Tereb.*, Verat. a.

Beer-like: Ars., Aspar., Benz. ac., Bry., Coloc., Myr. c., *Puls.*, *Sulph.*

Brandy like: Benz. ac.

Brown or brownish: Ant. t., *Arn.*, Ars., Aspar., Aur., Baryt. c., Benz. ac., Bell., Bry., Calc. c., Card. m., Caust, Chelid., Cimex, Dig., Graph., Kreos., Lach., Lac. ac., Lyc., Mancin., *Merc. cor.*, Nat. m., Nit. ac., Op., Petr., Phos., Plumb., Podo., Puls., Sep., *Sulph.*, Uva. ur.

Butter milk: **Ph.** ac.,

Changeable: Benz. ac., Chim., Sang.

Clay-like: Cham., Sars., Sep.

Clear: Alum., Amb., Anac., Apoc., Arg. m., Arg. n., Ars., Ced., Chelid., Cina, Cocc., Coloc., Con., Ferr., Gels., Graph., Ham., Helon., Hep., Hyos., *Ign.*, Kali nit., *Lact. ac.*, Lyc., Mag. p., Mosch., *Murex*, **Ph.** *ac.*, Plant., Ptel., Puls., Sars., Sep., Sulph., *Tereb.*

and copious: *Æth.*, *Anth.*, Ars., *Equis.*, *Gels.*, Helon., Ign., Kali nit., Lyc. v., Mosch., Murex, Ph. ac., Rumex, Sang., Sulph., Vib. op.

in diabetes: Ph. ac.

relieving headache: *Gels.*, Ign., Sang.

Dark: *Acon.*, Æscul. h., *Ant. t.*, Apis, Ars., Asaf., Aspar., Bar. c., Bell., *Benz. ac.*,

COLOR, dark.

Bry., *Calc. c.*, Calc. ph., Camph., Cann. i., Cann. s., Canth., Carb. ac., Ced., Chelid., Chim., Chin., *Colch.*, Conv., *Crotal.*, Crot., Dig., Elat., Equis., Eupat. perf., Ferr. i., Glon., *Graph.*, *Hell.*, Hep., Iod., Ipec., Kali bi., Kali. c., Kali i., Lac. d., *Lach.*, Led., Lil. t., Lyc., *Merc.*, Nat. m., Nit. ac., Nux mos., Op., Osmi., *Plumb.*, Pod., Ptel., Rheum, Rhod., Rhus t., *Selen.*, Sep., Staph., Sulph., Tereb., *Verat. a.*,

coffee-like: Apis, Lach., Nat. m.

Green or greenish: Ars., Aur. met., *Camph.*, Carbol. ac., Chel., Chim., Colch., Cop., Dig., Kali c., Merc., *Merc. c.*, Nit. ac., Ruta, Sant., Verat. a.

yellowish: Crot., Iod.

High colored and scanty: Acon., Apis, Bapt., *Euqis.*, Ferr. iod., Lept., Lil. tig., Nux m.

Milky Apis, Alum., Calc. c., Cina, Coloc., Iod., Lil. t., Lyc., Mur. ac., Nat. m., Nit. ac., Phos., *Ph. ac.*, Sul.

Red blood-like: Berb., Calc. c., Canth., Cham., Crot., Hep., Kali i., Merc. c., Rhus t., *Sep.*, *Tereb.*

dark, deep: Æscul., Ant. t., Apis, Arg. n., Ars., Bell., Benz. ac., Carb. v., Cham., Chelid., Crot. t., Cupr. m., Ferr., Hep., Lach., Lact. ac., Lob., Mosch., Op., Par. br.,

COLOR, red, dark.

Phyt., Polyg., Puls., Scilla, Sep., Staph., Tereb.

backache, with: Kali bi.

White, whitish: Arn., Calc., Cann. s., Caust., Chelid., Chin., Dig., Dulc., Mancin., Merc. s., Phos., Ph. ac., Psor., Rhus t.

whey, like: Arg. met., Aur. met., Nat. s., Ph. ac.

Yellow: Agar., Barty. m., Chelid., Daph., Kali i., Kalm., Laur., Merc., Raph., Sep., Spong.

dark, deep: Æscul. h., Arg. nit., Ars., Ced., Chelid., Daph., Hep., Nat., Sang.

golden: Bell., Car. m., Chelid., Mang., Phos.

greenish: Chin., Crotal., Iod.

Micturition, troubles, before: Ant. t., Arn., Bor., Bry., Canth., Coloc., Dig., Gels., Meli., Nux v., Ph. ac., Puls., Rhus t., Sep., Sul.

in the beginning of: Acon., Merc.

during: Acon., Aloe., Ant. t., Apis, Arg. n., Bap., Cann. s., Canth., Clem., Colch., Con., Dig., Dulc., Fl. ac., Hell., Hep., Hyos., Ip., K. bi., Lil. t., Merc., Lyc., Merc. c., Nit. ac., Nux v., Phos., Ph. ac., Puls., Sars., Sep., Sul., Thuja, Verat. a.

at the close of: Canth., Equis., Mez.

After: Anac., Ant. t., Arg. n., Arn., Bell., Bor., Calc. c., Cann. i., Cann. s., Canth.,

MICTURITION. troubles, after.

Caps., Chin., Coloc., Con., Dig., Fl. ac., Hep., K. bi., Merc., Mez., Nat. c., Nat. m., Nit. ac., Nux v., Par., Petrol., Petros., Phos., Puls., Ruta, Sele., Sep., Staph., Sul., Thuja, Zinc.

SEDIMENT:

Bloody: Apis, Puls., Sep.

brickdust: Cocc. c., Nat. m., Sep.

brown: Apis, Coloc., Crot. tig.

clay-coloured: Ferr. met., Sep.

crust-forming: Phos., Sep.

crystals-forming: Coloc.

greasy: Aspar.

red or reddish: Apis, Aspar., Cimex, Daph., Nit. ac., Puls., Sep.

sand: Lyc., Sep.

stains vessel red: Lach.

Black: Hell., Lach.

Blood-clotted: Alumen, Apis, Ars. hy., Cact. gr., Canth., Chim., Ham., Tereb.

Bloody-mucus: Canth., Puls.

Bloody slime: Rheum, Sulph. Uva ur.

Bluish: Ars. hy., Prun. s.

Brick-dust, like: Ant. t., Arn., Ars., Benz. ac., Bry., Caust., Chin., Chin. sul., Cop., Dig., Lob., Lyc., Merc. c., Nat. m., Nat. s., Nux v., Op., Par. br., Phos., Plant., Puls., Sep.

Casts, containing: Merc. c.

cylindrical tubes, tubular with: Apis, Canth.; Merc. c. Tereb.

CASTS.

epithelial: Apis, *Ars.*, *Merc. c.* Nat. ars., Phos.

Chalk-like: Phos.

Clay-like: Alumen, Amm. c., Amm. m., Anac., *Berb.*, Chin sul., Sars., Sep., Zinc.

Coffee-ground, like: *Apis, Hell.*, Lach., *Tereb.*

Cowdung, like: Ars.

Crystals: *Chin. sul.*, Lyc., Par br.

Flaky, flocculent: Benz. ac., *Berb.*, Cann. s., Canth., Cham., Coca, Coloc., Hep., *Merc. cor.*, Merc., Mez., Nit. ac., *Phos.*, Petr., Phos. ac.

gelationous: *Berb.*

greasy: Crot. tig.

Gravel-like: Calc c., Lach., Sars.

Greyish: *Berb.*

Mahogony color, like: Laur.

Membraneous: Alumen, Merc., Uva ur.

Milky: Ant. t., Coloc., Ferr. iod., Lyc., Phos., Ph. ac., Sec. cor.

Moss, like masses of: Asclep. t.

Mucus: Aloe., Alum., Ant. c., Aur. met., Benz. ac., *Berb.*, Bry., Canth., Chelid., Chim. *Dulc.*, Equis., Eupat. pur., Kali bi., Kali c., Kali nit., Lyc., Merc., Merc. cor., Mosch., Nat. c., *Nat. m.*, Nit. ac., Petr., Phos., Ph. ac. *Puls.*, Sars., Senecio, *Sep.*, Sulph., Tereb.

bloody: Dulc., Puls.

Muco-purulent: Benz. ac., Chim., Dulc., Kali c., Lyc., Puls.

SEDIMENT.

Mucus ropy, stringy: Chim., Hydrast., Kali bi., Ph. a^.

Mucus shreds, threads: *Berb.*, Canth.

pus and: Arn., Ars., *Canth.*, Clem., Merc., Nux v., Uva ur.

thick: *Berb.*, Chim., *Coloc.*, Cop., Dulc., Ham., Hydr., Kali c., Lyc., Merc. c., Merc. s., Nux, Par. br., Phos., Phos. ac., Psor., Sep., Spong., Ter.

tenacious, tough: Alumen, Berb., Dulc., Nux v.

Red: Bell., *Berb.*, *Canth.*, Carb. v., Card. m., Chelid., Chin., Cimex, Cocc., Con., Cop., Dulc., Graph., Ipec., Kreos., Lac. can., Lact. ac., Lith. c., Lob., Lyc., Mag. s., Mang., Merc. c., Mez., *Nat. m.*, Nat. s., Nit. ac., Nux v., Op., Osm., Par. br., Paris q., *Petr.*, Phos., Ph. ac., Psor., Puls., Scilla, *Selen.*, Sep., Sil., Still., Sulph., *Val.*, Verat. a.

Sandy, gravelly: Actea. r., Ant. c., Arg. n., Ars., Aspar., Calc. c., Canth., Chelid., Chin. sul., Cocc. c., Lach. *Lyc.*, Nat. m., Nat. s., Nit ac., Par. br., Phos., Puls., Ruta, Sars. Selen., Sep., Sil.

red: Ars., Chin., *Lyc.*, Nit. ac., Par. br., Phos., Puls., *Selen.*, Sep.

gray: Lyc., Phos., Sars.

white: Sars.

yellow: Lyc., Sil., Sep.

White: Alum., Berb., Canth., Caust., Chin., Coloc., Graph., Hep., Phos., *Sep.*

MALE GENITALIA.

AILMENTS, common:

Atrophy, penis: Agr. n., Berb., Cann. i., *Ign.*, *Lyc.*

Atrophy, testes: Aur., Caps., Carb an., Gels., Iod., *Kali i.*, Lyss., Meph.

sexual excesses, following: Staph.

Cancer: Carb. an., *Con.*

scrotum: Carb. an., Ph. ac.

testes: Spong.

Condylomata: Arg. n., Aur. m., Calc., Cinnab., Fl. ac., *Hep.*, Lyc., *Nat. s.*, *Nit. ac.*, Phos., Ph. ac., Sabin., Sars., Sep., Staph., Thuja.

penis: Apis, Calc., *Cinnab.*, Hep., Lyc., Merc., Nat. s., Nit. ac., Ph. ac., *Sabin.*, *Sep.*, Staph., Sulph., *Thuja.*

prepuce: Aur., Aur. mur., *Cinnab.*, Lyc., Nit. ac., Sabin., Sep., *Thuja.*

scrotum: Aur., Aur. mur., *Thuja.*

Eruptions:

penis: Crot. t., Rhus t.

prepuce: Ars. h., Calc., Caust., Graph., Merc., *Nit.* ac., Petr., Rhus t., Thuja.

scrotum: Ars. i., Calad., Crot. t., *Graph.*, Hep., *Petr.*, Rhus t., Rhus v.

scrotum, vesicular: Chel., *Crot. t.*, Petr., Rhus t., Rhus v.

ERUPTIONS.

syphilitic: Ars. i., *Nit. ac.*

Gangrene: Canth.

penis: Ars., Canth., Kali i., Kreos., *Lach.*, Laur.

paraphimosis, from: Lach.

scrotum: Fl. ac.

Hydrocele: *Apis*, Arn., Calc., Calc. p., Carb. s., Dig., Fl. ac., *Graph.*, Hell., Hep., *Iod.*, Lyss., Merl., Nat. m., Nux v., Psor., *Puls.*, *Rhod.*, *Sil.*, Spong., Sulph.

boys, of: Abrot., Ars., Calc., Calc. s., Graph. Kali chl., *Puls.*, *Rhod.*, *Sil.*, Sulph.

Masturbation: *Anan.*, *Bufo.*, *Lach.*, Nux v., *Orig.*, Phos., Ph. ac., *Plat.*, Staph., Stram., Tub., Ust.

Phimosis: Arn., Calc., Cann. s., Canth., Cinnab., Dig., Ham., Hep., Lyc., *Merc.*, *Nit. ac.*, Rhus t., Sulph.

paraphimosis: Coloc., Lach., *Merc.*, Merc. c., *Nit. ac.*, Rhus t.

Seminal emissions: Agar., Agn., Alum., Amm. c., Anac., Arg. m., Arg. n., Aur., Bar. c., Bar. m., Bell., Berb., Bism., *Bor.*, Bov., Bufo, *Calc.*, Calc. p., Carb. an., Carb. v., Carl., Cast., Caust., Cham., *Chin.*, Cic., Cimex, Cob., Cocc., Con., Cycl., *Cupr.*, Dig., Dios., Ery. a.,

SEMINAL EMISSIONS.

Ferr., Form., Gels., Graph., Hep., Kali br., Kali c., Kali p., Lach., Lyc., Mag. m., Merc., Mosch., Nat. a., Nat. c., Nat. m., Nat. p., Onos., Orig., Phos., Ph. ac., Pic. ac., Plat., Psor., Puls., Sabad., Sars., Sel., Sep., Sil., Staph., Stram., Sulph., Tarent., Thuja, Viol. t.

Caresses, during: Con., Gels., Nux v., Phos., Sars., Sel.

dream, without any: Anac., Camph., Con., Cor. r., Dios., Graph., Ham., Pic. ac., Stann., Zinc.

erections, without: Cob., Dios., Gels., Graph., Nat. c., Nuph., Ph. ac., Sars., Sel.

night, every: Nat. m., Nat. p., Pic. ac.

feels better after emission: Calc. p., Lach.

onanism after: Alum., Chin., Dig., Graph., Nux v., Ph. ac., Puls., Sars., Sep., Staph., Tarent.

Ulcers: Ars., Lach., Merc., Phyt., Thuja.

penis: Ars. i., Cinnab., Hep., Kali bi., Merc., Merc. c., Merc. i. f., Nit. ac., Nux. v., Ph. ac.

chancres: Aur., Aur. mur., Aur. m. n., Cinnab., Hep., Kali bi., Lac. c., Lach., Merc., Merc. c., Merc. i. f., Nit. ac., Phyt., Staph., Sulph., Thuja.

elevated margins, with: Ars., Lyc., Merc., Nit. ac.

cheesy base: Hep., Kali bi.

hard: Cinnab., Merc., Merc. c.

ULCERS.

lardaceous base: Merc., Staph., Sulph.

mercurio-syphilitic: Hep., Lach., Nit. ac., Sil., Staph., Sulph.

splinter pains: Nit ac., Thuja.

COITION,, aversion to: Graph., Lyc., Psor., Rhod.

Enjoy, cannot: Agar., Anac., Calad., Graph., Nat. m., Sep., Plat.

COLDNESS: Agn., Lyc., Dios., Gels., Iris, Sulph.

penis: Agn., Lyc., Onos., Sulph.

Scrotum: Berb., Caps., Merc.

Testes: Agn., Merc.

ERECTIONS: Amm. c., Aur., Cann. i., Canth., Euph., Fl. ac., Iod., Kali c., Kali i., Kreos., Nat. c., Nat. m., Nux v., Op., Phos., Ph. ac., Pic. ac., Plat., Plb., Puls., Sep., Sil., Staph., Stram.

Coition, after: Sep.

Continued: Cann. i., Canth., Coloc., Graph., Kali br., Nat. c., Nat. m., Phos., Pic. ac., Plat., Puls.

Delayed: Bar. c., Calc., Sel.

Excessive: Aur. m., Canth., Fl. ac., Graph., Ph. ac., Pic. ac.

Incomplete: Agar., Agn., Bar. c., Calad., Calc., Camph., Cob., Con., Graph., Hep., Lyc., Nat. c., Nat. p., Nuph., Nux m., Nux v., Petr., Phos., Ph. ac., Sel., Sep., Sulph.

during coition: Camph. Con., Form., Graph., Lyc., Phos. Ph. ac., Sep., Sulph,

ERECTIONS.

Painful: Arg. n., Calad., Camph., Cann. i., *Cann. s.*, *Canth.*, *Caps.*, Colch., Cub., Dig., Kali chl., Nit. ac., Nux, Petros., Phos., Puls., Sil., *Ter.*, Thuja.

Strong: *Canth., Fl. ac.*, Graph., Lach., *Phos., Pic. ac.*,

Violent: Alum., Canth., Cham., Clem., *Fl. ac.*, Gels., Graph., Hyos., Kali chl., *Mez.*, Nat. c., Nit. ac., Op., *Phos.*, *Pic. ac., Plat., Plb.*, Sil., Stram.

Wanting: Agar., *Agn.*, Alum., Arg. n., *Bar. c.*, Bufo, *Calad.*, Calc., *Calc. s.*, Camph., Caust., *Chin.*, Cob., Coc. c., *Con.*, Ferr., Graph., Ham., Hell., Iod., Lach., *Lyc.*, Nat. c., Med., Nit. ac., Nuph., Nux m., *Nux v.* Onos., Op., Phos., Ph. ac., Phyt., Plb., Psor., Puls., *Sel.*, Sep., Stann., Staph., *Sulph.*, Thuja.

penis relaxed, when excited: *Calad.*

penis, small and cold: Agn., Bar. c., *Lyc.*, Sulph.

FLACCIDITY: *Agn.*, Calad., Dios., Gels.

Penis: *Agn.*, Calad., Bar. c., Cann. i., *Lyc.*, Mur. ac., Nux m., Nux v.

HAIR, falling of: *Nat. m.*, Nit. ac., Ph. ac., Selen., Zinc.

INDURATION:

Penis: Sep.

Testes: Arg. m., Aur., Bar. c., Calc., Calc. f., Carb. an.,

INDURATION, testes.

Cinnab., Clem., Con., Cop., Graph., Iod., Kali i., *Med.*, Merc., Merc. i.r., Nux v., Puls., *Rhod.*, Sil., Spong., Staph., Sulph., Viol. t.

Epididymis: Aur., Med., Rhod., Spong.

INFLAMMATION: Apis, *Ars.*, Canth., Merc., Rhus t., Spong.

Penis: Arn., Ars., Kali i., Psor., Sulph.

Scrotum: Ars., Rhus t., Rhus v.

Spermatic cords: Berb., *Puls.*, Rhod., Spong., Syph.

Testes: Acon., Arg. n., Arn., Ars., Aur., *Bapt.*, Bell., Berb., Clem., Con., Kali i., Lyc., Merc., Nat. m., Nit. ac., Nux v., Phyt., Plb., *Puls., Rhod., Rhus t.*, Spong., Staph.

Epididymis: Aur., Chin., Med., *Puls., Rhod., Spong.*

ITCHING OF THE SCROTUM: Ambr., Apis, Aur., Calc., Calc. p., Carb. s., Caust., Chel., Cist., Cocc., Crot. t., Graph., *Kali c.*, Kali chl., Kali s., Lyc., Mag. m., Mang., Merc., Mur. a, *Nat. m.*, Nit. ac., Nuph., Nux v., *Petr.*, Rhod., Rhus t., Sars., Sel., Sil., Staph., Urt. u., Viol. t., Zinc.

SEXUAL PASSIONS:

Diminished: Agn., Alum., *Bar. c.*, Clem., Dios., Ferr., *Graph.*, Hep., Ign., Kali c., Kali i., Kali p., *Lyc.*, Mag. c., Mur. ac., Nat. m.,

SEXUAL PASSIONS:

Nit. ac., Nuph., Ph. ac., Psor., Rhod., Sep., *Sil.*, *Staph.*, Sulph.

Increased: Agar., All. c., Amm. ., Anac., *Anan.*, Ant. c., Aur., Bar. m., Bufo, *Calc.*, *Calc. p.*, Camph., *Cann. i.*, Can. s., Canth., Cast., Chin., Cinnab., Cocc., Coc. c., Coff., *Con.*, Croc., Dios., Ferr., Fl ac., Gels., Graph., Hep., Hyos., Ign., Iod., Kali bi., Kali c., Kali i., Kali n., Lac. c., Lach., Laur., *Lyc.*, *Lyss.*, Merc., Mez., Mosch., Nat. c., Nat. h., Nat. m., Plb., Nat. s., Nat. p., Nit. ac., *Nux v.*, Op., *Phos.*, Ph. ac., *Pic. ac.*, *Plat.*, *Puls.*, Sabin., Sep., *Sil.*, Stann., *Staph.*, Stram., Tarent., Thuja, *Tub.*

Erection, without: Agar., Agn., Alum., Amm. c., Anan., Arg. m., Arg. n., Aur., *Calad.*, Calc., Camph., Chin., *Con.*, Dig., *Graph.*, Lyc., Nat. m..

ERECTION, without.

Nat. p., Nux v., Phos., Ph. ac., Psor., Sel., Sep., Sil., Staph.

Violent: Anac., *Anan.*, Bufo, *Cann. i.*, *Canth.*, Fl. ac., Graph., Kali br., Lyss., Nat. h., *Phos.*, *Pi. ac.*, *Plat.*, *Sil.*, Stram., Tarent., *Tub.*, *Zinc.* sexual mania: *Phos.*, Tarent.

Wanting: Agn., Arg. n., Berb., Camph., Caps., *Carb. s.*, Carb. v., Graph., Hell., Ign., Iod., *Kali bi.*, Kali br., Kali c., Lyc., Nat. m., Nit. ac., Nuph., Onos., Ph. ac., Plb., Psor. Sulph.

SHRIVELLING:

Scrotum, of: Crot. t.

Spermatic cord, of: Caps.

SWEAT, PERSPIRATION:

Aur., Bell., Calad., Calc., Canth., Carb. v., Cor. r., Fl. ac., Gels., Merc., Petr., Puls., *Sel.*, *Sep.*, Sulph., *Thuja.*

FEMALE GENITALIA.

AILMENTS, common:

Abortion: Alet., *Apis*, Arn., Asar., *Bell.*, Bry., Calc., Canth., Caul., *Cham.*, Chin., Cimic., Cocc., *Croc.*, Ferr., Ferr. i., Hep., Hyos., *Ip.*, Iris, Kali c., Lyc., Mill., *Nux m.*, Nux v., Plat., *Puls.*, Rhus t., *Sabin.*, *Sec.*, *Sep.*, Sulph., Vib.

month, second: Apis, Kali c.
month, third: Sabin., Sec.
month, fifth to seventh: Sep.
last months: Opium.

Cancer: Arg. m., Arg. n., *Ars.*, *Ars. i.*, Bufo, Calc., Carb. an., Carb. v., *Con.*, *Graph.*, *Hydr.*, Iod., *Kreos.*, *Lach.*, Merc. i. f., *Murex*, Nat. c., Nat. m., Nit. ac., *Phos.*, Phyt., Sec., *Sep.*, *Sil.*, Staph., *Thuja*, Zinc.

vagina: *Kreos.*

Condylomata: Calc., Lyc., Merc., Sabin., Sars., Staph., *Thuja.*

uterus: Calc., *Kreos.*, Merc., Nit. ac., *Thuja.*

vagina: Nit. ac., Phos., Staph., Thuja.

Displacement of uterus: Amm. m., *Bell.*, *Calc.*, Calc. p., Caul., Cimic., Ferr. i., *Lach.*, *Lil. t.*, Mag. m., Merc., Murex, *Nat. m.*, Nit. ac., Nux m., Nux v., Plat., Podo., *Sep.*, Thuja.

AILMENTS, common.

Excrescences: *Kreos.*, *Nit. ac.*, *Thuja.*

uterus: Kreos., *Nit. ac.*, *Thuja.*

cauliflower: Graph., Kreos., Phos., *Thuja.*

Leucorrhœa: *Æsc.*, Alet., *Alum.*, Amm. c., Amm. m., Arg. n., *Ars.*, Ars. i., Aur. m., Bar. c., Bar. m., Bor., Bov., *Calc.*, Calc. p., *Calc. s.*, *Carb. an.*, Carb. s., Carb. v., *Caust.*, Chin., Cimic., Cinnab., Cocc., Con., Ferr., *Graph.*, Hep. Hydr., Iod., Kali ar., Kali bi., *Kali c.*, Kali chl., Kali i., Kali p., Kali s., *Kreos.*, Lac. c., Lach., Lyc., Mag. m., *Merc.*, Merc. c., Mur. ac., Nat. a., Nat. c., *Nat. m.*, Nat. p., *Nit. ac.*, Nux m., Orig., Pall., Petr., Phos., Ph. ac., *Plat.*, Podo., Psor., *Puls.*, Sabin., Sars., Sep., Sil., *Stann.*, Sulph., Sul. ac., Tarent., Thuja, Zinc.

albuminous: Alum., Amm. m., *Bor.*, Bov., Calc. p., Mez., *Nat. m.*, Petr., Plat., Podo., Sep., Stann., Sul. ac.

bloody: Alum., Ant. t., Arg. m., Arg. n., Ars., Ars. i., Bar. c., Calc. s., Carb. v., *Chin.*, *Cocc.*, Con., Iod., Kreos., Lyc., Merc., Merc. c., *Nit. ac.*, Phos., *Sep.*, Sil., Sul. ac., Ter., Tril.

LEUCORRHŒA.

cream-like: Calc. p., Nat. p., Puls., Sec., Tril.

girls, in little: Cann. s., Cub., Merc., Puls., Sep.

gonorrhœal: Aur. m., Cann., s., Nit. ac., Puls., Sep., Thuja.

greenish: Arg. n., Asaf., Bov., Carb. ac., Carb. v., Kali i., Kali p., Kali s., Lach., Merc., Murex, Nat. c., Nat. m., Nat. s., Nit. ac., Sec., Sep.

gushing: Calc., Cocc., Gels., Graph., Lyc., Sep., Sil.

milky: Amm. c., Bor., Calc., Calc. p., Crab. v., Con., Ferr., Kali chl., Kreos., Phos., Puls., Sep., Sil., Sulph., Sul. ac.

offensive: Aral., Arg. m., Ars., Carb. ac., Chin., Kali ar., Kali p., Kreos., Nat. a., Nat. c., Nit. ac., Nux v., Psor., Pyrog., Sabin., Sang., Sec., Sep., Sil., Sulph., Ust.

ropy: Asar., Bor., Bov., Caust., Coc. c., Croc., Graph., Hydr., Kali bi., Nat. c., Nit. ac., Phyt., Sabin.

Masturbation, disposition: Calad., Grat., Lach., Orig., Plat.

Metrorrhagia: Acet. ac., Acon., Agn., Apis, Apoc., Arg. n., Arn., Ars., Ars. i., Bell., Bov., Bry., Calc., Canth., Carb. an., Carb. s., Carb. v., Card. m., Caul., Cham., Chin., Chin. s., Cimic., Cina, Coc. c., Coff., Colch., Croc., Erig., Fer., Ferr. i., Ferr. m., Ferr. p., Ham.,

METRORRHAGIA.

Helon., Hep., Hyos., Ign., Iod., Ip., Kali br., Kali c., Kali chl., Kali fer., Kreos., Lac. c., Lach., Lyc., Med., Merc., Mill., Nat. c., Nat h., Nit. ac., Nux m., Nux v., Phos., Plat., Psor., Puls., Rat., Sabin., Sec., Senec., Sep., Sil., Stram., Sulph., Tril., Ust.

black: Carb. v., **Cham.**, Croc., Elaps, **Ferr.**, Helon., Kreos., *Plat.*, Puls., Sec., Sul. ac.

bright red: Arn., Bell., Calc., Cinnm., Ham., *Ip.*, Mill., Phos., Sabin., Sang., Tril

climacteric period: Alet., Aloe., Calc., Carb. v., Croc., Ferr., Lach., Med., Murex, Nux v., Plb., Puls., Sabin., Sang., Sec., Sep., Tril., Ust.

coition, after: Arg. n., Arn., Ars., Hydr., Kreos., Sep

gushing: Bell., Cham., Ham., Ip., Mill., Phos., Sabin., Puls., Sec., Ust.

labor, during and after: Arn., Bell., Cham., Chin., Cinnm., Croc., Ferr., Hyos., Ip., Phos., Plat., Sabina, Sec., Ust.

motion aggravates the condition: Bry., Coff., Croc., Helon., Ip., Sabin., Sec.

nursing the child, while: Sil.

paroxysms, in: Cham., Puls., Sabin., Carb. v., Chin. s., Ham., Kali fer., Sec.

polypus, from: Calc., Con.

METRORRHAGIA.

profuse: Arn., Bell., *Calc.*, Cham., Chin., *Ip.*, Kreos., Nux v., *Phos.*, Sabin, Sec.

scrawny women: Sec.

stop, after every: *Ambr.*

string blood: *Ust.*

tall women: Phos.

Placenta, retained: Agn., Ars., Bell., *Canth.*, Caul., Puls., Sabin., Sec., *Sep.*

Prolapsus uterus: Æsc., Alet., Aloe., Alum., Alumn., Apis, *Arg. m.*, Arg. n., Arn., *Aur.*, Bell., Benz. ac., Bry., Calc., Cal. p., Carb. an., Chin., Con., Ferr., Ferr. i., Graph., Helon., Kali bi., Kali c., Lach., Lil. t., Lyss., Murex, *Nat. h.*, Nat. m., Nit. ac., Nux m., Nux v., *Pall.*, Petr., Phos., Plat., Podo., Puls., *Rhus t.*, Sabin., Sec., *Sep.*, Sil., Stann., Sulph., Thuja.

crossing legs ameliorates: Lil. t., Murex, Sep.

Sterility: Alet., Amm. c., Aur., Bar. m., *Bov.*, Calc., Coff., Con., Ferr., Ferr. p. Graph., Iod., Kreos., Lach., Merc., Nat. c., Nat. m., Orig., Phos., Phyt., Plat., *Sep.*, Sil., *Sul. ac.*, Zinc.

Sub-involution: Bell., Calc., Caul., *Cimic.*, Hydr., Kali bi., Kali i., Lil. t., Nat. p., Op., *Puls.*, Sabin., Sec., *Sep.*, *Sulph.*, Ust.

Tumours: Calc., Lyc.

encysted: Graph., Sabin., Sil.

erectile: Carb. an., Carb. v., Lach., Nit. ac., Phos., Thuja.

TUMORS.

ovarian: *Apis*, Ars., Bar. m., Calc., Coloc., Iod., *Lach.*, *Lyc.*, Plat., Podo.

right: Apis, Iod., *Lyc.*, Podo.

left: *Lach.*, Podo.

cysts: Apis, Bov., Bufo, Coloc., Iod., Lach., Plat., Rhus t.

fibroids: Podo.

uterine fibroids: Apis, Aur. m.n., *Calc.*, Calc. f., Calc. p., Calc. s., Con., Kali c., Lach., Lyc., Merc. c., *Phos.*, Sil.

vaginal cysts: Lyc., Puls., Sil.

Vaginismus: Acon., Bell., Berb., *Cact.*, Canth., Ferr. p., Ham., Ign., Lyc., Nat. m., *Plb.*, Puls., Sil.

COITION, aversion to: Agn., Caust., Clem., Graph., Kali br., Lach., Med., *Nat. m.*, Petr., Phos., Psor., Rhod., Sep.

Enjoyment, absent: Berb., Brom., *Caust.*, Ferr., Ferr. m., Graph., Med., Nat. m., Phos., *Sep.*

DESIRE, increased: Ant. c., Apis, Ars., Ars. i., Asaf., Bar. m., Bell., Calad., *Calc.*, Calc. p., Camph., Canth., Carb. v., Coff., Con., Fl. ac., Gels., *Grat.*, Hyos., Ign., Kali br., Kali p., Lac. c., *Lach.*, Lil. t., Merc., Mosch., Murex, Nat. a., Nat. c., Nux v., Op., Orig., Phos., Pic. ac., *Plat.*, *Puls.*, Raph., Sabin., Sil., Stan., Stram., Tarent., *Verat.*, Zinc.

insatiable: Calc. p., Lach., Plat., Sabin., Zinc.

DESIRE, increased.

   lying-in-women, in: Chin.

   violent: Ars., *Calc.*, Calc. p.,
   Gels., Hyos., Lach.,
   Mosch, *Murex*, Orig.,
   Phos., Plat., Sabin., Sil.,
   Stram., Tarent., Zinc.

   involumtary orgasm, with:
   Arg. n., Ars., Calc., Lil.
   t., Nux v., *Plat.*

   masturbation, driving her to:
   Gels., Grat., Nux v.,. Orig.,
   Plat., Zinc.

   virgins, in: Con., *Plat.*

   widows, in: *Apis.*

FLATUS COMING FROM
VAGINA: Bell., *Brom.*,
Calc., Lac. c., *Lyc.*, Mag. c.,
Nat. c., Nux m., Nux v., *Ph.
ac.*, Sang., Sep.

MENSES, black: Amm. c.,
Amm. m., Bell., Carb. an.,
Carb. v., Chin., Cocc., Croc.,
Cycl., Elaps, Ferr., Ign.,
Kali n., *Lach.*, Lyc., Mag. c.,
Mag. m., Nat. p., Nux v.,
Ol. an., Plat., *Puls.*, Sang.,
Sec., Stram., Sulph.

   Copious, aggravated during exertions: Ambr., Bov., *Calc.*,
   Calc. p., Nit. ac.

   Delayed appearance of the first
   menses in girls: Aur., Bar. c.,
   Calc., Calc. p., *Caust.*, Con.,
   Ferr., *Graph.*, *Kali c.*, Kali
   p., Lyc., Mag. c., Mang.,
   Nat. m., Petr., *Puls.*, Sabin.,
   Senec., Sep., Sulph., Zinc.

   Membraneous: *Bor.*, Bry., Calc.,
   Calc. p., Canth., Cham.,
   Cycl., Kali bi., *Lac. c.*, Phos.

   Offensive: *Bell.*, *Bry.*, Carb. an.,
   Carb. v., Caust., Cham.,

MENSES, offensive.

   Croc., Ign., Kali ar., Kali c.,
   Kali p., *Kreos.*, Lil. t., Plat.,
   Psor., *Sabin.*, Sang., Sec.,
   Sil.

   Painful dysmenorrhœa [menstruation]: Acon.,
   Amm. c., Ars., *Bell.*, Berb.,
   Bor., Cact., Calc., *Calc. p.*,
   Caul., Caust., *Cham.*, Cimic.,
   Cocc., Coff., Coloc., Con.,
   Croc., Cycl., Dulc., Gels.,
   Graph., Ign., Kali ar., *Kali
   c.*, Kali i., Kali p., Kali s.,
   Lac. c., Lach., Lil. t., *Meli.*,
   Merc., Nat. c., Nux v., Phos.,
   Plat., Puls., Rhus t., Sabin.,
   Sec., Senec., Sep., Sulph.,
   Verat. Xanth.

   Pitch-like: Cact., Cocc., Graph.,
   Mag. c., Plat.

   Return after having ceased the
   periods: Calc., Kreos.,
   Lach., Nux v.

   excitement, from: Calc.

   Scanty, at day time: Bov.,
   Mag. c.

   morning, flow only in: Sep.

   Short duration: Alum., Amm.
   c., Asaf., Bar. c., Berb.,
   Carb. s., Cocc., Con.,
   Dulc., Graph., *Lach.*,
   Mang., Merc., Nat. m.,
   Nux v., Phos., Plat., *Puls.*,
   Sep., *Sulph.*, *Thuja.*

   one day, only: Alum., Apis,
   Arg. n., *Sep.*

   Sleep, only during: Mag. c.

   gushes in: Coca.

   Suppressed: Abrot., Acon.,
   Agn., Amm. c., Ant. c.,
   Apis, Arg. n., Ars., Aur. m.,
   Bar. c., *Bell.*, Brom., Bry.,
   Calc., Carb. a, Carb. s.,

MENSES, suppressed.

Caust., Cham., Chin. a.,
Cocc., Coc. c., *Con.*, Cupr.,
Cycl., Dig., *Dulc.*, Ferr.,
Ferr. ar., *Ferr. i.*, Ferr. p.,
Gels., *Graph.*, Hell., Hyos.,
Kali ar., *Kali c.*, Kali n.,
Kali s., Kalm., *Lach.*, *Lyc.*,
Mag. m., Nat. m., Nit. ac.,
Nux m., Phos., *Puls.*, Rhod.,
Rhus t., Sabad., Senec., Sep.,

MENSES, suppressed.

Sil., Staph., Stram., Sulph.,
Ust., Val., Verat.

Tenacious: *Croc.*, Cup., Mag.
c., Plat., Puls.

SENSITIVE:

Vagina: Bell., Berb., Coff.,
Ferr., Kreos., Nat. m., *Plat.*,
Sep., Sil., *Staph.*, Thuja.

UPPER EXTREMITIES.

ARTHRITIC COMPLAINTS:
Bry., Hep., Lach., Lyc.,
Merc., Petr., Phos., Rhod.,
Rhus t., Sabin., Sars., Spig.

Elbows and wrists: Grat., Mag.
s.

Fingers and finger joints: Ant.
c., Bry., Carb. an., Clem.,
Grat., Hep., Lyc., Mang.,
Nicc., Nit. ac., Ox. ac.,
Petr., Rhod., Rhus t., Sars.,
Sep., Spig.

Forearms: Merc.

right: Nit. ac.

wrists, left: Gua., Mag. s.

Shoulder:

left: Gua., Merc. c., Sulph.
right: Iris, Lob., Lyc.,
Pallad., Sang.

ARTHRITC NODES: Ant. c.,
Apis, Aur., *Benz. ac.*, Bry.,
Calc., Calc. s., Caust., Cic.,
Clem., Colch., Dig., Form.,
Graph., Gua., Kali i., Led.,
Lith., *Lyc.*, Merc., Puls.,
Rhod., Rhus t., Sil., Staph.,
Sulph., Urt. u.

ATAXIA: Agar., Arg. n., Calc.,
Caust., Cocc., Fl. ac., Gel.,
Graph., Hell., Lil. t., Nux v.,
Onos., Phos., Sil., Stram.,
Zinc.

ATROPHY: Iod., Lyc., Plb.

arm, upper: Nit. ac.
forearm: Phos.
fingers: Sil.

ATROPHY.

hand: Phos.
thumb: Thuja.
wrist: Plb.
Exostoses: *Calc. f.*, Sil.
forearm: Dulc.
fingers: Calc. f.

CALLOSITIES, HORNY, on
hands: Amm. c., *Graph.*,
Sulph.

CORNS: Acet. ac., Amm. c.,
Ant. c., Arn., B . c.,, Bor.,
Bry., Calc., Calc. s., Carb.
an., Caust., Cur., Graph.,
Ign., *Lyc.*, Nat. m., Nux v.,
Petr., Ph. ac., Phos., Ran. s.,
Rhus t., *Sep.*, *Sil.*, Sulph.

Felon (Onychia, Paronychia,
Panaritium etc): Phyt., Rhus
t., *Sil.*, Sulph.

cold application ameliorates:
Apis, Fl. ac., Led., *Nat
s.*, *Puls.*

bones are affected: Lach.,
Sil.

gangrenous: Ars., Lach.

hangnails:, from: Nat. m.

injury, from: Led.

itching: *Apis.*

lymphatics inflamed: Bufo,
Hep., Lach.

maltreated: Hep., Sil., Sulph.

panaritium: All. c., Amm. c.,
Amm. m., Anac., Anthr.,
Apis, Benz. ac., **Bufo**,
Calc., Caust., Cist., *Fl*

FELON, panaritium.

    ac., *Hep.*, *Hyper.*, *Iod.*, Iris, Lach., *Lyc.*, Merc., Nat. c., Nat. h., Nat. m., Nat. s., *Nit. ac.*, Phyt., Rhus t., Sang., Sep., *Sil.*, Sulph., *Tarent. c.*

    run around: Apis, Caust., Fl. ac., Hep., Mer., Nat. h., Nat. m., Nat. s., Sang., Sil.

    vaccination, after: Thuja.

    sloughing: *Anthr.*

    stinging pains: *Apis*, *Lach.*, Sil.

    suppurative stage: Calc. s., *Hep.*, Sil.

    winter, every: *Hep.*

Ganglion:

    hand, back of: Ph. ac., Sil.

    wrists, on: Calc., Sil.

Gangrene: *Ars.*, Carb. v., Chin., Crot. h., *Lach.*, Phos., Plb., *Sec.*

    fingers: Sec.

    hand: Arn., Lach., Sec.

    shoulder: Crot. h.

Hang nails: Calc., Merc., *Nat. m.*, Rhus t., Sil., *Sulph.*, Thuja.

In co-ordination: Merc., Onos.

Paralysis: Acon., *Agar.*, Apis, Ars., Bar. c., Bell., Calc., *Cann. i.*, Caust., Cocc., Dulc., Hell., Kali c., Nit. ac., Nux v., Op., Plb., *Rhus t.*, Stann., Sulph.

    right: Æsc., Amm. c.

    tongue, of: Caust.

    left: *Dig.*

    apoplexy: *Phos.*

    coldness, with: Dulc., Rhus t.

    diphtheria, after: Caust.

PARALYSIS.

    insensibility, with: Rhus t.

    pain in heart, with: Nat. m.

    sensation of: Abrot., Æsc., Alum., *Amm. m.*, Ars., Chin., *Cocc.*, Colch., Cycl., Ferr., Gran., Ign., Iod., Lith., Nux v., Phos., Sep., Sil., Tab., Verat., Zinc.

    shocks, with: *Nux v.*

Varices: Nux v., *Puls.*

Warts: Calc., Caust., Nat. s., Sep., Sil.

    hands: Ant. c., *Bar. c.*, *Calc.*, *Caust.*, *Dulc.*, Ferr., Lach., Lyc., Nat. c., Nat. m., *Nit. ac.*, Ph. ac., Psor., Rhus., Sep., Sulph., Thuja.

    flat: *Dulc.*, Sep.

    horny: Ant. c., Caust., Sep., itching: Sep.

    large: Dulc.

    sensitive: Nat. c.

BURNING:

    Arms: Agar., Alum., Berb., Bry., Phos., Plat., Puls., Rhus, Rhus rad.

    Humeri: Rhus t.

    Shoulder: Carb. veg., Graph., Rhus, Stront., Tabacum.

    Upper arm: *Agar.*, Berb., Sulph. elbow: Alum.

    Forearm: *Agar.*, Sulph.

    Hand: Bry., Carb. veg., Led., Nat. s., *Phos.*, Plat., Rhus, Sec. c., Sep., Stan., Tarent.

    Wrist: Nat. c.

    Palms of hands: Lach., Lyc., Petr., *Phos.*, Sang., Sep., Stann., Sulph.

BURNING.

Fingers: Agar., Alum., Borax, Croc., Kali c., Mosch., Nat. c., Oleand., Plat., *Sil.*, Teucr. finger-tips: Mur. ac.

CHILL BEGINS AND SPREADS FROM ARMS: Hell.

In right arm: Hell.

left hand: Carb. veg.

During the pain in hand and fingers: Nux.

CLENCHED THUMBS: Æth., Apis, Camph., Caust., Cham., Cocc., *Cupr.*, Glon., Sec.

Epilepsy, in: Bufo, Caust., Cic., Lach., Stann.

Fight, after: Ign.

COLDNESS: *Bell.*, Calc., Camph., Caust., Dulc., Led., Mez., Op., *Phos.*, Plb., *Puls.*, Rhus t., Sil.

Cough, during: Hep., Rhus t.

Paralysed arm: Dulc., Rhus t.

Rheumatism, in: Sang.

Shoulder, epilepsy in: Caust.

Upper, arm, burning, with: Graph.

Forearm, icycold: *Brom.*

Hands: Acon., Agar., Ant. t., Apis, Arg. n., Arn., *Ars.*, Ars. i., *Aur.*, Bar. m:, Bov., Brom., Cact., Calc., *Calc p.*, Camph., Carb. s., Carb. v., Caust., Cedr., *Chel.*, Chin., Chin. s., Cina, Croc., Cycl., Dig., Dros., Eup. per., *Ferr., Ferr. i., Ferr. p.,* Gels., Hell., *Iod., Ip.,* Kali ar., *Kali c., Kali p., Lach.,* Led., *Lyc.,* Mang., Med., Meny., Merc., Mez., *Mur. ac., Nat. c., Nat. m.,* Nat. p., Nit. ac.,

COLDNESS, hands.

Nux m., Nux v., *Olnd.,* Op., Pall., *Samb.,* Sang., *Sec.,* Sep., Stram., Sulph., Sumb., Tab., Thuja, *Verat., Verat. v.,* Zinc.

abdomen, cutting and tearing in, with: Ars.

hot face, with: *Arn., Stram.,* Thuja.

Icy: Acon., Arg. n., Cact., Camph., Carb. v., Caust., Eup. p., Manc., Meny., Nat. c., *Nux m.,* Nux v., Ph. ac., Plb., *Verat.*

Menses, during: Arg. n., Graph., Phos.

One hot, other cold: Chin., Dig., Ip., Mosch., **Puls.**

Fingers: Calc., Calc. p., **Carb. s.,** Cham., *Chel.,* Dig., **Hell.,** *Kali c.,* Lac. c., **Lac. d.,** Meny., Ph. ac., Rhus t., **Sep.,** *Tarax., Thuja.*

CONTRACTION: Calc., **Hydr.** ac., Ip., Rhus t.

Spasmodic: Ipecac.

Upper arm: Nat. m.

tendons: *Caust.*

Elbow: Apis, Caust., Puls.

Forearm: Caust., Meny.

Hand: Anac., Caust., Nux v., Sec., Sil.

Fingers: Ant. t., Apis, Ars., Calc., *Caust.,* Cupr. ac., Ferr., Graph., Merc. c., Nat. c., Plat., Sec., Sil.

CONVULSIONS: *Bell.,* Cham., Cic., Cocc., Ign., Iod., Ip., Op., Plat., Sec., Sil., Stram., Sulph.

Forearm: Chin., Sec., Zinc.

CONVULSION.

Wrist: Nat. m.

Hand: Bell., Iod., Stram.

Fingers: Bell., Calc., Chel., Cic., Cupr., Ign.

Thumb: Cocc.

CRACKED HANDS: Æsc., Alum., Amm. c., Aur., Aur. m., *Calc.*, Carb. s., Cist., Graph., Hep., Lach., Lyc., Merc., Nat. c., Nat. m., Lyc., Merc., Nat. c., Nat. m., *Nit. ac., Petr.*, Psor., Puls., Rhus t., *Sars.*, Sep., *Sil.*, Sulph., Zinc.

CRAMPS: *Amm. c., Calc.*, Jatr., Nat. m., Tab.

Shoulder: Plat.

Upper arms: Ph. ac.

Forearm, on holding something in hand: Rhus t., Valer.

Wrist: Ph. ac.

out-stretched when arm is: Cina.

Hand: Agar., *Bell., Calc.*, Coloc., Cupr., Graph., Kali bi., Kali s., Nat. m., Phys.

cholera, in: *Cupr.*, Sec.

grasping: *Dros.*

writing: Anac., Cycl., Nat. p.

Fingers: Arn., Carb. v., Chel., Cupr. a., Nat. m., Stann., Sulph.

cholera, with: Colch., *Cupr.*, Sec., *Verat.*

periodical: Phos.

pick up a small object, on attempting to: Stann.

playing piano or violin: Mag. p.

writing, while: Mag. p., *Stann.*

CRIPPLED, finger nails: Caust., *Graph.*, Nit. ac., Sabad., Sep., *Sil.*, Thuja.

DISTORTED NAILS: Fl. ac., *Graph.*, Sep., *Sil.*

EMACIATION: Iod., Lyc., Plb.

Shoulder: Plb., Sumb.

Upper arm: Nit. ac.

Forearm: Phos.

EXTERNAL AND FLEXED ALTERNATELY (arms): Cupr., Tab.

EXTENSION OF FINGERS, difficult: Ars., Camph., Coloc., Cupr. ar.

FLEXED:

Upper limb: Acon., Carb. o., Hydr. ac., Morph., Plb., Stry., Tax.

Fingers: Ars., Plat., *Plb.*, Stram.

HEAT:

Hands: *Agar., Ant. t., Bar. c., Bell.*, Carb. v., Cham., *Chel.*, Cycl., Fl. ac., Glon., Graph., Gua., Iod., Kali bi., Kali c., Kal. p., *Lach., Led.*, Lil. t., *Lyc., Nat. c., Nit. ac., Nux m.*, Nux v., *Op.*, Petr., Ph. ac., *Phos.*, Plan., Psor., *Puls., Rhod.*, Sabad, *Sep.*, Spig., Stann., Staph., *Sulph., Tarax.*

back of hands: Apis, *Nat. c., Rhus t.*

coldness of feet, during: Nux m., Sep.

or hot feet and hands: Sep.

flushes, in: *Sulph.*

beginning in hands: Phos.

Palm: *Acon., Asar.*, Bor., Bry., Calc., Eup. per., Ferr., Fl. ac., Gels., *Ip., Lach.*, Lil. t., *Lyc., Mur. ac.*, Nux v., Petr., *Phos.*, Samb., Sep., Stann., *Sulph.*

HEAVINESS, tired limbs feel: Agar., Alum., Amm. c., Amm. m., Ang., Ant. t., Apis, *Arg. n.,* Arg. m., Calc., Carb. ac., *Caust.,* Con., Cur., Ferr., *Gels.,* Glon., Ham., Lach., Led., Nat. c., Nat. m., Nux m., Onos., *Phos.,* Pic. ac., *Plb., Puls.,* Sabad., Sil., Stann., Stram., Sulph., Sumb.

Right: *Amm. m.,* Apis.

Left: Dig.

Ascending steps: Nux v.

Exertion, on: Pic. ac.

Motion, on: Stann.

ameliorates: Apis.

Playing piano aggravates: Cur., Gels.

Walking, while: Anac., Ang.

Writing, while: Carb. v.

Shoulder: Ferr., Nat. m., Nux m., Puls.

Elbow: Chin. a., Samb.

Forearm: *Arg. n.,* Croc., Mur. ac., Tell.

Hand: Alum., Ars., Bar. c., *Bell.,* Bov., Caust., Lyc., Phos., Zinc.

INDURATION OF MUSCLES, upper limbs: Mag. c., Tab.

Forearm: Sil.

Hands: Ars., Sulph.

palm: Cist., Lyc.

Fingers: Caust.

INFLAMMATION: Rhus t.

Erysipelatous: Apis, Kali c., Ph. ac., *Rhus t.*

Upper arm (erysipelatous): Bell.

Elbow: Ant. c., Lac. ac., Lach., Sulph.

Forearm: Ars., Rhus t.

Wrist: Euph., Rhus t.

Hand: Anthr., Crot. h., Kalm., Lach., Lyc., Rhus t., Sil.

INFLAMMATION, hand.

palm: Bry.

Fingers: Apis, Cupr., Hep., Mag. c., Sil.

bone: Staph.

joints: Lyc.

bursitis: Ruta.

nails: Kali c.

around: Nat. m., Nat. s.

root of: Hep.

INJURIES, shoulders: Ferr. m., Rhus t.

Wrist: Arn., Calc., Rhus t., Ruta, Stront.

Hand:

contusion: Arn.

fracture with laceration: Hyper.

lacerations: Calend.

sprain: Arn., Calc., Rhus t., Ruta.

Fingers:

amputed stump painful: Staph.

dissecting wounds: Apis, *Ars., Lach.*

nails of: Hyper, Led.

lacerations: Hyper.

splinter of glass: Sil.

JERKING: Alum., Arg. n., Bar. m., Cic., Cupr., Graph., Hyos., Ign., Ip., Puls., *Stram.,* Sulph., Thuja, Zinc.

Shoulder: Ars., Alum., Puls.

Upper arm: Anac., Meny.

Elbow: Stram.

Forearm: Cic., Hyper., Jal.

Wrist: Anac., Arund., Pall.

Hand: Cina, Cocc., Coff., Cupr., Merc., Nat. m., *Stram.*

Fingers: Calc., Cic., Cocc., Nat. c.

LAMENESS: Brom., Calc., Cinnab., Cocc., Cycl., Ferr., Fl. ac., Mag. c., Phyt., Psor., Rhus t., Sep.

Shoulder: All. c., Fl. ac., Lach., Nat. m., Rhus t.

Upper arm: Abrot., Agar., Bry., Colch., Com., Iris, Puls, Thuja, Zinc.

Elbow: All. c.

Hand: Cupr., Kali bi., Zinc.

writing, while: Sil.

Fingers: Sep.

second: Cimic., Rhus t.

third: Bry.

NUMBNESS:

Upper limbs: Acon., Æth., Alum., Alumn., Ambr., Apis, Bar. c., Bufo, Carb. s., Carb. v., Cham., Cocc., Con., Croc., Cupr., Cur., Dulc., Fl. ac., Graph., Hep., Kali c., Kali s., Lach., Lyc., Nux v., Onos., Ox. ac., Pall., Phos., Plb., Puls., Rhod., Rhus t., Sec., Sep., Sulph., Urt. u.

Forearm: Acon., Carb. s., Cham., Cocc., Cupr., Glon., Kali c., Nat. m., Nit. ac., Op., Pall., Plb., Sulph.

grasping anything, while: Plb., Zinc.

measles, in: Zinc.

Hands: Acon., Apis, Ars., Calc., Camph., Carb. an., Carb. s., Carb. v., Caust., Coca, Cocc., Colch., Con., Dulc., Ferr., Fl. ac., Graph., Hyos., Hyper., Kali ar., Kali c., Kali s., Lach., Lyc., Mez., Nat. m., Nit. ac., Nux v., Onos., Op., Phos., Plb., Puls., Sec., Sil., Zinc.

NUMBNESS, hands.

grasping anything, while: Calc., Cham.

anything ameliorates: Spig.

menses, during: Graph.

motion, on: Bapt.

motion, ameliorated by: Apis, Ferr.

sewing, when: Crot. h.

writing, on: Zinc.

Fingers: Acon., Amyl. n., Apis, Ars., Bar. c., Calc., Carb. an., Carb. s., Carl., Caust., Cic., Cimex, Con., Cupr., Dig., Ferr., Ferr. i., Graph., Hep., Iod., Kali ar., Kali chl., Kreos., Lyc., Mur. ac., Par., Phos., Plb., Rhus t., Sec., Sep., Sil., Sulph.

chest affections, with: Crab. an.

tips of, during whooping cough: Spong.

PAIN: Æsc., Ars., Bol., Bry., Cact., Caust., Cham., Coff., Eup. per., Gels., Glon., Hep., Kalm., Led., Meph., Nat a., Nux v., Phos., Phyt., Puls., Ran. s., Rhus t., Sang., Sulph., Verat.

Motion: Ant. t., Bry., Cham., Colch., Nux v., Phyt., Ran. b.

Motion, ameliorated by: Puls., Rhod., Rhus t.

Upper arm: Anac., Bell., Iod., Kali c., Kalm., Mang., Rhod., Rhus t., Sang., Verat.

Elbow: Alum., Bry., Caust., Corn., Gua., Iod., Kali bi., Lyc., Rhus t., Sil.

Forearm: Æsc., Colch., Mez., Nit. ac., Podo., Rhod., Rhus

PAIN.

Wrist: Ant. c., Calc., Caul.,
Eup. per., Gua., Hep., Kali
bi., Kalm., Lyc., Puls.,
Rhod., *Rhus t.*, Ruta, Sabin.

Hand: Act. s., Calc., Colch.,
Dig., Gua., Hep., *Rhus t.*,
Staph., Sulph.

joints of: *Anac.*

Finger: Acon., Calc., Carb. an.,
Caul., Dios., Hep., Nat. a.,
Nit ac., Plb., Rhus t.

PULSATION:

Upper limbs: Kali c.,
Shoulder: Coloc., Kali c., Led.
Upper arms: Kali c.
Elbow: Sil.
Wrist: Lach.
Fingers: Amm. m., Sulph.
Thumb: Hep., *Amm. m.*

ROUGHNESS:

Hands: Graph., *Hep.*, Petr.,
Rhus t., Sulph., Zinc.
Finger nails: Graph., *Sil.*
tips: *Petr.*

SENSITIVENESS,   shoulder:
Apis.
Fingers: Lac. c., Led., Sec.
tips: Staph.
nails: Nat. m., Sil.

SHAKING, upper limbs: Agar.

SHOCKS, upper limbs: Agar.,
Arg. m., *Cic.*

Fingers, when he touches anything: Alum.

SHRUNKEN, shrivelled: Ars.,
Camph., Lach., Lyco., *Merc.*,
Phos., Verat.

STIFF, upper limbs: Amm. c.,
Caust., Cham., Ferr., Ham.,
Nux v., Rhus t., Sep.

Shoulder: Calc. s., Cupr., Fl. ac.,
Ham., Ind., Lyc., Nat. c.,
Petr., *Rhus t.*

Elbow: *Bry.*, Calc., Chel., Kali
c., Sep.

Forearm: Caust., Rhus t.

Wrist: Apis, Bell., Chel., Lyc.,
Phos., Puls., *Rhus t.*, Sabin.,
Sep., Sulph.

Hands: Agar., Ars., Calc., Calc.
p., Calc. s., Carb. an., Coloc.,
Cupr., Ferr., Nux v., Stict.

Fingers: Agar., Apis, Ars.,
Calc., Calc. s., Carb. an.,
Carb. s., Caul., Caust., Cupr.,
Dros., Ferr., Led., Lyc.,
Manc., Merc., *Rhus t.*, Sil.

SWELLING:

Upper limbs: Anthr., Apis,
Aran., Ars., Bell., Bry.,
Bufo, Cur., Ferr. p., Hydr.,
Lach., Mez., Phos., *Rhus t.*,
Sulph.

Shoulder: Coloc.

Upper arm: Apis, Bry., Graph.
hard and hot: Sulph.
painful: Puls.
vaccination: *Sil.*,   Sulph.
Thuja.

Elbow: Bry., Coloc., Merc.

Forearm: Ars., Ferr. p., Graps.,
Lach., Merc., Rhus t.

Wrist: Act. s., Apis, Bufo,
Calc., Crot. h., Lach., Merc.,
Rhus t., Sabin.

Hand: Agar., Apis, Ars., Aur.,
Bell., Bry., Bufo, Cact.,
Calc., Cocc., Colch., Ferr.,
Lach., Lyc., Merc., Nit. ac.,

SWELLING, hand.

> Phel., Phos., Psor., Sec., Sulph.

> Fingers: Apis, Ars., Bry., Cic. v., Dig., Graph., Lyc., Mag. c., *Rhus t.*, Thuja.

TINGLING:

> Upper limbs: Acon., Alum., Ambr., Aur., Carb. an., Carb. s., Cocc., Dig., *Graph.*, Sec., *Sil.*

> side lain on: Bar. c., Calc., Carb. v., Graph., Lach., Phos., *Puls.*, *Rhus t.*

TREMBLING, upper limbs:

> Agar., Arg. n., Calc. p., Carb. s., Cocc., Cupr., Hyos., Plb., *Nit. ac.,* Op., Phos., Rhus t., Sil., Spig., Stram.

> Hands: Acon., *Agar.,* Amyl. n., Anac., *Ant. t.,* Arg. n., Ars., Ars. i., Calc., Calc. s., Carb. an., Carb. h., Carb. s., *Caust.,* Chin., Cocc., Coff., Crot. h., Ferr., Gels., Glon., Hyos., Ign., Iod., Kali p., Lach.. *Merc.,* Nat. m,. *Nit. ac.,* Nux m. *Nux v,* Onos., Op., Phos., Phyt., Plat., Plb., Psor., Puls., Sil., Stann., Stram., *Sulph.,* Thuja, Zinc.

TWITCHING, upper limbs:

> Ant. t., Asaf., Caust., Chel., Cic., Coff., Cupr., Kali c.. Lyc.. Merc., Merc.

TWITCHING.

> c., Nux v., Op., *Thuja,* Valer.

> Shoulder: Lyc.
> resting, while: *Dros.*

> Upper arm: Lyc., Ran b.

> Forearm: Led., Tarax.

> Hand: Asaf., Cina, Cocc., Coff., Cupr., *Hyos.,* Nux v., Op., Stram.

> Fingers: Acon., Agar., Alum. Anac., Chin., Cic., Cimic., Cina, Cocc., Merc., Nat. c., Osm.

WEAKNESS, upper limbs:

> Acon., All. c., Alum., Amm. c., Anac., Apis, Ars., *Bell.,* Bism., Calc., Calc. s., Carb. s., Caust., Chel, Chin., *Cic.,* Con., Crot. h., Cupr., Cur., *Dig.,* Gels., Glon., Gran., Gua., Iod., *Kali c.,* Kalm., Lach., Lyc., Nat. m., Petr., Ph. ac., Phos., Rhod., Rhus t., Sil., *Stann.,* Stapl., Thuja.

> Shoulder: Com.

> Upper arm: Phos., Sulph., Thuja.

> Forearm: *Bell.,* Dig., *Rhus t.*

> Wrist: Carb. v., Caust., Cur., Glon., Merc., Plb., Sil.

> Hand: Bov., Cina, Fl. ac., Kali bi., Merc., *Mez.,* Nat. s., Nit. ac., Ruta, Stann.

> Fingers: Bov., Carb. v., Nat. m., *Rhus t.*

LOWER EXTREMITIES.

AILMENTS, common:

Abscess: Anan., Ars., Bel., Calc., Guaj., Hep., Iod., Merc., Ph. ac., Sil., Sulph.

Arthritic: Bufo, Calc., Graph., Kali i., Led., Nat. s., Nux v.

Atrophy (emaciation): Abrot., Apis, Arg. n., Ars., Calc., Sanic.

hip: Calc.

thighs: Calc., Nit. ac., Sel.

leg: Abrot., Apis, Bov., Calc., Caps., Nux v., Rhus v.

foot: Ars., Caust.

Callosities:

soles: Ant. c., Ars., Calc.

soles, tender: Alum., Nat. s.

toes: Graph.

Carbuncles: Arn., Ars., Hep., Lach., Sil., Sulph.

thigh: Arn., Hep.

Caries of bones: Sil.

hip: Ang., Arg. m., Ars., Asaf., Aur., Bell., Bry., Calc., Calc. p., Calc. s., Canth., Caps., Carb. v., Car. m., Caust., Cham., Chin., Coloc., Fl. ac., Hep., Kali c., Kali p., Kali s., Lach., Lyc., Merc., Nat. m., Nit. ac., Nux v., Petr., Ph. ac., Phos., Phyt., Rhus t., Sil., Stram., Sulph., Tub.

CARIES.

femur: Calc., Sil., Stron.

knee: Sil.

tibia: Asaf., Aur., Calc. Gua., Lach., Phos., Si

fibula: Sil.

ankle: Calc., Gua., Puls. Sil.

foot: Hecla, Merc., Sil.

toes: Sil.

Chorea:

legs: Cocc.

Corns: (see upper extremities)

Dropsy: Apis, Apoc., Ars. Ars. i., Aur. m., Cact. Calc., Carb. ac, Carb. s. Chel., Chim., Chin., Colch Dig., Dulc., Ferr., Fl. ac Graph., Hell., Hippoz Hydr., Kali c., Led., Lyc Mag. m., Merc., Phyt., Rhu t., Samb., Senec., Zinc.

albuminuria, in: Apis, Ars Calc. ar., Ferr., Lach Sars., Ter

Exostoses: Calc. f., Sil.

tibia: Ang., Cal. p., Cinnb Dulc., Nit. ac., Phyt.

Gangrene: Ars., Carb. v Chin., Crot. h., Lach., Phos Plb., Sec.

thigh: Sec.

knee: Phos.

leg: Anthr., Sec.

foot: Lach., Sec.

toes: Sec.

GANGRENE.

toes, senile: Ph. ac., Sec.

Inco-ordination: Agar., *Alum.*, Calc., *Con.*, Cupr., Gels., *Nux m.*, Onos., *Phos.*, Stram., *Sil.*, Zinc.

Ingrowing toe-nails: Caust., *Graph.*, *Mag. acet.*, Nat. m., Nit. ac., Phos., Sil., Sulph., *Teucr.*, Thuja.

ulceration, accompanied by: Nit. ac., *Sil.*, Teucr..

unhealthy granulation: Lach.

Paralysis: Abrot., *Agar.*, Alum., *Arg. n.*, *Ars.*, Bell., Calc., Camph., Caps., Carb. ac., Cic., Cocc., Con., Cupr., Dulc., Gels., Kali c., Lach., Lith., Myg., Nux m., *Nux v.*, Olnd., Op., Phos., Pic. ac., *Plb.*, Psor., *Rhus t.*, Sec., Sil., Stram., Sulph., Thal., Verat.

anger, following: Nat. m.
apoplexy, following: Nux v., Phos.

parturition, after: Caust., Plb., *Rhus t.*

post diphtheritic: *Ars.*, Cocc., Con., Lach., Phos., Plb., Sec., Sil.

sexual excesses, after: Nat. m., *Nux v.*, Phos.

vaccination, after: Thuja.

Ulcers: Ars., Asaf., Calc., Carb. s., *Carb. v.*, Cist., Com., Crot. h., Ferr. m., Graph., Grind., Hydr., Kali c., Kali i., Lac. c., *Lach.*, Lyc., Merc., Mez., Mur. ac., Nat. c., Nat. m., Phyt., Puls., Rhus t., Sabin., Sep., *Sil.*, Sin. n., Sulph.

ULCERS.

thigh: Calc., Mez., Nat. s., Zinc.

knee: Calc., Phos.

leg: Anthr., *Ars.*, Asaf., Calc., Calc. s., *Carb. s.*, *Carb. v.*, Cist., Crot h., Ferr. m., Graph., Grind., Kali ar., Kali bi., Kali c., Kali i., Lac. c., *Lach.*, *Lyc.*, Merc., Mez., Mur. ac., Nit. ac., Ph. ac., Phyt., Psor., Puls., Rhus t., *Sil.*, Sin. n., Sulph.

ankle: Calc. p., Hydr., Syph.

foot: Anan., Carb. ac., Fl. ac., Graph., Kali bi., Psor., Puls., Sulph., Zinc.

toes: Ars., Bry., Graph., Petr., Sep., Sil., Sulph.

AWKWARDNESS:

Stumbling, when walking: Agar., Calc., *Caust.*, Colch., Con., Ign., Lach., Nat. m., Phos.

COLDNESS: Ars., Ars. i., *Bell.*, Calad., Chel., Lac. c., Led., Mez., *Nit. ac.*, Op., Ox. ac., Phos., *Puls.*, Sec., Sep., Stram., Sulph.

leg: Apis, Arg. n., Ars., *Calc.*, Calc. p., Camph., Carb. an., Carb. s., *Carb. v.*, Caust., Cham., Chel., Chin., Chin. a., Chin. s., Colch., Cupr., *Dig.*, Ferr., Hep., *Lach.*, Laur., Led., Med., Meny., Merc., Naja, Nat. c., Nat. p., Nit. ac., Nux m., Nux v., Op., Ox. ac., Petr., Ph. ac., Phos., Rhus t., Sec., Sep., *Sil.*, Stram., Sulph., Stry., Tab., *Verat.*

COLDNESS.

foot: Acon., Ambr., Amm. c., Anac., *Ant. c., Ant. t.*, Apis, Arg. n., Arn., *Ars., Ars. i., Aur.,* Bar. c., *Bell.*, Brom., Cact., *Calc.,* Camph., Canth., Caps., Carb. an, *Carb. s.,* Carb. *v., Caust.,* Cham., Chel., *Chin.*, Chin. a., Cimex, Cina, Cist., Cocc., Colch., *Con.*, Crot. t., *Cupr.,* Dig., Dros., Elaps, *Ferr.,* Ferr. i., Ferr. p., Gels., Glon., *Graph.,* Hell., Hep., Iod., *Ip.*, Kali ar., *Kali c., Kali n., Kali p., Kali s., Kreos., Lach., Lyc.*, Med., *Meny.,* Merc., Merc. c., Mur. ac., *Nat. c., Nat. m.,* Nat. p., Nat. s., *Nit. ac.*, Nux m., Nux v., Ox. ac., *Par., Petr.*, Phos., *Ph. ac.*, Phyt., Pic. ac., Plb., Podo.,Psor., *Puls., Rhod.,* Rhus t., *Ruta*, Sabin., Samb., Sars., *Sep., Sil., Squil., Stram., Sulph.,* Tarent., *Thuja*, Verat., Verat. v., Zinc.

fever, during: Arn., Lach., Stram., Sulph.

headache, during: Arg. n., Bell., Calc., Carb. v., Ferr., Gels., *Mel.*, Naja, Psor., *Sep.*, Sulph.

hot face, with: Asaf., Sep., *Stram.*

hot head, with: Arn., Bell., Cact., Calc., Ferr., Nat. c., Ph. ac.

icy cold: Apis Camph., Carb. v., Cupr., Elaps, Eup. per., Gels., Hep., Lach., Lyc.,

COLDNESS, icy-cold.

Merc., Merc. c., Nux m., Phos., *Psor.*, Sep., *Sil* Sulph., Verat.

menses, previous to: Lyc., Nux m.

when the flow is on: Arg. n., Crot. h., Graph., Nux m., Phos., *Sil.*

menses, following: Carb. v., Chin. s.

pregnant women, in: Lyc., *Verat.*

decrease of volume, shortening.

CONTRACTION: Amm. m., Bar. c., *Caust.*, Coloc., Gua., Phos., Rhus t.

Thigh: Rhus t.

bend of: Caust., Rhus t.

bend of, while walking: Rhus t.

hamstrings: Ambr., Amm.m., Calc. p., *Caust.*, Cimex, Gua., Lyc., *Nat. m.,* Phyt., Rhus t., Ruta.

hamstrings, after abscess: Lach.

hamstrings, while walking: Nux v., Rhus t.

Knee: *Amm. m., Caust.*, Cimex, Graph., Gua., Mez., Nat. c., Nat. m., Rhus t., Staph., Sulph., Tell.

Leg: *Amm. m.*, Aster., Cic., Nat. m., Phyt.

tendo achillis: Calc., Cann. s., Carb. an., Graph., Kali. c., Sep.

Toes: Ferr., Sec.

drawn down: Ars.

drawn up: Camph., Lach.

CONVULSION: Cocc., Cupr., Hyos., Ign., Ip., Lach., Op., Sec., Sulph., Stram.

alternately flexed and extended: Cupr.

Leg: Jatr.

Foot: Calc., Curp., Nat. m., Nux v., Zinc.

tetanic: Camph., Nux v.

Toes: Chel.

CRACKED FEET: Aur. m., Sars.

Heel: Lyc.

Toes: Graph., Hydr., Lach., Nat. m., Sil.

CRACKING: Benz. ac., Cham., Sep.

CRAMPS: Calc., Ferr., Ferr. m.
Hips: Arg. m., Coloc., Ph. ac., Sep.

Thighs: Asar., Cannab., Coloc., Hyos., Sulph.

walking, while: Sep.

walking, in open air: Verb.

Knee, bend of: Calc., Cannab.

Leg: Ars., Bov., Calc., Carb. an., Carb. s., Carb. v., Cham., Colch., Coloc., Cupr., Ferr., Jatr., Kali chl., Mag. p., Nat. m., Ph. ac., Puls., Rhus t., Sulph.

extension, on: Calc.

menses, during: Gels., Graph.

stool, during: Sulph.

urinate, on attempting to: Pareira.

calf: Acon., Alum., Ambr., Anac., Arg. n., Ars., Calc., Calc. p., Camph., Caust., Cham., Colch., Coloc., Con., Crot. h., Cupr., Ferr., Graph., Hep., Iris, Kali c.,

CRAMPS, leg, calf.

Nat. c., Nat. m., Nit. ac., Nux v., Ph. ac., Phos., Plb., Rhus t., Sec., Sep., Sil., Sulph., Verat., Verat. v., Zinc.

cholera in: Ant. t., Camph., Colch., Cupr., Jatr., Kali p., Mag. p., Sulph., Verat.

coition, during: Graph.

coition, after: Coloc.

coition on attempting: Cupr.

dancing, while: Sulph.

menses, before: Phos.

pregnant women, in: Sep.

walking, on: Anac., Calc. p., Sulph.

walking, after: Rhus t.

Foot: Acon., Agar., Ang., Asc. t., Bell., Calc., Camph., Carb. s., Caust., Colch., Coloc., Jatr., Lac. c., Lyc., Nat. c., Nat. m., Petr., Ph. ac., Rhus t., Sec., Sep., Sil., Stram., Sulph.

cholera, in: Cupr., Verat.

Toes: Amm. c., Ars., Asaf., Bar. m., Calc., Caust., Cham., Chel., Crot. h., Cupr., Cupr. ar., Ferr., Hep., Kali c., Lyc., Nux, Ph. ac., Sec.

DRAWING PAIN: Acon., Agar., Ang., Bapt., Bar. c., Bry., Carb. v., Caust., Cham., Chel., Ferr., Gels., Graph., Hep., Lyc., Merc., Nat. c., Nat. m., Nit. ac., Nux v., Puls., Rhus t., Sep., Sil., Stront., Sulph., Tub., Valer., Zinc.

Motion, on: Gels.

Motion, ameliorated by: Rhus t., Tub., Valer.

EMACIATION (see atrophy)

HEAT: Bar. m., Calc. p.,
Chel., Ham., Kali bi., Lach.,
Lyc., Meph., Mez., Nat. s.,
Sulph., Thuja.

Foot: Apis, Caust., *Cham.*,
Glon., Kali bi., Lyc., Nat. s.,
Nux v., Petr., Psor., *Puls.*,
Ruta, Sec., Sep., Sil., *Sulph.*

burning: Agar., Graph., Lyc.,
Med., Nat. s., *Ph. ac.*,
Puls., Sang., Sec., Sep.,
Sulph., Zinc.

burning, uncovers them:
Cham., *Med.*, *Puls.*, Sang.,
Sanic., *Sulph.*

flushes: *Sulph.*

one foot, coldness of the other:
Lyc.

HEAVINESS: Agar., *Alum.*,
Aran., *Arg. m.*, Arg. n., Arn.,
Ars., Bell., *Berb.*, Calc.,
Carb. s., Carb. v., Chel.,
Cimex, *Cocc.*, Con., Dulc.,
Gels., Graph., Ham., Hep.,
Ign., Kali ar., Kali c., Lyc.,
Mag. m., *Med.*, Merc.,
Merc. i. f., Mez., *Nat. c.*,
Nat. m., Nit. ac., Nux m.,
Nux v., Onos., Petr., Phos.,
Pic. ac., Plat, Puls., *Rhus t.*,
Ruta, Sabad., Seneg., Sep.,
Sil., Stann., Sulph., Thuja,
Zinc.

Exertion, after: *Con., Gels.*,
Rhus t.

Menses, previous to: Con.,
Graph.

Menses, when the flow is on:
Amm. c., Graph., Sep.,
Zinc.

suppression of: Graph.

Walking, while: *Berb.*, Calc.,
Con.

HEAVINESS, walking.

after: *Arg. m.*

Hip: Con.

Thigh: Agn., *Ang.*, Arn., Bry.,
Calc., Chin., Gua., Ip., Kali
c., Lyc., Merc., Puls., Sep.,
Stann., Thuja.

Knee: Con., *Nux m.*, Plat.,
Stann.

Leg: Æth., Agar., *Alum.*, Arg.
n., Bell., Bry., Calc., Calc p.,
Camph., Carb. ac., Carb. s.,
Carb. v., Cham., Chel., Chin.,
Cimex, Colch., Coloc., Ferr.,
Gels., Graph., Kali bi., Kali
c., Mag. m., Med., Merc.,
Nat. c., Nat. m., *Nux m.*,
Nux v., Onos., Petr., Phos.,
Phyt., Pic. ac., Plb., Puls.,
Rhus t., Sil., Sulph.

Foot: Agar., Agn., *Alum.*, Arn.,
Ars., Ars. i., Aur., Bell.,
Bov., Calc., Cocc., Cyc.,
Graph., Ign., Kali ar., Kali
c., Led., Nat. c., Nat. m.,
Ol. an., Petr., Phos., Pic. ac.,
Plat., *Puls.*, Sab., Sec., Sep.,
Sil., Sulph.

INFLAMMATION:

Psoas muscle: Calc.

Thigh: Sil.

periosteum of femur: Aur.,
Mez., Phyt.

Knee: Apis, Arn., Bar. m.,
Bry., Calc., Cocc., Fl. ac.,
Gua., Iod., Led., Nux v.,
Phyt., Psor., *Puls.*, Rhus t.,
Sars., Sulph.

erysipelatous: *Rhus t.*

Leg: Acon., Bor., Calc.

erysipelatous: *Apis*, Bor.,
Calc., Hep., Hydr., Lach.,

INFLAMMATION, leg, erysipelatous.

Nat. c., Rhus t., Sil., Sulph., Ter.

periosteum: Asaf., Kali bi., Phos.

tibia: Ph. ac., Phos.

Foot: Bry., Com., Merc., Puls., Rhus v., Sulph.

erysipelatous: Apis, Arn., Bry., Rhus t.

periosteum: Aur. m., Gua.

sole: Puls.

Toes:

erysipelatous: Apis.

frost-bitten: Agar.

INJURIES:

Hips: Rhus t.

Ankle: Arn., Calc., Rhus t., Ruta, Stront.

LAMENESS: Colch., Plb., Rhus t.

Suppressed perspiration: Colch., Rhus t.

Hip: Abrot., Amm. c., Arg. m., Bry., Cocc., Dios., Fl. ac., Rhus t., Zing.

left: Fl. ac.

Thigh: Ars., Arg. m., Carb. v., Calc., Chin., Iris, Kali c., Merc., Stann., Zinc.

Knee: All. c., Bar. c., Calc., Kali c., Spong.

rising from a seat: Berb.

Ankles: Arn., Ruta.

Foot: Aur., Colch., Rhus t.

Toes: Aur.

NUMBNESS: Alum., Ambr., Apis, Arg. m., Arg. n., Calc. p., Canth., Carb. an., Carb. v., Chel., Chin. s., Con.,

NUMBNESS.

Graph., Kali c., Kali s., Lyc., Nux v., Onos., Petr., Phos., Puls., Rhod., Rhus t., Sec., Sep., Spong.

Menses, during: Kali n., Puls., Sec.

Sitting, when he is: Ant. c., Ant. t., Calc. p.

Walking, while: Alum., Plb., Rhus t., Sep., Thuja.

Nates: Cal. p.

sitting, while: Alum., Calc. p., Sulph.

Hips: Apis.

Thigh: Ars., Calc., Con., Ferr., Fl. ac., Graph., Keros., Lac. d., Plb., Spong.

Knee: Coloc., Plat.

Leg: Acon., Alum., Ant. c., Apis, Arg. m., Arg. n., Calc., Calc. p., Carb. an., Carb. s., Caust., Cocc., Coloc., Con., Crot. h., Eup. pur., Graph., Ham., Hyper., Lyc., Merc., Merc. c., Nat. m., Nux v., Onos., Op., Phos., Phys., Phyt., Plat., Puls., Rhus t., Sil.

Ankles: Lac. c., Sulph.

Foot: Acon., Alum., Apis, Arg. m., Arg. n., Ars., Bapt., Calc., Carb. an., Carb. s., Carb. v., Caust., Cocc., Coloc., Con., Graph., Kali ar., Lyc., Nit. ac., Nux v., Phos., Ph. ac., Plat., Plb., Puls., Sec., Thuja.

soles of foot: Alum., Ars., Cann. i., Cocc.

Toes: Acon., Ars., Calc., Caust., Cham., Chel., Con., Graph., Phos., Sec.

PAIN: *Agar.*, Apis, Arg. m.,
Ars., Ars. h., Bell., Bol.,
Bry., Calc., Calc. p., Carb.
v., Caust., Cham., Chel.,
Coloc., Ferr., Gels., Kalm.,
Lac. c., Lil. t., Mag. p.,
Med., Merc., Nat. c., Nat.
m., Nux v., Petr., Phys.,
Phyt., Plb., Puls., Ran. b.,
Rhus t., Sep., Sil., Sulph.,
Tarax., Valer., Zinc.

Chill, during: Ars., Chin.,
Ferr., *Nux v.*, *Pyrog.*, Puls.,
Rhus t.

previous to: Nux v.

Cold relieves the pain: Apis,
Coff., Lac. c., *Led.*, *Puls.*,
Sec.

Hang down, while allowing the
limbs to: Con.

Menses, before: Caul.

Menses, during: Cham.

Motion aggravates the pain:
Apis, *Bry.*, Lac. c., Led.,
Merc., Nux v., Phyt.,
Ran. b.

relieves the pain: Agar., Arg.
m., Bell., Calc., Coloc.,
Ferr., Kali bi., *Kali s.*,
Lyc., Merc., Mur. ac.,
Nat. s., Ph. ac., *Puls.*,
Rhod., *Rhus t.*, Sep.,
Tarax., *Tub.*, Valer., Zinc.

Move, on beginning to: Caust.,
Ferr., Kali p., Petr., Plat.,
Rhod., *Rhus t.*

Sciatica: Arg. n., Arn., Ars.,
Bell., *Bufo*, Calc., Calc. p.,
Calc. s., Carb. s., Caust.,
Cham., Cimic., Coff.,
Coloc., Dios., Elaps, Elat.,
Ferr., Ferr. ar., Gels.,
Graph., Gua., Ign., Indig.,
Iris, Kali ar., Kali bi., *Kali*

PAIN, sciatica.

i., Lac. c., Lach., Led.,
Lyc., *Mag. p.*, Nat. m., Nux
m., *Nux v.*, Ol. j., Petr.,
Phos., Phyt., Plb., Podo.,
Puls., Rab. b., *Rhus t.*,
Ruta, Sep., Staph., *Tell.*,
Valer., Verat.

Nates: Calc., Puls., Sulph.

Hip: Acon., Æsc., Agar.,
Anag., Arg. m., Arn., Ars.,
Ars. i., Aur., Bar. c., Bell.,
Berb., Bry., Calc., Calc. p.,
Calc. s., Canth., Carb. an.,
Card. m., Caust., Chel.,
Cimic., *Colch.*, Coloc.,
Crot. t., Euph., Ferr., Ferr.
i., Fl. ac., *Hep.*, Hydr., Iod.,
Kali ar., Kali c., Kali p.,
Kali s., Kalm., Kreos., Lac.
d., Lach., *Led.*, Lyc., Merc.,
Murex, Nat. h., Nat. s.,
Phos., Ph. ac., Phyt.,
Puls., Rhus t., Sars., Sep.,
Sil., Stram., Sulph., Valer.

Thigh: Agar., Alum., *Anac.*,
Ars., Aur. m., Bell., Berb.,
Bry., Cact., Carb. s., Carb.
v., Chin., Chin., Cimic.,
Cimex, Cist., Coloc., Dulc.,
Gua., Hep., Hyper., Indig.,
Kali bi., Kali c., Kali i.,
Kalm., Led., Lyc., Merc.,
Mez., Murex, Nat. a., Nat.
m., Nit. ac., Petr., Ph. ac.,
Pyrog., *Plb.*, Rhus t., Sars.,
Sep., Staph., Sulph., Thuja,
Verb.

Knee: Acon., Æsc., All. c.,
Ang., Ant. t., Apis, Arn.,
Ars., Ars. i., Aur., Bar. c.,
Bell., *Benz. ac.*, *Calc.*,
Calc. p., Calc. s., Canth.,
Caust., Chel., Cinnab., Cocc.,
Coloc., Com., Con., Cop.,
Gels., Iod., *Kali c.*, Kalm.,
Lach., Led., Lyc., Merc.,

PAIN, knee.

Mez., Myrtus, Nat. s., Nux
v., Phos., Phyt., Pyrog.,
Psor., Puls., Rhod., Rhus t.,
Rhus v., *Verat.*, Verb.

Leg: *Agar.*, Alum., Apoc.,
Arn., Ars., Bell., Caps.,
Caust., Coff, Dulc., Eup.
per., Gels., Gua., Hydr.,
Kali bi., Kali c., Kali i.,
Kali n., Kalm., Kreos.,
Lach., Led., Lyc., Merc.,
Mez., Nux v., Petr., Phos.,
Phyt., Plat., Plb., Puls.,
Pyrog., Rhod., *Rhus t.*,
Rhus v., Sang., Sep., Stann.,
Staph., Sulph., Syph., Tub.,
Verat.

Ankle: All. c., Ant. t., Arn.,
Bol., Carb. an., Caul.,
Caust., Cham., Chel., Cop.,
Kalm., *Led.*, Lith., Lyc.,
Mez., Phyt., Sal. ac.

Foot: Anac., Apis, Arn., Ars.,
Aur. m., Calc., Cann. s.,
Caul., Caust., Coloc., Dig.,
Dulc., Gua., Lach., Led.,
Lith., Lyc., Mez., Nat. m.,
Nat. s., Nux v., Petr., Phyt.,
Plb., Rhod., Ruta, Sil.,
Syph., Thuja, Verat.

Toes: Aur., Benz. ac., Calc.,
Caul., Caust., Coloc., Lith.,
Lyc., Phos., Phyt, Plat.,
Sil., Stict., Sulph., Syph.,
Zinc.

PULSATION:

Hip: Coloc., Ign.
Thigh: Sil.
Knee: Acon.
Toes: Asaf., Gamb.

RESTLESS: Anac., *Ars.*, Bell.,
Calc. p., Caust., Chin. a.,
Kali c., Lyc., Mez., Nat. m.,

RESTLESS.

Phos., Phyt., Plat., *Rhus t.*,
Sep., *Tarent.*, Zinc.
Thigh: Anac., Camph., Mag.
m., Plat.
Knee: Rhus t.

Leg: *Amm. c.*, Anac., Arg. n.,
Ars., Bell., Calc., Calc. p.,
Camph., Carb. v., Caust.,
Chin., Chin. a., Cimex, *Ferr.*,
Glon., Graph., Kali c.,
Lach., Lyc., Mag. c., *Med.*,
Meph., Mez., Mosch., Nat.
m., Nit. ac., Nux m., Phos.,
Plat *Rhus t.*, Sep., Sulph.,
Tarax., *Tarent.*, Zinc.

Feet: Alum., Ars., Cham.,
Lil. t., *Med.*, Meph., Nat. m.,
Puls., *Rhus t.*, Stram.,
Sulph., Tarent., Zinc.

SENSITIVENESS: Agar.,
Mag. m., Petr.

Hip: Coloc.
Thigh: Agar., Gels., Merc.
Knee: Lach., Sars., Sep.
Leg: Calc.
tibia: Puls.
calf: Nat. m.

Foot: Kali c., Lach., *Lyc.*,
Mez., Merc. i, r., Petr., Sil.,
Staph.
sole: Alum., *Kali c.*, Lyc.,
Med., Staph.
Toes: Calc., Carb. an.

SHOCKS: Agar., Ars., Phos.,
Verat.

SHUDDERING:

Leg: Graph.
STIFF: Acon., Arg. m., *Atro.*,
Aur. m., *Berb.*, Bry. Calc.,
Carb. s., Carb. v., Cic.,
Cina, Cocc., Coc. c., *Eup.*

STIFF.

per., Ferr., Ham., Hydr. ac., Lac. c., Lith., Mag., p., Mang., Merc., Nat. m., Nat. s., *Nux v.*, Petr., *Plat.*, *Rhus t.*, Sep., *Sil.*, Spong.. Verat., Zinc.

SWELLING: Bar. m., Berb., Calc., Chel., Kali a., Kali c., Led., Lyc., Phos., Rhus t., Sep., Sil., Sulph.

Nates: Coloc.

Thigh: Ham., Lach.

femur: Mez., *Sil.*, Stront.

glands of: Calc.

Knee: Æsc., Anthr., Apis, Arn., Ars., Ars. i., Bar. m., *Berb.*, *Bry.*, *Calc.*, Calc. p., Chin., Cic., Clem., Cocc., Colch., Cop., *Hep.*, Iod., Kali c., Lach., *Led.*, *Lyc.*, Nat. m., Nux. v., *Phyt.*, *Puls.*, *Rhus t.*, Sal. ac., Sars., Sil., Sulph., Tub.

Leg: Acon., *Ars.*, Aur., Aur. m., Bad., Bry., Cact., Calc., Caust., Colch., Hell., Kali bi., Kali chl., Lach., *Led.*, *Lyc.*, Merc., Puls., *Samb.*, Syphil., Zinc.

Ankle: *Apis*, Ars., Asaf., Cact., Chel., Coloc., Dig., Eup. per., Ferr., Hep., Hydr., Lac. c., Lach., Lyc., *Med.*, Phos., Phyt., Psor., Puls., Rhus t., Ruta.

Foot: Apis., Arn., *Ars.*, Ars. i., Aur., *Bry.*, Cact., Calc., Calc. ar., Canth., Carb. an., Carb. s., Caust., Chin., Cocc., Colch., Dig., Elaps, Ferr., Glon., Graph., Hyos., Kali c., Lach., *Lyc.*, *Med.*, Merc., Nat. a., Nat. m., Nit. ac., Petr., Phos., Phyt., *Puls.*,

SWELLING, foot.

Rhus t., Samb., Sec., Sep., Sil., Stict.

TINGLING: Alum., Carb. s., Graph., *Kali c.*, Lyc., Petr.

TOTTERING: Agar., *Alum.*, Ambr., Amm. m., Anac., Apis, Arg. m., Ars., *Aur.*, Bar. c., Calc., Carb. ac., Carb. v., *Caust.*, Cocc., Con., Gels., Glon., Hell., Iod., Lith., Nat. c., Nat. m., *Nux v.*, Op., Ph. ac., *Phos.*, Pic. ac., *Rhus t.*, Sars., Sil., Sulph.

TREMBLING: Agar., Ambr., Arg. m., *Arg. n.*, Calc. Caust., Cimic., Crot. h., Glon., *Lach.*, Lith., Led., Merc., Nat. m., *Nit. ac.*, *Nux v.*, Phyt., Verat.

Coition, after: *Calc.*

Walking, when: *Nux v.*

ameliorates: Nat. m.

Thigh: Anac., Con., Plat.

Knee: Alum., Anac., Camph., Chel., Glon., Led., Puls., Ruta.

Leg: Cycl., Nat. m., Phos., Plat., Puls., Ruta., Sil.

Foot: Bar. c., Cupr., Hydr., Hyos., *Merc.*, Nat. m., Plat., Psor., *Puls.*, Stram., Sulph., Tab., Thuja.

TWITCHING: Alum., Cupr., Hell., Nux v., Op., Rhus t., Stront., Verat.

UNSTEADY: Acon., Nux v., Verb.

WEAKNESS: Æsc., Agar., *Alum.*, Amm. m., Anac., Apis, *Arg. m.*, *Arg. n.*,

WEAKNESS.

Ars., Aur., Bry., Bufo, *Calc.*, Carb. ac., Carb. s., Carb. v., *Caust.*, Chin., Chin. a., Cina, *Cocc.*, Con., Crot. t., Cupr., Ferr. i., Gels., *Glon.*, Hell., Hydr., Kali ar., Kali c., Kali n., Kali p., Nit. ac., Mag. m., Mez., Mur. ac., Nat. a., Nat. c., Nat. m., Nux m., Op., Nux v., Petr., Ph. ac., Phos., *Pic. a.*, *Plb.*, Rhus t., Sars., Sec., Sep., Sil., Stann., Sulph., Sul. ac., Stront., Zinc.

Child, late, learning to walk: *Calc.*

Coitiom, after: Calc.

Exertion, after: *Calc., Gels., Rhus t.*

WEAKNESS.

Menses, during: Cocc., Nit. ac., Zinc.

Standing, while: Anac., Bry., *Nux m.*

Walking, after: Æsc., *Arg. m.,* Bry., *Calc.*, Calc. s., *Con.*, Mur. ac., Plb., Rhus t., Sil.

Ankle: *Carb. an.*, Caust., Ferr., Lac. d., *Nat. a.*, *Nat. c.*, Nat. m, *Nat. p.*, *Nat. s.*, Nit. ac., Rhus t., Rhus v., Sep., *Sil.*, Sulph., Sul. ac.

Foot: *Ars.*, Bov., Calc., Cham., Chin., Hell., Lach., Lyc., Nat. m., Ol. an., Olnd., Phos., Plat., Puls., Rhus t., Sil., Sulph., Tab.

SLEEP

COMA: Agar., Agn., Ant. c., Ant. t., Apis, *Arg. n.*, Arn., Ars., Asaf., *Bapt.*, Bar. c., *Bell.*, Bor., Bry., Bufo, Calad., Camph., Caust., Chin., Chlor., Cic., Cimic., Colch., Con., *Croc.*, Crot. h., Cupr., Dig., Dor., Hell., Lach., Laur., Lyc., Led., Nat. m., *Nux m.*, *Op.*, Ph. ac., Phos., Plb., Puls., Rhus t., Sec., Stram., Sulph., *Verat.*, Zinc.

DEEP: Alum., *Ant. t.*, Apis, *Arg. n.*, Arn., Ars., *Bapt.*, Bar. c., *Bell.*, Bry., Calad., Calc., Camph., *Carb. h.*, *Carb. o.*, *Carb. s.*, *Carb. v.*, Carl., Caust., Chel., Chin., Cic., Cina, Colch., Con., *Croc.*, Crot. h., Cupr., Cycl., Fl. ac., Gels., *Graph.*, Hell., Hep., Hyos., Ign., Kali n., Lach., Led., Lyc., Mer. c., Naja, Nat. m., *Nux m.*, *Nux v.*, *Op.*, Ph. ac., Phos., Phys., Plb., Podo., *Puls.*, Rhod., Rhus t., Sec., Seneg., Stram., Sulph., Valer., *Verat.*, Zinc.

Heat, during: All. c., *Apis*, Arn., Calad., Mez., Nux v., *Op.*, Phos., *Rob.*

Menses, during: *Nux m.*, Phos.

FALLING ASLEEP:

Answering while: *Arn.*, *Bapt.*, Hyos.

Heat, during: Ant. t., Apis, *Calad.*, *Eup. per.*, *Lach.*,

FALLING ASLEEP, heat during.
Mez., *Nat. m.*, Nux m., *Op.*, *Podo.*, *Rob.*, *Samb.*

Mental exertion, from the slightest: *Ars.*, *Hyos.*, Kali c., Nux v.

FALLING ASLEEP LATE: Ars., Bry., Calc., Carb. an., Carb. v., Chin., Ferr., Kali c., Lach., Lyc., Merc., Nux, Phos., Puls., Ran. b., Rhus t., Sep., Stan., Staph., Sulph., Thuja.

SLEEPINESS:

Overpowering: Aur., Cor. r., Lach., Mez., *Nux m.*, Nux v., *Op.*

Pregnant women, in: Helon., Nux m.

SLEEPLESSNESS: Acon., Agar., Aloe., Apis, *Arg. n.*, Arn., *Ars.*, *Ars. i.*, Arum. t., Atro., Aur., Bapt., *Bell.*, Benz. ac., Bor., *Bry.*, *Cact.*, *Calc.*, Calc. p., Camph., Canth., Carl., Carb. s., Carb. v., Caust., *Cham.*, *Chin.*, Ch. a., Chin. s., Cic., Cina, Cic. v., Cocc., *Coff.*, Coloc., Con., Cupr., *Cycl.*, Dig., Dros., Dulc., Ferr., Ferr. ar., Fl. ac., Gels., Glon., Graph., Gua., Hell., *Hep.*, Hyos., Ign., Iod., Ip., Jal., *Kali ar.*, Kali bi., Kali br., *Kali c.*, Kali i., Kali s., Kreo., Lac. c., *Lach.*, Lachn., Led., Lyc., Mag. c.,

SLEEPLESSNESS.

Mag. m., Mag. s., Med., *Merc.*, *Merc. c.*, Nat. c., Nat. m., Nat. p., Nat. s., Nit. ac., Nux m., *Nux v.*, *Op.*, Ph. ac., *Phos.*, Plat., *Plb.*, *Puls.*, *Rhus t.*, Rumex, Sec., Sel., Senec., *Sep.*, *Sil.*, Stann., *Staph.*, *Sulph.*, Syph., Tab., Tarent., Thuja, Valer.

Anxiety, from: *Cocc.*, *Ars.*

Excitement, from: Ambr., *Coff.*, Colch., Hep., Lach., *Nux v.*, Puls.

SLEEPLESSNESS, sleepiness

with, from thoughts: Æsc., Bry., *Calc.*, Calc. s., Chin., Cocc., *Coff.*, Ferr., Fl. ac., Gels., Graph., *Hep.*, Hyos., Kali c., Lach., Lyc., Nat. m., *Nux v.*, Pic. ac., Psor., *Puls.*, Pyrog., Sep., Sil., Staph., Tub., Sulph., Zinc.

UNREFRESHING: Alum.,

Amm., c., Arg. n., Ars., Bar. c., Bell., Carl., Chin., Clem.,

UNREFRESHING.

Cob., Cocc., Cycl., Dig., Gua., *Lach.*, Lyc., *Mag. c.*, Mag. m., Nat. m., *Nit. ac.*, Nux v., Op., Petr., *Phos.*, Podo., Puls., Sep., Sil., Spig., Sulph., Zinc.

SWEATING, perspiration, dur-

ing: Ars., *Op.*, *Podo.*, Puls., *Rhus t.*

YAWNING:

Chill, during: Bry., *Elat.*, *Eup.*, *per.*, Meny., Mur. ac., *Nat. m.*, Olnd., Sep.

previous to: Eup. per.

Frequent: Acon., Brom., Caps., *Chel.*, Cic. v., Cocc., Cupr., *Graph.*, Ign., Lyc., Merc. c., Olnd., *Sulph.*

Menses, during: Amm. c., Carb. an.

previous to: *Puls.*

Vehement: Cor. r., Ign., Plat.

POSTURES IN SLEEP.

LYING ABDOMEN, on: Bell., Calc., Cocc., Coloc., Stram.

Arms and hands over head: Calc. c., Coloc., Nux v., Plat., *Puls.*

Arms and hands under head: Ars., Bell., Cocc., Coloc., Meny., Nux v., Plat.

Arms and hands abdomen, on: Puls.

Back, on: Acon., Ant. t., Aur., *Bry.*, Calc. c., Chin., Cic., Coca, Coloc., Dig., Dros., Ferr., Ign., Lyc., Nux v., Phos., Plat., *Puls.*, *Rhus t.*, Sul., Vio. o.

Head inclined forward: Staph.

LYING ABDOMEN, on.

Head inclined backward: Bell., Cic., Cina. Hep., Hyos., Ign., Sep., Spon.

Head inclined one side: Cina. hanging low down: Arn., Hep., Spon.

Knees bent: Vio. o. spread apart: Cham., Plat.

Leg crossed: Rhodo. drawn up: Carb. v., Plat., Stram. stretched out: Bell., Plat., Puls., Rhus t.

Side on: Alum., Bar. c., Caust., Colch., Merc., Nat. c., Nux v., Phos., Sabin., Spig., Sul.

DREAM.

ABSURD, inconsistent: Glon., Sulph.

ACCIDENTS: *Ars.*, *Graph.*, Nux v.

ANGER: Arn., Bry., Mag. c., *Nux v.*, Phos., Staph.

ANIMALS: Amm. m., *Arn.*, Merc., Nux v., Phos., Puls. Black: Puls.

Cats: Daph.

ANOTHER PERSON LYING IN BED WITH HIM: Petr.

Arrests, of being arrested: Clem., Mag. c.

AWAKE, while: Acon., Ign., Nux v., Op., Phos., Sil., Sulph.

BATTLES: Allium cepa.

BLIND, that he was: Phys.

BURIED ALIVE, being: Arn.

BUSINESS: Bry., Chel., Cur., Lach., Lyc., *Nux v.*, Puls., *Rhus t.*, Sil.

COMICAL: Glon., Sulph.

DANGER: Ars., Cann. i., Hep., Lach.

DEAD, of those that are: Anac., Arg. n., Arn., *Ars.*, Calc., Crot h., Graph., Kali c., *Mag. c.*, Med., Phos., Sulph., *Thuja*.

DEATH: Calc., *Lach.*, Sulph.

DISEASE: Calc., Kreos., Lyc., Nux v.

FALLING, of: Amm. m., *Bell.*, Cact., Dig., Gua., Hep.,

FALLING, of.
Kreo., Merc., Puls., Sars., Sulph., *Thuja*.

FEAST, of being at a: Mag. s., Ph. ac.

FIRE: *Anac.*, Ars., Bell., Calc. p., Carb. ac., Croc., Cur., Hep., Kreos., *Laur.*, *Mag. c.*, *Mag. m.*, Mag. s., Meph., Nat. m., Phos., Rhus t., Sulph.

FLYING: Apis.

JOURNEY: Apis, Calc. p., Carb. ac., Crot. h., *Kali n.*, Lach., Mag. c., Nat. c., Op., Rhus t., Sil.

MURDER: Arn., Kreos., Nat. m., Petr., Sil., Sulph.

NIGHTMARE: Acon., Alum., Amm. c., Bapt., Bor., Bry., Calc., Camph., Cann. i., Cham., Cinnab., Con., Cycl., Ferr., Gua., Iod., Led., Nat. c., Nit. ac., Nux v., *Pæon.*, Sil., *Sulph.*, Zinc.

ROBBERS: *Alum.*, Arn., Aur., Kali c., *Mag. c.*, Merc., *Nat. m.*, Sanic., Sil., Zinc.

And will not sleep unless the house is searched: *Nat. m.*

SHOOTING: Amm. m., Merc.

STORMS: Ars., Sil.

URINATING: Kreos., Seneg., Sep.

WATER: All. c., All. s., Amm. m., Ars., Bell., Dig., Ferr., Graph., Lyc., Meph., Merc., Sil., Verat. v.

FEVER.

CHILL:

Aggravated drinking, by: Ars., Caps., Elaps, Eup., Lob., Nux, Rhus t., Ver.

eating, after: Bell., Graph., Kali c., Rhus t.

motion, by: Acon., Ant. t., Apis, Bry., Canth., Cur., Hep., Kali c., Nit. ac., Nux, Rhus t., Sep., Sil.

stove, near a warm: Apis.

uncovered: Acon., Amm. m., Cyc., Nit. ac., Nux, Thuja.

Ameliorated:

heat of hot irons: Caps., Lachn.

held, by being: Gels.

held, firmly, by being: Lach.

lying down, after: Kali c., Kali n., Mag. m., Merc., Rhus, Sul.

Commencement of, in:

abdomen: Apis, Bry., Ign.

ankles, between knees and: Cinch., Lach., Puls.

arms: Bell., Hell., Ign.

arm, right: Merc.

arm, left: Nux.

back: Caps., Eup., Eup. p., Gamb., Lach., Lyc., Polyp., Sep.

lumbar region: Eep. p., Lach., Natr.

chest: Apis, Carb. an., Sep.

CHILL, commencement of.

lumbar region, in front of: Apis.

lumbar region, right side of: Merc.

face: Caust.

feet: Chel., Natr., Nux., Sep.

fingers: Bry., Natr., Sep.

fingers and toes: Med.

fingers, tips of: Bry.

hands: Chel., Gels., Nux.

hands and feet: Natr.

hand, left: Carb. v.

hand, right: Merc.

head: Bar.

knees: Apis.

knees and thighs: Thuja.

legs: Cinch., Nux m.

lips: Bry.

mouth, around the: Bry.

neck, neck and back: Val., Kali m.

nose: Sabad., Zinc., Tub.

shoulders, begins on: Lach.

shoulders, between: Sarr.

scalp, in: Mosch.

scapulæ, sometimes between the: Rhus t.

scrobiculus cordis: Calc.

stomach: Berb., Bry. Cahinca.

thighs: Thuja.

thigh, in one: Rhus t.

thorax: Lith.

vertex: Arum. t,

CHILL.

Location of:

abdomen: Æth., Apis, Calc., Ign., Meny., Merc., Mez., Op., Par., Puls., Sec., Ter.

arms: Bell., Camph., Caust., Hell., Mez., Puls., Sil.

arm, left: Carb. v., Nux m.

arm, right: Merc.

axilla: Astacus.

back: Cac., Camph., Canch., Canth., Eup., Eup. p., Gels, Lach., Led., Lob., Lyc., Natr., Nux, Polyp., Puls., Stram., Sul.

axilla, running down the, with shaking and chattering—the teeth, without external coldness: Nat. s.

interscapular region, in the: Caps., Polyp., Sep.

interscapular region, in the, like a piece of ice: Lachn.

body, all over the: Camph., Carb. v., Chin. s., Cinch., Ign., Lach., Lyc., Meny., Merc., Mez., Nux m., Nux v., Petr., Puls., Rhus t., Sec., Sep., Staph., Stram., Sul. ac., Ver., Ver. v.

chest: Apis, Ign., Merc., Sul.

coldness, external: Agar.

coldness, internal, as if frozen: Aran.

descends: Phos., Ver.

fingers, on the: Bry., Meny., Ph. ac.

genitals, icy coldness of: Sulphur.

hands: Cac., Camph., Canth., Carb. v., Chel., Hep., Hyos., Lyc.,

CHILL, location of, hands.

Meny., Mez., Natr., Nux, Op., Phos., Sec., Ver.

knees: Apis, Carb. v., Phos., Sil.

legs: Caust., Meny., Nux, Rhus, Sec., Sil., Stram., Sul.

leg, left: Carb. v., Caust., Stan., Thuja.

leg, right, icy coldness of: Chel., Sab., Sep.

leg, right, as if standing in cold water: Sab., Sep.

loins: Asaf., Camph., Puls.

parts, single, of: Amb., Calc., Caust., Cham., Ign., Led., Mez., Puls., Sep., Sil., Spig., Thuja.

stomach, pit of: Arn., Bell., Calc.

Symptoms, during:

alternate flushes and chilliness: Lachn.

arms, distention of the veins of: Chel.

back, lumbar region, aching in: Myr.

back, pain in: Caps., Chin. s., Eup., Nux, Polyp.

blood, feeling as though cold: Lyc., Rhus.

bones, aching in: Arn.

bones, pains in: Aran., Arn., Ars., Eup., Eup. p., Natr., Nux, Polyp., Rhus, Sabad., Tub.

breath, cold: Carb. v., Ver.

cheek, heat in one: Acon.

breath, desire to take a long: Cimex.

breath, hot: Rhus.

bruised, feeling as if: Arn., Bapt.

CHILL, symptoms, during.

cheek, redness of one: Cham.

cheek, heat and redness of one: Arn.

cheek, redness of one, the other pale and cold: Acon.

cheek, one pale and hot, the other red and cold: Mosch.

cheeks, cold: Cina, Petr., Rhus.

chest, oppression of: Apis, Bry., Mez., Natr., Puls.

cough: Bry., Psor., Rhus, Sabad., Samb.

covered, cannot bear to be: Camph.

covering, not relived by: Nux, Phos.

delirious: Ars., Elat., Phos., Rhus., Ver.

dyspnœa: Apis, Natr.

epistaxis: Kreos.

extremities, cold and blue: Camph., Ver.

extremities, icy cold: Camph., Canth., Ced., Meny., Natr., Nux, Phos., Stram., Ver.

face, blueness of: Nux, Stram.

face, cold: Camph., Cina, Dros., Hep., Nux, Petr, Puls., Sec., Stram., Ver.

face, red: Acon., Amm. m., Bell., Hyos., Ign., Rhus.

feet, icy coldness of: Ant. c., Calad., Meny., Phos., Ver.

feet, icy coldness of, soles: Nit. ac.

feet, icy coldness of, right limb, as if standing in ice water: Sab.

fingers, blueness of: Natr., Nux, Petr., Tar.

fingers, cold: Apis, Cac., Calad., Natr.

CHILL, symptoms, during.

shrivelled like a washer woman's: Canth.

gaping: Elat., Nux.

gaping, with a sound resembling the neighing of a horse: Elat.

goose flesh: Ang., Hell., Lyc., Merc., Natr., Nux.

hair, bristling of: Bar., Meny.

hands, blueness of: Nux, Stram.

hands, cold: Arn., Cac., Camph., Canth., Carb. v., Chel., Dros., Ferr., Hep., Hyos., Ipec., Led., Lyc., Meny., Mer., Mez., Natr., Nit. ac., Nux, Op., Phos., Polyp., Puls., Rhus, Samb., Sec., Sep., Stan., Tarax., Thuja, Verat.

head, hot: Arn., Bell., Stram.

head, heat in, rest of the body cold: Arn.

headache: Aran., Bell., Eup. p., Natr., Puls., Sep., Sul.

headache ceases entirely in open air: Aran.

heart, palpitation of: Gels., Lil., Phos.

heart, icy coldness about: Arn., Camph., Helod., Kali c., Natr., Oleand., Petr.

held, desire to be: Gels., Lach.

held, desire to be, firmly: Lach.

horripilation: Bar., Meny.

hunger: Cina, Sil.

hot drinks, craving for: Casc., Ced.

ice, lying on, feeling as though: Lyc.

CHILL, symptoms, during.

irritability: Cina, *Ign.*, N.t. ac.

knees, cold: *Apis, Carb. v.*, Ign., *Phos.*, Sil.

lachrymation: *Elat.*

lassitude: Amb., Aran., Carb. v., Caust., Merc., Natr.

legs, coldness of, excessive: *Meny.*

legs, gooseflesh of: Chin., Ars.

legs, numbness of: Eup. p., Nux.

lie down, desire to: Lach., Sep,. Sil.

lie down, desire to be near the fire and: *Lach.*

limbs, coldness of: Bell., *Meny.*, Mez., Nux, Op., Puls., Rhus, *Sec.*, *Stram.*

limbs, pain in: Eup., Mez., Nux, Puls., Rhus, Sabad.

lips, blue: Chin. s., Eu. p., *Natr.*, Nux, Sec.

liver, pain in the region of: Cinch., Nux, *Pod.*

loins, pain in: Ars., Kreos., Lach., Nux, Ver.

loquacity: *Pod.*

moaning: Eup.

muscular pains intense, must walk about for relief: Pyrog., Rhus.

nails bule: Asaf., Carb. v., Cinch., Dros., Eup. per., Petr., Thuja.

nausea: Ars., Lyc., Natr., Sabad.

nausea, drinking after: Ars., Eup.

nausea, relieved by swallow

CHILL, symptoms, during.

noise, dread of: Bell., Caps., Hyos.

neighing like horses: Elat.

nose cold: Polyp., Tarax.

tip of nose cold: Ced.

nose, red: Bell.

nose, sweat on, cold: Cina.

pain, in parts rested on: Bap., Pyrog.

respiration difficult: Apis, Thuja.

restlessness: Ars.

shivering, with: Clem., Kali br., Mur. ac., Sul. ac., Sab., Zinc.

shuddering with goose flesh: Sab., Zinc.

skin, blue: Arn., Cad. s., Cinch., Mez., Natr., Nux. m., Nux v.

skin, blue and mottled: *Nux v.*

skin, coldness, icy of: *Sec.*, Stram.

sleep: *Apis*, Kali i., Mez., Natr., *Nux m.*, Op.

sleep, deep snoring: *Op.*

sleepiness: Kali i., Natr., Nux m., *Op.*

spleen, pain in the region of: Bry., *Chin. s.*, Eup., Pod.

staggering: Caps.

streaching: Eup., Rhus.

sun, desire for the heat of: Con.

sweat, cold, from beginning of chill: Tar.

thirst: Alum., *Apis, Arn.*, Ars., Bry., Calc., *Caps.*,

THIRST, chill during.

>Eup. p., Ferr., *Ign.*, Led., Natr., Plumb., Rhus, Sec., Sep.. *Ver.*

thirst, much: Alum., Apis, Arn., *Bry.*, Caps., Eup., Ign., Natr.

thirst, for large quantities of water, giving relief: *Bry.*, Natr.

thirst, without: Ang., Ant. c., Ant. t., Aran., Bell., Cocc., Camph., Canth., Carb. an., Ced., Cham., Cina, Cinch., Coc., Dros., Gels., Ipec., Puls., Staph.

toes, coldness of: *Ferr.*, *Meny.*

toothache: *Carb. v.*

trembling: Agn., Cina, Eup., Par., Petr., Zinc.

unconsciousness: Bell., Hep., Natr.

urticaria: *Hep.*

veins distended: *Meny.*

vomiting, in all stages: *Eucal.*

vomiting: Ars., *Eup.*, Ipec., Ver

vomiting, of blie: *Eup.*

vomiting of ingesta: *Ferr.*

warmth, desire for, but does not relieve: Cic., Con., Lach.

warmth, desire for, specially heat of sun: *Con.*

yawning: Bry., Cina, *Elap.*, *Eup.*, Gamb., *Meny.*, Mur. ac., *Natr.*, Oleand.. Polyp.

Followed by:

sweat: *Ars.*, Bry., Caps., *Caust.*, *Eup.*, Ign., *Ipec.*, *Mez.*, *Nux*, *Petr.*, *Puls.*, Ver.

CHILL, followed by.

thirst: *Ars.*, Cim., Cinch., *Dros.*, Sabad.

urticaria: *Apis.*

vomiting: *Eup.*, Lyc., *Natr.*

ETIOLOGY:

Acids, abuse of, or after taking: Lach.

Alcohol, abuse of: Nux.

Anger: Nux.

Arsenic, abuse of: Ipec.

Coffee, abuse of: Cham., Nux.

Diet, indiscretions in: Ipec.

eating pork, rich fat food: *Puls.*

Dissecting wounds: Anth.. *Ars.*, Lach., *Pyr.*

Exposure: Acon., Aran.. Calc., Ced., Chin. s.

basements, cellars, living in: Ant. t., *Aran.*, Ars., Nat. s., *Ter.*

margins of streams or ponds, from living in: *Natr.*

sleeping in damp rooms or beds, from: Aran., Carb. v., Rhus.

soils freshly turned, to: Natr.

water, standing: Calc.

working clay: *Calc.*

wet, from getting: Bry., *Rhus*, Sep.

working in the rain, from: Aran., *Rhus.*

sea-shore, residing at: Natr., Nat. s.

sun, to: Cac., *Glon.*

Fright: Acon., Gels., Op.

Grief: Gels., *Ign.*

Joy, excessive: *Coff.*

Mechanical injury: Arn., Bellis, Calend., Ham., Hep., Mill., Rhus,

ETIOLOGY.

Perspiration, suppressed from: Sil.

Perspiration, suppressed from a draught: *Acon.*

Perspiration, suppressed from feet: Cup., *Sil.*

Post-mortem infection: Anth., *Ars., Lach., Pyr.*

Pus, absorption: Anth., Ars., Lach., Pyr.

Quinine, abuse of: Arn., Ars., Carb. v., Ipec., Lach., Natr., Puls., Stan.

Sewer gas: Anth., Bov., Op.

Tobacco, abuse of: Bell., Gels., Ipec., Nux, Phos., Sec.

HEAT ABSENT: Amm. m., Agar., Aran., Benz., Bov., Cac., Camph., Caps., Caust., Cimex, Coc., Dios., Hep., Lyc., Mag. c., Mez., Ph. ac., Rhus., Sabad., Staph., Sulph., Thuja, Ver.

HEAT AGGRAVATED BY:

Carriage, when riding in a: *Psor.*

drinking: Calc., Coc.

eating, after: *Caust.*

exercising, when: Camph., *Cinch,* Sep.

motion, by: Camph., *Cinch.,* Sep.

night: Cina, *Sil.*

sleep, after: Lach.

smoking, by: Cic., Coff., Ign.

warmth, by: *Apis,* Agn., Puls.

warmth, of room, by: Apis.

Ameliorated by:

heat, artificial: *Ign.*

HEAT, ameliorated.

motion, by: *Caps.*

sitting, while: *Bry.*

uncovering: Acon., Ars., Bor., Bov., Ign., Puls., Sulph.

HEAT, characteristics of:

anticipating: *Nux.*

aversion to uncovering: Eup., *Hep., Nux, Psor., Stram., Tub.*

back, from small of, in all directions: *Bap.*

body, left side of: *Mez.*

burning: Acon., Arn., *Apis, Ars.,* Bell., Elaps, Hep., Hyos., Op., *Puls., Tub.*

burning with internal chilliness: Hell.

burning even when bathed in sweat: *Op.*

burning without external redness: Hyos.

chest, in or on: *Apis.*

chilliness, with: Apis, Arn., Caust., Elaps, *Kali b.,* Merc., Nux, *Puls.,* Rhus, Sil.

chilliness, during the day: *Dros.*

chilliness, from putting hands outside the covering of the bed: *Nux, Stram, Tub.*

dry: Acon., Apis, *Ars.,* Bell., Bry., Hep., Hyos., *Nux,* Phos., Puls., Samb.

evening: Berb., *Cinch.,* Hep., Psor., *Sil.,* Sulph.

face, on: *Lyc.*

face, flushes in or over: Bap., Calc., Kali bi., *Kali c., Kali i., Nit. ac.,* Sul.

HEAT, characteristics of.

    face, flushes in or over, end-
        ing in sweat always:
        Amm. m.

    face, flushes in or over in sud-
        den towards evening: Nat.
        's., Sul. ac.

    face, flushes in or over with
        desire to be fanned: Zinc.

    flushes every afternoon: *Tub.*

    intense: Acon., Ant. t., Ars.,
        Bell., *Mez., Natr.,* Nux,
        Op., *Rhus,* Sec., *Sil., Tar.*

    internal: Acon., Arn., Ars.,
        Bell., Puls., Rhus, Sabad.

    internal, wants to uncover:
        Mur. ac.

    internal, burning, external
        chilliness: *Mez.*

    long lasting: Acon., *Ant. t.,*
        Sec., *Sul.*

    midnight, at: *Stram.,* Sul.

    midnight, before: Ant. c.

    midnight, after: *Ars.*

    midnight and noon: Stram.

    morning: *Arn.,* Nux, Sul.

    night: *Alum.,* Cal., *Phos.,*
        Puls.

    noon: *Stram.,* Sul.

    predominating: Ant. t., *Ipec.*

    shivering, with: Apis, *Arn.,*
        Card., Elaps, Gels.,
        Mal., Nux, Sul.

    shivering, drinking, from:
        Caps., *Nux.*

    shivering, motion from: Arn.,
        Nux.

    shivering, uncovering, from:
        Arn., Bar., *Nux.*

    short: *Ant. t.*

    spot, in one, which is cold to
        the touch: Arn.

    sweat, with: *Alum., Ant. c.,*
        Con., Kali i., *Mez., Op.,*

HEAT, characteristics of, sweat
with.

        Phos., Pod., Psor., Puls.
        Rhus, *Tub., Ver.*

    warmth, over whole body
        except the head: Ang.

HEAT, followed by:

    chill: Bell., Bry., Calad.
        Calc., Caust., Hell., Mal.
        Nux, Phos., *Puls.,* Sep.
        Stann., *Tub.*

    colic: Hell.

    debility: Aran., Hyd.

    drowsiness: Casc.

    exhaustion: Ars., Mal., Pyr.
        Tub.

    headache: Carb. v., *Eup.*
        Natr.

    hunger: *Cimex, Eup.*

    sleep: Eup., Op.

    thirst: Cinch.

    vomiting: Eup.

HEAT, in general: *Acon., Æsc.*
    Ant. t., Apis, Arn., *Ars.*
    Bap., *Bell.,* Bry., *Cac.*
    Casc., Chel., *Chin. s., Cinch.*
    Cur., Elap, *Eup.,* Ferr.
    Gels., Graph., Hell., Ign.
    Ipec., Kali i., Lach., *Lyc.*
    Merc., *Mez.,* Natr.
    Nit. ac., *Nux,* Op., Phos.
    Puls., Rhus, Samb., *Sec.*
    Sep., Sil.

    Symptoms, during:

        abdomen, coldness in: Zinc.

        abdomen, coldness in, after
        midnight with hot feet
        Calad.

        abdomen, burning in: Coca

        abdomen distended: Ars.

        abdomen rumbling in: Lachn

        abdomen, heat in: Cac., Cic

        abdomen, pain in: Rhus.

HEAT, symptoms, during.

abdomen, puffed up sensation in: Calc. ar.

pulsation in: *Kali c.*

air, sensitive to cold: Bar., Coc.

air, of room intolerable: *Apis.*

air, sensitive to warm: Coc.

anguish and oppression, excessive: *Acon.*

apples, desire for: Ant. t.

back, pain in: Eup., *Nux.*

back, pressure in, and forehead: Lyssin.

beer, desire for: Nux.

besotted: Gels.

blood, feeling as though hot: Ars., Bell., *Rhus.*

body, red: Canth.

body, purple: Curare:

body is too heavy, clothes seem burdensome: Euphor.

bones, pain in: Eup., Eup. p.

brandy, longing for: Ail., Asar., Psor.

breathing, anxious and rapid: Acon.

breathing, difficult, as if no air is in the room: Plant., Sul.

breathing, oppressed: *Apis,* Cim., Ipec., *Kali c.*

breathing, short: Sil.

bruised, feeling as though: Arn., Bap., Bellis, Pyrog.

burning intense: Gels.

cheeks, heat and redness of one: Ign., Ipec.

cheek, red spot on the left: Lyc.

cheek, red spot on the right: Lachn.

HEAT, symptoms, during.

cheeks, redness of one, the other pale: Cham., Ipec., Puls.

cheeks, burning and dark red: Chel., Eup., Lach., Merc.

warm: *Cinch.*

chest, burning in: Apis.

chest, oppression of: *Apis,* Lach.

chest, stitches in: Bry., Kali c.

coma: Arn.

consciousness, with almost loss of: Ph.ac.

convulsions: Hyos., *Nux,* Stram.

cough: Acon., Bry., *Ipec.*

conjunctiva, jaundiced hue of: Chin. s.

delirium: *Arn.,* Chin. s., *Natr., Pod.,* Psor., *Stram., Sul.,* Ver.

diarrhœa: *Cina,* Rhus.

diarrhœa, constant on the day, free fever: *Iod.*

drinking, repugnance to: Con., Hell., Nux.

drinks, feel too cold: Bell.

drinks, little at a time: *Ars.,* Cinch., Lyc.

drinks, warm, desire for: Casc., Eup. p.

dyspnœa: *Apis,* Arn., Kali c.

ear, heat and burning of one: *Ign.*

ear, heat of: Caps, Meny.

ears, coldness of: Ipec.

ears, redness of: Camph., Ign.

ears, roaring in: Nux.

epigastrium, fullness in: Ars.

HEAT, symptoms during.

eyelids, cannot open: *Gels.*

eyelids, swelling of upper: *Kali c.*

eyes, pupils contracted: Gels., Laur., Op., Phys., Ter.

eyes, pupils, dilated: Bell., Hell.

eyes, weakness of: *Natr.*

face, hot: Cina, Eup., Lyc., Mag. c., Polyp., Samb., Sarr., Ver.

face, paleness of: Ipec.

face, red: *Bell.*, Cac. Carb. v., Chin. s., *Cinch.*, Croc., *Ferr.*, Ign., Lachn., Patr., Polyp., Puls., Sep., Sil., Stram., Sul.

face, redness of, dark: *Lachn.*, *Sil.*

face, redness of, mahogany: Eup.

face, yellow: Ars., Cina, Eup., Natr.

fainting: *Acon.*, *Arn.*, *Natr.*

fainting, when rising up: *Acon.*

falling, fear of: *Gels.*

fanned, desire to be: *Carb.*

feet, coldness of: Arn., Samb., *Stram.*, *Sul.*

feet, hot: Led.

feet, soles burning: Ferr., Lach., Sul.

forehead, coldness of: Cina, Cinch., Puls.

forehead, hot: Stram.

forehead, sweat on: *Ver.*

gagging: *Cimex.*

hands, cold: Arn., Thuja.

hands, heat of: Led., Mag c., Nit. ac., Nux, *Puls.*, *Sul.*

HEAT, symptoms during.

hands, heat of, one, the other cold: Dig.

hands, palms of, hot: Ferr., Lach., Polyp., *Sul.*

hands, veins of, distended: Bell., Cinch., Hyos., *Led.*

head hot: Bell., Calc., Mag. c., Petr.

Headache: Ang., *Arn.*, Ars., *Bell.*, Cinch., *Eup.*, Hep., Ign., *Natr.*, Pod., Rhus, Sil.

heart, beats violently: Æsc., Kali mur.

heart, constriction about: Lil. t.

heart, palpitation of: Bar.

hunger: Cina., Cinch., Phos.

hunger canine or aversion to food: *Cinch.*

icecream, desire for: *Phos.*

irritability: Anac., Cham.

leg, pain in one: Gels.

legs, coldness of: *Stram.*

legs, heat in: *Led.*

legs, veins of, distended: *Chin. s.*

lie, still, wants to: Bry., Gels.

limbs cold: Stram.

lips, fever blister on: Hep., Ign., Natr., Nux, Rhus.

lips, fever blisters on, upper: Rhus.

lips, licks them but does not drink: *Puls.*

loquacity: Carb. v., *Lach.*, Mar. v., Pod.

moaning: Eup., *Puls.*

moaning, during sleep: Eup.

mouth, burning in: Æsc., Petr.

mouth, dryness of: Ars., Nux m.

HEAT, symptoms during.

mouth, frequent spitting of mucus: Æsc.

mouth, open: Op.

mouth, paleness around: Cina.

mouth, yellow inside: Plumb.

nausea: Carb. v., Elat., Ipec., Natr., Nux, Thuja.

noise, sensitive to: Bell., *Caps.*, *Ther.*

numbness: *Ced.*, Sep.

œsophagus, pressure in: Cimex.

painfulness of body when touched: *Stram.*

pains, on uncovering, violent: Stram.

photophobia: Hep., *Psor.*

position, desire to change: Arn., Bapt., Rhus.

position, desire to change because bed is hard: *Arn.*, Pyrog.

position, desire to change to relieve the pain: Rhus.

position, desire to change, move to a cool part of the bed: Bap., Op.

restlessness: Acon., Arn., *Ars.*, Cham., Gels., Puls., *Rhus*, Sec.

saliva, profuse discharge of watery: Æsc., Dros.

saliva, forthy: Rob.

saliva, stringy: Con., Kali bi., Mez.

scapula, pain under the right: Chel., Nux, Pod.

scapula, pain under the left: Sang.

shiverings, from uncovering: Nux.

HEAT, symptoms during.

shoulders, pain between: Rhus.

skin, hot: Hyos.

skin, itching of: Ign., Rhus.

skin, itching of, worse from rubbing: Rhus.

burning and pricking of: Merc. c.

skin, pricking in: Gels.

sleep: Ant. t., Cinch., *Eup.*, Gels., *Lach.*, *Mez.*, Natr. Nux m., *Op.*, *Pod.*, Rob., Samb.

sleep, at climax of heat: *Pod.*

sleep, deep snoring: Ign., Lach., Op., Rob.

sleep, soporous: *Op.*, Rob.

sleep, starting in: Cham., Chin. s.

sleep, starting in, when beginning to sleep: Ign., Puls.

sleepiness: Gels., *Ver. v.*

smothering, sensation of: *Apis.*

sneezing: Chin. s.

somnolency: Natr.

spine, painful to pressure: *Chin. s.*

spleen and liver, pain in the region of: Nux.

sweat: Alum., Amm. m., Ant. c., Anth., Calend., Camph., Caps., Colch., Con., Hell., Mag. c., Nicc., Stann., Stap.

sweat, profuse: *Colch.*, Psor.

sweat, on forehead: Mag. s.

sweat, on head: Bell.

temperature, subnormal: Pyr.

thirst: Acon., Arn., *Ars.*, Bell., Bry., Ced., Cham., China, Cina, Cinch., Coff., Eup. p., Hep., Mag. c.,

HEAT, symptoms during.

> Natr., Nux, Psor., Puls., Rhus, Sec., Sil., Thuja.

thirst, hot drinks, desire for: Ced., Casc., Eup. p.

thirst, large quantities of water, desire for: Acon., Natr.

thirst, large quantities of water, which relieve: Natr.

thirst, desire for, but unable to drink: Cimex.

thirst, much: Arn., Ars., Bry., Hep., Natr.

thirst, vomiting after drinking, with: Ars., Phos.

thirst, wanting: Æth., Alum., Ant. t., Apis, Calc., Camph., Caps., Carb. v., Caust., Cimex, Cinch., Dros., Ferr., Ign., Led., Nux m., Puls., Samb., Sep., Tar.

trachea, dryness of: Petr.

uncovered, desire to be: Acon., Ars., Cinch., Eup., Hep., Lach., Natr., Op., Petr., Puls.

uncovered, aversion to be being: Apis, Arg. n., Bell., Hell., Hep., Mag. c., Nux, Samb., Stram., Stront.

uncovered, chilliness when: Cinch., Nux.

urine, brick-dust sediment, with: Lyc., Phos., Sars.

urine, whitish sediment: Phos., Sep.

urine, pale: Ced., Cham.

urine, pale, frequent, large quantities of watery: Phos. ac.

urine, profuse: Cham., Eup. p., Phos.

HEAT, symptoms during.

urine, red: Nux.

urine, suppressed: Cact.

urine, turbid: Berb., Phos.

urticaria: Apis, Ign., Rhus.

urticaria, during heat, disappearing with sweat: Ignatia.

uterus, pain in the region of: Cac.

veins, blood burns in: Ars., Hyos.

veins, blood runs cold in: Ver.

veins, as from hot water running through: Rhus, Pyrog.

veins distended: Agar., Bell., Camph., Chin. s., Cinch., Hyos., Led., Merc., Puls.

vertex, hot sensation on: Nat. s., Sul.

vertigo: Carb. v., Natr., Sep., Stram.

vomiting: Cham., Cina, Eup., Ipec., Lyc., Natr.

voice weak: Hep.

warmth, of bed, intolerable: Led., Puls.

warmth, external, intolerable: Apis, Puls., Sep.

warmth, external, pleasant: Ign.

weakness: Arn., Ars., Natr., Rob.

yawning: Chin. s., Rhus.

SWEAT AGGRAVATED:

air, in open: Bry., Carb. an., Caust., Cinch., Psor.

covered, on being: Bell., Cinch.

eating: Carb. an., Carb. v.

exertion, mental: Kali c., Psor., Sep., Sul.

eyes, upon closing the: Con.

SWEAT, aggravated.

motion: Carb. an., Caust.,
Cinch., Coc., *Hep.*, Kali
c., Mer., Natr., Phos.,
Psor., *Sep.*, Sil., Sul., Ver.

sitting, during: Kali bi.

sleep, during: *Con.*, Mez.,
Phos., *Thuja.*

sleep, in first: Cal.

stool, after every: Ver.

waking on: *Samb.*, *Sep.*, Sul.

Ameliorated:

drinking, after: Chin. s.

motion, by: Caps.

sleep, in: Samb.

walking, on: Puls., Thuja.

wine, drinking: Sul. ac.

Character of:

acrid: Caps.

bloody: Crot., *Cur.*, *Lach.*,
Lyc., Nux m.

bloody, staining red: *Lach.*

chill, after the: Ant. c., Caust.

chill, after the, without previous
heat: Caps.

chill, alternating with: Nux.

chill, simultaneously: Ant. c.

chilliness with: *Eup.*, Natr.,
Nux, *Tub.*

coldness, with, on motion:
Eup., *Nux.*

clammy: *Ars.*, Ferr., Phos.

cold: *Ant. t.*, *Anth.*, *Ars.*,
Camph., Cina, *Cur.*, *Hep.*,
Ipec., *Lyc.*, *Sep.*, *Stram.*,
Ver.

cold, on forehead: Ver.

debility, not causing: *Rhus*,
Samb.

debilitating, from least movement: *Stan.*

exhausting: *Benz.*, *Cinch.*

SWEAT, character of.

easy: Cal., Lyc., *Natr.*, *Sep.*,
Sul., Sul. ac.

flies, which attracts the:
Calad., Sumbul.

hot: *Æsc.*, *Op.*

oily: *Bry.*, Cinch., Mag. c.,
Mer., Stram., *Thuja.*

partial: Cinch., *Petr.*, *Thuja.*

profuse: Ant. t., Bar., Benz.,
Bry., Calc., Carb. an.,
Casc., Caust., Ced., *Chin.
s.*, Dig., Ferr., *Hep.*,
Ipec., Kali bi., **Lach.**,
Lyc., *Mal.*, Mag. c., **Mer.**,
Natr., Nit. ac., Nux, Op.,
Ph. ac., Phos., Polyp.,
Psor., *Pyr.*, Samb., Sec.,
Sep., *Sil.*, Sul., *Tarax.*,
Thuja, *Tub.*, *Ver.*

profuse, on uncovered parts,
except head: Thuja.

smelling, fetid: Psor.

smelling, musk-like: Sul.

smelling offensive: Arn., Bar.,
Carb. an., Carb. v., Carb.
ac., Dul., *Graph.*, Lach.,
Lyc., Merc., *Mez.*, Nit.
ac., Nux., Psor., *Pyr.*,
Rhus, *Sep.*, *Sil.*

smelling, sour: *Arn.*, *Bry.*,
Caust., Cham., Colch.,
Hep., Ipec., *Lyc.*, Mag. c.,
Nit. ac., *Psor.*, Sep., Sil.,
Sul.

smelling, like urine: *Canth.*,
Nit. ac.

Followed by:

chill: *Carb. v.*, Mal., *Nux.*

chill, then sweat: *Nux.*

chill, then sweat, with heat:
Nux.

cough: Eup., Sil.

diarrhœa: Puls.

heat and thirst: Ant. c.

SWEAT, followed by.

hunger: Cina, Staph.

prostration: Ars., Kali br.,
Tar., Ter.

relief, of all complaints:
Calad., Natr., Psor., Val.

thirst: Lyc.

thirst, much: Lyc.

vomiting: Cina.

Location of:

abdomen: Anac., Dros.

arms: Merc.

axilla: Benz., Bov., Kali c.

back: Cinch., Sep., Sul.

body, all over the: Ant. t.,
Benz., Caust., Lyc.,
Merc., Natr., Nit. ac.,
Phos., Sil., Stram., Tarax.,
Thuja.

body, all over the, except the
head: Thuja.

body, but not in the face:
Rhus, Sec.

body, front of: Calc., Sel.

body, upper part of: Cham.,
Rheum, Sul. ac.

chest: Agar., Aanac., Benz.

face: Agar., Dros., Psor.,
Puls., Sam., Sil., Stram.

face, on, in beads: Arg. n.

face, all over excepting the:
Rhus, Sec.

face, right side of: Alum.

feet: Carb. an., Petr., Sil.

feet, profuse on the: Sab.

feet, profuse, offensive
Graph., Psor., Sil., Zinc.

feet, soles of: Nit. ac.

forehead: Cina, Ver.

genitals: Petr.

genitals, male: Sep.

genitals, profuse, offensive, of
the: Hydr.

SWEAT, location of.

hands: Cina, Kali bi., Sticta.

hands, palms of: Psor.

head: Op., Sil.

head, occipital region: Sul.

head, only: Sil.

knees: Cal.

hollow of: Carb. an.

legs, on the: Euphor.

neck: Stan.

neck, nape of: San., Sil.,
Stan.

nose: Cina.

parts affected: Ant. t., Amb.

parts, on affected side, worse:
Amb.

parts, covered: Acon., Bell.

parts, pressed by the clothing:
Chin. s.

parts, single: Acon., Cal.,
Lyc., Psor., Pyr., Sel.,
Sep., Stan., Sul., Thuja,
Tub.

parts, upper: Fl. ac.

parts, uncovered: Thuja.

perinæum: Hep., Kali c.,
Psor., Thuja.

scalp: Puls., Rheum, Rob.

scrotum: Thuja.

side affected: Amb.

side, left: Bar., Puls.

side, in, not lain on: Benz.

side, on, one: Amb., Bar.,
Nux, Puls.

side, on, he lies: Acon.,
Nit. ac.

side, right: Puls.

sides, both: Merc.

thighs: Carb. an., Hep., Sep.

thighs, inner surface of:
Thuja.

thighs, nowhere except on the:
Euphor.

SWEAT.

Predominates: *Carb. an.*, Cinch., *Merc.*, Nit. ac., *Psor.*, *Samb.*, *Ter.*, Thuja.

day, during the: *Ferr.*

evening, in the: Bar., Samb., Sul., Tub.

morning, in the: *Mag. c.*, Nit. ac., *Psor.*, Rhus., Sep.

night at: *Carb. an.*, Carb. v., Cinch., *Kali c.*, *Mez.*, Nit. ac., *Psor.*, Pyr., *Sil.*, *Sul.*, *Tarax.*, *Thuja*, *Tub.*, Val., Ver.

Produced by:

covering, on lightest: *Cinch.*, Spig.

headache: Ferr.

anger: Staph.

sleep, on going to: Cinch., *Con.*

sleep, after 3 a.m.: Merc.

sleep, only ceases on waking: Plat.

thirst: Coff., Thuja.

Symptoms during:

abdomen, distension of: Stram.

alternating with dryness: Act.

anxiety: Arn., Benz. ac., Berb., Bry., Calc., Coc., Ferr., Merc. c., Nat. c., Nux, Phos., Plumb., Puls., Sep., Sul.

anxiety, relieved: Acon., Bar., Natr.

body, lower part of, hot and dry: Op.

body, red, hot and dry: Stram.

body, hot and dry on going to sleep: Samb.

chill, alternating with: Glon.

chest, pain in: Bry.

SWEAT, symptoms during.

colic: Nux, Stram.

cold and hot and hot and cold: Ced.

convulsions: Nux.

cough: *Arg. n.*, Ars., *Dros.*

covered, desire to be: Acon., *Nux*, Samb., Stram., Stront.

diarrhœa: Acon., Chin. s., Stram., Sul.

diarrhœa, nightly: Chin. s.

dyspnœa: Anac., Cac., Mez.

epistaxis: Sul. ac.

exhaustion: Benz., Camph., Carb. an., Cinch.

eyes, burning in: Cinch., Stram.

face, dry: Kali bi.

face, paleness, deathly of: *Ver.*

fainting: Apis.

feet, pain in: Nit. ac., Staph.

soreness of: Sil.

feet, soreness of the balls: Nit. ac.

fingers, shrivelling of: Ant. c., Mer., *Ver.*

forehead cool, objectively and subjectively: Cist.

headache: Ant. c., Eup., Ferr., Natr., Rhus, Thuja.

headache, commencing with: Ferr.

headache, relieved gradually: *Natr.*

headache, relieved by thirst: Chin. s.

heart, palpitation of: Ced., Mez.

hunger: Cimex, Cina.

limbs, cold: Sec.

SWEAT, symptoms during.

limbs, cold and livid: Lys.

loquacity: *Puls.*

mouth, open: Op.

nails blue: *Nit. ac.*

nausea: Dros., Ipec.

nausea relieved: Glon.

pains, relieved: Arn., Lach., Nat. m., Nux.

pains, except headache, all: Eup.

pains, except gradually: *Natr.*

respiration, hurried: Ced.

respiration, short, anxious: Mang.

restlessness: Bry., Lachn.

sleep: *Op., Pod.,* Puls., *Rhus.*

sleep, restless: Sul.

symptoms, aggravated while sweating: Ferr., *Ipec.*, Merc., Op.

symptoms, ameliorated while sweating: Fl. ac., Natr., Psor.

symptoms, cessation of previous: Æsc., Natr., *Psor.*

symptoms, cessation, gradual: *Natr.*

thirst: Ars., Ced., *Cinch.*, Chin. s., *Natr.*, *Stram.*

thirst, wanting: Apis, Cal., Caps., Cimex, Cina., Ign., Nux, Samb., Ver.

toes, soreness of: Nit. ac.

toothache: Coff.

toothache, relieved by holding cold water in the mouth, returns when the water becomes warm: *Bry.*, Coff.

uncovered, desire to be: Acon., Eup., Natr., Op.

SWEAT, symptoms during.

urine, copious: Acon., **Dul.**, Phos.

urine, high colored and scanty: Ced.

urine, milky: Phos.

urine, transparent: Dul.

urine, turbid: Ipec.

urticaria: Apis, Rhus.

veins, swell up: Agar.

vomiting: Ars., Dros., Eup.

weakness: *Merc.*,   **Phos.**, *Psor.*

PRODROME:

abdomen, distention of: Ars. h.

appetite, loss of: **Hydr.**

backache: Eup., *Pod.*

backache, severe in lumbar region: Æsc., *Pod.*

billious, symptoms strongly marked: *Pod.*

bones, pains in: Eup.

bowels, pain in: Ars., Elat., Eup.

chest, pain in, cutting: Ars.

chest, pain in, erratic: Plant.

chest, oppression of: Ars. h.

chilliness: Elat., Thuja.

cough: *Rhus.*

cough, dry, hacking, in spells: Eup. p.

cough, deep, dry for half an hour with thirst and nausea. Samb.

covered, likes to be: *Eup.*

dreads the attack: *Natr.*

diarrhœa: Ars., Puls.

diarrhœa, in early morning: *Ferr.*

drink, cannot, enough: Eup.

PRODROME.

drink, desire to, sometime before: Caps., Eup.

drinking causes nausea and hastens chill: Eup.

drinking, chilliness and crawling, after: Ars.

drinking, vomiting after: *Eup.*, Natr.

drinking, refreshes: Arn.

excitement, mental: *Ced.*

epigastrium, entire goneness feeling five days before attack: *Hydr.*

eyes, blue margins around: *Cina*, Phos.

face, florid, animated: *Ced.*

face, pale: Ars., Cina., Ferr.

fever, evening without chill: Sulphur.

gastric disturbances: Ant. c., Ipec.

gastric disturbances, eating pork, fat, rich food, from: *Puls.*

head, heat of: *Stram.*

head, heaviness of: Calc.

headache: Æsc., *Bry.*, Natr., Thuja.

heat: Ced., Nux, Sul.

hunger: Cina, Cinch., Eup., Staph.

joints, aching in knee, ankles, elbows, and wrists: Pod.

languor: Bapt.

limbs, pain in: Eup., Nux, Rhus.

limbs, bearing in hands, feet and kidneys: Natr.

melancholy: *Ant. c.*

nausea: Cinch., Eup., *Ipec.*

paroxysm, always better before the: *Posr.*

suddering: Ars., *Ign.*

PRODROME.

shuddering after drinking: *Caps.*

sleep, restless, night before paroxysm: *Cinch.*

sleepiness: Ars., Corn., Puls.

sleeplessness: Amm. m.

sleeplessness, night before: Cinch.

sore, bruised feeling: Arn.

stretching: Ars., Eup., Natr., Nux.

sweating: Ver.

taste, bitter in mouth, hours before: Hep.

thirst: *Arn.*, Bry., Caps., *Cinch.*, *Eup.*, Gels., Puls., Sulph.

tonsils, pressure in: Ars. h.

urticaria, itching, stinging: Hep.

vomiting: Eup., Ferr., Natr.

weakness: Ars.

weakness, weariness and inclination to lie down: *Bapt.*

woeful: *Ant. c.*

TIME:

autumn: Ars., *Colch.*, Eup., Nux, *Psor.*, Sep., Ter.

autumn, hot days and cool nights: Acon., Colch., Mal., Mer.

autumn and spring: *Psor.*, Sep.

bed, in: Alum., Hep., Mer., *Phos.*

bed, in, in morning: Chin. s., Graph., Nux.

bed, in, at night: Cinch.

day, all: Alum., *Sil.*

day, all, at any time: *Ars.*, Plant.

TIME.

evening: Alum., Amm. m., Arn., *Ars.*, Bov., Calad., Calc, Cina, Gamb., *Hep.*, Ign., Kali c., Lach., Lyc., Mag. m., Nit. ac., Nux, Petr., *Phos.*, Psor., *Puls.*, *Rhus*, Sep., *Sul.*

evening, at sunset: Ign.

evening, in bed: Dros., Nat. s., *Phos.*, Sul.

evening, in bed, going off in bed: Natr. s.

evening, with the pains: Cycl., *Puls.*

forenoon: Arn., *Eup.*, *Natr.*, *Nux.*

midnight: *Sul.*

midnight, before: Cad. s.

midnight, after: Ars., Kali c., Op., Thuja.

Morning: Bry., Eup., Ferr., Hep., Lyc., *Natr.*, *Nux*, *Pod.*, Sep., Spig., Sul.

morning, early in: Chin. s., Natr. m., *Nux*, *Ver.*

morning, to noon: Eup., Natr.

night, at: Alum., Apis, Kali i., *Mer.*, *Nux*, Phos., Sars., Sul.

noon, at: Ant. c., Elat., Eup. Lach., Lob., Sul.

noon, after: Arn., *Ars.*, Bor., *Lyc.*, Natr., Nux, *Puls*, Ran.

paroxysm returning at:

paroxysm 1 a.m.: *Ars.*, Canth., Puls., Sil.

paroxysm, 1 to 2 a.m.: Aloe., Ars.

paroxysm, 2 a.m.: *Ars.*

paroxysm, 2 to 4 a.m.: Bor., Kali c.

paroxysm, 3 a.m.: *Thuja.*

TIME.

paroxysm, 4 a.m.: Alum., *Ced.*

paroxysm, 5 a.m.: Cinch., Natr., Polyp.

paroxysm, 5 to 8 a.m.: Sul.

paroxysm, 5-30 to 6-30 a.m.: Hura.

paroxysm, 6 to 9 a.m.: Bov., Chin. s., Eup., Nux.

paroxysm, at 7 a.m.: Bov., Eup., Nux., *Pod.*

paroxysm 7 to 8 a.m.: *Eup.*, Pod.

paroxysm, 7 to 9 a.m. one day, 12 a.m. next day: *Eup.*

paroxysm, 8 a.m.: Bov., *Eup.*

paroxysm, 8-15 a.m.: Hura.

paroxysm, 8 to 9 a.m.: Asaf., Eup.

paroxysm, 8 to 10-30 a.m.: Arn., Eup., Ipec., Natr.

paroxysm, 8-30 to 9 a.m.: Asaf.

paroxysm, 9 to 10 a.m.: Eup., Ferr. i., Rhus.

paroxysm, 9 to 11 a.m.: Natr., Stan.

paroxysm, 10 a.m.: *Natr.*, Polyp., *Stan.*

paroxysm, 10-30 a.m.: Lob., Natr.

paroxysm, 10 to 11 a.m.: *Natr.*

paroxysm, 10 to 2 p.m.: Chlor., Mer., Sul.

paroxysm, 1 to 3 p.m.: Sil., Sul., Tub.

paroxysm, 11 a.m.: Bap., *Cac.*, Chin. s., Ipec., *Natr.*, *Nux*, Polyp., Sep.

paroxysm, at 11 a.m. one day, 4 p.m. next: Calc.

TIME.

paroxysm, 11 a.m. to 12 p.m.: *Cac.*

paroxysm, 11 a.m. to 12 p.m.: Cac., Lach., Med.

paroxysm, 11 a.m. to 4 p.m.: *Cac.*, Gels.

paroxysm, 12 p.m.: Kali c., Lach., Sil., Sul.

paroxysm, 12 to 1 p.m.: Ars., Ferr. i., Lach.

paroxysm, 12 to 1-30 p.m. Mer., Sul.

paroxysm, 12 to 2 p.m.: Ars., Kob., Lach., Sul.

paroxysm, 1 p.m.: *Ars.*, Cina, Lach., *Puls.*

paroxysm, 1 to 2 p.m.: Ars.

paroxysm, 2 p.m.: Ars., Calc., Eup.

paroxysm, 2 to 4 p.m.: Gels.

paroxysm, 2 to 6 p.m.: Bor.

paroxysm, 2-30 p.m., at: Led.

paroxysm, 3 p.m., at: *Ang.*, *Ant. t.*, *Apis*, Canth., Ced., *Chin. s.*, Staph., Thuja.

paroxysm, 3 to 4 p.m.: Apis, Asaf., Canth., Med., Lach., Polyp., Puls.

paroxysm, 3 to 5 p.m.: Coc., Con.

paroxysm, 3 to 6 p.m.: Ars., Eup., Ferr.

paroxysm, 4 p.m., at: *Apis*, Ced., Hep., *Lyc.*, *Puls.*

paroxysm, 4 to 5 p.m.: Lyc., Puls.

paroxysm, 4 to 7 p.m.: Kali i., Natr., Rhus.

paroxysm, 4 to 8 p.m.: *Bov.*, Hep., *Lyc.*

paroxysm, 4 to 10 p.m.: Phel.

paroxysm, 5 p.m., at: Ced., *Kali c.*, Rhus, *Thuja.*

paroxysm, 5 to 8 p.m.: Alum., Arn., Carb. an., Gamb., Natr., Rhus.

paroxysm, 6 p.m., at: Ant. t., *Hep.*, *Kali c.*, Rhus, Sil.

paroxysm, 6 to 7 p.m.: Hep., Rhus.

paroxysm, 6 to 8 p.m.: Gamb., Hep., Kali i., Sul., Rhus t.

paroxysm, 6 to 7-30, p.m.: Clem.

paroxysm, 6 to 12 p.m.: Lachn.

paroxysm, 6-30 p.m., at: Canth., Rhus.

paroxysm, 7 p.m., at: Bov., *Hep.*, *Lyc.*, *Rhus*, Sul., Thuja.

paroxysm, 8 p.m., at: Bov., Rhus, Sul.

paroxysm, 8-30 p.m., at: Chin. ars.

paroxysm, 9 p.m., at: *Ars.*, Bov.

paroxysm, 10 p.m., at: Bov., Chin. s., Kali i.

paroxysm, 10 p.m., at: *Cac.*

paroxysm, 12 p.m., at: Ars.

anticipates 2½ hours every day: Aran. sc., Chin. s.

anticipates, one hour every other day: Ars., Cinch., Ign., Natr., Nux.

regular intervals: Aran. s., Chin. s.

regular intervals of two days: Brom.

TIME.

regular intervals of seven days: *Amm. m.*

regular intervals of fourteen days: Ars., Calc., Cinch. Puls.

sunset: Puls.

yearly: Ars., Carb. v., Lach., Sul.

fever, without chill returning at—

midnight: Stram., Sul.

12 to 3 a.m.: *Ars.*, Kali c., Med.

12 to 2 a.m.: Ars.

1 to 2 a.m.: Ars.

2 to 4 a.m.: Kali c.

3 a.m.: *Ang.*

4 a.m.: Arn.

6 to 10 a.m.: Rhus.

7 a.m.: Pod.

8 a.m. to 2 p.m.: Doryph.

9 a.m.: Kali c., Meny.

9 to 12 a.m.: Cham.

9 a.m. to 3 p.m.: Meny.

10 a.m.: *Natr.*, Rhus.

10 to 11 a.m.: Nat., Thuja.

11 a.m.: Bap., Natr.

12 a.m.: Stram., Sul.

12 to 1 p.m.: Sil.

1 to 2 p.m.: Ars.

1 to 4 p.m.: Lac. ac.

2 p.m.: *Puls.*

2 to 3 p.m.: Cur.

3 p.m.: Ant. t., Ars., Coff., Cur., Ferr., Lyc., Nicc.

3 to 4 p.m.: *Apis.*

4 p.m.: *Anac.*, Apis.

4 p.m. lasting all night: Ars., Hep., Puls., Stan.

4 to 8 p.m.: Lyc,

TIME.

5 p.m.: Con., Kali bi., Kali c., Petr., Sab., Stan.

5 and 5-30 p.m., pricking in the tongue: Ced.

5 to 6 p.m.: *Hell.*

5 to 6 p.m. very ill-humoured: Con.

6 p.m.: *Nux.*

6 p.m. to 7 p.m.: Calc., Nux.

6 to 12 p.m.: Lachn.

6 p.m. lasting all night: Nux.

6 to 8 p.m.: Ant. t., Caust.

6-30 p.m.: Ced., Hura.

7 p.m.: Calc., *Nux*, Rhus.

7 to 8 p.m.: Amb.

7 to 12 p.m.: Æsc.

8 p.m.: Ant. t., Cof., Ferr., Hep., Mur. ac., Sulph.

9 p.m.: Mag. s.

9 p.m. to 10 p.m.: Mag. s.

9 p.m. to 12 p.m.: Amm. c.

10 p.m., at: Ars.

11 p.m., at: *Calc.*

twice a day and 3 to 4 p.m.: Apis.

different times of a day: Eup., Tub.

TYPE:

Anticipating: *Ars., Bry., Chin. s., Cinch., Gamb., Nat., Nux.*

Autumnal: Æsc., *Bry.*, Cinch., Colch., Eup., *Nat., Ver.*

Bilious: Bry., *Chel., Ipec., Pod.*

Cerebrospinal: Act., **Bell.**, Bry., Gels., Nat. s., **Nux.**, Tub., Zinc.

Congestive: Arn., Camph., Lyc., *Nux, Psor., Ver.*

TYPE.

Intermittents, acute: Ars., Bry., Chin. s., Gels., Natr., Nux.

Intermittents, chronic: Psor., Sul.

Malarial: Arn., Chin. s., Cinch., Mal., Psor.

Malignant: Anth., Ars., Crot., Mur. ac., Pyrogen.

Menses, after the: Nux, Psor.

Monthly: Nux.

TYPE, paroxysm irregular: Ars., Ipec., Nux, Psor., Puls.

Periodicity marked: Aran., Ced., Chin. s., Cina, Gels.

Postponing: Gamb., Ipec.

Pernicious: Apis, Arn., Camph., Cur., Nux, Psor., Ver.

Quartan: Arn., Ars., Hyos., Iod., Meny., Nat., Nux, Puls., Sabad., Ver.

double: Bell., Cinch., Elat., Graph., Stram., Sul.

Relapsing: Psor., Sul.

Remittent: Ars., Psor.

prone to become typhoid: Ant. t., Ars., Bap., Mur. a., Psor., Rhus, Sec.

TYPE.

Septic: Anth., Ars., Carb. ac., Crot., Lach., Pyr.

Tertian: Apis, Aran., Ars., Bell., Bry., Canth., Ced., Chin. s., Cinch., Eup., Ipec., Lyc., Mez., Natr., Nux, Pod., Polyp., Puls., Rhus, Sabad.

fever, with no chill: Gels.

Typhoid: Ars., Bap., Bry., Crot., Elaps, Gels., Hyos., Lach., Lyc., Mur. ac., Op., Ph. ac., Psor., Pyr., Rhus, Stram., Sul. ac.; Ter., Zinc.

Typhus: Aran., Ars., Lach., Mur. ac., Op., Ph. ac., Psor., Pyr.

Yellow-fever: Ars., Cad. s., Camph., Canth., Carb. v., Carb. ac., Crot., Natr. s., Nux, Psor., Ter., Ver.

Zymotic: Arn., Ars., Bar., Bry., Cad. s., Crot., Cur., Hyos., Lach., Lyc., Mur. ac., Pyr., Sul. ac.

PULSE.

ABNORMAL: *Acon.*, Ant. t., Arg. n., Arn., *Ars.*, *Ars. i.*, *Bell.*, Bry., Camph., Carb. s., Carb. v., Chin., Con., *Cupr.*, Dig., Gels., Glon., Hep., *Hyos.*, *Iod.*, Kali c., *Kreos.*, *Lach.*, Laur., Merc., *Op.*, *Phos.*, *Ph. ac.*, Rhus t., Sec., Sep., *Sil.*, *Stram.*, Sulph. *Verat.*

AUDIBLE: Ant. t.

BOUNDING: Ars., Benz. ac., Camph., Cann. i., Canth., Chin. s., Eup. per., Glon., Iod., Kali chl., Lil. t., Naja, Plan., Raph.

CONTRACTED: Asaf., Kali bi., Sec.

DOUBLE: Phos., Stram.

FLUTTERING: Arn., Ars., Crot. h., Kali bi., *Nux v.*, Phos.

FREQUENT, rapid: *Acon.*, Æth., Agar., Ail., Ant. t., *Apis.* Arg. n., *Arn.*, *Ars.*, *Ars. i.*, Asaf., *Aur.*, Aur. m., Bapt., Bell., Benz. ac., *Berb.*, *Bry.*, Camph., Canth., Cham., Chin. s., Cina, Colch., *Con.*, Crot. h., *Cupr.*, *Dig.*, Echi., Ferr., Ferr. p., *Gels.*, *Glon.*, Hell., Hyos., Hyper., Ign., *Iod.*, Lach., Laur., Lycops., Manc., *Merc.*, Mez., Mosch., Mur., ac., Naja, Nat. c., *Nat. m.*, Op., *Phos.*, *Ph. ac.*, Phys., Phyt., Plat., Plb., Pul., *Pyrog.*, Ran. s., *Rhus t.*,

FREQUENT, rapid

Rhus v., Sang., *Sec.*, Sep Sil., Spig., Spong., *Stann* Stram., *Sulph.*, Tab., Tel Valer., Verat., *Verat. v.*

And intermittent: Aur., Dig Nux v., Sulph.

And small: *Acon.*, Ars., Aur Aur. m., Camph., Con., Dig Hell, Iod., Lach., *Laur* Mur. ac., Nux m., *Nux v* Sil., Stram., Verat.

FULL: *Acon.*, All. c., *Ant. t* Arn., *Bell.*, Berb., *Bry* Canth., *Chel.*, Chin., Cupr Dig., Dulc., Eup. per., *Gels* Glon., Hep., *Hyos.*, Ign Kali c., *Kali n.*, Lach., Led Merc., Mez., Mosch., Naja Nux v., Op., Petr., Phos Ph ac., Sabin., Sep., Sil Spig., *Stram.*, Sulph., Tab Verat., Verat. v.

HARD: *Acon.*, All. c., Ant. Arn., Bar. c., *Bell.*, Benz. a *Berb.*, *Bry.*, Cact., Canth *Chel.*, Chin., Cina, Cupr Dig., Dulc., Ferr., Hep Hyos., Ign., Ka. c., Kali r Kreos., Lach., Led., Merc Mosch., Nit. a., Nux v Phos., Sep., Sil., Stram Sulph., Ter.

HEAVY: Phos., Stram.

IMPERCEPTIBLE: *Acon* Ars,. Cact., Canth., Car ac., *Carb. v.*, Cocc., *Colch* Cupr., Ip., Merc., Naj Op., Sec., Sil., *Verat.*

IMPERCEPTIBLE.

Almost: *Acon.*, Apis, Ars., *Camph.*, Dig., *Gels.*, Ip., Lach., Laur., Merc., Naja, Podo., Puls., Rhus t., Spong., Stram., Tab., Verat.

INTERMITTENT: Acon., Æth., Agar., Arg. n., Ars., Aur., Bry., Canth., Caps., Carb. v., Cedr., *Chin.*, Cimex, Colch., Con., Crot. h., *Dig.*, Gels., Hep., Iod., Kali c., Kali i., Kalm., Lach., Laur., Lil t., *Merc.*, Merc. c., *Nat. m.*, Nit. ac., Op., Ox. ac., *Ph. ac.*, Plb., Rhus t., Samb., *Sec.*, Sep., Stram., Sulph., Tab., Zinc.

IRREGULAR: Acon., Agar., *Ant. c.*, Arg. n., *Ars.*, Ars. i., Asaf., Aspar., Aur., Bry., Cact., Caps., *Chin.*, Chin. a., Cimic., Colch., Con., Crot. h., *Dig.*, Gels., Hep., Hyos., Kali bi., Kali c., Kali i., Kalm., *Lach.*, Lycops., Merc., Merc. c., Naja, *Nat. m.*, Olnd., Op., *Ph. ac.*, Phos., Phyt., Plan., Plb., Rhus t., Samb., *Sec.*, Sang., Sep., Sil., Spig., Stil., *Stram.*, Sulph., Tab., Verat., *Verat. v.*

And slow: Acon., Agar., Amyg., Ant. t., Aspar., Bell., *Berb.*, Camph., *Cann. i.*, Cann. s., Canth., Caps., Chel., Chin. s., Con., Crot. h., Cupr., *Dig.*, Gels., Hell., *Kalm.*, Laur., Lob., Lycps., Manc., Naja, Nux m., *Op.*, Podo., Sang., Sec., *Sep.*, *Stram.*, Tab., Verat., Verat. v.

SMALL: *Acon.*, Agar., Ant. t., *Ars.*, Ars. i., Aur., Aur. m., Bell., *Camph.*, Carb. v., Cham., Chin., Cocc., Colch., Con., *Cupr.*, Dig., Dulc., *Gua.*, Hell., Hyos., Iod., Kali c., Kreos., Lach., *Laur.*, Lobel., Merc., Mur. ac., Nux m., Op., Phos., Ph. ac., Plat., Raph., Samb., *Sec.*, Sil., Stan., Stram., Sul. ac., Sulph., *Verat.*

SOFT: Acon., *Ant. t.*, Ars., Aur., Carb. ac., *Carb. v.*, Colch., *Cupr.*, Dig., Gels., Gua., Kalm., *Lach.*, Lob., Merc., *Mur. ac.*, Ox. ac., Phos., Plat., Sang., Spig., *Stram.*, Tab., *Ter.*, *Verat.*, Verat. v.

STRONG: Bell.

TENSE: Amm. m., Ant. t., Mez.,

THREADY: Ars.

TREMULOUS: Ant. t., Ars., Bell., *Calc.*, Cic., Hell., Kreos., Rhus t., Sabina, Sep., Staph., *Spig.*

WEAK: *Ant. t.*, Arn., Ars., Aspar., *Aur.*, *Berb.*, Camph., Canth., *Carb. v.*, Chin., Chin. a., Cimex, *Crot. h.*, Cupr., Dig., *Gels.*, Glon., Ign., Iod., Ip., Kali bi., Kali br., Kalm., *Lach.*, *Laur.*, Lycops., Manc., Merc., Merc. c., Mur. ac., *Naja*, *Ph. ac.*, Phos., Puls., Rhus t., Sang., Sec., Spig., Staph., Stram., Tab., Verat. v.

SKIN.

CHAPPING: Æsc., Calc., Cycl., Graph., Hep., Kali c., Lach., Puls., Rhus t., Sars., Sep., Sulph.

CICATRICES: the scar of a wound.

Break open: Bor., Carb. an., Caust., Crot. h., Iod., Lach., Nat. m., Phos., Sil.

Painful, becoming: Carb. an., Hyper., Lach., Nat. m., Nit. ac., Sil.

CRACKS: Æsc., Ant. c., Arn., Aur., Bad., Calc., Calc. s., Carb. an., Carb. s., Cham., Cycl., Graph., Hep., Kali s., Kreos., Lach., Lyc., Mang., Merc., Nat. c., Nat. m., Nit. ac., Petr., Psor., Puls., Rhus t., Sars., Sep., Sil., Sulph., Zinc.

Deep, bloody: Merc., Nit. ac., Petr., Sars., Sulph.

mercurial: Hep., Nit. ac., Sulph.

Winter, in: Calc., Calc. s., Carb. s., Graph., Petr., Psor., Sep., Sulph.

DISCOLORATION:

Blackish: Apis, Arg. n., Ars., Carb. h., Lach., Plb., Sec.

Bluish: Ant. t., Apis, Arg. n., Bapt., Bell., Brom., Camph., Carb. s., Carb. v., Crot. h., Cupr., Dig., Hydr. ac., Kali br., Lach., Laur., Nux m., Nux v., Op., Ox. ac., Phyt., Sec., Stram., Tarent., Verat., Verat. v.

DISCOLORATION.

Green spots: Arn., Bufo, Con Lach.

Spots, coppery: Ars., Carb. an Cor. r., Kreos., Lach., Mez Nit. a., Rhus t., Verat.

white: Apis, Ars., Fl. ac Kali c.

yellow, jaundice etc: Acon Aloe, Ambr., Amm. m Ant. t., Ars., Aur., Bell Berb., Bry., Calc., Cale p., Canth., Carb. v., Care m., Caust., Cham., Chel Chin., Chin. a., Chion Crot. h., Dig., Ferr., Fern i., Hep., Hydr., Ign., Iod Lach., Lept., Lyc., Merc Merc. c., Nat. m., Nat. s Nit. ac., Nux v., Op Phos., Plb., Pod., Ptel Puls., Sang., Sec., Sep Sil., Spig., Sulph.

ECHYMOSIS: Arn., Bry., Carb h., Ferr., Hep., Lach., Nu v., Ph. ac., Phos., Puls Sec., Sul. ac., Sulph., Taren

ERUPTION:

Boils: Anac., Ant. c., Apis Arn., Ars., Ars. i., Bar. c Bell., Calc., Calc. s., Con Crot. h., Euph., Graph Hep., Hyos., Iod., Kali i Lach., Led., Lyc., Merc Nat. m., Nit. ac., Nux v Petr., Phos., Ph. ac., Phyt Psor., Rhus t., Sec., Sep Sil., Sul. ac., Sulph., Thuja.

ERUPTION.

Boils, cold boils: Bell., Calc., Iod., Led., Lyc., Mur. ac., Nat. m., *Phos.*, *Sil.*

(1) Carbuncle: Apis Anthr., *Arn.*, *Ars.*, Bell., Bufo, Crot. h., Echi, Hep., Hyos., Lach., Rhus t., Sec., *Sil.*, Sulph.

burning: *Anthr.*, Apis, Ars.

Chickenpox: *Ant. c.*, Ant. t., Bell., Carb. v., Led., Merc., *Puls.*, Rhus t., Sep., *Sulph.*, Thuja.

Coppery: Ars., Ars. i., Calc., *Carb. an.*, Kali i., Kreos., Lyc., Merc., Mez., Nit. ac., Rhus t., Verat.

Crusty: Agar., Alum., Anac., Anan., Anthr., *Ant. c.*, *Ars.*, Aur. m., Bar. c., Bell., Bry., *Calc.*, *Calc. s.*, Carb. an., Carb. s., Caust., Chel., Cic., Cist., Clem., *Con.*, *Dulc.*, Fl. ac., *Graph.*, Hep., Jug. c., *Kali s.*, Lach., Lappa, Led., Lith., *Lyc.*, *Merc.*, Merc. i. r., *Mez.*, Mur. ac., *Nat. m.*, Nit. ac., *Olnd.*, *Petr.*, Phos., Phyt., Psor., Puls., Ran. b., *Rhus t.*, Rhus v., Sabad., Sars., Sep., *Sil.*, Spong., Staph., *Sulph.*, Viol. t.

honey-colored: **Carb. v.**

horny: *Ran. b.*

moist: Anthr., Ars., **Bar. c.**, Calc., *Carb. s.*, Cic., Graph., Hell., Hep., *Lyc.*, Merc., *Mez.*, Olnd., Rhus t., Sil., *Staph.*, Sulph.

Eczema: *Ars.*, *Ars. i.*, *Bar. m.*, Calad., Calc., *Calc. s.*, Carb. v., Caust., Cic., *Crot. t.*, *Dulc.*, Graph., Hep., Iris, Jug. c., Kali ar., Kali chl., *Lap. m.*, Lith., Lyc., Merc.,

ERUPTION, eczema.

Mez., Nat. s., *Olnd.*, *Petr.*, Phyt., *Psor.*, Ran. b., *Rhus t.*, Sars., Sep., Sil., Staph., Sulph., *Sul. i.*, Thuja, Vio. t.

Hairy parts, on: Lith., **Merc.**, Nat. m., *Rhus t.*

Herpetic, circinate: Bar. c., Calc., **Eup.** per., Graph., Lith., **Nat. c.**, *Nat. m.*, Phyt., Sep., *Tell.*, *Tub.*

scarly: *Calc.*, Clem., Con., **Dulc.**, Graph., Lyc., *Merc.*, **Phos.**, Psor., Sep., **Sulph**

suppurating: Dulc., Lyc., Merc., Nat. c., Petr., *Rhus t.*, *Sep.*

(3) (4) zoster, zona: Ars., Clem., Graph., Hep., *Iris*, Kali bi., Kali chl., *Merc.*, *Mez.*, Nat. m., Petr., *Ran. b.*, *Rhus t.*, Sil., Thuja, Vario.

itching, warmth aggravating: Alum., Caust., Clem., Led., Lyc., *Merc.*, Mez., Psor., Puls., Sulph.

itching, warmth of bed aggravating: Alum., Clem., Kali a., *Psor.*, Puls., Rhus t., *Sulph.*, *Til.*

Pemphigus: Anac., Ars., Crot. h., Dulc., *Lach.*, Lyc., Merc., Nat. m., Nat. s., Nit. ac., Psor., Rhus t., Sars., Sep., Sil., Sulph.

Psoriasis: Ars., *Ars. i.*, Calc., Calc. s., Canth., Chin., Clem., Iris, Kali ar., Kali c., Lob., *Lyc.*, Mang., Merc., Nit. ac., Petr., Phos., *Phyt.*, Psor., Puls., Rhus t., Sarr., **Sars.**, Sep., Sil., Sulph.

ERUPTION, psoriasis.

syphilitic: Ars., *Ars. i.*, Cor. r., *Merc.*, Nit. ac., Phyt., Sars.

Pustules: Ant. c., *Ant. t.*, Ant. s., *Ars.*, Aur., Bell., Calc., Calc. s., **Carb. ac.**, Carb. s., Carb. v., **Caust.**, Chel., Cic., Clem., Con., Crot. h., Crot. t., Dulc., **Hep.**, Hydroc.. Hyos., Iris, Kali bi., Kali br., Kali i., Keros., Merc., Mez., Nat. m., Nit. ac., Petr., Psor., Puls., *Rhus t.*, Sars., Sep., Sil., *Staph.*, Sulph.

black: *Anth.*, *Lach.*, Mur. ac.

malignant: *Anthr.*, *Ars.*, Bell., Bufo, Carb. v., Crot. h., *Lach.*, Ran. b., Rhus t.. Sec., Sil., Tarent. c.,

Scabies: Ant. c., *Ars.*, Aster., Bar. m., Calc., *Carb. s.*, *Carb. v.*, Caust., Clem., Cupr., Dulc., Graph., Hep., *Kali s.*, Keros., Lach., **Lyc.**, Mang., Merc., Nat. c., **Ph.** ac., *Psor.*, Sel., *Sep.*, Sil., Sul. ac., *Sulph.*, Verat., Zinc.

Scarlatina: *Ail.*, *Amm. c.*, **Apis**, Ars., Arum. t., *Bell.*, Bry., Calc., Carb. ac., **Carb. v.**, Cham., Crot. h., Cupr., Gels., Hyos., *Lach.*, Lyc., *Merc.*, *Nit. ac.*, Phos., **Ph.** ac., *Rhus t.*, Stram., Sulph., Zinc.

Smallpox: Ant. c., *Ant. t.*, Apis, Ars., Bell., Bry., Carb. ac., *Merc.*, Nat. m., Puls., *Rhus t.*, Sulph., Thuja, Zinc.

black: *Ars.*, Bell., Lach., Mur.. ac., *Rhus t.*, **Sec.**

Syr ilitic: *Ars. i.*, Aur., **Fl. ac.**, Gua., Hep., Kali bi., *Kali i.*, Lach Lyc., *Merc.*, **Merc. c.**,

ERUPTION, syphilitic.

Merc. i, f., *Merc. i. r.*, Nit. ac., Phyt., Sil., Syph., Thuja.

Urticaria: Acon., Ant. c., **Apis**, Ars., *Ars. i.*, Bov., Bry., Calad., *Calc.*, Calc. s., **Carb. s.**, Carb. v. Caust., Chin. s., *Chlor.*, Con., Cop., Crot. h., Cupr., Dulc., Elat., Graph., *Hep.*, Kali ar., Kali br., Kreos., *Led.*, Lyc., Mez., *Nat. m.*, Nat. p., Nux v., Petr., Phos., Psor., Puls., *Rhus t.*, Sep., Sul. ac., *Sulph.*, Sul. i., Til., *Urt. u.*, *Verat.*

night: *Apis.*, Bov., Chlor., Cop., Nux v., Puls.

bathing, after: Phos., Urt. u.

chill, previous to: Hep.

chill, during,: Ars., *Nat. m.*, *Rhus t.*

chill, after: Elat., Hep.

cold air, in: Nit. ac., *Rhus t.*, Sep.

Fever, during: *Apis*, *Ign.*, *Rhus t.*, Rhus v., Sulph.

Vesicular, washing aggravating: *Clem.*, Dulc., Psor., *Sulph.*, Urt. u.

Vesicular, washing, aggravating in cold water: Clem., Dulc.

ERYSIPELAS: Acon., Amm. c., Anac., Anthr., *Apis*, Arn., Ars., *Ars. i.*, Aur., *Bell.*, Bor., Bry., Calc., **Camph.**, Canth., Carb. an., **Carb. s.**, Cham., Chin., Clem., **Crot. h.**, Echi., *Euph.*, **Graph.**, Hep., Iod., Ip., Jug. c., *Kali c.*, Kali chl., Kali p., Lach., *Lyc.*, *Merc.*, Nat. ac., Ph. ac., Phos., Puls., Rhus t., **Ruta**, Sil., Sulph., Tarent. c., Ter., Thuja.

RYSIPELAS.

Erratic: Mur. ac., Puls.

Gangrenous: Anthr., Apis, Ars., Bell., Camph., Carb. v., Lach., Mur. ac., Rhus t., Sabin., Sec., Sil.

Smooth: Apis, Bell.

Swelling, with: Acon., Apis, Arn., Ars., Bell., Calc., Graph., Hep., Lach., Merc., Rhus t., Sulph., Thuja, Verat. v.

Vesicular: Anac., Ars., Bell., Canth., Carb. s., Euph., Graph., Hep., Kali chl., Lach., Rhus t., Sep., Sulph.

XCRESCENCES:

Condylomata: Apis, Aur., Aur. m., Calc., Cinnab., Euphr., Hep., Kali chl., Kali i., Lyc., Med., Merc., Merc. c., Nat. s., Nit. ac., Ph. ac., Phos., Sabin., Sars., Sep., Staph., Sulph., Thuja, Teucr.

horny: Thuja.

moist: Apis, Nit. ac., Thuja.

pedunculated: Caust., Lyc., Nit. ac., Ph. ac., Thuja.

sticking pain: Nit. ac.

suppurating: Thuja.

syphilitic: Cinnab., Merc., Nit. ac., Thuja.

Fungus, cauliflower: Ant. c., Ars., Con., Kreos., Lach., Nit. ac., Sil., Staph., Thuja.

hæmatodes: Ars., Carb. an., Carb. v., Kreos., Lach., Lyc., Merc., Nat. m., Nit. ac., Phos., Sil., Sulph.

Freckles: Amm. c., Ant. c., Calc., Dulc., Ferr., Graph., Lyc., Mur. ac., Nat. c., Nit. ac., Phos., Puls., Sep., Sulph.

EXCRESCENCES.

Gangrene, from burns or gangrenous sores: Agar., Asaf., Canth, Carb. v., Caust., Kreos., Rhus t., Stram.

cold: Ars., Asar., Canth., Carb. v., Euph., Lach., Plb., Sec., Sil., Squil.

senile: Carb. v. -

GOOSEFLESH: Acon., Ang., Ars., Bell., Bry., Calc., Camph., Cann. s., Caust., Chin., Croc., Hell., Led., Lyc., Nat. m., Nat. s., Nux v., Par., Phos., Sabad., Sil., Thuja, Verat.

HARD, like collosities: Ant. c., Dulc., Graph., Ran. b., Rhus t., Sep., Sil.

Parchment, like: Ars., Chin., Lith., Lyc., Sars., Sil.

thickening, with: Calc., Dulc., Lach., Ran. b., Rhus t. Sep.

ICE or iced cold needles, sensasation of: Agar., Ars.

ITCHING:

Perspiring parts: Cham., Lyc., Mang.

Scratch until it bleeds, must: Alum., Arg. n., Ars., Bar. c., Bor., Chlor., Puls.

Scratching aggravates: Alum., Anac., Arg. m., Ars., Bism., Bov., Calad., Caps., Caust., Con., Led., Mez., Puls., Rhus t., Sil., Staph., Stront., Sulph., Til.

Scratching ameliorates: Agn., Asaf., Brom., Bry., Calc., Canth., Cina, Crot. t., Cycl., Dros., Gua., Ign., Jug. c.,

ITCHING, scratching ameliorates.
Kali c., Kreos., Mag. c.,
Mur. ac., Nat. c., Phos.,
Plb., Ruta, Sars., Sep.,
Sulph., Thuja, Zinc.

Smarting: Arg. m., Graph.,
Plant., Rhus t., Sep., Sulph.,
Zinc.

Stinging: Apis, Arn., Bar. c.,
Bry., Caust., Chlor., Cocc.,
Con., Cop., Cycl., Dros.,
Graph. Kali c., Merc., Mur.
ac., Nat. m., Puls., Rhus t.,
Sabad., Sep., Sil., Spig.,
Spong., Stann., Staph., Sulph.,
Thuja, Til., Urt. u., Viol. t.

Undressing aggravates: Cocc.,
Dros., Nat. s., Olnd., Rumex, Staph., Tuber.

Voluptuous: Merc., Sil., Sulph.

Wandering: Agar., Bar. c.,
Canth., Con., Merc., Puls.

Warm, on getting: Æth., Alum.,
Dol., Kali ar., Led., Lyc.,
Merc., Nat. a., Psor., Puls.,
Sulph., Urt. u.

Warm, on getting, in bed: Æth.,
Alum., Anac., Ant. c., Apis,
Bov., Calc., Carb. s., Carb.
v., Clem., Cocc., Cycl.,
Gels., Graph., Kali ar., Kali
bi., Kali s., Led., Lyc.,
Merc., Mez., Nat. m., Nat.
p., Phos., Psor., Puls., Rhus
t., Sec., Sulph., Til., Urt. u.

LUPUS: Ars., Bar. c., Carb. ac.,
Carb. v., Caust., Cist.,
Hydroc., Kali bi., Kali chl.,
Kali s., Kreos., Lyc., Nit. ac.,
Phyt., Psor., Sil., Thuja.

NETWORK OF BLOOD VES-
SELS: Carb. v., Caust.,
Crot. h.

STINGS OF INSECTS: Apis,
Arn., Bell., Calad., Carb. ac.,
Led., Nat. m., Urt. u.

ULCERS, black: Anthr., Ars.,
Asaf., Carb. s., Carb. v.,
Con., Lach., Lyc., Mur. ac.,
Plb., Sec., Sil., Sulph., Sul.
ac.

Bleeding: Arg. n., Ars., Ars. i.,
Asaf., Calc., Carb. v., Con.,
Crot. h., Graph., Hep., Iod.,
Kali c., Lach., Lyc., Merc.,
Mez., Nit. ac., Phos., Ph. ac.,
Puls., Ran. b., Sec., Sil.,
Sulph., Sul. ac.

menses, during: Phos.

edges: Ars., Lyc., Merc., Sil.

Bluish: Ars., Asaf., Aur., Carb
v., Con., Hep., Kali i., Lach.,
Lyc., Mang., Merc., Sil.

Burning: Anthr., Ars., Bufo,
Carb. s., Carb. v., Caust.,
Cham., Clem., Con., Dros.,
Hep., Hydr., Kali c., Kreos.,
Lyc., Merc., Mez., Nat. a.,
Nat. c., Nit. ac., Phos., Plb.,
Puls., Ran. b., Rhus t., Sil.,
Staph., Sulph., Thuja.

Cancerous: Ambr., Ars., Ars. i.,
Bufo, Calc. c., Carb. ac.,
Carb. an., Carb. s., Carb. v.,
Graph., Hep., Hydr., Kali i.,
Kreos., Lach., Lyc., Merc.,
Nit. ac., Phos., Petr., Ph. ac.,
Phyt., Rhus t., Sep., Sil.,
Staph., Sulph., Thuja.

ULCERS, deep: Agar., Ant. c.,
Anthr., Ars., Asaf., Aur.,
Bell., Bov., Calc., Calc. s.,
Carb. v., Com., Con., Hep.,
Hydr., Kali bi., Kali i., Lach.,
Lyc., Merc., Merc. c., Mur.
ac., Nit. ac., Petr., Psor.,
Puls., Sep., Sil., Sulph.,
Syph.

ULCERS.

Dirty: Arn., Ars., *Lach.*, Lyc., *Merc.*, *Nit. ac.*, Sulph.

Discharges albuminous: Calc., Puls.

blackish: Anthr., Sulph.

bloody: Anthr., *Ars.*, Ars. i., *Asaf.*, Carb. v., Caust., Con., Dros., Hep., Kali c., Lyc., *Merc.*, Nit. ac., Petr., Puls., Sars., Sil.

cheesy: Merc.

corrosive: *Ars.*, Carb. v., *Caust,* Fl. ac., Graph., Hep., Iod., Kali bi., Lyc., *Merc.*, Nit. ac., Petr., Phos., Ran. b., Ran. s., *Rhus t.*, Sil., Squil., Staph.

green: Ars., Asaf., Carb. v., Caust., Kali i., Lyc., Nat. s., Nux v., Phos., Puls.. Sil., Sulph.

tenacious: Bov., Con., Graph., Hydr.

Dry: *Kali bi.*

Elevated, indurated margins, with: Apis, Ars., Hep., Kali ar., Kali bi., *Lyc.*, Merc., Nit. ac., Petr., Phos., Puls., Sil., Sulph.

ULCERS, fungus: Arg. n.. *Ars.*, Calc., Carb. an., Carb. s., Carb. v., Cham., Hydr., Lach., Merc., Nit ac., Petr., Sep., Sil., Sulph., Thuja.

Gangrenous: Anthr., *Ars.*, Asaf., Bapt., Carb. v., Chin., Cinnab., Con., Crot. h., Kreos., *Lach.*, Lyc., Mur. ac., Sec., Sil.

Indurated: Alumn., Arg. m., Ars., Asaf., Aur., Bell.;

ULCERS, indurated.

Bry., *Calc.*, Carb. an., Carb. s., Carb. v., Chin., Clem., Con., Dulc., Fl. ac., Hep., Hydr., Kali bi., Lach., Lyc., Mang., Merc., *Puls.*, Sil.

margins: Ars., Asaf., *Calc.*, Carb. an., Carb. v., Caust., Com., Fl. ac., Hep., Lach., Lyc., *Merc.*, Nit. ac., Phos., Puls., Sang., *Sil.*, Sulph.

Lardaceous: Ars., Hep., *Merc.*, Nit. ac., Phyt.

Mercurial: Asaf., Aur., Carb. v., Cist., *Hep.*, Kali bi., Lach., Lyc., *Nit. ac.*, *Ph. ac.*, *Phyt.*, Sars., Sil., Sulph.

Phagedenic: Anthr., Ars., Calc., *Carb. v.*, *Caust.*, Crot. h., Graph., Hep., Hyper., Kali ar., Kali c., Lach., *Lyc.*, *Merc.*, Merc. c.. Merc. i. r., Mez., Nat. c., Nat. m. *Nit. ac.*, Petr., Puls., Ran. *b.*, *Ran. s.*, Rhus t., Sep., *Sil.*, Sulph., Sul. ac.

Serpiginous: Ars., Merc., Phyt., Sars., Sil.

Stinging, stitching: Apis, *Ars.*, Asaf., Bell., Bry., Carb. an., Cinnab., Graph., Hydr., Lyc., *Merc.*, Nat. c., *Nit. ac.*, Petr., *Pul.*, Rhus t., Sep., Sil., Staph., *Sulph.*, Thuja.

splinters, as from: Hep., *Nit. ac.*

ULCERS, syphilitic: *Ars.*, Aur., Aur. m., Aur. m. n., Carb. v., Cist., Hep., *Iod.*, Kali bi., Kali chl., *Kali i.*, Lach., Merc., Merc. c., *Merc. i. r.*, Nit. ac., Petr., *Phyt.*, Sars., Staph., Still., Syph., *Thuja.*

ULCERS.

Varicose: Ars., Calc., Carb. v., *Caust.*, Fl. ac., Lach., *Lyc.*, *Puls.*, Rhus t., Sil., Sulph., Zinc

WARTS: Ant. c., Ars., Aur., *Bar.* c., *Bell.*, Benz. ac., *Calc.*, *Calc. s.*, *Caust.*, *Dulc.*, Hep., Kali chl., Lach., *Merc. c.*, Nat. c., *Nat. s.*, *Nit. ac.*, Ox. ac. Ph. ac., Psor., Rhus t., Sep., *Sulph.*, *Thuja.*

WARTS.

Bleeding: *Caust.*, Nit. ac., Rhus t., *Thuja.*

Horny: *Ant. c.*, Calc., Caust., Nit. ac., Sep., Sulph.

Indented: Ph. ac., Thuja.

Jagged: *Caust.*, *Nit. ac.*, Sep., *Thuja.*

Sensitive to touch: Caust.. Cupr., Nat. c., *Staph.*, Thuja.

DESIRES AND AVERSIONS.

DESIRE For:

Alcoholic drinks: *Ars.*, Asar., Aur., *Caps.*, *Crot. h.*, Hep., Iod., Kreos., *Lach.*, Led., Lyc., Med., Mur. ac., *Nux v.*, Op., Phos., Psor., Puls., Sel., Sep., Spig., Staph., *Sulph.*, Sul. ac., Syph.

beer: *Acon.*, Bell., Bry., Caust., Cocc., Coloc., Graph., Kali bi., Lach., Merc., Nat. c., Nat. m., Nat. s., *Nux v.*, Petr., Phell., Puls., Rhus t., Sabad., Spig., Stront., *Sulph.*

brandy: Hep., *Nux v.*, Op., Petr., Phos., Sel., Sep., Spig., Staph., Sulph., Sul. ac.

whisky: Arn., Ars., Carb. an., *Lac c.*, Lach., Phos., Sel., Spig., *Sulph.*

wine: Acon., Æth., Ars., Bry., Calc., Cic., Hep., Lach., Mez., *Phos.*, Sep., Spig., *Sulph.*

Bread: Ars., Aur., Cina, Coloc., Ferr., Mag. c., Merc., Nat. m., Plb., Stront.

and butter: Ferr., Mag. c., *Merc.*

Cheese: Cist.

Coffee: Alum., *Ang.*, Ars., Aur., Bry., Caps., Carb. v.,

DESIRE for.

Chin., Con., Mez., Nux m., Sel.

Eggs: Calc.

Fat: *Nit. ac.*, Nux v., Sulph.

Fish: Nat. m.

Fruit: Alum., Ant. t., Ign., Mag. c., *Ph. ac.*, Sul. ac., *Verat.*

Highly seasoned food: *Chin.*, Hep., Lac. c., Nux v., *Phos.*, Sang., *Sulph.*, Tarent.

Ice: Elaps, Med., *Verat.*

Ice-cream: Calc., Eup. per., *Phos.*

Indigestible things: Alum., Calc., Calc. p.

Juicy things: *Ph. ac.*, Sabad.

Lemonade: *Bell.*, Jatr., Nit. ac., Sabin., Sul. i.

Lime, slate pencils, earth, chalks, clay, etc: Alum., Calc., Cic., *Nit. ac.*, Nux v.

Meat: Ferr. m., Kreos., Lil. t., Mag. c., Meny.

smoked: Calc. p., *Caust.*, Kreos.

Milk: Apis, Ars., Aur., Bry., Calc., Chel., Elaps, Merc., Nat. m., Nux v., Ph. ac., *Rhus t.*, Sabad., Sil., Staph., Stront.

Oysters: Bry., Calc., *Lach.*, Lyc., Nat. m., Rhus t.

Pickles: Ant. c., Lach., Sulph Sul. i.

DESIRE for.

Pork: Crot. h., Tub.

Salt things: Aloe., *Arg. n.*, Calc., Calc. p., *Carb. v.*, Caust., Con., Cor. r., Lyss., Manc., Med., *Nat. m.*, Nit. ac., *Phos.*, Plb., Sanic., *Verat.*

Sand: *Tarent.*

Smoked things: *Caust.*, Kreos.

sour, acids, etc: Ant. c., Ant. t., Apis, Arn., Ars., Bor., Brom., Bry., Calc., Carb. v., Cham., Cist., Con., Cor. r., Ferr., Ferr. m., Fl. ac., *Hep.*, Ign., Kali ar., Kali c., Lach., Mag. c., Med., Nat. m., Phos., Podo., Puls., Sabad., Sabin., Sec., Sep., Squil., Stram., Sulph., Sul. i., *Verat.*

Sweets: Amm. c., *Arg. n.*, Bry., Calc., Calc. s., Carb. v., *Chin.*, Ip., Kali c., Kali s., Lyc., Mag. m., Med., Nat. c., Plb., Rheum, Rhus t., Sabad., Sec., Sep., *Sulph.*

Tobacco: Staph., *Tab.*

Vegetables: Alum., Mag. m.

AVERSION TO ACIDS: Bell., Cocc., Ferr., Sabad., Sulph.

Alcoholic stimulants: Hyos., Rhus t.

beer: Alum., Cham., *Chin.*, Clem., Cocc., Cycl., Ferr., Nat. s., *Nux v.*, Phos., Rhus t., Stann., Sulph.

brandy: Merc.

Bread: Chin., Con., Cycl., Kali c., Lyc., *Nat. m.*, Nat. p., Nat. s., Nit. ac., Nux v., Phos., Ph. ac., Puls., Sep.

AVERSION to.

Butter: Chin., Cycl., Merc., Phos., *Puls.*

Coffee: Bell., Bry., *Calc.*, Cham., Chin., Coff., Dulc., Lyc., Merc., Nat. m., *Nux v.*, Phos., Spig., Sul. ac.

Fats and rich food: Ars., Bry., Carb. an., *Chin.*, Colch., Cycl., Hep., Merc., Nat. m., *Petr.*, *Ptel.*, Puls., Sep., Sulph.

Fish: Colch., Graph., Phos., Zinc.

Food: Acon., Alum., Ang., Ant. c., Arg. n., Arn., *Ars.*, Asaf., Bar. c., Bell., Bry., Cact., Canth., Carb. an, *Chin.*, Chin. a., Chin. s., *Cocc.*, Colch., Coloc., Cycl., Dig., Dulc., *Ferr.*, Ferr. ar., Glon., Grat., Gua., Hell., Hydr., Ign., Iod., *Ip.*, Kali c., Laur., *Lil. t.*, Mag. c., Mag. s., Merc., Merc. i. f., *Nux v.*, Op., Pic. a, Plat., Podo., Puls., Rhus t., Sabad., Sep., Staph., Tarent., Tub.

smell of: *Cocc.*, Colch., *Ip.*, Podo.

Garlic: Sabad.

Meat: Alum., Ang., Arn., Ars., Aur., Bry., Cact., *Calc.*, Cann. s., Carb. v., *Chin.*, Chin. a., Cycl., Ferr., Ferr. ar., Ferr. m., *Graph.*, Ign., Kali ar., Kali bi., Kali c., Lap. a., Lyc., Merc., Mez., *Mur. ac.*, Nat. m., Nit. ac., *Nux v.*, *Petr.*, Phos., Plat., Ptel., Puls., Rhus t., Sabad., *Sep.*, *Sil.*, Sulph., Syph., Tub. Zinc.

Milk: Æth., Ant. t., Arn., Bry., Calc., Calc. s., Carb. v.,

AVERSION to.

Cina, Gua., Ign., *Lac. d.*,
Nat. c., Phos., **Puls.**, Sep.,
Sil., Sulph.

Onions: Sabad.

Oysters: Phos.

Pork: Colch., Dros., Psor.,
Puls.

Salty food: Carb. v., *Cor. r.*,
Graph., Nat. m., Selen., **Sep.**

Solid food: Ferr., Staph.

Sweets: Ars., Caust, *Graph.*,
Merc., Phos., Sin. n., Sulph.,
Zinc.

Tea: Phos.

AVERSION to.

Tobacco: *Calc.*,   Camph.,
Canth.,   Carb. an.,   Ign.,
Lach., Lyc., Nat. m. *Nux v.*,
Op., Phos., Puls., Sulph.

smoking: Arn., Brom., Calc.,
Camph., *Ign.*, Lyc., Puls.,
Sulph.

Vegetable: Hell., Mag. c.

Water: Apis,   Bell.,   **Bry.**,
Calad., Canth., *Hyos.*, Lyss.,
Nat. m., *Nux v.*, Phys.,
Puls., Stram.

Wine: Ign., Merc., Rhus t.,
Sabad., Sulph., Zinc.

COUGH.

ABDOMEN:

Diarrhœa sensation in abdomen as from, on coughing: Ferr.

Drawing in of, with whooping cough, cough so frequent can scarcely breathe, wakes at 7 a.m.: Dros.

Griping in, and feeling as if he would vomit, from the cough, when expectoration was incomplete or difficult: Dros.

Hypochondriac region, aching in right, at night, during cough: Sulph.

cramps in, with cough: Zinc.

pain in, from cough: Ambr., Amm. c., Amm. m., Arn., Ars., Bry., Dros., Hell., Hyos., Hepar, *Lach.*, *Lyc.*, Nit. ac., Nux v., Oena., *Phos.*, Sepia, Sulph.

pain in, as if ulcerated, when coughing: Lach., Puls.

Pressure in, with cough: Acon., Cocc., Ambr., Spong., Valer.

stitches in, when coughing: Acon., Amm. m., Ars., Bry., Lyc., Nitr. ac., Phos., Sabad., Samb., Sulph., Sul. ac.

stitches in, left, when coughing: Amm. m., Bell., Carb. v. Con., Sulph., Zinc.

stitches in, right, when coughing: Bry., Carb. v., Eup. p., Kali c., Merc., Nat. m., Sep.

ABDOMEN.

support it, must, with hands, when coughing: Dros.

Hypogastric region, contraction of, with cough: Dros., Squil.

Hypogastric region of, bruised sensation in, on coughing: Hyos.

Hypogastric region of, constriction in, on coughing: Lach.

Hypogastric region of, contraction in, on coughing: Squil.

Hypogastric region of, pain in, on coughing: Hyos., Nux v., Squil., Sulph.

Pain in, and chest, with coughing, in open air: Phos.

Pain in, to chest on coughing: Coloc.

Protrude, dry, violent coughs, morning on rising, shaking as if contents would (must support it with hands): Carb. an.

pain in side, as if intestines would, on coughing and waking: Squil.

Shaking of, from cough: Kreos.

as if everything wauld fall out, must hold abdomen and sit, from severe, dry cough, in morning on rising, and nearly all day: Carb. an.

Umbilicus, colic as if, would be torn out, with continual cough; heat in face and sweat on forehead; after walking in open air and when lying morning and evening: Ipec.

AFTERNOON, cough in: Agar., All. c., Alum., Amm. c., Amm. m., Ant. t., Arn., Ars., Asaf., Bad., *Bell.*, Bry., Caps., China, Coc. c., Gamb., Kali c., Laur., Lyc., Mag. c., Mez., *Mosch.*, Mur. ac., Nat. c., Nux v., Phos., Stann., Staph., Sulph., Thuja, Zinc.

1 to 2 p.m.: Ars.

3 p.m.: Coc. c.

4 to 8 p.m.:Lyc.

hacking cough: Kali c.

inclination to cough in: Bapt.

inclination to cough, aggravated in: Sulph.

inclination to cough, aggravated at 7-30 p.m., on attempting to speak: Cimic.

AIR, close, or dust aggravate, dry cough at night: Natr. ars.

Cold, excites or aggravates cough: Acon., Amm. m., *Ars.*, Aur., Bar., Bry., Bov., Carb. an., Carb. v., *Caust.*, Cepa, Cham., Cimic., Cina, Cist., Cupr., Dulc., Hepar., Hyos., Hyper., Ipec., Kali c., Kali i., *Lach.*, Mez., Nit. ac., Nux m., Nux v., *Phos.*, Ph. ac., Rhus, Rumex, Sabad., Samb., Sep., Sil., Spong., Squil., Stram., Sulph.

Damp cold, aggravates cough: Ant. t., Calc., Carb. an., Carb. veg., Chin., Dulc., Lach., Mag. c., Mosch., Mur. ac., Nit. ac., Sulph., Sul. ac., Verat., Zinc.

Warm room, going from, to cold air, or vice versa, causes coughing: Sepia, Nux v., Nit. ac.

Night, aggravates cough: Merc.

AIR.

Open, excites or aggravates cough: Acon., Alum., Ang., Ars., Bar., Bry., Calc., Carb. v., Cham., Cina., Cocc., Coff., Dig., Ferr., Ipec., Kali bi., *Lach.*, Lyc., Mosch., Nit. ac., Nux v., Osm., *Phos.*, Ph. ac., Rhus, Rumex, Seneg., Sil., Spig., Staph., Stram, *Sulph.*, Sul. ac.

AIR, open ameliorates cough: Dulc., Nux v., Sulph.

AIR PASSAGES, burning in, with cough: Ant. c., Carb. v., Caust., Cina, Iod., Lach., Mag. m., *Spong*, Sulph., Zinc.

dryness of, causing cough: Carb. an., Lach., Merc, Petr., Puls.

sore, pain as if, with cough: Alum., Ambr., Amm. c., Bell., Calc., Carb. v., Caust., Chin., Cina, Hep., Lach., Lyc., Mag. m., Merc., Nat. c., Nux m., Nux v., Phos., Sep., Sil., Spig., Spong., Stann., Sulph.

tickling in, causing cough: Acon., Amm. c., Amm. m., Ant. t., Arg. n., *Arn.*, Asaf., Bar., Bell., Bor., *Bov.*, *Brom.*, Bry., Caps., *Carb. an.*, *Carb. v.*, *Caust.*, Cham., Cina, Coc. c., Colch., Con., Cupr., Dig., Ferr., Graph., Hepar, Ign., Iod., Ipec., *Kali b.*, Kali c., Lach., Lact., Laur., Led., Mag. c., Mag. m., Merc., Marum, Mur. ac., Nat. c., Nat. m., Nux v., *Phos.*, Prun., Puls., Rumex, Sabin., Sant., Seneg., Sep., Sil.

H. M. M.—65

AIR PASSAGES, tickling in.
Spong., Stan., Staph., Verat., Zinc.

Warm aggravates cough: Ant. c., Cocc. c., Iod.

ANGER, coughing from: Acon., Ant. t., Arg. n., Ars., Cham., Chin., Ign., Nux v., Sep., Staph., Verat.

ANUS, pain in, with cough: Lach.

ANXIOUS BEFORE AN ATTACK OF WHOOPING COUGH: Cupr.

ANXIETY WITH COUGH: *Acon.*, Cina, *Coff.*, *Dros.*, Eup. per., *Hepar.*, *Iod.*, Rhus, Samb., Spong., Stram.

APHONIA, cough with: Amm. caust., Phos., Spong.

ARMS, becoming cold, cough from: Ars., Calc., Ferr., *Hepar*, Kali c., *Rhus*, Sil.

Putting out of bed, or becoming cold, causes coughing: Hepar, Rhus, Sil.

Stretching out, causes coughing: Lyc.

ASCARIDES, spasmodic cough in persons troubled by: Mag. s.

ASLEEP, before getting cough: Calc., Merc.

On falling, at night, coughing: Lach., Petr.

ASTHMATIC AFFECTIONS (dyspnœa, obstructed respiration etc.) with cough: Acon., Alum., Bell., Brom., Hepar, Kreos., Lach., Led., Nux m., Sep., Sil.

ATMOSPHERE, from change of, coughing: Rumex.

Stormy, aggravates cough: Phos., Rhod., Sil.

AUTUMNAL COUGH: Verat.

BACK, aching in, on coughing: Amm. c., Merc., Nit. ac., Puls.

And limbs, stiff with hard tickling cough, worse evening till midnight, on lying: Rhus t.

BACK, lying on, aggravates cough: Amm. m., Iod., Nux v., Phos., Plumb., Rhod., Rhus, Sil.

Midsternum through to, cough with pain from: Kali bi., Rumex.

Small of, pain in, with cough: Amm. c., Kali bi., Merc., Nit. ac., Sulph.

stitches in, on coughing: Acon., Amm. c., Arn., Bell., Bry., Caps., Nit. ac., Sep., Sulph.

BARKING cough: Acon., All. c., Bell., Brom., Cimex, Clem., Coc. c., Coral., Cub., *Dros.*, Hepar, Hipp., Lach., Nit. ac., Phos., *Rumex*, Spong., Stann., Stram., Sulph.

day and night: Spong.

BATH, after, cough aggravates: Ant. c., Calc., Nit. ac., Rhus.

BED, compelled by the cough to spring up immediately and involuntarily: Bry.

lying in, excites or aggravates cough: Anac., Ant. t., Aralia, Ars., Bry., Cact., Cham., Coc. c., Dolic., Dros., Euphr., Ferr., Hep.

ED, lying in.

> Ignat., Indi., Kreos., Lach., Lachnan., Mag. c., Mag. m., Staph., Natr. m., Nux v., Puls., Rhus, Samb., Sep., Staph., Squil., Verb., Vib.

Warm, on becoming, in, excites or aggravates cough: Ant. t., Brom., *Caust.*, Cham., Dros., Led., Merc., Nat. m., Nux m., Nux v., Puls., Verat.

Warm, on becoming, in, ameliorates cough: Cham.

EER, drinking aggravates cough: Mez., Nux v., Rhus, Spong.

ENDING BACKWARDS A G G R A V A T E S COUGH: Cupr.
forwards aggravates cough: Dig.

LADDER, pain in, from cough: Caps.

READ, eating, aggravates cough: Kali c.

REAKFAST, cough ameliorates after: Kali c.

REATH OFFENSIVE, stinking, with cough: Ambra, Arn., Caps., Dros., Graph., Mag. s., Mez., Plumb., *Sang.*, Sep., Stann., Sulph.

RIGHT OBJECTS, looking at, excites cough: Stram.

ACHECTIC COUGH: Nux v., *Phos.*, Puls., Stan.

ARDIAC REGION, tearing, sensation in, with cough and expectoration of black blood: Elaps.

CATARRHAL COUGH:
Acon., Arn., Ars., Bry., Cact., Calc., Caps., Carb. v., Caust., Cham., Chin., Cina, *Dros.*, Dulc., Euphr., Hyos., Ign., Ipec., Kali b., Lach., Lip., Lyc., Merc. c., Nux v., *Phos.*, Ph. ac., Puls., Rhus, Sep., Sil., Sin. n., *Spig.*, Squil., Stann., Staph., *Sul.*, Verat., Verb.

CHEEKS, drawing in the, with chilliness and desire to cough, evening: Carb. v.

CHEST, aching in, when coughing: Chin., Kali c., Mang., Raph.

> Bruised, pain as if, in, caused by cough: Arn., Ferr., Verat., Zinc.

> Burning in, with cough: Ambra, Amm. c., *Ant. c.*, Carb. v., Caust., Cina, Ferr., Iod., Led., *Mag. m.*, *Mag. s.*, Phos., Ph. ac., Sang., Zinc.

CHEST, clavicle, pain extending from, through, on coughing: Apis.

> Left, stitches beneath, at every pulsation, aggravated by cough, deep inspiration and emotion: Lyc.

> Emptiness in, hollow feeling, after cough: Kali c., Sep., Stan., Zinc.

> Expand, effort to, causes cough: Iod.

> Gargling downwards in, audible, with cough: Cina, Mur. ac.

> Itching in, excites cough: Ambra, Ars., Coc. c., Con., Iod., Mag. m., Phos., Puls., Sep., Stann.

CHEST.

Looseness of everything in, sensation of, with cough: Mez., Rhus.

Mammæ, beneath right, stitch on coughing: Sulph.

Mediastinum, posterior, sensation of mucus in, causing cough: Nitrum.

Middle, crawling from, up into throat, excites cough: Kreos.

Mucus, excites cough: Ant. t., Arg., Ars., Arum t., Asar., Baryt., Carl., Caust., Cham., Cina, Euphr., Graph., Gua., Ipec., Nat. m., Puls., Sepia, Stan., Sulph.

Oppression of, with cough: Amm. c., Ars., Asar., Aspar., Aur., Brom., Chin., Cocc., Con., Dros., Graph., Grat., Iod., Kali b., Lach., Mur. ac., Nat. m., Nicc., *Phos.*, Rhod., Rhus, Seneg., *Stan.*, Tarent., *Verat.*

Pain in, during cough: Acon., Ambr., Amm. m., Ant. c., Arn., Ars., Bell., Bor., Brom., Bry., Calc., Carb. a., Carb. v., Caust., *Chin.*, Cina, Con., Dig., Dros., Eup. per., Ferr., Ferr. m., Gad., Iod., Kali bi., Kali c., Kali hyd., Kreos., Lach., Lachnan., Led., Lyc., Mag. m., Mang., *Merc.*, Mur. ac., Nat. c., *Nat. m.*, *Nitrum*, Nit. ac., Nux m., Nux v., Ox. ac., Petr., Phos., Ph. ac., Puls., Ran. b., Rhus, Rumex, Sabad., Sang., Seneg., Sep., Sil., Spig., Spong., Squil., Stan., Staph., Sulphur, *Verat.*, Zinc.

CHEST.

Pain in, with circumscr ed redness of the chee coryza and then diarrhœ Sanguinaria.

drawing and stitching, exte ing from left side, n nipple through to scapula, aggravated coughing, sneezing, e Rhus t.

from abdomen to, on cou ing: Coloc.

in side, during cough: A Puls., Sulph., Taren.

in sternum, cough with stitc in chest, lumbar region; uterus, with tightness chest and rattling of mu in chest: Bell.

violent in, with morning co and green expectorati Lyc.

Pressure on, relieves pain cau by cough: Arn., Bor., B *Dros.*, Eup. per., Kre Merc., Nat. s., Nat. Phos., Ran. b., Sep.

Rattling in, when cough Angust., Ant. t., Bell., C Calc., Caust., Cham., Ip Lycop., Op.

Side of, stitches in, on cough Acon., *Arn.*, Ars., A Bor., Bry., *Caps.*, Ca Chel., Clem., Coff., C Kali c., Lyc., Merc., Nat Nitrum, Phos., Puls., R Rumex, Sabad., Sepia, Sq Sulph.

Soreness in, from cough: Ac Alum., Arn., Ars., Bar Bell., Calc., Carb. s., C v., *Caust.*, Cina, Cocc., C Dig., Dros., Eugen., F per., Ferr., Gamb., C

HEST, soreness in.

Guare, Hepar, Ipec., Kali b., Kreos., Lach., Lyc., Mag. c., Mag. m., Meph., Merc., Mez., Mur. ac., Nat. c., Nat. s., Nit. ac., Nitrum, Nux m., *Nux v.*, Phos., Ratan., Rumex, Rhus, Seneg., Sep., Sil., Spig., Spong., Stann., Staph., Stront., Sulph., Thuja.

HEST, stitches in, on coughing: Acon., Amm. c., Amm. m., Ant. c., Ant. ox., Arn., *Ars.*, Bell., Bor., Bry., Cact., Calc., Cann., Caps., Carb. an., Carb. v., Chel., Coff., Con., Cupr., *Dros.*, Dulc., Ferr., Iod., Kali. b., Kali c., Kreos., *Lyc.*, Mez., Nat. m., Nat. s., Nit. ac., Nitrum, Nux m., Nux v., *Phos.*, Petr., Psor., Puls., Rhus. Rumex, Ruta, Sabad., Seneg., Sep., Sil., Squil., Stront., Sulph., Verat., Zinc.

HICKEN-POX, cough following the: Ant. cr.

HILL, accompanied by cough: Acon., *Ars.*, Bor., *Bry.*, Calc., Cham., *Chin.*, Con., Hepar, Hyos., Ipec., Kali c., Kreos., Lach., Lyc.. Nux m., Nux v., Phos., *Puls.*, Rhus, Sabad., Sep., Spong., Sulph., Thuja.

Accompanied by cough, with expectoration: *Acon.*, Ars., Bell., Bry., Carb. v., Cham., Cimex, China, Hepar, Hyos., *Ipec.*, Kali c., Lach., Nux m., Nux v., Phos., Puls., Rhus, Sabad., Sep., *Spong.*, Sulph.

Before and continuing after, a day teasing cough: Rhus t.

CHOKING COUGH, of a croupish nature and rattling: Hepar.

Croupy cough at night (in fat children): Ipec.

Cough on inspiration: Cina.

CHINA, cough following abuse of: Arn., Ferr.

COLIC, cough with: Con.

CONSCIOUSNESS, loss of, with cough: Cina.

CONSTIPATION, with cough: Bry., Nat. c., Podo., Sepia.

CONTINUOUS COUGH, dry cough for years: Lyc.

cough, while lying: Hyos., Puls.

short, dry, suffocative cough: Acon.

violent cough: Ipec.

violent cough till relieved by vomiting: Mezereum.

CONVULSIVE COUGH: Agar., Ambra, Amm. caust., Ars., Arum t., Asc. t., *Bell.*, Bov., Cact., *Carb. v.*, Chel., Chlo., Der., *Hyos.*, Ipec., Kali c., Lact., Meli., Merc. c., Oena., Osm., Pod., Petr., *Phos.*, Plumb., *Rumex*, Sep., Sil., Stram., Stry., Tabac., Thuja.

CORYZA WITH COUGH: Acon., Alum., Ambr., Ars., Bar., Bell., Calc., Canth., Carb. an., Caust., Cepa, Cimex, Con., Dig., *Euphr.*, Gels., Graph., Ign., Kali c., Kali chl., Lach., Lyc., Mag. c., Meph., Merc., Nat. c., Nitrum, Nit. ac., Phos., Ph. ac.. Rhus, Rumex, Sang., Sep., Spong., Sulph., Sul. ac., Thuja.

CROUPY COUGH: Acon.,
Ant. t., Bell., Brom., Cham.,
Hepar, Iod., Kali b., Lach.,
Phos., Rumex, Spong., Stram.

Hoarse cough: Ant. t., Bell.,
Brom., Hepar, Lach.

CRYING DURING THE
PAROXYSM OF
COUGH: Ant. t., Arn.,
Ars., Bell., Cham., Chin.,
Cina, Hepar, Ipec., Lyc.,
Sep., Sil., Samb., Verat.

DAY, cough during: Alum.,
Amm. c., Amm. m., Anac.,
Ang., Arg., Bar., Bism.,
Bov., Bry., Calc., Cham.,
Chin., Cic., Coloc., Con.,
Cotyl., Euphr., Ferr., Gamb.,
Graph., Guai., Kali c., Lach.,
Laur., Lyc., Manc., Mez.,
Mur. ac., Nat. ar., Nat. c.,
Nit. ac., Nitrum, Nux v.,
Phos., Rhus, Sars., Sep.,
Sol. t., Stan., Staph., Sulph.,
Thuja, Zinc.

ameliorated in: Euph., Lach.,
Merc.

And night, cough during: Bell.,
Bism., Calc., Carb. an.,
Cham., Chinin., Cupr., Dulc.,
Euph., Hepar, Ign., Ind.,
Lyc., Mez., Mur. ac., Nat.
c., Nat. m., Nitrum, Nit. ac.,
Phos., Rhus, Sep., Sil.,
Spong., Stan., Sulph., Zinc.

Every other, violent cough:
Nux v.

third, cough: Anac., Lyc.

Hour, cough at the same, every:
Lyc., Sabad.

Only during the, cough: Arg. n.,
Euphr., Lach.

Suffocative cough, between 2
and 4 a.m.: Chin.

DAY.

Suffocative cough, at 5 a.m.
from dryness in laryn
Kali c.

DAYBREAK, dry cough fro
midnight to: Nux v.

DEBAUCH, cough after
Stram.

DEBILITY WITH TH
COUGH: Ars., Chin., Fer
Lach., Op., Psor., Sta
Verat.

DEGLUTITION, every emp
excites cough: Nat. m., Op

EXERTION, cough durir
Calc., Cham., Cina, Hy
Rhus.

Tardy and often attended
convulsions and a loose ra
ing cough: Calc.

DIAPHRAGM AN
STOMACH, affected
night cough, must before s
set: Lyc.

DIARRHŒA, cough acco
panying: Op., Puls., Rum
Sang., Sars., Sul. ac.

Involuntary, with cough: Ph
Verat.

Cough with coryza, then: Sa

with belching of wind a
Ambr., Sul. ac., Verat.

worse at night with: Pu
Sang.

DINNER AFTER, cou
Agar., Anac., Arg. n., B
Carb. v., Coc. c., Ferr.
Kali b., Nux v., Ph
Sulph., Tab., Thuja, Zin

DREAD OF COUGH, pain
soreness in chest from: Pl
although it relieves: Mag.

DRINK, cold excites cough, warm relieves: Ars., Rhus, Sil.
relieves cough: Caust., Coc. c., Cupr.

DRINKING, after cough is dry, after eating cough is loose: Nux m., Staph.

Ameliorates dry cough: Coc c., Iod., *Spong.*

Cough from: Acon., Amm. caust., Amm. m., Ant. t., Arn., *Ars., Bry.,* Calc., Carb. v., *China,* Cina, Cocc., Dig., Dros., Ferr., Hepar, Hipp. m., Hyos., *Lach.,* Laur., Lyc., Manc., Meph., Nat. m., Nux v., Op., *Phos.,* Psor., Rhus, Sil., Squil, Tell., Verat.

Beer aggravates or excites cough: Mez., Rhus, Spong.

Coffee aggravates cough: *Caps.,* Caust., Cham., Cocc., Ign., Nux v.

Cold fluids, excite or aggravate cough: Amm. m., Calc., Carb. v., Dig., Hepar, Kali c., Lyc., Rhus, Sil., Spong., Squil., Staph., Stram., Sul. ac., Verat.

ameliorate cough: Borax, Coc. c., Cupr., Op., Sul.

Milk, after, aggravates cough: Ambr., Ant. t., Brom., Kali c., Spong., Sul. ac., Zinc.

Tea, aggravates cough: Ferr., Spong.

Vinegar, aggravates cough: Ant. c., Sep., Sil.

Warm fluids, aggravate cough: Ambr., Ant. t., Coc. c., Laur., Mez., Stan.

ameliorate cough: Ars., Alum., Lyc., Nux v., **Rhus, Sil., Spong., Verat.**

DRINKING.

Wine, aggravates cough: Acon., Bor., Lach.

Sour aggravates cough: Ant. cr.

Without thirst, excites cough: Ars.

DRY COUGH: Acal., Acet. ac., Acon., Æsc., Agar., Aloe, All. sat., Alum., *Ambra,* Amm. c., Amm. m., Anac., Ang., Ant. c., Ant. ox., Ant. t., Apoc. c., Aqua. p., Arg., Arg. n., Arn., *Ars.,* Arum. t., Arum. i., Asaf., Asar., Asc. t., Aur., Aur. m. n., Bar., Bell., Benz. ac., Berb., Bov., *Brom.,* Bry., Bufo, Calc., Carb. v., Caust., Cham., Chin., Cina, Coc. c., Coff., Croc., Cupr. a, Hyper., Kreos., Merc. s., Nit. ac., Nux m., Plat., Plumb., Psor., Puls., Rhus, Seneg., Spong., Squil, Stan., **Staph.,** Sulph.

afternoon: Amm. m., **Kali** bi., Mez., **Phel., Sulph.,** Thuja.

at 3 p.m.: Calc. p.

at 4 p.m.: Chel.

at 5 p.m.: Nat. m.

at 7 p.m.: Bry., Grat., Spira.

DUST, cough from: Nat. a.

DYSPNŒA WTIH COUGH: see asthmatic cough.

EAR, aching, in throat or, with every coughing spell, or in distant parts, as leg, bladder etc: Caps.

Pain in, from cough: Caps., **Nux v.**

EATING, excites or aggravates cough: Amm. m., Bry., Calc., Carb. v., Caust., Cham., Chin., Cocc., Ipec., Dig., Ferr., Hyos., ipec., Kali c., Laur., Mag. m., Mosch., Nux v., Phos., Puls., Rhus, Sep., Staph., Thuja, Verat.

After, a cough: Agar., Amm. m., Anac., *Ant. t.*, *Ars.*, Bell., *Bry.*, Calc., Carb. v., Cham., *Chin.*, Ferr., Hepar, Kali b., Kali c., Lach., Laur., Nux m., Nux v., Op., Phos., Puls., Ruta, Rhus, Sep., Sil., Staph., Sulph., Thuja, Zinc.

Acrid or biting food, cough aggravates as from: Thuja.

Ameliorates cough: Amm. c., Anac., Euphr., Ferr., Spong.

whooping cough: Tabac.

Solid food, aggravates cough: Cupr.

Sour things aggravate cough: Ant. c., Brom., Con., Lach., Nat. m., Nux v., Sep., Sulph.

Sugar ameliorates cough: Sulph.

Sweetmeats, cough from: Zinc.

Vinegar aggravates cough: Ant. c., Sep., Sulph.

ERUCTATION, abundant, accompanying cough: Ambra, Arn., Sul. ac., Verat.

Of food, after cough: Sul. ac.

ERUPTIONS, suppressed, cough from: Dulc.

EVENING COUGH (or aggravated in): Acon., Agar., Ail., Alum., Ambr., Amm. c., Amm. m., Anac., Ant. t., Apis, Arg. n., Arn., Ars.,

EVENING COUGH.

Arund., Aspar., Bad., Bar., Bell., Bism., Bov., Bry., Calc., Caps., *Carb. an.*, Carb. v., Caust., Cepa, Cham., Chin., Chin. s., Cina, Cocc., Cocc. c., Coloc., Con., Croton. t., Dros., Eugen., Eupat. per., Euphr., Ferr., Fluor. ac., Graph., Hepar, Ign., Indig., Iod., Ipec, Kali c., Kali i., Kreos., Lach., Laur., Led., Lith., Lycop., Mag. c., Mag. m., Mag. s., Marum, Merc., Mez., Mosch., Mur. ac., Naja, Nat. c., *Nat. m.*, Nicc., Nit. ac., Nux m., Nux v., Olean., Ox. ac., Par., Pet., Phos., Ph. ac., Psor., Puls., Ran. b., Rheum, Rhod., Rhus, Rumex, Ruta, Sang., Seneg., Sep., Sil., Sin. n., Spong., Squil., *Stan.*, Staph., Sticta, Stront., Sulp. Tarent., Thuja, Upas., Verat., *Verb.*, Zinc.

at 4 p.m.: Calc. f., Kali b.

between 4 and 8 p.m.: Lyc.

at 5 p.m.: Sol. t.

at 6 p.m.: Rhus.

between 6 and 7 p.m.: Sepia.

at 9 p.m., on going to bed: Sil.

at 10 p.m.: Bell.

between 11 and 12 p.m. in bed: Hepar.

aggravated in bed: Agn., Amm. c., Amm. m., Anac., Ars., Bell., Bor., *Calc.*, Carb. an., Carb. v., Cocc., Coff., Con., Dros., Ferr., Graph., Hepar, Ipec., Kali c., Kreos., Lach., Lyc., Marum, Merc., Nat. m.,

EVENING COUGH, aggravated in bed.

> Nit. ac., Nux m., Nux v., Petr., Phos., Ph. ac., Puls., Rhus., Sep., Sil., Stram., Staph., Verb.

exhausting: Ipec., Kali c.

at 7 p.m.: Ipec.

at 2 p.m.: Laur.

at 3 p.m.: Calc. p.

at 7-15 p.m. from tickling in trachea, on entering a warm room: Com.

aggravated after lying down: Sil.

ameliorated after lying down: Amm. m.

Cough, irritation to, in larynx toward evening: Merc. c.

irritation in larynx and trachea at 2 p.m.: Coca.

irritation to, in larynx from tickling at 7 p.m.: Cimic.

irritation to, pain in right lung, 8 p.m.: Dios.

loose: Mur. ac.

loose at 7 p.m.: Spire.

paroxysmal, 1-2 p.m.: Aqu. p.

paroxysmal, 1-30 p.m.: Phel.

paroxysmal, 2 p.m.: Ol. an.

paroxysmal 3 p.m.: Phel.

paroxysmal, 4 p.m.: Chel., Coca.

paroxysmal, 5 p.m.: Cupr.

paroxysmal, 6-15 p.m.: Ol. an.

paroxysmal, 7 p.m.: Grat.

paroxysmal, 11 p.m. after lying down: Rumex.

racking at 10 p.m.: Nat. m.

racking, short, 2 p.m.: Laur.

EVENING COUGH.

racking, short, 5 p.m.: Nat. m.

racking, short, 11 p.m., from tickling behind upper sternum: Rhus.

racking, tickling, 3 p.m.: Hepar.

racking, tickling, 6 p.m.: Sulph.

EXERTION, aggravates or excites cough: Arn., Bar., Bry., Dulc., Ferr., Iod., Ipec., Lyc., Merc., Mur. ac., Nat. a., Nat. m., Nux v., Ox. ac., Sil., Spong., Squil., Verat.

EXHAUSTING (fatiguing, wearying) cough: Ail., Alum., Aqu. p., Arg. n., Benz. ac., Carb. v., Chel., Croc., Coral., Cupr., Graph., Hyos., Ipec., Kali bi., Kali c., Lip., Lyc., Mag. s., Merc. c., Merc. s., Nat. c., Nux v., Phos., Plumb., Rhod., Rumex, Sang., Sil., Stan., Sulph., Sul. ac., Tarent., Thuja, Verat.

hand laid on pit of stomach ameliorates: Croc.

EXPECTORATION AMELIORATES, severe and long coughing spells: Lob. in.

evening cough without, but with dyspnœa: Ars.

EXTREMITIES, cold with suffocating, exhausting cough, evening: Ipec.

EYE BLOODSHOT AND BLEEDING FROM NOSE, with cough: Arn.

Lachrymation with cough: Acon.: Agar., Brom., Calc., Carb.

LACHRYMATION, cough with.
v., Cepa, Chel., Cina, Euph., Hepar, Ipec., Kali c., Kreos., Merc., Nat. m., Puls., Rhus, Sabad Squil., Staph., Sulph.

EYELIDS, dull shock behind right, from cough: Sul. ac.

pain in: Kali b., *Kali c.*, Kali hyd., *Lach.*

swelling of upper eyelid with whooping cough: Kali c.

FACE BLUISH: Acon., Ars., Bad., Bell., Carb. v., Cina, Cupr., Dros., Hyos., Ipec., Kali c., Lach., Nux, Op., Sil., Staph., Verat.

Bluish red: Bell., Con., Staph.
Pain in bones of face: Kali b.
Puffiness of: Acon., Ars., Bell., Dros., Hyos., Ipec., Kali c., Mag. c., Meph.

Red: Acon., Bell., Bry., Caps., Con., Eup. per., Ferr., Hepar, Hyos., Ipec., Kali c., Lyc., Mur. ac., Nit. ac., Sabad., Samb., Sil., Squil., Staph., Stram., Sulph.

Redness, alternating with paleness: Acon., Caps.

of one cheek: Acon., Cham., Ipec., Mosch.

Yellow: Caust., Lyc., Mag. m., Puls., Sep., Verat.

FASTING AGGRAVATES COUGH: Kali c., Mag. m.

FEVER, cough with expectoration during: Alum., Arg., Ars., Bell., Bism., Bry., Calc., Carb. v., Cic., Chin., **Dig.;** Dros., Dulc., Ferr., Iod., Kali c., Ruta, Seneg.,

FEVER, cough with expectoration during.
Sep., Sil., Spong., Squil., Stan., Staph., *Sulph.*, Thuja.

without expectoration during: Acon., Ang., Ant. cr., *Apis, Arn., Ars.,* Bell., Brom., *Bry.,* Cupr., Carb. v., Caust., Cham., Calc., Chim., Cina., Coff., Con., Dros., Hepar, *Hyos.,* Ign., Ipec., Kali c., Lach., Lyc., Nat. m., Nit. ac., Nux m., Nux v., Op., Petr., Phos., Plat., Puls., Rhus., Sabad., Samb., Sep., Spig., Spong., Squil., Staph., Sulph.

FLATUS, dry cough wakes patient, must sit up; ceases only when sits up and passes flatus up and downwards: Sang.

FOREIGN BODY, in larynx seems to excite cough: Bell.

FOREHEAD, pain in, from cough: Asc. t., Kali b.

FORENOON, cough in the: Agar., Alum., Amm. c., Amm. m., Bell., Bry., Chin. s., Coc., Hell., Kali c., Mag. c., Nat. c., Nat. m., Rhus, Sabad., Sars., Seneg., Sep., Sil., Stan., Staph., Sul. ac.

at 1 a.m.: Coc. c.

at 2 a.m., from scratching larynx: Zinc.

at 1-4 a.m., prickling in larynx: Bufo.

at 2 a.m.: Phos., Cocc., Rum.

at 2 or 3 a.m.: Ant. t., Merc.

at 3 a.m.: Amm. c., Bapt., Cupr., Kali c., Mag. c., Mur. ac., Nitrum.

COUGH.

at 3-4 a.m.: Amm. c., Lyc.

at 4 a.m.: Anac., Nit. ac., Nux v.

at 5 a.m.: Arum. t., Kali c., Rum.

at 6-7 a.m.: Arum. t., Cal. p.

at 8 a.m.: Ham., Ol. an.

at 8-9 a.m.: Sil.

at 9 a.m.: Sep., Tarent.

at 10 a.m., from rawness in airpassages while lying: Coc. c.

at 10 to 12 a.m.: Nat. m.

at 11 a.m., from rush of blood to chest: Raph.

between 10 and 12 a.m.: Coc. c.

ameliorated on sitting up: Euphr.

BRIGHT, cough after: Acon., Bell., Rhus, Stram., Samb.

GAGGING COUGH, morning after rising: Cina, Sepia.

fetching or vomiting with cough: Ant. t., Brom., Bry., Cocc., Coral.

GAYETY WITH COUGH: Verat.

GONORRHŒA, long continued dry cough after suppressed: Benz. ac.

GRIEF AND CARE AGGRAVATE THE COUGH: Ph. ac.

HEAD, aching (includes pain etc.): Acon., Alum., Ambr., Anac., Ang., Apis, *Arn.*, Ars., Aur., Bad., Bell., Bry., *Calc.*, Cact., Caps., Carb. v., Caust., Chin., Chel., Con.,

HEAD, aching.

Ferr., Hepar, Ign., Ipec., Iris. v., Kali b., *Kali c.*, Lach., Led., Lyc., Mag. s., Mang., *Merc.*, Nat. m., Nitrum., Nit. ac., Nux v., Oena., Ol. m., Phos., Ph. ac., *Puls.*, Rhus, Rumex, *Sabad.*, Sang., Sars., Sep., Spig., Spong., Squil., Sulph., *Stan.*, Taren.

HEAD, brain, sensation of looseness of the, with cough: Acon., Sep., Sul. ac.

Fly to pieces, feels as if it would, from the cough: Bry., Calc., Caps., Kali b., Merc., Nat. m., Nux v., Phos., Ph. ac., Sep., Sulph.

Forehead, aching in, with cough: Asc. t., Brom., Chel., Spong.,

pain in, relieved by cough: Arg. mur.

Occiput, aching in, on coughing: Tarent.

pain in, from cough: Anac., Carb. an., Ferr., Mag. c., Merc., Mosch., Sulph., Sep.

Pain in temples with cough: Ambr., Caust., Cina, Kali c., Kreos., Lyc., Puls., Rhus, Verb.

in vertex on coughing: Con., Cupr., Sabad., Squil.

violent, in centre of, from coughing or sneezing: Sulph.

Parietal bones, darting in, from cough: Mang.

Perspiration on, with cough: Ant. t., Calc., Ipec., Sil., Tar.

Shocks in, from cough: Ars., Calc., Ipec., Lach., Lyc., Mang., Nat. m., Rhus, Seneg., Spig., Sul. ac.

HEAD.

Stitches in, when coughing:
Alum., Anac., Arn., Bry.,
Calc., *Carb. v.*, Caust., Chel.,
Cina, Con., Hyos., Kali c.,
Mez., Nit. ac., Phos., Ph.
ac., Ruta, Sabad., Sulph.,
Sul. ac., Verb., Zinc.

Stretching back, excites cough:
Lyc.

Stupefying pain in, cough
awakens him at 3 a.m. with:
Nitrum.

HEARING IMPAIRED BY COUGHING: Chel., Dulc., Seneg.

HEART, affections of, with cough: Ars., Lach., Laur., Naja, Mosch.

Palpitation, with cough: Arn.,
Calc., Kali b., Nitrum., Puls.,
Spong., Stan.

HICCOUGH, during cough: Ang., Tabac.

HOARSENESS, with cough:
Acon., Amm. c., *Ant. t.*,
Arg. n., Asaf., Bad., *Bell.*,
Bry., Brom., Calc., Caps.,
Carb. an., Carb. v., Caust.,
Cham., Chin., Cina, Cupr.,
Dig., Dros., *Dulc.*, Ferr.,
Hepar, Iod., Kali b., Kali c.,
Kali hyd., Lach., Laur., Lyc.,
Mag. m., Mang., Merc.,
Mez., Mur. ac., Nat. c., Nat.
m., Nit. ac., Nitrum, *Nux
v.*, Phos., Ph. ac., *Puls.*,
Rhus, Rumex, *Samb.*, Seneg.,
Sep., Sil., Spong., Stan.,
Staph., Sulph., Sul. ac.,
Thuja, Verat., Verb., Zinc.

HUNGER, violent, with cough and coryza: Sul. ac.

INGUINAL REGION, pain in the, on coughing: Borax.

INSPIRATION (inhaling, inspiring) aggravates or excites cough: Acon., Asaf., Asar., Benz. ac., Calc., Cina, Con., Coral., Croc., Graph., *Hepar*, Ipec., Kali b., Mag. m., Meny., Meph., Merc. iod., Olean., Op., Puls., Squil., Sitcta, Verb.

INSPIRING COOL AIR, aggravates cough: All. c., Cist., Cupr., Rhus., *Rumex*, Staph.

INVOLUNTARY COUGH: Amyl. n.

JAW, pain in, when coughing, not on touch: Amm. c.

LABOR, dry cough following difficult labour or abortion, with backache and sweat: Kali c.

LABORED cough: Agar.

LARYNX, burning in, causing cough: Acon., Bell., Mag. s., Phos., Seneg.

Cold sensation in, on inspiration:
Brom.

Consant desire to clear the throat
and: Crot. t.

Irritation to cough felt in:
Acon., Alum., Amm. c.,
Amm. m., Arn., Ars., Bar.,
Bell., Bov., Bry., Calc.,
Calc. f., Canth., Carb. an.,
Carb. v., Caps., Caust.,
Cham., Chel., Cimic., Cina,
Coc. c., Cocc., Colch.,
Coloc., Con., Dig., Dros.,
Euphr., For., Guare., Hepar,
Hydr. ac., Iod., Ipec., Ign.,
Kali b., Kali c., Kali chl.,
Lach., Lachn., Laur., Mag.

LARYNX, irritation to cough, felt in.

c., Mang., Manc., Merc. cor., Mez., Mur. ac., Naja, Nat. c., Nux v., Olean., Osm., Puls., Rumex, Sabad., Sabin., Seneg., Sep., Sil., Spong., Staph., Stront., Sulph., Sul. iod., Tab., Tarax.

Itching in, cough from: Ambr., Cact., Carb. v., Dig., Laur., *Nux v.*, Puls.

Mucus in, excites or aggravates cough: Arg., Arg. n., *Brom.*, Caust., Crot. t., Dulc., Euphr., Kali b., Kreos., Mang., Osm., Seneg.

Painfulness of, with danger of suffocating when touching or turning neck, or coughing or drawing a long breath: Bell.

Pressure upon, causes cough: Chin., Cina, Lach., Rumex, Tarax.

LAUGHING COUGH: *Arg.*, Ars., Bry., *China*, Cupr., Dros., Kali c., Lach., Mur. ac., Nit. ac., Phos., Sin. n., Stan., Zinc.

LEUCORRHŒA, cough with: Nux v., Stan.

Succeeded by hoarseness and cough: Con.

LIVER, deepseated, heavy pain in region of, worse from pressure, cough, laughing or deep inspiration: Pœor.

Painless twitching in, or cough: Lyc.

LOOSE COUGH: Agar., Ant. t., Arum. d., Asaf., Calc., Cal. ac., Carb. an., Cal., Cham., Chel., Chin., Chin. ar.,

LOOSE COUGH.

Cina, *Coc. c.*, Cocc., Coloc., Con., Cupr., Dig. Elaps, Eugen., Euph., Eupion., Ferr., Graph., Hepar, Hydr., Ign., Jabr., Kali c., Lap., Mag. s., Merc., Merc. c., Nat. ar., Nat. c., Nat. s., *Phos.*, Podo., Puls., Sabad., Secale, Sepia, Still., Sulph., Tarent., Tel.

LUNGS, burning in, when coughing: Arum. t.

Loose sensation, as of something loose and fluttering in, during cough: Phos.

LYING EXCITES OR AGGRAVATES COUGH: All. c., Ambr., Amm. m., Apis, *Ars.*, Bell., Bry., Calc., Caps., Carb. v., Cham., Cinnab., Cocc., Con., Dros., Euphr., Ferr., Hyos., Ign., Ipec., Lach., Lact., Lith. c., Lyc., Mar., Meph., Merc., Mez., Nat. m., Nicc., Nit. ac., Nux v., Par., Petr., Phos., Ph. ac., Puls., Rhus, Rumex, Ruta, Sabad., Sang., Sep., Staph., Stann., *Sulph.*, Thuja, Verb.

afternoon, 2 p.m., hacking cough: Laur.

Ameliorates, cough: Acon., Amm. m., Euphr., Mang., Sep., Zinc.

MEASLES, cough after: Ant.c., Bry., Camph., Cham., *Coff.*, Con., Dros., Dulc., Eupat. per., Gels., Hyos., Ign., Nux v.

MENSES, at beginning of, exhausting cough: Phos.

MENSES.

Before, cough, evening, in bed, ameliorates by sitting up: Sulph.

During, aggravation of cough: Amm. m., Graph., Rhod., Zinc.

During, hoarseness and dry morning cough: Copaiva

MIDNIGHT, cough about:
Amm. c., Ant. t., Ars Bar., Bell., Bry., Calc. a., Caust., Cham., Coff., Dig., Hepar, Kali c., Manc., Mag. c., Mag. m., Mez., Nit. ac., Nitr., Nux v., Phos., Rhus r., Samb., Zinc.

MORNING COUGH: Acon.,
Alum., Amm. c., Amm. m., Anac., Ang., Ant. t., Arn., Arg., Ars., Aur., Bar., Bell., Bov., Bry., Cala., Calc., Calc. f., Canth., Carb. an., Carb. v., Caust., Cham., Chel., *Chin.*, Cina, Coca, Cocc., Cod., Coloc., Coral., Crot. t., Cupr., Dig., Dros., Erio., Euphr., Ferr., Grat., Gymno., Hepar, Ign., *Iod.*, Ipec., *Kali b.*, Kali c., Kreos., Lach., Led., *Lyc.*, Mag. c., *Mag. s.*, Mang., *Meph.*, Merc., Mur. ac., Naja, Nat. c., Nat. m., Nat. s., Nitrum, Nux m., Nux v., Osm., Par., Phos., Ph. ac., Puls., Pyrus., Rhod., Rhus, Sars., *Selen.*, Seneg., Sep., Sil., Spig., Squi, Stan., Staph., *Sulph.*, Sul. ac., Tab., Thuja, Verat.

MORTIFICATION, cough:
after, with stitches inside and frothy bloody expectoration: Puls.

MOUTH, bleeding from with
cough: Dros., Ipec., Merc., Nux v.

Herpetic eruption around, with cough: Ars., Nat. m., Rhus.

MOVEMENT EXCITES OR AGGRAVATES COUGH:
Arn., Ars., Bar., Bell., Brom., Bry., Bufo., Calc., Carb. v., China, Dros., Eupat. per., Ferr., Iod., Ipec., Kali c., Kreos., Lach., Laur., Led., Lyc., Merc., Mez., Mosch., Mur. ac., Nat. m., Nitrum, *Nux v.*, *Phos.*, Sep., Sil., Spong., Stan., Squil., Staph., Sul. ac.

Ameliorates violent dry cough, felt while lying or sitting: Phos.

MUCUS COUGH: Kali c.

MUSIC EXCITES COUGHING: Ambr., *Calc.*, Cham., Kali c., Kreos., Ph. ac.

NAUSEA, with cough: Ant. t.,
Ars., Aspar., Bry., Cajup., Calc., Caps., Coloc., Dros., Elaps, Hepar, Hydr., Ign., Ipec., Iod., Kali b., Kali c., Lach., Merc., Natr. c., Nit. ac., Petr., Ph. ac., Pic. ac., Puls., Ruta, Sabin., Sars., Sep., Squil., Thuja, Verat.

NERVOUS COUGH: Plumb.

Fram tickling in larynx: Lach.

When anyone enters the room: Phos.

NIGHT COUGH: Acon.,
Agar., Alum., *Ambr.*, Amm. c., *Amm. m.*, Anac., Ant. t., Apis, Arg. n., Arn., Ars., Asar., Aur., Aur. mur., Bar., Bell., Bism., Bor., Bry., Calad., Calc., *Caps.*, Carb.

NIGHT COUGH.

an., Carb. v., Cast., *Caust.*, Cham., *China*, Cina, Cocc., Cocc. c., Coff., Colch., Coloc., Con., Coral., Cupr., *Cycl.*, Dig., Dros., Dulc., Eugen., Ferr., Gamb., Graph., *Grat.*, Guai., Hepar, Hipp., Hyos., *Ign.*, Indig., *Ipec.*, Kali b., Kali c., *Kreos.*, Lach., Lact., Led., Lepi., Linu., *Lyc.*, *Mag. c.*, *Mag. m.*, Meph., Merc., Mez., *Nat. m.*, Nat. s., Nicc., Nit. ac., Nitrum, *Nux v.*, Ol. an., Ol. jec., Op., Par., Petr., Phell., Phos., Puls., Rhod., *Rhus*, Rumex, Ruta, Sabad., Sang., Seneg., Sep., Sil., Sol. t., Spig., Squil., Stan., Staph., Sticta, Stront., Sulph., Thuja, *Verat.*, *Verb.*, Zinc.

Whooping cough at: Ambr., Anac., Ant. t., Arn., Bar., Bry., Carb. v., *Cham.*, China, Coc. c., Coral., Cupr., Dros., Dulc., Hepar, Hyos., Meph., Mez., Mur. ac., Nat. m., Nit. ac., Puls., Samb., Seneg., Sep., Sil., Spong., Sulph., Sul. ac., Verat.

NOSE, bleeding of, with cough: Acon., Ars., Bell., Bry., Carb. v., Carb. an., China, Cupr., Dros., Dulc., Ferr., Hyos., Indigo, Iod., Ipec., Kreos., Led., Merc., Mosch., Mur. ac., Nat. m., Nit. ac., Nux v., Phos., Puls., Rhus, Sabad., Sep., Sil., Spong., Sulph., Sul. ac.

PAROXYSMAL COUGH:

Acon., *Agar.*, Alum., Ambr., Ang., Aqu. p., Arum t., Bell., Bry., Calad., Cann. s.,

PAROXYSMAL COUGH.

Carb. v., Carb. h., *Caust.*, *Chel.*, China, Cimex, Cina, Coc. c., Coff., Con., Coral., Croc., *Cupr.*, Dros., Ferr., Ferr. mur., Gins., Hepar, Hyd. ac., Hyos., Ign., Jatr., Kali ch., Kreos., Lact., Laur., Lina, Lobel., Lyc., Mag. c., Mag. m., Mang., Merc., Merc. c., Merc. i. r., Morph., Nat. m., Nicc., Nit. ac., Nitrum, Nux v., Op., Phos., Plumb., *Puls.*, Rumex, Sabad., Sep., Sil., Stann., Sulph., Sul. ac., Tarent., Verat., Zinc.

PARTURITION, cough after: Rhus.

PENIS, darting in, as from congestion, on coughing: Ign.

Erection of, while coughing: Cann. s., Canth.

PEPPER, cough from eating: Cina.

PERIODIC COUGH: Ars., Cocc., Cocc. c., Colch., Lach., *Nux v.*

speaking or smoking from: Atro.

PERSISTENT COUGH: Acon., Am. caust., Bell., Cub., Cupr., Dios., Hyos., Ipec., Jatr., Lyc., Merc., Mez., Nitrum, Rumex, Sang., Squil.

PERSPIRATION, dry cough with: Acon., Ant. t., Apis, Arg. n., Bell., Bry., Carb. an., Caust., Cham., Cimex, Coff., Con., Dros., Dig., Hepar, Hyos., Ign., Ipec., Led., Lyc., Merc., Mur. ac., Nat. c., Nitrum, Nit. ac.,

PERSPIRATION, dry cough with.

> Nux v., Phos., Puls., Rhus, Sabad., Samb., Sepia, Stront., Sulph., *Verat.*

> On forehead, with cough: Ant. t., Ipec.

> On head, with cough: Ant. t., Calc., Ipec., Sil., Tarent.

> Inclination to: China, Psor.

PHARYNX, burning in, excites cough: Ars., Caust., Ph. ac.

> and soreness in, from cough: Sulph.

PREGNANCY, cough during: Calc., Con., Ipec., *Nux m.,* Phos., Puls., Sabin., Sep.

PRESSURE ON CHEST, relieves pains from the cough: Arn., Bor., Bry., Cimic., Dros., Eup. per., Kreos., Merc., Nat. m., Nat. s., Phos., Ran. b., *Sep.*

PTYALISM WITH COUGH: Ambr., Merc., Mez., Staph., Verat.

READING AGGRAVATES COUGH: Cina, Mang., Ment. pi., Meph., *Nux v.,* Phos.

RESPIRATION DIFFICULT, coughing after: Ars., Phos.

> Every cause desire to cough: Ipec.

> Interrupted (short stoppage of etc.) with cough: *Acon., Alum.,* Amm. c., Anac., Ant. t., Aralia, Arg. n., Arn., Ars., Bar., *Bell.,* Brom., Bry., Calad., Calc, Carb. an., Carb. v., Caust., Cina, Cocc., Clem. Con., Cupr., Dolich., Dros., Euphr., Ferr., Gua., Hepar,

RESPIRATION, interrupted.

> Ign., Iod., Ipec., Kali bi., Kali chl., *Kreos.,* Lach., Led., Lyc., Merc., Mosch., Natrum m., Nat. s., Nicc., Nit. ac., Nitrum, *Nux m.,* Nux v., Op., Phell., Phos., Puls., Rhus, Sep., Sil., Spig., Squil., Spon, Verat., Zinc., Zing.

REST AGGRAVATES COUGH: Ambr., Ars., Caps., Coc. c., Dros., Dulc., Euphr., Euphorb., Ferr., Hyos., Mag. c., Mag. m., Nux v., Phos., Ph. ac., Puls., Rhus r., Rhus t., Sabad., Samb., Seneg., Sep., Sil., Stan., Sulph., Verb., Zinc.

RIDING AGGRAVATES COUGH: Sul. ac.

RIGIDITY, body of, with cough: Bell., Cina., *Cupr.,* Ipec., Led., Mosch.

RINGING (clear) cough: Acon., All. c., Ars., Dros., Stram.

RUBS, child constantly rubs eyes, nose, and face with his fist during coughing spell: *Squil.*

RUNNING AGGRAVATES COUGH: Cina, Iod., Merc., Seneg., Sil., Stan., Sul. ac.

SACRAL REGION, pain in, with cough: Amm. c., Merc., Nit. ac., Sulph.

SHATTERING COUGH: Ant. ox., *Rhus,* Sil., Stann.

SHIVERINGS with cough: Grat., Kreos.

SHOULDERS, pain in, with the cough: Amm. c., Ars., China, Bry., Dig., Lach., Phos., Puls., Thuja.

SHUDDERING, coughing when:
Puls.

SIBILANT AND DRY
COUGH, like a saw driven
through a pine board: Spong.

SINGING AGGRAVATES
OR EXCITES COUGH:
Dros., Meph., Phos., Spong.,
Stan., Stram.

SITTING, cough when: Alum.,
Euphr., Ferr., Guai., Kali
c., Mag. c., Mag. m., Nat.
c., Phos., Ph. ac., Puls.,
Rhus, Sabad., Sep., Zinc.

SKIN TROUBLES WITH
COUGH: Bell., Con., Lach.,
Lact., Puls.

SLEEP, cough during: *Acon.*,
Arn., *Bell.*, Calc., Carb. an.,
Cham., Hipp., Hyos., *Lach.*,
Kreos., Merc., Samb., Sep.,
Stram., Verb.

SMOKING TOBACCO
EXCITES COUGH:
Acon., All. c., Brom., Bry.,
Carb. an., Cham., Clem.,
Cocc., Coc. c., Coloc., Dros.,
Euphr., Ferr., Hell., Hepar,
Ign., Iod., Lach., Mag. c.,
Ment. pi., Nux v., Osm.,
Petr., Spig., Spong., Staph.,
Sul. ac., Thuja.

SNORING WITH COUGH:
Ant. t., Arg., Bell., Caust.,
Ipec., Nat. c., Nat. m., Nux
v., Puls., Sep.

SOCIETY, strangers of, excites
cough: Acon., Agar., All. c.,
Ambr., Bad., Bell., Brom.,
Bry., Cact., Calc., Carb. v.,
Cast., Chel., China, Cina,
Con., Coral., Cupr., Dig.,
Dros., Ferr., Ferr. ac., *Hepar,*

SOCIETY, strangers of, excites
cough.

Hyos., *Ign.*, Ipec., Kali b.,
Kali c., *Kreos.*, Lach., Lact.,
Laur., Led., Lyc., *Mag. c.*,
Mag. m., Merc., Mez.,
Mosch., Nat. m., Nit. ac.,
Nux v., Osm., Phos., Ph. ac.,
Plumb., Puls., Rhus, Samb.,
Sep., Sil., Squil., Staph.,
Stram., *Sulph.*, *Verat.*, Zinc.

SPEAKING (talking) aggravates
or excites cough: Acon.,
Ambr., Anac., Arn., Ars.,
Bar., Bell., Bry., Calad.,
Calc., Carb. v., *Caust.*,
Cham., China, Cimic., Cupr.,
Euphr., *Hepar*, Ign., Iod.,
Ipec., *Lach.*, Mag. c., Mag.
m., Mang., Meph., Merc.,
Mez., Mur. ac., Nat. m., Nit.
ac., Phos., Ph. ac., Psor.,
Rhus, Rumex, Sil., Spong.,
Squil., *Stann.*, Stram., Sulph.,
Sul. ac., Verb.

STAIRS, ascending aggravates
cough: Arg. n., *Ars.*, Bar.,
Iod., Lyc., Mag. c., Mag.
m., Merc., Nitrum, Nux v.,
Seneg., Sep., Spong., Squil.,
Stan., Staph., Zinc.

STERNUM, aching behind, on
sitting bent forward, morning,
causing short cough: Rhus.

Aching in middle of, when
coughing: Nitrum.

in upper part, with catarrh
and cough: Ferr. ac.

Burning pain under the, and
stitches in sides of lungs, with
hacking cough: Clem.

in upper part after cough:
Ferr.

STOMACH, cold feeling in, with
dry suffocative cough: Lact.

SUFFOCATIVE (choking) cough: Acon., Anac., *Ant. t.*, Aqua. pe., Ars., . Bar., Brom., *Bry.*, *Carb. an.*, *Carb. Cham.*, Chin., Cina, Cocc., Con., Cupr., Cycl., Der., Dros., Euphr., Eupion., Gua., *Hepar*, Indig., Ipec., Kreos., Lach., Lact., *Led.*, Mang., *Nat. m.*, Nux m., *Nux v.*, Op., *Petr.*, Phell., Puls., Samb., *Sep.*, Sil., Spig., Spong., Squil., Sulph., Tabac., Zinc.

SWALLOWING aggravates or excites cough: Brom., Eugen., Kali hy., Op., Phos., Puls.

Ameliorates irriitation to cough: Eugen.

TASTE BAD AFTER THE COUGH: Cocc.

Bloody, when coughing: Amm. c., Bell., Elaps, Kali b., Nit. ac., Rhus.

Offensive with cough: *Caps.*

Sour, when with cough: Cocc.

Sweet with cough; Æth., Amm. c.

TEETH, cleaning the teeth provoked a violent cough, with vomiting of slimy fluid: Coc. c.

TESTICLES, pain in, when coughing: Zinc.

THINKING, cough worse when thinking of it: Bar., Ox. ac.

THROAT, irritation in, excites cough: *Acon.*, Ambr., Amm. c., Anac., Ant. c., Ant. t., Ars., Asaf., Asar., Bar., Bell., Bov., Brom., Bry., Calad., Carb. an., Carb. v., Caust., Cham., Chenop.,

THROAT, irritation in, excites cough.

China, Cocc., Coff., Coloc., Con., Croc., Dios., Dros., Ferr., Graph., Hepar, Hura, Hyd. ac., Hyos., Hyper., Kali c., Kali i., Lach., Laur., Lith. c., Lyc., Mag. c., Mag. m., Marum, Merc., Mez., *Nat. m.*, Nicc., Nit. ac., Nux v., Ol. an., Par., Petr., Ph. ac., Plan, Puls., Rhod., Rhus, Sabad., Sars., Sepia, Sil., *Squil.*, Staph., Stront., Sulph., Tab., Trom., Thuja, Verat., Verb., Zinc.

TOOTHACHE, coughing when: Lyc., Sepia.

TREMOR, cough with: Phos.

TROUBLESOME DRY COUGH: Ign.

ULCERS, cough excites pain in: Con.

URINE, involuntary discharge of, when coughing: Alum., *Ant. c.*, Bell., *Caps.*, Carb. an., Caust., Colch., Dulc., Hyos., Ign., Kreos., Laur., Mag. c., Nat. m., Nit. ac., Phos., Ph. ac., Puls., Rhod., Rhus, *Sepia*, Spong., Squil., Staph., Sulph., Verat., Zinc.

VEXATION, cough after: Acon., Ars., Bry., Cham., China, *Nat. m.*, Nux v., Sep., Staph., Verat.

VIOLIN, playing on, aggravates cough: Calc., Kali c.

VISION CLOUDY, when coughing: Coff., Kali c., Lach., Sulph.

VOMITING WITH, or from cough: Alum., *Anac.*, Ant. t., Arg. n., Arn., Bell., Bry.,

VOMITING, cough from.

Calc., Cann. s., Caps., *Carb. v.*, Coc. c., Con., Cupr., *Daph.*, Dig., Dros., Ferr., *Hepar*, Hyos., Indig., Iod., Ipec., Kali b., Kali c., *Lach.*, Merc., Merc. c., Mez., Mille., Nat. c., Nat. m., Nit. ac., *Nux v.*, Phos., *Ph. ac.*, Plumb., *Puls.*, Rhus, Sabad., Sep., *Sil.*, *Sulph.*, Sul. ac., Tarent., Thuja, Verat.

Acid, when coughing: Nat. c., Phos., Thuja.

acrid, morning, on coughing: Thuja.

Bilious (bitter): Carb. v., Cham., China, Cina, Cupr., Lach., Merc., Puls., Sabad., Sepia, Stram., Sulph.

Bloody: Arn., Carb. v., China, Cupr., Dros., Hyos., Ipec., Nux v., Sulph.

Of food, then of blood: Nux v.

Of ingesta: Anac., Ant. t., Arn., Ars., Bry., Calc., Carb. v., Cina, Dig., Dros., Eugen., Ferr., Hepar, Hyos., Ign., Iod., Ipec., Lach., Laur., Meph., Mez., Nat. m., Nit. ac., Phos., *Ph. ac.*, Rhus, Stann., Verat.

Milk: Chel., Spong.

Mucus: Carb. v., Cham., Cina, Coc. c., Con., Coral., Dros., Dulc., Hyos., Ipec., Mez., Nat. c. Puls., Sil., Seneg., Spong.

WALKING EXCITES COUGH: Alum., Ars., Carb. v., Cina, Dig., Ferr., Hepar, Iod., Lach., Nat. m., Rumex, Seneg., Stram., Stront., Sul. ac.

WASHING AGGRAVATES COUGH: Ant. c., Ars., Calc., Rhus, Stram., Sul. ac., Verat.

WHOOPING COUGH: Acon., *Ambr.*, *Anac.*, Ant. c., *Ant. t.*, *Arn.*, *Ars.*, Bar., *Bell.* *Bry.*, *Carb. an.*, Carb. v., *Cham.*, China, *Cina*, Coc. c., Con., *Coral.*, *Cupr.*, *Dros.*, *Dulc.*, *Euphr.*, *Guare.*, *Hepar*, *Hyos.*, Ign., Indig., Ipec., Kali c., Kali iod., Laur., *Led.*, Lobel., Lyc., Merc., *Meph.*, *Mez.*, Mosch., Mur. ac., Nat. m., Nit. ac., *Nux v.*, Op., Par., Phell., Phos., Podo., Puls., Rhus, Ruta, *Samb.*, Sang., Seneg., Secale, *Sep.*, *Sil.*, Spig., *Spong.*, *Sulph.*, *Sul. ac.*, *Tab.*, *Verat.*

WIND, belching of, after coughing: Sul. ac.

WRITING AGGRAVATES COUGH: Cina.

YAWNING EXCITES OR AGGRAVATES COUGH: Arn., Cina, Mur. ac., Nux v., Staph.

EXPECTORATION.

ACID (sour): Ambr., Ant. t.,
Ars., *Bell.*, Bry., Calc., Carb.
an., Carb. v., Cham., *China*,
Con., Graph., Hepar, Ign.,
Ipec., Kali c., Lyc., Mag. m.,
Merc., Nat. c., Nat. m., Nit.
ac., Nux v., Petr., Phos.,
Ph. ac., Plumb., *Puls.*, Rhus,
Sabin., Sepia, Stann., *Sulph.*,
Tarax.

ACRID: Alum., Amm. c., *Amm.
m.*, Anac., *Ars.*, Carb. v.,
Caust., Cham., Con., Ferr.,
Ign., Iod., Kreos., Lach.,
Lyc., Mag. m., *Merc.*, Mez.,
Nat. m., Nit. ac., Nux v.,
Phos., Puls., Sepia, *Sil.*,
Spig., Squil., Sulph., Sul. ac.

ALBUMINOUS: Amm. c.,
Amm. m., Arn., *Ars.*, Asaf.,
Bar., Bov., Bor., *China*,
Cocc., *Ferr.*, Kali b., *Laur.*,
Mez., Petr., Senega, Sil.,
Sulph., Stann.

ALMONDS, tasting like: Caust.,
Dig.

BITTER: Acon., Ail., Arn.,
Ars., Bry., Calc., Canth.,
Cham., China, *Cist.*, Coloc.,
Con., *Dros.*, Ign., Kali c.,
Lyc., *Merc.*, Nat. c., Nat.
m., *Nit. ac.*, Nux v., Puls.,
Sabad., *Sepia*, Stan., Sulph.,
Verat.

BLACKISH: Arn., Bell., China,
Elaps, *Kali b.*, Lyc., *Nux
v.*, Ox. ac., Puls., Rhus.

BLOODY: Acon., Ail., All. c.,
Aloe, Alum., Ambr., Amm.

BLOODY.

c., Amm. m., Anac., Ant. c.,
Ant. t., Arg. n., Arn., *Ars*,
Arum. m. n., Asar., Bad.,
Bell., Bism., Bond., *Bor.*,
Both., *Bry.*, Cact., *Calc.*,
Caust., *Canth.*, Caps., Carb.
ox., Carb. an., *Carb. v.*,
Cham., *China*, Cina, Cist.,
Con., Cop., *Croc.*, Crot. h.,
Cupr., Daph., Dig., *Dios.*,
Dros., *Dulc.*, Elaps, Erig.,
Eugen., Euphr., Ferr., Fluor.
ac., Gam., Gels., Graph.,
Guai., Ham., Hell., Hepar,
Hyd. ac., Hyos., Iod., Ipec.,
Jug. c., Kali b., Kali. c., Kal.
i., Kali hy., Kob., Kreos.,
Lach., Lachn., *Laur.*, Led.,
Lyc., *Mag. c.*, Mag. m.,
Mang., Merc., Merc. c.,
Mez., *Mill.*, Mur. ac., Nat.
c., *Nat. m.*, *Nit. ac.*, Nitrum,
Nux m., Nux v., *Op.*, Penth.,
Phos., Ph. ac., *Plumb.*,
Psor., Puls., *Rhus*, Ruta,
Sabad., *Sabin.*, Salic. ac.,
Sang., *Secale*, Selen., *Sepia*,
Sil., Sol. m., Squil., Stan.,
Staph., Sulph., *Sul. ac.*,
Tarax., Thuja, *Zinc.*

Black: Arn., Bism., Canth.,
China, Croc., Digit., Dros.,
Elaps, Kali b., Nit. ac., Nux
v., Ph. ac., Puls., Zinc.

Bright-red: Acon., Amm. c.,
Arn., Ars., Bell., Bry.,
Calc., Canth., Carb. an.,
Carb. v., China, Di., Dros.,
Dulc., Ferr., Hyos., *Ipec.*,
Kob., *Led.*, *Merc.*, Mill.,

BLOODY, bright-red.

Nitrum, Nux m., Nux v., *Phos.*, Puls., *Rhus*, Sabad., Sab., *Sec.*, Sep., *Sil.*, Zinc.

Coagulated: Acon., *Arn.*, *Bell.*, Bry., Canth., Carb. an., Caust., Cham., China, Coll., Con., Croc., Dros., *Ferr.*, *Hyos.*, *Ipec.*, Kreos., Mag. m., Merc., *Nit. ac.*, Nitr., Nux v., Ph. ac., Puls., Rhus, *Sab.*, Sec., Sep., Stram., Stront.

Dark: Acon., *Amm. c.*, Amm. m., Ant. c., *Arn.*, *Asar.*, Bell., Bism., *Bry.*, *Canth.*, Carb. v., Cham., *Chin.*, Con., Croc., *Cupr.*, Dig., Dros., *Elaps*, Ferr., *Kreos.*, Led., *Lyc.*, *Mag. c.*, Mag. m., Merc., Mur. ac., Nitr., Nit. ac., Nux m., Nux v., Phos., Ph. ac., *Puls.*, Sec., Sel., Sep., *Sulph.*, Sul. ac.

Frothy: *Arn.*, Dros., Ferr., *Led.*, Opium, *Phos.*, *Sil.*

BLOODY, hæmorrhage after suppression of menses: Acon., Ars., *Bell.*, *Bry.*, Con., *Ferr.*, Mill., Phos., Puls., Sep., Sulph.

in phthisical patients: *Acon.*, Arn., Ars., Cham., Dros., Ferr., Lach., *Mill.*, Phos., Puls., Sepia, Stan., Sulph., Sul. ac.

after wine: Acon.

hæmoptysis, tickling cough, tightness of chest, cannot lie down, mind calm: Ham.

during menses: Nat. m., *Phos.*,

during menses, and before, with dry cough, burning

BLOODY.

pain and soreness in chest, morning and evening: Zinc.

moon, during full: Nitrum.

after sea bath: Mag. m.

Streaked, while suckling a child: Ferr.

BLUISH: *Kali b.*, Nat. ar., Sulph.

BRICK-DUST COLOR: Bry., Phos., Rhus.

CHOCOLATE and milk, like: Hura.

COMPACT: Clem.

COOL: Bry., Calad., Cann. s., *Coral.*, Lach., Merc., Nit. ac., Nux v., *Phos.*, Rhus, Sulph.

COPPER, tasting like: Cupr., Kali c., Lach., Nat. m.

CORROSIVE: Iod.

DRINKING, ameliorates after: Amm. caust.

DUNG, tasting like: Calc., Carb. an., Cham., Merc., Sepia, Verat.

EARTHY, tasting: Ars., China, Ferr., Hepar, Ign., Merc., Phos., Puls.

EGGS, tasting like bad: Acon., Arn., Carb. v., Con., Hepar, Merc., Mez., Mur. ac., Phos., Ph. ac., Sepia, Stan., Sulph.

FATTY TASTING: Caust., *Mag. m.*, Mur. ac., Puls., Sil.

FACES, tasting like: Merc.

FETID: Arn., Ars., Bell., *Calc.*, Carb. v., Cocc., Cop., Guai., Led., Lyc., Nat. c., Nit. ac., Ph. ac., Puls., Sang., Sil., Stan., Sulph.

FISH, tasting like: Acon.

FLAT, tasting: Alum., Amm. m., Anac., *Ant. c.*, Ant. t., Ang., Ars., Aur., Bell., Bry., Calc., Caps., China, Cop., Euphr., Ipec., Ign., Kali c., Kreos., Lyc., Nat. c., Nat. m., Par., Petr., Phos., Ph. ac., Puls., Rhus, Sabad., Sabin., Sepia, Stan., Staph., Stron., Sul., Thuja.

FLESH, tasting like putrid: Ars., Bell., Bry., Carb. v., Dulc., Kali c., Lach., Nit. ac., Phos., Puls., Rhus.

FLIES forcibly out of mouth: *Bad.*, Chel.

GARLIC, odor like: Ars.

GELATINOUS: *Ang.*, Arn., Bar., China, Dig., Ferr., Laur.

GLAIRY: *Arn.*, Carb. h., Lip.

GREENISH. Arn., *Ars.*, Asaf., Aur., Benz. ac., Bor., Bov., Bry., Calc., *Cann. s.*, *Carb. an.*, *Carb. v.*, Coc. c., Colch., Cop., Dig., Dros., Ferr., Ham., Hyos., *Kali b.*, Kali c., *Kali i.*, Kreos., Led., *Lyc.*, Mag. c., Mang., Merc., Merc. i., Nat. c., Nitrum, Nit. ac., Nux v., Ol. jec., Ox. ac., Par., *Phos.*, Plumb., Psor., Puls., Raph., Rhus, *Sepia*, Sil., Stan., *Sulph.*, Thuja, Zinc.

HERRING, taste like: Anac.

INK, tasting like: Calc.

IRON, tasting like: Calc., Cupr., Sulph.

LOATHSOME: Dros., Puls.

LIE DOWN, profuse sputa of mucus, cannot lie down: Spong.

MEAT, tasting like: Ars., Bell., Bry., Carb. v., Dulc., Kali c., Lach., Nit. ac., Phos., Puls., Rhus.

MEMBRANEOUS: Amm. caust., *Brom.*, Hepar, Kali b., *Merc. c.*, Spong.

METALLIC, taste: Agnus, Calc., Cocc., *Cupr.*, *Ipec.*, Kali b., Kali c., Kreos., Nat. c., Nux. v., *Rhus*, Zinc.

MILKY: Amm. c., *Ars.*, Carb. v., Ferr., Plumb., Puls., Sep., Sil., *Sulph.*, Zinc.

MOUTHFULS of mucus at a time, raises: Phos., Lyc.

NAUSEOUS: Coc. c., Cop., Dros., Nux v., Tarent.

NIGHT, expectoration at, none during day: Alum., Amm. m., Arn., Calc., Kali c., Euphr., Led., Lyc., Phos., Raph., Rhod., Sabad., Sepia, *Staph.*, Sulph..

Bloody: *Ferr.*, Mez., Sulph.

Mucus: Agar., Calc., Cycl., Hepar, Sepia, Sil., Sulph.

Transparent: Calc. s.

Whitish: Sepia.

Yellow: Lyc.

NOON, bloody: Sil.

ONIONS, tasting like: Asaf., Mag. m., Sulph., Sul. ac.

ORANGES, tasting like: Phos.

PEPPER, tasting like: Acon., Ars., Mez., Sabad, Sulph.

PURULENT: Acon., Ail., All. s., Amm. c., *Anac.*, *Ant. t.*, Arg., Arn., *Ars.*, Asaf., Aur., Bell., Bry., Calc., Carb. an., Carb. v., Cham., China, Cic., Cimex, Cina., Cocc., *Cod.*, Con., Cop., Cupr., *Dros.*, Dulc., Ferr., Graph., Guai., Hepar., Hyos., Ign., Ipec., Kali b., Kali c., Kali i., Kreos., Lach., Led., Lyc., Mag. c., Mag. m,, *Merc.*, *Nat. c.*, Nat. m. *Nitr.*, Nit. ac., Nux m., Nux v., Oena, Phos., *Ph. ac.*, *Plumb.*, *Puls.*, *Rhus*, Ruta, Sabin., Samb., Sang., Sec., Sep., Sil., *Stan.*, Staph., Stront., Sulph., Verat., Zinc.

PUTRID TASTE: Acon., All. s., *Arn.*, *Ars.*, Bell., Bov., Bry., Calc., Carb. an., *Carb. v.*, Caust., *Cham.*, Cocc., Con., Cupr., Dros., Ferr., Ham., Iod., Ipec., Kali c., Kalm., Kreos., Led., Lyc., Merc., *Nat. c.*, Nux v., Phos., Ph. ac., *Puls.*, Rhus, Samb., Sep., Sil., *Stan.*, Staph., Sulph., Verat., Zinc.

RANCID TASTE: Ambr., Bar., Bry., Caust., Cham., Ipec., Lach, Merc., Mur. ac., Nux v., Phos., Puls.

REPULSIVE TASTE: Bry., China., Merc., Puls., Sabad., Sepia, Squil., Stan., Zinc.

ROPY: Cocc. c., Kali b., Lob.

RUSTY: Acon., Atro., Bry., Lyc., *Phos.*, Rhus, Sang., Squil.

SALTY: Acon., Agar., Alum., Ambr., Amm. c., Ang., Ant. t., Aralia, Ars., Bar., Bell.,

SALTY.

Bov., *Calc.*, Cann. s., Carb. v., *China*, Cocc., Con., Cop., Dros., Euph, Graph., Hyos., Iod., Kali b., Kalm., Lach., Lep., Lyc., Mac., Mag. c., Mag. m., *Merc.*, Merc. c., Mez., Nat. c., Nat. m. Nit. ac., *Nux m.*, Nux v., *Phos.*, Plan., *Puls.*, Raph., Rhus, Samb., *Sep.*, Sil., Stan., Staph., Sulph., Sul. ac., Tarax., Tarent., Theriod., Verat.

SIT UP, must, at night to raise the supta: Ferr.

On sitting up in bed, expectoration: *Phos.*

SLATE-COLORED: Kali b., Nat. ar.

SMOKY TASTE: Bry., Nux v., Puls., Rhus, Sep.

SOUR-SMELLING: Calc., Cham., Dulc., Merc., Nit. ac., Nux v., Sulph., Sul. ac.

STRINGY: Æsc., Agar., Arg., Arum t., Asaf., Coc. c., Ery. a., Ferr., Hydras., *Kali b.*, Lach., Lob., Ruta, Sticta.

SUGAR, tasting like: Calc., Lyc., Sepia.

SULPHUR, tasting like: Nux v., Phos., Ph. ac., Sulph.

SWEETISH TASTE: Acon., Alum., Amm. c., Anac., Ant. s., Ant. t., Apis, Ars., Asaf., Aur., *Calc.*, Canth., China, Coc. c., Cocc., Dig., Ferr., Hepar, Iod., Ipec., Kali b., Kali c., Kreos., Lob., Laur., Lyc., Merc., Mez., Nux v., Phos..

SWEETISH TASTE.

Plumb., *Puls.*, Rhus, *Sabad.*, Samb., Selen., Sep., Squil., *Stan.*, Sulph., Sul. ac., Zinc.

TAR, tasting like: Con.

TENACIOUS: Acet. ac., Aloe, Alum., Aqu. p., Arum t., Aspar., *Carb. v.*, Coc. c., Crot. t., Dig., Dulc., Hyper., Indig., *Kali b.*, Lept., Lact. ac., Lact., Lyc., Mag. c., **Mag. m.**, Merc., Merc. sul., Mez., Nat. c., Nat. m., Pæon., Par., *Phos.*, Raph., Ruta, Sang., Sec., Seneg., Sep., Sul. ac., Thuja, Uva ur., Zinc.

TICKLING: Caust., Iod.

TOBACCO JUICE, tasting like: Puls.

TOUGH: Æsc. h., Acon., Agnus, Ambr., Anac., Atro., Aur., Bov., Bry., Carl., Caust., Coc. c., Iris, Kali b., Kali c., Kob., Merc. i. r., Phos., Phyt., Puls., Sang., Senec., Sil., Tarent., Thuja, Verat., Vinc.

URINE, tasting like: Phos., Seneg.

VIOLETS, odor of: Phos., Puls.

VISCID (gelatinous, gluey): Acon., Agar., Agnus., Ail., Alum., Ambr., Amm. m., Ant. c., Ant. t., Arg., Ars., Asar., Bad., Bar., Bell., Bor., Bov., Bry., Cast., Calc., Calc. s., *Cann. s.*, *Canth.*, Carb. v., Caust., Cham., Chin, Cocc., Coc. c., Colch., Cupr., Dulc., Euphr., Ferr., Graph., Hell., Hepar,

VISCID.

Hyper., Iod., Kali b., Kali c., Kob., Kreos., Lycop., Mag. c., Mag. m., *Mez.*, Nat. ar., Nat. c., Nux v., *Paris*, Petr., *Phos.*, Ph. ac., Plumb., Puls., Rhus, Ruta, Sabad., Sabin., Samb., Seneg., Sep., Sil., Spig., Spong., Squil., *Stan.*, *Staph.*, Sulph., Ust., Verat., Zinc.

WAKING, after, in morning, thick expectoration: Lyc.

WALKING, in open air aggravates: Nux v.

Bloody expectoration while: Cham., Merc., Sul. ac.

WARM: Aralia.

WHITE, like white of egg: Amm. m., Arn., Ars., Bar., Bov., China, Coc. c., Ferr., Kali b., Laur., Mill., Petr., Seneg., Sil., Stan.

WHITISH: *Acon.*, Ail., Agar., Ambr., Amm. m., Ant. t., Arg., Arundo, Caps., Carb. an., *Carb. v.*, Chin., Chin. s., Chlo., Cina, Coc. c., Crot. t., Cupr., Ferr., Gad., Hyper., Illi., Iod., Kali b., Kali i., Kob., *Kreos.*, Laur., Lyc., Manc., Mer. i. r., Nicc., Ol. jec., Par., *Phos.*, Ph. ac., Plumb., *Puls.*, Puls. n., Raph., Rhus, Selen., Senec., Seneg., Sepia, Sil., Spong., Squil., Stront., *Sulph.*, Tarent., Tell., Thuja.

YELLOW: *Acon.*, Ail., Aloe, Alum., Ambr., Amm. c., *Amm. m.*, Anac., Ant. c., Arg., Arg. m., *Ars.*, Aur., Aur. mur., Bad., Bar., Bell., Bism., Bor., Bov.,

YELLOW.

Brom., *Bry.*, Cact. g., *Calc.*, Calc. ph., Calc. s., Cann. s., Carb. an., Carb. v., Caust., Cham., Chlor., Cic., Coca, Coc. c., Coloc., Con., Cop., Cupr., Daph., Dig., *Dros.*, Eugen., Ferr., Gels., Graph., Ham., Hepar, Hura, *Ign.*, Iod., Ipec., Kali b., Kali c., *Kreos.*, Lach., Linu, *Lyc.*, Mag. c., **Mag. m.**, Mang.,

YELLOW.

Merc., Merc. i. r., Mez., Mur. ac., Nat. ar., Nat. c., Nit. ac., Nux v., Oena, Op., Ox. ac., Par., Petr., Phos., Ph. ac., Plumb., Psor., Puls., Rumex, *Ruta*, Samb., Sabad., Sabin., Selen., Seneg., Sep., Sil., Spig., Spong., Stan., *Staph.*, *Sulph.*, Sul. ac., Tarent., *Thuja*, Verat., Zinc.

INDEX

INDEX OF REMEDIES.

PULSATILLA (Contd.)

flatulence, 611
fever, 612, 613
gastric symptoms, 368
gonorrhœa, 611
hallucinations, 605
headache, 60, 452, 606
phthisis, 709, 710
pregnancy, 227, 609, 610
prostate, 614
rheumatism, 614, 645
tinnitus aurium, 509
toothache, 223, 625, 607
urinary symptoms, 117, 503,
  612, 682, 747
vertigo, 60

PYROGEN, 615

constipation, 616
diarrhœa, 252
diphtheria, 615
female sexual system, 617
fever, 807
septicæmia, 615
typhoid, 354, 408, 561, 615,
  616

R

RADIUM BROMIDE, 619

boils, 620
skin, 619
vertigo, 620

RANA BUFO, 621

(See Bufo)

RANANCULUS BULB., 621

epilepsy, 88 622
hay fever, 621
herpes zoster, 622
hiccough, 622
pleurisy, 621, 622
pneumonia, 622
rheumatism, 622
skin, 622

RAPHANUS SATIVUS, 623

diarrhœa, 623
female genital organs, 623

RAPHANUS (Contd.)

flatulence, 623
toothache, 625

RATANHIA, 624

anal fissure, 584, 624
eyes, 625
pinworm, 625
toothache, 441, 625

RHEUM, 625

acidity, 625
diarrhœa, 343, 626
dysuria, 626

RHODODENDRON, 627

gout, 627, 628
neuralgia, 446, 627
rheumatism, 627, 628
scrotum, 627
toothache, 627, 628
vertigo, 627

RHUS AROMATICA, 628

diabetes, 628
dysuria, 629
hemorrhage, 629

RHUS GLABRA, 629

headache, 629

RHUS TOX., 630

cellulitis, 631
coryza, 643
delirium, 605 632
dysentery, 335
erysipelas, 112, 631, 632
eyes, 309, 635
fever, 154, 505, 592, 633,
  643, 648, 807
headache, 510, 511
injury, 65, 640, 727, 748
kidneys, 117
rheumatism, 277, 567. 630, 631
scarlatina, 634
skin, 244, 450, 622, 631, 644
toothache, 607
typhoid, 102, 334, 561, 633,
  634
vertigo, 635

INDEX TO REPERTORY.

Printed by Mr. W. R. Khan, at Karim Bux Bros.,
Government of India and General Printers,
9, Anthony Bagan, Calcutta.

Published by Mr. D. N. Chatterjee,
at the Presidency Homœopathic Pharmacy,
12, Lindsay Street, Calcutta.

Therapeutic Index[*]

*Compiled by Dr. I. Prabhakra Rao, Rajanagaram (A.P.)

Anemia

Acetic Acid, 6

Angina Pectoris

Aconite, 9
Angustura, 81
Arsenicum Album, 81
Asafoetida, 81
Aurum Mur., 99
Dioscorea, 272
Lactuca Virosa, 81, 415
Naja Trip., 494
Sambucus, 81
Sepia, 81
Veratrum Album, 81
Spongia, 705

Aphonia

Ammonium Caust., 35

Anus

Slag., 694
Causticum, 186
Ferrum Picricum, 300
Gelsemium, 309

Aphthae

Antim Crud., 753
Borax., 735
Hydrastis Can., 735
Mercurius, 735, 754
Mercurius Cyan., 753
Muriatic Acid, 754
Syphilinum, 753, 754

Apoplexy

Aconite, 95
Asterias Rubens, 95
Belladonna, 95, 112, 697
Formica, 303
Gelsemium, 308
Glonoine, 313
Lachesis, 727
Solanum Arr., 697
Strontiana Carb., 727
Sulphur, 727
Veratrum Vir., 95, 804

Arthritis

Causticum, 184, 187

Asciatic Cholera

Ricinis Communis, 636

Ascites

Apis Mell., 50, 56
Apocynum Can., 56
Senecio Aureus, 675
Senega, 675

Asphyxia

Camphora, 164

Asthma

Arsenicum. Alb., 82
Blatta Orientalis, 124
Colchicum, 228
Digitalis, 269
Ferrum Met., 82, 298
Gallicum Acidum, 304
Graphites, 82
Grindella, 327
Ipecac., 369
Kali Carb., 385
Kali Nitricum, 395
Lactuea Virosa, 415
Lobelia Inflata, 369
Mephitis., 464, 634
Natrum Sulph., 512
Nux Vomica, 529, 530
Ocimum Can., 532
Psorinum, 599
Pulmo Vulpis, 602
Rumex. 639
Sticta Pulm., 639
Sulphur, 735, 754
Zingiber Off., 830

Baldness

Arnica, 68

Blindness

Filix Mas., 301

Blood

Ammonium Carb., 32

Boils

Arnica, 67, 112, 161
Calcarea Picrica, 161
Picric Acid, 161
Radium Bromide, 620
Syphilinum, 751

Bone

Angustura, 41, 565
Asafoetida, 565
Aurum Met., 265, 565, 752
Calcarea Fluor., 157, 301
Calcarea Hypo., 159
Calcarea Phos., 159
Capsicum, 169
Capsicum, 169
Daphne Odorata, 265
Euphorbium, 290, 291
Fluoric Acid, 290, 301, 302
Hecla Lava, 332
Kali Iod., 752
Manganum, 565
Mercurius 265, 752
Mezerium, 265, 480, 481
Nitric Acid., 752
Phospharic Acid, 560
Phosphorus, 564
Phytolucca, 752
Salicylic Acid, 641
Silicea, 290, 301, 686, 687
Staphisagria, 265, 713
Syphilinum, 752

Brain

Lachesis, 411

Brain Fag

Scutellaria, 664

Bright's Disease

Terebinmina, 763

Bronchites

Carbo Veg., 47
Hippozaenium, 346
Ipecac, 47
Kali Iodatum, 47

Natrum Salicyli., 509
Phellandrium, 558
Pix Liauida, 575
Psorinum, 599, 660
Sanguinaria Nit., 363
Sulphur, 735

Broncho-pneumonia

Phosphorus, 564, 651
Bubo. Badiaga, 101 and Mer.
Iod. Rub., 477

Burns

Urtica Urens., 787

Calculi

Berberis Vulg., 120, 121

Cancer

Acetic Acid, 6
Arsenicum Alb., 85
Asterias Rub., 95
Cistus Can., 213
Condurango, 238
Hippozaenium, 346
Hydrastis Can., 348
Ornithogalum, 545

Carbuncles

Anthricinum, 42, 761
Arsenicum Alb., 761
Hippozaenium, 346
Kreosotum, 398
Lachesis, 762
Silicea, 686, 687
Tarentula Cub., 761

Carcinoma

Lapis Albus, 416

Caries

Strontiana Carb, 727

Cataract

Castor Equireum, 181

Catarrh

Allium Cepa, 23, 35, 716

Arsenicum Alb., 23, 35, 76
Arum Tryphyllum, 23, 35, 643, 716.
Eucalyptus, 286
Euphrasia, 23, 35, 716
Hydrastis Can., 348
Kali Iodatum, 390
Kali Mur., 394
Kali Sulph., 396
Menthol. 461
Merc. Iod. Flavus. 476
Myrica Cerifera, 492
Natrum Ars., 496
Natrum Mur., 502
Pulsatilla, 606
Senega, 675
Sinapis Alba, 693
Sticta Pulmanoria, 716, 717

Cellulitis

Rhus Tox., 631

Cerebro Spinal Affection

Paris Quadri., 552

Chancres

Merc. Iod. Rub., 477
Nitric Acid, 516, 517

Cholera

Aconite, 10, 796
Antim Tart., 48
Arsenicum Album, 84, 670, 797
Ars. Hydrogen, 87
Cadmium Sulph., 146, 147
Camphora, 163, 636, 797
Carbo Veg., 177, 670, 797
Cuprum Ars., 257, 258, 797
Cuprum Met., 163, 258, 260, 261, 636
Elaterium, 280, 369
Hydrocyanic Acid, 351, 797, 798
Secale Cor., 669, 670
Stramonium, 491, 723, 831
Veratrum Album. 128, 163, 795, 796

Chorea

Actea Rac., 490, 831
Agaricus Murc., 16, 491, 831
Artemesia Vug., 88
Arum Try., 92
Hippomanes, 345, 346
Ignatia 491, 831
Mygale 491, 831
Nux Moschata, 521
Pass.flora., 553
Tanacetum, 759
Tarentula Cub., 491, 761, 831
Veratrum Viride, 808, 809
Zizia 491, 831

Ciliary Neuralgia

Lac Felinum, 404

Circulatory Disturbance

Aconite, 650
Amyl Nitrosum, 650
Belladonna, 650
Opium, 651
Sanguinaria Can., 649, 650
Veratrum Viride, 650, 804
Zincum Met., 829

Climaxis

Amyl Nitrosum, 678
Carduus Mar., 180
Crotalus Horr., 678
Glonoine, 678
Jaborandi, 678
Kali Bichro., 678
Lachesis, 180, 678
Prunus Spinosa, 595
Sanguinaria Can., 678
Sepia, 678
Sulphur, 180
Sulphuric Acid, 678

Cold

Hepar Sulph., 643
Mercurius, 643
Sabadilla, 643

Coma

Stramonium, 722

Colic

Aconite Nap., 444
Actea Rac., 444
Aloe Socotrina, 234
Ammon., Mur., 444
Apis Mell., 444
Belladonna, 234
Bovista, 128, 129, 604
Carbolic Acid, 234
Castoreum, 182
Causticum, 188
Chamomilla, 234, 445
China Off., 234, 445
Cocculus, 234
Colchicum, 234
Colocynthis, 128, 129, 234,
    318, 444, 446, 586, 604
Cuprum Met., 234, 586
Dioscorea Vill., 234, 271,
    272, 586, 587
Dulcamara, 604, 605
Kali Bich., 445
Magnesia Phos,, 234, 443,
    444
Mancinella, 410
Ocimum Canum, 532
Platinum, 582
Plumbum Met., 445, 585,
    586
Pulsatilla, 446, 604
Senna, 677
Stannum, 235, 391, 708
Veratrum Album., 801

Condylomata

Mercurius Dulcis, 475

Constipation

Aletris Farinosa, 23
Aloe Socotrina, 26, 151, 662
Alumen, 28
Alumina, 30, 187, 343, 518,
    582, 655, 798
Ammon. Mur., 36, 48, 655
Anacardium 30, 343

Antim Crudum, 28, 481,
    682
Apis Mell., 481
Bryonia, 28, 482, 543, 674,
    828
Calcarea Carb., 151
Causticum, 30, 187, 343
Chelidonium, 197, 543, 754
Collinsonia., 231
Conium, 241
Crotallus Horr., 662
Graphites 30, 482, 518, 674,
    682, 754, 828
Hepar Sulph., 343
Ignatia, 359
Indium Met., 362
Lac Defloratum, 403
Lachesis, 28, 482, 754
Lycopodium. 429, 754
Magnesia Mur, 444, 655
Medorrhinum, 187
Mezerium 481, 754
Natrum Mur., 504, 506, 655,
    682, 754, 755
Nitric Acid, 518, 754, 755
Nux Vomica., 527, 528, 754,
    755
Opium, 532, 616, 674, 798
Platinum, 30, 343, 563
Plumbum Met., 28, 543, 587,
828
Pyrogen, 616
Sanicula, 151, 655, 661
Sarsaparilla, 662
Selenium, 151, 655, 673, 674
Sepia, 28, 151, 682
Silicea 30, 151, 343, 543, 548,
    582, 655, 673, 674, 682,
    690
Strontiana Carb., 727
Sulphur, 28, 662, 673, 674,
    828
Syphilinum, 754
Thuja, 543, 655
Veratrum Alb., 30, 343, 798
Zincum Met., 828

Consumption

Lycopus Virg., 436
Natrum Phos., 508

Convulsions

Aethusa Cyn., 15
Belladonna, 111, 353
Cicuta Virosa, 207
Hyosyamus, 354
Mille folium, 482
Solanum Vigrum, 696
Stramonium 88, 722, 723

Corns

Antim. Crud., 44
Graphites, 44
Hepar Sulph., 44
Silicea, 44

Coryza

Aconite, 8, 35, 136, 286, 716
Ammonium Carb., 643, 716
Ammonium Mur, 35, 643
Ars. Iodatum, 87
Belladonna, 286
Bryonia, 136
Jaborandi, 373
Justicia, 377
Lycopersicum, 426
Naphthalinum, 495
Nitric Acid, 515
Nux Vomica, 527, 643
Rhus Tox., 643
Sabadilla, 35
Sinapis Nigra, 694

Cough

Aconite, 9, 452
Allium Sat., 24
Ammonium Carb., 33, 676
Ammon. Mur., 452
Angustura, 42
Antim Tart., 9, 47, 274, 676, 800
Aralia Racemosa, 57
Badiaga, 101
Brayonia, 288, 514

Capsicum, 170
Causticum, 9
Conium, 242
Cuprum Met., 210, 220, 221, 259, 274
Eupatorium Perf,, 288, 289
Euphrasia, 291, 452
Glonoine, 220
Hepar Sulph., 9, 220, 221, 342, 704
Hyoscyamus 220, 221, 354
Indigo, 361
Iodium, 365
Ipecac, 220, 221, 377, 676
Kali Sulph., 376
Laurocerasus, 210, 417
Lycopodium, 220, 221
Mangunum, 451
Medorrhinum, 457
Mentha Piperita., 461
Mephitis, 220, 221, 464, 465
Myrtus Communis, 494
Natrum Mur., 220
Niccolum Met., 514
Phospharic Acid, 560
Phosphorus, 220
Psorinum, 601
Rumex, 220, 461, 465, 638 639
Sambucus, 9
Sanguinaria Can., 32, 220
Sarsaparilla, 220
Sepia, 452, 676
Silicea, 220
Sinapis Nigra, 694
Spongia 9, 220, 221, 703, 704
Squilla, 706
Sticta Pulm., 465, 717
Sulphur, 220, 221, 736
Sulphuric Acid, 678
Teucrium, 765
Thuja, 773
Veratrum Album, 32, 800
Verbascum, 812
Zincum Met., 452, 453, 829

Coxalgia

Solanum Mamm., 697

Cystitis

Dulcamara, 278
Mercurius Corr., 473
Tarentula Cub., 762

Debility

Abies Can., 1
Acetic Acid, 6
Arsenicum Alb., 570, 671
Calcarea Carb., 570, 571
Carbo. Veg., 176
China 371, 570, 571
Conium 570, 571
Gelsemium 1, 570, 571, 689
Iodium, 570, 571
Iridium, 371
Laurocerasus, 317, 416
Muriatic Acid, 489
Natrum Carb., 498, 570, 571
Phosphoric Acid, 570, 571
Phosphorus, 570, 571
Picric Acid, 350, 570
Selenium, 570, 571, 671
Silicea, 688
Stannum, 707
Sulphur, 570, 571

Delirium

Absinthium, 5
Agaricus, 586
Apis Mell., 52
Belladonna, 108, 586, 696, 327
Cantharides, 586
Cuprum Met., 586
Euphorbium, 603
Hyosyamus, 108, 352
Lachesis, 108
Lachnanthes, 352
Lyssen, 108
Plumbum Met., 585
Podophyllum, 352
Rhus Tox., 603, 632

Scutellaria, 108, 664
Selenium, 352
Solanum Nigrum, 696
Stramonium, 108, 721, 722
Tanacetum, 108
Teucrium, 352
Zincum Met., 353, 827

Delirium Tremens

Opium, 542

Delusion

Lac Caninum, 401, 722
Valeriana, 722, 791, 792

Dentition

Belladonna, 192, 592
Chamomilla, 192
Erigeron, 284
Podophyllum, 592
Zincum Met., 826

Diabetes

Argentum Met., 60
Bovista, 1 8
Calcarea Hypo, 160
Calcarea Phos., 160
Ferrum Iod., 294
Lactic Acid., 414
Lycopus Virg., 436
Lycopersicum, 426
Magnesia Sulph., 447
Moschus, 486
Picric Acid, 573
Rhus Aromatica, 628
Syzygium, 755
Uranium Nit., 784

Diarrhoea

Acalypha Indica, 5
Acetic Acid, 6
Aconite, 9
Aloe, 25, 26, 254, 282, 305. 326, 511, 591, 640, 655, 772, 778
Ammonium Carb., 128
Apis Mell., 52, 778, 779

Diphtheria

Acetic Acid, 6
Allanthus, 20
Amygdala Amara, 37, 113
Apis Mell., 21, 22, 486
Arum Try, 90
Bromium, 130
Carbolic Acid, 21, 22, 178
Grotallus Horr, 21, 22, 252, 495
Hydrocyanic Acid, 37
Kali Mur., 394
Lac. Caninum, 402
Lachesis, 21, 22, 405, 410, 495, 558
Lycopodium, 21. 22, 568
Mercurius, 467, 568
Mercurius Cyan, 21, 22, 474, 477
Merc. Iod. Flavus, 476
Merc., Iod. Rub., 477
Muriatic Acid, 490
Naja Trip., 494
Natrum Ars., 496
Nitric Acid, 21, 22, 515
Opium, 541
Phytolucca, 568

Dropsy

Acetic Acid, 6
Apis Mell., 50, 56
Apocynum Can., 56, 147, 268
Aurum Met., 268
Cainca, 147
Chimaphila, 268
China, 268
Digitalis, 268, 335
Fluoric Acid, 268
Helleborus Niger, 332, 335
Jaborandi, 373
Lycopodium, 268
Prunus Speniosa, 595
Terebinthina, 335

Dysentery

Aloe Socotrim, 335, 738

Arnica, 67
Belladonna, 116, 117
Cantharides, 168, 170
Capsicum, 170
Garbo Veg., 177
Chamomilla, 116
Colchicum, 335, 738, 739
Crotallus Horr., 252
Eucalyptus, 286
Hamamelis Virg., 331
Helleborus, 335
Ipecac., 368
Kali Mur, 394
Lyssin, 438
Mercurius, 67, 467, 468, 469
Mercurius Corr., 472, 473
Natrum Sulph, 511
Nitric Acid, 518
Podophyllum, 117
Rhus Tox., 335
Trombidium, 778

Dyspepsia

Abies Nigra, 2
Abratanum, 714
Anacardium, 39, 323
Angustura, 323
Argentum Nit., 62, 737
Arnica, 67
Bryonia, 663
Calcarea Carb., 2, 323, 501, 535, 637
Carbo Veg., 67, 175, 218, 636, 757
Carbolic Acid, 179
China, 2, 201, 535, 607, 637, 737
Cocculus, 218, 323, 683
Digitalis, 743
Graphites, 322, 323, 535
Hepar Sulph, 343
Hydrastis Can., 348
Hydrocyanic Acid, 350
Ignatia, 358, 359, 682, 683, 737
Kali Carb., 384, 682, 683

Kali Sulph.. 637
Lachesis, 175, 176, 507
Lactic Acid, 2
Lycopodium, 428, 522, 637, 663
Mercurius, 682, 683
Natrum Mur., 2, 15, 504
Natrum Phos, 507, 508
Nux Moschata, 522, 523
Nux Vomica, 2, 67, 176, 428, 522, 527, 555, 744
Opium, 744
Ornethogalum, 544
Petroleum, 323, 555, 682, 683, 737
Picric Acid, 350
Pulsatilla, 611, 663
Robinia, 631, 744
Salicylic Acid, 646
Sarsaparilla, 663
Selenium, 744
Sepia, 682, 710, 737
Stannum, 682, 683, 710
Staphisagria, 714
Sulphur, 176, 683, 736
Zincum Met, 2, 827

Dysphegia

Gelsemium, 309

Dyspnoea

Antim Ars., 43
Antim Tart., 47, 267
Carbo Veg., 175, 323, 507

Dysuria

Petroselinum, 557
Rheum, 626
Rhus Aromatica, 629

Earache

Plantago Major, 576

Ears

Calcarea Carb., 151
Causticum, 185, 734
China, 734

Dulcamara, 392
Graphites, 324, 734
Kali Iodatum, 391, 392
Kali Sulph, 392
Lycopodium, 392
Manganum, 451, 452
Nitric Acid, 372
Petroleum, 392, 734
Phospharic Acid, 734
Phosphorus, 392
Pilocarpus, 574
Salicylic Acid, 734
Sepia, 392
Sulphur, 734
Veratrum Album, 392
Violo Odorata, 817

Eclampsia

Artemesia Vulg., 88

Endocarditis

Aurum Mur, 99

Enteritis

Carbolic Acid, 178

Enterocolitis

Nuphar Luteum, 520

Enuresis

Belladonna, 577
Causticum, 577
Kreosotum, 577, 682
Lac Caninum, 577
Plantago Major, 576, 577
Senega, 577
Sepia, 577, 682

Epilepsy

Absinthium, 5
Agaricus Mus., 88, 587, 588
Alumina, 587, 588
Argentum Met., 60
Arsenicum Alb., 533
Artemesia Vul., 88, 89, 533 587, 588
Aurum Met., 533

Mercurius Corr., 472
Naphthalinum, 495
Natrum Mur, 502
Natrum Phos, 508, 509
Natrum Sulph, 511
Phosphorus. 566
Physostigma, 567
Pilocarpus, 574
Prunus Spinosa, 594
Pulsatilla, 606, 607
Ratanhia, 625
Rhus Tox., 309, 635
Ruta Grav. 640, 641
Santoninum, 656
Silcea, 689, 690
Spigelia, 304, 699
Staphisagria, 713
Sulphur, 324, 734
Syphilinum, 753
Tabacum, 756
Thuja, 771
Tilia Europia, 777
Viola Odorata, 818

Fainting

Aconite, 485
Agaricus, 486
Alumina, 486
Asafoetida, 486
Carbo Veg., 486
Conium, 486
Moschus, 485
Opium, 485
Phosphorus, 486
Podophyllum, 486
Sepia, 486
Sulphur, 486
Tnuja, 486

Felons

Anthracinum, 761
Arsenicum Album, 42
Lachesis, 42, 761

Female Genital Organs

Ammon. Mur., 36

Antim Crud., 45
Apis Mell., 52, 806
Arsenicum Alb., 85
Borax, 125
Cocculus, 218, 219
Colocynthis, 235
Digitalis, 269
Ferrvm Iod., 294
Gelsemium, 310
Hydrocotyle. 349
Hyosyamus 353, 544, 581
Ignatia, 359
Laurocerasus, 269
Lycopus and Virg., 436
Medorrhinum, 454, 458
Mel Cum Sale, 459
Murex Purpurea, 487, 488, 581
Natrum Carb., 498
Natrum Mur, 114, 502, 503, 504
Raphnus Sat., 623
Sanicula, 656
Sepia, 114, 128, 487, 488, 499
Spongia, 703
Stannum, 708
Staphisagria, 714
Ustilago Maidis, 741, 788
Veratrum Album, 544, 800
Veratrum Viride, 806
Viburnum Opulus, 815
Viscum Album, 821
Xanthoxylum, 822
Zincum Met., 828
Zizia, 831

Female Mammae

Phellandrium, 588

Female Sexual System

Actea Racemosa, 11, 114
Ambra Girsea, 32, 788
Ammonium Carb., 34
Aurum Met., 97
Aurum Mur Nat., 100
Baryta Mur, 106

Ledum, 419, 432
Muriatic Acid, 807
Natrum Mur, 100, 170, 206,
    288, 289, 333, 334, 505,
    506, 633
Natrum Sulph, 513
Nux Vomica, 67, 100, 155,
    190, 202, 505, 528, 529,
    670, 671, 699
Ocimum Canum, 532
Opium, 360
Phospharic Acid, 807
Podophyllum, 591, 592, 633
Psorinum, 633
Pulsatilla, 612, 613
Pyrogen, 807
Rhus Tox., 154, 505, 592,
    633, 643, 648, 807
Sabidilla, 633, 642, 643
Sabina, 190
Sambucus, 613, 633, 648
Santoninum, 657
Secale Cornutum, 670
Silicea, 691
Stramonium, 206
Sulphur, 206, 613, 739, 740

Fibroid Tumour

Kali Iod. 393, 394

Fidgitiness

Kali Bramatum, 381
Zincum Met., 381, 826

Fissure

Graphites, 548
Nitric Acid, 548, 624

Flatulence

Aloe 25, 26
Argentum Nit., 62
China, 200
Colocynthis, 611
Iodium, 62, 364
Ledum, 427, 428, 621
Nux Moschata, 62
Pulsatilla, 611

Gall Stones

Carduu. Mar., 180

Gangrane

Arsenicum Album, 86
Crotallus Horr., 252
Kreosotum., 398

Gastric Affections

Abies Canadensis, 1
Apocynum Can., 56
Argentum Met., 62, 535
Arsenicum Album, 83, 85, 368
Asafoetida, 93
Belladonna, 116
Bismuth, 123
Calcarea Phos., 535
Chamomilla, 193
Colchicum, 268, 323
Crocus Sativa, 248
Cuprum Met., 260
Doryphora, 273
Ferrum Met., 296, 535
Hydrastis Can., 737
Ipecac., 260, 296, 367, 368,
    714, 757
Iris Ver., 372
Kali Bich., 308, 378, 502, 536,
    689 700
Kreosotum, 39
Leptandra, 421
Lobelia Inflata, 267, 425, 682,
    683, 714
Morphinum, 484
Oleander, 535
Picrotoxin, 573
Pulsatilla, 368
Tabacum, 267, 714, 757
Thea, 766
Valeriana, 15

Gastric Irritation

Aethusa Cynapium, 15, 637
Antim Crudum, 15, 44, 368.
    535
Silicea, 15
Sulphur, 15, 93, 535

Gastrodynia

Oxalicum Acidum, 547

Glands

Bromium, 130
Carbo Ani., 172
Iris Ver., 371, 372, 373
Mercurius Cyan., 47
Solanum Oler., 697

Glaucoma

Commocladia, 237

Goitre

Eabis Albus 416

Gonorrhoea

Agnus Castus, 19
Argentum Nit., 611
Cannabis Indica, 556
Cannabis Sativa, 166
Cantharides, 556
Cinnabaris, 211
Copaiva, 243, 528
Cubeba, 256, 528
Doryphora, 273
Erechthites, 612
Mercurius, 556
Natrum Mur., 503, 504
Natrum Sulph., 511
Nitric Acid, 517
Nux Vomica, 528
Petroselinum, 556
Pulsatilla, 611
Sarsaparella, 612
Yucca Filamentosa, 824

Gout

Ammonium Benz., 32
Menyanthes, 462
Rhododendran, 624, 628
Sepia, 684
Silicea, 684
Urtica Urens, 786
Zincum Met., 462

Haemoptysis

Acalypha Indica, 5
Ferrum Iod., 294

Hallucinations

Cannabis Indica, 165
Kali Carb., 383, 384
Pulsatilla, 605

Hay Fever

Ars Iod, 88
Ranunculus Bulb, 621
Sinapis Alba, 693
Sticta Pulm., 717

Headache

Aconite, 8, 141, 308, 358, 459
Actea Racemosa, 11
Agaricus, 16
Ailanthus, 459
Aloe Socotrina, 25, 141
Alumina, 141
Ammonium Carb., 33
Amyl Nitrosum, 38, 109, 459
Antimonium Crudum, 700
Apis Mell, 141
Arania Diadema, 58, 59
Argentum Met., 60
Argentum Nit., 62, 462, 606
Arsenicum Album, 74
Aurum Met., 109
Badiaga, 101
Belladonna, 109, 141, 260, 459, 460, 689
Bryonia, 133, 134, 375, 511, 706
Cactus, 141, 176, 462
Capsicum, 169
Carbolic Acid, 178
Chelidonium, 375
China, 141, 201
Cina, 462
Cocculus, 217, 213
Coffea Cruda, 233, 606

Heart

Aloe, 26
Alumen, 28

Hemorrhoids

Antimonium Crudum, 44
Bromium, 26, 131
Collinsonia, 231
Hamamelis Vorg., 331
Ledum, 429
Muriatic Acid, 15, 26, 490
Nitric Acid, 515, 518
Nux Vomica, 528
Sepia, 682
Sulphur, 739

Hernia

Arsenicum Album, 800
Lachesis, 800
Sulphuric Acid, 746
Tabacum, 758
Veratrum Album, 800

Herpes Zoster

Ranunculus Bulb., 622

Hiccough

Ledum, 522
Nux Moschata, 523
Nux Vomica, 522
Ranunculus Bulb., 622

Hydrocephalus

Apis Mell., 50, 56
Apocynum Can., 56
China, 201
Kadi Iodatum, 390
Zincum Met., 826

Hydrophobia

Agaue Americana, 18
Belladonna, 109
Cantharides, 109
Coccinella, 215
Hoang-Nan, 347

Hysteria

Ambra Girrsa, 747

Asafoetida 92, 358, 747
Castor Equirum, 747
Cocculus, 358
Coffea Cruda, 223
Cubeba, 747
Hyoscyamus Niger., 354
Ignatia, 92, 358
Moschus, 358, 485, 486
Nux Moschata, 358, 521, 522,
   747
Scutellaria, 664
Sticta Puem., 718
Sumbul, 747
Tana Celum, 759
Tarentula Cub., 761
Theridion., 766, 767
Valeriana, 358, 791

Hydrothorax

Apis Mell., 50
Mercurius Sulph, 478

Impotence

Agaricus Musc., 672
Agnus Castus, 18, 310, 672
Argentum Met., 61
Aurum Met., 672
Caladium, 19, 148, 310, 672
Calcarea Carb., 672
Conium, 19, 310, 672, 673,
   828
Ledum, 19, 43, 672, 673
Moschus, 358, 485, 486
Nux Vomica, 310, 528
Onosmodium, 539
Phospharic Acid, 559
Phosphorus, 19, 672, 673
Selenium, 310, 559, 672
Sulphur, 19
Thuja, 19
Yohimbinum, 823

Indigestion

Allium Sativa, 24
Homarus, 317

Pnellandrium, 558
Pix Lialuida, 575
Pulsatilla, 709, 710
Rumex, 639
Sepia, 710
Silicea, 709
Theridion, 767

Piles

Carbo Veg., 15
Lachsis, 15
Phosphorus, 548
Verbascum Thapsus, 812

Pin Worms

Ratanhia, 625

Plague

Hippozaenium, 346
Naja. Trip , 494

Pleurisy

Aconite, 9
Apis Mell , 622
Bryonia, 136, 622
Cactus, 144
Jadorandi, 373
Kali Mur., 394
Ranunculus Bulb, 621, 622
Senega,676

Pleurodynia

Gaultheria, 306

Pleuro-Pneumonia

Squilla. 706

Pneumenia

Antim. Tart. 46, 106, 130,
278, 369, 697
Asclepias Tuberosa, 94
Bryonia, 94, 133, 136
Carbo Animalis, 172
Carbo Veg., 47
Chelidonium, 197
Iodium, 365, 366

Ipecac, 47, 369
Kali Iodatum, 47, 391
Kali Mur, 394
Kali Nitricum, 395
Natrum Sulph., 512
Nitric Acid, 515
Nux Vomica, 530
Opium, 541
Ranunculus Bulb, 622
Sanguinaria Can., 651
Sulphur, 735
Veratrum Viride., 651, 804,
807, 808

Polypus

Sanguinaria Can., 652
Teuerium, 765

Pregnancy

Belladonna, 183, 311
Calc. Carb., 153
Caulophyllum, 183
Cocculus, 227
Colchicum, 227
Cuprum Ars., 258
Cyclamen, 264
Ferrum Met, 298
Gelsemium 183, 310, 311
Gossypium, 318
Hamamelis Virg , 331
Ipecac., 227
Kali Carb., 227
Kreosotum, 227
Ledum, 430, 431
Lyssin, 438
Mitchella Repens, 483
Nux Vomica, 227, 529
Petroleum, 555
Pulsatilla, 227, 609, 610
Sinapis Alba, 694
Tabacum, 227, 228
Veratrum Album, 227, 228
Vcratrum Viride, 183

Prolapsus

Ignatia, 641

Muriatic Acid, 641
Ruta Grav., 641
Solanum Tub , 696

Prelapsus Recti.

Arnica, 67

Prostrate

Ferrum Pic., 300
Merc. Dul., 476
Pulsatilla, 614

Prouritus

Collinsonia, 231

Pruaitus Vulvae

Caladium, 148
Menthol, 461
Urtica Urens, 787

Ptosis

Alumina, 30
Gelsemium, 309
Kalmia Lat., 309

Pyorrhoea

Causticum, 628

Quinsy

Psorinum, 600

Repur Cussed Eruptions

Bryonia, 259
Calcarea Carb., 259
Causticum, 259
Cuprum Met., 154, 259
Cuprum Met., 154, 259
Gelsemium, 138, 164
Sulphur, 46, 259
Zincum Met., 138, 164, 259, 825

Respiratory Troubles

Aconite, 8, 651, 735
Baryta Carb., 105

Calcarea Carb., 153, 151
Calcarea Phos, 647
Chlorum 206, 207
Formalin, 303
Iodum, 647
Ledum, 431
Osmium, 546
Sambucus, 647
Sanguinaria Can., 649
Solanum Aceticum, 697

Rheumatesm

Abrotanum, 2
Aconite, 622
Actea Racemosa., 11
Actea Spicata, 13
Allium Sativa, 24
Ammonium Mur., 36, 645
Apis Mell., 50
Argentum Met., 60
Arnica, 622
Asofoetida., 273
Asclepias Tuberosa, 94
Aurum Met., 273
Aurummur Nat., 99
Benzoic Acid, 119
Bryonia, 133, 277, 567, 622
Caulophyllum 13, 183
Chelidonium, 196
Colchicum 13, 25, 119, 224, 228
Dulcamara, 277
Ferrum Met., 298, 642
Ferrum Picricum, 300
Formica. 304
Gaultheria, 304
Graphites, 645, 684
Kali Carb., 384
Kali Mur., 394
Kali Sulph, 614
K lmia Lat., 397, 568
Lac. Can., 401
Ledum, 418, 419, 645
Lithium Carb., 424
Lycopersicum, 426
Manganum, 451

Sleepiness

Phellandrium, 588

Small Pox

Hippozaenium, 346
Malandrinum, 448, 449
Sarracenia, 658, 659
Thuja, 771, 772
Varioinum, 793, 794

Sore Throat

Ailanthus, 20
Alumen, 28
Ammonium Carb., 33
Apis Mell., 21, 22
Arum Try., 90
Gymnocladus, 329
Kali Bichronicum, 377, 329
Lachesis, 21, 22, 405, 406
Ledum, 21, 22, 431, 432
Mercurius Cyan, 21, 22, 474
Nitric Acid, 21, 22, 515

Spasm

Cuprum Met., 258, 259

Spinal Meningitis

Oxalic Acid., 546

Spinal Irritation

Theridion, 766, 767

Spleen

Ferrum Iod., 294

Sprains

Ammonium Mur., 36
Strontiana Carb., 728

Stammering

Cicuta Virosa, 724
Euphrasia, 724
Spigelia, 724
Stramonium, 724
Cincum Met., 724

Sterility

Natrum Carb., 498

Stomatitis

Kali Chloricum, 386

Strabismus

Cina, 210

Stranguary

Prunus Spinosa, 595, 660

Sun Stroke

Natrum Carb., 498

Suppressed Eruptions

Antim Tart., 46, 138
Apis Mell., 46
Belladonna, 46, 138
Heloderma, 138

Supra Orbital Neuralgia

Kali Iodatum, 389

Suppression

Mercurius, 341, 470, 687

Suppuration

Calcarea Fluor, 156
Calcarea Phos., 156
Calcarea Sulph, 341
Guaiacum, 328
Hepar Sulph, 341, 470
Myristica Seb., 493
Silicea, 156, 157, 341, 471, 686

Sycosis

Antim Tart., 48
Ausum Mur., 99

Synovitis

Apis Mellifica, 50
Bryonia, 136, 137

Syphilis

Ars. Alb., 85

Aurum Met., 96, 97
Aurum Mur., 99, 328, 392
Corrallium Rub., 245
Fluoric Acid., 328
Guaiacum, 328
Hepar Sulph., 393
Hoang-Nan, 347
Kali Bichrom., 328, 329, 378
Kali Iodatum, 385, 390, 392
Mercurius, 328, 329. 393, 470
Mercurius Corr., 393
Mercurius Dulcis, 393
Merc. Iod. Rub., 393
Mezerium, 328
Nitric Acid, 328, 329, 393, 515, 516
Stillingia, 719
Viola Tricolor, 819, 820

Tabes Misenterica

Ioduim, 366
Oleum Jec, 537

Talkativeness

Eugenia Jambos, 287

Tape Worm

Cucurbita Pepo., 257
Filix Mas, 301
Granatum, 319

Testicles

Hamamelis Virg., 788
Ustilago Maidas, 789

Tetanus

Hydrocyanic Acid, 349, 350
Possiflora, 553
Scutellaria, 664
Strychninum, 730

Throat

Aconite, 113
Baryta Carb., 105, 106
Cantharides, 113
Gambogia, 305

Hepar Sulph, 113
Ignatia, 113
Mancinella, 450
Medorrhinum, 457
Spongia, 703
Sulphur, 113

Tinnitus Aurium

Cocculus, 509
Natrum Salicyli, 509
Phosphorous, 509
Pulsatilla, 509

Tonsilitis

Amygdala Amara., 37
Baryta Mur., 106
Calc. Carb., 105
Calcarea Phos., 105
Lac Caninum, 402
Mercurius, 467
Mercurius Cyan., 474
Psorinum, 600
Ustilago Maidis, 789

Toothache

Aranea Diadema, 59
Arsenicum Album, 77
Bismuth, 124, 223
Bryonia, 223
Calcarea Carb., 77
Causticum, 223
Chamomilla, 77, 625
Chenopodium, 198
Coffea Cruda, 223
Ignatia, 359
Kreosotum, 714
Lachesis, 77
Lyssin, 437
Magnesia Carb., 440, 441, 607
Magnesia Sulph., 447
Mercurius, 467
Mezerium, 481, 714
Natrum Sulph, 223
Nux Moschata, 625
Oleum Animale, 536
Phosphorus, 77, 607

Piper Meth, 575
Plantago Major, 576
Prunus Spinosa, 594
Pulsatilla, 223, 607, 625
Raphanus, 625
Ratanahia, 441, 625
Rhododendran, 627, 628
Rhus Tox., 607
Sanguinaria Can, 607
Sepia, 625
Staphisagria, 77, 625, 713
Theridion, 77
Thuja, 714

Torticollis

Lachnanthes, 413

Trauma

Arnica, 66
Bellis Perinnis, 119
Sulphuric Acid, 746, 748

Tuberculosis

Actea Racemosa, 12
Drosera, 275
Kali Carb., 385, 710
Phosphorus, 564, 709
Stannum, 709, 735
Tuber Culinum, 781

Tumour

Ars Iod., 88
Chimaphilla, 199
Conium, 240
Palladium, 449, 550

Typhoid

Alumina, 31
Ammonium Carb., 486
Antim Tart., 487
Arnica, 66, 102, 408, 561, 634, 748
Arsenicum Album, 80
Baptisia, 66, 101, 102, 334, 408, 561, 634
Borax, 745

Carbo Veg., 486, 487, 634
Cocculus, 2.8
Gelsemium, 102, 308, 309
Helleborus, 332, 333, 334
Hyosyamus Nig., 353, 354, 408
Ipecac, 486
Lachesis, 103, 407
Ledum, 432
Mercurius, 745
Methylene Blue, 478
Moschus, 486, 487
Muriatic Acid, 102, 136, 353, 408, 489, 634, 745
Nux Moschata, 532
Nux Vomica, 531
Opium, 155, 335, 408, 541, 543, 561
Phospharic Acid, 66, 334, 353, 559, 560, 634
Phosphorus, 486, 670, 671
Pyrogen, 354, 408, 561, 615, 616
Rhus Tox., 102, 334, 561, 633, 634
Sulphuric Acid, 745
Taraxacum, 760
Terebenthina, 764
Zincum Met., 827, 828

Typho-Pneumonia

Phosphorus, 564

Ulcer

Lachesis, 411
Ledum, 498
Natrum Carb., 497, 498
Uranium Nit., 784

Ulcerated Nipples

Castor Equirum, 181

Uremia

Jaborandi, 373

Uremic Coma

Terebinthina, 763

Vertigo

Absinthium, 5
Bromium, 130
Carbo Veg., 174
Causticum, 184
Conium, 239, 240
Curare, 263
Gratiola, 326
Ignatia, 355
Morphenium, 481
Petroleum, 555
Pulsatilla, 60
Radium Bromide, 620
Rhododendran, 627
Rhus Tox., 635
Theridion, 766

Warts

Ferrum Picric., 300
Magnesia Sulph, 447
Nitric Acid, 300, 517
Picric Acid, 300
Thuja, 300, 679, 769, 770

Whitlow

Myristica Seb., 493

Whooping Cough

Ambra Girsea, 31, 32, 220, 274
Anacardium, 220
Arnica, 32, 68, 220
Bromium, 274, 647
Cina, 210, 220, 221
Coccus Cacti. 220, 274
Corrallium Rub., 244, 274, 465
Drosera, 273, 274, 377, 416, 495
Justicia, 377
Naphthalinum, 495
Senega, 274, 675, 676

Worms

Cina, 510, 644, 764
Indigo, 361
Natrum Phos, 509
Santoninum, 656, 764
Teucrium, 644, 764

Wounds

Plantago Major, 578

R